MASSAGE THERAPY

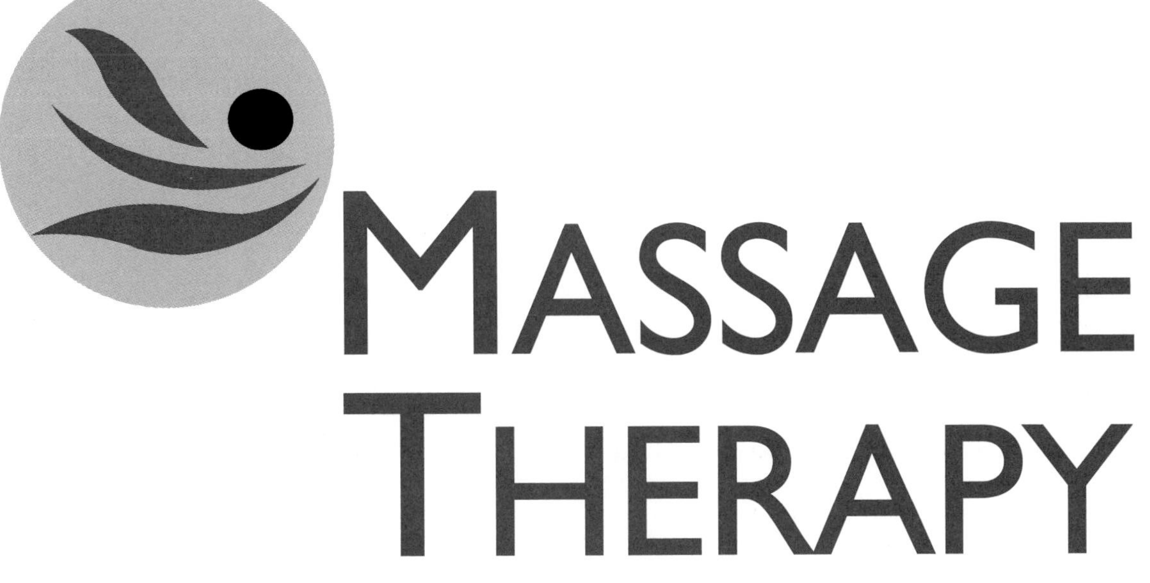

MASSAGE THERAPY

Principles & Practice

Susan G. Salvo, LMT, CI, BA
Co-owner, Director, and Instructor
Louisiana Institute of Massage Therapy
Lake Charles, Louisiana

W.B. SAUNDERS COMPANY
A Division of Harcourt Brace & Company
Philadelphia • London • Toronto • Montreal • Sydney • Tokyo

W.B. SAUNDERS COMPANY
A Division of Harcourt Brace & Company

The Curtis Center
Independence Square West
Philadelphia, Pennsylvania 19106

Library of Congress Cataloging-in-Publication Data

Salvo, Susan G.
Massage therapy: principles and practice/Susan G. Salvo.

p. cm.

ISBN 0-7216-7419-4

1. Massage therapy. I. Title.

RM721.S146 1999

615.8′22—dc21 98-8139

MASSAGE THERAPY:
Principles and Practice ISBN 0-7216-7419-4

Printed in the United States of America.

Last digit is the print number: 9 8 7 6 5 4 3 2 1

I would like to dedicate this book to Mike Breaux.
Thank you for being there and thank you for being you.

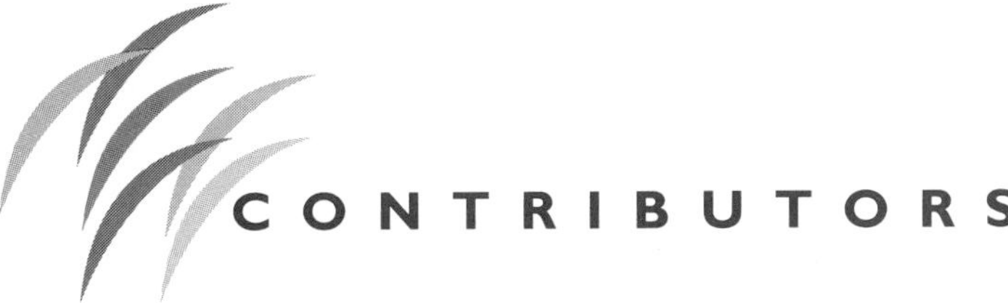

CONTRIBUTORS

Cathy Allen, LMT
Former Faculty, current part-time instructor of postgraduate courses, Swedish Institute of Massage; Private practice, New York, New York
Foot Reflexology

Sandra Kauffman Anderson, BA, LMT, NCTMB
Instructor and Chair, Anatomy and Physiology Department, Desert Institute of the Healing Arts, Tucson, Arizona
Indications/contraindications in all body systems chapters

Susie Ogg Cormier BSEd, BSN, RN, LMT, NCTMB
Coordinator, LGMC Massage Therapy Services, Lafayette General Medical Center, Lafayette, Louisiana
Professional Communication, Assessment, and Documentation

Michael J. Loomis, BSEd
Founder/Director, Sports Massage Certification Training, Florida School of Massage, Gainesville, Florida; Certified Instructor, Injury Evaluation and Orthopedic Assessment, Muscular Therapy Institute, Cambridge, Massachusetts
Website: http://www.massageonline.com
Sports Massage

Maria Mathias, MS, BA
Infant Massage Specialist, University of New Mexico Medical Center, Albuquerque, New Mexico
Website: http://www.infantmassageprograms.com
Infant Massage

Ralph R. Stephens, BSEd
Instructor, Helping Hands Seminars, Cedar Rapids, Iowa
Seated Massage

H. Micheal Tarver, PhD
Assistant Professor of World History, McNeese State University, Lake Charles, Louisiana
E-mail: MTARVER@ACC.MCNEESE.EDU
A Historical Perspective of Massage

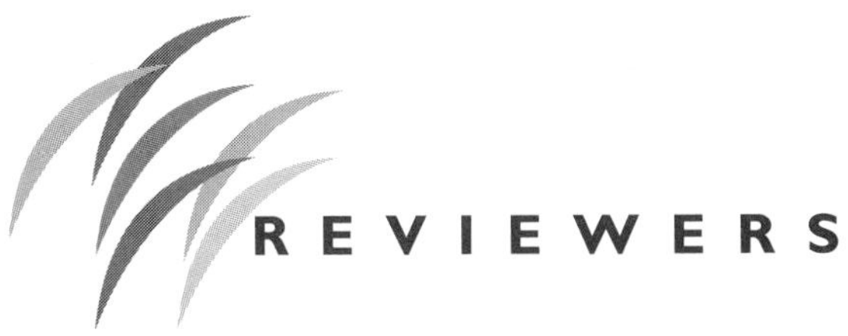

REVIEWERS

Sandra Kauffman Anderson, BA, LMT, NCTMB
Desert Institute of the Healing Arts
Tucson, AZ

JoAnn Bock, LMT, RPP
Florida School of Massage
Gainesville, FL

Iris Burman, LMT
Educating Hands School of Massage
Miami, FL

Gloria Ray Carpeneto, PhD, MST, NCTMB
Villa Julie College
Baltimore, MD

Lauren M. Christman, MFA, LMP
Brian Utting School of Massage
Seattle, WA

Nancy W. Dail, LMT, NCTMB
Downeast School of Massage
Waldoboro, ME

Patricia Marie Holland, BS, LMT
Desert Institute of the Healing Arts
Tucson, AZ

Kamalapati S. Khalsa, CSMT
Phoenix Therapeutic Massage College
Phoenix, AZ

Robert King
Chicago School of Massage Therapy
Chicago, IL

Jim McKnight, BA, LMT
Delta Junction, AL and Honolulu, HI

Carolyn A. Nelka, BA, CMT
Catonsville Community College
Catonsville, MD

Mary L. Puglia, MS, PhD
Phoenix Therapeutic Massage College
Phoenix, AZ

Frank Puglia, MBA, current AZ teaching certificate
Phoenix Therapeutic Massage College
Phoenix, AZ

June E. Schneider, NTCMB
Baltimore School of Massage
Baltimore, MD

Jan Schwartz, LMT, NCTMB
Desert Institute of the Healing Arts
Tucson, AZ

Dave Shahan, LMT
Desert Institute of the Healing Arts
Tucson, AZ

Sari Spieler, LMT
Seattle, WA

Dennis M. Walker, MD, FRCS(C), FAAOS
Lake Charles Memorial Hospital
Lake Charles, LA

Jerry Weinert, RN, NCTMB
Desert Institute of the Healing Arts and Southwest Wellness Educators
Tucson, AZ

Paul Wyman, BA, CMT
Denver, CO

John Yates
West Coast College of Massage Therapy
Vancouver, British Columbia

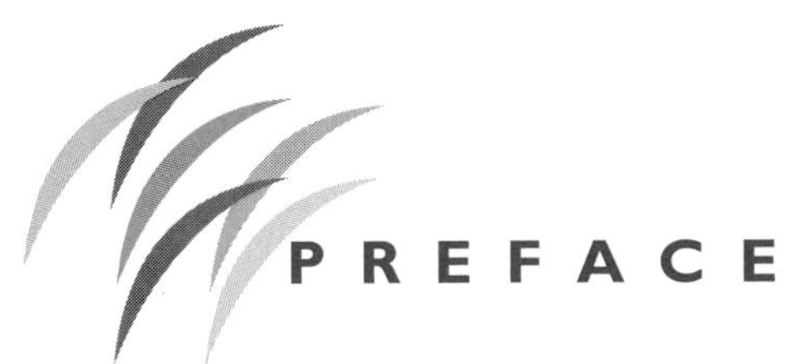

PREFACE

Massage is multidimensional—it is simultaneously an art and a science—and through learning it, you will become a sculptor, a technician, a confidante, a musician, a teacher, an actor, and a health care professional. As a health care profession, massage therapy is one of the fastest growing career fields in the country. Massage therapy programs are emerging quickly to respond to the increasing demand, and educational standards are on the rise. With these new energies of new programs come new ideas and a revolution in the concept of massage education. This textbook was written in the spirit of this massage revolution, and it is our intention that it lead the way into the new millennium.

This textbook combines the classically accepted ideology of the past with today's new concepts. We utilize modern educational techniques to bridge the gap between old and new, thus creating the highest quality educational and reference materials to be found in the field of massage therapy. Our primary aim is to provide the fundamental topics that massage therapy schools must teach students to prepare them for a career in massage therapy. Through careful organization we take the reader into the world of massage. Here is how this text is organized:

Unit One–Surveying the Territory: History, Professional Standards, Boundaries, Equipment and Supplies

Unit Two–Anatomy and Physiology for the Massage Therapist (separate chapters for muscle and bone nomenclature)

Unit Three–Massage: Health, Sanitation, and Safety; Massage Physiology; Table and Body Mechanics; Professional Communication and Assessment; and Adaptive Massage

Unit Four–Alternative and Adjunctive Therapies: Hydrotherapy, Reflexology, Seated Massage, Sports Massage, and Infant Massage

Unit Five–Business Practices

This book is an outgrowth of the need for innovative ways to teach massage therapy. We wanted to inform the reader in a way that is at once both interesting and entertaining, easy to read, easy to use, and highly informative. This book succeeds where other texts do not; it is the only textbook that combines content (derived from the author's years of practical massage experience as a therapist and a massage school instructor) with format (learned in formal university training in the field of education). An Instructor's Manual accompanies this text. Educational techniques are used to develop an interactive approach to massage therapy instruction, which is accomplished by using a variety of formats and features, including:

- **Interweaving massage with the anatomical sciences:** The culmination of our efforts has led to a work that, though broad in scope, successfully fuses the anatomical sciences with hands-on techniques. The anatomy and physiology chapters are written from a massage therapist's point of view. This book incorporates a general knowledge of anatomical science while focusing on the aspects that are most important to the massage practitioner. The science chapters include practical information such as specific benefits, contraindications, touch research, and adaptations of massage in regard to each individual body system. The massage application chapters refer back to and reinforce anatomical and physiological concepts found in the science chapters.
- **Emphasis on the musculoskeletal system:** In order to thoroughly cover the topic of muscles, their origins, insertions, actions, and innervations, the skeletal and muscular systems are divided into four chapters. Two cover each system in general. The other two chapters highlight each system by nomenclature, listing each muscle and bone individually with illustrations and important details.
- **Adjunctive and complementary therapies:** Besides the base of Swedish massage techniques, this text covers such modalities as sports massage, infant massage, reflexology, seated massage, and adaptations for special populations.

- **Mini-labs:** These short lab sessions within chapters are skill-building activities. They are designed so that left-brained and right-brained techniques reinforce each other. Direct student participation will enhance the learning process by stimulating creativity and imagination. The goal is to create an interactive text that pulls the reader out of passive reading into situations in which he or she will be asked to think about, experience, and discuss topics with classmates and to write down goals and dreams. We believe that students will love this book!
- **Personal vignettes and author's notes:** Unlike some other career fields, massage therapy is extremely personal in nature. We have infused this book with an individual touch, so that the reader will feel as if he or she has a personal relationship with the author. This is accomplished by the addition of author's notes and stories from actual massage sessions. We want readers to sense that they are learning from master practitioners who have a sense of humor and a passion for the subject.
- **Biographical sketches:** In addition to contributing our own stories, we have included biographies and candid interviews with many of the pioneers of massage therapy, both past and present.
- **FYI (for your information), tables, charts, and checklists:** Through these features, the book becomes more than an instructional text; it doubles as a practical reference guide—a welcome addition to the bookshelf of the practicing therapist. The reader can thumb through and take random bits of massage information.
- **Self-test:** We want you to pass your tests. Giving you anatomy information and teaching you massage routines is not enough if you cannot pass the licensing exams. Self-tests are included at the end of each chapter to assist the student in self-assessment, as well as studying for and taking tests. Yes, there is a skill involved, and, if you know and understand that skill, your test-taking ability will improve. We call it becoming "test-wise." We chose a multiple choice and matching format because this is the format used for most state and national tests. Hence, you can use this book as a study guide to prepare for and successfully pass state and/or national examinations. Other study tips include the use of mnemonic devices and an explanation of the prefixes, suffixes, and word roots of anatomical terminology.
- **Inspiration:** Besides providing intellectual stimulation, one of our goals was to have the book inspire students emotionally and spiritually. This is accomplished through the use of insightful and thought-provoking quotations throughout the book.
- **Visual enhancement:** For the reader's visual stimulation, we have lavishly illustrated this book with spectacular art by Theodore Huff and the professional photography of Mike LeBlanc.

Our final word of advice is to read this book three times: once during class, next as you are studying for licensing exams, and again as a reference when situations are presented to you in your practice. Remember that this book is a very small part of your education. In fact, quality massage therapy cannot be learned solely from a book—just as you cannot learn art, music, or cooking from a book. Good role models (teachers), a stimulating environment of fellow students, curiosity, compassion, and open-mindedness are essential components of the educational process. Congratulations on beginning your education as a massage therapist. Bear in mind that your learning experience does not end with graduation from a massage school. Classroom education is simply to provide basic training and competence. Excellence is achieved by working with the body itself, where you are your own textbook, laboratory, and teacher. The body is your guide—all you need to do is listen.

SUSAN G. SALVO
salvobreaux@usunwired.net

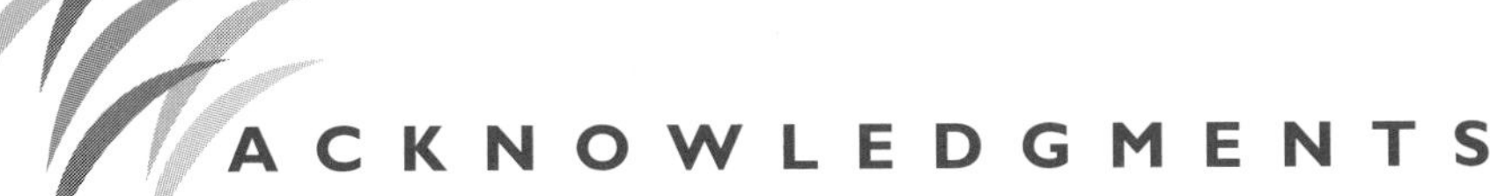

ACKNOWLEDGMENTS

I would like to acknowledge the following individuals who assisted me in writing this book: Teena Cole (my grammarian), H. Micheal Tarver, Susie Ogg Cormier, Cathy Allen, Ralph Stephens, Michael J. Loomis, Maria and Wayne Mathias, Sandra Kaufmann, Anne McDonald, Cheryl Navarre, Donny Kron, Mike Breaux, Rita Shirley, Theodore Huff, Mike LeBlanc; all the photo models (Sehoya Battise, Sehoke Bordelon, Chelsea Breaux, Ernest Cormier, Jr., Jamie Dowd, Melissa Dowd, Skylar Dowd, Loretta Fabacher, George Fondel, Christy Fontenot, Lisa Heindel, Hope Hernandez, Trina McDaniel, Kim Reeves, Peter Richard, Barbara Salvo, Angela Stevens, and Jennifer Tupper), Mark Brown, Tony Dupuis, Stewart Griffith, Monica Haynes, Tim Hebert, Jeanette Ritchey, Robin Zill, John Moreno, Kathy Lea, Robin Martin, Damon Ogle, Connie Modyelewski, Craig Parham, Stefanie Gore, Michael Kent, Dennis Walker, Belford Carver, Kevin Bernier, Ann Dunn, Linda Warner, Scott Weaver, Maureen Pfeifer, George King, John Fanuzzi, Ann Hawkins, Belinda Hughes, Karla Hunt, Edwin Hunter, Stephanie Ecker, and Cherie Sohnen-Moe. I would also like to thank all of my teachers and the students whom I have had the pleasure to teach.

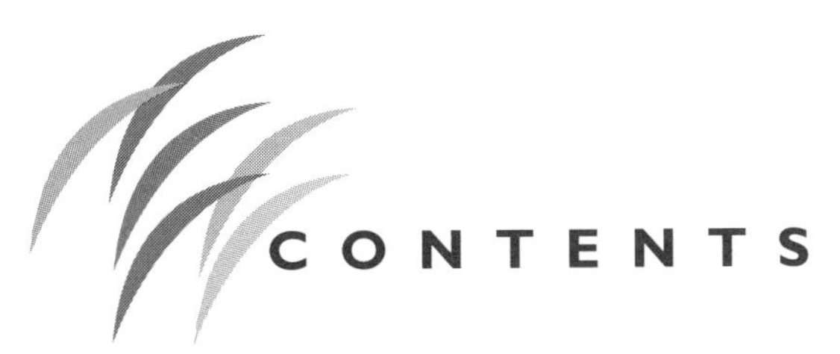

CONTENTS

UNIT ONE

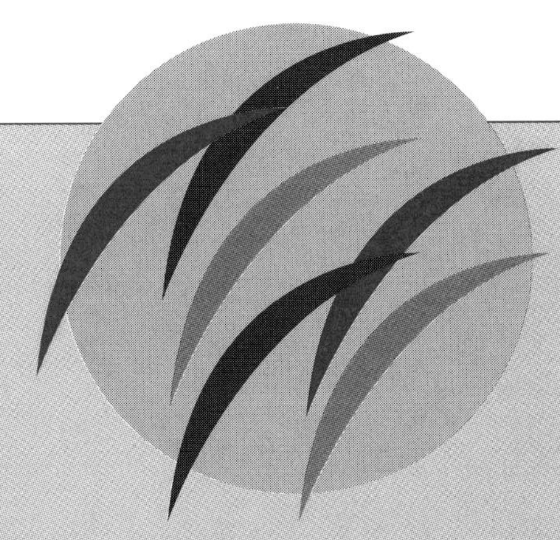

Surveying the Territory: History, Standards, Boundaries, and Equipment

Nature, being well-instructed, does what is needed without being taught.

—*Hippocrates*

H. Micheal Tarver

1 A Historical Perspective of Massage

Student Objectives

After completing this chapter, the student should be able to:

- Name the major figures in the development of medicine and specifically in massage
- Discuss the ancient views and uses of massage incorporating both Eastern and Western cultures
- Explain the role of the European Renaissance and Enlightenment on the professionalism of massage therapy and on medical gymnastics
- Distinguish the contributions of Pehr Henrik Ling from those of later physicians and therapists
- Reconstruct the development of therapeutic massage incorporating the various massage styles and key personnel involved
- Integrate recent developments in the field of therapeutic massage into the original framework of Pehr Ling and his students
- Define the term "massage" (including any variations)

INTRODUCTION

A complete history of massage (the systematic and scientific manipulation of the soft tissues of the body) is long and complex, as there are over 75 different types of massage and bodywork, a generic term used to describe massage and its various forms. Archaeological and historical evidence seems to indicate that therapeutic touch has been practiced for thousands of years in all regions of the globe. Massage is instinctive. It is a natural response to rub our aches and pains, whether or not we are familiar with the medical knowledge behind those actions. In modern health care, therapeutic massage has taken on an important role. It has been shown beneficial to reduce stress, enhance blood circulation, decrease pain, improve sleep, reduce swelling, enhance relaxation, and increase oxygen capacity of the blood. Massage has also been recognized as a nondrug treatment for cancer and postoperative pain.

In this chapter, we will briefly examine the history of massage from its earliest records to the present (Fig. 1–1). *The goals of this chapter are to provide the massage therapist with the information necessary to illustrate the path taken in the development of the profession and to instill in the therapist a sense of connection with those who preceded him or her.* Some names will be familiar, others will be quite foreign. You need not memorize every

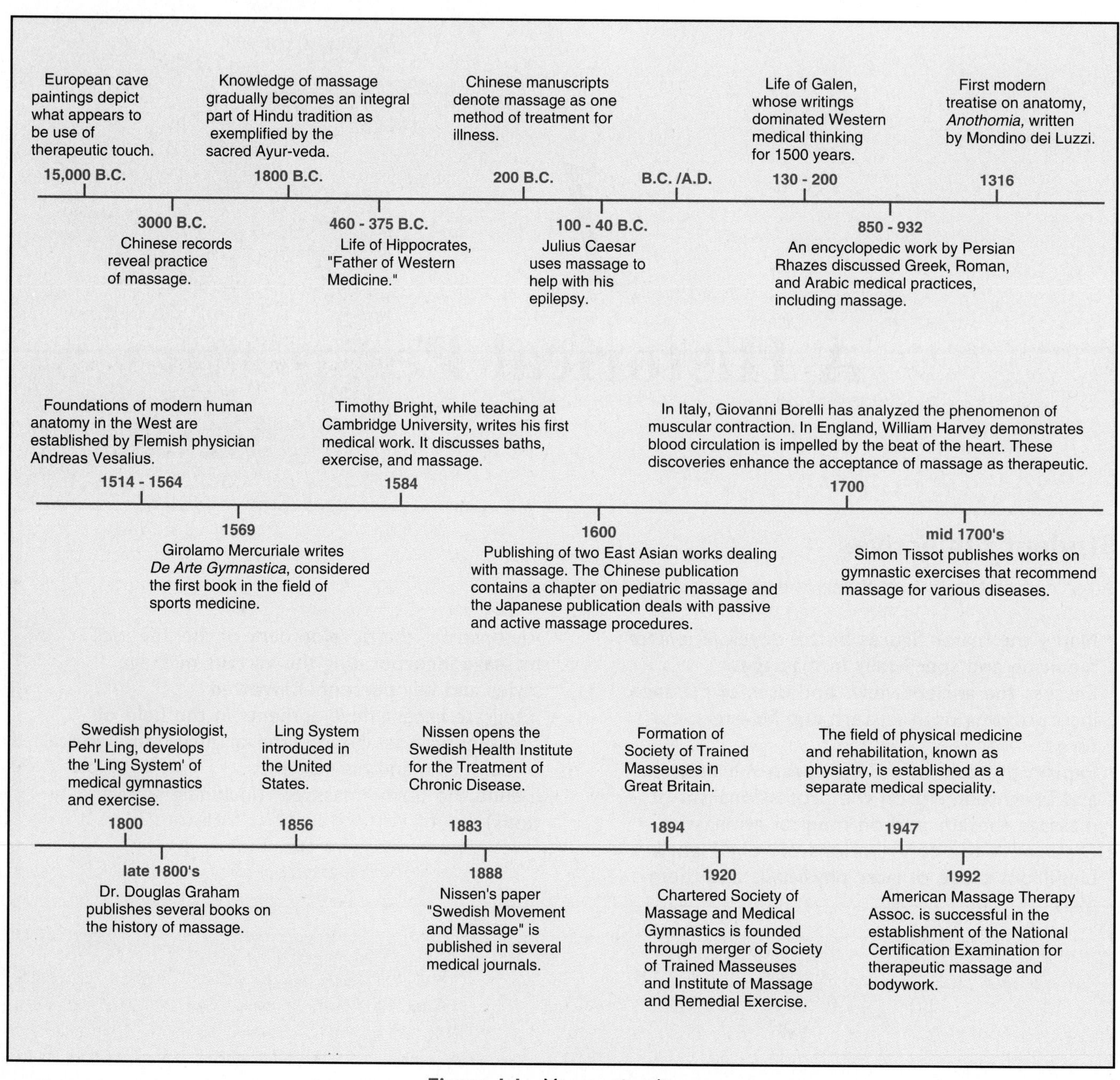

Figure 1•1 Massage time line.

name mentioned in the following pages, although some are important enough that you should know them (ask your instructor). What the names with their different nations of origin tell us is that the development of massage therapy was a global endeavor; people from around the world contributed to the knowledge base that transformed massage from folk remedy to scientific treatment. It should be noted that from the beginning of this chapter the word "massage" is used to refer to soft tissue manipulation, even though the term did not come into use until the middle of the 19th century. The origin of the word "massage" is unclear, but it can be traced to numerous sources: the Hebrew word "mashesh," the Greek roots "masso" and "massin," the Latin root "massa," the Arabic root "mass'h," the Sanskrit word "makeh," and the French word "masser."

THE PREHISTORIC WORLD

In prehistoric times (i.e., before written records) evidence supports the position that massage was practiced by several groups around the world. Archaeologists have found artifacts that depict the use of massage in a number of world cultures. Although there is no direct prehistoric evidence that verifies the use of massage for medical reasons, the indirect evidence clearly intimates that it was used in this manner. European cave paintings (c. 15,000 B.C.), for example, depict what appears to be the use of therapeutic touch. In the historic period, however, extensive written and pictorial records show the use of massage.

THE ANCIENT WORLD

In the ancient East, a concern with illness has been documented in China for millennia, and records have revealed that the practice of massage goes back as early as 3000 B.C. However, it was in the period between the second century B.C. (i.e., 200–101 B.C.) and the first century A.D. (i.e., A.D. 1–100), that Chinese medicine began to take on its basic shape. Manuscripts found in China dating from the second century B.C. discuss massage as one of the various methods of treatment for illnesses. It should be noted, however, that acupuncture was not referred to (although it was mentioned in Chinese medical writing from 90 B.C.). Using their knowledge of massage and later acupuncture (Fig. 1–2), the Chinese developed a style of massage that they termed "amma" or "anmo." The Chinese had developed the art of massage so well that they were the first to train and employ blind masseurs.

As early as the first century A.D., various schools of medical thought had been founded and had already begun to produce diverging ideas. These various ideas and beliefs were compiled under the name of the mythical Yellow Emperor and have become the classic scripture of traditional Chinese medicine, the **Huang-ti nei-ching.** Although the exact date of the original writing of the work is unknown, it was already in its present form by approximately the first century B.C. The work, commonly known as **Nei Ching,** contained descriptions of therapeutic touch procedures and their uses. There is some debate over the actual date of this work, as some historians argue that it was written around 2760 B.C. However, leading Chinese medical historians tend to date the work as noted above. By A.D. 700, there was a Chinese ministry of health and a public health system.

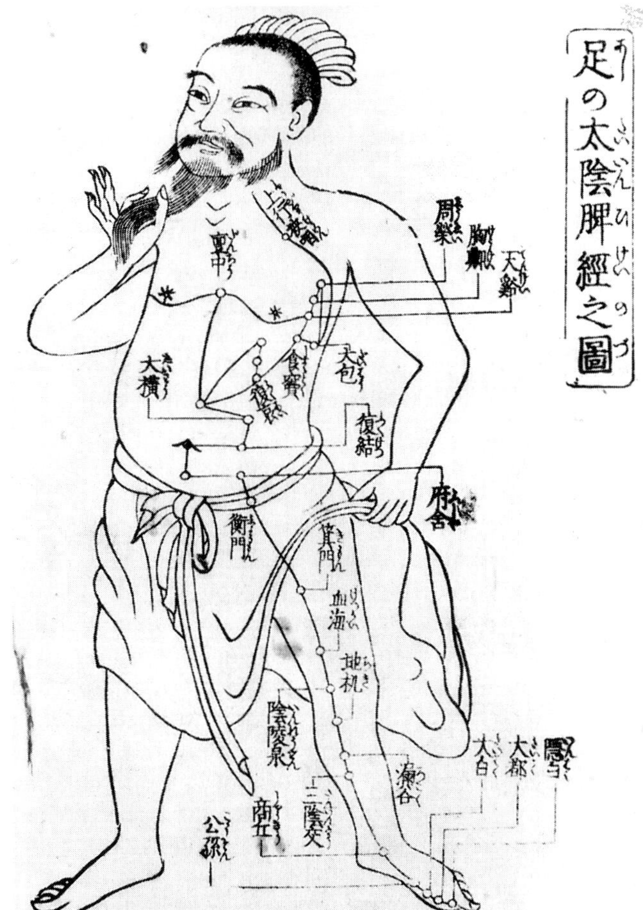

Figure 1•2 Chinese acupuncture chart. (Courtesy of the U.S. National Library of Medicine, Bethesda, MD.)

By the sixth century, the techniques and use of massage were well established in China and found their way into Japan. In general, the Japanese methods of massage were basically the same as the Chinese. In Japan, we see the Chinese amma, referred to as "anma," which means massage in Japanese. Shiatsu, literally meaning finger pressure, is considered a component of anma. It is a Japanese modality based on the Asian concept that the body has a series of energy points, or *tsubu.* When pressure is properly applied to these points, circulation is improved and nerves are stimulated. There are numerous tsubu points along the body, each having different purposes. The shiatsu practitioner massages the tsubu to bring balance between mind and body. Like the Chinese, the medieval Japanese employed blind masseurs.

FYI FOR YOUR INFORMATION

In the Pergamon Museum in Berlin, there is a 2,000-year-old alabaster relief depicting a massage treatment.

In addition to the Chinese and Japanese, other Asian cultures practiced massage. On the Indian subcontinent, the practice of massage has also existed for over 3,000 years. Knowledge of massage had probably been brought to India from China, and gradually it became an integral part of Hindu tradition, as exemplified by the inclusion of massage treatments in the sacred Ayur-Veda (c. 1800 B.C.). The Ayur-Veda (literally, a "code of life"), deals with rebirth, renunciation, salvation, soul, the purpose of life, the maintenance of mental health, and the prevention and treatment of diseases. As for medicine, the most important Ayurvedic texts are the samhitas. A later work, the ***Manav Dharma Shastra*** (c. 300 B.C.), also mentions therapeutic massage. In addition to the above-mentioned Eastern cultures, the Polynesians have also been documented as practicing therapeutic massage.

The concept of health and medicine in the West began to take shape during the seventh and sixth centuries B.C. During that time, the legendary Greek physician **Æsculapius (Asclepius)** evolved into a god responsible for the emerging medical profession. His holy snake and staff still remain symbols of the medical profession. Around 500 B.C., the various ideas of healing and treatments in Greece merged into a **techne iatriche,** or healing science. During this process, two individuals, Iccus and Herodicus, concerned themselves with exercise and the use of gymnastics. Among the numerous followers of this new science was **Hippocrates of Cos** (460–375 B.C.) (Fig. 1–3).

With his emphasis on the individual patient and his belief that the healer should take care not to cause any additional harm to the patient, Hippocrates is generally recognized as the father of modern Western medicine. Although we know little about him, he is reputed to have been a fine clinician, as well as a founder of a medical school and the author of numerous books, though most of the works attributed to him were written by other members of the Hippocratic school. These works are collectively known as the **Corpus Hippocraticum,** which summarized much of what was known about disease and medicine in the ancient world. During the four centuries following the development of the techne iatriche, several debates occurred within the healing profession, one of which placed great stock in the value of therapeutic massage.

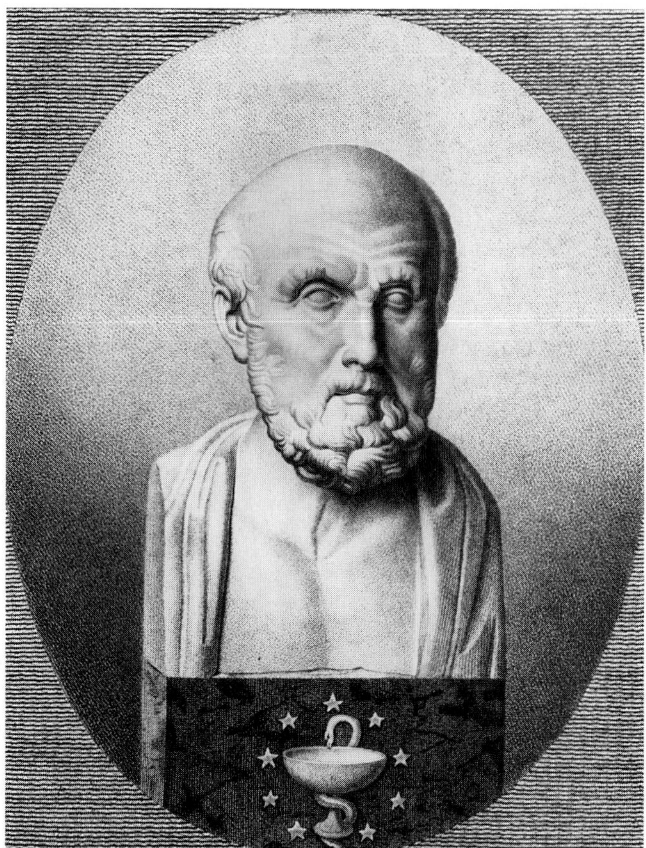

Figure 1•3 Hippocrates of Cos. (Courtesy of the U.S. National Library of Medicine, Bethesda, MD.)

A group of Greek physicians residing in Rome, known as the **Methodists,** supported a simplistic view of healing and restricted their treatments to bathing, diet, massage, and a few drugs. This is not to say that the earlier practitioners and other groups did not recognize the importance of touch. The founder of this school of thought was **Asclepiades.** Among his many contributions to Roman medicine was a treatise on friction (massage) and exercise. Although the work is no longer in existence, it was cited by Aulus Aurelius Cornelius Celsus (c. 25 B.C.–c. A.D. 50) in his writings on friction. In his essay *περι αρθρων* (On Joints), Hippocrates wrote, "*πολλῶν ἔμπειρον δεῖ εἶναι τὸν ἰητρόν, ἀτὰρ δὴ καὶ ἀνατρίψιος*" ("the physician must be skilled in many things and particularly friction") (section IX, lines 25–26). Hippocrates also noted that following the reduction of a dislocated shoulder, the friction should be done with soft, gentle hands (section IX, lines 31–33). Obviously, Hippocrates was a proponent of therapeutic massage.

During the transitional period between Greek and Roman dominance in the ancient world, there were a few individuals who helped pass on the medical knowledge of the Greeks and helped incorporate it into Roman medicine. One such individual was **Aulus Celsus,** who is regarded by many to be the first important medical historian. His ***De Medicina*** is an outstanding account of Roman medicine, and it bridges the gap between his times and those of the Hippocratic corpus. During this period, massage had gained such acceptance that Julius Caesar (c. 100–44 B.C.) used massage to help with his epilepsy.

A later follower of Hippocratic medicine was **Galen of Pergamon** (c. A.D. 130–c. 200)(Fig. 1–4). Galen was a Roman physician who studied medicine in Alexandria (Egypt) and who became personal physician to the Roman emperor Marcus Aurelius. In at least 100 treatises, Galen synthesized and unified Greek knowledge of anatomy and medicine; his system continued to dominate medicine throughout the Middle Ages and until relatively recent times. Among his many works, Galen's *De Sanitate Tuenda* considers exercise, the use of baths, and massage. Following the division of the Roman Empire into eastern and western halves, the decline in learning was much more rapid and severe in the Roman west than in the Greek east (Byzantium).

Farther east of the Romans, the ancient Slavs reportedly used massage. In the Americas, the Mayas and Inca have been documented as practicing joint manipulation and massage. The Inca also used the application of heat in their treatments of joint maladies, through the use of the leaves of the chilca bush. It should come as no surprise that the South American Inca developed procedures for joint manipulation and massage. They had a higher success rate for **trepanation** (surgical procedure involving the removal of a segment of the skull) in 2000 B.C. than the Europeans did in A.D. 1800. In addition, records indicate that the Cherokees and Navajos utilized massage in their treatments of colic and to ease labor pains.

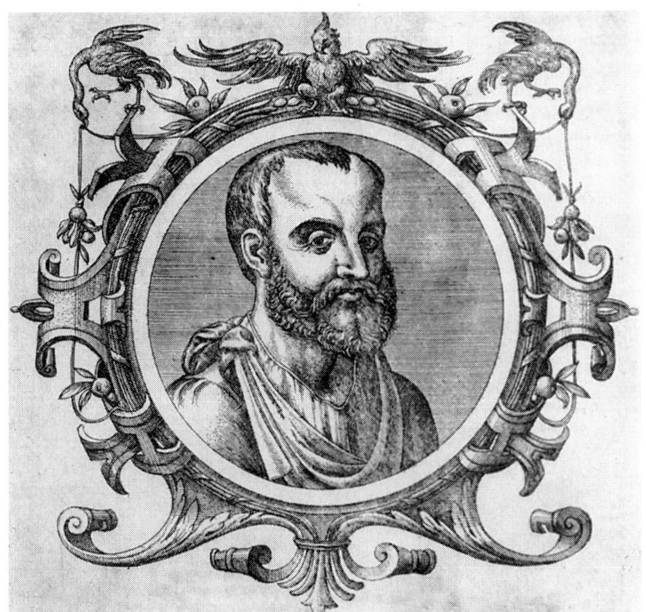

Figure 1•4 Galen of Pergamon. (Courtesy of the U.S. National Library of Medicine, Bethesda, MD.)

THE MIDDLE AGES

After the collapse of the Roman Empire (476), Western medicine experienced a period of decline. In reality, it was only because of the writing efforts of a number of Western physicians (such as Oribasius and Alexander of Tralles) that the ancient medical knowledge of the Greeks and Romans was preserved. Among the last of the Greco-Roman writers to consider treatment by mechanical means (as opposed to drug therapy or surgery) was **Paul of Aegina** (625–690), who advocated the bending, stretching, and rubbing of paralyzed limbs. As a consequence of his writings, Galen became the central medical authority in the West for centuries. It should be noted that Galen had written extensively on the topic of massage and its administration. After the decline of Rome, the Hippocratic-Galenic tradition survived in the Greek-speaking East. Following the fall of Alexandria (642), knowledge of Greek medicine spread throughout the Arabic world.

Following the expansion of the Islamic world in the seventh and eighth centuries, the comprehensive body of Greco-Roman medical doctrine was adopted, together with extensive Persian and Hindu medical knowledge. One such example of this synthesis of knowledge was an encyclopedic work *(Kitabu'l Hawi Fi't-Tibb)* by the Persian physician **Rhazes** (Abu Bakr Muhammad ibn Zakariya al-Razi)(c. 850–932), which discussed Greek, Roman, and Arabic medical practices, including massage. Another important work was that by the Persian physician Abu-Ali al-Husayn ibn-Sina (980–1037), generally known as **Avicenna.** He also authored numerous medical books which remained standard until the 17th century. His *Canon of Medicine* was an especially famous medical text, which compiled the theoretical and practical medical knowledge of the time. The work illustrates the tremendous influence of Galen on the medical knowledge of the time; the text makes numerous references to the use of massage. In fact, by the end of the ninth century, almost all of Galen's lengthy medical texts had been translated into Arabic. In general, it appears that the Islamic physicians of the European Middle Ages were more interested in developing and commenting on the truths learned from the Greeks and Romans than they were in discovering new knowledge. The Muslims simply incorporated Greco-Roman medical knowledge into the Islamic framework. It was through Latin translations of these Arabic authors that most of the knowledge of Greek medicine was revived in the Christian west (i.e., Europe).

For the most part, Western medical practitioners of the Middle Ages abandoned massage in favor of other treatments. Massage did, however, remain an important procedure for folk healers and midwives, and its procedures were passed on as an art form. Subse-

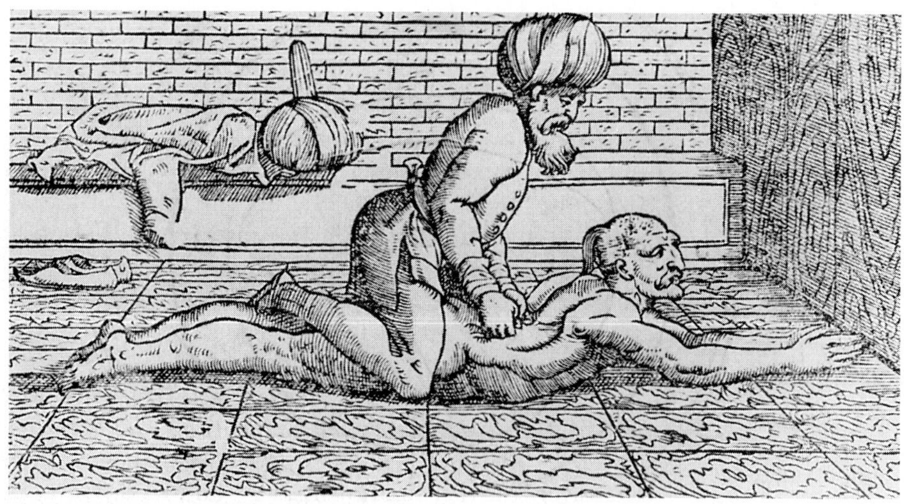

Figure 1•5 Print of woodcut of massage therapy. (Courtesy of the U.S. National Library of Medicine, Bethesda, MD.)

quently, no early compilation of the techniques and procedures was undertaken. It is also very likely that monastic clergy used massage in their *hospitale pauperum,* for they would have had copies of earlier Greco-Roman medical writings.

During the course of the later Middle Ages, the collection, preservation, and transmission of classical medical knowledge occurred (Fig. 1–5). After the 12th century, medieval medical knowledge in the West expanded, thanks in part to the existing works by the Muslims, who had earlier translated Greek and Latin medical texts into Arabic. By the 13th century, medical knowledge had advanced to the point that three major European centers (Montpelier, Paris, and Bologna) were offering degrees in medicine. In 1316, Mondino dei Luzzi wrote ***Anothomia,*** the first modern treatise on anatomy.

With the revival of classical Greek learning during the Renaissance, Western medicine was revitalized by new translations of old Greek and Latin texts. Among the newly revived texts was Aulus Celsus's *De Medicina,* which once again came into circulation, thanks to the newly invented printing press.

> *When you steal from one author, it's plagiarism; if you steal from many, it's research.*
>
> —Wilson Mizner 1876–1933

THE EUROPEAN RENAISSANCE AND ENLIGHTENMENT

The **Renaissance** (c. 1250–c. 1550) was an exciting period in the history of medicine and medical treatments. The word "renaissance" means "rebirth," and it was during that time that the foundations of modern human anatomy (in the West) were established by the Flemish physician **Andreas Vesalius** (1514–1564). His ***De Humani Corporis Fabrica*** (1543) is considered one of the most important studies in the history of medicine. In addition, the foundations of chemical pharmacology—as opposed to herbal remedies—were laid by the Swiss physician Philippus von Hohenheim (1493–1541), better known as **Paracelsus.** New surgical procedures were also established, particularly those by the French military surgeon **Ambroise Paré** (c. 1510–1590) (Fig.1–6). In addition to inventing several surgical instruments, Paré was among the earliest modern physicians to discuss the therapeutic effects of massage, especially in orthopedic surgery cases. Paré even went so far as to classify various types of massage movements.

Two other notable Renaissance physicians were **Gi-**

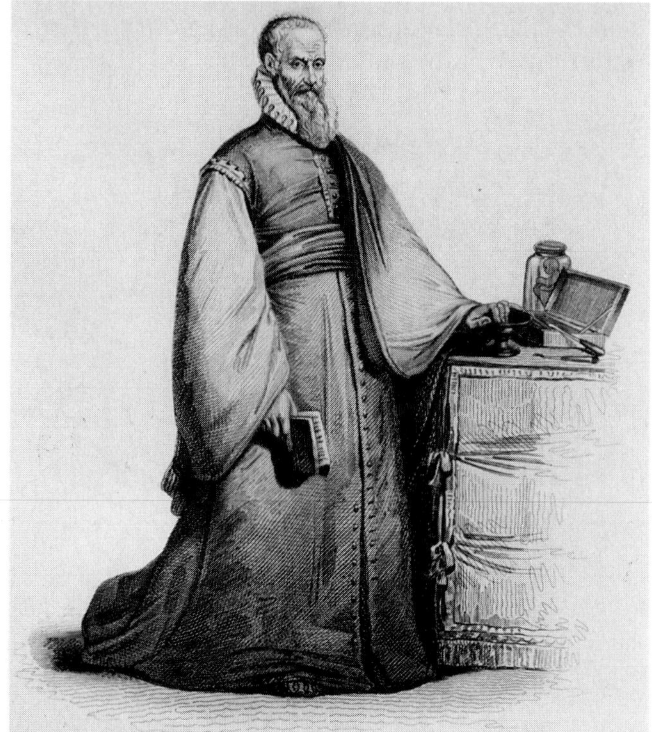

Figure 1•6 Ambroise Paré. (Courtesy of the U.S. National Library of Medicine, Bethesda, MD.)

rolamo **Mercuriale** (1530–1606) and **Timothy Bright** (c. 1551–1615). Mercuriale spent several years in Rome examining the manuscripts of the ancient writers. His extensive knowledge of the attitudes of the Greeks and Romans toward diet, exercise, and their effects on health and disease is evident in ***De Arte Gymnastica*** (1569), considered to be the first book in the field of sports medicine. The work compiled the history of gymnastics up to that time, synthesizing all that had been written on the use of exercise (for both the purpose of health and the treatment of disease).

Bright's first medical work (c. 1584) was divided into two parts, *Hygienina on Restoring Health* and *Therapeutica on Restoring Health.* In this work, Bright discussed baths, exercise, and massage, and the book supports the position that he was teaching these same techniques to his classes at Cambridge University.

Around the 16th century, we see two important East Asian works that dealt with massage. The Chinese published ***Chen-chiu ta-ch'eng,*** which contained a chapter on pediatric massage, and the Japanese published ***San-tsai-tou-hoei,*** which mentioned both passive and active massage procedures.

By the end of the 17th century, Western medicine had experienced a revolution in both ideas and knowledge. In Italy, **Giovanni Alfonso Borelli** (1608–1679) carried out extensive anatomical dissections and had analyzed the phenomenon of muscular contraction. In England, **William Harvey** (1578–1657) had demonstrated that blood circulation in animals is impelled by the beat of the heart through arteries and veins (Fig. 1–7). This discovery enhanced the acceptance of massage as a therapeutic measure. Another crucial development during the 17th century was the realization that it was necessary to compile complete clinical descriptions of disease, generally at bedsides, and to develop specific remedies for each specific disease. In this area, the English physician **Thomas Sydenham** (1624–1689) was most prominent. At the same time these scientific advances were being made, massage was reemerging as a therapy acceptable to the medical profession and as a therapeutic practice for health and disease.

The 18th century in the West introduced medicine to the Enlightenment. What emerged was an optimistic outlook concerning the role and benefits of medicine. It was widely believed that health was a natural state to be attained and preserved. Within this new philosophy, massage came to be viewed as a popular treatment in Europe. **Simon André Tissot** (1728–1797), an important figure in physiotherapy, published several works on gymnastic exercises that recommended massage for various diseases and that gave indications for its use. The 18th century also saw the creation of new medical "systems," which incorporated the anatomical, physiological, and chemical discoveries of the previous 200 years. These comprehensive systems were necessary to provide a rationale for and guidance to clinical activities. Some believed that the compilation and synthesis of this new knowledge would add prestige to the medical profession and help weed out the "quacks."

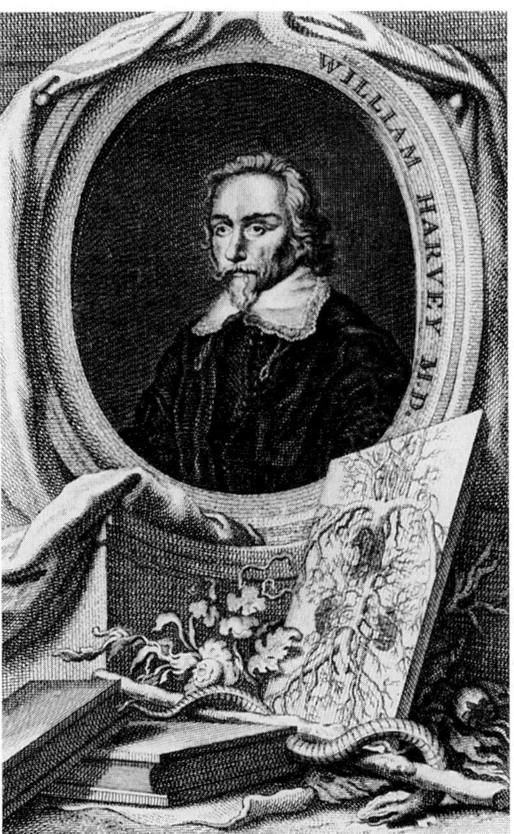

Figure 1•7 William Harvey. (Courtesy of the U.S. National Library of Medicine, Bethesda, MD.)

THE MODERN ERA

The era of modern massage began in the early 19th century, when a wide variety of authors were advocating massage and developing their own systems. The most important of these writers was **Pehr Henrik Ling** (1776–1839), a Swedish physiologist and gymnastics instructor. Through his experiences at the University of Lund and the Swedish Royal Central Institute of Gymnastics, Ling developed his own system of medical gymnastics and exercise, known as the Ling System, Swedish Movements, or Swedish Movement Cure. The primary focus of Ling's work was on gymnastics applied to the treatment of disease and/or injury. In this regard, Ling was a proponent of **Medical Gymnastics,** a subject that was promoted over 2,000 years earlier by Herodicus, the teacher of Hippocrates. According to Ling, medical gymnastics were gymnastics "by which, either alone, in a suitable position, or with the assistance of others, we try by means of influencing movements to alleviate or overcome the sufferings that have arisen through abnormal conditions."

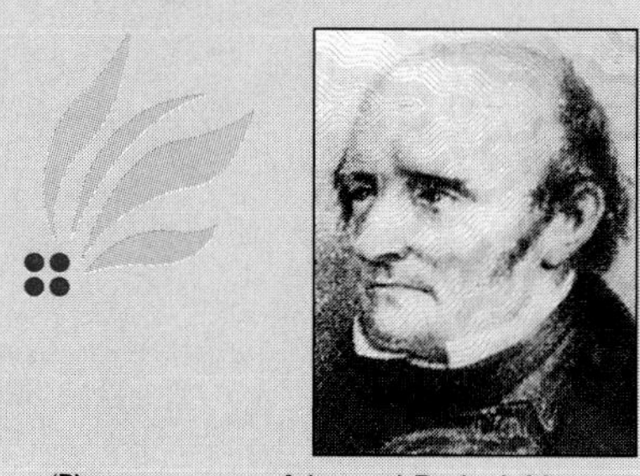

(Photo courtesy of Armand Dedrick Maanum, the last Master-Master Masseur-Teacher of the Sjuk Gymnastiken Passiva Rorelser Massage of Pehr Henrik Ling, MD)

Pehr Henrik Ling

1776–1839
Father of Physical Therapy
Father of Swedish Massage

Born in Smaaland, one of the southern provinces of Sweden, Pehr Henrik Ling led a very interesting life. After being expelled from school for disciplinary problems, Ling traveled through Europe and eventually returned to Sweden where he learned fencing (the art of using a sword). In 1804 he accepted a post at the Lunds Universitet (University of Lund), where he taught fencing and gymnastics. At the same time, he studied anatomy and physiology. In his teaching of fencing techniques, he noted that often the movements he wanted his pupils to make were hindered by motions that the student had learned from habit. Ling, therefore, resolved to teach the movements of the body in a systematic manner. For Ling this training was important for military concerns, and he viewed fencing as an important part of Military Gymnastics ("by which we try, through some object exterior to ourselves, i.e., weapons, or by our own physical power, to subject a second exterior will to our own will"). What he meant was that the brain could be taught to use and move muscles in ways that were new to his students.

At the same time, Ling also developed what is referred to as Medical Gymnastics, through which we "try by means of influencing movements to alleviate or overcome the sufferings that have arisen through abnormal conditions." These gymnastics comprised only a few stretching movements done by the student alone (active movements), performed by another pupil (passive movements), or resisted by another pupil (duplicated movements). In Ling's system, there was very little, if any, mechanical apparatus involved.

In 1813 Ling opened the Swedish Royal Central Institute of Gymnastics, where he further developed his own system of medical gymnastics and exercise, known as the Ling System, Swedish Movements, or the Swedish Movement Cure. The primary focus of Ling's work was on gymnastics applied to the treatment of disease and/or injury. Massage was viewed as a component of Ling's overall system. Known commonly as Swedish massage, Ling and his followers used a system of long, smooth, slow strokes that created a very relaxing experience. In general, they used massage in tandem with the movements described above. The active and passive movements of the joints promote general relaxation, improve circulation, relieve muscle tension, and improve range of motion.

Ling was not a physician, and his system of medical gymnastics was bitterly opposed by many within the medical profession during much of his lifetime. However, many of his students were physicians, and these individuals spread his teachings and began to publish success stories of his techniques in respectable medical journals. Ling's influence was so great that by 1851 there were 38 schools located throughout Europe teaching his system of gymnastics and massage.

After years of failing health, Pehr Henrik Ling died in 1839. His legacy is seen today throughout the health professions, especially in the teachings of massage therapy, physical therapy, kinesiology, and gymnastics.

Ling's system classified movements into three types: active, passive, and duplicated. Active movements were those performed by the patient/client (i.e., exercise). Passive movements were movements of the patient/client performed by the gymnast/therapist (e.g., range of motion). Duplicated movements were those performed by the patient/client with the cooperation of the gymnast/therapist. In this manner, the actions of the patient were in opposition to the actions of the gymnast (i.e., resistive exercises).

Massage was viewed as a component of Ling's overall system and was known commonly as Swedish Massage. Ling (the father of Swedish massage) and his followers used a system of long, smooth, slow strokes that created a very relaxing experience. In general, these followers used massage in tandem with the movements described above. Its active and passive movements of the joints promoted general relaxation, improved circulation, relieved muscle tension, and improved range of motion. For Ling, massage was a form of passive gymnastics, done *on* the body part, as opposed to *with* the body part (as is range of motion). As you read the chapter on classifying massage movements, try to imagine how Pehr Ling would have categorized them.

From 1813 to 1839, Ling taught these techniques at the Royal Central Institute of Gymnastics, which he founded with governmental support. While Ling is considered the father of physical therapy (physiotherapy), actually his students would be responsible for the spreading of his ideas throughout the world. Among the more important cities with established schools teaching Ling's methods were St. Petersburg, London, Berlin, Dresden, Leipzig, Vienna, Paris, and New York. Within 12 years of his death (1839), there were 38 institutions in Europe teaching the Swedish Movements system. Included in these students were numerous medical doctors who became convinced of the usefulness of massage and of therapeutic exercise in the practice of medicine. Medical doctors could complete Ling's medical gymnastics program in one year, as compared to two to three years for nonphysicians. As more physicians trained, massage became more and more acceptable as a traditional medical procedure and practice.

Another key individual in the history of massage was the Dutch physician **Johann Mezger** (1839–1909), who was born the same year Ling died. Mezger is generally given credit for making massage a fundamental component of physical rehabilitation; he has been credited for the introduction of the still-used French terminology into the massage profession (e.g., effleurage, petrissage, tapotement). The French translated several of the Chinese books on massage, and this probably explains why the French terminology for the procedures has become so common in massage texts. Unlike Pehr Ling, Mezger, being a physician, was much more able to promote massage using a medical and scientific basis. In this regard, Mezger was quite successful getting the medical profession to more readily accept massage as a bona fide medical treatment for disease and illness. A number of European physicians began to use massage therapy and to publish scientifically the positive results of the modality. What occurred was the inclusion of the art of massage in the science of medicine.

The Swedish Movement system was introduced into the United States in 1856 by two brothers, **George Henry Taylor** and **Charles Fayette Taylor.** The Taylors had studied the techniques in Europe and returned to the United States where they opened an orthopedic practice with a specialization in the Swedish Movements. The two physicians published a number of important works on Ling's system, including the first American textbook on the subject in 1860. A third prominent American follower of the Swedish Movement was **Douglas O. Graham.** Not only was Dr. Graham a practitioner of the system, he also authored, from 1874 to 1925, several works on the history of massage.

Another prominent practitioner in the United States was **Hartvig Nissen,** who in 1883 opened the Swedish Health Institute for the Treatment of Chronic Diseases by Swedish Movements and Massage (Washington, D.C.). Nissen presented a paper titled "Swedish Movement and Massage" in 1888, which was subsequently published in several medical journals. The result of publication was numerous letters from physicians who wanted to know more about Ling's system, and this inquiry led him to publish *Swedish Movement and Massage Treatment* in 1888. Taken together, Nissen's book and Graham's *A Treatise on Massage, Its History, Mode of Application and Effects* (1902) are generally credited with arousing interest in the U.S. medical profession in the benefits of massage.

While the Taylor brothers, Graham, and Nissen were convincing the medical community of the benefits of massage and medical gymnastics, several other individuals were busy convincing the general public. Among the most famous of these was **John Harvey Kellogg** (1852–1943). Kellogg (of Battle Creek, Michigan) wrote numerous articles and books on massage, and published *Good Health,* a magazine that targeted the general public. Efforts by men such as Kellogg helped popularize massage in the United States.

The end of the 19th and beginning of the 20th centuries witnessed important changes in the use of massage, the most important of which was the development of the field of physical therapy. Physical therapy, or physiotherapy, developed from the physical education segment, which was responsible for the training of women to work in hospitals, where they used massage and therapeutic exercise to help patients recover. These women were frequently trained in mechanotherapy, which is the healing of the body by means of manipulations (massage and special exercises).

World War I provided countless opportunities for the use of therapeutic massage, exercise, and other physiotherapeutic methods (electrotherapy and hydrotherapy) in efforts to rehabilitate injured soldiers. During the course of treating war casualties, the earlier ideas of **Just Lucas-Championniere** (1843–1913) were eventually recognized. Briefly, what Dr. Lucas-Championniere advocated was the use of massage and passive motion exercises after injuries, especially fractures. What changed, however, was that more and more physicians were frequently administering the treatments (some of which were new, such as electrotherapeutics).

By the beginning of the 20th century, massage had

begun to be used throughout the West. Once the procedures of massage were accepted, what developed was the profession of massage. In Great Britain, the Society of Trained Masseuses (1894) was formed by several women who realized the need for the standardization and professionalization of their trade. The organization was successful in several key areas: establishing a massage curriculum; accrediting massage schools, which had to undergo regular inspections; requiring qualified instructors for the massage classes; and establishing a board certification program. By the end of World War I (1918), the Society had nearly 5,000 members.

In 1920, the Society merged with the Institute of Massage and Remedial Exercise, and the new group became known as the Chartered Society of Massage and Medical Gymnastics. This new group also took some important steps at professionalism. Among the new membership requirements were the requirement for physician referrals and the issuance of certificates of competence to those who passed the required tests. By 1939, the membership in the organization numbered approximately 12,000.

Following World War I, medical organizations such as the American Society of Physical Therapy Physicians also formed. In the 1920s and 1930s, programs for physical therapists were becoming standardized, while at the same time physicians were being trained in the field. **John S. Coulter,** in 1926, became the first full-time academic physician in physical medicine at the Northwestern University Medical School. By 1947, the field of physical medicine and rehabilitation, known as physiatry, was established as a separate medical specialty.

While many masseurs and masseuses frowned upon the encroachment of the medical profession on their art form, the events just described can be viewed with excitement. By the early part of the 20th century, the Western medical profession had begun to realize what the Chinese and masseurs/masseuses had long preached: therapeutic rubbing had an important place in the treatment of illnesses and diseases. The professionalism of medical gymnastics (as physical therapy) simply meant that in addition to learning the art of massage the therapist needs also to acquire the scientific background necessary to understand human anatomy and physiology. As this textbook illustrates, the editor also believes in a well-educated, well-trained massage therapist.

As technology and medical advances caught up with the profession, a simple massage became less crucial on its own, but rather it became one procedure in the arsenal of rehabilitation. As a consequence, the British Chartered Society of Massage and Medical Gymnastics changed its name to the Chartered Society of Physiotherapy. At about the same time, the American Association of Masseurs and Masseuses was formed in the United States; the group would later change its name to the American Massage Therapy Association. Over time, the American Massage Therapy Association came to represent the professional masseurs and masseuses, properly called massage therapists. The organization, with chapters in all 50 states, has nearly 25,000 members.

NEW METHODS

Over the past 50 years, several new massage styles and techniques have entered the profession. While space limitations prohibit detailed discussions of all of these procedures, several deserve some attention. As a general rule, these new techniques go beyond the original concepts of Swedish massage, and most were developed in the United States since 1960.

Esalen massage (developed at the Esalen Institute) is designed to create a deeper state of relaxation and general well-being. Compared with the Swedish system, Esalen massage is slower and more rhythmic and focuses on the whole individual (mind and body). Many massage therapists actually use a combination of Swedish and Esalen techniques.

Rolfing, developed by Dr. Ida Rolf, involves a form of deep tissue work, which loosens adhesions in the flexible tissue (fascia) surrounding our muscles. In general, the style aligns the major body segments through the manipulation of the fascia.

Deep tissue massage uses slow strokes, direct pressure, and/or friction. As the name implies, the procedure is applied with greater pressure and to deeper layers of muscles than Swedish massage.

Sports massage is massage that has been adapted to the needs of the athlete and consists of two categories: maintenance (as part of a training regimen) and event (pre-event and postevent). Sports massage is also used to promote healing from injuries. For more discussion, see Chapter 26.

Reflexology, also known as zone therapy, is based on the Oriental idea that the stimulation of particular points on the surface of the body has an effect on other areas of the body. Using deep finger pressure, massage therapists treat specific areas on the extremities (hands and feet) to normalize functions in the body. For more discussion, see the chapter on reflexology.

Neuromuscular massage is a form of deep massage that applies concentrated finger pressure to specific muscles. This form of massage helps to break the cycle of spasm and pain and is used on trigger points, which are intense knots of muscle tension that refer pain to other parts of the body. *Trigger point massage* and *myotherapy* are varieties of neuromuscular massage.

Bindegewebsmassage, or *connective tissue massage,* developed by Elizabeth Dicke, is a type of myofascial release technique that is concerned with the layer of connective tissue (fascia) located between the skin and muscles. The followers of Bindegewebsmassage believe that massage of the connective tissue will affect vascular and visceral reflexes relating to a number of pathologies and disabilities.

SUMMARY

In the past 25 years, massage has risen in popularity in the United States. Especially important in this rise of popularity are those individuals who are looking for alternative therapies (diet, exercise, herbal remedies, acupuncture, acupressure, and massage) to supplement their medical treatments, and thus help them with their lives and health. Massage, as one method of alternative therapy, has been shown to be beneficial for many people.

As a consequence of this increase in popularity, the profession has also grown during that time. In 1988, the American Massage Therapy Association pushed for the development of national certification, which finally came about in 1992 with the National Certification Examination for Therapeutic Massage and Bodywork. As such, massage therapy has become a respected and much used allied health care profession. According to the American Massage Therapy Association, massage therapy was the third most prevalent type of alternative/complementary medicine used by adults in the United States in the 1990s.

By no means is this study of massage history complete and exhaustive. A detailed history of massage would take volumes and entail years of research. This chapter should have given you a thorough sense of how the profession developed and in what direction we seem to be headed. There are over 75 different varieties of massage and bodywork. This chapter has given you a glimpse of how they first began.

SELF-TEST

Multiple Choice • Write the letter of the best answer in the space provided.

_______ 1. The first written accounts of therapeutic rubbing (massage), are found in
A. China C. Japan
B. India D. Greece

_______ 2. The father of modern Western medicine is generally recognized as being
A. Iccus C. Galen
B. Hippocrates D. Paré

_______ 3. The systematic and scientific manipulation of the soft tissues of the body is called
A. acupressure C. massage
B. mobilization D. gymnastics

_______ 4. According to Pehr Henrik Ling, gymnastics by which we try to alleviate or overcome the sufferings that have arisen through abnormal conditions are known as
A. pedagogical gymnastics
B. military gymnastics
C. medical gymnastics
D. aesthetic gymnastics

_______ 5. Western massage texts tend to use French terminology, primarily because of the efforts of one individual,
A. Pehr H. Ling C. Hippocrates
B. Ambroise Paré D. Johann Mezger

_______ 6. Which of the following would **not** be considered a recent development in alternative medicine?
A. Esalen massage C. acupuncture/pressure
B. Rolfing D. Bindegewebsmassage

_______ 7. The medical field of physical medicine and rehabilitation is known as
A. physiology C. psychology
B. physiatry D. psychiatry

_______ 8. His 11th-century *Cannon of Medicine* was an especially famous medical text that compiled the theoretical and practical medical knowledge of the time.
A. Ambrose Paré C. Avicenna
B. Galen of Pergamon D. Rhazes

_______ 9. The scientist who demonstrated that blood circulation in animals is impelled by the beating of the heart through arteries and veins was
A. Timothy Bright C. John S. Coulter
B. William Harvey D. Simon André Tissot

_______ 10. Who founded the ancient Greek "Methodist" school of thought, which supported a simplistic view of healing and restricted treatments to bathing, diet, massage, and a few drugs?
A. Iccus C. Galen of Pergamon
B. Hippocrates of Cos D. Asclepiades

_______ 11. The work generally credited as being the first book in the field of sports medicine was
A. *De Arte Gymnastica*
B. *Chen-chiu ta-ch'eng*
C. *Swedish Movement and Massage Treatment*
D. *A Treatise on Massage*

_______ 12. The different kinds of movements which are used in Ling's System of Medical Gymnastics are
A. active, passive, duplicated
B. active, gymnastics, passive
C. active, passive, range-of-motion
D. active, resistive, duplicated

_______ 13. Reflexology is also known as
A. neuromuscular massage
B. zone therapy
C. sports massage
D. myotherapy

_______ 14. Trigger point therapy and myotherapy are methods of
A. connective tissue massage
B. sports massage
C. Esalen massage
D. neuromuscular massage

_______ 15. Electrotherapy and hydrotherapy are methods of

A. physiotherapy C. zone therapy
B. Bindegewebsmassage D. reflexology

_______ 16. The Swedish Movement System was introduced into the United States by
A. Johann Mezger
B. Douglas Graham and Hartvig Nissen
C. Just Lucas-Championniere
D. George and Charles Taylor

_______ 17. The healing of the body by means of manipulations is known as
A. zone therapy C. hydrotherapy
B. mechanotherapy D. physiotherapy

_______ 18. Sports massage is specifically tailored to the athlete and consists of two main categories
A. maintenance and event
B. maintenance and pre-event
C. maintenance and postevent
D. all of the above

_______ 19. Active movements are those
A. performed by the therapist/gymnast
B. performed by the patient/client
C. performed by both the therapist and the client
D. all of the above

_______ 20. Which of the following statements is **not** true, regarding Esalen massage and Swedish massage.
A. Swedish massage is more rhythmic than Esalen massage
B. Swedish massage focuses more on the whole body
C. Esalen massage is designed to create an overall sense of well-being
D. none of the above

References

Basham, A. L. The Practice of Medicine in Ancient and Medieval India. In *Asian Medical Systems.* ed. Charles Leslie, pp. 18–43. Berkeley: University of California Press, 1976.

Buikstra, Jane E. Diseases of the Pre-Columbian Americas. In *The Cambridge World History of Human Disease.* Kenneth F. Kiple et. al. (eds.). pp. 305–317. New York: Cambridge University Press, 1993.

Castiglioni, Arturo. *A History of Medicine.* Translated by E. B. Krumbhaar. New York: Alfred A. Knopf, 1947.

Coulter, John. *Physical Therapy.* New York: Paul B. Hoeber, Inc., 1932.

Fryback, Patricia, and Bonita Reinert. "Alternative Therapies and Control for Health in Cancer and AIDS." *Clinical Nurse Specialist,* 11(2): 64–69, 1997.

Goldberg, J., D. Seaborne, S. Sullivan, and B. Leduc. "The Effect of Therapeutic Massage on H-Reflex Amplitude in Persons with a Spinal Cord Injury." *Physical Therapy* 74(8): 728–37, 1994.

Liddel, L. *The Book of Massage: The Complete Step-by-Step Guide to Eastern and Western Techniques.* New York: Simon and Schuster, 1984.

McMillan, Mary. *Massage and Therapeutic Exercise.* Philadelphia: W. B. Saunders, 1921.

Means, Philip Ainsworth. *Ancient Civilizations of the Andes.* New York: C. Scribner's Sons, 1931.

Meintz, Sharon L. "Alternatives and Complementary Therapies: Whatever Became of the Back Rub?" *RN* 58(4): 49–50+, 1995.

Mulliner, Mary Rees. *Mechano-Therapy: A Text-book for Students.* Philadelphia: Lea & Febiger, 1929.

Nissen, Hartvig. *Practical Massage in Twenty Lessons.* Philadelphia: F. A. Davis Co., 1905.

Rahman, Fazlur. *Health and Medicine in the Islamic Tradition: Change and Identity.* New York: Crossroad, 1987.

Salmon, J. Warren, ed. *Alternative Medicine: Popular and Policy Perspectives.* New York: Tavistock Publications, 1984.

Solomon, Walter. "What Is Happening to Massage?" *Archives of Physical Medicine* (August): 521–523, 1950.

Acute Pain Management in Adults. Operative Procedures. Quick Reference Guide for Clinicians. Rockville, MD: United States Department of Health and Human Services, 1992.

Management of Cancer Pain: Adults. Quick Reference Guide for Clinicians. Rockville, MD: United States Department of Health and Human Services, 1994.

Unschuld, Paul U. "History of Chinese Medicine." *The Cambridge World History of Human Disease.* Kenneth F. Kiple et. al. (eds.). pp. 20–27. New York: Cambridge University Press, 1993.

Veith, Ilza. *Huang Ti: Nei Ching Su Wen.* Baltimore: Williams & Wilkins, 1949.

Wanning, Thomas. *Healing and the Mind/Body Arts: Massage, Acupuncture, Yoga, Tai Chi, and Feldenkrais.* AAOHN Journal, 41(7): 349–351, 1993.

White, Jennifer. "Touching With Intent: Therapeutic Massage." *Holistic Nursing Practice* 2(3): 63–67, 1988.

Wide, Anders G. *Hand-Book of Medical and Orthopedic Gymnastics.* New York: Funk & Wagnalls, 1905.

Zyzk, Kenneth G. *Religious Healing in the Veda.* Transaction of the American Philosophical Society 75: 7, 1985.

Good fences make good neighbors.
—Robert Frost

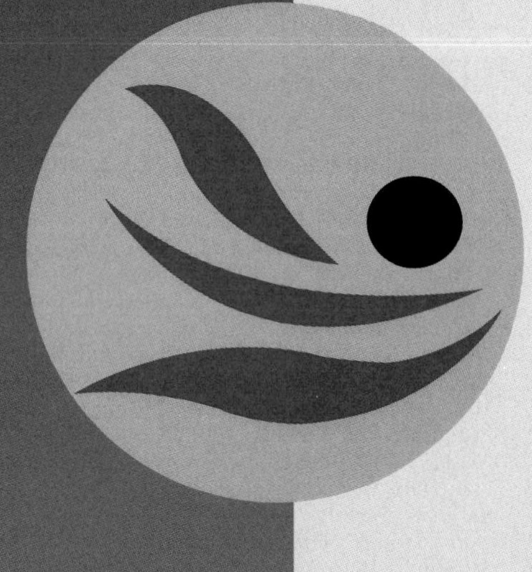

2

Professional Standards and Boundaries

Student Objectives

After completing this chapter, the student should be able to:

- Define the massage therapist's scope of practice
- List at least 15 different standards of conduct from the Code of Ethics
- Define confidentiality, and give examples of exceptions to it
- Define the concept of boundaries as they relate to your personal and professional life
- Write a set of personal and professional boundaries for yourself
- Create procedures for handling "fire drills" and identifiable scenarios of client conflict
- Describe when it is appropriate to terminate the massage session if a client violates your personal or professional boundaries

INTRODUCTION

The prevailing guidelines for the massage therapy profession can be divided into two areas: professional standards and boundaries. *Professional standards* consist of the boundaries that are set by the massage profession itself in order to promote consistency and integrity. These standards apply to all massage therapists in a given jurisdiction and define how the individual therapist relates to the profession as a whole. While geographically these standards may vary widely, they include a number of vital elements: educational requirements; professional scope of practice; a code of ethics; professional conduct guidelines; confidentiality; and state and municipal laws.

The second area, *boundaries,* consists of our individual standards in interactions with our clients and all relationships. For our purposes, boundaries may be personal or professional, but vary with the individual therapist according to personal need. As the Robert Frost quotation reminds us, fences (a type of physical boundary) can enhance our relationships with others. Boundaries in relationships impart a sense of self, a personal or professional space to grow, and a sense of protection. As we explore the topic of boundaries, we will discuss personal boundaries, professional boundaries, issues of client abuse and neglect, how to handle problem situations, issues of intimacy, inappropriate behavior and its consequences, session termination procedures, and incident reports (Fig. 2–1).

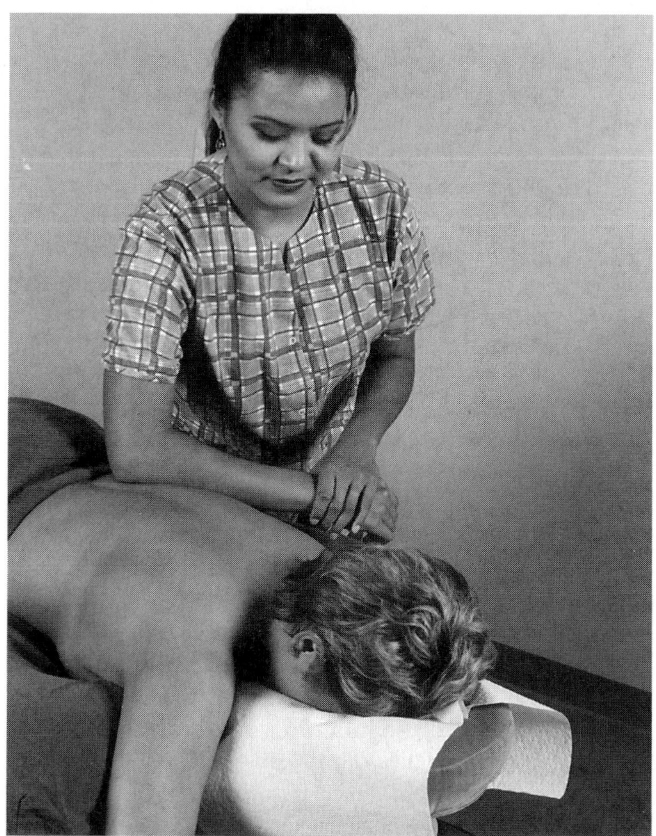

Figure 2•1 The massage therapist is a professional.

PROFESSIONAL STANDARDS

In general, professional standards help to define and distinguish our profession from that of other health care professions. As our profession grows, more distinct borders, which give our profession limitations, are defined. We can call these parameters our professional standards. These standards include the requirements for education, testing and licensing, scope of practice, the code of ethics, and principles of professional conduct.

What's in a Word? The Educational Requirements

The terms "licensed," "certified," "registered," and "nationally certified" are all adjectives used to describe educated massage therapists. Credentials and identifying titles are important parts of professional image and allow you to promote yourself as qualified and competent to the general public. These adjectives are often confusing because different agencies who issue the right to use these descriptions often have different requirements. Each region (e.g., state, county, parish, city) may have its own rules and regulations for the practice of massage therapy.

Massage therapy schools today teach certification courses that range from 100 to over 2,000 hours. At the time of this writing the national average of formal training in the United States is 500 hours. The terms "masseur" and "masseuse" were dropped in favor of "massage therapist." In some areas, this was done to move from the gender-specific French terms to a title that is not gender specific. In other areas of the country, the change in terminology was made to differentiate between individuals who were apprentice trained and those who received classroom training in anatomy and physiology. These educated therapists were described by a confusing variety of terms and titles because there was no national standard. These titles included certified massage therapist (C.M.T.), registered massage therapist (R.M.T.), licensed massage therapist (L.M.T.), and simply massage therapist (M.T., Ms.T., or M.Th.).

According to *Webster's New Collegiate Dictionary,* one meaning of the word "certify" is "to attest authoritatively as to the validity of" something. Therefore, to certify a massage therapist means to attest the training, knowledge, and skill of a practitioner. Such verification is usually made by a nongovernmental institution, such as a trade school, massage school, or professional organization. Since the students choose voluntarily to take the classes in the massage field, the certification itself is only as good as the reputation and credentials of the certifying body. A massage therapy school therefore **certifies** that the student has completed a course in massage therapy and may grant the title of Certified Massage Therapist or C.M.T. This certification usually involves completion of a required number of hours of classroom instruction in combination with other educational requirements: apprenticeship; internship; and successful passing of exams that cover science and applied skills. In many states, one must obtain a state license as well as receiving an official certificate of successful completion of a course of study, in order to practice massage therapy legally.

The word "licensing" means that "permission has been granted by a competent authority for a person to engage in an occupation which would otherwise be considered to be unlawful." It is a government body, such as a state, province, or municipality, that grants the license to practice massage therapy as a means of regulating the profession according to law. Licensure is a mandatory (or nonvoluntary) process because it is passed into law by a legislative body. Everyone who wants to practice massage therapy must complete the licensing process in states that require it. Once a therapist has been qualified (through certification) to take the licensing exam, successfully passing the exam leads to a **license;** the massage therapist is then known as a Licensed Massage Therapist or L.M.T. once this, and perhaps further requirements (i.e., paying a license fee), are met.

The massage profession appears to have a broad range of usage of the word "registered." Two definitions of "register" are "to make a record of" or "a book or system of public records." *Webster's New Collegiate Dictionary* defines a registered nurse as "a graduate trained nurse who has been licensed by a state authority after passing qualifying examinations for registration." When the state of Texas created its massage therapy law, it chose to use the designation "registered" instead of "licensed" massage therapist. According to the American Massage Therapy Association, "registered" is generally "somewhat less restrictive than licensing," but each state varies in its use of "registered."

The American Massage Therapy Association (AMTA) also had a registered massage therapist program that sought to elevate standards by creating a higher tier of professional. This program required successful completion of certain education, experience, and testing standards. This R.M.T. program and testing for entry into the association were eventually abolished.

In 1987, with the purpose of promoting higher standards for massage therapists, a joint organization was created consisting of representatives from the AMTA, the American Oriental Bodywork Therapy Association (AOBTA), the American Polarity Therapy Association (APTA), the Rolf Institute, and the Trager Institute. Together the various groups formed the National Certification Board for Therapeutic Massage and Bodywork. By 1992, the National Certification Board for Therapeutic Massage and Bodywork (NCBTMB), a nonprofit organization that is governed by an elected board of directors, was established. This independent national board was accredited by the National Organization for Competency Assurance (NOCA) in 1993. The goal of the NCBTMB was to define and implement high standards for the massage therapy profession through the successful completion of a nationally recognized test.

The NCBTMB has been quite successful, and, while it has not been accepted unanimously in all states, some states with licensing laws accept the national exam in lieu of their own state written licensing exam. There is an NCBTMB national code of ethics and a disciplinary board for processing grievances filed against nationally certified practitioners.

In summary, massage therapy schools certify students. The majority of the states license their massage therapists through a testing procedure. Some states opt to use "registered" to define massage therapists in their regions. National certification is a process designed to raise professional standards and create additional professional recognition for those who can complete it.

The Scope of a Massage Therapy Practice

Scope of practice, often derived from the legal definition of massage, defines the working parameters of a particular profession, and is solely a matter of state law, which may vary from state to state. Scope of practice defines what services can be provided by massage therapists; it may also list specific practices that massage therapists may not offer because a separate type of license (such as ultrasound treatments) is required. Professional massage therapy associations and certifying bodies, such as massage therapy schools, workshops, and national organizations, may also have their own requirements. However, superseding any other conflicting legal definitions and professional parameters, state law defines scope of practice as the minimum standard by which massage therapists must practice (Fig. 2–2).

It is important to obtain a copy of your state law and to know your scope of practice.

1. It may include the application of any form of manual treatment of bodily soft tissues for the purposes of general relaxation, of improving the health of the client, and of maintaining or restoring the client to proper health. The term "soft tissue" denotes the various layers of the integument, the muscles, tendons, ligaments, fascia, cartilage, nerves, blood vessels, viscera, and membranes of the body. The

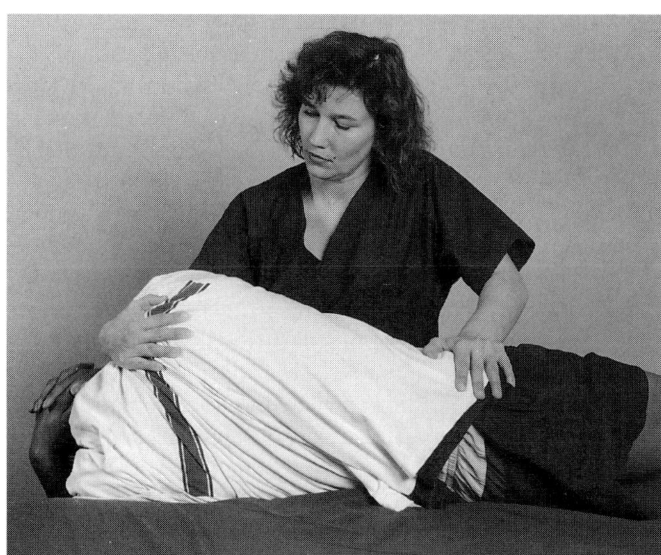

Figure 2•2 Massage therapists' scope of practice is determined by state law.

term "manual treatment" includes all forms of therapy whereby the soft tissues of the client's body are treated with direct or indirect contact of the massage therapist's hands, feet, elbows, knees, and forearms. *Direct* contact may include the application of pressure to the tissues and may introduce movement to the joints in order to affect surrounding tissues. Direct contact may also include various devices, such as mechanical vibrators or handheld pressure bars for applying static pressure. *Indirect* contact may be energetic in nature; that is, it may not necessarily involve actual touch as much as sensitivity to the energy fields surrounding the body.

2. Scope of practice includes the general assessment of the client's condition by interview, palpation, and consultation with the client's other health care providers. Assessment is needed to determine treatment goals, contraindications, and the need for referral to other health care professionals. "General assessment" refers to the massage therapist's ability, based upon past training and experience, to recognize specific pathologies and to formulate an appropriate treatment based upon established protocol.
3. Scope of practice does not include diagnosis of illness or injury. While it may include joint mobilizations and range of motion, it does *not* include performing spinal or joint manipulations. Prescribing or advising the use of medication, or rendering a prognosis, all of which are in the domain of medical and chiropractic physicians, is also omitted. Instead of a prognosis, massage therapists can give an estimated duration of treatment or opinion regarding the client's progress.
4. Due to the popular use of massage therapy as "recreational," massage therapists have open access to the public. A doctor's prescription is *not* required for someone to see a massage therapist. However, in cases involving insurance reimbursement for treatment of illness or injury, the massage therapist must have a written diagnosis and referral from a medical or chiropractic physician.
5. Scope of practice may include the use of hydrotherapy and aromatherapy. Hydrotherapy encompasses the therapeutic use of ice packs, heat packs, whirlpools, saunas, and steam baths. Aromatherapy includes the use of essential oils to heighten the relaxation effect of the therapy.

Code of Ethics

When you enroll in a massage therapy school, you agree to accept certain rules and standards. Likewise, when you enter into the profession in a state that requires licensure, you also inherently accept the massage therapy laws and ethical standards of that state. Typically the licensing board of your state is responsible for creating and distributing its code of ethics. Professional massage therapy organizations may have their own codes of ethics, which you as a member are expected to incorporate into your practice.

A **code of ethics** is a set of guiding moral principles that governs one's course of action. Most licensed health care professions have a code of ethics that members of those professions are expected to follow when working within their scope of practice. Most codes of ethics for massage therapists include governing principles for therapeutic relationships, for professional behavior, for business policies, and even for guidance in decision making. An ethical decision is required to solve a problem that has long-term implications. For example, most state laws do not require therapists to post a list of fees for a given service, nor do states require that the therapist equally charge every client. No one will argue with a therapist who gives a discount to senior citizens, the disabled, or the economically disadvantaged. But how will a therapist be judged if an attorney or a doctor is charged more than the normal fee? While it may be legal to do so, it is not ethical.

Most people have a personal code of ethics that governs their behavior. Many of us acquired our codes during interactions with family, members of our religious congregation, and members of our community. When you are acting unethically, you are acting in contradiction to a generally accepted standard of conduct set forth by your peers or your profession.

In addition to a code of ethics, many health professions publish a list of principles of professional conduct. While similar in many ways to a code of ethics, the principles of professional conduct serve as another guide to ensure high performance standards of the massage profession. Examples of a code of ethics and principles of conduct follow.

The National Certification Board for Therapeutic Massage and Bodywork Code of Ethics

The Code of Ethics of the National Certification Board for Therapeutic Massage and Bodywork (NCBTMB) specifies professional standards that allow for the proper discharge of the massage therapist's and/or bodyworker's responsibilities to those served, that protect the integrity of the profession, and that safeguard the interest of individual clients. It was adopted in 1995.

Those practitioners nationally certified in therapeutic massage and bodywork in the exercise of professional accountability will conduct themselves as follows:

1. Have a sincere commitment to provide the highest quality of care to those who seek their professional services.
2. Represent their qualifications honestly, including education and professional affiliations, and provide only those services which they are qualified to perform.
3. Accurately inform clients, other health care practitioners, and the public of the scope and limitations of their discipline.
4. Acknowledge the limitations of and contraindications for massage therapy and bodywork, and refer clients to appropriate health professionals.
5. Provide treatment only when there is reasonable expectation that it will be advantageous to the client.
6. Consistently maintain and improve professional knowledge and competence, striving for professional excellence through regular assessment of personal and professional strengths and weaknesses and through continued educational training.
7. Conduct their business and professional activities with honesty and integrity, and respect the inherent worth of all persons.
8. Refuse to unjustly discriminate against clients or other ethical health professionals.
9. Safeguard the confidentiality of all client information, unless disclosure is required by law, court order, or absolutely necessary for the protection of the public.
10. Respect the client's right to treatment with informed and voluntary consent. The NCTMB practitioner will obtain and record the informed consent of the client, or client's advocate, before providing treatment. This consent may be written or verbal.
11. Respect the client's right to refuse, modify, or terminate treatment regardless of prior consent given.
12. Provide draping and treatment in a way that ensures the safety, comfort, and privacy of the client.
13. Exercise the right to refuse to treat any person or part of the body for just and reasonable cause.
14. Refrain, under all circumstances, from initiating or engaging in any sexual conduct, sexual activities, or sexualizing behavior involving a client, even if the client attempts to sexualize the relationship.
15. Avoid any interest, activity, or influence which might be in conflict with the practitioner's obligation to act in the best interests of the client or the profession.
16. Respect the client's boundaries with regard to privacy, disclosure, exposure, emotional expression, beliefs, and the client's reasonable expectations of professional behavior. Practitioners will respect the client's autonomy.
17. Refuse any gifts or benefits which are intended to influence a referral, decision, or treatment that are purely for personal gain and not for the good of the client.
18. Follow all policies, procedures, guidelines, regulations, codes, and requirements promulgated by the National Certification Board for Therapeutic Massage and Bodywork.

Massage Therapist's Principles of Professional Conduct

Principle 1. Massage Therapists shall conduct themselves in a manner compatible with a code of ethics set forth by a municipal, county/parish, or state governing board under which they practice or a professional organization with which they are affiliated.

Principle 2. Massage Therapists shall continually improve their knowledge of the human body and massage therapy by attending and participating in academic pursuits and professional activities and will share this information with their colleagues.

Principle 3. Massage Therapists shall always take appropriate measures to protect the health, safety, right to privacy, and confidentiality of their clients and shall treat their clients with dignity and respect.

Principle 4. Massage Therapists shall provide services to members of the community regardless of gender, race, national origin, ancestry, religious affiliation, creed, marital status, political affiliation, disability, sexual orientation, and social or economic status.

Principle 5. Massage Therapists shall apply only those modalities in which they are qualified and proficient, as long as such modalities do not violate their scope of practice as determined by the laws in the state in which license is issued.

Principle 6. Massage Therapists shall always represent their qualifications honestly.

Principle 7. Massage Therapists shall act independently as well as collaboratively with other health care professionals in the implementation of professional services.

Principle 8. Massage Therapists shall not render a medical diagnosis, but due to their skill, experience, and knowledge shall provide the client and other allied health care providers with specific visual and palpatory findings, as well as other insights that are relative to the care of the client.

Principle 9. Massage Therapists shall report all unethical conduct and illegal professional activities of their colleagues to the proper authorities.

Principle 10. Massage Therapists shall model optimal health and hygiene practices for their clients by following a regimen of good hygiene and health-promoting activities.

The Good Samaritan Law

Every state in the United States has a Good Samaritan law to protect individuals who give medical aid in emergency situations from criminal and civil liability. Within each state, the law concerning the Good Samaritan may vary slightly, but in general, if a health care professional renders help to an individual in need, such as performing CPR, she is not held liable for any harm to the individual as a result of her decision to help in the emergency.

Confidentiality and Its Exceptions

All information exchanged between the client and therapist is confidential. **Confidentiality** is the nondisclosure of privileged information; that is, it may not be divulged to a third party without the client's written permission. Confidentiality is an important part of the client-therapist relationship.

There are two basic exceptions to the confidentiality rule. The first exception is when clients give permission for the massage therapist to reveal their name or specific personal information to a third party. This may occur when the therapist is part of a therapy team, working in connection with a client's mental health counselor, doctor, attorney, or other involved professional. Release of information may also involve a family member, such as a parent of a minor client or the adult child of an elderly client. Other third-party involvement can include a translator for someone with a language barrier or a relative who has power of attorney for a disabled client.

The second exception occurs when keeping information confidential would cause harm to either the client or to a third party. These situations might involve a client who, taking the massage therapist into his confidence, discusses plans of suicide or actions that will harm others (e.g., homicide). In these cases, the therapist should contact the client's psychotherapist or medical doctor if known or may contact the emergency contact person listed on the client intake form. Reporting the situation initiates a process, often an investigation. In some areas, the massage therapist may be required to report situations of child abuse, elder abuse, or any criminal activity to law enforcement. Call the local district attorney's office or the massage therapy board to find out which agency in your area is appropriate for each situation.

You may also be required to report cases of communicable diseases, such as tuberculosis or hepatitis, to your public health department to make sure that you and others are not at risk of infection from contagions. Contact your local health department and inquire what your responsibilities are as a health care provider.

Terms of Reference—How Do We Refer to Our Patrons?

There has been a great deal of discussion over whether the patrons of massage therapy should be referred to as clients or patients. If your state law specifies the use of client or patient, then the language of the law supersedes any professional preference. When the law does not specify, or if your state currently does not require licensure, how we refer to our patrons may be strictly situational. For example, if you are in private practice or are employed by a nonmedical establishment such as a salon or a spa, "clients" is the appropriate reference for your patrons. If you work in a medical setting, such as a hospital, a physical therapy office, or a chiropractic clinic, the preferred terminology is "patients." The major difference is that "patients" denotes that our patrons are under medical supervision of another health care professional.

Discrimination

It is the right of either party to decide not to engage in or maintain the therapeutic relationship. The therapist's right of refusal is covered in detail in Chapter 20, Professional Communication.

The therapist has the right to refuse any client as long as there is a justifiable reason for the refusal of service, and the therapist must inform the client of the reason for refusal. A justifiable reason may include health-related issues such as contraindicated conditions, improper hygiene, and personal safety. The therapist may not refuse a client for reasons of race, creed, political affiliation, disability, religion, gender, marital status, national origin, ancestry, sexual orientation, or social or economic status. The massage therapist should perform her work in an unbiased, nonjudgmental, and professional manner.

Moshe Feldenkrais

May 6, 1904–Feb. 9, 1984

"We settle for so little! As long as we can get by, we let it go at that."

Moshe Feldenkrais's father sold bits of forests . . . sort of like the owner of a modern-day timber and logging operation, but that's about the only thing that is ordinary about the man, his work, and his background. Feldenkrais was reared in the Talmudic tradition and came from a long list of rabbis. His great-great-grandfather was a famous rabbi who is still quoted today. Feldenkrais changed his nationality three times before he left home at 13: first it was Polish, then German, then Russian. In 1918, at age 14, he walked with a group of people from Poland to Turkey. It was the end of WWI and his parents stayed behind. He never saw his father again.

His doctorate was in science and he had degrees in both mechanical and electrical engineering. Feldenkrais worked on the French atomic research program as well as the British antisubmarine program.

As a boy of 16 in Palestine, Feldenkrais was part of a group called the Haganah, which means self-defense force. They learned some basic jujitsu, which didn't prove successful. It was then that Feldenkrais realized that the only way to learn was to start at the beginning—with the first move.

> *And I built this system of defense for any sort of attack where the first movement is not what you think to do, what you decide to do, but what you actually do when you are frightened. And I said, "all right, let's see now, we will train the people so that the end of their first spontaneous movement is where we must start."*
>
> — "Moshe on Moshe on the Martial Arts." From Feldenkrais Journal 12, Issue #2

Feldenkrais published an instructional book on the subject, which gained him admission to his first judo exhibition.

The Japanese minister of education was so taken with Feldenkrais and what he had accomplished without any formal training, that he asked him to introduce judo to Europe. Feldenkrais refused, explaining that he couldn't devote himself to such an enterprise and continue his university studies at the same time. But the minister was determined, and soon it was agreed that an expert would come to France and work with Feldenkrais when time would allow.

Thus, Feldenkrais became the first European to hold a black belt in judo. He was also a fierce soccer player. In fact, it was a soccer injury that flared up during the German invasion of France that prompted him to pull from his martial arts experience as well as his engineering and mechanical background to explore the relationship between the nervous system and body function. (A 50-50 chance that surgery would correct the problem wasn't good enough odds for Feldenkrais.)

The result of his work is pure genius. And what is so awesome about Feldenkrais's legacy? He believed in—and made a difference to—the potentiality of humankind. He helped men and women become more *themselves.* He saw the infinite possibilities, since he, like Descartes, viewed the human being as a tabula rasa ("clean slate").

The problem is that much of what we have learned is harmful to our system because it was learned in childhood, when immediate dependence on others distorted our real needs. Long-standing habitual action feels right. Training a body to be perfect in all the possible forms and configurations of its members changes not only the strength and flexibility of the skeleton and muscles, but makes a profound and beneficial change in the self-image and quality of the direction of the self.

—From: "Mind and Body." Moshe Feldenkrais.

Feldenkrais believed that habitual patterns are imprinted in the nervous system—good or bad—and that verbally directed exercises and manipulation could help the brain/body learn movements that would free bodily limitations and instill our natural birthright, a sense of grace.

His methods led to what could be considered incredible results. People with multiple sclerosis and cerebral palsy gained a new lease on life, and athletes without any obvious physical limitations sought his therapy.

A typical session consists of an instructor leading a group in various exercises or manipulating an individual through small repeated movements. This creates a new awareness or spatial reality, which the brain recognizes as being immediately right or better than the original impeded movement.

The sensations experienced in these sessions bring into focus the tension and stress that make our movement inefficient, and prepare us to learn new patterns that permit the body to function at a level much closer to its full human potential. Feldenkrais was big on the concept of learning. He thought it was the gift of life, inextricably tied to personal growth and the key to body/mind health.

My way of learning, my way of dealing with people, is to find out, for that person who wants it, what sort of accomplishment is possible for that person. People can learn to move and walk and stand differently, but they have given up because they think it's too late now, that the growth process has been completed, that they can't learn something new, that they don't have the time or ability. You don't have to go back to being a baby in order to function properly. You can, at any time of your life, rewire yourself, provided I can convince you that there is nothing permanent or compulsive in your system, except what you believe to be so.

—From: "Movement and the Mind." Moshe Feldenkrais and Will Shutz.

Practitioners worldwide are achieving dramatic results with Functional Integration and Awareness Through Movement. In North America alone, there are 1,500 certified practitioners. Training takes about three years and since Feldenkrais believed the only way he could teach his work was to experience it, graduates leave not only with a diploma and opportunity for a promising career, but also improved posture, flexibility, coordination, and ease of movement (at any age), freedom or reduction of pain, profound psychological and emotional growth, improved physical well-being and vitality, and the ability to understand how to "learn" effectively and enjoyably in any area of life.

BOUNDARIES: THE EXTENT OF OUR ROLE AS MASSAGE THERAPISTS

A boundary can be defined as "a set of parameters that indicates a border or limit." In this section, "boundaries" will include not only boundaries that pertain to our profession but also personal and emotional boundaries. Violation of someone else's boundaries represents a situation of abuse or neglect. We will also explore issues of intimacy and personal disclosure with clients, consequences of misconduct, and how to handle problematic situations.

Boundaries represent the limits we establish between others and aspects of our lives. Thereby we establish our personal space, our emotional separateness, and our professional distance. Let's look at various boundaries as they occur in real estate. A property line exists between two lots and is generally respected by neighbors, even though the line is typically unmarked. Repeated violations of this invisible boundary may cause feelings of anger or anxiety. The walls and doors of our homes are also boundaries that shut or open. A home with open doors (or even unlocked doors) may be considered an unsafe situation; without an invitation such as a knock, it would be difficult to control who entered. Professional boundaries are very similar.

In her work *Exploring Boundaries,* Pat Ogden, developer of Hakomi Integrative Somatics, offers a very comprehensive description of boundaries. She states that boundaries are:

> ■ *Infinitely flexible and changeable, depending, moment to moment, upon both inner and outer conditions. A healthy sense of boundaries indicates that we can connect with the experience or sense of ourselves as both separate and in unity with the world. A "holding environment" for one's own presence, a container for our individual sense of self, of who we are, is established through healthy boundaries. We are aware of our differences, yet we can sense the interconnectedness of all beings. We can maintain both differentiation and connection.*
>
> *Through boundaries we are able to screen input from the world, to know what input is appropriate to let in and assimilate, and what input we need to keep out. With healthy boundaries, we keep ourselves from accepting subtle or overt kinds of abuse, and we also are sensitive to and respect the rights and boundaries of others.* ■

Imagine that you are always surrounded by a semipermeable membrane and this membrane can expand or contract depending on the person or situation you encounter. You are able to choose (either consciously or unconsciously) how close, both physically and emotionally, to allow the other person (or situation) to be to you. This may be difficult if you have never been exposed to the concept of boundaries. Some relationships do not honor or respect (therefore do not teach or reinforce) good healthy boundaries. In these cases, the therapist is encouraged to obtain as much information as possible on boundaries.

In this section, we will explore the concept of boundaries as they relate to our personal and professional lives. Perhaps the most important part of Ogden's description is her statement about healthy boundaries: "With healthy boundaries, we keep ourselves from accepting subtle or overt kinds of abuse. . . ." Boundaries are about self-protection.

The next section of Odgen's statement reads, "And we also are sensitive to and respect the rights and boundaries of others." It is from this aspect of healthy boundaries that the majority of our professional boundaries as massage therapists are derived. By respecting the boundaries of others, we instill a sense of dignity and respect to our clients, to our profession, and to ourselves.

Personal Boundaries

Personal boundaries are boundaries that you create to protect yourself, nurture yourself, make your life less stressful, and maintain a healthy sense of your separateness from others. Many people get by without having to commit them to paper, but writing down your personal boundaries is a good idea. The very act of writing these boundaries down helps to anchor them in the conscious and unconscious mind. Remember that boundaries are extremely personal decisions that are unique to the individual based upon their personal belief system, needs, and environment. Examples of healthy boundaries may include:

1. I will recognize and respect the boundaries of others. I realize that I may not be able to meet their every need but I will be sensitive to them, meet the needs I can, and when someone says stop, I will comply.
2. I will say no when I am at my limit. I realize, in some occasions, I have gone out of my way to please others. While it's okay to do favors out of love and kindness for other people, I have overcommitted myself in the past and have become resentful. When solicited for help, time, or money, I will take 24 hours to think about it before giving the person an answer. This reduces my stress level and often prevents me from making impulsive decisions.
3. If someone is being verbally abusive, I can state my feelings about the situation and ask him or her to stop. While I cannot change the person, I can always remove myself from the situation by leaving.

The aforementioned boundaries were thought out and planned, but boundaries can be inherent as well. You may recognize some of these boundaries as things you do naturally. For example, when you get into a crowded elevator with strangers, everyone's physical boundaries are necessarily compressed. As a coping mechanism for the physical closeness, the normal reaction is to emotionally distance yourself from the other passengers. This is usually accomplished through silence and by staring at the numbers of the floors going by. Our physical boundaries are different for different people. Some people are not comfortable touching at all; others warrant a handshake, still others a hug, and some a kiss.

Personal boundaries can surround privacy issues such as nudity, doors being closed, telephone conversations, mail, journals, and diaries. They may be about personal space in a variety of situations with friends, strangers, family, lovers, and people who smoke, wear too much fragrance, or who are noisy. Personal boundaries also encompass our mental, emotional, and spiritual beliefs. We may choose with whom we share our feelings, beliefs, decisions, and spirituality; all these help us define who we are as individuals. Many people with unhealthy boundaries find themselves taking on the likes, dislikes, belief systems, and even the personalities of those with whom they are in a relationship. The following list contains illustrations of unhealthy boundaries. Unhealthy boundaries are usually not chosen by the individual, but occur as we model the inappropriate behavior of others in our environment or as a coping mechanism that may have worked during childhood but is no longer valid for us as adults.

1. I tell my problems to anyone who will listen, even extremely personal information concerning my body, my sexuality, or my problems with my spouse and family. I make no distinction about whether I talk about these things in private or on a crowded subway.
2. I really don't like to go to action movies with my spouse, but I never tell him that I would rather see a romance or drama instead. Usually I just sit through it with him, resenting that I'm wasting my time, and treating him coldly for the rest of the evening.

These types of behaviors often lead to self-dissatisfaction and depression. People with poor boundary systems typically find themselves being either totally vulnerable or totally intrusive. With healthy boundaries comes security and the ability to give as well as receive in relationships.

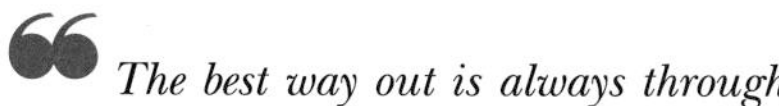
The best way out is always through.

—Robert Frost

Professional Boundaries

Professional boundaries, like massage therapy itself, relate to the integrity of the therapist. Integrity comes from the word "integer" or to integrate. **Integrity** is the condition of being whole and undivided. To have a character with integrity, you must deal honestly with yourself and with others. Webster defines integrity as the "firm adherence to a code of moral or artistic values." Integrity is central to our work as massage therapists.

The majority of the professional boundaries will be client focused so that, according to Ogden, "we also are sensitive to and respect the rights and boundaries of others." In a healthy therapeutic relationship there is a balance between safety and objectivity and between care/compassion and distance. There is no formula for achieving this balance, but healthy boundaries can provide the foundation on which the therapist builds his professional relationship with the client. Remember that boundaries are always contextual; they are interpreted in the context of the therapeutic relationship.

The following list contains several suggestions for professional boundaries. Notice that they include issues of time, appointment scheduling, relating, draping, hugging, and other professional issues. Each item can be used as a topic for group discussion, or the list may be used by therapists to form their own "professional conscience" regarding their practice. The purpose of the following list is to begin examining ways to prevent situations of boundary violation, abuse, or neglect to both the client and the therapist.

1. Schedule a minimum of 15 to 30 minutes between client appointments; you will then have the flexibility of dealing with late clients, time to extend appointments from 60 to 90 minutes if requested, and time to return calls or take a break.
2. Make house calls or out-calls to hotels only to clients who have been referred by an existing client, or set up some safeguards. You should only make out-calls to reputable hotel chains, and check in at the front desk when you arrive. Be sure and let the staff know that you will be coming by to check out when the session is complete. When you get to the room, call the front desk and let them know that you are starting your massage and that you will be checking back in with them in about an hour (or length of the session). This should be done in the presence of your client, so that she is aware that others know your location.
3. Always provide a basket for the client's jewelry and personal items so that nothing valuable gets misplaced or stolen.
4. Avoid asking the client personal questions that have nothing to do with the massage treatment.
5. Respect the client's physical appearance. Large or unusual scars, tattoos, body piercing, birth defects, body hair, and body size should not be referred to rudely or disrespectfully. There are times when you may be surprised by a scar, tattoo, or other anomaly.
6. Avoid using high-pressure tactics to sell the client vitamin supplements, to sell health foods, or to make commitments to long-term massage treat-

ments. Many therapists believe it is unethical for them to sell products as it invites a dual relationship; one aspect of the relationship is as a therapist and the other is as a salesperson.

7. Provide adequate draping to ensure the client's privacy and your professionalism. Avoid drapes that are semitransparent, and respect the boundary of the drape.
8. Avoid hugging your client until permission is granted. Hugging your client is acceptable only if hugs are solicited by the client *after* she is dressed and off the table and *only* if the therapist also is comfortable with giving and receiving hugs.
9. Refrain from making sexual innuendos, sexual jokes, or propositions, and flirting or giving physical compliments.
10. Always respect a client's comfort level. Respond immediately to his requests for a change in pressure applied to his body, for a change in the room temperature, for omission of a certain part of the massage therapy routine, or for extra work in a problem area if there is time within the session.
11. Always dress professionally while engaging in the practice or promotion of massage therapy. Definitions of professional dress may vary greatly, from suits to scrubs to casual wear, depending on the occasion. How we dress carries a message. There is a big difference between casual attire and revealing attire.
12. Avoid inflicting pain on the client in any way, especially after the client has made the therapist aware that the technique being used is painful. Once aware of client sensitivity, the therapist is legally bound by the informed consent agreement to lighten the pressure or change the technique. If a level of comfort cannot be found, then the area should be avoided altogether.
13. Avoid dating your clients. Don't ask a client out on a date or accept a date if she asks you. If you are contemplating a possible romantic relationship with a client, it is best to terminate the therapeutic relationship first. Many professions require that a specified amount of time should pass between termination of the professional relationship and the beginning of a personal/romantic relationship. This may vary from 6 months to 10 years. Check the state law and code of ethics in your area to see if a specific time frame is required.
14. Never engage in sexual activities with any client. This means avoiding any activity that is directed at sexually stimulating either the client or the therapist. Additionally, the American Massage Therapy Association recommends that therapists avoid placing their own pelvis, breasts, chest, hair, lips, or face in contact or proximity to the client. For the purpose of most therapeutic massage, the therapist should touch the client only with his hands, forearms, or elbows. Some Eastern forms may also make use of the feet and knees of the therapist. Occasionally, you may use the sides of your hip to stabilize a client during a mobilization.
15. Always respect a client's confidentiality. Never reveal a client's name, physical condition, and any information from the client's conversation while on the table or written on the intake forms. Do not leave client forms out for others to read.
16. When purchasing client gifts, choose inexpensive to moderately priced presents that relate to massage therapy or relaxation.
17. Do not accept expensive gifts from clients. Expensive gifts often strain the therapeutic relationship.

Client Abuse and Neglect

When any professional, whether doctor, attorney, minister, or massage therapist, does not recognize or respect the rights and boundaries of the client, the result may be client abuse or neglect. **Client neglect** is defined as physical or emotional harm sustained by the client due to lack of knowledge or sensitivity on the therapist's behalf. An example of a neglectful act might be a therapist who mistakes a cyst for a trigger point, causing tissue damage through prolonged pressure. Another example might be a therapist who, rather than providing emotional support for the client, oversteps his training, slips into a "counselor" role, and gives unsolicited and/or untrained advice. In neither of the above cases did the therapist intend to harm the client, and yet it happened. Negligent treatment is often spawned by ignorance. Our chief tools in the prevention of negligence are (1) a cautious and professional attitude and (2) providing ourselves with continuing education.

Client abuse is defined as physical or emotional harm sustained by the client due to *deliberate* acts of the therapist. An abusive therapist is one who makes a conscious decision to take advantage of a client physically, sexually, financially, or emotionally.

Emotional abuse typically occurs in a relationship where there is an imbalance of power and when the person who wields the greater power does not recognize or respect the boundaries of the other. The therapeutic relationship between a client and the massage therapist is particularly vulnerable to this type of abuse situation. In relationship to the client, the massage therapist has the authoritative position. The client has entered into the relationship because the massage therapist has a particular skill, knowledge, and experience. The relationship may be considered intimate because it involves skin-to-skin contact. The client may feel vulnerable both physically and emotionally because she is usually lying down and draped, whereas the therapist is standing and clothed. Often when someone removes her clothing, she becomes emotionally naked as well. It is because of the vulnerability of the client that the therapist must have good professional boundaries.

Fire Drills—A Boundaries Concept

When you were in elementary school, your teachers marched you in a single file down the halls and out a prescribed exit during a fire drill. Why? Because when you establish a habit by performing an action when you have time to think clearly, you will most likely react to threatening situations by repeating the ingrained habit. Had there been an actual fire, you and your classmates would have known what to do.

So what do fire drills have to do with massage therapy? Most uncomfortable situations can be handled tactfully if we prepare for them with "fire drills." Remember, the idea is to form a rational plan of action so that you act instead of react at the time of stress. The fire drill should consist of the situation and three possible ways of resolution. These steps should be in order from simple to complex. The simplest usually reflects the most gracious means of handling an uncomfortable situation, whereas the most complex or drastic usually focuses on protecting the therapist physically and emotionally. The therapist should use the most gracious means first and should try other means if resolution does not occur.

Fire drills are designed to act out the situation in a safe environment with a fellow classmate (under the direction of an instructor or with a colleague). Let's say the topic for the fire drill is "Client makes a pass [romantic overture] toward the therapist." The sample fire drill for this situation might look like this.

Problem: Client tests the boundaries of the relationship by making a pass toward the therapist; specifically, he asks the therapist if she is married.

Step 1. The therapist informs the client that she is married and tries to redirect the conversation by changing the subject. She might say, "Yes, my husband and I have been married for five years. We just had a wedding anniversary and went to New York to see Broadway plays. Do you like theater [or do you like to travel]?" Client responds, "I'd like anything with you. You said you're married, but are you *happily* married?"

Step 2. At this point the client has made it clear that he does not respect the boundary of marriage, and the therapist must take control of the conversation. She might say, "I'm very happy with my married relationship, but I'm not happy with the trend of this conversation. Let's keep *our* relationship on a professional level."

The client presses the issue by asking the therapist out to dinner.

Step 3. The therapist informs the client that she is not interested in anything outside of their therapeutic relationship, states that she is feeling uncomfortable with the direction of the conversation, and tells the client that the massage will be terminated if the conversation continues in the direction it is heading.

The client drops the subject at this point, but had he continued, the last steps would look like the following:

Step 4. The therapist terminates the session according to an established plan. A session termination form is given to the client, who is left alone in the massage room to get dressed. An example of the session termination form is provided in the chapter.

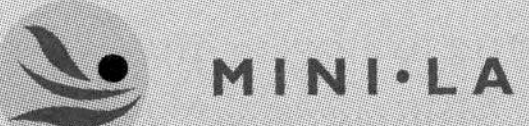

Make a list of five or more situations to create fire drills. They can be repeats of past unpleasant experiences or situations that constitute the most uncomfortable or frightening scenarios that could happen to you as a massage therapist. For example, it could be that a client goes into heart failure on the table, you accidentally undrape a client, or someone makes a pass at you.

Act out each situation with a classmate in front of the class. Once the situation is complete, ask the class and/or instructor for other options. Revise the fire drill if necessary. This activity will help you become more prepared to handle difficult situations.

By using the fire drill approach to reestablish violated boundaries, you can protect yourself from many types of abuse. Even subtle abuse may take its toll on the body, mind, and spirit. It is important that we understand the effects of abuse both personally and for our clients.

Issues of Intimacy: Just How Friendly Can a Massage Therapist Become?

Being friendly is good for business. No one ever lost a client or customer by smiling and by being nice and polite. The problem is that being *too* friendly can harm the therapeutic relationship. If we are attracted to the majority of our clients and develop friendships or dating relationships with them, we are assuming dual roles. We may unconsciously take advantage of our clients. We may become unclear about where to draw the line between clients and friends or clients and lovers.

It is helpful to realize that the therapeutic relationship is not a friendship. In a friendship, the relationship is 50-50; there is a certain amount of give and take between parties. In a friendship, your friend knows as much about you as you know about her. This is not the case in a therapeutic relationship; it is not an equal partnership. The therapeutic relationship exists to benefit the client! In some ways, the therapeutic relationship can be compared with the parent-child relationship. The relationship is one-sided. The therapist has the more powerful position, but it is the power to serve.

Intimacy is an innermost sensual (meaning an experience of the senses) bond to another in which the following elements exist: choice, mutuality, reciprocity, trust, and delight. This definition of intimacy is generally true for those to whom we are closest, usually family and friends. The element of choice is present in that we can choose to be in the relationship; we cannot be forced into intimacy. Mutuality goes hand-in-hand with choice. There is balance in the fact that the other person chooses to be in the relationship as well. Reciprocity is the knowledge that if I choose to be in the relationship, over a period of time I will receive as much from the relationship as I give to the relationship. Trust is the result of continued risk taking. We can choose to trust blindly, without a history of trust, but we are more likely to get hurt. Finally, delight is the sensual experience that the relationship brings to us because of these first four elements: choice, mutuality, reciprocity, and trust.

The therapeutic relationship, then, is very similar to an intimate relationship with a few important differences. Choice and mutuality exist, or there would be no relationship. Trust is built from the continued risk taking of subsequent sessions. Delight may even be experienced at times by both parties. It is for these similarities that people often confuse the closeness of a love relationship with the closeness of the therapeutic relationship. But the key element missing is reciprocity. The roles are not equal. The massage therapist is getting paid to be in this relationship. And while it may be argued that what the client is receiving is worth the money exchanged, the relationship is at best one-sided. While the massage therapist is caring and compassionate, he also keeps a therapeutic distance from personal involvement outside the therapy room with his clients.

In fact, what you may soon discover is that it is the distance that makes the therapeutic relationship safe for the client's experience. Let us consider Chapter 11 of the *Tao Te Ching:*

Thirty spokes share the wheel's hub;
It is the center hole that makes it useful.
Shape clay into a vessel;
It is the space within that makes it useful.
Cut doors and windows for a room;
It is the holes which make it useful.
Therefore profit comes from what is there;
Usefulness from what is not there.

Lao Tsu

When the space is provided for clients to relax and be themselves, healing is more likely to occur. If we fill up the space in the relationship with too much conversation, with our own agendas, or with our own concerns, the client does not have the opportunity to come out from behind her wall (often in the form of muscular tension). The distance we can provide, like the pauses in a symphony, are often the places we can feel peace, sanctity, and oneness. This is a gift not often acknowledged. This is the gift of the therapeutic relationship and why it is so important to protect it by not entering into dual relationships with our clients (Fig. 2–3).

In some cases, the client wishes for more of a relationship with the therapist. Psychotherapists have long been taught about a phenomenon of personalization that often takes place between counselors and their clients. These phenomena are referred to as **transference** and **countertransference.** The *Miller-Keane Encyclopedia & Dictionary of Medicine, Nursing, & Allied Health* defines these terms: Transference is "the unconscious tendency to assign to others in one's present environment feelings and attitudes associated with significant persons in one's early life, especially the patient's transfer to the therapist of feelings associated with a parent." Countertransference is "a reaction of the psychotherapist to the patient; an emotional reaction that is generally a reflection of the therapist's own inner needs and conflicts but also may be a reaction to the client's behavior." The feelings that are projected in both the transference or countertransference process

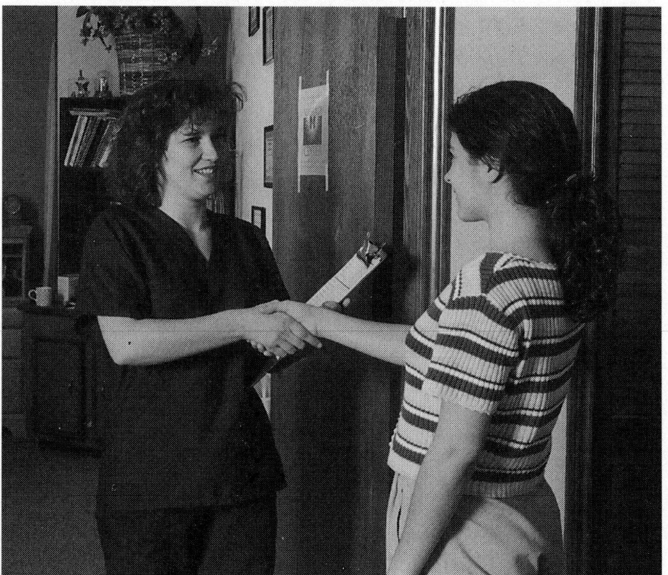

Figure 2•3 The massage therapist and the client have a therapeutic relationship.

may be affectionate, which results in a positive transference situation, or they may be feelings of hostility or animosity, which creates a negative transference situation.

Massage therapists and their clients are just as susceptible to these phenomena as are counseling professions; massage therapists are not always trained or prepared to recognize and deal with the problems. Transference occurs when the client begins to personalize the professional relationship. This is usually due to the fact that some personal needs (touch, empathy, support, comfort, acceptance) that were not being met in his personal relationships are now being met in the professional relationship. A blurring of reality occurs. Instead of seeing that he is a client paying a therapist to perform a specific service, the perception is that the therapist is a caring friend, confidant, or possible lover.

This is not to suggest that the relationship should be cold and sterile. Some of the most successful massage therapists are those who are extremely personable and friendly. People like to give their business to someone who truly cares about them. There simply needs to be an element of reality that a business relationship exists. It is the responsibility of the massage therapist to maintain this balance.

Countertransference occurs when the therapist has trouble maintaining her professional "detachment" from the client. The therapist may reverse roles and try to get her needs met through the intimacy of the professional relationship. The therapist may take a personal interest in the client, become overly responsible for the client's recovery, think about the client between appointments, and in more extreme cases may get into sexual fantasizing.

If the transference-countertransference process is allowed to continue once it has been identified, these feelings may progress into sexual behavior. It is important that massage therapists be able to recognize these situations and take appropriate steps to set firm boundaries with the client who wants to personalize the relationship. If boundaries are not firmly identified, the client's behavior may be progressive. If countertransference develops unnoticed by the therapist, the result may be emotional and sexual intimacy. Ultimately, the situation damages the therapeutic relationship and removes the focus of healing from the client.

So what can a massage therapist do if he suddenly finds himself in such a situation? The first step is to tell someone of the relationship. This can be done by going to a licensed counselor, a closed support group for professionals only, or to another massage therapist who can be unbiased, nonjudgmental, and supportive. The act of breaking the secret brings the situation out into the light of reality where it can be examined. The supporting counselor, support group, or colleague may then ask questions and offer feedback on handling the situation. If the relationship has progressed so far that countertransference has occurred, it is generally best to terminate the professional relationship and to refer the client to another massage therapist. This prevents the dynamic from progressing to a sexual/emotional relationship, which is detrimental to both the client and the therapist.

The dynamics of the situation should be explained to the client, and she should be told by the therapist that "I have a personal issue that prevents me from providing you with the best possible care." The massage therapist should then take a close look at his own needs and examine which ones are not being met. It is typical that this pattern will repeat itself with other clients as long as the therapist is not getting his own needs met. At this point, the massage therapist should consider going to a licensed counselor who can help him to identify his needs and to develop appropriate ways of getting them met.

What about friends who become clients? In order for a therapeutic relationship to occur, boundaries must be established, and both parties should understand their individual position and responsibilities. The massage therapist will provide massage therapy, for which the client will pay the requested fee. It's best to keep the massage therapy conversation focused on the massage session.

Consequences of Inappropriate Behavior and Sexual Misconduct

Part of understanding boundaries means accepting the consequences when we choose to cross them. It is therefore necessary that every massage therapist understand the consequences of inappropriate behavior, particularly sexual misconduct. Becoming sexual with a client, even if it is in a dating situation and not the massage room, is considered to be sexual abuse. This is true because the power dynamic between client and therapist does not empower the client easily to say no to the therapist. Therapists should be taught to look for warning signs in themselves and their colleagues and should learn how to help clients handle complaints about other therapists.

Inappropriate behavior and sexual misconduct are forms of client abuse because therapists take advantage of their more powerful positions in the therapeutic relationship to meet their own emotional or sexual needs. The professional relationship is considered a business arrangement between therapist and client, which benefits the client through healing touch and massage. When a therapist violates the boundaries of the therapeutic relationship through severe misconduct, the consequences associated with the violation are often of a corresponding severity. Possible consequences of this type of behavior include loss of income, loss of reputation, loss of marriage, loss of friendships, loss of relationship with peers and colleagues, loss of license, loss of membership in professional organizations, loss of insurance coverage, lawsuits for damages, criminal charges, fines, attorney's fees, court costs, and time in jail.

Remember that the therapist is *always* responsible and liable for her actions, even if the client initiated the situation. Do not depend upon professional liability insurance to cover any damages. While your insurance company may well provide an attorney to assist in your defense, it typically does not cover damages due to sexual misconduct.

This is not to say that sexual feelings are wrong or unhealthy. American culture has a history of being both obsessed and repressed about nudity and sexuality. Noted psychotherapist Terry Kellogg stated that one of the most perverse teachings in America today is that "sex is evil, dirty, nasty, sinful and wrong, so we have to save it for the one we love." We are all sexual beings. Our sexuality is a large part of our self-esteem and our identity. We simply need to keep some healthy separateness between our sexuality (which is part of our personal life) and our profession.

At one time or another you may feel an attraction to one of your clients, and sometimes it will be sexual. There is nothing wrong with this; it is natural and healthy. When we experience sexual feelings toward a client, we can honor this feeling by acknowledging it to ourselves and to a supportive colleague (not to the client). Having done so, we then focus on the job at hand and put our minds back in professional mode. Again, it is not the attraction that is dangerous; it is acting out the attraction.

When Clients Break the Rules

Occasionally you may run into a client who wants to go beyond a professional relationship. This may be someone who has an honest attraction to you as a person, or it could be someone who believes that massage therapy is related to sexual service. This violates not only your professional space, but your personal space as well. Fortunately, these situations tend to be the exception rather than the rule. Clients may approach the therapist in one of two ways: covertly or overtly.

Clients acting covertly typically begin by testing your boundaries. The word "covert" suggests that their approaches will be subtle and sneaky rather than honest and direct. Clients may hint about their loneliness and failed loves. Sometimes the client may ask personal questions about you and your love life. He may "accidentally" expose himself. Or he may "accidentally" brush his hands up against you while you are working. Inform the client that you are in the business of therapeutic massage and that his behavior is unacceptable. In most cases, your directness will put an end to his subterfuge.

As stated earlier, overt behavior is obvious, and there is no doubt what the client has in mind. Overt violations leave no doubt as to the client's intentions and may include grabbing the therapist sexually or verbally propositioning the therapist for sex, or the client may be intentionally stimulating himself on the massage table. Do not compromise yourself under these circumstances. Every incident of overt behavior must be confronted. Some therapists think that ignoring the situation will make it go away. Silence and nonaction are the wrong responses in cases like these; silence is often taken as permission. Even in ordinary conversation, silence is generally accepted as agreement with the speaker. Disagreement is expressed verbally and through action. If the overt behavior is not harmful, such as a client's asking you out on a date, then he needs to understand the boundaries of the therapeutic relationship. If the overt behavior is harmful physically or emotionally, then take control of the situation by initiating the session termination procedure.

Session Termination Procedure

Rarely does it happen that a massage therapist will have to terminate a session due to some inappropriate statement or action by the client. But if it does happen, the therapist must be prepared to deal with the situation by standard procedure. Usually this involves three steps.

1. *Notifying the client of the session termination.* If the client commits some faux pas or inappropriate behavior that the therapist judges to be mild, subtle, or covert, the therapist has the option of providing the client with an initial verbal warning that, if the behavior is repeated, the session will be terminated. If the behavior is overt, such as sexual touching or a direct proposition, then a warning is not necessary. The therapist should terminate the session immediately. The therapist may want to vocalize the termination by using one of the following statements: "I do not believe anything therapeutic is going on. This session is now over," or "I do not feel comfortable with your behavior, and this session needs to end." If the therapist is uncomfortable with verbalizing the termination, he or she should find a reason to leave the room. Once out of the treatment room, the therapist writes a general account of the incident and makes a copy of it. The actual termination can be accomplished by handing the client the session termination notice (Fig. 2–4) and promptly leaving the room.
2. *Have the client leave the premises, thereby reestablishing therapist safety.* Once the client has been notified of

SESSION TERMINATION NOTICE

You have been handed this notice due to the use of language or behavior that the massage therapist perceives to be inappropriate.

This is to notify you that your massage session has been terminated at the therapist's discretion. You should dress and leave.

Charges for the entire session will be collected at the business office.

OR

You will receive a bill for the entire session.

The language or behavior constituting session termination is recorded on this form below and is confidential between the therapist, coordinator, and department manager.

You may request an incident review by calling (a persons name) at (phone number).

Future appointments will not be accepted without an incident review and resolution of the situation.

Date: ______________ Client Name: ______________________

Time: ______________ Therapist's Name : ______________________

Place: ______________________________________

Therapist's Perceptions of Incident:

Actions Taken:

Proposed Resolutions:

Reviewed and Resolved:

Date: ______________

Time: ______________

Place: ______________________________________

Those in attendance:

Figure 2•4 A sample session termination notice. (Permission is hereby granted to reproduce this form in its entirety, including the copyright notice, for commercial or instructional use but not for resale.)

the session termination, the therapist should leave the room and take steps to ensure her own safety. Each situation will have to be judged independently. If you work with others, get a coworker to stay with you until the client has left the building. If you work alone or if you are physically intimidated by the client, use the phone to make contact with a colleague, friend, or family member. The therapist should inform the person contacted that she will call again as soon as the client has left, usually within three minutes. If the friend does not receive a call back, the friend is instructed to alert the proper authorities. If the therapist feels that she may be harmed physically by the client, the therapist may choose to dial 911 and have a police unit sent to the premises to escort the client out. The therapist must use her discretion to determine which situations are potentially threatening from those that are merely nuisances.

3. *Documenting the session termination in writing.* A session termination form is simply a document to record the events as they took place from the therapist's point of view. The first copy that was handed to the client should just be a brief statement of the problem. The office copy should be a total replay of the entire incident. The main purpose of this form is to have a written record that can be used as a reference should the case go to court. It is important for the therapist to document every detail of the situation that led her to terminate the session. If it was sexual improprieties, document the statements verbatim or describe actions that gave that impression. For more information on documentation, see the section on Client Incident Reports.

One other situation merits mention here, and that is the *house call* or *out-call.* In business arrangements, where the massage therapist makes trips to the client's home or hotel, the session termination may have to be handled differently. During a house call, you are on the client's turf with your equipment. The most straightforward response is to tell the client that the massage is over and that you will be leaving. If for any reason the client tries to intimidate you, it is best to simply leave your equipment behind and come back for it with the authorities (hotel security or the local police). It is still in your own best interest to record the cir-

INCIDENT REPORT FORM

Date:__________ Client Name: ____________________________________

Time:__________ Therapist's Name: ________________________________

Place:____

Therapist's Perceptions of Incident:

Actions Taken:

Proposed Resolutions:

______________________________ ________ ______________________________ ________

Signature of Massage Therapist Date Signature of Client Date

Reviewed and Resolved:

Date:________________ Time: ________________

Place: ____

Those in attendance:

Figure 2•5 A sample incident report form. (Permission is hereby granted to reproduce this form in its entirety, including the copyright notice, for commercial or instructional use but not for resale.)

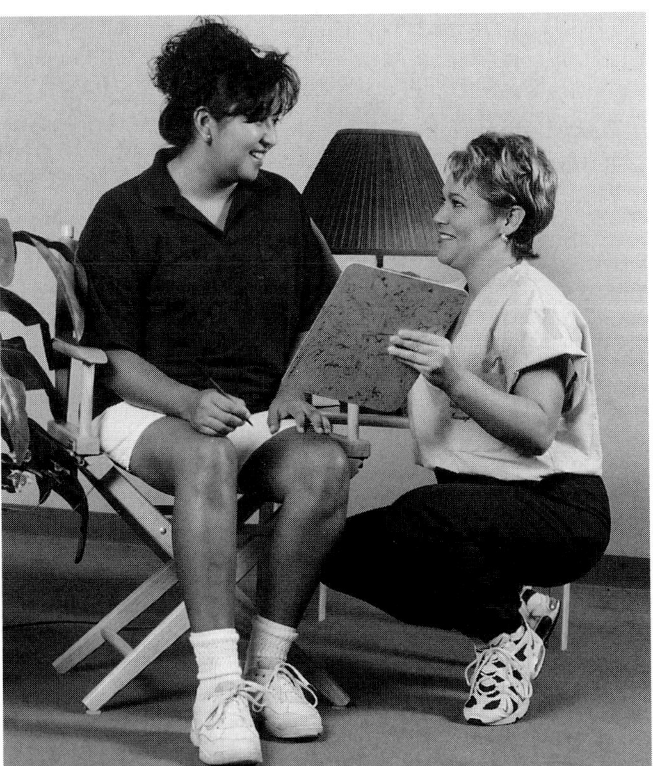

Figure 2•6 The incident report form should be reviewed with the client, then signed by both the massage therapist and the client.

cumstances surrounding the session termination. You may ask for a credit card number in advance to secure your fees if a situation develops.

Hopefully, the use of session termination forms will be minimal. This form is merely another useful tool in establishing client and therapist boundaries and in preserving the therapeutic relationship.

Client Incident Reports

Incident reports are also known as *accident reports* or *unusual occurrence reports* (Fig. 2–5). Regardless of how small the accident or unusual episode, a report should be filled out and retained to document the unusual things that happen to a client, in the same way that the session termination form documents unusual things that happen to the therapist. Incident reports most often involve a client who slips and falls, who misplaces belongings, or who becomes ill during a massage session. The incident report should include the date, time, and exact location of the occurrence, who was present, and what was done to alleviate the problem. If physical injury was involved, the report should include the condition of the client when he departed from your establishment. If possible, obtain signatures from all individuals who were present during the incident (Fig. 2–6).

SUMMARY

The professional image and behavior of a massage therapist can be divided up into the areas of professional standards and boundaries.

Professional standards are set from within the profession itself and govern the actions of the individual practitioners. This is done by defining a certain scope of practice, educational requirements, code of ethics, and principles of conduct. These may all vary slightly from state to state, but share the same common belief in professional, client-centered care.

Boundaries are our personal and professional parameters that specify how we will interact with others, including our personal space, our professional conduct, and our emotional boundaries. Having healthy boundaries also means respecting the boundaries of others, even if their standards are different than our own. Observing boundaries prevents client abuse, client neglect, becoming too intimate, or disclosing too much personal information to our clients. Understanding boundaries means accepting the consequences for our actions when we choose to disregard boundaries. It is therefore necessary that every massage therapist understand the consequences of inappropriate behavior and sexual misconduct. Likewise, when clients behave inappropriately, the therapist must be prepared to terminate the session.

SELF-TEST

Multiple Choice • Write the letter of the best answer in the space provided.

_______ 1. The voluntary process of completing training in knowledge and skill by a nongovernmental institution such as a trade school is called

A. certification
B. registration
C. accreditation
D. licensure

_______ 2. The certification process usually involves which of the following?

A. completion of a required number of hours of classroom
B. apprenticeship and/or internship
C. successful passing of exams covering science and applied skills
D. all of the above are involved in the certification process

_______ 3. Within a year after establishment, NCBTMB was accredited by the

A. Occupational Safety and Health Administration (OSHA)
B. National Organization for Competency Assurance (NOCA)
C. American Massage Therapy Association (AMTA)
D. Associated Bodywork and Massage Professionals (ABMP)

_______ 4. Often including principles for therapeutic relationships, professional behavior, and business policies, which one of the following is a set of guiding moral principles that influence one's course of action?

A. code of ethics
B. principles of professional conduct
C. scope of practice
D. Patient's Bill of Rights

_______ 5. Nondisclosure of privileged information is referred to as

A. integrity
B. communication skills
C. transference
D. confidentiality

_______ 6. Unless your local law specifies, whether you use the term "client" or "patient" when referring to your patron has to do with if you are working in a

A. private practice
B. medical or nonmedical establishment
C. spa or health club
D. hospital or medical clinic

_______ 7. According to Pat Ogden, healthy boundaries are

A. connecting with the experience or sense of ourselves as both separate and in unity with the world
B. keeping ourselves from accepting subtle or overt kinds of abuse
C. remaining sensitive to and respecting the rights and boundaries of others
D. all of the above

_______ 8. Physical or emotional harm sustained by the client due to lack of knowledge or sensitivity on the therapist's behalf is called

A. client carelessness
B. client neglect
C. client abuse
D. therapeutic relationship

_______ 9. Which of the following elements of intimacy does *not* exist in the therapeutic relationship?

A. choice
B. mutuality
C. reciprocity
D. trust and delight

_______ 10. An emotional reaction of the therapist to the client's act of transference, often marked by a difficulty in maintaining professional detachment from the client is called

A. integrity
B. disassociation
C. countertransference
D. projection

_______ 11. A typical session termination procedure would include which of the following?

A. notifying the client of the session termination
B. asking the client to leave the premises, reestablishing therapist safety
C. documenting the session termination in writing in an incident report
D. all of the above would be included in a session termination procedure

_______ 12. Which of the following should *not* be included in an incident report?

A. date, time, and exact location of the occurrence
B. who was present at the reported incident
C. the social security number of all persons involved
D. what was done to alleviate the problematic situation at the time

References

Baron, Robert A. *Psychology,* 2nd ed., Boston: Allyn & Bacon, 1992.

Carnes, Patrick, Ph.D. *Out of the Shadows, Understanding Sexual Addiction.* Minneapolis: CompCare, MI, 1983.

Credentials Used for the Massage Therapy Profession. The American Massage Therapy Association's Internet Publication on the World Wide Web, 1997.

Fritz, Sandy, Dr. M. James Grosenbach, and Kathy Paholsky, Ph.D. "Ethics and Professionalism." *Massage Magazine* Jan/Feb, 1997.

Ignatavicius, Donna D. and Marilyn Varner Bayne. *Medical-Surgical Nursing.* Philadelphia: W. B. Saunders, 1991.

Johanson, Greg and Ron Kurtz. *Grace Unfolding, Psychotherapy in the Spirit of the Tao-te ching,* New York: Harmony Books, 1991.

Kasl, Charlotte Davis. *Women, Sex and Addiction, A Search for Love and Power.* New York: Ticknor and Fields, 1989.

Kellogg, Terry, Ph.D. Sex and Sexuality, a Workshop. Dallas, TX.

Kurtz, Ron. *Body-Centered Psychotherapy, the Hakomi Method.* Mendocino, CA: LifeRhythm Books, 1990.

Miller-Keane Encyclopedia & Dictionary of Medicine, Nursing, & Allied Health. 6th ed. Philadelphia: W. B. Saunders, 1997.

National Certification Board for Therapeutic Massage and Bodywork. Code of Ethics: Adopted 2/17/95.

Ogden, Pat. *Boundaries II* or *Somatic Psychology,* Hakomi Integrative Somatics, 1995.

Torres, Lillian S. *Basic Medical Techniques and Patient Care for Radiologic Technologists,* 4th ed. Philadelphia: J. B. Lippincott Company, 1993.

Tsu, Loa. *Tao Te Ching.* Translation by Gia-Fu Feng and Jane English. New York: Vintage Books, 1972.

Webster's New World College Dictionary. Springfield, MA: G. & C. Merriam Co., 1995.

What Are Certification, Licensing and Accreditation? The American Massage Therapy Association's Internet Publication on the World Wide Web, 1997.

Whitfield, Charles L., M.D. *Boundaries and Relationships, Knowing, Protecting and Enjoying the Self.* Deerfield, FL: Health Communications, 1993.

All labor that uplifts humanity has dignity and importance and should be undertaken with painstaking excellence.
—Martin Luther King, Jr.

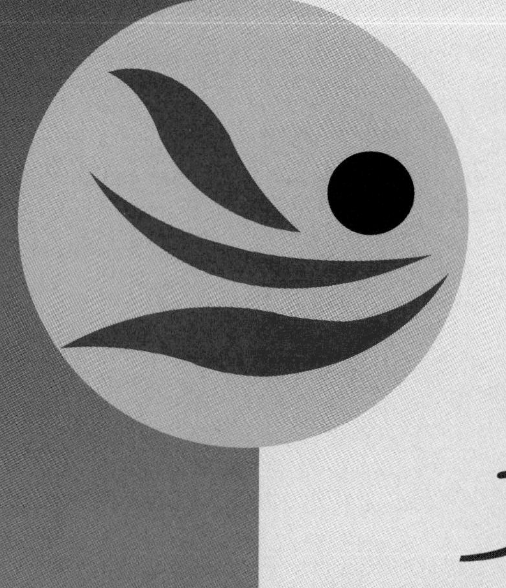

3
Tools of the Trade and the Massage Environment

Student Objectives

After completing this chapter, the student should be able to:

- Identify and discuss three massage table features
- Choose the correct massage table
- Apply fabric care to the massage table top
- Discuss differences in massage media and aromatherapy
- Design a massage room

INTRODUCTION

Your career as a massage therapist not only depends on your education and skills training but also on your ability to use wisely the tools of the trade. Like any other skilled artisan, these tools will be used to implement the massage work itself. The finished product depends both on the quality of the tools and how well the artisan uses them. The tools of the massage therapist include the massage table and related equipment, the massage lubricants, and even the room environment itself. In this chapter we will open the therapist's toolbox and examine each item in detail. Practical suggestions are included to assist the massage therapy student in making wise decisions when choosing equipment or designing a room.

First of all, we need to distinguish between a massage *room* and a massage *office.* A massage room is the place where the massage service itself is actually performed. This room contains the massage table, lubricant, and any other incidentals that are required for the actual massage. The massage room is often referred to as a massage *studio.* This chapter will concern itself with the massage room and all the objects that may be found there.

The massage office, also known as the paper office, is where massage appointments are scheduled, phone calls are placed, and records are kept. All "business" activities take place in the office. These activities are necessary for your massage practice to run smoothly and efficiently. Equipment such as the telephone, answering machine, computer, files, and accounting supplies is located in the massage office.

Before you start buying furniture and equipment for your massage room, spend some time evaluating yourself and your prospective clientele. The following list of questions may help you gain a clearer picture of who you are as a massage therapist and what you want to convey to your clients.

1. *What style of massage work are you most attracted to? Why?*

2. *Describe the kind of massage environments in which you feel most comfortable.*

3. *How much physical space do you need to practice comfortably?*

Let's explore each question further.

1. *What style of massage work are you most attracted to? Why?*

The kind of massage you want to offer and past experiences of massage rooms will play a part in how your room looks and feels. If orthopedic massage is what you will be doing, your massage room may look more like a doctor's office with anatomical charts, little or no music, lightly colored walls, and white massage linens.

The room of a sports massage therapist may have sports-type paintings or photographs, reference books on sports-related problems, and a single free-standing locker for clients' garments. A sports massage therapist is more likely to own a portable massage table to be used when his or her services are needed at sports events.

A massage therapist who focuses on stress-reduction massage will want to create a relaxing environment. The walls may be painted in warm colors; only natural or subdued lighting may be used, with a hint of lavender scent in the air. Knowing who you are and what you want to accomplish will help you decide how to create the most appropriate massage room environment.

2. *Describe the kind of massage environments in which you feel most comfortable.*

When describing the massage environment, think in terms of details. Distinguish the colors, smells, objects, music, linens, furniture, and other specific items that make it comfortable. Many massage therapists choose a theme or motif to accent their massage room and office. Examples of a decorative theme are Southwest, Eastern, oceanside, rain forest, or eclectic (borrowing from many different influences). This may help you determine colors, furnishings, and even music. An interior decorator or a space designer can help you plan before costly mistakes are made. Even if you know exactly what you would like to create, a designer can help you with additional suggestions.

3. *How much physical space do you need to practice comfortably?*

The size of your room will have a determining factor on the size and type of equipment you plan to purchase. Wall shelving units may be preferred over floor shelving units if your massage room is small. Oversized chairs and folding screens can be used if the room is large. Wall colors can also make a room

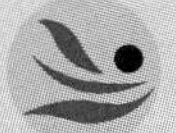

MINI•LAB

If possible, receive massages from a variety of therapists. After the experience, write a summary on how you felt about the massage environment. Use this information when deciding not only the type of equipment you will use, but the decor as well. This mini-lab can be expanded to include the therapist's interviewing skills and the massage technique used.

MASSAGE TABLE CHECKLIST

TYPE OF MASSAGE TABLE

☐ Stationary Massage Table ☐ Portable Massage Table

☐ Electric Lift Table ☐ Hydraulic Lift Table

MASSAGE TABLE FEATURES

Frame	☐ Aluminum		☐ Wood-Type: ______	
Width	☐ 26" ☐ 28" ☐ 30" ☐ 32"		☐ Custom Width: ______	
Height	☐ Standard Height		☐ Custom Height: ______	
Length	☐ Standard Length		☐ Custom Length: ______	

PADDING

Layering	☐ Single Layer		☐ Multiple Layering System		
Density	☐ Light		☐ Medium		☐ High
Thickness	☐ 1½"	☐ 2"	☐ 2½"	☐ 3"	☐ Other
Fabric	☐ Vinyl		☐ Textured Vinyl		☐ Vinyl Suede
	☐ Velour		☐ Cotton Velvet		☐ Ultra Leather

Color: ______

Other Options: ______

______

ACCESSORIES FOR YOUR MASSAGE TABLE

Face Rest: ☐ Standard ☐ Deluxe

☐ Arm Shelf ☐ Side Extenders ☐ Foot Rest

☐ Carrying Case ☐ Table Skates

BOLSTERS AND SUPPORTIVE DEVICES

☐ Round Bolster (6"X27") ☐ 2 Half Bolsters (8"X27")

☐ Round Bolster (8"X27") ☐ Soft Neck Bolster

Figure 3•1 Massage table checklist. Use this to compare the features of several massage tables. (Permission is hereby granted to reproduce this form in its entirety, including the copyright notice, for commercial or instructional use but not for resale.)

appear bigger or smaller. Again, interior decorators or space designers can help you make the most of your designated space.

WHAT IS THE "RIGHT" KIND OF EQUIPMENT?

Massage equipment refers to the objects or machinery used in the successful execution of massage therapy services. When considering the purchase of massage equipment, there are several things to keep in mind.

First, will it ergonomically support you, the therapist, by reducing stress? **Ergonomics** is the scientific study of individual anatomy, physiology, and psychology relating to humans' work and adjusting the environment and equipment to support the alignment and balance of the body in its daily activities. If your back, neck, or wrist is in pain after performing one or more massage sessions, chances are that your equipment is *creating* stress. Use the section on table features to help you better understand table mechanics and assist you in altering your equipment to better suit your body. If it is not the massage equipment, then you need to look at your body mechanics. Use the chapter on body mechanics to assist you in correcting inefficient body postures you may be using.

Second, will your massage equipment add comfort to the client? Does the padding support the client's body, and are the physical dimensions of the table comfortable? For example, a table that is too narrow may not allow the client's arms to rest comfortably at his or her side. This may create a feeling of unease in the client.

Third, how long can you expect this piece of equipment to last? Most table manufacturers offer a 5-to-10-year warranty. However, top-quality tables last much longer, especially if you are willing to remove and replace worn padding and top fabric. Eventually, you may want to have a stationary table for your office and a lightweight, portable table for home visits. This prolongs the life of both tables. It's like rotating two pairs of shoes; both pairs last longer.

And last, is it a wise investment? Since your equipment, especially your massage table, is an investment in your business, resist the urge to buy impulsively. Ask veteran massage therapists which equipment they use and why. Why did they choose a particular table width or padding? Besides other therapists, contact several table companies and ask them to mail you product catalogs. If possible, go to a massage school or a massage convention where you can see and lie on tables from several different manufacturers. If you can compare, you will have a better understanding about table features. This will help you make an informed decision (Fig. 3–1).

Ergonomics, client comfort, durability, and workmanship are all important factors in purchasing massage equipment. Because these four elements are so important, we will discuss these factors throughout the chapter.

One word of caution: Some therapists resort to building their own massage tables or to having their tables made by well-meaning friends or family members. Some table companies offer table kits that you can assemble. This may not be a good idea in the long run because the only tables that can be guaranteed by a reputable table manufacturer are those that are assembled by the table manufacturer. With a homemade table or a table kit, you may be held liable if table failure occurs during a massage. Should something happen to your table, it's preferable to have a table manufacturer who can stand behind their materials and workmanship. In addition, all table companies make accessories that can be purchased to add to the comfort or transportability of their massage tables.

MASSAGE TABLES

The two most popular styles of massage tables sold to massage students and massage therapists are stationary tables and portable tables. Stationary tables are made to stay in a massage room. Portable tables are designed to be folded in half and carried, like an oversized suitcase, from one location to another.

Portable tables account for 90 to 98 percent of all table sales by table manufacturers with prices ranging from $300 to $600. Some advantages of portable tables are that the therapist is able to make home or office visits (going to the client), the table can be moved if the therapist is utilizing multiple office locations, and, if the massage therapist shares office space with other therapists, he or she can easily move the portable table out of the office. Most therapists start out with a portable massage table, often practicing their skill in a home setting.

Whether you purchase a portable or stationary table, buy the one you want, not the least expensive. Massage therapists must feel totally confident in their equipment, and your massage table is the fundamental tool of your business and will be a major expenditure. When your table arrives, take the packing slip that has your table style, dimensions, color, and table company with address and phone number, and attach it to the bottom of your table with a sheet of adhesive laminate. This information should also be kept in your office in case the massage table is lost or stolen. Then you will always have the information at your fingertips when you want to order additional equipment or supplies (such as table pads or linens). As you will see, there are many table features to choose from.

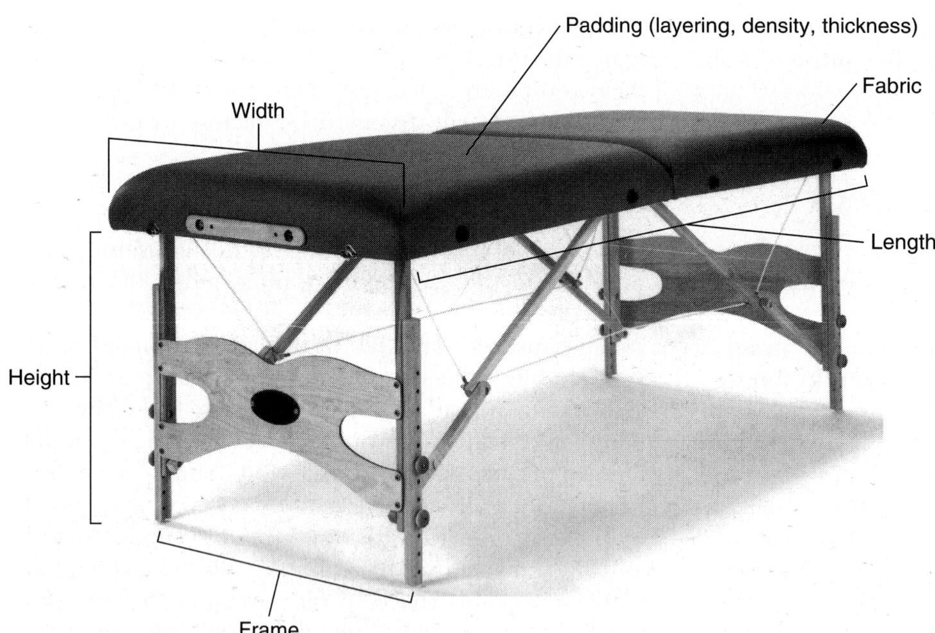

Figure 3•2 A typical massage table.

Massage Table Features

When you are considering the purchase of a stationary or a portable massage table, most table manufacturers let you decide the specifications on features such as width, height, length, frame, padding, and fabric (Fig. 3–2). To assist you in this task, let's look at a few guidelines.

Width. Most massage tables sold are between 28 and 31 inches wide. In most cases, the width of the table depends on the height of the therapist. Shorter therapists should consider tables that are 28 and 29 inches wide as it is easier to reach across the table, safeguarding proper body mechanics. Taller therapists usually can work with a wider table (30 to 31 inches wide). Other considerations are your clients. For example, if your table is less than 28 inches wide, your large-framed clients may feel uneasy when they are lying supine, as their arms tend to hang off the sides of the table. If your table is wider than 31 inches, it may be difficult for you, as the therapist, to reach across the table. Wider portable tables are taller (when folded up), and heavier, which is a consideration because they are lifted and carried from location to location. It is helpful to massage several body styles on a range of table widths before choosing which table width to purchase.

Height. Almost all portable and stationary tables have an adjustable height range, which is usually between 22 to 34 inches high. Adjustment is achieved, usually in half-inch increments, by lengthening or shortening the four legs of the table. The optimum working height of the massage table is determined by the height of the practitioner and by his preferred style of massage.

For Swedish massage, there are three generally accepted methods for determining the height of the table top.

- Stand by the massage table, arms to your side, and extend your wrist in a 90-degree angle. Take care to relax your shoulders fully to get an accurate measurement. The height of where your fingertips slightly brushes against the table represents the appropriate table height for you (Fig. 3–3A).
- Or stand by the massage table, arms to your side, and make a fist with your hand. Using this method, the table height is where the table touches your fist or proximal set of knuckles (Fig. 3–3B).
- As you stand by a massage table, extend your open palm inferiorly and laterally. The proper table height is where the table rests under your palm (Fig. 3–3C).

For several massage sessions, try both of these methods for deciding table height. Notice how your body feels. If your arms or shoulders feel achy, the table is probably too high. If your lower back feels stiff after giving a massage, most likely your table is too low. After a massage, the therapist should feel anywhere from relaxed to energized. Raise or drop the table top by small increments until optimal table height is achieved. Remember to let the comfort level of your body decide the most appropriate table height for you.

Many deep-tissue therapists prefer to adjust their table heights slightly lower than normal to take mechanical advantage of their body weight behind downward pressure. Conversely, many massage therapists who

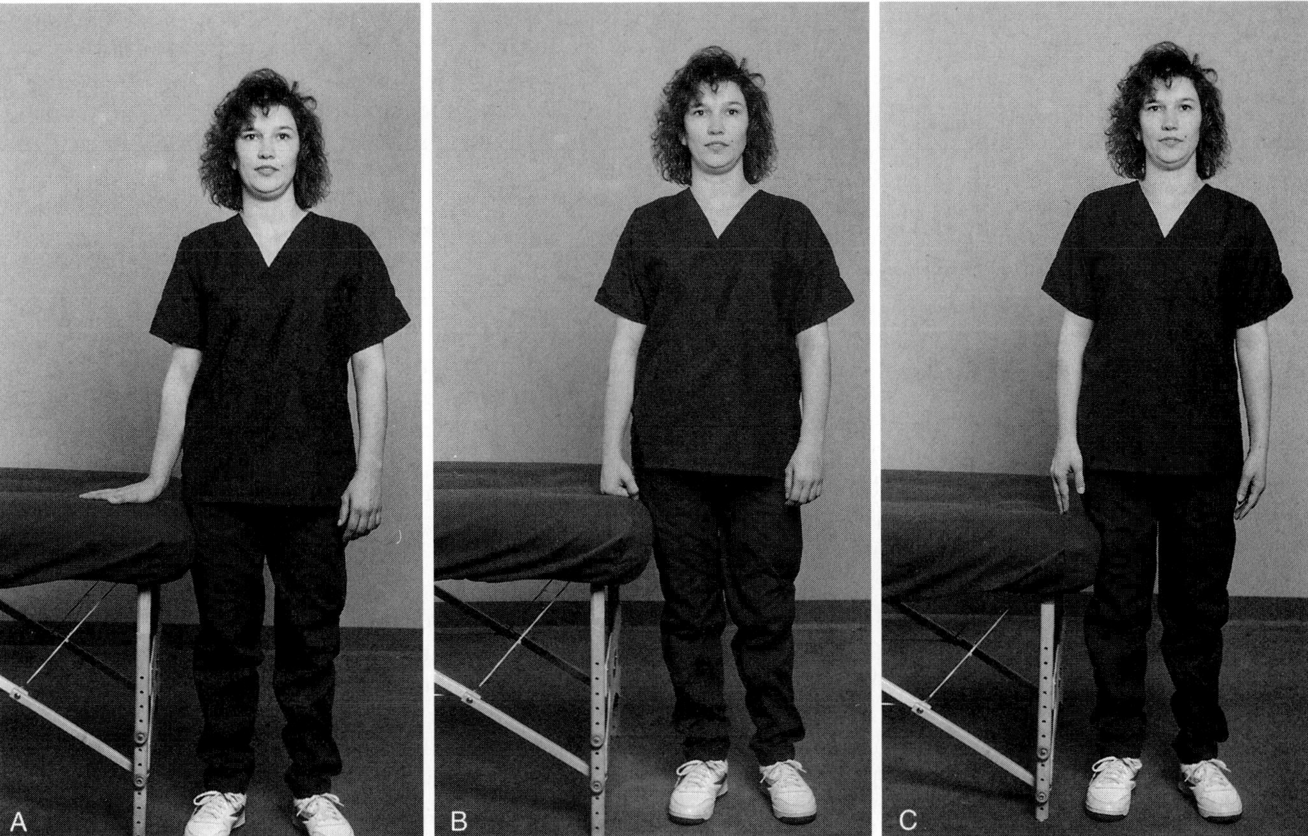

Figure 3•3 Three methods of determining the correct height for a massage table.

practice Trager or craniosacral therapy like a higher table because it is most comfortable for them.

Length. Most massage tables are either 72 or 73 inches long, but custom lengths are offered by many table manufacturers. Because most massage therapists use face rest extensions and bolsters, your over-6-foot-tall client will have ample room. This is because a face rest adds 10 to 12 inches to your table, and a 6- or 8-inch-wide bolster will shorten the client's leg length when placed under the knees or ankles. Using bolsters can increase your table length by 3 to 5 inches.

Frames. Table frames are made of either wood or aluminum, the most popular being wood. The major difference between wood and aluminum is that wood frames are heavier. Welded aluminum frames have a slight advantage in lateral stability over wooden frame tables, but this difference probably will not be noticed with a high-quality wooden table. Beware of aluminum-framed massage tables that are fastened with rivets, as they can become loose and are difficult to tighten. The chief reasons for buying aluminum tables are its light weight and strength. Small-framed massage therapists often purchase aluminum-frame tables because they are easier to transport. Some workers who are conscious of body energy fields avoid aluminum, citing that the metal interferes with the energy field of the body.

If the table you are thinking about purchasing has a single-knob attachment, make sure the leg extensions are attached to the table legs by a tongue-and-groove mechanism. A two-knob attachment or a tongue-and-groove system is more stable and increases the table-to-table leg integrity. If the table leg has only one knob without a tongue-and-groove system, that knob can become the pivot point when lateral pressure is applied to the table. This feature is even more important with massage styles such as Trager, Feldenkrais, and some Eastern styles, when considerable movement occurs during the session or when you are working on a high table. Whether you have one or two leg knobs, tighten them up at the beginning of every week. This ensures that the table is as strong and stable as possible.

Many table manufacturers also offer an inverted truss system. The theory behind this frame option is to offer added resistance against bending at the hinged midpoint of the table. However, most massage table companies claim that this adds little, if any, extra support. Inverted truss systems also add approximately 5 pounds to table weight and usually ensures an additional cost. Table manufacturers offer inverted truss systems because they are offered by competing table manufacturers. Also, some companies offer a "deep tissue" upgrade, which is often more of a marketing campaign gimmick. Any high-quality table should be expected to support the weight of both the client and the therapist during a deep-tissue session.

Padding. If you ask clients what they remember about being on your massage table, they will more than likely mention padding. This material adapts and supports your client's body. When selecting a pad for your massage table top, decisions must be made regarding layering, foam density, and thickness. Let's look at these areas.

- **Layering.** Some tables are padded with a single layer of foam, whereas other manufacturers pad their tables with multiple (two or three) layers. In the multiple-layer system, the densest foam is on the bottom. The lower layers of foam support the bony structure and prevent the body from "bottoming out" on the wood plate of the table. The upper layers are less dense to conform to the contours of the body. Multiple-foam layering usually outlasts single-foam layering and is much more comfortable to the client, especially when the therapist is performing deep-tissue or sports massage.
- **Density.** Most foam pads are divided into three grades of density—light, medium, and high. High-density foams generally have better memory, which is the ability of the foam to return to its original height after its surface has been disturbed. Higher-density foams are heavier and will add weight to your massage table; they are typically not found on a table designed for lightness. High-quality tables use a medium- to high-density foam because light-density foam does not have enough memory, even when used as a top layer.
- **Thickness.** Foam thickness typically ranges from 1½ (firm) to 3 inches (plush). Deep-tissue practitioners traditionally work on tables with firm foam thickness. Using a firm padding prevents loss of the therapist's energy when downward pressure is applied. Without a firm pad, the client sinks down into the foam. If you like to work beneath the client's body, a plush foam top is best. Plush foam is preferred by stress-reduction therapists because it is more comfortable. You may also hear the term "loft" used to describe foam thickness. Loft is the height of the foam with no added surface weight.

Author's Note

Because of government regulations, all table manufacturers use padding that is fluorocarbon-free. This manufacturing process does not damage our fragile ozone layer.

Table Fabric. Table fabric covers the foam padding of your massage table. The most common fabric choice is vinyl because it is long lasting and easy to clean and disinfect. Other fabrics available are textured vinyl, vinyl suede, velour, cotton velvet, and ultra leather.

Vinyl fabrics also resist oil, perspiration, and makeup stains; however, they also tend to be stiff, retain the cold, and are not as comfortable as velour, cotton velvet, or ultra leather. Vinyl is sensitive to changes in environmental conditions and may become dry and brittle and may crack, especially if you leave your massage table in your car between appointments (see fabric care recommendations below). Vinyl fabrics can be easily punctured by keys, hairpins, jewelry, and pets. Massage linens have a tendency to slip on the slick surface.

Ultra leather is soft and resists punctures better than vinyl fabrics. All ultra leather products offered by table manufacturers are imported because the process used to make ultra leather is unsafe for the environment. If you make decisions according to how a product affects the environment, you will probably not choose ultra leather as your table fabric.

The cloth fabrics such as cotton velour, velour, and other textured fabrics are very soft and provide the utmost in client comfort. Unfortunately, they are difficult to clean and impossible to disinfect. Many state laws require therapists to use surfaces that can be disinfected such as vinyl.

Vinyl Fabric Care. The most important thing to know about the care of your table vinyl fabric is to keep it clean. For daily cleaning, simply wipe down the table surface with a mild cleaner, such as a solution of liquid dishwashing detergent and water. Dry with a soft, lint-free towel or old T-shirt. Avoid using vinyl conditioners or protectants because they are unnecessary and may damage the vinyl top coat.

The three worst substances for the vinyl surface of the table are the very things that you might expect it to come in contact with (oils, isopropyl alcohol, and chlorine bleach). Body oils or massage oils can erode the protective top coat, which is specially designed to keep the fabric soft. When the top coat is damaged by oil, the plasticizers that give the vinyl its softness, suppleness, and resilience are broken down. The other two substances, isopropyl alcohol and chorine bleach, are often used in the disinfecting process. Use the chlorine bleach and water solution (ten parts water to one part chlorine bleach) to disinfect the vinyl surface *only* when it comes into contact with bodily fluids. All three substances will shorten the life of the vinyl by causing it to become dry and brittle, making it susceptible to cracking or splitting.

Vinyl table fabrics are like fine wine: They do not like wide temperature ranges. This becomes a problem only if you keep your massage table outdoors or in your car. After a home or office visit, put the table back in your office or your home. If your table fabric does get cold, allow it to return to room temperature before you begin your next massage. Direct sunlight can also break down vinyl and cause it to become dry and crack, and high temperatures can soften it; again, allow the table to return to room temperature before using it. Pressure on a hot table may cause permanent damage by leaving a "stretch mark."

Avoid table fabric wear and tear by transporting your portable table in a carrying case. It is virtually impossible to keep your table top unblemished when you have to haul the table from your office or home, to the car, to your client's home, back to your car, back to your office or home, then to your—*whew!* If you are going to move your table around, get a carrying case. Your table is certainly worth it.

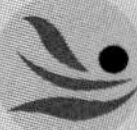

MINI•LAB

If you are fortunate enough to have several manufactured tables on display at your school, try these three tests before you finalize your purchase.

1. **One-Knee Test.** Kneel down and place your weight on one-knee and see if you "bottom out." This will indicate the integrity of the foam and what a client might be feeling when he or she is pressed into the table.
2. **The Bounce.** Lean your body weight against the massage table and lay your forearm on the table top. Gently bounce up and down. Notice how much the table flexes when you jump. The ideal table will resist you as you bounce. If the table top is not firm, some of the energy you use pressing into the client's muscles will be lost. This also translates into conserving the therapist's energy!
3. **Table Rock.** Rock the table back and forth to check for lateral stability. If the table wobbles, the integrity of the table should be questioned (or the joints should be tightened).
4. **Ready, Set, Go!** Fold the massage table, and close it securely. Holding it by the handles, lift the table and walk around the room. Unfold the table and set it up on its four legs, noticing the ease or difficulties you encounter.

ACCESSORIES FOR YOUR MASSAGE TABLE

Face Rest. A face rest, or face cradle, allows clients to keep their heads and necks relatively straight while they are lying prone. The face rest extends the functional length of the table by 10 to 12 inches. The face rest consists of two parts, a cushion and a frame (Fig. 3–4). The cushion is generally attached to the frame by Velcro strips. This enables the crescent-shaped cushion to be spread or narrowed to accommodate a wide variety of facial structures. The cushion fabric is usually the same fabric as that on the massage table.

The face cradle frame may attach to the massage table in several ways. It may connect with support rods that insert into grommets at either or both ends of the table or by a brace that slides laterally in a channel connected to the table. It is more convenient for the therapist to have face rest attachments at *both* ends of the table.

Standard face rests allow the head and neck to be in only one position—parallel to the table top. Adjustable models can be purchased that allow the head and neck to be moved into two or three dimensions. The more positions available to the client and therapist, the more opportunities there are for relaxation and muscle release. Adjustable face rests also add comfort for clients, especially when working with elderly clients, large clients, and clients who are physically challenged.

Other face rest options include a face hole with plug and the prone pillow (see Fig. 3–4). The face hole is an oval opening in the table surface that allows the client to lie face down looking through the table. The hole can be closed with a fitted plug when the client is lying supine. The prone pillow is contoured foam covered with vinyl, which sits on top of the table and supports the face comfortably above the table surface.

Arm Shelf. An arm shelf provides a place for the arms to rest in the prone or supine position. The arm shelf model used in the supine position looks like a pair of bolsters connected by a wide strap. Also referred to as an arm support or side extension, this option simply widens the table. During the massage, this type of arm shelf has a tendency to slide around the table top. Other models slide into grommets located in the sides of the table. Make sure you have enough room in your studio to maneuver around the table with its additional width.

Another model of arm shelf is a small platform suspended below the face cradle. This particular arm shelf is solely for use in the prone position (Fig. 3–5). Arm shelves that attach to the table frame seem to be more stable than those that suspend from the face rest, but because they are permanently attached, they are usable at only one end of the table and usually cannot be adjusted in height. The arm shelf that suspends from the face rest may become unclipped or may tilt, swing, or slip, especially if the client presses down on the arm shelf when it is time to turn over. Both models come in a full range of fabrics and colors

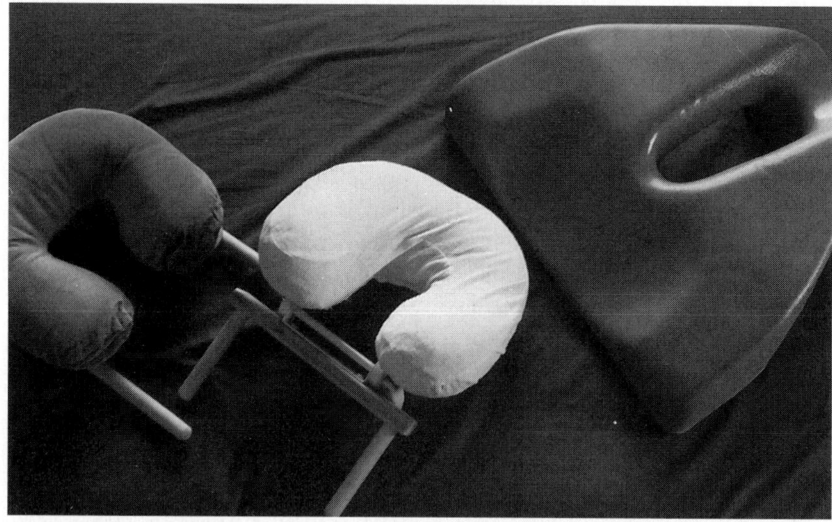

Figure 3•4 Standard and adjustable face rests and a prone pillow.

to match your massage table. Either style is preferable to having a client's arms "fall asleep" from nerve compression when lying prone with arms hanging off the sides of the table.

Foot Rest. A foot rest is basically a padded platform covered with table fabric. The same width as your massage table and extending from one end, the rest attaches to the table by either sliding rods or by a locking hinge mechanism. Using a foot rest can increase the length of your massage table by 10 to 12 inches, depending on the length of the foot rest. When it is not in use, it can either fold down or slide out of the grommets.

Carrying Case. A carrying case helps to protect your table fabric from being damaged during transport, while adding a few handles, pockets, and padded straps, which makes the table easier to lift and carry. Many massage therapists consider a carrying case absolutely necessary if the table is placed in a vehicle's trunk. Most cases are made of tough synthetic fabrics, such as Cordura nylon. Buy table carrying cases that zip both on the top and down the sides, as they are easier to maneuver onto your table.

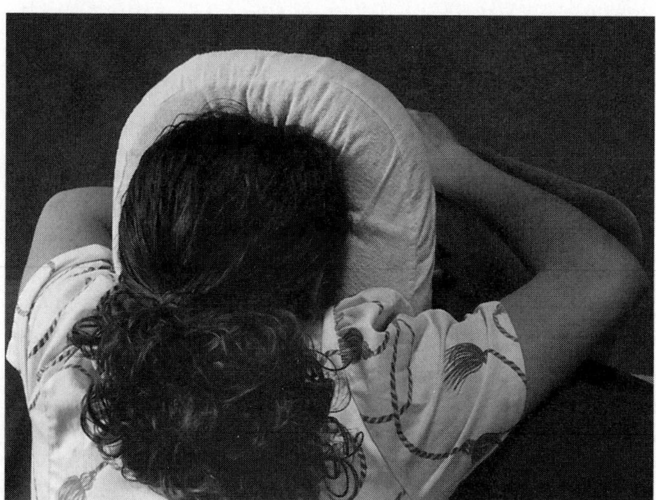

Figure 3•5 Client is shown using a face rest and an arm shelf.

Table Skates and Carts. If you move your table often, table skates or a table cart can save your back and shoulders from ache and injury, as well as help you conserve your energy. These rolling devices allow your table to be rolled across the floor instead of being lifted and carried. Table skates and carts are made by using two high-quality casters mounted on a strip or two of thick plywood board. The boards are attached to the folded table by means of an adjustable quick-clip strap. Once skates are attached, the table can be easily pushed. This accessory makes transporting your table much easier in some ways, but you will still need to lift the table over curbs and up stairs.

Bolsters and Supportive Devices. If client comfort is a priority for your massage practice, you will want to use bolsters and supportive devices to enhance relaxation of the client's muscles and spine. These cushions come in a variety of sizes and shapes and are used to support your client on the massage table. Pillow shapes include tubular, square, rectangular, and wave-shaped (orthopedic); they support the neck, ankles, and knees (Fig. 3–6). These pillows can be made of foam or stuffed with feathers or seeds, such as buck seed or flaxseed.

A soft, tubular pillow is typically used for the neck while the client is in the supine position. Always cover the neck pillow with a pillowcase, which should be laundered after each use. Besides your neck pillow, it's a good idea to keep four to six regular-sized bed pillows on hand, which can be used when positioning the client in a side-lying posture.

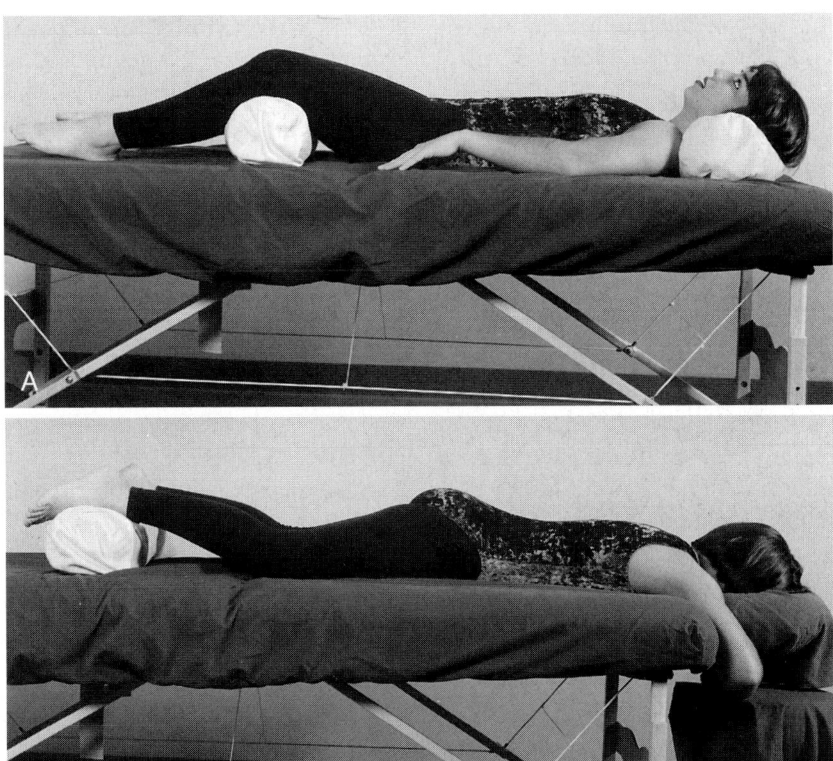

Figure 3•6 A, B, Bolsters are used to support the client's neck, ankles, and/or knees.

The two most popular sizes of knee and ankle bolsters are 6 × 27 inches and 8 × 27 inches. Flat-bottomed bolsters tend to stay in place; they reduce the actual height of the bolster. All knee and ankle bolsters are covered with vinyl, making them easy to clean and disinfect. Most manufacturers offer a variety of styles; full-round and half-round bolsters are available. It is recommended that both sizes be available for your clientele. More elaborate cushion systems can be purchased for your massage practice.

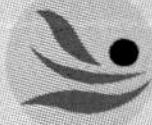

MINI•LAB

Obtain a 6 × 27 inch bolster and a 8 × 27 inch bolster or two that are very close to these two sizes. Lie on your back (supine position) and place the 6 × 27 inch bolster behind your knees for 2 minutes. Next, place the 8 × 27 inch bolster behind your knees for 2 minutes. On a sheet of paper, note the differences you feel in your back, hips, knees, ankles, and feet. Repeat the procedure, but this time, lie on your abdomen (prone position) and place the bolsters under your ankles for 2 minutes. Again, noting the differences in specific body joints, jot down your findings on a sheet of paper. This will help you understand why bolsters are used in your massage practice and why it is preferable to include both sizes. One will usually feel more comfortable than the other, but this will vary from person to person. Both sizes need to be offered to the client.

The fabric surfaces of body cushions, bolsters, and supportive devices must be wiped down with mild cleanser and draped with a clean cloth or paper cover before the start of each massage. Because of the damage caused by disinfecting chemicals, disinfect the fabric surfaces only when they come into contact with body fluids, for sanitation (client coughs and sneezes), and client comfort.

STATIONARY MASSAGE TABLES

The stationary table is usually slightly larger and much heavier than the portable table. Stationary tables are also more stable and offer greater support because they have fewer movable joints. Costing more than portable tables, stationary tables are visually appealing for your clients: they look more secure. Various options include table shelves, storage drawers, built-in music systems, tilting backs for facials, as well as other options available for portable tables. Height adjustment can be manually adjusted or is fully automatic through the use of hydraulics or electric lifts. Let's examine both electric lift tables and hydraulic tables.

Electric Lift Tables. Many massage table companies only offer electric lift massage tables. Electric lift tables use low amperage and require a standard 110-volt circuit. To operate the electric lift, a foot pedal or handheld switch is used to activate the motor. Make sure the manufacturer uses a code-approved, thermally protected motor. With this feature, the motor will turn itself off when it becomes overheated. A good electric motor will last about 10 years, but it is warranted for about 3 years.

When the motor is in use, a mechanical gear box is activated. The action in the gear box causes a large screw to extend or contract, moving the table top up or down, similar to a car jack lifting a car. Instead of manually turning a rod to jack up the car, the table uses the motor to operate the screw drive either forward or backward to vary the table height. Most electric lift tables can raise a load of 550 to 750 pounds.

The downside of the electric lift table is the motor noise created while changing height. Contact the table manufacturer and inquire about the noise level of the motor. Make sure to install a surge protector, and plan the electric cord location to minimize tripping hazards. The ideal location for the electrical outlet is in the floor, under the massage table.

Hydraulic Lift Tables. Requiring only a 110-volt outlet, a hydraulic massage table also uses an electric motor to raise and lower the table top quickly and easily, depending on the needs of the client or practitioner. In recent years, the medical community has turned away from hydraulic tables because these tables had a bad habit of leaking hydraulic fluid from worn-out seals, fittings, and hoses. Leakage created a maintenance and housekeeping problem, especially in hospitals and surgical centers where sterile procedure and hydraulic fluid do not mix. The medical community began replacing hydraulic tables with electric lift tables. Although modern hydraulic technology has greatly improved, the change to electric tables is so widespread that going back to hydraulic equipment does not appear to be happening. So why would a massage therapist consider purchasing a hydraulic table? Read on.

Most electric tables lift the table top up with a pedestal or central post, while most hydraulic tables raise the table top using four points, one located in each corner of the table. This makes for a stronger and smoother ride. Four points also translates into a more stable table top because the points of lift are wider; most hydraulic tables can lift 2,000 pounds (compared with the lifting capacity of electric tables of 550 to 750 pounds). Because there is more "hardware" in the table, hydraulic lift massage tables are more expensive than electric lift tables. Hydraulic tables are also heavier and more expensive to ship. In hydraulic tables, an electric motor turns a pump to create the pressure in the cylinders. As the screw extends into the fluid-filled cylinder, the pressure of the hydraulic fluid is increased in the cylinder and the piston is driven upward, extending the table height. As with electric lift massage tables, ask the company about the noise level of the motor when it is in use. The new technological advances in hydraulics have created an improved product, but the real test is the test of time.

CLEANING MASSAGE EQUIPMENT

Maintainance of massage equipment involves daily cleaning and periodic disinfecting. Cleaning removes dirt, body oil, and massage lubricants from the equipment surfaces. Disinfectants are used to kill viral, bacterial, and fungal agents. If you work in a hospital setting, your equipment must be cleaned in accordance with hospital policy and state law.

All massage equipment is draped during the massage session and all draping material is laundered after each massage; therefore, vinyl surfaces need only be cleaned at the start of each workday. Cleaning includes face rests, arm rests, bolsters, and the massage table top. Place special emphasis on the surfaces that come in contact with the client. Use a mild cleanser, such as liquid hand soap or dish soap.

A disinfectant will chemically remove pathogenic organisms when applied to equipment surfaces. Because frequent disinfectant use will damage the vinyl, disinfect the massage equipment only when necessary. For example, if your client has a contagious skin condition, has a local or general infection, or if any body fluid seeps, cleaning and disinfecting are required after the client leaves the room. Note that most situations that require immediate cleaning and disinfecting are also contraindications for massage. Many massage therapists periodically disinfect the vinyl surfaces every month as well as following an incidence of contact with viral, bacterial, or fungal agents.

Choose good-quality cleaning and disinfecting agents, both of which are available in either liquid or aerosol form. Using disposable towels, apply the agent to the equipment surface. Disposable or single-use towels are preferred over cloth towels because they are more sanitary and can be discarded after each use. Using a circular motion, wipe the equipment, beginning with the least soiled area, and move toward the most soiled area. This prevents the areas that are clean from being contaminated by the areas that are heavily soiled. If you are ever in doubt whether a piece of equipment or a supply is clean, do not use it until it has been properly treated.

MASSAGE LINENS

Massage linens consist of the following: a top and bottom sheet for the massage table, bolster covers, face rest covers, pillowcases, eye pillow covers, towels, arm shelf covers, and blankets. All linens used on massage tables or to cover equipment must be clean prior to the massage, then removed and laundered after the massage. The amount of linens needed will depend on the number of clients you see per day; a two-day supply on hand is recommended. Replace the linens whenever they become stained or threadbare. If washing and folding linens is something you do not wish to do, locate a linen service in your area.

Popular linen fabrics are flannel, cotton, cotton blends, and percale. Be cognizant of the weight and thickness of the fabric. Many inexpensive linens, such as cotton-polyester blends, are too see-through to be appropriate draping material. If you find yourself in this predicament, a blanket over the top drape can remedy the problem. If you choose to use flannel sheets, you can buy sets of single-sized (twin) fitted and flat sheets or purchase sheets from the table manufacturer that are designed for your table. Many therapists drape with bath-sized towels or bath sheets. Whichever type of drape you choose, have an alternative drape available if your client makes a request.

White, off-white, or soft pastels look great and these colors bleach well. Darker colors may show oil stains too easily. Some massage oil manufacturers sell a product that is added to the wash water to help remove the appearance and smell of oil from massage linens. If you are using oil as your primary medium, this product would be an asset.

Towels are often used as draping material. They are heavier than sheets, provide good client coverage, and provides access to the abdominal region when the client is supine. Other reasons massage therapists cite for using towels are that towels are easier to maneuver than sheets and oil stains are less obvious on towels than on sheets. Draping material is a matter of personal preference; client comfort should determine which type of draping material you offer.

Blankets. Have at least two cotton or woollen blankets to drape over your client on cold days, should he or she become chilled. As the body begins to relax, blood pressure is lowered, circulation returns to the core (the circulation pattern change from the skeletal muscles to the internal organs). With this change, the body often feels cooler, and a blanket may cause an even greater feeling of relaxation. Many times the weight of the blanket adds a feeling of comfort and security for the client during the massage. Make sure the blankets you choose are machine washable and that they can be tossed in the dryer. Always drape a blanket *over* the original drape used to cover the client. The blanket does not replace the original drape.

MASSAGE MEDIA—OILS, LOTIONS, CREAMS, AND POWDERS

The primary purpose of massage media is to reduce the friction between the therapist's hands and the client's skin. However, other factors must be considered when choosing a good quality lubricant. There are a few basic guidelines that can be used when deciding what medium works best for you and your clients.

1. *Does the lubricant nourish the skin?* Ingredients such as cold-pressed vegetable, nut, and seed oils and plant essences are good for the skin, whereas ingredients like mineral oil and isopropyl alcohol can clog the pores and deplete nutrients from the skin. Even though stearyl and cetyl alcohol do not nourish the skin, they are safe for the skin and are often used as emulsifiers and stiffening agents in various creams and lotions. Always read the ingredients list to ascertain the contents of a massage lubricant.
2. *How will my client's skin react to the lubricant?* Some skin types will be sensitive to certain products and not to others. During the massage consultation, inquire about allergies to nuts or other products that act as ingredients in massage lubricants. If the client indicates that she has a skin condition, this must be taken into consideration when choosing a lubricant. Since lubricant sensitivity cannot always be predetermined, keep a bottle of hypoallergenic cream or lotion available to use upon request or when you are unsure about how a client will react to your primary lubricant. However, the word "hypoallergenic" does not mean that your client will not have an allergic reaction to the product. Hypoallergenic generally means that the product has undergone lengthy testing and that the majority of the subjects in the study did not have an allergic reaction to the product tested. Scented lubricants often increase allergic reactions. Many skin conditions are exasperated by massage lubricants. Allow the client to read the contents on the lubricant container to see if she recognizes any potential problems in the ingredients.

Author's Note

Allergic Reaction to Lubricant. If you notice or if the client reports that a massaged area is discolored, or if the topography has changed, he probably had a reaction to the massage lubricant. If this occurs, wash and dry the area immediately. You and your client may decide to finish the massage over the top drape or use talc as a massage lubricant. However, many allergic reactions to topical agents do not show up for

24 to 48 hours after the agent comes into contact with the skin. This means that most allergic reactions will not be apparent until a day or two following treatment! This is another argument in favor of hypoallergenic lubricants.

---

3. *Will the lubricant easily stain my massage linens?* Oil-based products are more likely to stain linens than water-based products. Creams and lotions are typically water based. Massage linens like bolster covers and bottom sheets are more susceptible to staining and may have to be replaced more frequently. Conversely, top sheets and face rest sheets, especially those made of terry cloth and flannel, are the least likely to become stained by oily products. Do not use linens that are stained. Even if clean, stained linens appear unsanitary, which may reduce client confidence.

The amount of lubricant you use will depend on the type of massage lubricant, the dryness of the client's skin, and the intention of the massage. In Swedish massage, the hands' ability to glide across the skin is important, and a fair amount of lubricant is required to accomplish this task. When performing some types of deep-tissue massage such as myofascial release, the ability to grasp superficial layers of skin and fascia is important, so very little lubricant is needed. In general, excessive amounts of lubricant will prevent you from manipulating tissue, and inadequate amounts of lubricant will pull and irritate the skin. Experience will teach you how much lubricant is the right amount. Less is better; you can always add more lubricant if necessary.

When choosing a lubricant dispenser, make sure the dispenser contents do not become contaminated when applying and reapplying the lubricant to the client's skin. A pump or squeeze container works best. The downside to pumps is that they break easily if dropped. The dispenser can be placed on the massage table between the knees for easy access and to prevent the dispenser from being knocked off the massage table. Placing the dispenser on the floor requires the therapist to continually bend over or squat in between lubricant applications. Squeeze dispensers that are smooth and round are hard to grasp and easier to drop. Lubricant "holsters" are also available; they allow the lubricant and dispenser to be worn around the therapist's hips.

Never apply the lubricant directly on the client's skin. Place the proper amount in your own hands, warming it by rubbing the fingers and palms together to create friction. Apply lubricant only on the area you will be massaging, never on adjacent areas. If too much lubricant is accidentally used, wipe off the excess with a paper towel.

It is preferred to have both unscented and scented lubricant available. Ask the client to state her preference. If you discover that your client has numerous allergies, she may be sensitive to scented lubricants. If allergies are not a consideration and the client chooses the scented lubricant, place a small amount on the back of the client's hand before the massage begins so she may approve the scent. Avoid using a scent that offends the client. Even if aromatherapy is one of your specialties, have unscented massage lubricant available for your clients.

Oils. Massage oils are the most traditional and most commonly used lubricant. Nut and seed oils are the best because they are the most nutritive. Healing agents, such as vitamin E, may be added to the oil. Vitamin E also acts as a preservative, which is important, because natural, cold-pressed oils can become rancid. Some therapists mix their oil with a lotion in a 50-50 solution. They will separate, so blend the mixture before use by stirring or shaking the container.

The use of massage oils stains not only massage linens but clothing as well. The best preventive method for reducing linen and clothing stains is not to overapply your massage oil. You may choose to inform your clients about the possibility of oil stains on their garments when they call and schedule the massage appointment so they can plan accordingly. This usually involves wearing loungewear to the session or bringing a change of clothes to be used after the massage session. Offer the client a hand towel to wipe any excess oil from the skin. A shower after the massage may remedy this problem.

Avoid mineral oil, as it is a known **carcinogen** (substance that causes or is suspected to cause cancer). Mineral oil, or liquid petroleum, is not miscible in body oils and adds no nutritive value to the skin because it does not penetrate the skin. Often, mineral oils serves as a barrier that may clog the pores. Most brands of body lotions and creams contain mineral oil because it is inexpensive and has an infinite shelf life.

Lotion. Lotions are preferred by deep-tissue massage therapists because of the limited amount of glide they afford. When you do not want to slip and slide over the skin's surface, lotion is a good choice. This gives you more control over the lubricant because glide can be decreased by working longer. Lotion will not leave the skin feeling greasy. However, lotion does not have the staying power of oil or cream and is quickly absorbed into the skin. Therefore, you will use more lotion than oil or cream, but lotion is generally less expensive.

Cream. Creams are more emollient than lotion, but less greasy than oils. Since they cannot be spilled like oils or lotions, creams are less messy than any other massage medium because they are more viscous. This quality also gives them a staying power almost equal to that of massage oils. Creams are less likely to stain clothing. They are typically the most expensive massage medium.

Cocoa Butter Sticks. Cocoa butter sticks provide precise lubrication application and are frequently used in deep-tissue work because they allow more control and are easily absorbed by the skin. A small amount will cover a large area on the body because the client's body temperature will melt the cocoa butter. Allergic reactions to cocoa butter are rare.

Powder. Baby powder, talc, powdered chalk, or cornstarch may be used to reduce the friction between the therapist's hands and the client's skin, but it is not as efficient at friction reduction as other forms of massage media. Occasionally you may have a client who may request powder or a client who does not want any topical agents used that will leave a residue. Powder may be used as an alternative lubricant and is the lubricant of choice for therapists who practice manual lymphatic drainage. Be careful when applying powder to the skin because the powder particles can enter the nasal passages and cause the client or therapist to sneeze or cough.

AROMATHERAPY

The use of scents for therapeutic purposes is called aromatherapy. Aromatherapy can be used in baths, candles, candle-lit diffusers, massage lubricants, incense, and specially designed aromatherapy diffusing units or heating units. Massage and aromatherapy are often combined to enhance the therapeutic value of each other. How aromatherapy works will be discussed in the respiratory system chapter.

Essential oils are concentrated essences of aromatic plants. They have been used for thousands of years for their healing properties. For use in massage therapy, essential oils can be used to scent a room and scent the massage medium. Before using any of these essential oils, read the product label carefully for precautions and warnings. For example, many essential oils are not recommended for use on pregnant women. Other essential oils are contraindicated for some skin conditions because of the possibility of irritation. As a rule, most fair-haired, fair-skinned people have sensitive skin. In these cases, use essential oils sparingly (only a few drops at a time) or avoid them altogether. Essential oils, used safely, can enhance your client's health and well-being.

According to a manufacturer of massage products and essential oils, the 12 most popular essential oils are lavender, clary sage, eucalyptus, sandalwood, rosemary, tangerine, vetiver, peppermint, lemon, juniper, chamomile, and ylang-ylang. If you wish to use aromatherapy in your massage practice, these essential oils are recommended to begin your collection. To obtain a more complete list of essential oils, purchase a book on aromatherapy.

1. **Lavender.** The most widely used essential oil, it combats insomnia, calms and balances the mind and emotions, and helps to ease irritability.
2. **Clary Sage.** This essential oil acts as an antidepressant. It is said to calm and balance the mind and emotions. Because of its calming effect, it is great before and during menstruation, but is not recommended during pregnancy.
3. **Eucalyptus.** Highly used for respiratory congestion, eucalyptus helps to bring comfort when experiencing loss and grief. This oil is also used during periods of physical and mental fatigue and exhaustion. Use sparingly, as it can irritate the skin.
4. **Sandalwood.** Sandalwood promotes deep relaxation, abates depression, and quiets the mind and emotions.
5. **Rosemary.** Aiding in stimulating mental clarity, concentration, and memory, rosemary promotes cerebral activity. Rosemary also brings balance by helping to detoxify the mind and body. Do not use during pregnancy or on epileptic clients.
6. **Tangerine.** Tangerine is said to clear away negativity and opens up the heart by inspiring sensitivity and empathy. It also helps to calm an overactive nervous system.
7. **Vetiver.** Vetiver promotes a sense of balance by activating a feeling of security and stability, as well as by erasing worries.
8. **Peppermint.** Peppermint adds a sense of excitement and enthusiasm. It is great when you need a little "get up and go" or after a long period of depression. This oil is used for headaches, nausea, and motion sickness. Do not use during pregnancy. If your client is taking homeopathic remedies, avoid using peppermint because it can act as an antidote.
9. **Lemon.** Lemon is used for added energy to the mind and body, and a sense of clarity, which makes it useful during times of indecisiveness. Lemon essential oil may irritate the skin.
10. **Juniper.** This scent promotes a sense of strength and well-being. Juniper can ease the pain in muscles and joints. Avoid during pregnancy.
11. **Chamomile.** Chamomile helps to ease depression, stress, anger, tension, and irritability. It can also restore the mind and body after a long illness.
12. **Ylang-ylang.** This oil can calm the nervous system, ease depression, and reduce frustration. Used topically ylang-ylang can irritate the skin.

MASSAGE SUPPLIES

Massage supplies are items such as paper towels and lubricants that are bought and used frequently. They

MASSAGE SUPPLY CHECKLIST

	Facial Massage Supplies:
☐ Lubricant	☐ Make-up Remover
☐ Liquid Antibacterial Soap	☐ Cleansing Cream
☐ Vinyl Gloves and Finger Cots	☐ Toner/Astringent
☐ Cleaning and Disinfectant Supplies	☐ Moisturizing Cream
☐ Box of Tissues	☐ Clay Masque
☐ Paper Towels	☐ Other:__________
☐ Toilet Paper	☐ Other:__________
☐ Cotton Balls	__________
☐ Disposable Cups	
☐ Hairspray	
☐ Contact Lens Solution	

Figure 3•7 Massage supply checklist. (Permission is hereby granted to reproduce this form in its entirety, including the copyright notice, for commercial or instructional use but not for resale.)

are needed to provide a clean, sanitary, and comfortable massage environment. Some massage supplies are not necessary for direct massage services but should be considered as minor accompaniments, such as hair spray, disposable cups, and cotton balls. Use the checklist (Fig. 3–7) when shopping for your massage supplies and incidentals. Extra lines have been added to the checklist for you to write in your own massage items.

FURNISHING THE MASSAGE ROOM

The furnishings and fixtures you choose for your massage will help you create the best setting for you and your clients. These items include a mirror, a clock, water dispenser, wastebasket, supply cabinet, chairs and stools, a place for your client's clothes and personal items, and wall hangings. Window treatments, light sources, and floor and wall treatment are important also. Most furnishings are intended to increase client comfort and to provide minor conveniences. Some suggestions for your massage room can be seen in Figure 3–8.

Mirror. A mirror is an essential for massage rooms. Clients use mirrors to groom themselves after their massage to make sure they are presentable when returning to work or home. Therapists use full-length mirrors to aid in assessing body posture with clients. Mirrors come in various sizes, ranging from wall-size to handheld. Mirrors are also used to reflect light and to make a room appear larger.

Clocks. Wall clocks or desk clocks are needed to keep the therapist on schedule and to time certain treatments such as ice packs or facial masks. There are two standard types of clocks, the digital and the analog. The digital clock displays the time numerically, whereas the analog clock has the numbered circular face with hour, minute, and sometimes second hands. The digital clocks are more convenient if the therapist does a lot of small timed treatments during the session. It is often easier to watch the numbers click from 2:35 to 2:38 for a 3-minute treatment than it is to estimate the analog clock's hand movement from across the room. The clock should be more visible to the therapist than to the client, for whom it may be a distraction.

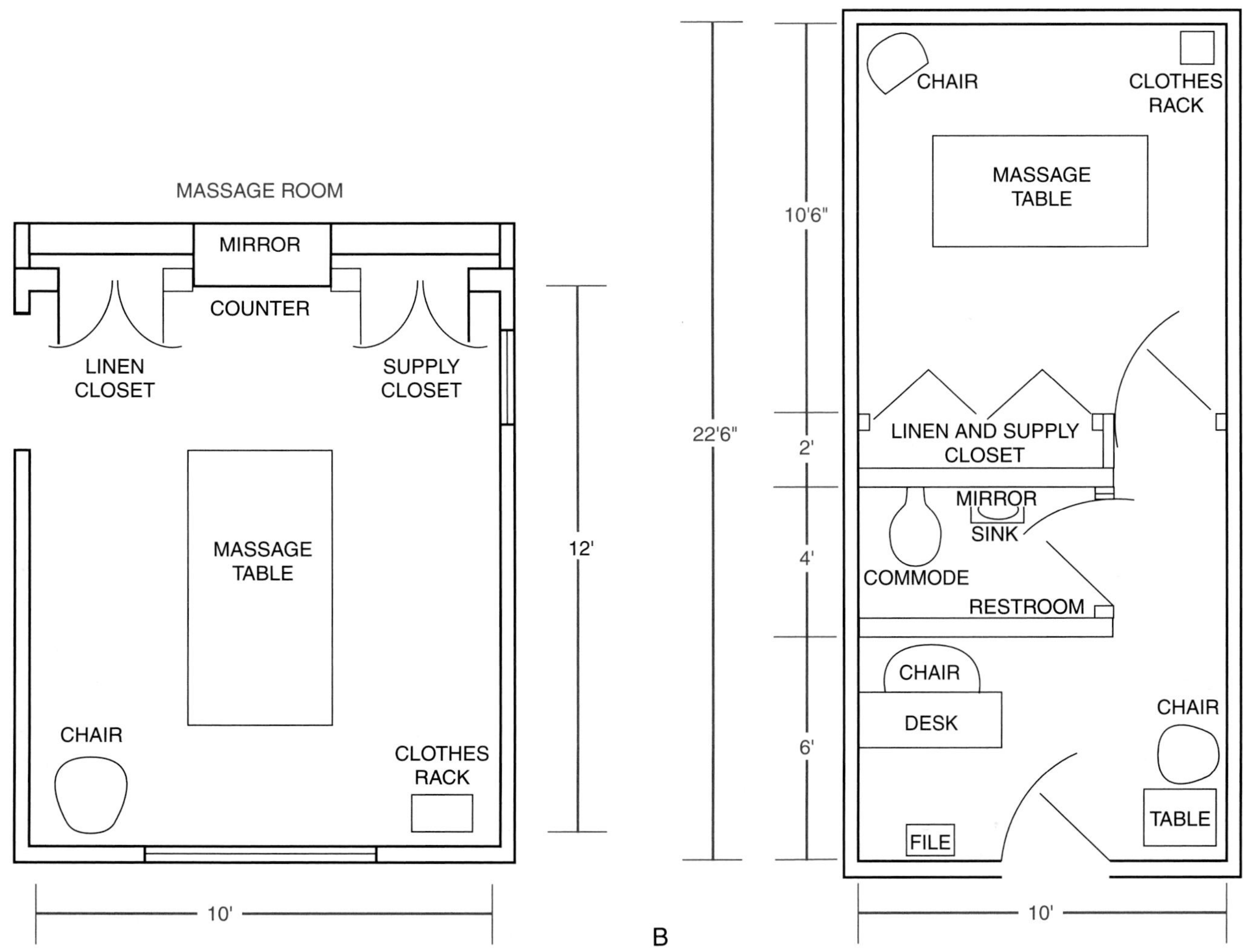

Figure 3•8 A, B, Possible room layouts for a massage practice.

Water Dispenser. Clean, pure drinking water is an important element in maintaining health. Most people do not drink enough fluids. A water dispenser makes it easy to get the water your body requires. Clients will want to take advantage of a water dispenser as well. Part of your massage service can include offering each client a cup of fresh water before and after each massage.

Wastebasket. A wastebasket is needed in the massage room for paper towels, tissue paper, disposable gloves, and other items. Most states require that the wastebasket have a lid to close the basket top. The lidded wastebaskets that lift by a foot pedal are preferred to ones that must be opened by lifting the lid by hand, because of the possibility of hand contamination. Clean daily and disinfect the wastebasket once a week.

Supply Cabinet. A supply cabinet with hinged doors is preferred to open shelves because supply items are kept out of sight. A supply cabinet can be used to store your massage linens. Cabinets or closets fitted with louvered doors allow linens to breathe, reducing the formation of a rancid odor. These types of doors also hide stereo speakers while still allowing sounds to move through the slats. Line the top surface of your shelves with laminate (Formica), which resists stains from lubricant dispensers and linens and is easy to clean and disinfect. Be sure to provide a place to store soiled linens separately from clean ones.

Chairs and Stools. A chair provides a place for the client to sit while removing trousers, stockings, shoes, and socks. Depending on available space and personal taste, you may choose a simple straight-back chair, a plush oversized chair, a chaise longue, or an ottoman. Upholstery fabrics are available in a wide variety of textures and colors, and contribute to creating the desired atmosphere by bringing in color, texture, and patterns.

A stool is often used by the therapist when performing massage on the head, neck, hands, or feet. Sitting on a stool takes the place of kneeling on the floor or sitting on the massage table. The best stool design is one that can be raised or lowered for the best administration of different massage techniques. One height does not fit all circumstances! Remember, all massage equipment, including furniture, should ergonomically support the therapist. There are all kinds of different height adjustment mechanisms, from hydraulic to screw-type. The hydraulic type can be quietly adjusted while the therapist is sitting on the stool. The screw-type mechanisms often require the therapist to remove himself from the stool first. Some screw-type mechanisms are noisy and time consuming if you need a great change in height. Many therapists also use a large inflatable physio-ball as a stool.

A Place for Clothes and Personal Items. For the application of most massage techniques, the client will remove some or all of his garments, glasses, and jewelry. A designated place should be provided for all articles of clothing, including coats, hats, and umbrellas. The most common devices are wall hooks, a coat tree, free-standing locker, or a valet. If a place for clothes and personal items is not specified by the therapist, the client may feel confused and disoriented.

Often, a small desk or table is placed next to the designated clothing area for the client's personal items. A small dish or basket can be provided for clients to place items such as keys, pocket change, wallet, eyeglasses, wristwatches, and jewelry. In this way, clients can easily take their personal property with them if they move from one location to another. Make sure these items are safe and secure and are not accidentally misplaced. It would be unfortunate if the client reports to you that she has misplaced her jewelry or coin purse while in your establishment.

Wall Hangings. Most massage therapists use wall hangings in their massage studios for four reasons. First, wall hangings can add ambiance to the room. Second, wall hangings can be used to inform and educate the client. Third, some wall hangings provide acoustical properties to help achieve a quieter room. Fourth, certain wall decor will add a sense of professionalism to the room.

When choosing a wall hanging for ambiance, consider color and content. Warm or soft colors, such as peach and beige, are calming and tranquil. Bright, intense colors, such as red and yellow, stimulate our central nervous system and typically do not provide a relaxing environment.

In selecting art such as paintings or prints, nature scenes of waterfalls and open meadows help provide a relaxing environment. Save your battle scene pictures of the American Civil War for your living room. A picture or painting of an ocean or sunset adds a serene, tranquil feeling to your massage atmosphere. Keep art simple—if it is too busy, it may distract the client from the massage experience. You want your art to make a statement, not an exclamation. When choosing art, before you make the purchase it is often a good idea to get the opinion of at least three people who will give you honest feedback.

Anatomical charts, trigger point charts, or acupuncture meridian charts are often used by massage therapists as wall hangings. These charts provide a quick reference for locating muscles, bony markings, trigger points, acupressure points, and other important areas of the body. They are also used for educating the client about her musculoskeletal anatomy and mechanisms of pain and discomfort. These charts are perfect if you are striving for a clinical look and feel to your studio. If you use anatomical charts but do not want to use them wall mounted, there is an alternative. Many chart companies now offer flip charts in specially designed notebooks. These can be stored on a bookshelf and referred to as needed.

Framed diplomas, certificates, and awards help instill a sense of confidence in your clients. Achievement papers are a reminder that you are accomplished, experienced, and committed to your profession. Many massage therapists prefer to hang their diplomas and awards in their offices and to keep the studio atmosphere artistic and relaxing; the studio space belongs to your clients. Other professional documents to display include a photographic collage of you working on clients, receiving awards, or giving lectures. Display all of your academic achievements and professional affiliations where you feel they are appropriate.

Window Treatments

Windows treatments, also known as window dressings, include vertical and horizontal blinds, shades, and an assortment of drapes. Window treatments have four main functions: they provide wall decoration, they insulate from sound and outside temperature variations, they block or filter light, and they provide privacy for clients.

Window treatments can be simple or can be an addition to your wall ornamentation. When choosing window treatments as a form of decoration, the color and shade of the walls and floor must be taken into consideration. For example, window treatment fabrics with a pattern usually do not look good with a printed wallpaper. Ask someone who has talent or training in interior decorating to assist you in this selection.

For privacy, all windows that provide a view *into* the studio should be covered by a window treatment. Heavy drapes absorb more sound than shades or blinds; a combination of blinds, drapes, and shades is

I love being a mother, and I love Southwest art. One reason why I love Southwest art is because I went to school in Albuquerque, New Mexico. The Southwest is noted for its wonderful paintings, sculpture, and pottery. My massage establishment is decorated in Southwest style because of my massage education roots.

One day, I found a beautiful R. C. Gorman print in a local frame shop. It was of a woman nursing her child. In this phase of Gorman's career he was using soft, muted colors. The print would be a wonderful addition to my collection. Or so I thought.

I presented the print to a few close friends and asked them what they felt when they looked at it. One woman felt sad because she could not nurse any of her three children, one woman loved it, and one woman was upset because she was unable to have children. The men I showed it to liked it or felt neutral about it. I quickly decided that this picture should not hang on the walls in my massage room or office.

often used to create the right effect. Massage therapists prefer window treatments that are light blocking over those that are light filtering because it is easier to add more light than to try to reduce it. Fabric-covered blinds are more attractive than the vinyl and aluminum versions but are also more expensive. Window treatments come in a wide variety of styles, weights, and colors, but all may be stained by being touched by oily hands.

Flooring and Walls

Carpet is the best choice for flooring in your massage room. As an insulator, carpet provides warmth and absorbs sound. Carpeted floors also provide safety for clients; oily feet can pose a liability risk on hard flooring. If your massage room has vinyl or hardwood flooring, a thick throw rug that takes up the majority of the room will suffice.

To reduce further unwanted sounds from outside the massage room, interior walls can be insulated, or sound-absorbing panels can be placed in the room. Textured wallpaper, hanging pictures, and other large decorations on the walls will minimize the echoing sounds. Hollow-core doors can be replaced with solid-core doors to reduce further undesired sound.

Where the spirit does not work with the hand, there is no art.

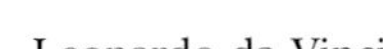

—Leonardo da Vinci

THE MASSAGE ROOM ENVIRONMENT

Beyond your professional appearance, one of the most important factors for "client appeal" is the atmosphere of your massage studio. The surroundings of the room set the tone for the massage session. Ideally, you want a place that is quiet, private, easy to heat or cool, and draft-free. The room must also be free of tobacco and incense smoke, pet dander, and the smell of cleaning solutions. All supplies such as bolsters, blankets, lubricants, and pillows should all be within easy reach. Convenient access to a bathroom is desirable. However, local ordinances may dictate part of the massage environment; check with the proper authorities.

The importance of atmosphere cannot be overemphasized. The symbol for space in Chinese is the symbol for gate in Japanese. Open the gates to relaxation and healing by creating a space for this to occur. If possible, atmosphere should begin when the client drives up to your office and should be maintained all the way to your treatment room. Atmospheric considerations include lighting, music, temperature, and room color. The examples here are given to stimulate your imagination and to help you set your goals. Whenever you can, purchase items to increase both client and therapist comfort, to offer new services, and to improve the esthetics of your studio.

The dining-room metaphor is one way of explaining why the massage room ambiance is so essential. When you are serving a specially prepared meal, adjustments are made to make the dining experience extraordinary. The table is set using attractive linens, plates, cups, flatware, and flowers. Soft music is playing in the background, and the lights are dimmed. Give your massage clients the same kind of care and consideration. Let them feel, through the environment you create, that they are honored guests in your establishment. The food makes the meal, but the setting can greatly enhance the experience.

Light Sources and Lighting. Lighting serves several purposes in a massage setting. First, you must provide adequate lighting so your clients can read, remove garments, maneuver around the room, get on the massage table, get off the massage table, redress, and exit the office. This same lighting can be used for the therapist visually to assess the condition of the skin before and during a massage. Second, most massage therapists lower the lights during the massage to assist the client in achieving relaxation.

The best light source is provided by Mother Nature—sunlight. Natural light coming in a window can be controlled through your window treatments. If you live in a predominantly sunny climate, you can also tint exterior windows on the east and west side of your massage room to create the best lighting for massage therapy.

Even if you use sunlight as your main light source, other forms of light will have to be used on overcast days or after sunset. Indirect lighting is best. Indirect lighting means that the bulbs are obscured from view by means of opaque shades or baffles. A pattern of reflected light is visible but not the bulbs themselves. A similar effect can be achieved by placing floor lamps in the corners of the room or by using recessed ceiling lights at the corners of the rooms.

Incandescent bulbs are the next best choice, and they can be used in a variety of lamps and fixtures. The higher the wattage of the bulb, the more light it will emit. However, many lamps require a medium- to low-wattage incandescent bulb. The intensity of many lamps and light fixtures can be adjusted by using a special switch known as a rheostat or dimmer. Your lighting needs will vary from time to time, depending on if you are assessing the client or if you are performing a stress-reduction massage. Have several lighting possibilities available.

The two other forms of light bulbs used are halogen and fluorescent lights. Even though both types of bulbs use very little energy, a few problems should be noted. There have been a few reported incidents of exploding halogen bulbs. Fluorescent lights often emit a humming noise and a bluish color, which may contribute to the onset of headaches. The bluish tint of fluorescent lights also gives a bluish color that can distort the color of your client's skin and your intended wall color. If your office already has fluorescent lighting, you may want to leave it turned off and use table or floor lamps or replace the fluorescent bulbs with a "full spectrum" tube.

There are still other mood lighting suggestions that can be accomplished rather inexpensively. Line a window, a corner, or a beam with strings of clear Christmas lights (not the twinkle kind). Try placing a night-light behind a large object, such as an oversized vase. Many massage therapists include the use of candlelight in their practice. Although candles are unbeatable for creating a relaxing ambiance, they also create a fire hazard. No matter how careful you are, candle wax spills as well as soot deposits occur on shelves and walls. However, you may decide the benefits are worth the risks.

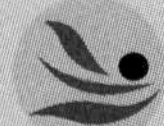

MINI•LAB

Lie on your massage table in the prone and the supine positions. Get the client's perspective. Notice what the major issues are: visual stimuli, odor, sound, etc.

Music. Since "music soothes the savage beast," it stands to reason that it be included in creating an environment conducive to massage therapy. Music is art for the ears, and most massage therapists will tell

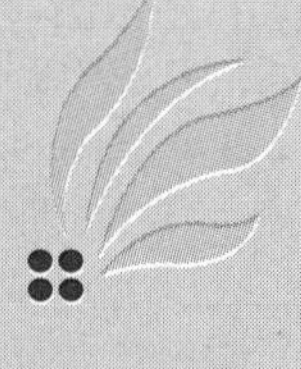

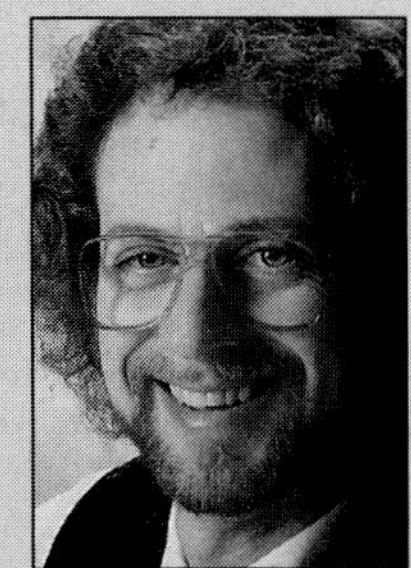

Steven Halpern, Ph.D.

Born: April 18, 1947

"Mother Nature gave us eyelids. She didn't give us ear-lids or body-lids."

As the true pioneer in the field of relaxation music, Steven Halpern is far from being simply a gifted musician. His eternal thirst for knowledge has genuinely benefited the field of massage therapy, and any therapist who has used any of his music can attest to this undeniable fact. His extensive research has taken music to a scientific level and beyond.

His interest in music actually began as a toddler growing up in Long Island, New York. Surprisingly, his parents never played music in the home. In fact, it wasn't uncommon for him to crawl down the hallway of his apartment building to the doors of neighbors playing music. This allowed him to follow his heart and listen to music that he truly enjoyed at a very young age. A short while after starting in the school music program, he found himself becoming bored with just playing "little black dots written by dead white composers." This led to his involvement in jazz, which allows a great deal of improvisation.

While in college in the late '60s his curiosity about music led to his revolutionary research on the effects of certain rhythms on the human body. At the time it was practically a virgin field. There were very few schools that would allow such research, but fortunately he was introduced to the University of California at Sonoma. Here he had access to biofeedback equipment and did thorough investigations on the effects of music consisting of subtle rhythms, gentle tones, and nontraditional harmonics. The result has been the hallmark of his approach to composition. He says:

continued on the following page

"One of the most fundamental responses of the human organism is that it is easily rhythm entrained to an external rhythmic stimulus. In other words, if there is a steady beat, your heart and pulse will naturally synchronize to that rhythm." This explains why music that has a beat faster than a resting heartbeat is impossible to relax to.

This theory instantly made Dr. Halpern's music popular with massage therapists and clients. After hearing this new type of music, people actually hired him to play live as they were receiving massages. Many massage professionals claimed that as a result of listening to his music, clients were actually relaxing before they even placed a hand on them. Thus, therapists had much less resistance to deal with, which in turn resulted in making their work much easier.

Although music is important, Dr. Halpern reminds us not to forget about other forms of sound. Having a great deal of control over her environment, a therapist needs to be very aware of the noises that are often taken for granted. He says he is amazed at how many therapists have a loud ticking clock or a noisy air conditioner. These factors should be taken care of before music can even be considered. There are certain sounds that many of us have conditioned ourselves to block out. Dr. Halpern states, "Mother Nature gave us eyelids. She didn't give us ear-lids or body-lids." Whether we are consciously aware of it, our entire body is picking up and responding to all sounds.

Dr. Halpern notes that "while listening to true relaxation music, an altered state can be entered. . . . whereas dancers say they become one with the music, a massage therapist can become one with the massage. This state allows therapists to consciously lose track of the exact strokes they are going to do next, yet they always seem to do exactly the right ones." He claims that some of the best massage professionals he has talked to say that such music has helped them reach this zone in which the realm of massage lives and a wonderful healing energy can be tapped into. He admits that this phenomenon has yet to be scientifically documented, but after hearing it from so many people he feels that it must be true. He invites all massage professionals to keep their awareness and hearts open to this because it can be of great service and benefit to their clients. "Music is much more powerful, and the effects of music are much more pronounced than most people realize," says Halpern. "In the past 25 or 30 years, people have forgotten how to listen in a lot of respects, but I now start to see people come back." Steven Halpern's words are as powerful as his music. Perhaps if we all consciously listened with more than our ears, we could tap into infinite amounts of wisdom and give credit due to this incredible man.

you that it makes a difference in how clients relax (if the music is soft and slow). Music also helps the therapist in keeping a rhythm with massage movements.

Music systems can range from a transportable box style with a handle to a multicomponent system. The most convenient feature on a cassette player is an "auto reverse" or a "repeat" button on a compact disc player. This allows uninterrupted massage time, since your time will not be spent turning the tape over or restarting it. It is helpful to listen to the mechanical sounds of the music system during its operation. Many units are quite noisy when loading the tape or compact disc or when the tape is reversing direction.

If you have detachable speakers, place them at your client's ear level when he or she is lying down on your massage table. Small, hidden speakers are preferred to overly large speakers that look like furniture. Thanks to technology, small high-quality speakers are available. Most music systems can accommodate as many as four speakers.

Have a variety of cassette tapes or compact discs available for your client's (and your own) listening pleasure. Some therapists encourage clients to bring their own music selections to the session. Although music, like room decor, is a matter of taste, most therapists like a slow, even melody. Most classical selections are not appropriate because of an ebb and flow of crescendos and decrescendos. Be careful of New Age music, because most selections have jumpy melodies and are too stimulating. Music companies are now subdividing New Age music—a category called "minimalism" is suitable for massage. Nature sounds, such as waves breaking on the shore, whale songs, and thunderstorms, combined with orchestral music, are also a good choice. Beware of trickling water sounds; they may induce some clients to request a visit to the bathroom during the massage.

Author's Note

In my opinion, the massage therapist should not talk loudly in the massage room. Clients respond well to a soft voice, and normal or loud talking is usually unnecessary. Also, there is nothing so disturbing to a client than a loud noise once relaxation is achieved. Some clients prefer total silence, with no talking by the therapist.

As my massage career evolved and I began to design studio space, I found myself becoming more and more concerned with sound. Music systems became more elaborate, and insulating the massage room from outside noises also become more important. My latest massage studio has insulated interior walls and a solid-core door. I also advocate something that has come to be called "door etiquette."

During the massage, you may have to open a cabinet or door. Leave the door to the cabinet closed, but not closed tight. When you go to open the cabinet or closet door, you can do so without noise.

When you are entering or exiting the massage room, turn the door handle, close the door, then release the handle slowly. In this way, the dreadful "click" is avoided. Think I am oversensitive? I might be, but try it and see how your clients react. Let your clients have a few moments of peace before they come back to the "real world."

Temperature of the Massage Room. The ideal temperature range for your massage room is between 68° and 75°F. Clients may have difficulty relaxing if the room temperature is not comfortable. As the massage progresses, the parasympathetic nervous system is activated, and pulse rate, respiration rate, and blood pressure decrease. This is why clients often become chilled during the massage, even though they felt comfortable at the beginning of the massage. Always ask the client if he is warm enough halfway through the massage session.

Once your room temperature is set, there are several ways to keep your client warm as her body physiology changes. One of the functions of draping is to provide warmth. A small portable heater can be placed in the room if additional warmth is needed. Make sure that no one is in danger of touching the heating element on the unit. In winter months, a heating blanket can be added to the massage table top. Blankets can be placed on top of the client for warmth as well. Many clients express that the room temperature is fine, but their feet feel cold. Clients may elect to bring and wear socks while on the massage table, or an extra blanket can be draped over their feet for added warmth.

The massage therapist may become warm during the massage because of physical exertion. If you become overheated easily, try wearing clothes made of natural fibers and that fit loosely to allow air to evaporate active and insensible perspiration. A small oscillating fan can be placed on the floor and the airflow directed at the therapist's feet. No matter where the therapist is standing, the air will reach him as the fan turns. The fan should not interfere with keeping the client warm. Make sure the fan or fan cord is not in a location to create a safety hazard. If the room has vertical blinds, be sure they are not in the path of the fan, otherwise the breeze will disturb them, creating both an audible distraction and an invasion of privacy.

Color. Colors used for your massage room can be divided into two categories—warm and cool. Warm colors naturally bring a feeling of warmth, but also stimulation; cool colors can make a room feel cool, but they are also relaxing. Shade of a particular color also has the most impact on what you are trying to achieve. This concept can be illustrated by using an effleurage stroke. A light effleurage has a small impact on circulation of blood, and a deep effleurage has a greater impact on circulation of blood. The same stroke produces different levels of effect.

Warm colors are reds, browns, yellows, and oranges; cool colors are blues, violets, and greens. White is the

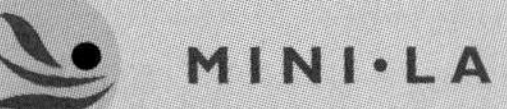

MINI•LAB

Using all the elements discussed in this chapter, sit down and design your massage room.

absence of color, and black is the combination of all colors. You can choose what you like; if you do not have a strong preference, go with the color most of your clients like. Color can also open up a small room or make a large room appear smaller and cozier.

The most important color considerations in your massage room are the walls, floor, window treatments, and linens. Choose colors that contrast well, such as tan walls and sage green linens, or green walls and burgundy linens. Neutral colors work best because they do not overwhelm clients.

SUMMARY

Career success depends not only on education and skills but also on your ability to use wisely the tools of the trade. Tools or massage equipment includes the massage table, face rests, arm shelves, carrying cases, table skates, linens, bolsters, and massage lubricants. Equipment should be chosen with consideration to ergonomics, client comfort, longevity, and wise investment.

Your massage table is your most important tool. When purchasing a stationary or a portable massage table, most table manufacturers let you decide the specifications of features such as width, height, length, frame, padding, and fabric.

It is essential that the therapist understand the procedures and frequency of simple cleaning and disinfecting each piece of equipment.

Massage linens include towels, sheets, blankets, pillowcases, bolster and face rest covers, etc. Popular linen fabrics are flannel, cotton, cotton blends, and percale.

Massage media or lubricants include oils, creams, lotions, and powders. Good lubricants should nourish the skin. They should not cause allergic reactions or stain clothing and linens.

Finally, the massage room environment ties everything together. Considerations should be made for temperature, lighting, color, music, decorations, and client comfort.

This information is really quite simple; using these recommendations can produce a great savings of time and money, as well as improve the quality of the beginning therapist's work.

SELF-TEST

Multiple Choice • Write the letter of the best answer in the space provided.

_______ 1. In choosing the right kind of equipment, the following is *not* an important consideration

A. ergonomically supporting the therapist
B. adding comfort to the client
C. color of the equipment matching the window treatment
D. how long will the equipment last

_______ 2. Massage tables that are too wide make it difficult for the therapist to

A. sit on the massage table
B. lower the massage table
C. apply pressure on tight muscles
D. reach across the massage table

_______ 3. The three *worst* substances for your table and accessory vinyl are

A. soap, water, and oil
B. soap, alcohol, and chlorine bleach
C. oils, alcohol, and chlorine bleach
D. oil, vinegar, and massage linens

_______ 4. Which table accessory allows your client to keep his head and neck relatively straight when lying prone?

A. face rest
B. arm shelf
C. foot rest
D. table skate

_______ 5. Disinfect your massage table

A. after each client
B. when it comes in contact with body fluids
C. once a week
D. once a month

_______ 6. Massage linens must be changed and laundered

A. at the start of each workday
B. after each client
C. only when oil stained
D. when the fabric is threadbare

_______ 7. The primary purpose of a massage lubricant is to

A. soothe and soften the skin
B. stain massage linens
C. reduce skin friction
D. remove blemishes

_______ 8. The amount of massage lubricant is determined by the intent of the massage and the

A. dryness of the skin
B. temperature in the massage room
C. type of massage lubricant
D. A and C

_______ 9. The ideal massage room temperature is between

A. 60° and 70°F
B. 70° and 80°F
C. 78° and 85°F
D. 68° and 75°F

_______ 10. The most popular table style is

A. a portable massage table
B. a stationary massage table
C. an electric massage table
D. a hydraulic massage table

References

McClure, Vimala Scheider. *Infant Massage Instructor Handbook.* Self-published manuscript. 1997.

Tisserard, Robert. *The Art of Aromatherapy Handbook.* Healing Arts Press, 1977.

UNIT TWO

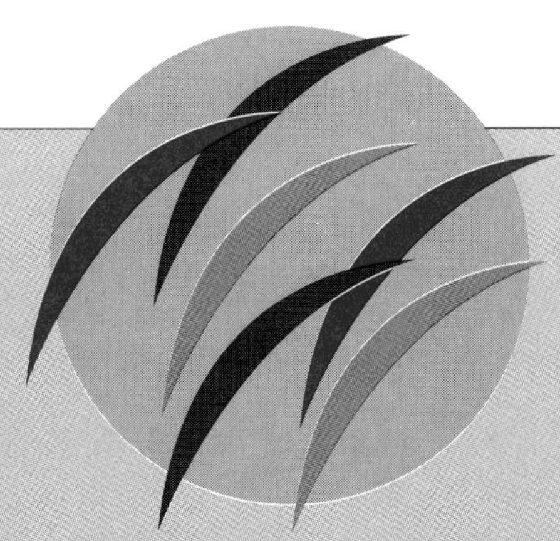

Anatomy and Physiology for the Massage Therapist

When health is absent . . .
Wisdom cannot reveal itself
Art cannot become manifest
Strength cannot be exerted
Wealth is useless and
Reason is powerless. . . .
—*Heraphilies, 300 B.C.*

4

Introduction to the Human Body: Cells, Tissues, and the Body Compass

Student Objectives

After completing this chapter, the student should be able to:

- Define anatomy, physiology, and homeostasis
- Identify the parts of a cell and discuss their functions
- Describe passive and active cell processes
- Discuss the four basic tissue types and their individual classifications
- Explain the three types of membranes
- State ten main body systems and discuss their basic functions
- Indicate the planes of the body
- Differentiate the main body cavities and the organs contained within them
- Name the directional terminology used in anatomy and physiology. Use it to locate structures of the body
- Identify the anterior and posterior body landmarks

INTRODUCTION

You are about to embark on an unforgettable journey—a new path of self-discovery—into your own interiors. But first you have to learn some new language and definitions. The basic anatomical terminology is crucial to your understanding of the anatomy that follows, and, to be an effective massage therapist, a thorough knowledge of this material is essential.

A clear visual picture of the many possible arrangements of cells and tissues will help you truly feel what is beneath your hands. As massage therapists, you will be manipulating and comparing many types of tissues. You will be compressing and stretching fascia (connective tissue), kneading gluteus maximus (muscle tissue), chucking metacarpals (connective tissue), and feathering the epidermis (epithelial tissue). Remember, all these terms will be reinforced many times during your studies. This is only the beginning, an initial step through the door.

Anatomy and physiology are inseparable. Structure is determined by function and function is carried out through structure. Another way of looking at this concept is that "form follows function." For example, consider the form (or structure) of the lungs, thin-tissued paired organs with no muscle tissue present in their linings. Lung tissue is best suited for gas exchange. What organ (structure), with its thick, muscular walls, is suited for pumping fluids (function)? You are right—the heart!

Our bodies are all physiological masterpieces. As you read this, your heart is pumping blood, your lungs are moving air, your pupils are adjusting to reading conditions, and your nerves are monitoring both the internal and external environments. These processes occur within us at every moment. During your study of anatomy and physiology, these many wonders will be revealed. The philosopher Plato once noted that the "acquiring of knowledge is just a form of recollection." Learning anatomy and physiology is just becoming aware of what you already are.

This chapter is designed to serve as a reference as you continue your studies in anatomy and physiology. Here you'll learn about cells, tissues, and their membranes (thin sheets of tissue) and will be introduced to the organ systems. Also, you will learn terms used to negotiate your way around the body. This reference for directional terminology, structural landmarks, and body cavities is known as the *body compass.*

INTRODUCTION TO ANATOMY AND PHYSIOLOGY

There are two ways to approach the study of the human body: *regionally* and *systemically.* The regional approach is typically used in medical schools, especially in laboratory classes. In the cadaver lab, the student learns the regional structures of the body such as the arm, leg, and chest as well as the skin's many underlying structures. The most common approach for anatomy and physiology study in a lecture setting is the systemic approach, in which each body system is explored individually. This approach will be used in the following chapters to explore nine of the ten body systems. In a different manner, the regional approach will be used in Chapters 7 and 9 to cover skeletal and muscular nomenclature. A laboratory class format is the best way to approach the information presented in these two chapters. Both approaches are valid, and although we can look at each system individually or by region, it is important to remember that the body functions as an interrelated whole and that all the systems balance and support one another.

Almost everyone has some understanding of basic anatomy and physiology, if not from prior education classes then from practical experience of one's own body. As we begin our study, it is important to get a good definition of anatomical terms based upon the medical model so that everyone speaks a common language. **Anatomy** is the study of the structures of the human body and their positional relationship to one another (the head bone is connected to the neck bone, and so on). There are two divisions of human anatomy, *gross* and *microscopic.*

Gross anatomy (macroscopic) is the study of larger body *structures,* such as bones, muscle, nerves, blood vessels, visceral organs, and glands. **Microscopic anatomy** is the study of the smaller structures of the body, such as cells and tissues, that make up the larger structures (cellular tissues can best be seen through a microscope). **Physiology** is the study of how the whole body and its individual parts *function* in normal body processes. Anatomy is always related to physiology because form follows function. If you want something to work a certain way (physiology), you must work on design (anatomy).

Homeostasis is a relatively stable condition of the body's internal environment within a very limited range. Even when the outside conditions change, the body's internal environment is relatively constant. Homeostasis is maintained by adjusting the *metabolism* of

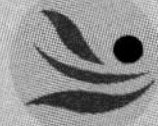

MINI•LAB

In small groups or as a class, discuss the concept of "alive." Use a board or overhead projector to list all the ideas that accumulate. As you will discover, the concept of being alive is a very complex set of ideas.

the body. **Metabolism** is the total of all the physical and chemical processes that occur in a given organism (i.e., those that are considered to be signs of life). To maintain homeostasis the body adjusts several different metabolic functions, including heart rate, blood pressure, respiratory rate, growth, body temperature, hormone production, glandular secretions, energy generation and consumption, the digestion and absorption of food, and the elimination of wastes.

The human body can be thought of as a universe, made up of very small parts organized to function as a unit. These smaller structures can be divided into six basic levels: chemical, cellular, tissue, organ, organ system, and organism levels. The chemical level encompasses the biochemistry of our body. The cellular level deals primarily with cells, which are the smallest basic living units of the body. Cells are composed of chemicals from the chemical level and can perform all the functions vital to life. The tissue level is composed of groups of cells that perform a specific function. There are four basic kinds of tissues, each possessing its own unique properties. The organ level is composed of two or more specialized groups of tissue that have one or more specific functions, for example, the stomach, liver, and the brain. Related organs with complementary functions arrange themselves into organ systems that can perform certain necessary tasks, such as respiration and digestion. The organism level is the highest level of organization. All of our organ systems work together to promote life: The total of all structures and functions is a living individual.

Think of these levels like the building materials of a house. The cells are similar to the individual parts, such as nails, studs, tiles, bricks, and mortar. These materials are put together to make walls, floors, and ceilings, which correspond to the tissues of the body. Then put tissues together, and you get a room, which is similar to an organ. Several rooms may function as an organ system; the bedrooms might constitute one organ system, while the bathrooms and kitchen consti-

Biological Prefixes

a-, an- lacking, without, not – atypical
ab- away from, absent, decrease – abduct
ad- toward, near to, increase – adduct
ante- front, before, toward – anterior
anti- against; opposed – antifungal
auto- self – autoimmune
bi-, di- twice, double, two – bifocal, diencephalon
bi- also means "life" – biology
cephal- head – cephalitis
contra- opposite, against – contraindication
cryo- extreme cold – cryotherapy
cyto- cell – cytoplasm
de- separate, away from, down – decapitate
dia- through – diaphragm
dis- apart, away – dislocation
dys- difficult, bad, labored – dysfunction
ecto-, exo-, ex- on the outer side – ectoplasm
endo-, em-, en- within, inside – endometrium
epi- upon, over, in addition to – epidermis
eu- good, well, normal – euphoria
glu-, gly- sugar, sweet – glucose
histo- tissue – histology
hydro- water or hydrogen – hydromassage
hyper- over, above, excessive – hypertrophy
hypo- under, below, deficient – hypodermic
hyster- uterus, womb – hysterectomy
infra- under, below, beneath – infraspinatus
inter- between, together, midst – intercondylar
intra- within – intravenous
mastoid- breast-shaped or nipple-like – mastectomy
meta- beyond, after, change, transformation – metacarpals
mono- one, single – mononuclear
narco- sleep, numbness, stupor – narcolepsy
necro- death – necrosis
ophthalmo- eye – ophthalmologist
ot- ear – otitis
para- by the side of, alongside, beside – parasympathetic
patho- disease – pathophysiology
ped- foot – pedicure
peri- around, about – periosteum
post- rear, after, behind – posterior
pre-, pro- before, front – prenatal, protuberance
re- again, back – realign
recto- straight – rectum
retro- backward – retroperitoneal
sub- under, beneath, below – subscapular
super-, supra- above, over – superficial, supraspinatus
syn-, sym- together, with, joined – synarthrotic, symbiotic
therm- heat – thermotherapy
trans- across, over, beyond, through – transverse
tri- three – triceps

Biological Suffixes

algia- pain – fibromyalgia
ate- use, action – articulate
blast- germ cell or bud – blastocyte
clast- to break – osteoclast
cyte- cell – hemocyte
ectomy- excision or to cut out – tonsillectomy
emia- blood condition – hyperemia
ia, osis, ism- state or condition – anemia, cyanosis, embolism
iatry- healing – psychiatry
itis- inflammation – arthritis
oid- shaped – rhomboid
ology- study of – urology
osis- condition – lordosis
otomy- incision or to cut into – colostomy
pathy- disease – neuropathy
scopy- to view or examine – orthoscopy
stasis- control, stopping – homeostasis
trophy- nourishment, to grow, development – atrophy

tute another. These systems are all linked together into one home, which is akin to the organism level. To understand the body, we will examine the smallest components first as we proceed to the organism level. Let's take a look at our cellular level.

THE CELL

In the late 1600s, Robert Hooke was examining plant tissue samples through a primitive microscope. He identified structures that reminded him of the long rows of cell rooms in a monastery: he named these cubelike biological structures cells. The **cell** is the fundamental unit of all living organisms and is the simplest form of life that can exist as a self-sustaining unit. Cells are the building blocks of the human body (Fig. 4–1).

Scientists estimate that there are between 75 and 100 trillion active, living cells in the body. Cells consist of four elements: carbon, oxygen, hydrogen, and nitrogen, plus trace elements such as iron, sodium, and potassium. These trace elements are very important for certain cellular functions: Calcium is needed for blood clotting (among other things); iron is necessary to make hemoglobin, which carries oxygen in the blood; and iodine is needed to make thyroid hormone, which controls metabolism. Besides the four primary elements, water makes up about 60 to 80 percent of all cells.

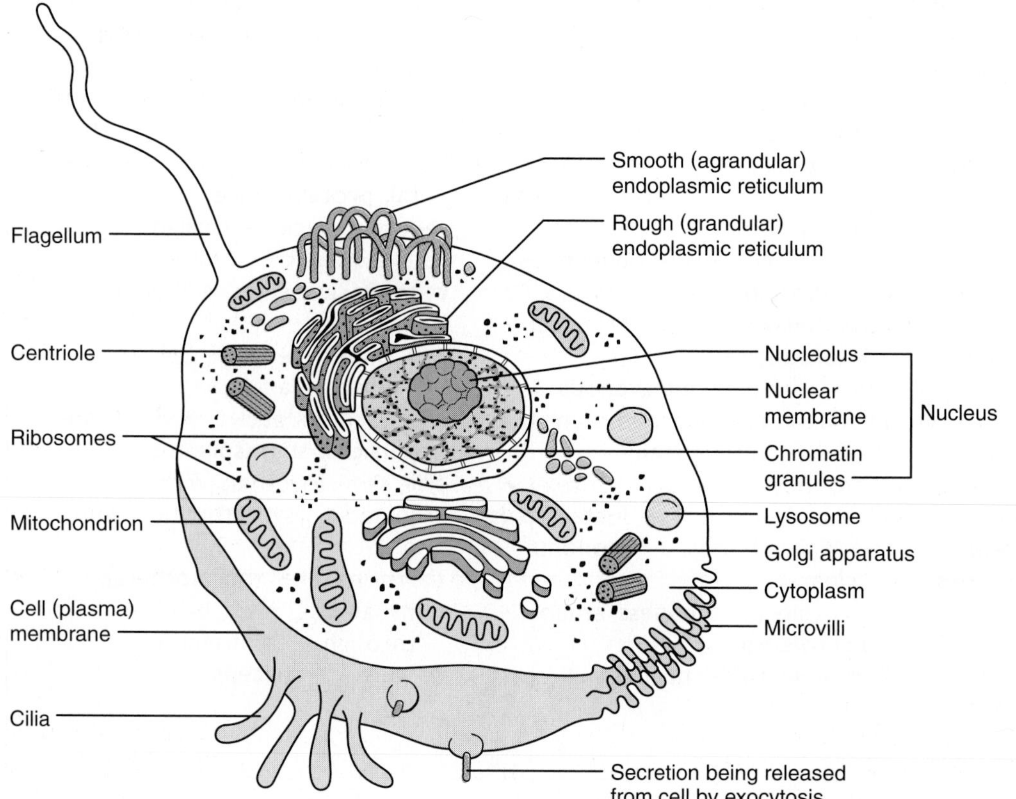

Figure 4•1 A cell.

The basic components of a cell are the cytoplasm, nucleus, nucleolus, and the cytoplasmic organelles (i.e., mitochondria, ribosomes, endoplasmic reticulum, Golgi apparatus, lysosomes, centrioles). The entire cell is surrounded by a cell membrane. The specialized nature of bodily tissues reflects the specialized function of their cellular makeup.

Cell Membrane

The **cell (plasma) membrane** separates the cytoplasm (intracellular) from the surrounding external environment (extracellular). The membrane creates a semipermeable boundary (some materials can freely pass and others cannot) that governs exchange of nutrients and waste materials and that responds to stimulation. The cell membrane is a gatekeeper; once your identification is checked, you may or may not be allowed passage. The cellular membrane often contains projections such as *microvilli, cilia,* or *flagella,* which help protect the cell and aid in mobility.

Cytoplasm

Consisting primarily of water, **cytoplasm** is the gel-like intracellular fluid within the boundaries of the cell membrane. Within the cytoplasm are many small cellular structures called *organelles,* which provide special functions. Most cellular metabolism occurs within the cytoplasm.

Within the cell are **cytoplasmic organelles,** which are necessary for metabolism. Each organelle possesses a distinct structure and function within the cell. Some function in reproduction, some store materials, and some metabolize nutrients. Types of organelles are the nucleus, ribosomes, endoplasmic reticulum, Golgi apparatus, mitochondria, lysosomes, and centrioles.

Nucleus

The **nucleus,** the largest organelle in the cytoplasm, is the control center of the cell, directing nearly all metabolic activities. All cells have at least one nucleus at some time in their existence. Red blood cells lose their nuclei (enucleate) as they mature, and skeletal muscle cells possess many nuclei (multinucleated). The shape of the nucleus is usually spherical and it is enclosed in a double-layer nuclear membrane. Within this membrane are pores that allow molecules of ribonucleic acid or RNA to pass from the nucleus to the cytoplasm.

Each nucleus consists of **nucleoli,** which are clusters of protein, DNA and RNA, and chromatin. **Chromatin** is a threadlike mass of chromosomes (genetic material arranged in a specific order) in a nondividing cell. Humans possess 23 pairs of chromosomes, although abnormalities can exist. The nucleolus does not contain an enclosing membrane, and the number of nucleoli within the nucleus varies from one to four.

Ribosomes

Ribosomes are small granules of RNA and protein in the cytoplasm. They function to synthesize protein for use within the cell and also produce other proteins that are exported outside the cell.

Endoplasmic Reticulum

A complex network of membranous channels within the cytoplasm is the **endoplasmic reticulum.** This structure frequently extends from the cell membrane to the nuclear membrane and may extend to certain organelles. The endoplasmic reticulum functions in the synthesis of protein and lipids and assists the transportation of these materials from one part of the cell to another. Endoplasmic reticula are classified as rough or granular (ribosomes attached to the surface) or as smooth or agranular (ribosomes are absent).

Golgi Apparatus

The **Golgi apparatus (Golgi complex)** is a series of four to six horizontal membranous sacs typically located near the nucleus and attached to the endoplasmic reticulum. Referred to as the "packing and shipping" plant of the cell, the Golgi apparatus is associated with altering proteins and lipids (from the endoplasmic reticulum) to enhance their properties. Once this process is complete, they are wrapped in a piece of Golgi apparatus membrane and jettisoned to become secretory vesicles (saccules). These vesicles find their way to the cell wall and release their contents into the extracellular spaces.

Mitochondria

An oval organelle, the **mitochondrion,** lies within the cytoplasm and is considered the cell's "power plant" because it is a site for cellular respiration, which provides most of a cell's adenosine triphosphate (ATP), which is the energy molecule of organisms. Mitochondria consist of an inner and outer membrane; the outer shell is smooth and the inner, convoluted one contains many projections called *cristae.* These chambers increase the surface area to enhance the mitochondrion's metabolic properties. Mitochondria contain their own DNA and are self-replicating.

Lysosomes

Membrane-bound organelles containing various digestive enzymes are the **lysosomes.** These digestive enzymes, which have been altered by the Golgi apparatus, function in both intracellular and extracellular digestive processes. Functioning within the cell, lysosomes can engulf bacteria, cellular debris, and other organelles and digest them, after which any reusable matter is returned to the cytosol for reuse. The lysosome can also cause self-digestion of the cell when the reduction of cells in an organ is needed, such as reduction in the size of the uterus following childbirth. In extracellular functions, the lysosomes release their digestive enzymes at injury sites to help dispose of cellular debris. Most abundant in liver and kidney cells, lysosome enzymes also help to protect the cell by destroying invading bacteria.

Centrioles

Contained within the **centrosomes** (dense areas located near the nucleus), **centrioles** are rod-shaped paired structures. These structures, which appear as tiny cylinders positioned at right angles to each other, are associated with cell division.

PASSIVE AND ACTIVE CELL PROCESSES

In order for a cell to survive, it must be able to carry on a variety of functions. In a majority of these processes, substances are exchanged across the cell membrane, which allows for the assimilation of oxygen, nutrients, and water, the elimination of pathogens, and the excretion of waste products. These processes can be classified as *passive* or *active processes.* The passive processes occur naturally by means of gradients of temperature, pressure, or concentration. It is the *gradient* or *difference in levels* of temperature, pressure, or concentration that drives the exchange of particles or fluid through the membrane. Involving no active expending of energy by the cells, passive cell processes include diffusion, osmosis, and filtration.

Active processes are those that require an expenditure of energy (ATP) by the cell itself to transport the products across the membrane. Active processes include active transport and endocytosis.

Passive Processes

Simple and Facilitated Diffusion

The process of diffusion involves the movement of solutions, which are solid particles dissolved in a liquid medium. Dissolved particles may be atoms, ions, or entire molecules. **Diffusion** is the movement of dissolved substances from a region of higher concentration to a region of lower concentration. This action, which requires no expenditure of cellular energy or ATP, will continue until the strength of the solution is equal in all areas (Fig. 4–2).

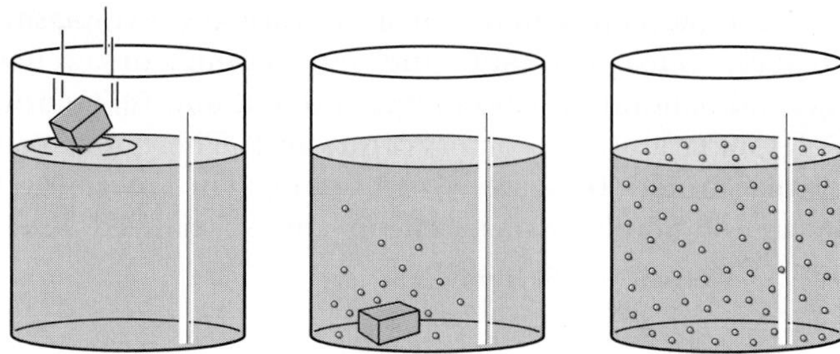

Figure 4•2 Simple diffusion.

Diffusion can be easily demonstrated by filling a long baking pan with cool water and setting it somewhere where there is no vibration or movement to disturb the pan. Open a packet of colored soft drink mix (i.e., Kool-Aid) and gently sprinkle the powder in one corner of the pan. Even though there are no true currents in the pan, the colored powder will diffuse across the pan.

This same process can occur on a cellular level, and diffusion may even occur through the cell membrane, which is semipermeable (semipermeable refers to the ability of a membrane to allow passage of some substances and to exclude passage of others). Simple diffusion involves the movement of dissolved substances. When the kinetic energy, or speed, of the particles is increased (by raising the temperature, for example), the rate of the diffusion process increases as well. The diffusion process is directly proportional to heat, pressure, and the concentration gradient. Simply put, as heat, pressure, and the concentration gradient increase, so does the rate of diffusion. The concentration gradient is the difference in concentration of two solutions. The greater the difference, the higher the gradient, and the faster the rate of diffusion. Try the Kool-Aid experiment with a pan of hot water and see how the rate of the diffusion process increases.

Facilitated diffusion is a special type of diffusion that uses a *carrier molecule* of protein to facilitate the diffusion process. Carrier molecules are contained in the cell membrane. Sometimes there are molecules in solution that are too large to cross the cell membrane. When the solution outside the cell membrane has a high concentration of large molecules, the carrier molecules contained in the cell membrane assist the large molecules in crossing the membrane. Facilitated diffusion is limited by the number of available carrier molecules.

Filtration

Filtration is the movement of particles across the cellular membrane due to pressure. A pressure gradient across a cell membrane is the force that drives the filtration process. The air filter on your furnace or central air unit is a good example. The vacuum created by the suction of the fan lowers the pressure behind the filter. The atmospheric pressure in the room is then greater than that behind the filter. The air flows through the pores of the filter, which is selective and traps the larger particles of dust, pet hair, and smoke.

Osmosis

Unlike filtration, **osmosis** does *not* depend upon pressure, but rather upon the concentration of dissolved elements that lie in the solutions on each side of the cell membrane. When the solutions contain particles that are too large to cross the membrane, diffusion cannot occur. Even though a cell membrane does not permit the solution to pass through its walls, the solvent fluid is still able to permeate the membrane. The fluid from the less concentrated solution (usually water) moves across the cell membrane. Osmotic movement of water is always from the lowest concentration (most dilute) to the highest concentration (least dilute). This action continues until the two concentrations equalize.

Active Processes

Active Transport

Active transport moves important atoms and molecules such as ions against the concentration gradient from low levels to high levels in order to maintain such vital processes as nerve conduction. The mechanisms of active transport are both chemical and physical. The chemical part of the mechanism involves the breakdown of ATP within the cell. Scientists estimate that at least 40 percent of the ATP in the human body is used solely for active transport.

An ion is attracted to a protein molecule, which is part of the cellular membrane. The outside wall of the protein molecule opens like a clamshell, and the ion is drawn inside and binds to it. The binding causes the chemical breakdown of ATP, which again transforms the shape of a protein molecule. The clamshell closes; then the opposite side of the protein molecule opens again to release the ion to the inside of the cell membrane. This process is much like an air lock, in that only one door can be open at a time.

Endocytosis

Endocytosis is a process that moves large particles across the cell membrane into the cell. The two main types of endocytosis are *phagocytosis* and *pinocytosis,* both of which are vital to the immune defense systems of the body.

Phagocytosis, or "cell eating," is the process by which specialized cells engulf harmful microorganisms

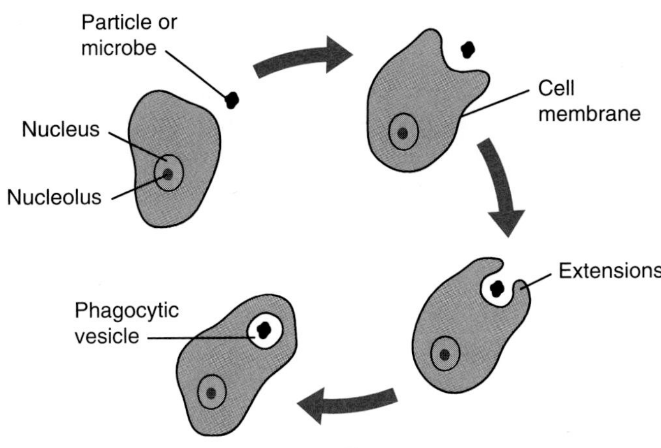

Figure 4•3 Phagocytosis.

and cellular debris, break them down, and expel the harmless remains back into the body. Phagocytosis is chiefly characteristic of leukocytes and macrophage cells found in the blood. The process has several steps. First, the leukocyte is chemically attracted toward the microbe targeted for destruction. Second, the leukocyte adheres itself to the microbe. Next, the leukocyte or macrophage forms extensions, surrounds, and ingests the microbe much like an amoeba engulfs its food. Fourth, the leukocyte produces enzymes that destroy and digest the microbe. Finally, the tiny remains are encapsulated, recycled, or expelled (Fig. 4–3).

Pinocytosis, or "cell drinking," is almost identical to phagocytosis except that the targeted object is liquid. In this process, the cell develops a saccular indention, drawing the molecule inside and then enclosing it. Pinocytic cells are more common than phagocytic cells.

Exocytosis

Exocytosis is the movement of large particles to the outside of the cell. Secretory vesicles form inside the cell and fuse with the plasma membranae, then release their contents into the extracellular fluid. Examples of exocytosis are neurons that release neurotransmitters, cells that produce and secrete digestive enzymes or hormones, and the minute materials that remain after destruction of pathogens.

EMBRYONIC CELL LAYERS: ECTODERM, MESODERM, AND ENDODERM

All tissues of the body develop from one of three cell (germ) layers, the formation of which is one of the first events of embryonic development. From superficial to deep, these are the ectoderm, mesoderm, and endoderm. As the embryo develops, these layers begin to specialize to form the four main types of tissues, from which all organs and glands are derived.

The outermost of the three cell layers is the **ectoderm,** which gives rise to the structures of the nervous system, including the special senses (e.g., ears, eyes), the mucosa of the mouth and anus, the epidermis of the skin and epidermal tissues such as fingernails, hair, and skin glands.

The middle layer is the **mesoderm**—the muscles and connective tissues of the body such as fascia, tendons, retinaculum, ligaments, cartilage, bone, mesenteries, dermis, and hypodermis. Vascular and lymphatic tissues, as well as the pleurae of the lungs, the pericardium, and peritoneum are all derived from the mesoderm.

The innermost cell layer is the **endoderm.** From this embryonic cell layer arise the lining of the alimentary canal, the lining of the respiratory passages, and all tissues of the organs and glands (e.g., lungs, urinary bladder, pancreas). Thus, the endoderm comprises the lining of the body's passages and the covering for most of the internal organs.

BODY TISSUES

Tissues are defined as a group of similar cells that act together to perform a specific function. The study of tissues is known as histology. There are only four major types of tissues in the human body: epithelial, connective, muscle, and nervous.

All four tissue types have special purposes and correspondingly have varying rates of cellular regeneration. The cells of epithelial tissue, which makes up the skin, are constantly being renewed through the process of cell division called **mitosis.** At the opposite end of the spectrum, nervous tissue regenerates very slowly, if at all. Bone tissue, muscle tissue, and the various forms of connective tissue all heal at different rates, but generally heal in direct proportion to blood supply. Bone tissue and adipose connective tissue are highly vascular and heal quickly. Muscle tissue takes a little longer to regenerate, and the less vascular forms of connective tissue, such as ligaments and tendons, are even slower. Cartilage, an avascular tissue, is among the slowest to heal.

Finally, the tissues organize into organs. Organs are defined as a group of two or more tissue types that act together to perform a specific common function and have a consistently recognizable shape. In order to understand better the structure and functions of our body's organs, it is beneficial first to study the tissues that comprise the organs.

Epithelial Tissue or Epithelium

Epithelial tissue lines or covers the internal and the external organs of the body, lines blood vessels and body cavities, and lines the digestive, respiratory, urinary, and reproductive tracts (Fig. 4–4). The functions of this tissue include protection, absorption, filtration, secretion, excretion, and diffusion. Epithelial tissue is typically avascular and receives nutrition by diffusion from blood vessels in underlying connective tissues. Epithelium reproduces and regenerates quickly.

Because epithelium lines or covers body surfaces, there is one free or exposed surface and one surface that is bound to connective tissue. The attaching surface is called a noncellular **basement membrane.** Epithelium is classified according to its shape and number of layers. Epithelium in different parts of the body is made of either squamous (flat), cuboidal (cube-shaped), or columnar (tall and narrow) cells. Simple epithelium is one layer of cells. Stratified epithelium, which is multilayered, is more durable and provides more protection than simple epithelium.

Simple Squamous Epithelium

Also called pavement epithelium, **simple squamous epithelium** is a single layer of thin, flat cells that are close together, attaching at their edges. This tissue type is well suited for cellular processes such as diffusion and filtration (e.g., alveoli of the lungs, areas of the kidney, capillary walls).

Simple Cuboidal Epithelium

A single layer of cube-shaped cells, **simple cuboidal epithelium** possesses more volume, as well as more cytoplasmic organelles, than simple squamous epithelium. This type of tissue is well suited for secretion and absorption and is found in the ovaries, kidney tubules, thyroid gland, pancreas, and salivary glands.

Simple Columnar Epithelium

Simple columnar epithelium is a single layer of cells that is taller than wide, in which the nuclei are located toward the bottom portion of the epithelial cell (near the basement membrane). This tissue offers some protection to underlying structures and is found in stomach and intestines. The free surface typically possesses tiny projections called **microvilli** (to increase surface area) or **cilia** (to move secretions along the free surface).

Pseudostratified Columnar Epithelium

Pseudostratified columnar epithelium has the appearance of being stratified, but it is actually a single layer of tissue. The cells possess different heights, and not all cells reach the free surface. This type of epithelium is found in portions of the respiratory tract and the male reproductive tract.

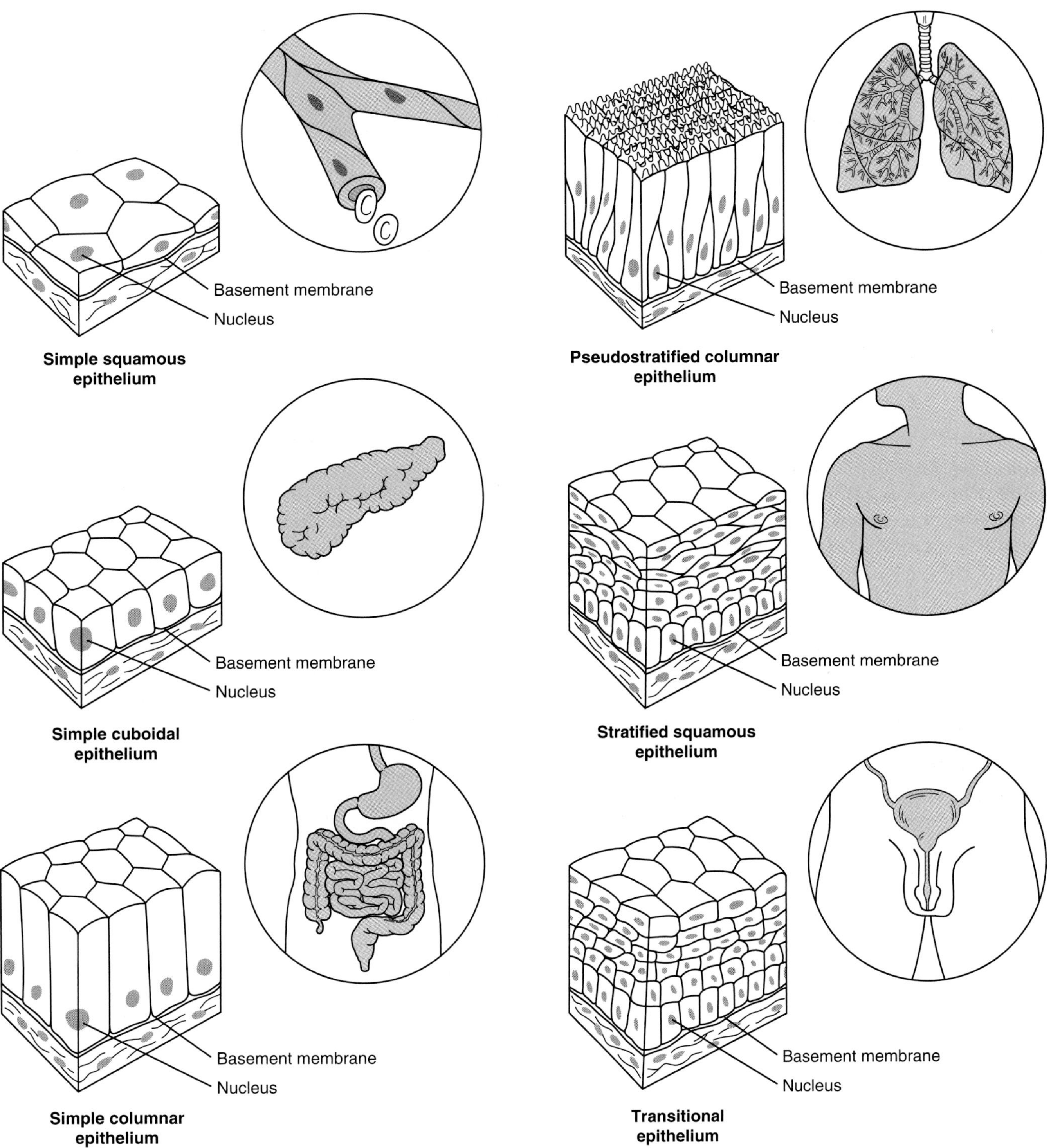

Figure 4•4 Types of epithelial tissue.

Stratified Squamous Epithelium

The most common epithelium, **stratified squamous epithelium,** is packed closely together, is arranged in layers over the external surface of the body (e.g., skin), and lines most of the hollow structures (e.g., oral cavity). Cells in the lower layers undergo cell division and are soon pushed toward the free surface. As the cells approach the exterior, they become thinner, die, and are sloughed off.

Transitional Epithelium

Transitional epithelium is stratified but can stretch in response to pressure. The appearance of transitional epithelium varies depending on whether it is relaxed or expanded. When relaxed, it is columnar-shaped, but as pressure is applied, it changes to cuboidal-, and finally to squamous-shaped. This alteration in shape allows distention and prevents the organs supplied by transitional epithelium from rupturing; this tissue type is found in the urinary bladder.

Glandular Epithelium

A specialized type of epithelium, **glandular epithelium,** produces and secretes substances the body needs. These tissue cells lie below the surface of a gland, usually in clusters, and secrete their products either into ducts (exocrine glands) or directly into the bloodstream (endocrine glands).

Connective Tissue

Connective tissue is the most abundant and ubiquitous tissue of the body. This tissue serves a wide variety of functions. Some connective tissue types serve as nutrient transport systems, some defend the body against disease, some possess clotting mechanisms, and others act as a supportive framework and provide protection for vital organs. It is important to remember that all of the following connective tissue structures are interconnected and that all participate in a connective tissue network (Fig. 4–5).

Connective tissues are composed of cells and matrix. The cells do not generally touch each other like the epithelial tissues, but are separated from each other by the matrix. Made up of ground substance and fibers, the matrix may be liquid, fibrous, gelatinous, or calcified and is secreted by the cells of the connective tissue.

Most types of connective tissue are well vascularized; some are not. There are five different classifications of connective tissue, some of which contain more than one division or type of tissue: liquid connective tissue (blood), bone or osseous tissue, cartilaginous tissue, loose connective tissue, and dense connective tissue.

Liquid Connective Tissue

Also known as hemopoietic or vascular tissue, **liquid connective tissue** consists of blood. Blood contains three formed elements, two of which are cells (erythrocytes or red blood cells and leukocytes or white blood cells) and one of which are cell fragments (thrombocytes or platelets). The fluid medium in which these elements exist is called plasma. Blood aids in transportation and immunity.

Bone

The hardest and most solid of all connective tissue, **bone** (osseous tissue) consists of compact tissue, a spongy cancellous tissue, collagenous fibers (for strength), and mineral salts (for hardness). Bone is infused with many blood vessels and nerves through a membranous sheath surrounding the bone called the *periosteum.*

Cartilaginous Tissue

Cartilage is an avascular, tough, protective tissue capable of withstanding repeated stress. Cartilage is the slowest tissue to heal because it has no direct blood supply. Cartilage is typically found in the thorax, the joints, and certain rigid tubes of the body (e.g., trachea). Cartilaginous tissue can be divided into three subcategories: hyaline cartilage, fibrocartilage, and elastic cartilage.

Hyaline cartilage (gristle) is an elastic, rubbery, smooth type of cartilage that covers the ends of bones (epiphysis), connects the ribs to the sternum (costal cartilage), is part of the larynx and the nose, and forms the C-shaped rings of the trachea. The skeleton of a fetus is mostly hyaline, which is replaced by osseous tissue by the time the baby is born (except for the fontanels or “soft spots” on the baby’s head).

Fibrocartilage has the greatest tensile strength of all three cartilage types. It is found in the intervertebral disks, in the meniscus of the knee joint, and between the pubic bones (pubic symphysis).

Elastic cartilage is soft and more pliable than hyaline or fibrocartilage and gives shape to the external nose and ears and to internal structures, such as the epiglottis and the auditory tubes.

Loose Connective Tissue

Loose connective tissue is regarded as the packing material of the body. It attaches the skin to underlying structures, serves to wrap and support the body cells, fills in the spaces between structures (i.e., organs, muscles), and helps to keep them in their proper places. In general, loose connective tissue is pliable and consists of a loose network of elastic and collagenous fibers, interspersed with many cells. Loose connective tissue is extremely vascular and as such heals quickly. There are three types of loose connective tissue.

Areolar connective tissue is one of the most widely distributed. It has several types of cells: macrophages, fibroblasts, mast cells, plasma cells, adipocytes, and a few white blood cells. Along with adipose tissue, areolar connective tissue forms the hypodermis (superficial fascia). This layer of tissue attaches the skin to the underlying tissues and structures.

Adipose tissue is specialized for fat storage. This connective tissue also insulates the body against heat loss, provides fuel reserves for energy, and provides a cushion around certain structures (e.g., heart, kidneys, and some joints). Cells of adipose tissue are called *adipocytes.*

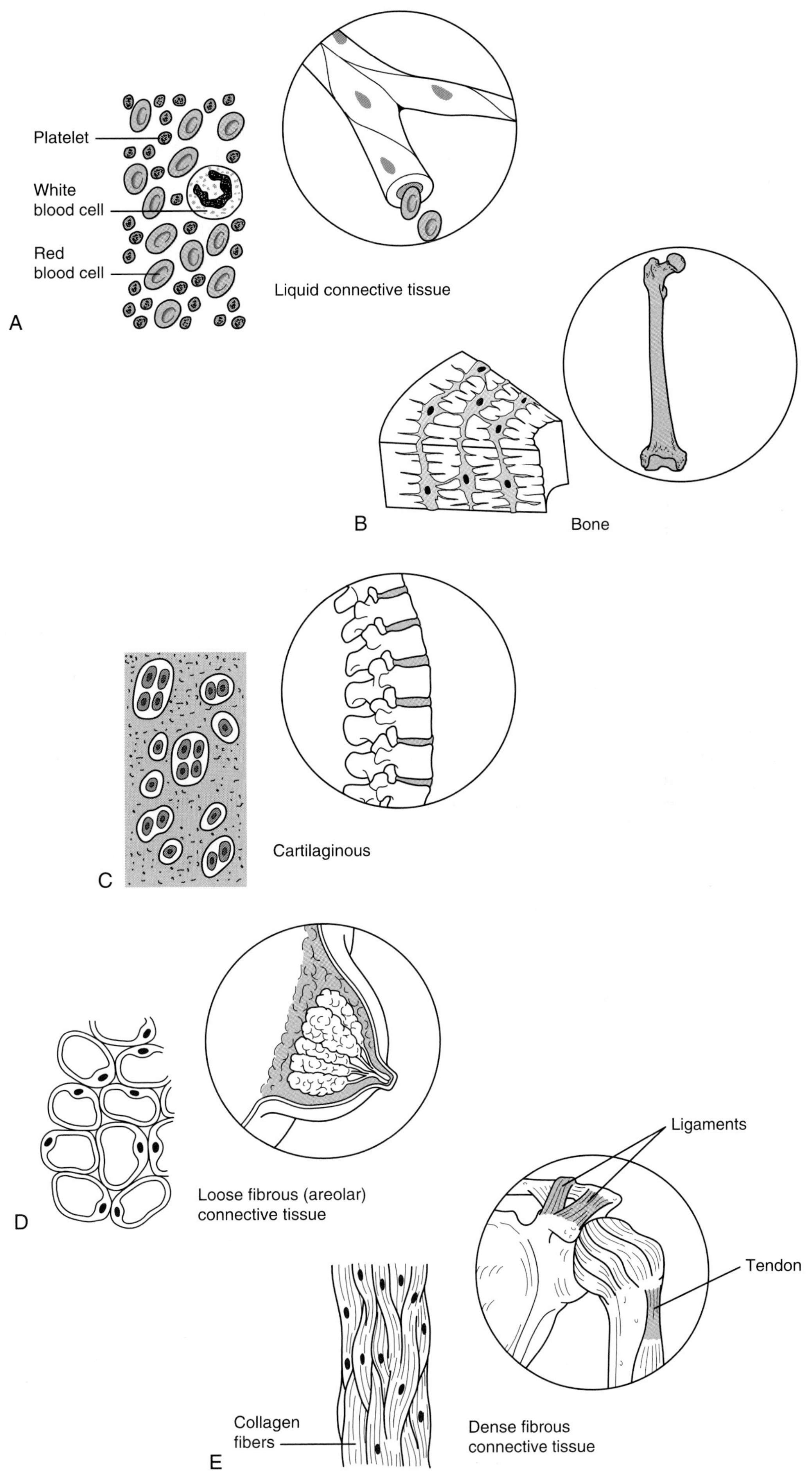

Figure 4•5 Types of connective tissue.

Reticular connective tissue forms the framework of certain organs as well as providing support.

Dense Connective Tissue

Dense fibrous connective tissue consists of densely packed, strong collagenous fibers with fewer cells than loose connective tissue. This tissue type is not very vascular, so is slow to heal. There are three types of dense connective tissue.

Dense regular connective tissue has bundles of collagen fibers in an orderly parallel arrangement that gives great strength and can resist pulling forces in one direction.

Elastic connective tissue has an abundance of elastic fibers, which allows it to be stretched and restored to its natural shape. It is found in vocal cords and in the ligaments connecting adjacent vertebrae.

Dense irregular connective tissue has collagen fibers that are ordinarily irregularly arranged. It can resist pulling forces in several different directions. The following are examples of dense irregular connective tissue.

1. *Tendons*—fibrous bands of tissue that attach muscle to bone
2. *Aponeurosis*—a thin strong sheet of fibrous connective tissue that serves as a tendon connecting muscle to muscle or muscle to bone
3. *Ligaments*—white, shiny bands of fibrous tissue binding bones together across joints
4. *Dermis*—the deeper layer of the skin below the epidermis
5. *Periosteum*—a dense, fibrous, vascular connective tissue sheath around the bone, except at the ends of the bone
6. *Deep fascia*—lines the body wall and limbs and holds muscles together and separates them into muscle groups. Fascia is of extreme importance to the massage therapist because it is often thought of as an organ of structure. Like muscle, fascia can develop tight bands of fibers, restrict normal movement, and harbor trigger points.

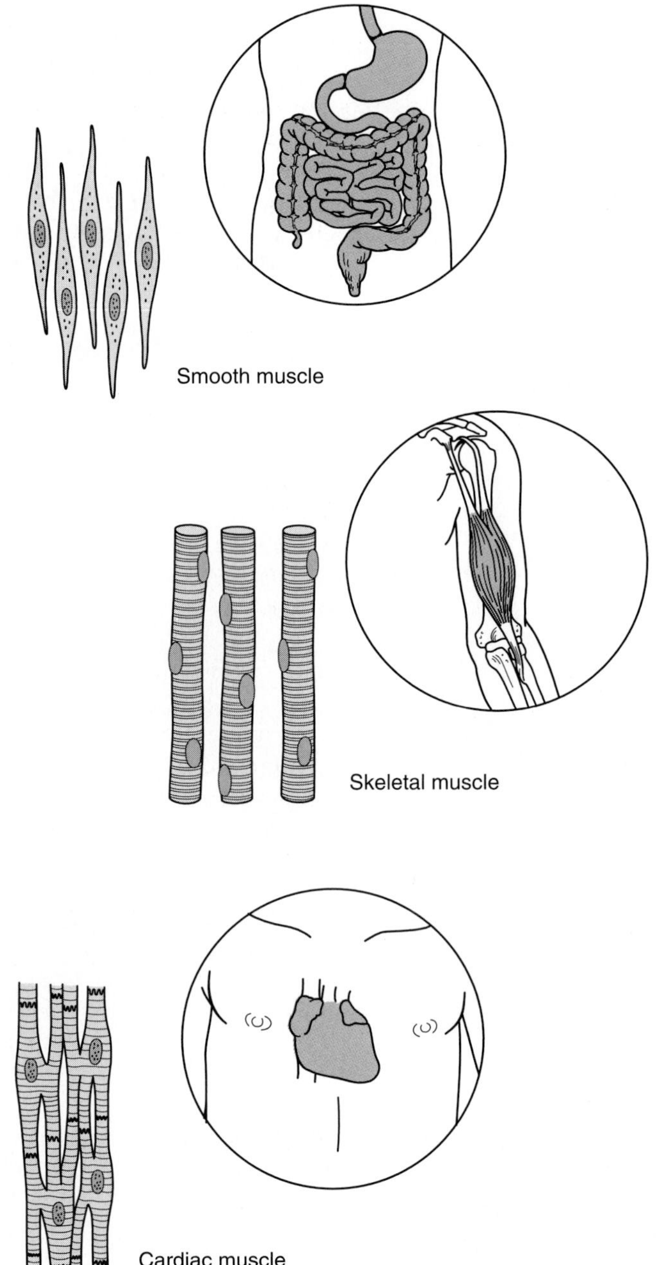

Figure 4•6 Types of muscle tissue.

Muscle Tissue

Extremely elastic, **muscle tissue** is very vascular and has the unique ability to shorten (contract) and to elongate to produce movement. Because of their shape, muscle tissues are made up of muscle fibers and are usually arranged in bundles surrounded by connective tissue called fascia. The three types of muscle tissue are skeletal, smooth, and cardiac (Fig. 4–6.) Generally speaking, skeletal muscle causes bones to articulate (move), smooth muscle causes the contents of a tube to move, and cardiac muscle causes the heart to contract, forcing blood to move.

Stimulated by a nerve impulse to contract, *skeletal muscle* (voluntary and striated) attaches to bones via their membranes and to fascia and other muscles. These muscle fibers are cigar-shaped and are multinucleated; many nuclei are located near the periphery of the cell. Each skeletal muscle fiber contains bands of red and white material, causing it to appear striped or striated under a microscope.

Smooth muscle (involuntary muscle or visceral muscle) forms the walls of hollow organs and tubes, such as the stomach, bladder, uterus, and blood vessels. Consuming very little energy, these muscle cells are adapted for long, sustained contractions. The muscle cells are spindle-shaped (pointed at both ends) and each contains one oval nucleus.

Cardiac muscle is located in the heart wall (myocardium) and is shaped like the letters "Y" or "H." These shapes allow the cells to fit together like clasped fingers and help create the spherical shape of the heart. Cardiac muscle is said to be striated because of its alternating light and dark bands. Between each cardiac muscle cell is a structure known as the intercalated disk. These disks assist in the transmission of a stimulus from cell to cell.

Nervous Tissue

Nervous tissue consists of oddly shaped cells called neurons, which can pick up and transmit electrical signals by converting stimuli into nerve impulses. Located in the brain, spinal cord, and peripheral nerves, nervous tissue possesses characteristics of excitability and conductability. Neurons detect changes both inside and outside the body, interpret the perceived information to provide a response (e.g., muscular contractions or glandular secretions), and are involved in higher mental functioning and emotional responsiveness.

The three principal parts of a neuron are the cell body (containing the nucleus and other standard cell machinery), the dendrites (which transmit impulses to the cell body), and the axon (which transmits impulses away from the cell body).

Neuroglial (glial) cells are connective tissue that supports, nourishes, protects, and organizes the delicate neurons. These cells are smaller than neurons and are unable to transmit impulses (Fig. 4–7).

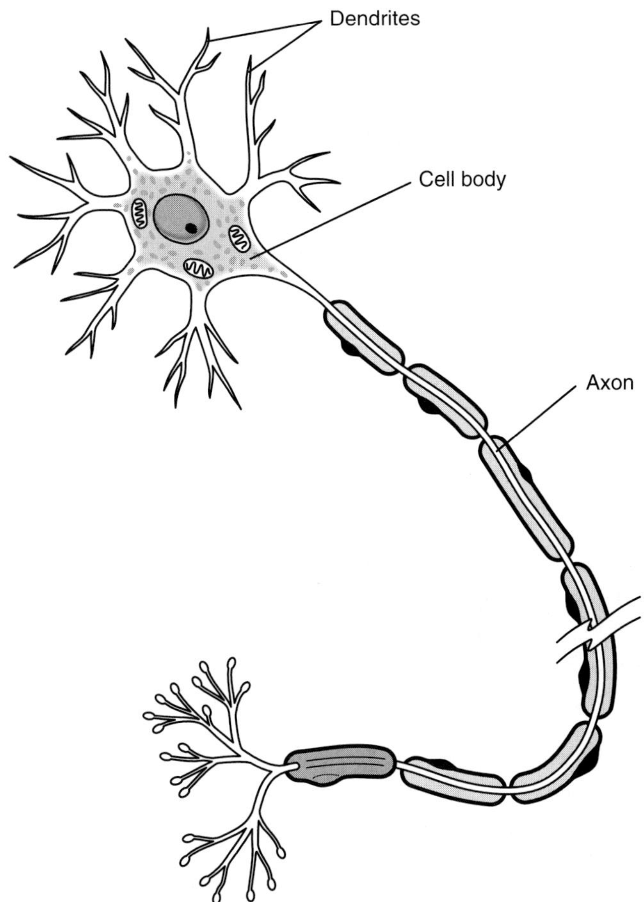

Figure 4•7 A nerve cell.

Tissue Repair

Tissue healing consists of a series of processes that restore traumatized tissue to its near-original health. There are three physiological phases in the healing process, which follows trauma to the tissue: The first is *inflammation,* a bodily defense mechanism to stabilize the traumatized area; the second is *regeneration,* in which the actual tissue repair takes place; last is *remodeling,* a phase of scar tissue maturation.

Inflammation

Inflammation, one of the body's reactions to soft tissue injury, is a protective mechanism, and its purpose is to stabilize and prepare the damaged tissue for repair. It occurs in response to trauma from physical injury, burns, chemical irritation, and invasion by viruses and bacteria. The intensity of the inflammation is directly proportional to the extent of the trauma to the tissue. The primary symptoms of inflammation are local *heat, swelling, redness, pain,* and *decreased function.* When tissue trauma occurs, the body reacts by releasing histamine and kinins. These chemicals cause vasodilation at the site of the trauma and increase the permeability of the capillary walls. Vasodilation increases local blood circulation; thus, there is an increase in heat and redness. The changes in the capillary walls allow blood plasma to cross into the interstitial fluid of the tissue cells; this excess fluid results in swelling. As the tissue pressure increases, the nociceptors fire, resulting in the symptom of pain. The sensation of pain, combined with the swelling, limits the range of motion.

As the plasma fills the tissue, several things happen. Phagocytes and white blood cells are attracted to the trauma site. The phagocytes engulf damaged cellular debris, foreign objects, and any hostile invaders. The plasma cleanses the area with its flushing action and dilutes any toxic substances in the trauma site. Clotting proteins construct a clot that seals any break in the skin and form walls within torn tissues to isolate the wound.

Regeneration

Regeneration, which follows the cleanup of the trauma site, is the process by which the traumatized tissue is repaired or rebuilt. This process can occur in a variety of ways, depending upon the type of tissue and the severity of the trauma.

One of these methods is *resolution,* which is a normal replacement of damaged tissue when the trauma is mild and when the tissue has the ability to replicate itself by mitosis. The replacement of skin after a mild sunburn is an example of tissue repair by resolution.

Regeneration occurs when damaged tissue is replaced with new tissue of the same type. Again, the tissue has to be able to reproduce itself; however, damage can be more severe. A fall that produces a skinned knee or elbow is a good example of regeneration. The open wound becomes sealed with a scab, and the surrounding healthy epithelial cells divide until the skin beneath the scab has been reproduced completely. At this point the scab is sloughed off.

The last type of tissue repair is **fibrosis (scar formation),** which replaces the original tissue type with a different kind of tissue. Fibrosis occurs when the damage is so severe that there are not enough healthy cells to reproduce the tissue required or when the damaged tissue does not have the ability to readily reproduce itself. Skeletal muscle, cardiac muscle, and central nervous system tissues do not readily regenerate and thus are generally repaired by fibrosis. The scar tissue formed by fibrosis is usually stronger than the original tissue; scarring is, in a sense, a patch. Since scar formation is not the original tissue, there is usually some loss of function.

Muscle is highly vascular tissue, and trauma to an area results in oxygen deprivation to the tissue. Restoration of oxygen is achieved by the growth of a new capillary network, a process known as *neovascularization* or *angiogenesis.* Buds form on capillaries neighboring the wound and then extend into the wound area. These buds proliferate and combine with other offshoots to create a new capillary network. As oxygen is returned to the area, fibroblasts produce collagen fibers, which become the basis of the scar. Remember that the word "scar" applies not only to a visible mark on the skin but to any place where scar tissue has formed to weave torn tissue back together. The regeneration phase is complete when enough collagen has been produced to repair the trauma site. Repair is marked by the disappearance of fibroblasts in the area.

Remodeling

The collagen fibers in the scar tissue are formed randomly and are consequently poorly organized. The scar may be bulky and soft or fibrous and tough. When fibrosis occurs, some changes must occur within the scar tissue if it is to be somewhat pliable and function efficiently. This process is call the **remodeling** or **scar maturation phase.** At this time the body is continually restructuring the scar tissue by a simultaneous destruction and creation of collagen fibers. The new fibers reorganize themselves along the axis of muscle fiber movement. What this means to massage therapists is that mobilization of a joint, contraction and relaxation of the affected muscle, and cross-fiber friction applied to the scar can aid in the restructuring process. These massage techniques increase scar pliability and strength while reducing bulk and breaking adhesions to surrounding tissue. Without any intervention from the massage therapist, tissue will heal fully, but normal muscle function may be impaired.

BODY MEMBRANES

Membranes are thin, soft, pliable sheets of tissue that cover the body, line tubes or body cavities, cover organs, and separate one part of a cavity from another. Using this definition, the skin itself can be considered a membrane and is known as the *cutaneous membrane.* An entire chapter has been devoted to the skin (integumentary chapter).

There are three basic types of membranes in the body: mucous, serous, and synovial. Mucous and serous membranes are classified as epithelial membranes; synovial is considered a connective tissue membrane.

Mucous Membrane

Membranes that line openings to the outside of the body are called **mucous membranes,** or **mucosae.** This type of membrane is found in the respiratory, digestive, reproductive, and urinary tracts. Mucous membranes secrete a viscous, slippery fluid called *mucus.* Many of these mucous membranes provide protection for underlying structures. The mucous membrane lining the digestive tract also aids in the processes of digestion and absorption.

Serous Membrane

Serous membranes line closed body cavities that do not open to the outside of the body. These membranes consist of two layers: a parietal layer, which lines the wall of body cavities, and a visceral layer, which provides an external covering to organs in body cavities. Examples of serous membranes are the pericardium (heart), the pleural membranes (lungs), the peritoneum (the abdominal organs), and the mesenteries (double folds of serous membranes that suspend or support the small and large intestines). Serous membranes secrete a thin, serous fluid between the parietal and visceral layers. This fluid lubricates organs and reduces friction between the organs in the thoracic or abdominopelvic cavities.

Synovial Membrane

Lining the joint cavities of freely moving joints (e.g., shoulder, hip, and knee) are the **synovial membranes.** These membranes secrete synovial fluid, a viscous liquid that provides nutrition and lubrication to the joint so it can move freely without undue friction. This fluid can also be contained in bursa sacs located around the joint cavity or in synovial sheaths surrounding a tendon of a muscle.

BODY SYSTEM OVERVIEW

There are ten organ or body systems discussed in this unit; all are interrelated and interdependent. Each system, except the reproductive system, will be discussed in its own chapter.

Circulatory System

Within the circulatory system are two divisions, the cardiovascular and the lymphvascular components. The anatomical structures of the circulatory system are the heart, blood and blood vessels, lymph and vessels, and lymph glands (e.g., tonsils, spleen, thymus). The functions of the circulatory system are many.

1. Transportation and distribution of respiratory gases, such as oxygen and carbon dioxide, nutrients from the digestive tract, antibodies, waste materials, and hormones from endocrine glands
2. Protection of the body from disease
3. Prevention of hemorrhage by clotting mechanisms, which prevents loss of body fluids from damaged vessels
4. Regulation of body temperature by moving heat from active muscles to the skin, where it can be dissipated through the mechanisms of perspiration and vasodilation

Skeletal System

The anatomical structures of the skeletal system are the bones, cartilage, ligaments, and joints. The functions of the skeletal system are as follows:

1. It supports the body through a bony framework.
2. It protects the body's vital organs.
3. The skeleton gives leverage through muscle attachment.
4. The bones house the mechanism of hemopoiesis, or the forming of blood cells. Producing both red and white blood cells, and platelets in the marrow of long bones.
5. Fats are stored in bone marrow to be released when needed. Osseous tissue acts as a reservoir for minerals such as calcium phosphate, calcium carbonate, phosphorus, magnesium, and sodium, which are stored and released when the body needs them.

Integumentary System

The anatomical structures of the integumentary system are the skin, hair, nails, oil glands, and sweat glands.

1. One of the primary functions of the skin is protecting the organism by acting as a physical, biological, and chemical barrier.
2. The skin has limited properties of absorption. Substances that can be absorbed by the epidermis are lipid-soluble substances, such as oxygen, carbon dioxide, fat-soluble vitamins (A, D, E, and K), steroids, resins of certain plants (poison ivy and poison oak), organic solvents (such as paint thinner, which can cause brain and kidney damage), and salts of heavy metals such as lead (Pb), mercury (Hg), and nickel (Ni).
3. The skin is considered an extension of the nervous system because it receives stimuli such as pressure, touch, pain, and temperature from the external environment and transports this information to the central nervous system for further instructions.
4. The skin regulates body temperature.
5. The skin functions as a miniexcretory system, eliminating wastes through perspiration.
6. Located in the skin are modified cholesterol molecules that are converted by the ultraviolet rays in sunlight to vitamin D.

Respiratory System

The anatomical structures of the respiratory system are the nose, nasal cavity, pharynx, larynx, trachea, bronchi, bronchioles, alveoli, lungs, and the respiratory diaphragm. Our respiratory system serves us in many ways:

1. Exchanging oxygen and carbon dioxide
2. Detecting smell (olfaction)
3. Producting speech
4. Regulating pH

Reproductive System

The anatomical structures of the reproductive system are the gonads (ovaries in females and testes in males), ducts (fallopian tubes in females and spermatic duct in males), and gametes (ova in females and spermatozoa in males). Other reproductive structures are the uterus and vagina in females and the penis and urethra in males. The primary function of the reproductive system is to produce offspring and propagate the species.

Muscular System

The anatomical structures of the muscular system are the skeletal muscles, tendons, smooth muscle, and cardiac muscle.

1. Skeletal muscles create movements we can see, which include both motion and locomotion. *Motion* is defined as a change in position resulting from movement; *locomotion* is movement from one place to another.

2. Smooth muscle produces internal mobility, which is the movement resulting from the contraction of smooth muscles (motility).
3. All muscle contractions produce and release heat, which is important to preserve correct body temperature. Additionally, when the body becomes chilled, skeletal muscles begin to rapidly contract and to produce heat; this is called shivering.
4. To maintain static positions, such as sitting and standing, the skeletal muscles contract to hold us in these postures. Muscles also contribute to joint stability.
5. As skeletal muscles contract, lymph vessels are compressed and lymph fluid is displaced. Lymph flow can also be stimulated by peristaltic action of the gastrointestinal tract, by arterial pulsations, and by contraction of the diaphragm.

Endocrine System

Anatomical structures of the endocrine system are the endocrine glands (pituitary, pineal, thyroid, parathyroids, thymus, adrenals, pancreas, and gonads, placenta, and some cells of the digestive tract) and the products of these glands, known as hormones. The functions of the endocrine system are complex:

1. It produces and secretes hormones.
2. It regulates body activities, such as growth, development, metabolism, and fluid balance.
3. It maintains the body during times of stress, such as infection, trauma, dehydration, emotional stress, and starvation.
4. It contributes to the reproductive process.

Nervous System

The anatomical structures of the nervous system include the brain, spinal cord, meninges, cerebrospinal fluid, cranial nerves and spinal nerves, and the special sense organs, such as the eyes and ears. Our nervous system serves us in many ways.

1. The nervous system receives sensory input from sensory receptors of the body by detecting changes such as pressure, temperature, and motion, both inside the body and out.
2. This system interprets and integrates all stimuli. After sensing changes, the nervous system interprets the perceived information to provide a response.
3. The nervous system initiates motor output; once the nervous system has received and interpreted the stimuli, a motor response is activated in the form of muscular contractions or glandular secretions.
4. The nervous system is also responsible for mental processes (i.e., cognition and memory) and emotional responses (i.e., anger and anxiety).

Urinary System

The anatomical structures of the urinary system are the kidneys, ureters, urinary bladder, and urethra. The urinary system does many things.

1. It eliminates metabolic wastes that are produced by cellular metabolism and released in the urine.
2. The urinary system regulates blood pH and its chemical composition through specialized cells located in the kidney.
3. The kidneys regulate blood volume and fluid balance by controlling the amount of water reabsorbed back into the circulatory system.
4. The urinary system continuously monitors blood pressure and helps to maintain a normal range by secreting enzymes that stimulate vasoconstriction.
5. With the removal of metabolic wastes, the urinary system helps to maintain homeostasis by regulating the chemical composition of the blood, by regulating blood volume, and by maintaining fluid balance and blood pressure.

Digestive System

The anatomical structures of the digestive system are the teeth, tongue, the alimentary canal (tube from mouth to anus), and related accessory glands (e.g., liver, gallbladder, pancreas, salivary). There are four processes of the digestive system.

1. *Ingestion* is the process of orally taking materials into the body such as food, liquids, and oral medications.
2. *Digestion* is the mechanical and chemical processes that occur as food is mixed with digestive enzymes and converted into an absorbable state.
3. *Absorption* is the process by which the products of digestion move into the bloodstream or lymph vessels and then into the body's cells.
4. *Defecation* is the process of eliminating indigestible or unabsorbed material from the body.

> *The body's life is the life of sensation and emotions. The body feels real hunger, real thirst, real joy in the sun or snow, real pleasure in the smell of roses or the look of a lilac bush; real anger, real sorrow, real tenderness, real warmth, real passion, real hate, real grief. All these emotions belong to the body and are only recognized by the mind.*
>
> —D. H. Lawrence

THE BODY COMPASS

Every good travel map will always have a compass drawing to indicate which way is north, south, east, and west. The map will also have some distance reference, such as a scale of miles per a specific measure.

Any map without these items is of little or no use. Imagine trying to read a map if you cannot understand the definitions of the words "north," "south," "5 miles," "1 block," or "by the lake." Think of the anatomical drawings as your map, and consider this section of the book your body compass. You will learn new terms that constitute medical directional terminology to help you find your way around the body. These terms will include names for planes of the body, locations that are relative to the body planes, regional terms for different aspects of the body, and the body cavities.

To avoid confusion when discussing anatomical directions, all parts of the body are described in relation to other body parts using a standard body position, called the **anatomical position.** In this position, the body is erect and facing forward, the arms are at the side, the palms are facing forward with the thumbs to the side, and feet are slightly apart with toes pointing forward.

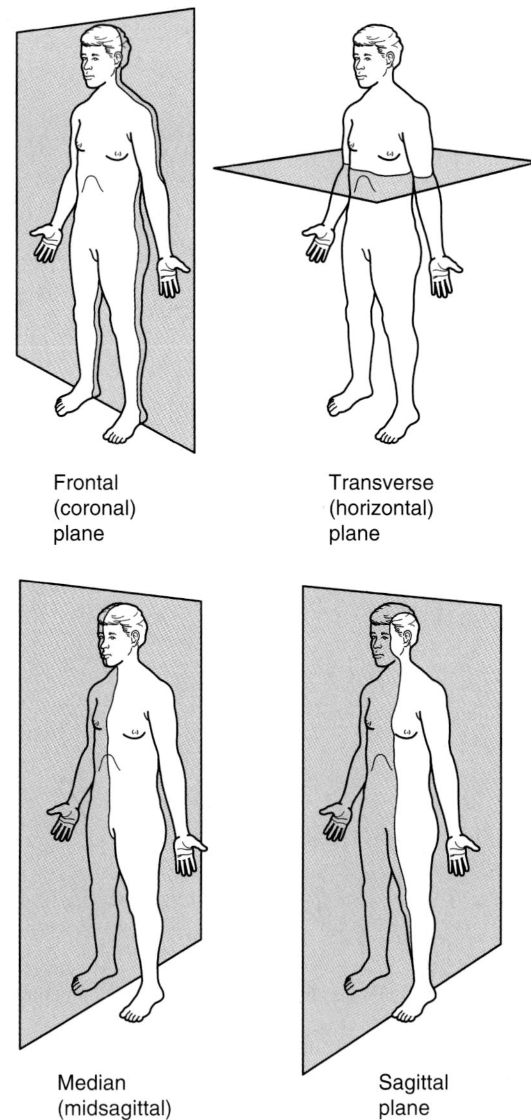

Figure 4•8 Planes of the body.

Planes of the Body

We live in a three-dimensional structure: Our height, depth, and width help to describe volume in space. It is easy to think of ourselves as flat; mirrors and photographs give us the illusion that we are two dimensional, but we have sculpted fullness, curves, and angles. Since the body is three dimensional, we can refer to three planes or sections that lie at right angles to each other. These planes do not necessarily divide the body into halves, but can be referred to in a variety of locations within the plane itself (Fig. 4–8).

The **midsagittal** or **median plane** runs longitudinally or vertically down the body, anterior to posterior, dividing the organism into right and left sections, creating a right lateral and a left lateral portion of the body. When a plane passes through the body parallel to the median plane, we have the **sagittal plane.** The **frontal** or **coronal plane** passing through the body side-to-side to create anterior (ventral) and posterior (dorsal) sections. The **transverse** or **horizontal plane** passes through the body and creates superior (cephalic or cranial) and inferior (caudal) sections.

Body Cavities

The body contains organs and other structures in closed spaces called cavities; the two main cavities are the *dorsal* and the *ventral.* The **dorsal (posterior) cavity,** located on the back or posterior aspect of the body, is further divided into the *cranial cavity* (containing the brain) and the *spinal* or *vertebral cavity* (containing the spinal cord). The larger **ventral (anterior) cavity,** located anteriorally to the dorsal cavity, is further divided into the **thoracic cavity** and the **abdominopelvic cavity.** The thoracic cavity contains the right and left **pleural cavities** (the lungs) and the mediastinum (containing the pericardium, the heart, the great vessels such as aorta and vena cava, the esophagus, and the trachea).

The abdominopelvic cavity is further divided into the abdominal cavity and the pelvic cavity. The abdominal cavity contains the digestive system and its accessory organs. The pelvic cavity contains the organs of the reproductive and urinary systems, as well as the rectum of the digestive system (Fig. 4–9).

The healthcare profession requires specific directional terminology in reference to the human body in order for professional communication to occur without confusion. Most of these terms will be used to describe the location of a certain body part, in relation to an adjacent body part.

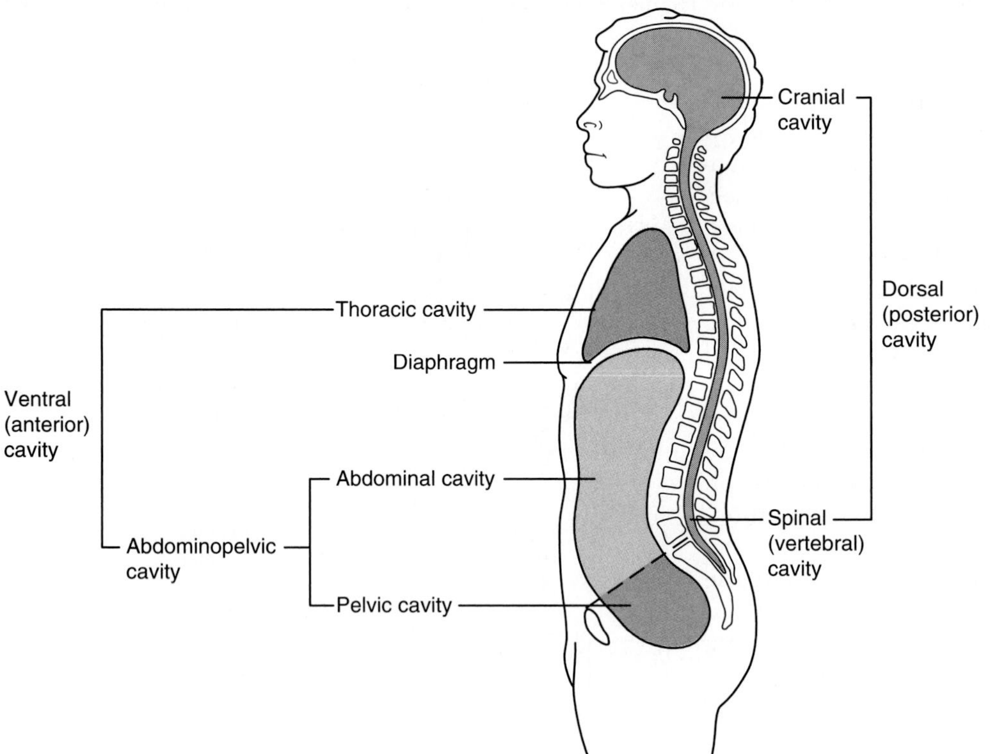

Figure 4•9 The body cavities.

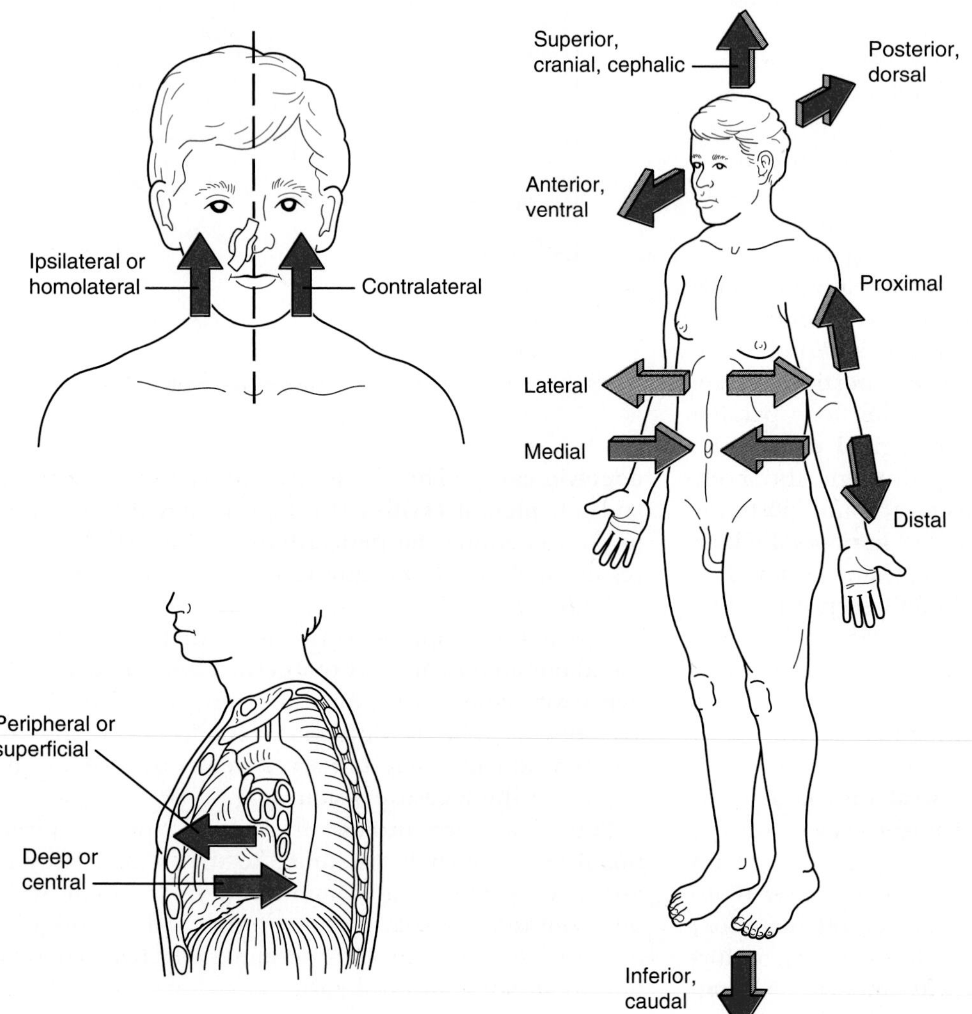

Figure 4•10 Directional terminology.

Directional Terminology

In this section we will define directional terminology (Fig. 4–10).

- **Prone:** lying face or belly down in a horizontal, recumbent position
- **Supine:** lying face or belly up in a horizontal, recumbent position
- **Superior, cranial,** or **cephalic:** situated above or toward the head end; the jaw is superior to the navel
- **Inferior** or **caudal:** situated below or toward the tail end; the sacrum is inferior to the skull
- **Anterior** or **ventral:** pertaining more to the front side of a structure; the navel is anterior to the vertebral column
- **Posterior** or **dorsal:** pertaining more to the back of a structure; the vertebral column is posterior to the lungs
- **Medial:** oriented more toward or near the midline of the body; the nose is medial to the ears
- **Lateral:** oriented farther away from the midline of the body; the ribs are lateral to the vertebral column
- **Homolateral** or **ipsilateral:** related to the same side of the body; the right hand is homolateral (ipsilateral) to the right foot
- **Contralateral:** related to opposite sides of the body; the right foot is contralateral to the left foot
- **Proximal:** nearer to the point of reference, usually toward the trunk of the body; the hip is proximal to the knee
- **Distal:** farther from the point of reference, usually away from the midline or a central point; the foot is distal to the hip
- **Central:** pertaining to or situated at a center of the body, is often referred to as deep; the heart is centrally located, and the heart is deep to the rib cage
- **Peripheral:** pertaining to the outside surface, periphery, or surrounding external area of a structure, is often referred to as superficial; the skin is superficial (peripherally located) to the bones
- **Internal:** nearer the inside (within) of a body cavity; the stomach is an internally located organ
- **External:** nearest the outside of a body cavity; the skin is located on the external surface of the body
- **Parietal:** referring to the walls of a cavity or an organ; the parietal peritoneum lines the abdominopelvic cavity
- **Visceral:** pertaining to the outer coverings of a body cavity or hollow organ; the visceral pericardium lines the heart

Regional Terms

In this section, we will identify both anterior and posterior landmarks of the body (Figs. 4–11 and 4–12).

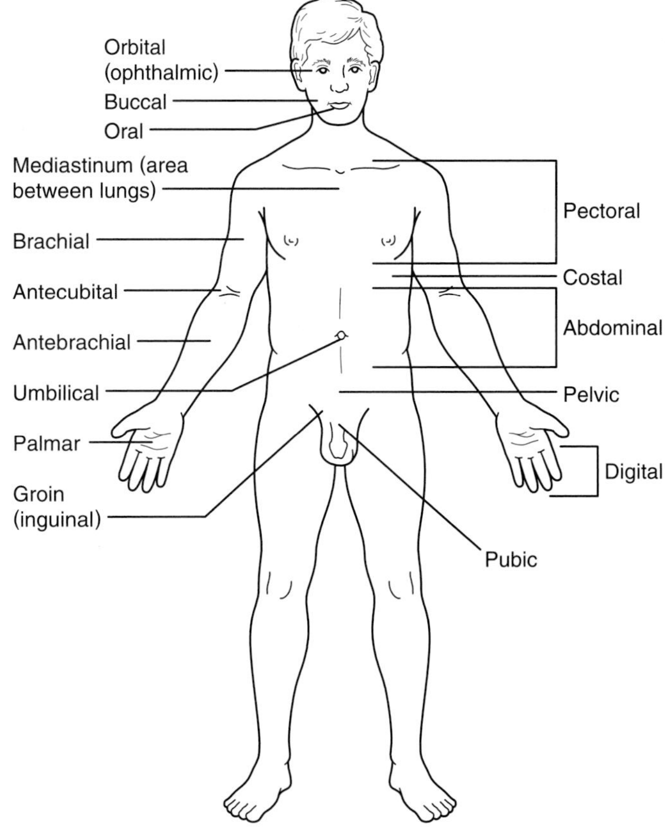

Figure 4•11 Anterior body landmarks.

Anterior Body Landmarks

- **Abdominal:** anterior trunk; between the thorax and the pelvis
- **Antebrachium:** pertains to forearm; between the wrist and elbow
- **Antecubital:** the space in front of the elbow or at the bend of the elbow
- **Axillary:** armpit; pyramid-shaped area formed by the underside of the anterior and posterior aspects of the shoulder
- **Brachial:** refers to the upper arm; between the shoulder and the elbow
- **Buccal:** pertaining to the cheek area
- **Cervical:** pertaining to the neck area
- **Costal:** referring to the ribs; the space near a rib or on a side close to a rib
- **Cubital:** pertains to the elbow
- **Digital:** pertaining to a digit; fingers or toes
- **Femoral** (crural): pertaining to the femur or the thigh area; between the hip and the knee
- **Groin** (inguinal): the area where the thigh meets the abdomen
- **Inguinal:** see **groin**
- **Pectoral:** pertaining to the thorax or chest area
- **Mediastinum:** a portion of the thoracic cavity occupying the area between the lungs

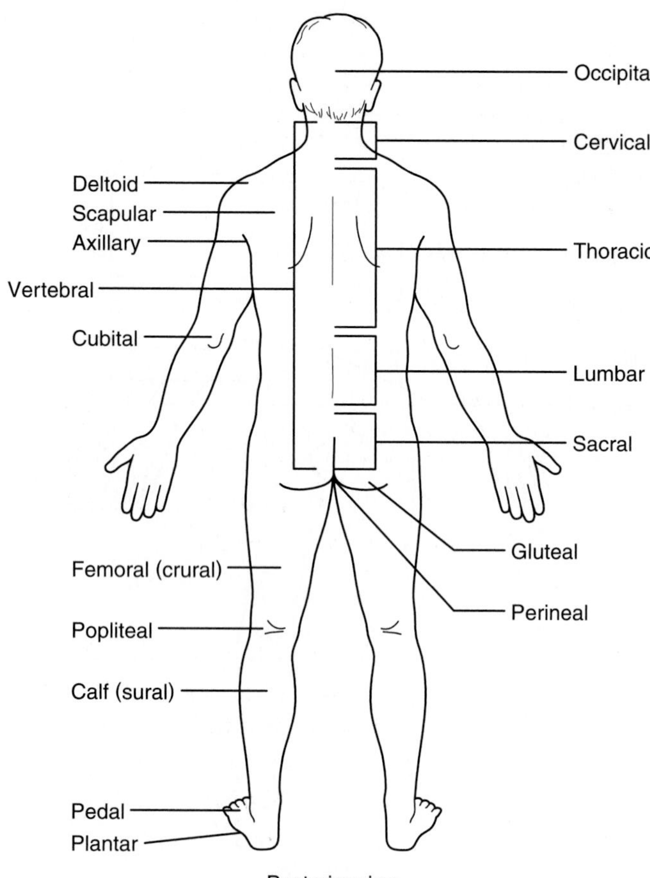

Figure 4•12 Posterior body landmarks.

- **Oral:** pertaining to the mouth region
- **Orbital** (ophthalmic): pertaining to the eye area
- **Palmar:** refers to the anterior surface or the palm of the hand
- **Pelvic:** inferior region of the abdominopelvic cavity
- **Pubic:** pertaining to the region of the pubic symphysis or the genital area
- **Thoracic:** the chest area; between the neck and the respiratory diaphragm, or between the neck and the low back
- **Umbilical:** referring to the area of the midabdomen or navel (the scar left from the umbilical cord)

Posterior Body Landmarks

- **Calf** (sural): pertaining to the calf area of the lower leg
- **Crural** (femoral): pertaining to the femur or the thigh area; between the hip and the knee
- **Deltoid:** the curve of the shoulder and upper arm formed by the large deltoid muscle
- **Gluteal:** the curve of the buttocks formed by the large gluteal muscles
- **Lumbar:** pertaining to the area of the back between the ribs of the thorax and hips of the pelvis
- **Occipital:** posterior surface of the head; situated near the occipital bone
- **Perineal:** the region between the anus and the genitals; inferior pelvic cavity
- **Pedal:** referring to the foot/feet
- **Plantar:** pertaining to the bottom surface of the foot or sole
- **Popliteal:** the area located on the posterior aspect of the knee
- **Sacral:** pertaining to the sacrum or sacral area of the spinal column
- **Scapular:** referring to the shoulder blade area
- **Sural:** see **calf**
- **Vertebral:** pertaining to one or more vertebrae of the vertebral or spinal column

SUMMARY

An introduction to the human body includes a study of the basic structural building blocks of the body, their functions, and the directional terminology based upon the medical model.

The first of these building blocks is the cell, the simplest form of life that can exist as an independent self-sustaining unit. Each cell is made up of a combination of the following structures: the cell membrane, cytoplasm, nucleus, mitochondria, ribosomes, endoplasmic reticulum, Golgi apparatus, and lysosomes. Cells function through the exchange of fluids, nutrients, chemicals, and ions, which are carried out by passive and active cell processes. Examples of passive processes are simple and facilitated diffusion, osmosis, and filtration. Active processes include active transport, endocytosis, and exocytosis.

Cells organize to form tissues; the study of tissues is known as histology. There are four divisions of body tissues: epithelial, connective, muscle, and nervous. Some tissues present themselves as membranes that protect organs or separate body cavities. The three types of bodily membranes are mucous, serous, and synovial.

Tissues organize to form organs, which are classified according to organ systems. The ten organ systems of the body are the circulatory, the skeletal, the integumentary, the respiratory, the reproductive, the muscular, the endocrine, the nervous, the urinary, and the digestive.

In order to negotiate these body systems, it is necessary to learn the language of the body itself. Our map consists of anatomical directional terminology, planes of the body, body cavities, and regional body landmarks. All of these are based on the medical model.

SELF-TEST

Multiple Choice • Write the letter of the best answer in the space provided.

_______ 1. The study of the structures of the human body and their positional relationships to one another is known as

A. physiology
B. homeostasis
C. anatomy
D. metabolism

_______ 2. The human body's internal environment, which remains relatively constant within a very limited range, is referred to as

A. physiology
B. homeostasis
C. anatomy
D. metabolism

_______ 3. The total of all the physical and chemical processes that occur in a given organism is

A. physiology
B. homeostasis
C. anatomy
D. metabolism

_______ 4. How the body functions in normal body processes is called

A. physiology
B. homeostasis
C. anatomy
D. metabolism

_______ 5. The simplest forms of life that can exist as independent self-sustaining units are

A. cells
B. tissues
C. organs
D. atoms

_______ 6. Which of the following are basic components of a cell?

A. cytoplasm
B. mitochondria
C. nucleus
D. all of the above

_______ 7. The control center of the cell that directs nearly all metabolic activities is the

A. ribosome
B. endoplasmic reticulum
C. nucleus
D. mitochondrion

_______ 8. The oval-shaped organelle that lies within the cytoplasm and is considered the cell's "power plant" is called

A. a lysosome
B. a mitochondrion
C. a nucleus
D. endoplasmic reticulum

_______ 9. A series of four to six horizontal membranous sacs, which is referred to as the "packing and shipping" plant of the cell because it is associated with altering proteins and lipids, is the

A. Golgi apparatus
B. endoplasmic reticulum
C. nucleolus
D. Golgi tendon bodies

_______ 10. The movement of particles across the cellular membrane due to the force of pressure is called

A. diffusion
B. osmosis
C. filtration
D. cellular mobility

_______ 11. Movement of dissolved substances from a region of highest concentration to a region of lowest concentration that requires no expenditure of energy is known as

A. diffusion
B. osmosis
C. filtration
D. cellular mobility

_______ 12. Movement of important atoms and molecules such as ions against the concentration gradient from low levels to high levels, in order to maintain such vital processes as nerve conduction, is called

A. facilitated osmosis
B. reverse diffusion
C. cellular mobility
D. active transport

_______ 13. Tissue that lines the internal and the external organs of the body and lines the vessels and body cavities is the

A. connective tissue
B. epithelial tissue
C. covering tissue
D. serous tissue

_______ 14. The most abundant and widely distributed tissue of the body is

A. connective tissue
B. epithelial tissue
C. covering tissue
D. serous tissue

_______ 15. Also called pavement epithelium, _______ is a single layer of thin, flat cells that are close together, attaching at their edges.

A. pseudostratified columnar epithelium
B. transitional epithelium
C. glandular epithelium
D. simple squamous epithelium

_______ 16. Which of the following epithelium has the appearance of being stratified because the cells possess different heights, so that not all cells reach the free surface?

A. pseudostratified columnar epithelium
B. transitional epithelium
C. glandular epithelium
D. simple squamous epithelium

_______ 17. The most widespread epithelium that is arranged in layers over the skin and that lines most of the hollow structures (e.g., oral cavity) is called

A. stratified squamous epithelium
B. transitional epithelium
C. glandular epithelium
D. simple squamous epithelium

_______ 18. Which of the following is *not* a classification of connective tissue?

A. liquid C. cartilaginous
B. areolar D. smooth

_______ 19. The hardest, and most solid, of all connective tissue is

A. cartilage C. muscle
B. bone D. tendons

_______ 20. A tough, dense material that has the greatest tensile strength and that is found in the intervertebral disks, in the meniscus of the knee joint, and between the pubic bones, is called

A. fibrocartilage C. hyaline cartilage
B. elastic cartilage D. osseous cartilage

_______ 21. Soft and pliable cartilage that gives shape to the external nose and ears and to internal structures such as the epiglottis and the auditory tubes, is known as

A. fibrocartilage C. hyaline cartilage
B. elastic cartilage D. osseous cartilage

_______ 22. The most widely distributed connective tissue, which is regarded as the packing material of the body, is the

A. loose connective tissue
B. cartilage
C. dense connective tissue
D. epithelial tissue

_______ 23. A specialized form of loose connective tissue that provides fuel reserves for energy expenditure, insulation for heat, and a cushion around certain structures, such as the kidneys, heart, and some joints, is called

A. reticular tissue C. insulative loose tissue
B. fascia D. adipose tissue

_______ 24. Which of the following tissue type is very vascular and has the special ability to contract and elongate to produce movement?

A. nervous C. epithelial
B. muscle D. connective

_______ 25. Thin, soft, pliable sheets of tissue that cover the body, line tubes or body cavities, cover organs, or separate one part of a cavity from another, are known as _______ tissue.

A. epithelial C. membranous
B. connective D. muscle

_______ 26. Which one of the following is *not* a type of membrane found in the body?

A. salivary C. synovial
B. mucous D. serous

_______ 27. Membranes that line openings to the outside of the body are called

A. epithelial membranes C. synovial membranes
B. mucous membranes D. serous membranes

_______ 28. Membranes that line closed body cavities that do not have openings to the outside of the body are the

A. epithelial membranes C. anterior membranes
B. mucous membranes D. serous membranes

_______ 29. Which of the following body systems is involved in protection of the body by acting as a physical, biological, and chemical barrier; in regulation of body temperature; and in synthesis of vitamin D?

A. circulatory system C. integumentary system
B. endocrine system D. nervous system

_______ 30. Which of the following body systems transports and distributes respiratory gases, nutrients, antibodies, and hormones, and protects the body through clotting mechanisms?

A. circulatory system C. integumentary system
B. endocrine system D. nervous system

_______ 31. Which of the following body systems is involved with oxygen and carbon dioxide exchange, the sense of smell, and speech production?

A. nervous system C. urinary system
B. circulatory system D. respiratory system

_______ 32. The body system that creates movement, internal mobility (motility), and heat is the

A. circulatory system C. skeletal system
B. endocrine system D. muscular system

_______ 33. The body system that involves the processes of ingestion, digestion, absorption, and defecation is the

A. respiratory system C. urinary system
B. digestive system D. endocrine system

_______ 34. The position in which the body is erect and facing forward, the arms are at the side, the palms are facing forward with the thumbs to the side, the feet are slightly apart, and the toes are pointing forward is called the

A. fundamental position C. reference position
B. essential position D. anatomical position

_______ 35. The plane that goes longitudinally down the body, anterior to posterior, dividing the organism into right and left sections, is the

A. midsagittal or median plane
B. transverse or horizontal plane
C. frontal or coronal plane
D. midline plane

_______ 36. Which of the following planes passes through the body side to side to create anterior and posterior sections?

A. sagittal or median plane
B. transverse or horizontal plane
C. frontal or coronal plane
D. midline plane

_______ 37. The two main body cavities are called the

A. abdominal and the pelvic cavities
B. dorsal and the ventral cavities
C. cranial and the spinal cavities
D. cranial and the ventral cavities

_______ 38. Which of the following cavities contains the brain and spinal cord?

A. ventral cavity C. anterior cavity
B. craniospinal cavity D. dorsal cavity

Matching I • Match the letter of the term with the phrase that best describes it.

A. anterior I. ipsilateral
B. prone J. superior
C. posterior K. medial
D. inferior L. proximal
E. supine M. visceral
F. lateral N. contralateral
G. distal O. parietal
H. peripheral

_______ 1. pertaining more to the back of a structure

_______ 2. referring to the walls of a cavity or an organ

_______ 3. lying face or belly up in a horizontal, recumbent position

_______ 4. oriented more toward or near the midline of the body

_______ 5. situated above or toward the head end

_______ 6. related to the same side of the body

_______ 7. oriented away from the midline of the body

_______ 8. pertaining more to the front of a structure

_______ 9. pertaining more to the outside surface, periphery, or surrounding external area of a structure and is often referred to as superficial

_______ 10. pertaining to the outer coverings of a body cavity or organ

_______ 11. situated below or toward the tail end

_______ 12. lying face or belly down in a horizontal, recumbent position

_______ 13. farther from the point of reference, usually away from the midline or a central point

_______ 14. nearer to the point of reference, usually toward the trunk of the body

_______ 15. related to opposite sides of the body; the right foot is contralateral to the left foot

Matching II • Match the letter of the term with the phrase that best describes it.

A. axillary	J. orbital
B. digital	K. antebrachium
C. pubic	L. femoral
D. oral	M. cervical
E. umbilical	N. palmar
F. pectoral	O. thoracic
G. abdominal	P. buccal
H. brachial	Q. costal
I. mediastinum	R. antecubital

_______ 1. pertaining to the mouth region

_______ 2. armpit; pyramid-shaped area formed by the underside of the anterior and posterior aspect of the shoulder

_______ 3. a portion of the thoracic cavity occupying the area between the lungs

_______ 4. space in front of the elbow or at the bend of the elbow

_______ 5. anterior trunk; between the thorax and the pelvis

_______ 6. pertaining to a digit; fingers and toes

_______ 7. pertaining to the femur or the thigh area; between the hip and the knee

_______ 8. pertaining to the cheek area

_______ 9. pertaining to the forearm; between the wrist and elbow

_______ 10. referring to the area of the midabdomen or navel

_______ 11. referring to the upper arm; between the shoulder and the elbow

_______ 12. referring to the ribs; the space near a rib or on a side close to a rib

_______ 13. pertaining to the neck area

_______ 14. referring to the anterior surface or the palm of the hand

_______ 15. pertaining to the thorax or chest area

_______ 16. pertaining to the eye area

_______ 17. pertaining to the region of the pubic symphysis or the genital area

_______ 18. the chest area; between the neck and superior to the respiratory diaphragm

Matching III • Match the letter of the term with the phrase that best describes it.

A. lumbar	G. pedal
B. deltoid	H. vertebral
C. calf	I. popliteal
D. gluteal	J. scapular
E. plantar	K. sacral
F. occipital	L. crural

_______ 1. pertaining to the calf area of the lower leg

_______ 2. posterior surface of the head

_______ 3. referring to the foot/feet

_______ 4. pertaining to the femur or the thigh area; between the hip and the knee

_______ 5. the area located on the posterior aspect of the knee

_______ 6. pertaining to the area of the back between the ribs of the thorax and hips of the pelvis

_______ 7. pertaining to the bottom surface of the foot or sole

_______ 8. the curve of the shoulder and upper arm formed by the large deltoid muscle

_______ 9. referring to the shoulder blade area

_______ 10. the curve of the buttocks formed by the large gluteal muscles

_______ 11. pertaining to the sacrum or sacral area of the spinal column

_______ 12. pertaining to one or more vertebrae of the vertebral or spinal column

References

Applegate, Edith J. *The Anatomy and Physiology Learning System: Textbook.* Philadelphia: W. B. Saunders, 1995.

Goldberg, Stephen. *Clinical Anatomy Made Ridiculously Simple.* Miami: Medmaster, 1984.

Gray, Henry, T. Pickering Pick, and Robert Howden. *Gray's Anatomy,* 29th ed. Philadelphia: Running Press, 1974.

Haubrich, William S. *Medical Meanings, A Glossary of Word Origins.* New York: Harcourt Brace Jovanovich, Publishers, 1984.

Juhan, Deane. *Job's Body, A Handbook for Bodyworkers.* Barrington, NY: Station Hill Press, 1987.

Kapit, Wynn and Lawrence M. Elson. *The Anatomy Coloring Book,* 2nd ed. New York: HarperCollins Publishers, 1993.

Kapit, Wynn, Robert Macey, and Esmail Meisami. *The Physiology Coloring Book.* New York: HarperCollins Publishers, 1987.

Lauderstein, David. *Putting the Soul Back in the Body: A Manual of Imaginative Anatomy for Massage Therapists.* Self-published manual. Chicago, IL: 1985.

Marieb, Elaine N. *Essentials of Human Anatomy and Physiology,* 4th ed. New York: Benjamin/Cummings Publishing Company, 1994.

Taber's Cyclopedic Medical Dictionary, 13th ed. Philadelphia: F. A. Davis Company, 1977.

Tortora, Gerald J. *Introduction to the Human Body: The Essentials of Anatomy and Physiology,* 3rd ed. New York: HarperCollins Publishers, 1994.

The skin is no more separate from the brain than the surface of a lake is separate from its depths. They are two different locations in a continuous medium. To touch the surface is to stir the depths.
—*Deane Juhan*

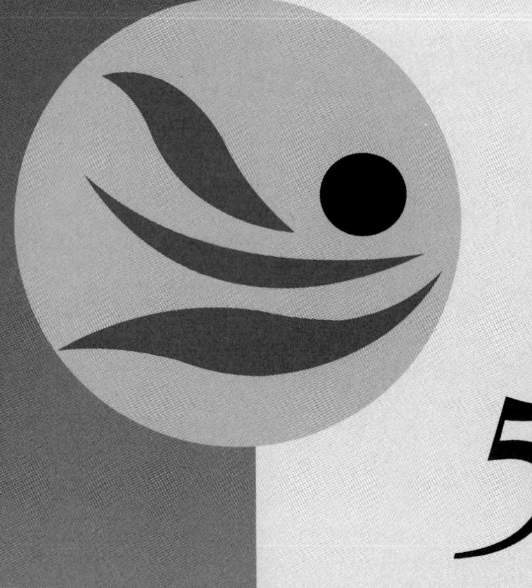

5 Integumentary System

Student Objectives

After completing this chapter, the student should be able to:

- Recall the six functions of the integumentary system
- Identify the epidermal layers
- Define several factors that contribute to skin color
- Name the main parts of a nail
- Differentiate between sebaceous glands and sudoriferous glands
- Identify three types of sudoriferous glands
- Name five types of skin conditions and give one characteristic of each
- Explain first-, second-, and third-degree burns
- Define three types of skin cancer
- Identify four ways to access moles for possible changes
- List all the known sensory receptors associated with the skin and name what type of sensation they detect
- Discuss the possible implications that touch research, as presented in this chapter, has on massage therapy

INTRODUCTION

The word "integumentary" is derived from the Latin word *integumentum* which means "a covering." The integumentary system consists of the skin and all of its derivatives; the hair, nails, and glands. By weight, the skin is the largest organ of the body. As you recall from the orientation chapter, an organ possesses at least two kinds of tissue that enable it to perform specific functions. It may be difficult to think of the skin as an organ, but its functions are vital to our existence.

The skin, like a cell membrane, defines our parameters. Housed within its layers are various tissues that carry out special functions, such as waste elimination and temperature regulation. The skin forms natural openings such as the mouth, external ear canal, nose, urethra, vagina, and the anus. These passageways to the digestive, respiratory, urinary, and reproductive systems can be seen as extensions of the external environment. No other body system is more easily exposed to infections, disease, pollution, or injury than our skin, yet no other body system is as strong and resilient.

The appearance of the skin reflects our physiology. At a glance you will know something about a person's nutrition, hygiene habits, circulation, age, immunity, parents (genetics), and environmental factors. These factors play a significant role in our skin's tone, color, and condition. Healthy skin is soft, flexible, moist, acidic, and blemish-free. People spend millions of dollars each year on products that profess to give them a more youthful appearance. Millions of dollars are also spent on surgical and nonsurgical procedures to darken the skin, remove wrinkles, lighten freckles, minimize scars, smooth out cellulite, remove unwanted hair, restore lost hair, and treat acne.

Not only does it reveal vital physiological data (e.g., circulation, fever), the skin also mirrors our emotional self, through muscular expression and neurological impulses. The skin has the power to reflect an ever changing stream of emotions. How we feel about ourselves and how we feel about others are reflected on the surface of our skin.

In this chapter we will examine the skin and its derivatives, their structure and function, as well as the concept of touch. By understanding the skin's embryonic origins and its connection with the nervous system, we can appreciate the relationship of "touch" and massage therapy.

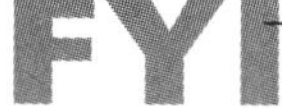

FOR YOUR INFORMATION

The skin covers an area of about 22 square feet and weighs approximately 9 pounds (or 7 percent of body weight). A piece of skin the size of a quarter contains more than 3 million cells, 100 sweat glands, 50 nerve endings, and 3 feet of blood vessels. The fingertips have approximately 700 touch receptors on 2 square millimeters of surface area. This is 2 square millimeters ⇨ □.

FUNCTIONS

The skin is a complex organ. The integumentary system illustrates this well, encompassing a vast variety of functions. It protects and provides immune functions for other body systems, absorbs certain substances, produce vitamins, and eliminates waste products. It also works as a body thermostat to control temperature. Most important for our purposes, it receives stimuli through touch.

1. **Protects.** One of the primary functions of the skin is protecting the organism by acting as a physical barrier, biological barrier, and a chemical barrier. The skin's physical barrier is essential for protecting the underlying tissues from abrasion. **Keratin,** a cordlike protein, provides protection by waterproofing the skin's surface. This function serves a dual purpose; keeping water in and water out. The skin also provides limited protection from ultraviolet radiation through specialized cells called melanocytes. As a biological barrier, intact skin is an effective barrier against many foreign agents, such as bacteria and viruses. The skin's acidic secretions inhibit the growth of these foreign agents by providing an "acid mantle." This surface acidity provides our skin with a chemical barrier.
2. **Absorbs.** The skin has limited properties of absorption. Substances that can be absorbed by the epidermis are lipid soluble substances, such as oxygen, carbon dioxide, fat-soluble vitamins (A, D, E, and K), steroids, resins of certain plants (poison ivy and poison oak), organic solvents (such as paint thinner, which can cause brain and kidney damage), and salts of heavy metals such as lead (Pb), mercury (Hg), and nickel (Ni). The use of medicated transdermal patches is based on these absorption properties of the skin.
3. **Receives Stimuli or Sensation.** The skin is considered an extension of the nervous system. It receives stimuli such as pressure, pain, and temperature from the external environment and brings this information to the central nervous system. The most fundamental of all the senses is touch. The very concept of touch encompasses emotional as well as physical aspects of well-being; we will cover the physical dimensions, such as sensory receptors, in the section titled "Skin and Its Sensory Receptors." A separate section of this chapter has been set aside

Terms and Word Roots Related to the Skin

acne vulgaris – common acne
contusion – bruise
corium – leather, skin
cutaneous – skin
cuticle – little skin
decubitus – lying down
dermis – skin
eczema – to boil out
epidermis – upon or over skin
follicle – sac, small
furuncle – boil
granulosum – grain, small
integument – a covering, to cover over
Krause's end bulbs – named after the German anatomist (1833–1910)
lacrimal – tear
Meissner's corpuscles – named after the German histologist (1829–1905)
melano – black
Pacinian's corpuscles – named after the Italian anatomist (1812–1883)
palpate – stroke or touch
papule – pimple
pruritus – itching
psoriasis – an itching
pustule – blister
Ruffini's end organs – named after the Italian anatomist (1864–1929)
scleroderma – hard, skin
seborrhea – tallow, to flow
sebum – grease, tallow
senile lentigo – old freckle
stratum – a layer, cover, or spread
sudoriferous – sweat, to carry or bear
verruca – wart

to examine touch in greater detail in the section titled "Skin and the Importance of Touch," especially as it relates to our emotional needs.

4. **Regulates Body Temperature.** An increase in blood circulation to the skin's surface changes its insulative properties into a mechanism of temperature regulation. As the blood moves to the skin's surface and the blood vessels dilate, heat is discharged into the atmosphere. In this way our bodies radiate to release internal heat. Heat can also be dissipated through the evaporation of perspiration produced by specialized glands called sudoriferous glands. Perspiration may be either insensible or active. Insensible perspiration, as the name implies, is the constant evaporative cooling of microscopic sweat beads from the skin surface. This process occurs without our knowledge during periods of low activity or in dry climates. Active perspiration usually accompanies heavy exertion and is common in humid or hot climates. When sweat accumulates faster than evaporation can take place, perspiration may run down our bodies and saturate our clothing.
5. **Eliminates Waste.** The skin functions as a mini-excretory system, eliminating wastes through perspiration. Sweat, a waste product, is a mixture of 98 percent water and 2 percent solids (salt ions, lactic acid, and other metabolic wastes). By contrast, urine is 96 percent water and 4 percent solids.
6. **Synthesizes Vitamin D.** Located in the skin are modified cholesterol molecules (also known as precursor molecules) that are converted by the ultraviolet rays in sunlight to vitamin D. Vitamin D is important because it stimulates the absorption of calcium and phosphorus from the food we eat. Very little ultraviolet light is required for this synthesis to occur. This should not be used as a reason to engage in prolonged sunbathing.

ANATOMICAL REGIONS AND STRUCTURES OF THE SKIN

The skin is divided into two distinct regions: the epidermis (superficial region) and the dermis. The epidermis consists of four or five layers. The dermis is located under the epidermis and contains the blood vessels and nerve receptors. Underneath the skin is a layer of tissue known as the subcutaneous layer. Let's look at these regions and layers closely.

Epidermis

The **epidermis,** or cuticle skin, is derived from ectoderm, the same embryonic cell layer that gives us the brain, spinal cord, and special senses. Contained in its epidermal layers are melanocytes, which contribute to the color of the skin and nails and absorption of ultraviolet light. The epidermis also contains pores; these openings allow passage for hair and specialized glands.

Composed solely of epithelial tissue, the epidermis does not contain blood vessels. Therefore, all oxygen and nutrients must reach the epidermal cells by diffusion of tissue fluids from the underlying dermis. The cells of the epidermis are formed in the stratum germinativum (basale layer), where they multiply and eventually push themselves up toward the surface, like a seedling or a budding tooth. As they move farther away from their source of nutrition, they become starved and eventually die. The superficial epidermal cells are constantly being sloughed off in an endless renewal process. The entire life cycle of skin cells from birth to their demise requires 21 to 27 days.

Epidermal Layers

There are typically four epidermal layers. However, in areas where friction is greatest, namely the soles of the feet and palms of the hands, there is an extra layer of skin. Cell production begins at the innermost layer of skin and moves upward to the surface layers as the cell matures. From deepest to most superficial, these layers are the stratum germinativum, the stratum spinosum, the stratum granulosum, the stratum lucidum, and the stratum corneum. The stratum germinativum and the stratum spinosum can collectively be referred to as the stratum malpighii. Let's examine these layers closer (Fig. 5–1).

1. **Stratum Germinativum.** Also known as the basale layer, this is the innermost layer or the matrix layer of the epidermis. The stratum germinativum undergoes continuous cell division and produces all other layers. This layer also contains Merkel's disks or tactile disks, which are nerve endings that give our skin the sense of touch.
2. **Stratum Spinosum.** The stratum spinosum, or "prickly layer," is a bonding and transitional layer between the stratum granulosum and the stratum germinativum because it possesses cells of both these layers.
3. **Stratum Granulosum.** A layer of cells containing an accumulation of keratohyalin granules distinguishes the stratum granulosum under a microscope. This layer is three to five cells deep, depending on the thickness of the skin. This layer marks the beginning of change before the drying or cornification of the tissue. The presence of keratohyalin granules and the degeneration of cell nuclei are indicative of the first step of keratinization.
4. **Stratum Lucidum.** In the thick skin of the hands and the feet, there is a translucent layer between the stratum corneum and the stratum granulosum. Like the stratum corneum, the stratum lucidum contains cells that are keratinized. In thin skin, the stratum lucidum is absent. Lucidum comes from the Latin word meaning "clear."
5. **Stratum Corneum.** This is the outermost layer of the skin. By the time these epithelial cells reach the surface, they are no longer living cells. The nuclei and other parts of the stratum corneum cells have been replaced with keratin. Keratin is an extremely tough, fibrous protein found in hair, nails, and the top three layers of the epidermis. Keratin is insoluble in water, and has the ability to waterproof the skin and contributes to the body's immune defenses. These keratinized cells of the stratum corneum appear scaly or horny, so this epidermal layer is often referred to as the "horny" layer. These cells

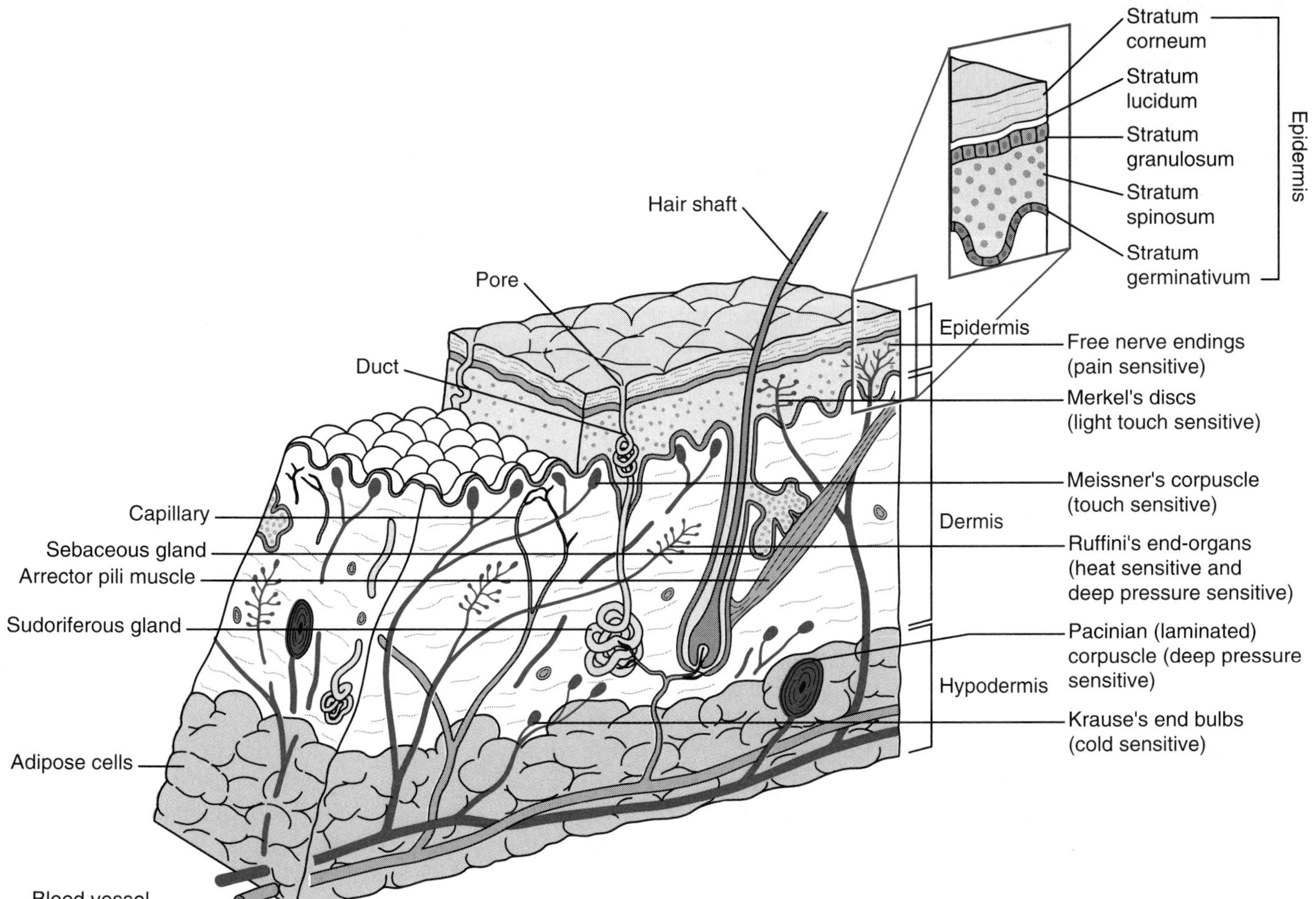

Figure 5•1 A cross-section of skin.

are dead and begin shedding, to be replaced by cells from a deeper layer.

Melanocytes

Melanocytes are specialized cells in the stratum germinativum and the stratum spinosum, where the yellow, brown, or black skin pigment, or melanin, is synthesized. **Melanin** contributes to the color of the skin but is also found in the hair and in the iris of the eye. Melanin granules serve to protect the underlying cells from ultraviolet radiation. Melanocyte-producing hormone from the pituitary, as well as genetics, determines the amount of melanin produced in an individual.

Ultraviolet light stimulates the formation of this pigment and causes darkening of the melanin granules. Melanin serves as a protective shield for the skin from the damaging effects of sunlight, especially due to suntanning. Freckles and moles are present when melanin is concentrated in one area.

Malignant melanoma is a group of melanocytes that have mutated into cancerous tissue. They are very dark, almost black, and may have some red or blue coloration. They may have a nodular surface and are more common in people with fair skin who have been overexposed to sunlight. Albinism is a genetic condition in which the individual cannot produce melanin. An albino's hair and skin appear white or pale and the iris of the eye appears pink or red because of the easy visibility of blood vessels. Vitiligo or leukoderma is the partial or total loss of skin pigmentation, which occurs in patches. This may be as the result of a deep burn or scar that damages the melanocytes in a given area of the body. The skin in this area remains white and will not tan.

Certain hormones, such as those secreted during pregnancy, can stimulate the synthesis of melanin. This can produce a dark line between the navel and the pubic area or give the childbearing woman a "mask of pregnancy" by darkening the skin of the face and throat.

Skin Color. Skin color variations are due to several factors including

1. the brown pigment, melanin
2. the amount of oxygen present in the capillaries of the dermis, which can give the skin a rosy cast ranging from erythema (dilation and congestion of the skin due to inflammation, nervousness, or mild sunburn) to the blue or purple cast of cyanosis (excessive amounts of deoxygenated blood)
3. the presence of the pigment bilirubin in the blood, which can produce the yellowish appearance of jaundice
4. the presence of the pigment beta carotene in the skin, which produces the yellowish appearance of Asians

Nails

Nails, an appendage of the skin, are a modification of the stratum corneum and the stratum lucidum. These epidermal layers are heavily keratinized and form the thin hard plates that are found on the dorsal surface at the distal ends of the fingers and toes. Nails are nonliving tissue.

The two main functions of the nails are protection of the ends of the fingers and use as a tool for tasks such as digging, scratching, and manipulation of objects. Nails are typically transparent but appear pinkish because of blood vessels present in the dermis below. If there is not sufficient oxygen in the blood, the nails will appear bluish, or cyanotic. Nail changes, like ridges and white spots, may occur as a result of poor nutrition or disease. The **body** of the nail is the main visible part of the nail. Other nail structures are the **nail bed,** nail root, lateral nail folds, eponychium (cuticle), lunula, free edge of the nail, and the hyponychium. The **nail root** is located behind and under the proximal nail fold. This portion of the nail is invisible and is imbedded in the matrix, where nail production takes place. Nail growth occurs at approximately 1 mm per week. The **lateral nail folds** are the edges of the nail where they meet the skin at the sides of the finger. This is the area where hangnails occur. The **eponychium,** or **cuticle,** is the tough ridge of epidermis (stratum corneum) that grows out over the nail from the proximal nail fold. Also located here is the **lunula,** which is the whitish half-moon shape at the base of the nail. The white coloration of the lunula is caused by the thickened layer of stratum basale under the nail, which obscures the view of the more vascular dermis tissue below the nail bed. The **hyponychium** is the thickened layer of the epidermis below the distal area of the nail. The most distal portion of the nail is the **free nail edge,** which is what we trim because of nail growth (Fig. 5–2).

Hair and Related Structures

Hair is an appendage of the skin made up of keratin filaments arising from a specialized follicle in the epidermis. Its function is primarily protection. Hair follicles are pouchlike depressions in the skin that enclose the hair shaft. Hair and hair follicles cover almost the entire body but most are barely visible to the naked eye. Hair is typically absent on the palms of the hands, sides of the fingers, soles and sides of the feet and toes, lips, the eyelid, the navel, and parts of the genitalia. Heavier concentrations of hair are found in the axillae, the scalp, on the external genitalia, and above the eyes and eyelids. Because of male hormones, men typically have extra hair growth on their face and chest.

Hair comes in a variety of sizes and shapes. Hair is

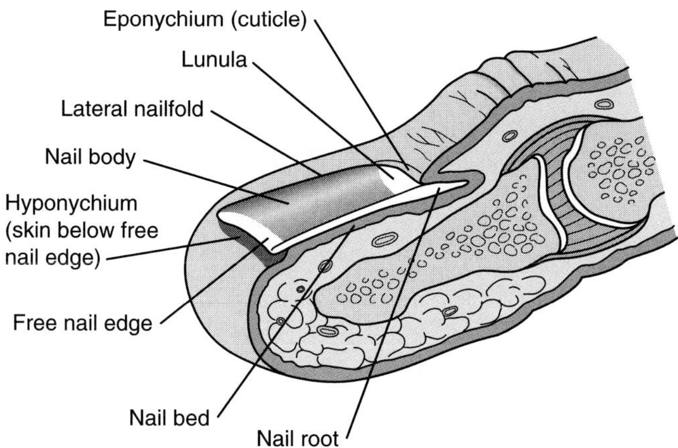

Figure 5•2 A cross-section of a nail.

short and stiff in the eyebrow, flexible and long on the top, sides, and back of the head. A round shaft of hair will produce straight hair. When the hair shaft is oval, the person usually has wavy hair. If the hair shaft is flat and ribbonlike, the hair is curly or kinky. In fine hair, no medulla (inner core) is present in the hair follicle. Genetics determine most of our hair characteristics, from hair color to texture.

All shades of hair come from one or a combination of the three colors of melanin: brown, yellow, and black. Red hair is a combination of brown and yellow pigment. White hair often is the result of air in the hair follicle itself. Gray hair occurs when the amount of melanin deposited in the hair decreases or becomes entirely absent. Aging, emotional distress, certain chemical treatments (chemotherapy), radiation, excessive vitamin A, and certain fungal diseases can cause both graying and/or hair loss.

Hair loss is common; most people lose about 70 to 100 strands of hair per day. Scalp baldness, which is more common in men than in women, does not mean that men are hairless, because frequently hair exists in the bald region. Hair in the bald region is usually colorless and very thin and may not even emerge from the follicle. Baldness may be the result of hair follicle degeneration, which is mainly due to

- genetic or hereditary factors
- an infection or other pathological condition
- the side effects of radiation or chemotherapy
- male hormonal output, namely androgens

Hair follicles can sometimes become irritated during a massage. This may be caused by

- having an allergic reaction to the massage lubricant
- pulling of the hair, which usually results in not using enough lubricant on the skin, causing undue friction

ARRECTOR PILI MUSCLE

Arrector pili are the muscles of the hair. It's hard to imagine that each strand of hair has its own muscle! Also known as arrectores pilorum, these muscles contract when you are cold or experiencing emotions, such as fright or anxiety. The hair is pulled upright, and a dimpling of the skin surface with goosepimples, goosebumps, or gooseflesh (cutis anserina) is noted. If an animal is cold, this creates an insulating layer of air in the fur. Since most humans do not have fur, this effect is relatively useless. If an animal is frightened, this added volume allows the animal to appear larger and possibly deter an enemy.

SEBACEOUS GLANDS

Sebaceous glands, also known as oil glands, are glands that possess ducts (exocrine) and are attached to the hair follicle. Sebaceous glands secrete sebum, a mixture of fats, cholesterol, proteins, and inorganic salts, which is mildly antibacterial and antifungal and which lubricates both the hair and the epidermis.

Overproduction of sebum, caused by hormones or disease, can make the skin appear oily; underproduction of sebum caused by nutritional factors and ultraviolet radiation makes the skin appear dry. Massage therapists can use massage to stimulate the production of sebum, which adds additional natural oils to the skin. The best massage movement for sebaceous gland stimulation is light friction.

Dermis

The **dermis** layer is also known as the corium, or your "hide." When you buy a leather product, you are buying the treated dermis of a mammal. The dermis contains adipose tissue, many blood vessels, and nerve endings, such as Meissner's and Pacinian's corpuscles, and it is generally thicker on the posterior aspect of the body. It is also thicker in men than in women; this may be due to the presence of certain hormones.

More specifically, dermis is thickest on the palms of the hands and soles of the feet and quite thin over the eyelids. The dermis and epidermis are firmly cemented together. However, a severe friction abrasion, such as the rubbing of an improperly fitting shoe, may cause the dermis and the epidermis to separate, resulting in a blister. The surrounding cells secrete a protective fluid to insulate themselves from the abrasive heat of the friction.

Collagen, the main component of connective tissue, is an insoluble, fibrous protein that constitutes about 70 percent of the dermis and offers supports to the nerves, blood vessels, hair follicles, and glands. Within the collagen fibers are pliable fibers called elastin, which gives the skin its elasticity, and resilience. As we age, fat is lost under the skin, which results in sags and wrinkles. So it is the loss of these protein elements, and not sagging muscles, that causes lines and wrinkles.

The loss of elasticity can be accelerated by excessive exposure of ultraviolet rays; perhaps one of the best things you can do to prevent premature wrinkling is to protect your skin from the sun. Although there is no way to avoid aging, good nutrition, drinking plenty of fluids, and daily skin care can retard the process.

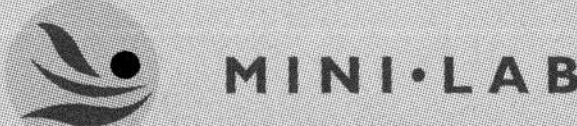

Spray the back of your hand with tap water. Blow on the damp surface and describe the sensation as the water evaporates. Speculate how evaporation of water (sweat) from the skin surface can regulate the temperature of the body. Repeat the experiment with alcohol, which evaporates at a lower temperature than water, and compare the results.

Sudoriferous Glands

Sudoriferous glands, located in the dermis, are exocrine glands that secrete sweat, or perspiration. They are regulated by the sympathetic nervous system and can be stimulated in response to excess heat or emotional arousal. Heat will generally stimulate sweat production on the forehead first. Emotions such as fear, anger, anxiety, or sexual arousal may produce a "cold sweat" beginning with the hands, feet, and armpits. The skin's surface possesses approximately 2 million sweat glands. There are two types of sudoriferous glands: eccrine glands and apocrine glands.

Eccrine glands, the most numerous of the sweat glands, are found in largest concentration in the palms of the hands, soles of the feet, and the forehead, and are absent in the nail beds, the tympanic membrane (eardrum), and parts of the external genitalia. These eccrine glands are not connected with the hair follicle and become stimulated to produce sweat during periods of high activity, high temperature, or sexual arousal. In the female, the secretions may fluctuate with the menstrual cycle. The perspiration produced by eccrine glands does not emit an offensive odor.

Apocrine glands are attached to the hair follicles and are located in the axillae, the groin, and the areola surrounding the nipples. Apocrine glands become active after puberty. Their secretions are viscous and odorless, but bacteria can quickly alter the chemical composition, producing an unpleasant odor. This "body odor" is basically caused by the decomposition of fat and proteins on the skin due to bacterial action.

The primary functions of sudoriferous glands are to regulate body temperature and to eliminate waste products. As perspiration evaporates, it carries large amounts of body heat away from the skin surface. The most rapid process of heat dissipation is evaporation of perspiration.

Approximately 1 pint of aqueous fluid and impurities is lost in each 8-hour period when a person is visibly sweating. When sweat production is high, replacement of lost minerals is essential. When the sweating is low, most of the sodium chloride present in the perspiration is reabsorbed in the skin. In this case, mineral depletion is minimal.

Hypodermis

Also known as the subcutaneous layer or superficial fascia, the hypodermis is *not* a true layer of skin. A layer of adipose tissue forms a continuous layer between the dermis and the underlying muscle called the panniculus adiposus. The thickness of the panniculus adiposus varies with age, sex, and health. Infants and children have a uniform fat layer under the skin. Females have an extra thickness of adipose over the breasts, hips, and inner thighs. Males have an accumulation of fat on the nape of the neck, the deltoid muscle, the triceps muscle, and the abdominal region of the body.

SKIN CONDITIONS AND CLINICAL TERMS

1. **Skin Pallor.** This term refers to an unnatural paleness or lack of color of the skin.
2. **Striae.** Striae, or stria, are silvery to white stretch marks characterized by linear scars. These streaks often result from extreme stretching of the skin. This can be due to pregnancy, body building, sudden weight gain, or severe swelling due to accident or surgical complications.

   Deep massage is contraindicated on stretch marks. Massage will not remove or reduce striae because they are not a buildup of scar tissue. They are tearing, thinning, or overstretching of skin that actually reduces its thickness.
3. **Contusion.** Also known as a bruise, a contusion is an injury that does not disrupt the integrity of or break the skin. It is caused by a blow and is characterized by swelling, discoloration, and pain.

   Local massage is contraindicated. However, massage around the contusion may help facilitate its healing by increasing nutrition to and removal of wastes from the area.
4. **Blisters.** A blister is a collection of fluid below the epidermis sometimes caused by pressure or friction. Draining a blister constitutes medical treat-

ment and therefore is not in the massage therapist's scope of practice.

Local massage is contraindicated.

5. **Pruritus.** Pruritus is severe itching of the skin caused by dryness, sweat retention on the skin, kidney failure, allergic reactions, fungi, or parasitic agents such as scabies or body lice. Pruritus can also be caused by bile salts in the skin, cancer, or psychogenic disorders, such as emotional stress.
6. **Papule.** This is a small, round, firm, elevated area in the skin varying in size from a pinpoint to that of a small pea. An example of a papule is a wart.

   Local massage may be contraindicated, depending on the cause. For instance, if it is a wart, it can be contagious.

7. **Pustule.** This skin condition is a small, raised elevation of the skin, often with a "head" containing lymph or pus such as a pimple.

   Local massage is contraindicated.

8. **Acne Vulgaris.** This type of acne is an infection of the sebaceous glands and hair follicles, caused by bacteria. It causes inflammation and pus formation. Acne usually begins at puberty and may continue through adolescence. Scarring from acne vulgaris is common. Whiteheads are accumulations of dead bacteria, cell debris, and dead white blood cells. Blackheads are accumulations of dried sebum and bacteria in the gland and its duct. The black appearance is due to oxidation of the sebum.

   Massage over the infected area is contraindicated if there is extensive inflammation. The client may prefer facial massage without oil. It is important that massage therapists wash their hands thoroughly before massaging areas with acne.

9. **Senile Lentigo.** Commonly known as liver or age spots, senile lentigo are tan or brown patches found on the skin of older people, especially those who have been exposed to excessive sun.

   Massage is fine for clients with age spots.

10. **Impetigo.** This is an inflammatory skin infection caused by staphylococci or streptococci bacteria. It is characterized by raised, fluid-filled sores that itch or burn. This condition is most common in children, and it occurs mainly around the mouth, nose, and hands. Impetigo is highly contagious and can be spread by hand contact and handling contaminated objects such as linens, doorknobs, and toothbrushes.

    Local massage is definitely contraindicated.

11. **Furuncle.** This is a boil or an abscess caused by the staphylococcal bacteria, resulting in necrosis (death) of a hair follicle.

    Local massage is contraindicated. Lymph nodes in the area may be painfully enlarged, so massage over them should be avoided.

12. **Eczema.** Eczema, also known as chronic dermatitis, is an acute or chronic superficial inflammation of the skin characterized by redness, watery discharge, crusting, scaling, itching, and burning (Fig. 5–3A). This disorder is not contagious.

    Massage is fine for clients with eczema. Massage over affected areas is contraindicated if there are open areas and watery discharge.

13. **Psoriasis.** Psoriasis is characterized by distinct red, flaky skin elevations (Fig. 5–3B). A chronic form of dermatitis, it is marked by periods of remission and exacerbations. In severe forms, psoriasis is a disabling and disfiguring affliction and can involve the scalp, elbows, knees, back, and buttocks. Often, it is genetic. This disorder is not contagious.

    Massage is fine for clients with psoriasis. Some of the scales may dislodge during treatment.

14. **Seborrhea.** Seborrhea is a topical (pertaining to the surface) disease of the sebaceous glands, marked by an increase in the amount of oily secretions (Fig. 5–3C). Also known as "cradle cap" in infants, seborrhea begins as a pink raised patch that gradually turns yellow and scaly. The crust or

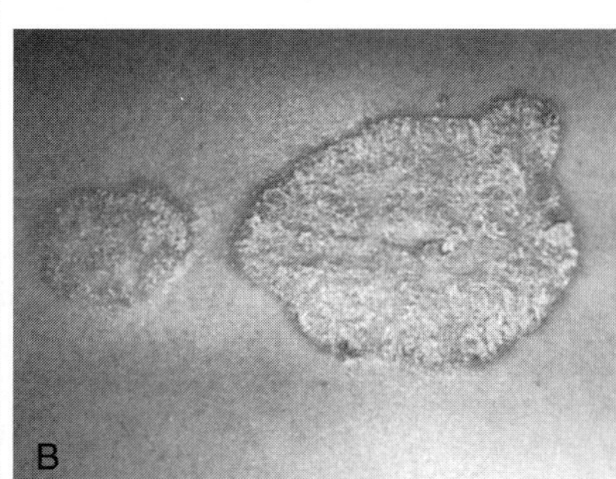

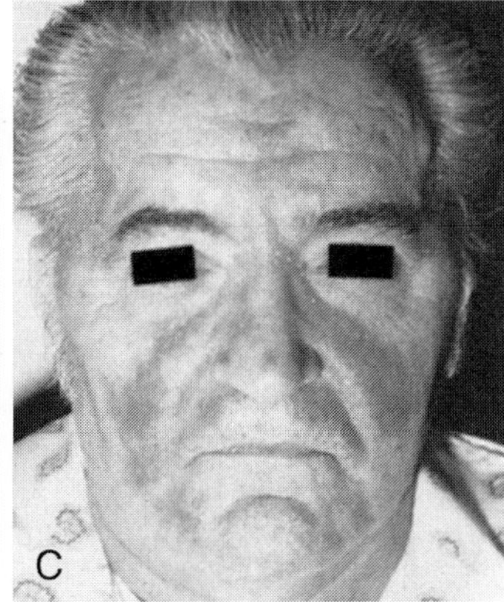

Figure 5•3 A, Eczema; B, psoriasis; and C, seborrhea.

scales can be removed by carefully washing or lubricating the area with oil, then gently brushing the hair to remove the buildup.

Local massage is contraindicated.

15. **Verruca.** Also known as a wart, verruca is a mass of cutaneous elevations caused by a contagious virus, papillomavirus. Most warts are not cancerous.

    Local massage is contraindicated because warts are contagious.

16. **Herpes Simplex.** Also known as cold sores or fever blisters, herpes simplex is a viral infection that has the ability to lie dormant for extended periods without expressing any signs or symptoms of disease. Cold sores are usually present at the site where mucous membranes meet the skin. The appearance of cold sores is associated with stimuli such as ultraviolet radiation from the sun, hormonal changes that occur during menstruation and pregnancy, or even emotional upset.

    Local massage is definitely contraindicated.

17. **Athlete's Foot.** Athlete's foot is a superficial fungal infection of the foot characterized by discoloration of the skin, a ring or ridge of red tissue (Fig. 5–4). The skin may also break, bleed, or ooze clear fluids. The infected foot often has an unpleasant odor. The same fungus may also cause jock itch or ringworm in other areas of the body.

    Local massage is contraindicated because this fungal infection is easily spread.

18. **Ringworm.** Ringworm is not a worm at all, but a group of fungal diseases characterized by itching, scaling, and sometimes painful lesions manifested as a raised red-ringed patch.

    Local massage is contraindicated because this is a contagious disorder.

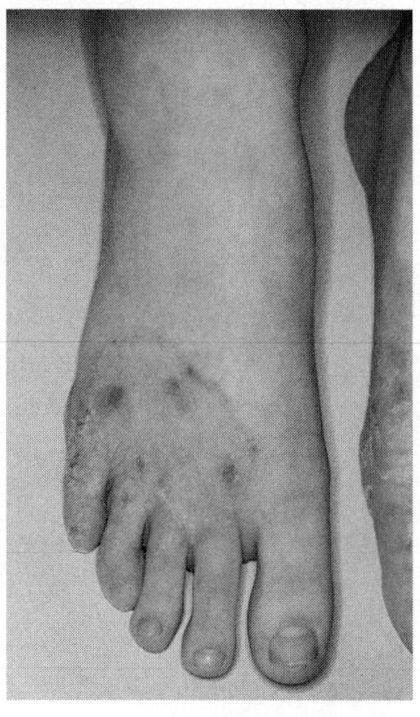

Figure 5•4 Athlete's foot.

19. **Decubitus Ulcers, Bedsores, Pressure Sores or Tropic Ulcers.** Decubitus ulcers are caused by constant deficiency of blood to tissues that have been subjected to prolonged pressure. This restriction of the normal blood supply to the skin results in cell necrosis. The weight of the body puts pressure on the skin (especially over bony projections), the cells die and ulcers form. Decubitus ulcers occur in bedridden patients who are not turned regularly, and in people who use wheelchairs, braces, or have casts.

    Local massage is contraindicated. Light massage in a wide area encircling the ulcer may be beneficial to increase blood flow to an area that has been deprived. Gentle active and passive range of motion exercises in bedridden clients will help with joint mobility. The client's caregiver should be advised of any redness, blistering, or ulcers the massage therapist notices.

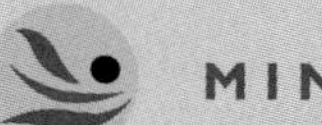

MINI•LAB

Take the bottom of a clear glass and press it into the heel of your hand. Describe the color changes and possible explanation for these changes. What would happen to the skin cells if the pressure were prolonged? How does this experiment reflect what happens to the skin when clients are bedridden? How can massage, with its circulatory effects, aid to prevent decubitus ulcers (bedsores)?

20. **Scleroderma.** Scleroderma is a rare autoimmune disorder affecting blood vessels and connective tissue. There is fibrous degeneration of the connective tissue of the skin, lungs, and internal organs. The skin tightens and becomes fixed to underlying tissues. Scleroderma may occur in a mild form with the person living 30 to 50 years, or there could be early death because of cardiac, renal, pulmonary, or intestinal involvement. There may be localized forms with just small patches of the skin involved. Scleroderma is not contagious.

    Massage is contraindicated for the severe forms. In less severe forms, massage can be beneficial. Friction and cross-fiber friction may help reduce adhesions. Deep strokes can increase local circulation and improve nutrition and drainage for the tissues. Passive and active range of motion can help retain joint mobility.

21. **Systemic Lupus Erythematosus.** This is also known as lupus. It is an autoimmune, inflammatory disease of connective tissue that occurs mostly in young women. It is not contagious. The cause of lupus is unknown, and its onset may be abrupt or

gradual. Symptoms include painful joints, fever, fatigue, weight loss, enlarged lymph nodes and spleen, sensitivity to light, and an eruption across the bridge of the nose and cheeks called a butterfly rash. There are periods of remission and exacerbation. Triggers for exacerbation include certain drugs, exposure to excessive sunlight, injury, and stress. Serious complications of the disease involve inflammation of the kidneys, liver, spleen, lungs, heart, and central nervous system.

Massage is contraindicated when clients have a flare-up. During periods of remission, a gentle full body massage is indicated. Clients may be on corticosteroids and anti-inflammatory drugs, so they may be more susceptible to bruising.

22. **Burns.** When the skin is damaged by heat, radiation, electricity, or chemical agents, skin cells perish. The damage that results is called a burn. Burns can be classified into three categories, depending on the severity of damage to the tissues and the area of involvement.

    - A first-degree burn is mild damage to the epidermis. Symptoms are redness and mild pain. An example of a first-degree burn is a mild sunburn, which typically heals in 2 to 3 days.
    - A second-degree burn damages the epidermis and the upper layers of the dermis. Some symptoms associated with second-degree burns are swelling, blistering, and pain. Hair follicles and sweat glands usually remain functional. Healing time can be from 7 days to 4 weeks. Once the burn heals, a mild scar remains.
    - A third-degree burn destroys the epidermis, the dermis, and the epidermal derivatives, like hair, nails, and associated glands. Because of the damage to the skin glands and hair follicles, the functions of the skin are reduced or nonexistent. Due to injury of the lymph capillaries and nerve endings, there is very little swelling and pain. A client with third-degree burns may experience limited mobility due to the restrictive effect of scar tissue. Almost all third-degree burns require skin grafting.

Massage should be performed only when tissue is fully healed and can withstand pressure. Unhealed skin is pink, thin, and delicate and should not be massaged. Gentle massage is indicated, and no movements should be forced. Friction and cross-fiber friction over healed and scarred tissue may help break up adhesions. Gentle range of motion can help increase mobility. Massage for clients with healed skin grafts should be to soften and loosen the graft and improve circulation. Massage over the graft should occur only after complete healing. Use a good quality lubricant, preferably one with cocoa butter, Aloe vera, and vitamin E.

23. **Skin Cancer.** Cancer of the skin is the most common form of cancer. It is also the least lethal because it is the most detectable. Ninety percent of all reported skin cancers can be abated through early detection and treatment. The best preventive measure anyone can take to reduce skin cancer is to avoid overexposure to the sun. This is more important for light-skinned people. Darker-skinned people have fewer incidents of skin cancer because they have more pigment, or melanin, to protect their cells from ultraviolet radiation. If you have to be in the sun, wear a sunscreen lotion with a sun protection factor (SPF) of 15 or more. The three most common types of skin cancer are basal cell carcinoma, squamous cell carcinoma, and malignant melanoma.

    Basal Cell Carcinoma. This accounts for about 75 percent of all cancers of the skin. This type of cancer is slow growing and is characterized by lesions that begin as small raised nodules that ulcerate (Fig. 5–5A). The primary cause of basal cell carcinoma is excessive exposure to ultraviolet radiation (sunlight). Basal cell carcinoma develops in the stratum germinativum (also known as the stratum basale) and rarely metastasizes.

    Squamous Cell Carcinoma. This type of cancer is more aggressive than basal cell carcinoma and accounts for about 20 percent of all cases of cancer. Squamous cell carcinoma also arises from the epidermis, beginning as a scaly pigmented area that may develop into a ulcerated crater (Fig. 5–5B). This type of cancer is common on sun-exposed areas like the face, neck, ears, and hands.

    Malignant Melanoma. One of the most malignant and lethal skin cancer types, melanoma is cancer of the melanocytes and begins as a raised dark lesion with irregular borders and appears uneven in color (Fig. 5–5C). It typically occurs in light-skinned people who are exposed to ultraviolet light radiation over many years. Melanoma is more likely to metastasize, or spread, than any other form of cancer. If you have a relative who has been diagnosed with melanoma, your risk factor is greater. Have any suspicious-looking moles checked by your personal physician.

Author's Note

Transdermal patches are used for conditions such as hormone replacement therapy and by clients who are trying to stop using tobacco products. Because the massage lubricant will weaken the adhesive, avoid up to 2 inches around the patch area.

If an area of complaint is under the transdermal

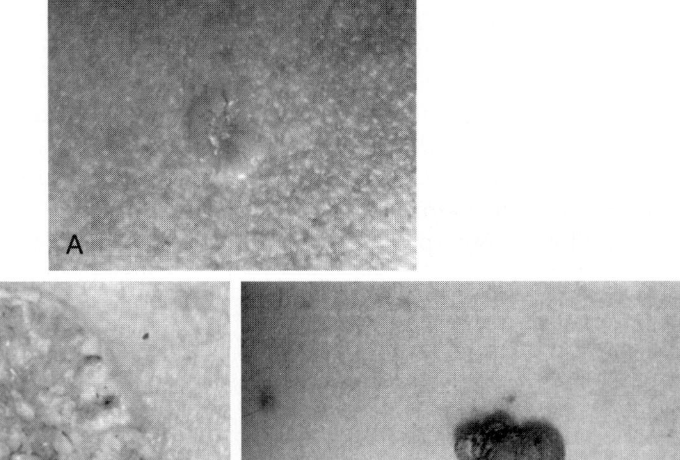

Figure 5•5 Any mole change must be brought to the client's attention. A, Basal cell carcinoma; B, Squamous cell carcinoma; C, Malignant melanoma.

patch, consult with the client's physician, and obtain permission to remove the patch. Proceed with the massage as usual. After the massage, clean the area with alcohol and reapply the patch.

Mole Changes

Observing any changes and reporting those changes to the client is an added service in massage therapy. Because our profession uses the skin as the primary organ of contact, we have the unique opportunity to notice any changes in the skin's surface. These changes are noted both visually and tactilely.

Mole changes may occur more frequently with people who are exposed to natural and artificial ultraviolet light. Mole changes may also be associated with friction or irritation from clothing (particularly bra straps), elastic waistbands, eyeglasses, or hard hats. Changes in moles should be noted and discussed with the client. A referral may be made to a medical doctor for diagnosis and possible treatment.

Common moles and melanoma do not look alike. Using the ABCD method of mole assessment listed below, you will be able to detect changing moles as they occur. Point these moles out to your clients and ask them to continue checking their moles at home. A mirror can be used for hard-to-see places on the body. If moles have any of the abnormal characteristics listed below, see a physician immediately.

Asymmetry. Asymmetry means that if a line were drawn down the middle, it does not create two equal halves. Common moles are symmetrical and round. Malignant moles are asymmetrical.

Border. The edges or borders of early malignant melanoma are uneven, often containing scalloped or notched edges.

Color. Different shades of brown or black are often the first sign of a problem. Common moles are evenly shaded brown. Black moles are darker than surrounding moles, and should be checked by a physician.

Diameter. Common moles are usually less than one-quarter inch in diameter (6 mm), the size of a pencil eraser. Early melanomas tend to be larger than common moles.

Other things to look for are changes in the texture

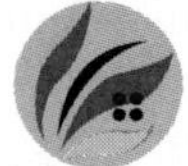

Rick, a weekly client for the past 4 years, had a large dark mole on the back of his left triceps. Annette, his massage therapist, noticed some subtle changes in the mole over a couple of weeks. She encouraged Rick to see his dermatologist or personal physician, just to be on the safe side.

Rick returned two weeks later with an adhesive bandage on his arm. The pathology report revealed malignant melanoma. Rick was elated; Annette's perceptiveness had enabled the doctors to catch the cancer in the early stages and he was going to be fine.

of the surface of a mole and a sore that does not heal properly.

SKIN AND ITS SENSORY RECEPTORS

The sense of touch is actually a complex composition of seven specialized receptors found in the skin. Touch is an amalgamation of many sensations and is the least understood of all the senses. Touch provides sensory input and physical information about our surroundings. This sense also warns the body of damage, such as the cooking pot is hot or your finger is in the way as you cut an orange with a sharp knife. Below is a list of all the currently known receptors and their functions.

1. **Meissner's Corpuscles.** These are receptors for light touch, responding to both the actual movement and the length of the movement across the skin. More specifically, Meissner's corpuscles monitor low-frequency vibration (the onset and removal of pressure), and adapt slowly. Meissner's corpuscles are located in the dermis just below the epidermis.
2. **Pacinian's (Laminated) Corpuscles.** Also known as corpuscles of Vater-Pacini, these pressure-sensitive receptors respond to skin displacement and high-frequency vibration. Unlike Meissner's corpuscles, Pacinian's corpuscles adapt quickly to all external stimuli. Notice how we quickly stop feeling an elastic band around our waist. The corpuscles are located in the deeper layers of the dermis and their shape resembles a fingerprint.
3. **Free Nerve Endings.** Free nerve endings are bare nerve endings that detect pain. They are also known as nociceptors and they are located in all parts of the body, especially in the skin. They can be stimulated by extremes in temperature, intense mechanical stimulation, and specific chemicals in extracellular fluid, including ones released by injured cells.
4. **Merkel's Disks.** Located in the epidermis (stratum germinativum), these bodies respond to skin displacement, somewhat like the Meissner's and Pacinian's corpuscles, but Merkel's disks have the capacity for a longer or more continuous response.
5. **Hair-Follicle Receptors.** Each hair follicle is wrapped by a nerve that responds briefly to hair movement. These receptors may alert us to "goosebumps" or a small breeze or an intrusive insect.
6. **Krause's End Bulbs.** Although the operating mechanism of Krause's end bulbs is not exactly known, they are believed to be stimulated by lowering temperatures and are found widely distributed in the hypodermis.
7. **Ruffini's End Organs.** These bodies alert us when the skin comes into contact with deep or continuous pressure. Some references indicate that these receptors detect the increase of temperature (i.e., warmth and heat). Ruffini's end organs are located in the subcutaneous tissue, principally at the junction of the dermis and the subcutaneous tissue.

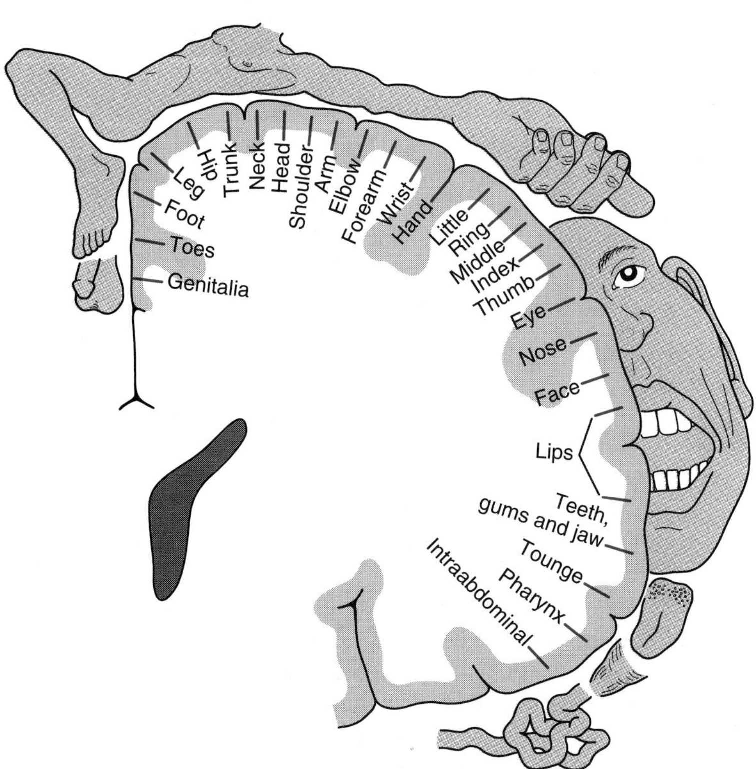

Figure 5•6 An illustration of the "homunculus," meaning "little man," in the postcentral gyrus.

In October of 1996, my husband and I journeyed to San Francisco to sit for the National Certification Exam for Massage Therapists and Bodyworkers. After completing the exam, we settled into a cable car tour of the city, but anatomy information was still predominant in my brain.

The sky was bright and clear, but the warmth of this Indian summer was canceled by the 30-mile-an hour wind coming off the bay. As I huddled under a blanket on the trolley, I began to wonder why Mike seemed oblivious to the cold. The popular theories hold that metabolism and body fat are responsible for differences in individuals. Metabolism also made sense, but I wondered if genetics could have something to do with it. What if the number of cold and heat receptor organs in the skin is an inherited condition? Could some people have a greater concentration of Krause's end bulbs, making them more "cold-natured"? Could my spouse just have more Ruffini's end organs than I? This may be a good research project someday.

The Brain's Role in Touch

The brain detects the sensation of touch in the parietal lobe of the cerebral cortex. The postcentral gyrus, an elevated area of brain tissue located in the parietal lobe, is where the axons that detect touch terminate. Keep in mind that the right postcentral gyrus represents the left side of the body and vice versa. It is interesting just how much gray matter is dedicated to each surface area (Fig. 5–6). The hand and face (mainly lips and jaw and tongue) take up about 80 percent of this neural space. The more space devoted to an area in the postcentral gyrus, the more sensory "touch" receptors are found in the corresponding part of the body. The more sensory receptors located in that part of the body, the more "sensitive" it is.

SKIN AND THE IMPORTANCE OF TOUCH

There are so many other forms of communication that can be and should be used. Not just pictures and melodies, but touch, dance, and food.

—Pete Seeger

While an intellectual comprehension of anatomy and physiology is vital to the understanding of the skin, it is the sense of touch itself that enables us to actually experience this knowledge. *The sense of touch is the massage therapist's main avenue used to affect another human being* and is the body's main method of gathering information about itself. In contrast, an artist uses the sense of vision, and a musician uses the sense of hearing to communicate with others. Touching can affect us physically, intellectually, psychologically, and emotionally.

Aristotle was the first to enumerate the five senses. Of all the senses, only touch involves the *entire body*. The other four senses reside in the head. Indeed, touch is not one sense, but many. Touch can detect deep pressure or light stroking. It can differentiate between the weight of a feather and immersion in water.

The skin is temperature sensitive. It can distinguish between the warmth of wooden bleacher seats on a summer day and the cool shade found beneath the live oaks lining the still bayous of the South. It communicates intrusions, from the tickle of a kitten's fur to the intense pain of a nail piercing your shoe sole.

Touch is the most primitive of all sensations. Among the many studies that have been conducted, touch is the earliest sensory system to become functional in the human embryo. When the embryo is less than 6 weeks old, measuring less than an inch long from crown to rump, light stroking of the upper lip or wings of the nose will cause bending of the neck and trunk away from the source of stimulation. At this stage of gestation, neither the eyes nor ears have developed.

The skin and the brain arise from ectoderm, the same cells that give rise to the entire nervous system, including the sense organs of smell, taste, hearing, and vision—all of which keeps the organism informed about what is going on in its environment. Because of the ectoderm connection, the skin is considered exposed neural tissue, and, in contrast, the brain is immersed skin. As you probably recall from earlier in this chapter, a large portion of parietal lobe in the brain is involved with touch or tactile stimulation. We can therefore regard the skin as a "superficial nervous system."

Perhaps the fact that touch is such a primal sensation is precisely what makes it such a powerful therapeutic tool. Our first lessons about love and tenderness are learned through the medium of touch. Whether breast- or bottle-fed, our first meals were touch centered. Touch communicated some of our early experiences with pain. Quite often, this sense played a major role in the physical and emotional healing of those same wounds. Everyone, whether nurse or patient, massage therapist or client, parent or child, lover or friend, can look back on a time when touch played a personal role that was extremely important.

Touch is our first means of communication, and the skin is our main organ of sensation. We can see, hear, and think about something, but it is through touch that the event becomes part of our personal experience. Touch can alter how we perceive the world. Touch can also stimulate us to action.

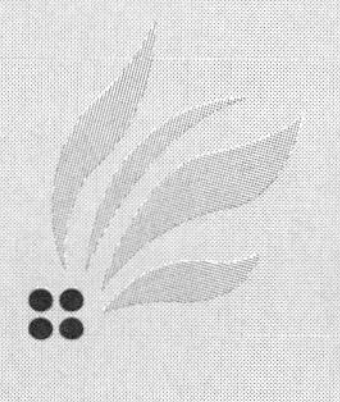

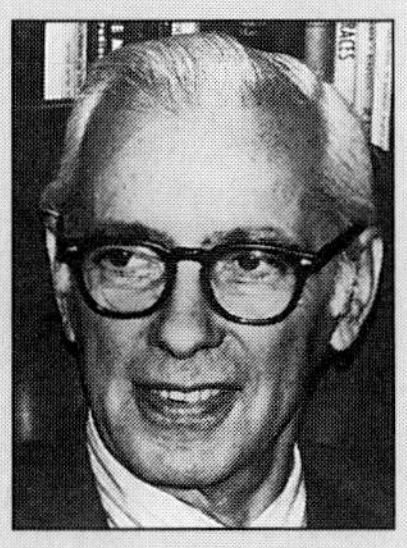

Ashley Montagu

Born: June 28, 1905

"To be kind, to be, to do, and to depart gracefully."

Ashley Montagu was born in London, England. After studying at the University of London and the University of Florence, he came to the United States in 1927. He earned his Ph.D. from Columbia University in 1937. That same year he published his first book *Coming into Being Among the Aborigines.* Between 1937 and 1988, he authored over 50 books, most of which are in their second or third editions. In 1940, he become a naturalized U.S. citizen. Montagu's long and distinguished academic career included positions at some of the most respected schools in the country. He was a professor of anatomy at Hahnemann Medical College and Hospital, Philadelphia, 1938–49, Chairman, Department of Anthropology, Rutgers University, 1940–55, and a lecturer at Princeton University from 1978 to 1983. During this period Montagu also held many other concurrent positions in education, professional associations, the United Nations, and the media. His listing in *Who's Who in America,* 1998, is over 5½ column inches long. Very few individuals have listings that are over 2 inches.

Ashley Montagu is one of the few scientists who has recognized that touch is an enormously important experience for every human being, not only from birth but from the moment that life begins in the womb. As a professor of anatomy and anthropology, he was inspired to begin researching the effects of touch and nurturing after reading an article on the effects of thyroid surgery on two groups of rodents. The first group had a 75 percent survival rate. They were cared for by a woman doctor who caressed each rodent at feeding time. In the second group, the animals all died very rapidly. They were cared for by a male lab attendant who threw food into the cages and roughly clanged the door. Although the article noted this, it attached no significance to it; Montagu did. In sharing this study with a class he was teaching, a student from a farming area told Montagu that everyone knows that newborn animals must be licked by their mother or they soon die. These were the clues that led him to begin his research on effective nurturing. As a scientist, Montagu solved, scientifically, the mysteries concerning the attributes that make up what we understand to be love. In his own words, "It [Love] is the communication to another, by demonstrative *acts,* of your profound involvement in their welfare."

His books, lectures, and papers have emphasized that a healthy mental state results from effective nurturing. He says, of his own findings, that "the most surprising of all things was that doctors had rarely understood this."

Most of Ashley Montagu's books deal in some way with the human condition. One of his most important to those of us in the health care professions is *Touching: The Human Significance of the Skin,* a must read for all massage therapists. He is also well known for his books *The Elephant Man* and *Man's Most Dangerous Myth, The Fallacy of Race,* now in its sixth edition.

In 1987 Ashley Montagu was honored with the Distinguished Achievement Award of the American Anthropological Association; in 1994, with the Darwin Award of the American Association of Physical Anthropologists; and in 1995, with the American Humanist of the Year Award. So far, he has received over a dozen major words and two honorary doctorate degrees during his long and prolific career. At this writing, Montagu is 92 years old. He continues to lecture, write, and to create updated editions of his books, extending and applying his findings about relationships between human beings and the planet.

When asked what he would like to tell future massage therapists he says, "to understand that what they are doing is very important indeed. That by caressing another human being's body, in which you are trained to do, I hope, by communicating this involvement in their welfare, what you are doing is what human beings should always be doing, all the days of their lives—caressing other people."

MINI·LAB

Write about a time in your life when touch was meaningful to you in a personal way. (Your essay will probably be longer than the space shown here.)

Our intention during a massage can alter the result of the session. If you approach the massage with too many personal or therapeutic agendas, you may not be able to listen to what the body is telling you. This is very similar to having a one-sided conversation with someone; when you do all the talking, all you hear is yourself! Sometimes in massage therapy our desire to "help" interferes with our actual ability to observe what the client needs to happen. It helps to be willing to approach the massage table totally empty and willing to "listen."

In massage, touch is not a monologue; it is a dialogue. It is a reciprocal exchange. The client's body leads you in a certain direction, and you follow. Your hands, in turn, communicate with the client's tissue, and it responds accordingly. Spoken communication and the tissue response you feel in the client's skin give you the information you need to create therapeutic impact. Your hands become sensitive miniature microphones sensing restrictions in the tissue. With this information, you can verify or discard your original therapeutic assessment and offer the client the fullness of your therapeutic abilities.

Then if we combine the approaches of the two preceding paragraphs, we can create a session that is client focused *and* experience led. In this time of being both full and empty, the massage therapist can actually bring awareness to the clients and initiate the dialogue that can effect positive change.

Touch Research

Many doctors, nurses, biochemists, and psychologists have developed studies on the effects of touch. These studies address physical, intellectual, psychological, and emotional themes. Several studies discussed here are considered groundbreaking and fundamental. Below are brief summaries from research that focus on touch as a medium of communication. As you read them and draw your own conclusions, apply the concepts you develop to your attitude about massage and to your role as a caregiver.

Harry Harlow. In 1958, Dr. Harlow, a pioneer in touch deprivation research, conducted experiments at the University of Wisconsin that involved the isolation of monkeys during their early developmental stages. After a period of time, these touch-deprived monkeys exhibited evidence of emotional and social impairment. The lack of touch during their early developmental years had left them neurotic and socially retarded. Most female monkeys refused mating by becoming hostile and aggressive when approached. The monkeys that did mate rejected or harmed their young. Harlow observed that during periods of isolation, the infant monkeys valued tactile stimulation more than they did nourishment. Harlow then created

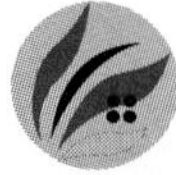

The Effects of Massage on the Integumentary System

1. Massage stimulates sebaceous glands of the skin, causing an increase in sebum production. This added sebum improves the skin's condition, texture, and tone.
2. Through increased circulation, massage strokes increase insensible perspiration by stimulating the sudoriferous glands located in the skin.
3. Creating increased circulation and heat, massage stimulates vasomotor activity in skin. As superficial blood vessels dilate, the skin appears hyperemic (reddish pink) and feels warm to the touch. This increased skin circulation will bring added nutrients to these tissues
4. Massage applied to scar tissue helps to reduce the formation of superficial keloids in the skin and reduce excessive scar formations in the soft tissues beneath the site of massage application.

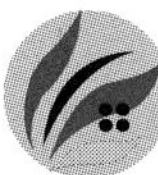

Effects of Massage on Connective Tissues

1. Theoretically, massage flattens out adipose globules located under the skin and makes the skin seem smoother. Cellulite, a type of adipose tissue, appears as groups of small dimples or depressions under the skin. Dimples are caused by an uneven separation of fat globules below the skin's surface, which is displaced by manual manipulation. Massage does not reduce the amount of cellulite present below the skin; instead, massage temporarily alters the shape and appearance of cellulite.
2. Deep massage displaces adhesions and rearranges scar tissue. Deep friction can create an appropriate scar that is strong, yet does not interfere with the muscle's ability to broaden as it contracts. Massage therefore helps to restore normal, pain-free motion of the affected joint if restrictions are due to adhesions.

two artificial surrogate "mothers." One was a bare wire sculpture of a monkey that housed a bottle of formula. The other was a fur-covered wire monkey that felt and smelled like other monkeys, but offered no food. The infant monkeys preferred to cling to the "mother" who provided a semblance of physical contact without nourishment rather than to the wire models that provided food (Fig. 5–7).

Author's Note

What is a double-blind study? The outcomes of scientific experiments can be distorted when either the scientist or the subject interjects their own prejudices, whether consciously or unconsciously. In order to prevent this from occurring, the double-blind study was developed. Using the double-blind format, both the scientists and the subjects are kept intentionally unaware of key factors of the experiment. These factors include which subjects belong to the group being tested, which subjects are in the control group receiving the placebo (nonmedicinal agent), what specific treatment or substance is being administered, and what the outcome of the study is attempting to prove.

Bernard Grad. Grad, a Canadian biochemist, conducted his groundbreaking touch research on mice and barley seedlings in the early 1960s. In the first of his double-blind studies, 300 mice were selected and injured in the same manner. One-third were allowed to heal without intervention, one-third were held by medical students who did not profess to heal, and one-third were held by a faith healer. After just 2 weeks, the mice held by the faith healer recovered remarkably faster than the mice in both of the other groups.

For the barley seed study, Grad soaked the seeds in a saline solution to get them off to a bad start. The seeds were then divided into three equal groups. The first group was watered with tap water. The second group was soaked using water held by disinterested students, and the last group was irrigated with water that was held by a renowned healer. The seeds that were watered by the healer sprouted faster, grew taller, and contained more green chlorophyll than either of the other two groups.

Dr. Delores Krieger. In the 1970s, Dr. Krieger, a professor at New York University, became interested in touch healing through studies like Grad's. She was fascinated with the idea that intent was so important in healing touch. Using noninvasive techniques, Krieger wanted to apply the concepts of Grad's work in a way that could help her patients.

Through Krieger's research a tangible relationship emerged between touching and healing. She was able to measure an increase in the hemoglobin content of the blood, which directly corresponded to levels of touching. Hemoglobin is the oxygen-carrying molecule in red blood cells. In Krieger's study, when a healthy person placed his hands on or near an ill person for 10 to 15 minutes, with the intent to heal, this was enough to cause the measurable increase.

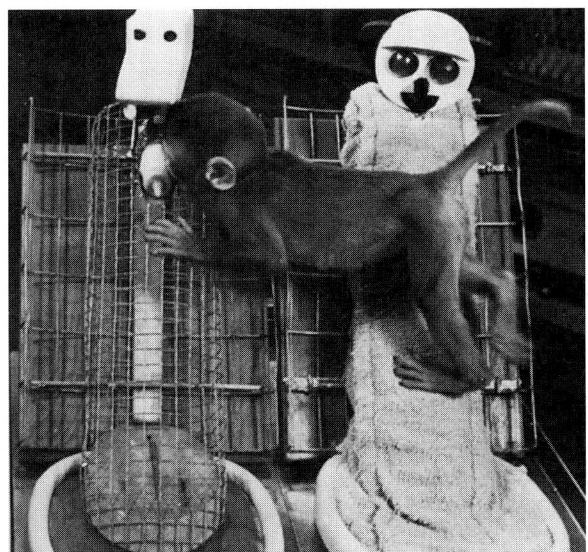

Figure 5•7 Harlow's monkeys. (Courtesy of Harlow Private Laboratory, Madison, WI.)

Dr. Tiffany Field. Tiffany Field Ph.D., professor of pediatrics, psychology, and psychiatry of the University of Miami School of Medicine, began a research project to study the effects of massage on 40 premature babies. Half of the group was massaged three times a day for 15 minutes for 10 days. The massaged infants gained 47 percent more weight. They spent less time in the hospital than the babies who were not massaged, even though both groups of babies had the same number of feedings and averaged the same intake per feeding. The massaged babies were also more active, alert, and stayed about 6 days less in the hospital. The massaged babies were also more socially active, more responsive, and had better coordination and motor skills than the nonmassaged babies. She published the results of this research in 1986.

In research published in 1997, Dr. Tiffany Field, at the Touch Research Institute in Miami, found that individuals who received a 15-minute seated massage twice a week showed increased cognitive ability, performed better on math tests, and completed problems with increased accuracy and speed. These individuals also experienced a significant decrease in tension over individuals who practiced traditional relaxation techniques without massage.

Wayne Dennis. In the 1950s, Dennis published his findings on what he called, infant and child "retardation." His research was based on his experience at an orphanage in Beirut, Lebanon. He found that the facility that contained the orphanage was more than adequate, but because of the orphanage's meager income, personnel was limited to one employee to ten infants. The children were only taken out of the cribs for feedings, diaper changing, and a daily bath. The children remained in the crib until they began to pull up on the sides. From that point, they were placed in a playpen during the daylight hours with two other children. Opportunities for touch were very limited. A large number of these children died, even though they were receiving adequate nutrition and hygiene. The children who did survive were dwarfed or deformed.

The explanation Dennis gave for his findings of marasmus (wasting away) combined with the tragic death rates of the Lebanese orphanages were the result of touch deprivation, lack of physical stimulation, and learning opportunities. The employees were so busy providing for their physical needs, they did not have time to hold and caress the infants. When aides were hired to rock and sing to these children, mortality rates dropped 70 percent.

Dr. Marc H. Hollender. In 1970, Hollender conducted a study at the Department of Psychiatry, Vanderbilt School of Medicine, Nashville, Tennessee, using a test group of 39 women. He found that the need for human contact varied from person to person. Furthermore, this need for touch changed from time to time. After conducting surveys and interviews with these women, he determined that more than 50 percent used sex as a way of getting their touch needs met and not because they desired the sexual act.

Hollender and his team of researchers commented that "the desire to be cuddled and held is acceptable to most people as long as it is regarded as a component of adult sexuality. The wish to be cuddled and held in a maternal manner is felt to be too childish. To avoid embarrassment or shame, women convert it into the longing to be held by a man as part of an adult activity, involving sexual intercourse."

Abraham Maslow. In the 1960s, Maslow, a renowned psychologist, placed the needs of human beings in a sequential order, from the most basic to the most ideal and abstract. He believed that these needs directed all human behavior and as these basic needs are met, other needs begin to emerge until the individual reaches what he terms "self-actualization." Maslow called this the Theory of Human Motivation.

Maslow states that we have five general needs, beginning from the biological needs of food, water, and sleep. The other levels, in order of importance are safety and security, love and belonging, self-esteem and the esteem of others and finally, self-actualization. Maslow characterized the self-actualized person as self-accepting, striving to help others, and engaging in activities that will help the person achieve the highest potential. His model was later redesigned, with the help of other psychologists, to a broader list of human needs. It is interesting to note that touching and skin contact are ranked very high on the list, just below the individual's needs for a safe shelter. Many massage therapists will attest to the fact that clients often receive massage to get their "touch needs" met.

A Hierarchy of Human Needs

(Compiled in part from Maslow, 1962; Miller 1981; Weil, 1973; Glasser, 1985.)

1. Survival
2. Safety
3. Touching, skin contact
4. Attention
5. Mirroring and echoing
6. Guidance
7. Listening
8. Being real
9. Participating
10. Acceptance
    - Others are aware of, take seriously and admire the Real You
    - Freedom to be the Real You
    - Tolerance of your feelings
    - Validation

Respect
Belonging and love
11. Opportunity to grieve losses and to grow
12. Support

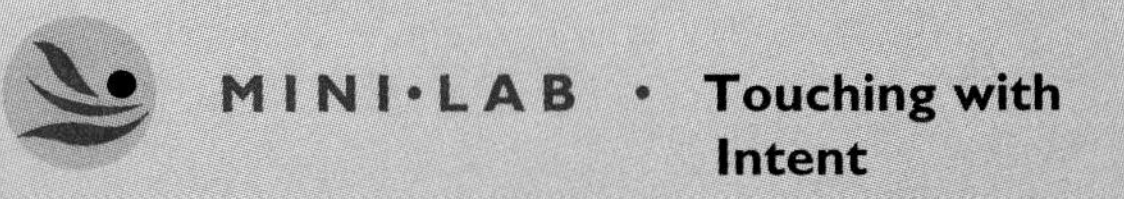

MINI•LAB • Touching with Intent

Props: None required.

Procedure

1. Locate a partner.
2. Assign one person as the "giver" and one person as the "receiver." Sit facing each other.
3. The receiver extends his or her hands, palms up. The giver places his or her hands on the receiver's hands, palm down. Both the giver and the receiver close their eyes.
4. The giver becomes unfocused, disinterested, and mentally distracted as the receiver stays open and passive for 2 minutes.
5. After that time, the giver becomes very aware, interested, and concerned about the receiver. This attitude is maintained for 2 minutes.
6. Reverse roles and repeat.
7. Share your experiences with each other. Some questions to ask are "Did you notice any differences when the attitudes changed?" "Does intent really alter how touch is received?" "How can I use this information during a massage therapy session?"

13. Loyalty and trust
14. Accomplishment
    Mastery, "Power," "Control"
    Creativity
    Having a sense of completion
    Making a contribution
15. Altering one's state of consciousness, transcending the ordinary
16. Sexuality
17. Enjoyment or fun
18. Freedom
19. Nurturing
20. Unconditional Love (including connection with a Higher Power)

SUMMARY

The skin is so much more than an external covering. It is a highly sensitive boundary between our body and the environment. It offers protection, heat exchange, vitamin synthesis, waste removal and serves as a membrane of interfacing. We can survive without sight, taste, smell, or hearing, but to lose our sense of touch would leave us walled off from our environment and from contact with others.

Touch offers us a sense of nourishment and a feeling of belonging. The need for touch intensifies during periods of stress and cannot be addressed without the participation of another person. Without touch, we experience profound psychological pain. If massage does nothing else than to nurture the human race through touch, our profession will be providing a great service.

SELF-TEST

Multiple Choice • Write the letter of the best answer in the space provided.

_______ 1. The largest organ in the body by weight is the

A. liver C. skin
B. brain D. bladder

_______ 2. The epidermis is made from which germ layer.

A. phisoderm C. mesoderm
B. endoderm D. ectoderm

_______ 3. The superficial layer of the epidermis is the

A. stratum corneum C. stratum lucidum
B. stratum spinosum D. stratum germinativum

_______ 4. Skin color variations exist due to the amount of oxygen and bilirubin in the blood and specialized cells in the stratum spinosum and stratum germinativum called

A. hemocytes C. erythrocytes
B. osteocytes D. melanocytes

_______ 5. Which structure is responsible for making our skin pigmentation darker?

A. keratin C. carotene
B. melanin D. sebum

_______ 6. What structure is heavily keratinized, forming thin hard plates and located on the distal ends of the fingers and toes?

A. nails C. carotene
B. melanin D. sebum

_______ 7. The main visible part of the nail is the

A. proximal nail fold C. body
B. lunula D. hyponychium

_______ 8. Which layer is known as the true skin?

A. epidermis C. melanocytes
B. dermis D. hypodermis

_______ 9. Collagen and elastin are fibers in cells of the

A. epidermis C. melanocytes
B. dermis D. A and C

_______ 10. Pouchlike depressions in the skin that enclose the hair shaft are called hair

A. cuticles C. follicles
B. muscles D. permanents

_______ 11. What is the hair muscle called?

A. arrector pili C. sebaceous glands
B. sudoriferous glands D. melanocytes

_______ 12. Irritation of the hair follicle can be caused by

A. pulling of the hair
B. not using enough lubricant
C. allergic reaction to lubricant
D. all of the above

_______ 13. What is another term used to describe the subcutaneous layer?

A. deep epidermis C. melanocyte
B. subdermis D. hypodermis

_______ 14. Which exocrine gland is associated with the hair follicle and secrete sebum?

A. arrector pili C. sebaceous glands
B. sudoriferous glands D. melanocytes

_______ 15. Which exocrine glands secrete sweat, or perspiration?

A. arrector pili C. sebaceous glands
B. sudoriferous glands D. melanocytes

_______ 16. By what mechanism does the skin help in regulating the body's temperature?

A. sweating C. tanning
B. digestion D. keratin

_______ 17. In which burn classification are both the skin and subcutaneous tissues destroyed?

A. first-degree C. second-degree
B. third-degree D. fourth-degree

_______ 18. According to Maslow's Hierarchy of Human Needs, touching skin contact is listed as having which order of importance?

A. first
C. third
B. second
D. last

_______ 19. The most lethal type of skin cancer is

A. basal cell carcinoma
B. epidemical carcinoma
C. squamous cell carcinoma
D. malignant melanoma

Matching • List the letter of the answer to the term or phrase that best describes it. One will be used twice.

A. Free nerve endings
B. Merkel's disk
C. Ruffini's end organs
D. Meissner's corpuscles
E. Hair-follicle receptors
F. Pacinian's (laminated) corpuscles
G. Krause's end bulbs

_______ 1. detects pressure, has a longer, more continuous response

_______ 2. pressure sensitive; responds to skin displacement and high-frequency vibration

_______ 3. responds to deep and continuous pressure and heat

_______ 4. detects light pressure

_______ 5. stimulation brings about erect hair

_______ 6. pain receptors

_______ 7. believed to respond to cold

_______ 8. also known as nociceptors

References

Applegate, Edith J., M.S. *The Anatomy and Physiology Learning System: Textbook.* Philadelphia: W. B. Saunders, 1995.

American Cancer Foundation. "The ABCD's of Moles and Melanomas," 1985.

Clarke, A. M. and A. D. Clarke. *Early Experience: Myth and Evidence.* London: Open Books, 1976.

Dennis, Wayne. Causes of Retardation Among Institutionalized Children. *The Journal of Genetic Psychology,* Vol. 96, 1960.

Field, Tiffany, Ph.D., Charles Bauer, and Jerome Nystrom. "Tactile/Kinesthetic Stimulation Effects on Preterm Neonates." *Pediatrics,* Vol. 77 No. 5., May 1986.

Gerson, Joel. *Standard Textbook for Professional Estheticians.* Albany: Delmar Publishers, 1992.

Gould, Barbara E. *Pathophysiology for the Health-Related Professionals.* Philadelphia: W. B. Saunders, 1997.

Grad, Bernard. "The Influence of an Unorthodox Method of Treatment on Wound Healing in Mice." *International Journal of Parapsychology.* Spring 1961.

Guyton, Arthur, M.D. *Human Physiology and Mechanisms of Disease,* 3rd ed. Philadelphia: W. B. Saunders Company, 1982.

Harlow, H. and M. Harlow. "Learning to Love." *American Scientist,* Vol. 54, 1966.

Haubrich, William S. *Medical Meanings, A Glossary of Word Origins.* New York: Harcourt Brace Jovanovich, 1984.

Hollender, Marc., L. Luborsky, and T. J. Scaramella. "The Wish to Be Held." *Archives of General Psychiatry,* Vol. 22, 1970.

Juhan, Deane. *Job's Body, A Handbook for Bodyworkers.* Barrington, NY: Station Hill Press, 1987.

Kalat, James W. *Biological Psychology,* 2nd ed. Belmont, California: Wadsworth Publishing Company, 1984.

Kendall, Florence and Elizabeth McCreary. *Muscles: Testing and Function.* Baltimore: Williams & Wilkins, 1983.

Kordish, Mary and Sylvia Dickson. *Introduction to Basic Human Anatomy.* Lake Charles, LA: McNeese State University, Self-Published Manual, 1985.

Krieger, Dolores. Therapeutic Touch: The Imprimatur of Nursing. *American Journal of Nursing,* Vol. 75 No. 5, 1975.

Marieb, Elaine N. *Essentials of Human Anatomy and Physiology,* 4th ed. New York: Benjamin/Cummings Publishing Company, Inc, 1994.

McAleer, Neil. *The Body Almanac.* Garden City, NY: Doubleday and Company, Inc., 1985.

Montagu, Ashley. *Touching: The Human Significance of the Skin,* 2nd ed. New York: Harper and Row Publishers, 1978.

Mosby's Medical, Nursing, and Allied Health Dictionary, 4th ed. St Louis: Mosby–Year Book, Inc., 1994.

Newton, Don. *Pathology for Massage Therapists,* 2nd ed. Portland: Simran Publications, 1995.

Olsen, Andrea and Caryn McHose. *BodyStories: A Guide to Experiential Anatomy.* Barrytown, New York: Station Hill Press, 1991.

Premkumar, Kalyani. *Pathology A to Z—A Handbook for Massage Therapists.* Calgary, Canada: VanPub Books, 1996.

Tabers Cyclopedic Medical Dictionary, 13th ed. Philadelphia: F. A. Davis Company, 1977.

Tortora Gerald J. *Introduction to the Human Body: The Essentials of Anatomy and Physiology,* 3rd ed. New York: HarperCollins Publishers. 1994.

Spitz, R. "Hospitalism: An Inquiry into the Genesis of Psychiatric Conditions of Early Childhood." *Psychoanalytic Study of the Child,* Vol. 2, 1945.

What a piece of work is man.
—Shakespeare

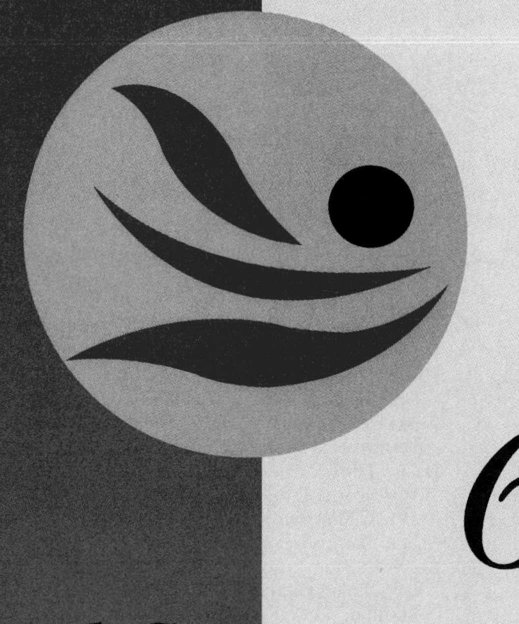

6 Skeletal System

Student Objectives

After completing this chapter, the student should be able to:

- Recall the five functions of the skeletal system
- Group the bones into four classifications, according to their shape
- Determine if a bone is part of the axial skeleton or the appendicular skeleton
- List and describe the surface markings on bones
- Compare synarthrotic, amphiarthrotic, and diarthrotic joints
- Identify the six types of synovial joints and give an example of each
- Demonstrate all the possible movements of the synovial joints

INTRODUCTION

The skeletal system is composed of bones, cartilage, ligaments, and joints. For those of you who have never thought much about your bones, you may be surprised. Not only do they provide protection and support movement, they also store minerals like calcium and phosphorus.

Bone is living tissue. Yes, our skeleton is alive. The skeletons we see in art classes, laboratories, and museums are the mineral salts that remain after death, representing approximately 65 percent of our total bony weight. The other 35 percent is a mixture of connective tissues in a watery ground substance, or matrix, containing many blood vessels and nerves. Bones are one of the hardest materials in the body, yet they are relatively light, somewhat flexible, and able to resist tension and other forces of stress. It cannot be emphasized strongly enough that bones must be physically stressed in order to remain healthy. The more you use them, the stronger they will become. When we remain physically active, when muscles and gravity exert force on our skeleton, the bones respond by becoming stronger.

There are 206 bones in the human body, or 210 bones if you count the sesamoid bones under each thumb and great toe. Bones are the "steel girders" of the body, forming our internal framework. Without our bony framework, we would crawl around on our bellies like worms or puddle up like a jellyfish out of water.

Mammals, ranging from humans to bats to elephants, have remarkably similar skeleton systems. For example, there are seven vertebrae in the human cervical spine; it may surprise you to discover that both the long-necked giraffe and the no-necked whale have seven cervical vertebrae as well.

The skeletal system is of the utmost importance to the massage therapist because it constitutes the road map for locating muscles. Muscles attach to bones at various bony markings known as origins and insertions. Because bones are hard, most markings are easy to palpate. Learn your bony markings well in the next chapter because they will guide you into locating the muscles that are causing your clients the most difficulty. Muscles are located between their attachment points.

The study of the skeletal system is multifaceted. Besides the basic structure and function of bone, we will also study movement and leverage, types of joints and articulations, abnormal conditions, and the general bony markings.

FUNCTIONS

The skeletal system serves a wide variety of functions. They are as follows:

1. It supports the body through a bony framework.
2. It protects the body's vital organs.
3. The skeleton gives leverage through muscle attachment.
4. The bones house the mechanism of **hemopoiesis,** or the forming of blood cells, producing both red and white blood cells, and platelets in the marrow of long bones.
5. Fats are stored in bone marrow to be released when needed. Osseous tissue, or bone tissue, acts as a reservoir for minerals such as calcium phosphate, calcium carbonate, phosphorus, magnesium, and sodium, which are stored and released when the body needs them. Skeletons in the earliest fish were external, or exoskeletons. Like the teeth, mineral deposits were a one-way process. Once minerals were deposited, they were as good as lost. With our endoskeleton, minerals vital to metabolism can be deposited, removed, replaced, or distributed throughout the body. All this is accomplished through vascular interfacing with the bones. In this way, our skeleton can act as a storehouse for minerals. Many physiologists claim that the metabolic properties of bones, like fat and mineral storage, are primary to their function of support.

HISTOLOGY AND STRUCTURES

The skeletal system is composed of five types of connective tissue: osseous tissue, cartilage, ligaments, periosteum, and bone marrow. Most of these tissue types have been introduced in Chapter 4. Osseous tissue can be classified according to its texture—spongy bone and compact bone—differing only in bone density. Spongy bone, which is the lighter of the two, is a lattice-like bony network found in the bony thin plate, or trabeculae, which is typically filled with red bone marrow. Compact bone forms the periphery of all bones and the majority of the shaft of long bones (Fig. 6–1). The rest of this section will introduce you to several microscopic tissues within the skeletal system, as well as structures associated with bones.

1. **Osteoblasts** are bone-forming cells found in the connective tissue sheath on the surface of the bone, known as the periosteum.
2. **Osteoclasts** are cells in bone whose function is to break down osseous tissue to maintain homeostasis and to repair bone.
3. **Osteocytes** are mature osteoblasts that soon become embedded in the bone matrix.
4. **Ossification** is the process by which bone develops. There are two types of ossification, intramembranous ossification, or the formation of bone from a membrane, and intracartilaginous ossification, or formation of bone from cartilage. Intramembranous ossification is found on the roof and sides of the

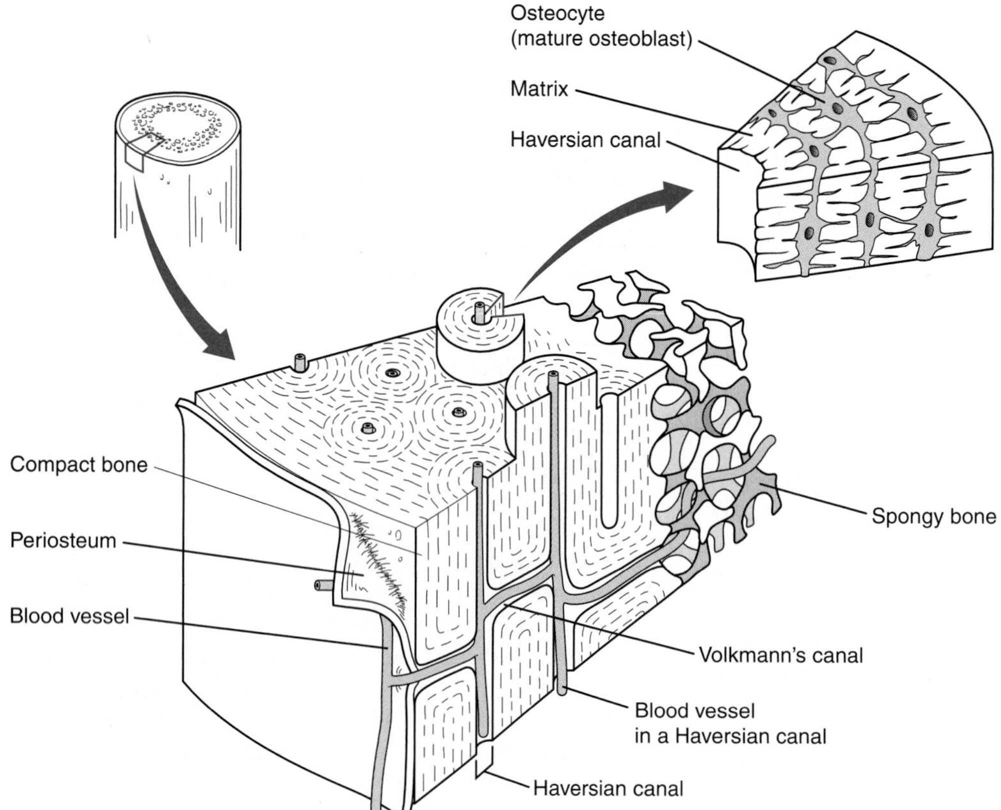

Figure 6•1 Haversian and Volkmann's canal, and periosteum.

skull and intracartilaginous ossification is found in the bones of the extremities.

5. **Haversian Canals,** or central canals, are minute vascular canals found in osseous tissue that run longitudinally through the bone.
6. **Volkmann's Canals** connect the longitudinal Haversian canals. These two canal networks complete the system of vascular canals in osseous tissue.
7. **Periosteum** is the fibrous, dense, vascular connective tissue sheath around the bone that penetrates the bone like nails, thus anchoring itself to the bone. Periosteum is the life support system of the bone; it contains blood and lymphatic vessels, nerves, and bone-forming cells for growth and fracture healing. Liken periosteum to the bark of a tree. Periosteum functions to secure tendons and ligaments to the bone, but is noticeably absent in the joint regions.
8. **Interosseous membrane** is a tough membrane that interconnects select bones (i.e., the ulna and radius) by attaching to their periosteum. This is also referred to as the interosseus ligament because it connects bone to bone.
9. **Ligaments** are connective tissues that connect bone to bone. Functionally, ligaments are an extension of the bone to allow lightness, flexibility, and added strength.

CLASSIFICATION OF BONES

Bones are scientifically classified according to their shape. These categories are long bones, short bones, flat bones, irregular bones, and sesamoid bones (Fig. 6–2). A brief description follows.

- **Long.** These bones are longer than they are wide. There is a shaft known as the **diaphysis** and one or more shaft endings, known as the **epiphysis.** Smooth hyaline cartilage covers the articular surface of the epiphysis. Between the diaphysis and epiphysis of growing bones is a flat plate of hyaline cartilage called the **epiphyseal plate,** or growth plate. This is the site of bone growth and is replaced by an **epiphyseal line** when growth is complete. All bones of the limbs, except wrist and ankle bones, are long bones.
- **Short.** Short bones are generally cube shaped, like wrist (carpals) and ankle (tarsals) bones.
- **Flat.** Flat bones are thin and flattened like pancakes. The sternum, ribs, scapula, and certain skull bones are flat bones.
- **Irregular.** Consider this a catch-all category for bones that do not fit in other categories. Irregular bones are certain cranial bones, facial bones, sutural bones, and the vertebrae. Sutural bones are

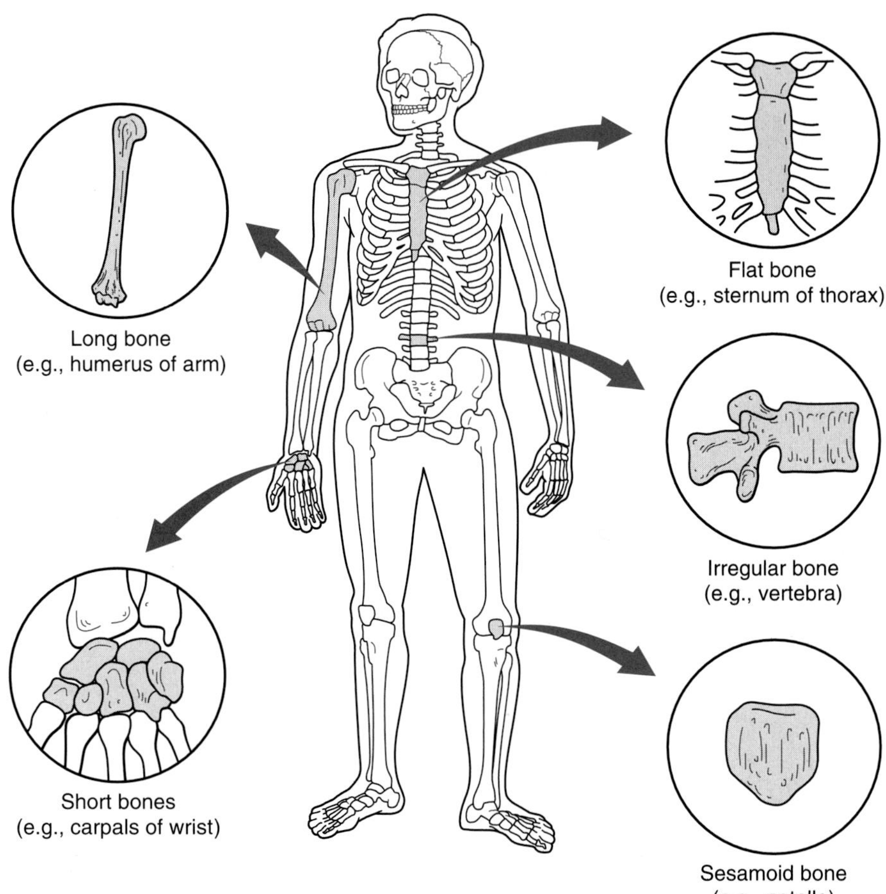

Figure 6•2 Examples of long, short, flat, irregular, and sesamoid bones.

bones that lie within the sutures of the cranium. A suture is a joint located between the bones of the skull.

- **Sesamoid.** Sesamoid bones are small, round bones that are embedded in certain tendons. Often, they are found in the hands and feet. The largest sesamoid bone is the patella (kneecap), which is embedded in the quadriceps femoris tendon.

SKELETAL DISTRIBUTION

To make our study of the skeletal system easier, we can divide it up into two distinct regions (Fig. 6–3). These regions are

- the axial skeleton, which consists of the bones associated with the central axis of the body (skull, vertebrae, ribs)
- the appendicular skeleton, which makes up the extremities (arms, legs, and girdles)

Axial Skeleton. There are 80 bones in the axial skeleton. They include the following:

1. **Skull.** Twenty-nine bones (eight bones in the cranium, fourteen bones in the face, six ear ossicles, and one hyoid bone)
2. **Vertebral Column.** Twenty-six bones in an adult and 31 or 33 unfused bones in the embryo, depending on how many bones are present in the coccyx
3. **Sternum.** One fused bone in the adult and three unfused bones in the embryo
4. **Ribs.** Twenty-four bones or 12 pairs of bones, which are located in the thorax

Extremities or Appendicular Skeleton. There are 126 bones in the appendicular skeleton. They are the following:

1. **Pectoral,** or **Shoulder Girdle.** The clavicle and scapula on both sides totaling four bones.
2. **Upper Limbs.** The 30 in each upper limb are the humerus, ulna, radius, 8 carpals, 5 metacarpals, and 14 phalanges, totaling 60 bones.
3. **Pelvic Girdle.** The pelvic girdle is often referred to as the "hip bone," and consists of a left and right ilium, ischium, and pubis. These two bones in the adult pelvis were once six unfused bones in the embryo.

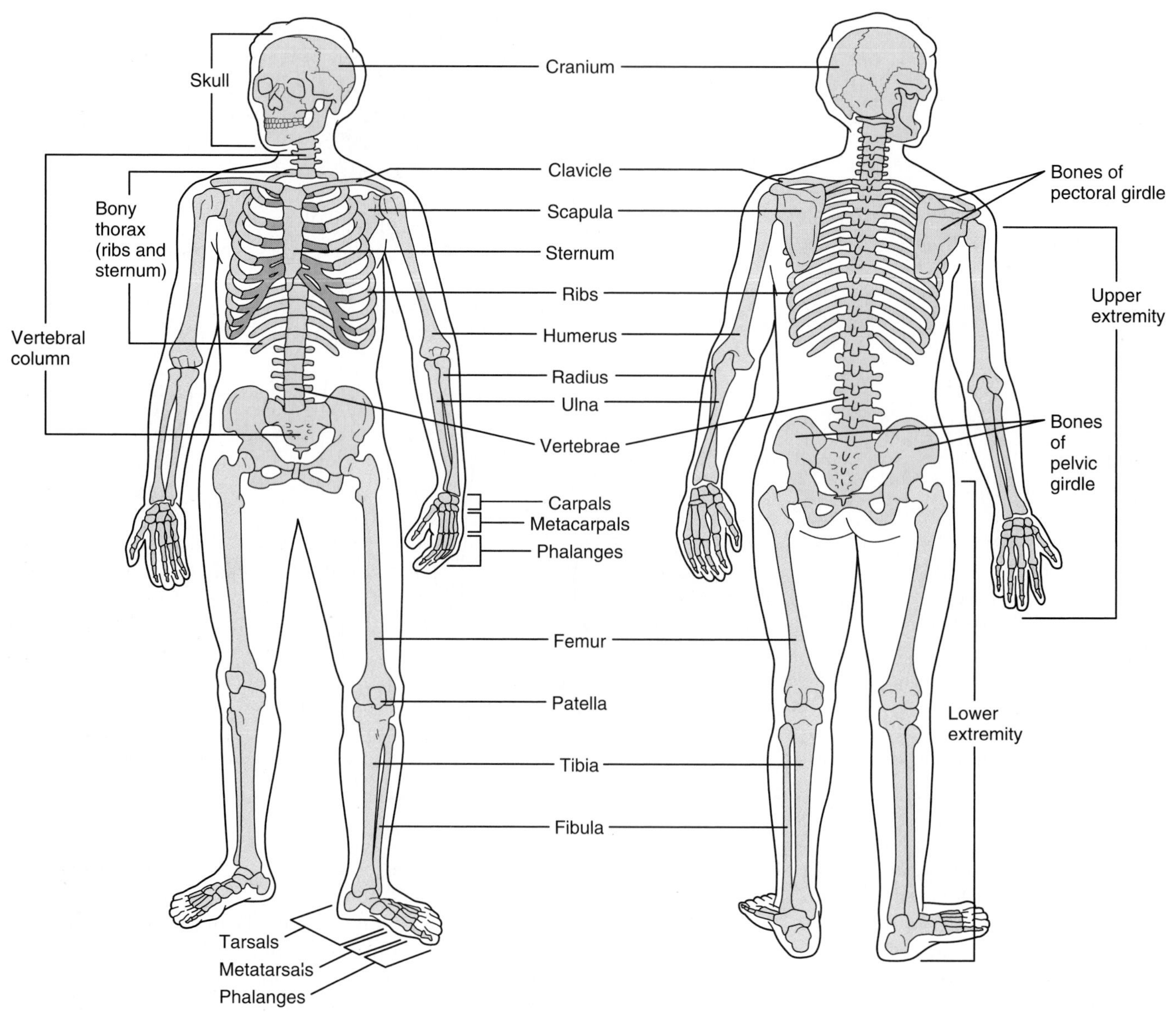

Figure 6•3 Skeletal bones with axial and appendicular divisions.

4. **Lower Limbs.** The 30 in each lower limb are the femur, patella, tibia, fibula, 7 tarsals, 5 metatarsals, and 14 phalanges, totaling 60 bones.

BONY MARKINGS

Bones are not smooth, but are marked with bumps, holes, and depressions. These markings are located where muscles, tendons, and ligaments attach and where nerve and blood vessels pass. These exterior marks are called **bony markings, bony landmarks,** or **surface markings.** Even though specific bones have not been introduced, examples for each surface marking are given to assist you in making the connection between the word and an example of a bony marking. Use this information to help you remember specific markings on bones when they are presented in the skeletal nomenclature chapter.

Bony marking are as follows:

1. **Process.** A general term for any prominence or prolongation from a bone. Example: styloid process of the radius
2. **Coracoid.** A bony projection resembling a crow's beak. Example: coracoid process of the scapula
3. **Mastoid.** A nipplelike or breastlike bony protrusion. Example: mastoid process of the temporal bone
4. **Styloid.** A sharp bony projection. Example: styloid process of the temporal bone
5. **Tubercle.** A rounded projection usually blunt and irregular. Example: greater tubercle of the humerus
6. **Tuberosity.** Large, rounded rough projection. Example: deltoid tuberosity

7. **Trochanter.** Large rough process found only on the femur. Example: greater trochanter
8. **Crest.** A very prominent linear elevation that forms a border or a ridge. Example: tibial crest
9. **Condyle.** Rounded projection that forms a joint; knuckle-shaped. Example: lateral condyle of the femur
10. **Epicondyle.** A projection over a condyle. Example: medial epicondyle of the humerus
11. **Spine.** A sharp, slender projection. Example: spine of the scapula
12. **Head.** The rounded, proximal end of a bone. Example: head of the fibula
13. **Fossa.** Shallow depression in a bone. Example: glenoid fossa of the scapula
14. **Foramen.** A hole or opening for blood vessels and nerves to pass. Example: foramen magnum of the occipital bone
15. **Meatus.** A tubelike opening in a bone that forms a tunnel or canal. Example: external auditory meatus of the temporal bone
16. **Facet.** Small, smooth, shallow depression articulating with another bone. Example: vertebral articular facet
17. **Ramus.** Long branchlike bony prolongation of a bone. Example: superior pubic ramus
18. **Notch.** A deep indention or a narrow gap in a bone. Example: sternal notch

ARTICULATIONS

Articulations, or joints, are the meeting places for bones. Every bone in the human skeleton articulates with at least one other bone, except the hyoid bone. Where a joint exists, so do joint movements. This movement may be limited, like sutures in the cranium. Or it may be very mobile like the ball-and-socket joint of the shoulder. Joints serve two purposes:

1. they hold the bones together via the ligaments, and
2. they allow a rigid skeletal system to become somewhat flexible by changing their relative positions to one another when acted on by muscles or outside forces.

Articulations can be classified according to how the joint *functions*.

Three Types of Articulations

These types of joints take into account the range or degree of movement that is allowed physiologically. The three classifications of joints are synarthrotic, amphiarthrotic, and diarthrotic (Fig. 6–4). Use the mnemonic phrase SAD to recall the terms *s*ynarthrotic, *a*mphiarthrotic, and *d*iarthrotic.

1. **Synarthrotic.** Movement in these joints is absent or extremely limited. Examples of synarthrotic joints are the sutures found in the cranium.

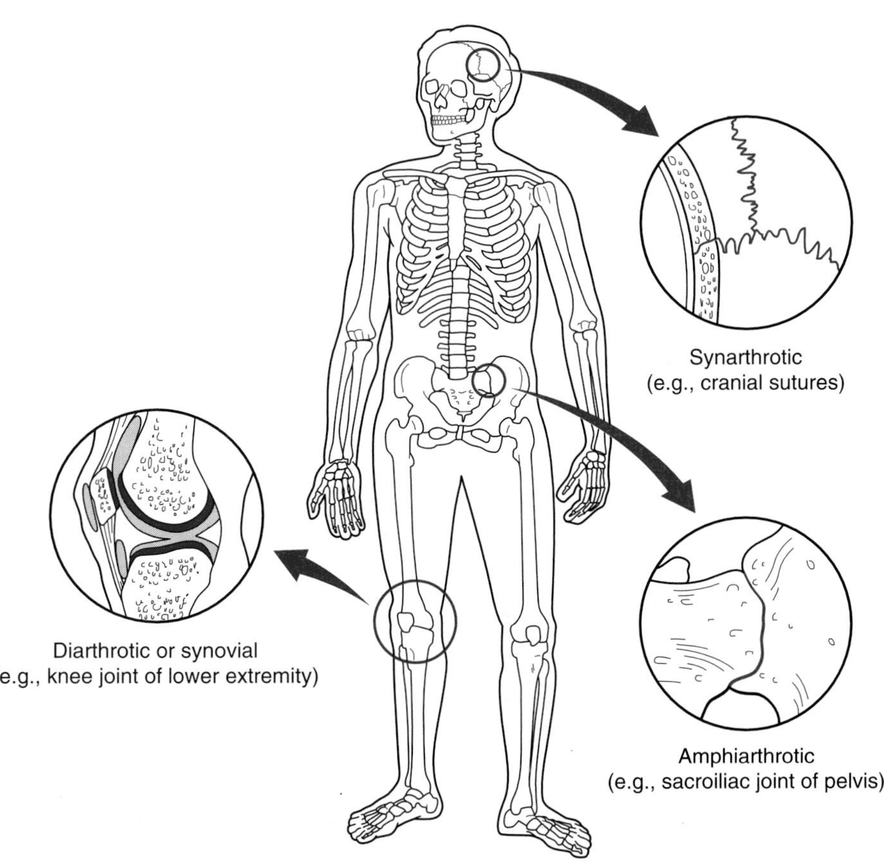

Figure 6•4 Functional classifications of joints.

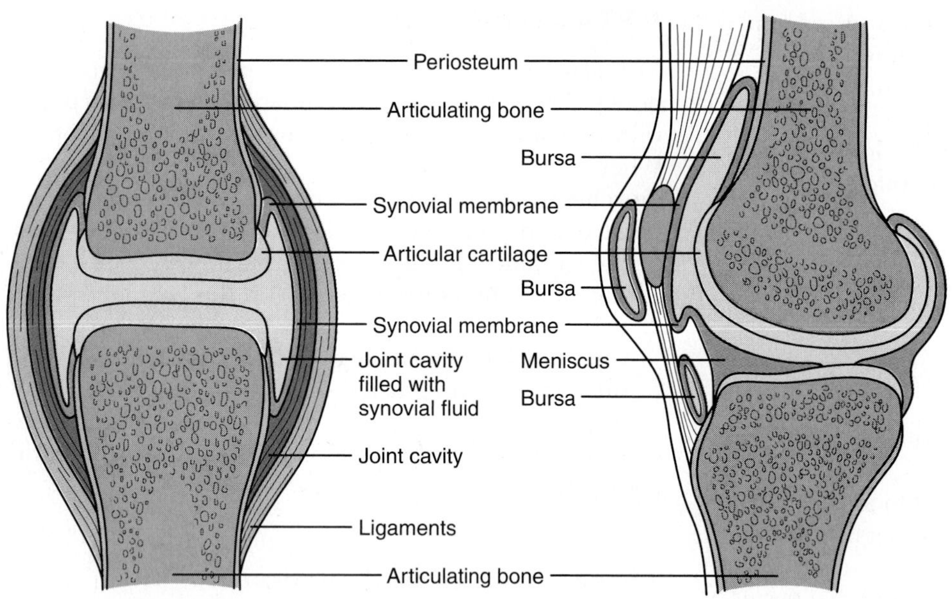

Figure 6•5 A joint.

2. **Amphiarthrotic.** These joints are slightly movable, like intervertebral joints or the sternoclavicular joints. These joints move apart only a few millimeters.
3. **Diarthrotic.** Also known as synovial joints, these are freely movable joints. Diarthrotic joints allow movement in one, two, or three dimensions. These joints also feature articular cartilage and synovial membranes. Many synovial joints also contain bursae sacs filled with synovial fluid. Examples of synovial joints include knees, elbows, hips, shoulders, wrists, and knuckle joints of the fingers and toes.

Diarthrotic/Synovial Joints

The joints of main concern for the massage therapist are diarthrotic or synovial joints (Fig. 6–5). The following structures are associated with synovial joints:

1. **Articular Cartilage.** The articulating surfaces of the bones that participate in the joint structure are covered with hyaline cartilage. This allows gliding movements to occur more easily.
2. **Joint Capsule.** Diarthrotic joints are enclosed with a joint capsule in the shape of a sleeve. The joint capsule is a continuation of the periosteum of the bones involved in the joint. The sleeve is lined with a synovial membrane that produces synovial fluid, hence the name synovial joint.
3. **Joint Cavity.** The joint cavity is the enclosed space between the bones of the joint filled with lubricating (synovial) fluid.
4. **Synovial Membrane.** The synovial membrane lines the interior of the joint capsule and the bursae sac. The function of the membrane is to secrete synovial fluid.
5. **Synovial Fluid.** Also known as synovia, this viscous fluid is found in joints, bursae sacs, and synovial sheaths. Synovial fluid provides *nutrition* and *lubrication* so the joint can move freely without friction. The amount produced depends upon the physical activity of the joints. Stiffness and reduction of movement will result in synovial fluid deficiency.
6. **Bursae.** A bursa is a collapsed saclike structure with a synovial membrane that contains synovial fluid. It looks like a deflated balloon, and many bursae sacs also have villi (additional folds within the bursae to increase the surface area). This provides a cushion that protects the tendon from rubbing against the bone during muscular contraction. Not all diarthrotic joints have bursae, such as the joints located in the ankles, fingers, and toes.
7. **Synovial Sheaths.** Synovial sheaths are similar to bursae sacs except, instead of being flat they are tubular. These structures surround long tendons (mainly found in the hands and feet).
8. **Reinforcing Ligaments.** Ligaments reinforce and stabilize the joint. Bursae sacs are often found between the ligaments and the joint capsule.

ACTION TERMINOLOGY

The following are the movements provided by the synovial joints of the body. Use the activity at the end of this section as an educational dramatization to assist you in learning these joint movements.

CLASSIFICATION OF LEVERS

For the muscular system to produce movement at joints, it uses the skeletal system for leverage. A lever (bone) is a rod that is moved by use of a fulcrum (joint). In order for a lever to be set in motion, it must be acted on by two forces. These forces are re-

Text continued on page 116

TYPES OF MOVEMENT

FLEXION bends or decreases the angle of a joint

EXTENSION straightens or increases the angle of a joint

HYPEREXTENSION is a continuation of extension beyond the anatomical position, as in bending the head backward

EXAMPLES:

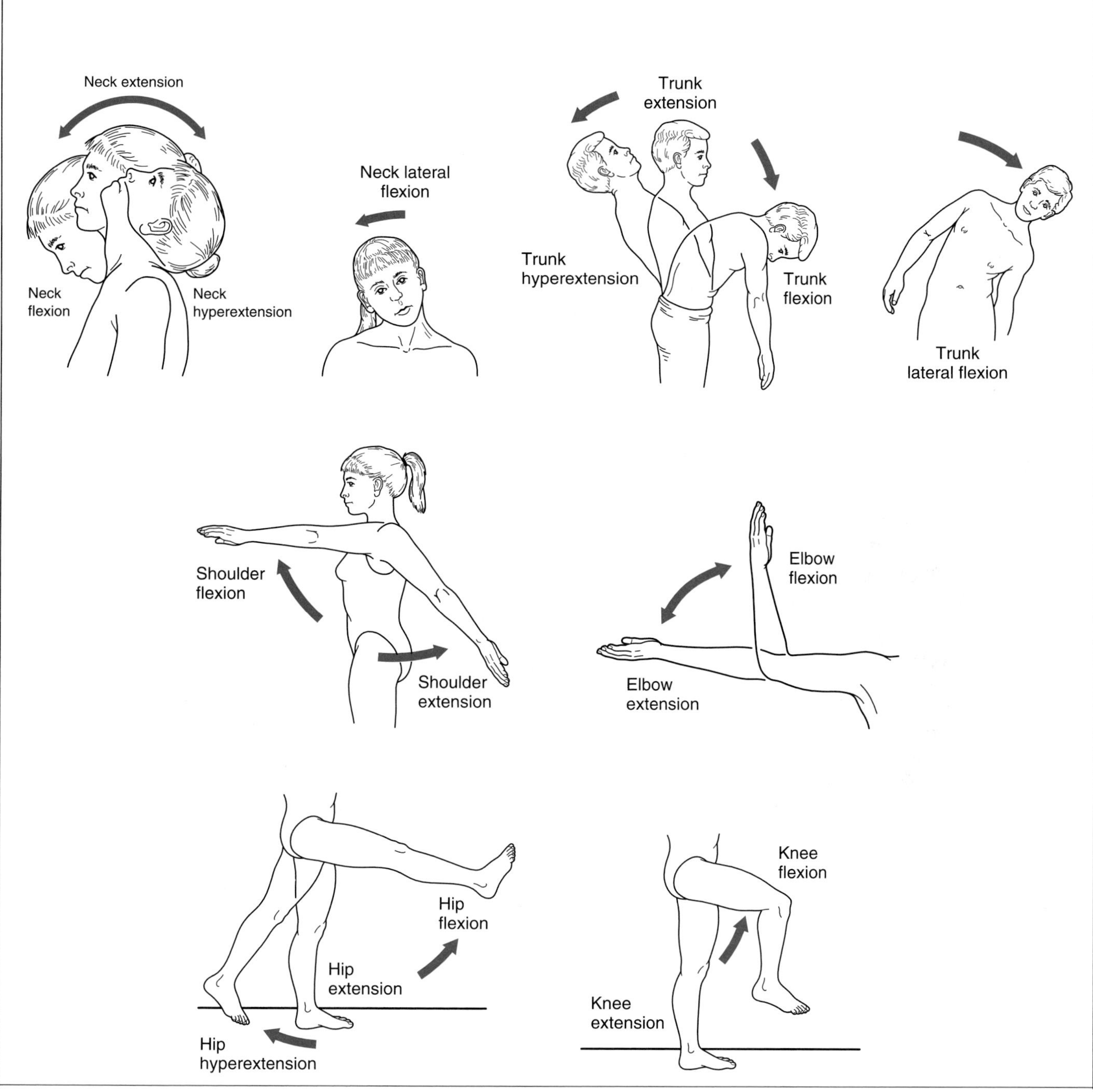

continued on page 114

ABDUCTION is movement away from the median plane. Note: The hand has its own midline: the middle finger. Spreading the fingers apart is called abduction.

ADDUCTION is movement toward the median plane

EXAMPLES:

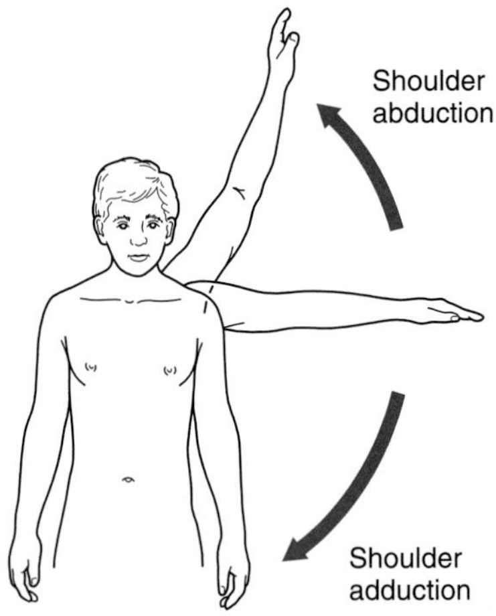

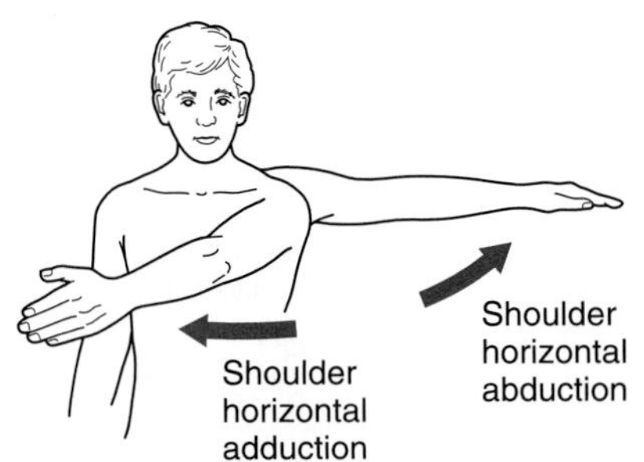

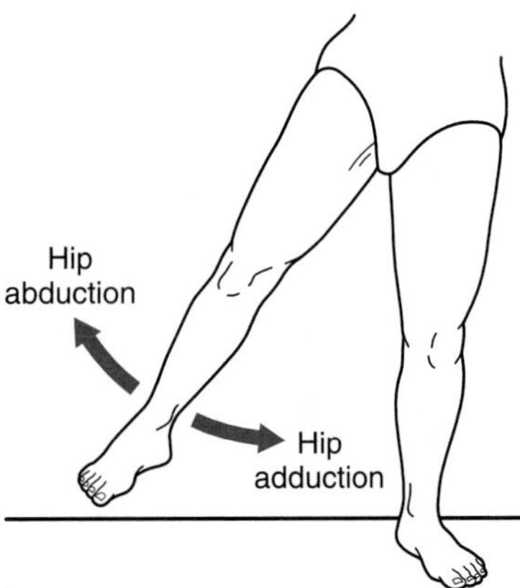

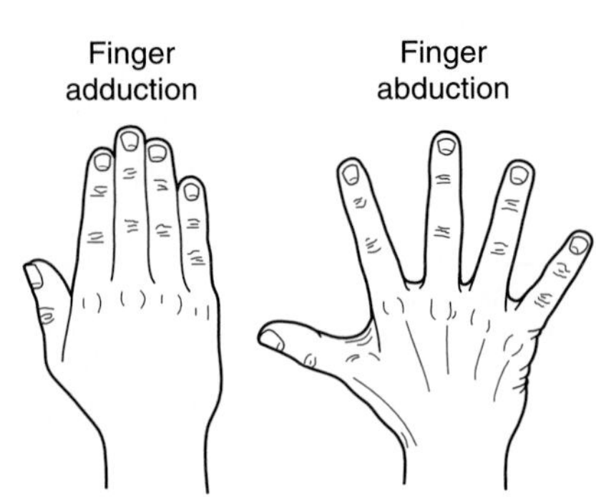

SUPINATION is a lateral rotation or outward rotation of the forearm; the hand is turned over so it can hold a cup of "soup."

PRONATION is medial rotation or inward rotation of the forearm.

EXAMPLES:

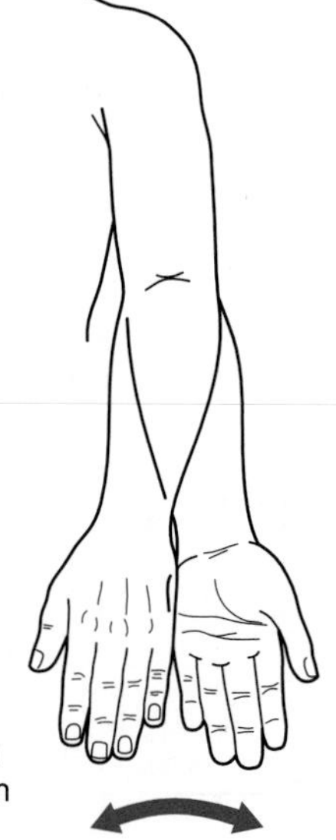

continued on page 115

TYPES OF MOVEMENT *continued*

PLANTAR FLEXION is extension of the foot so that the toes are pointing downward in the direction of the plantar surface of the foot; it increases the ankle angle anteriorly.

DORSIFLEXION is hyperextension of the foot; it decreases the ankle angle anteriorly more than the anatomical flexion, as in walking on the heels.

EXAMPLES:

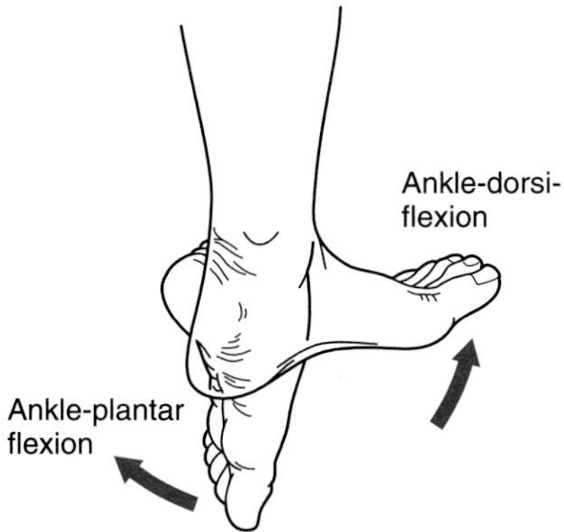

INVERSION is medial rotation or movement in which the sole is turned inward (or medially). When both feet are inverted, the soles of the feet face each other.

EVERSION is a lateral rotation or movement in which the sole is turned outward (or laterally).

EXAMPLES:

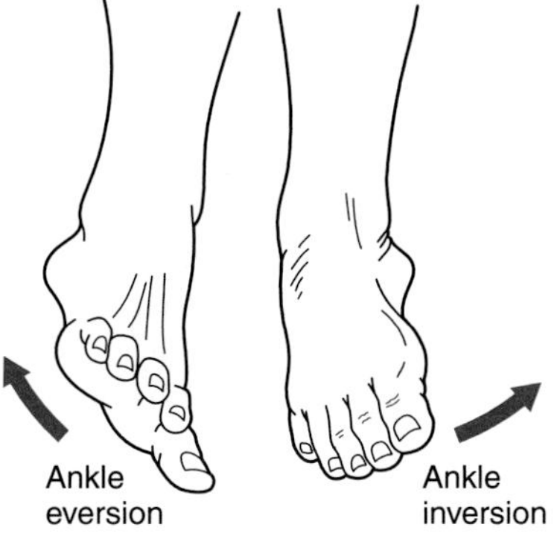

CIRCUMDUCTION occurs when the distal end moves in a circle and the proximal end is fixed; cone-shaped range of motion.

ROTATION is circular movement when a bone moves around its own central axis.

EXAMPLES:

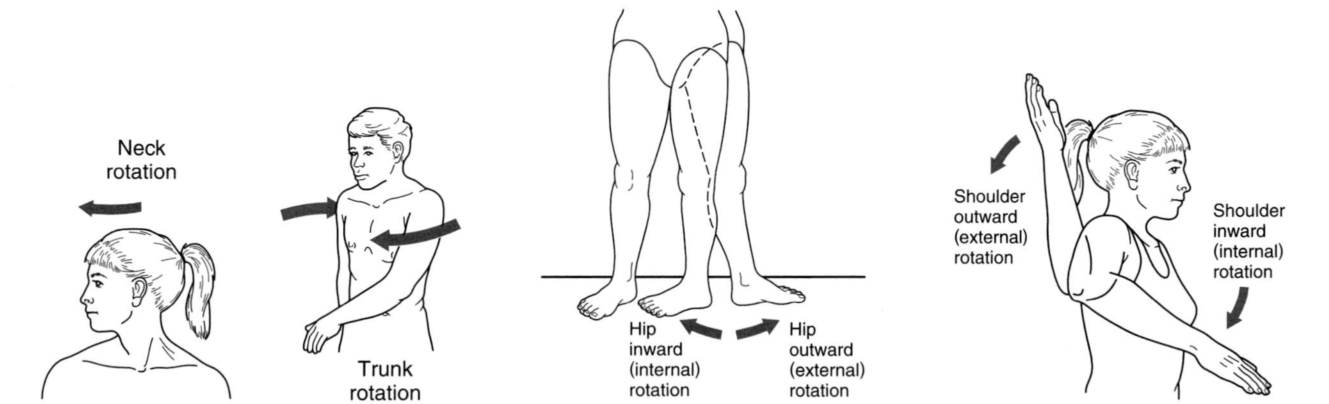

continued on page 116

TYPES OF MOVEMENT *continued*

ELEVATION is raising or lifting a body part.

DEPRESSION is lowering or dropping a body part.

EXAMPLES:

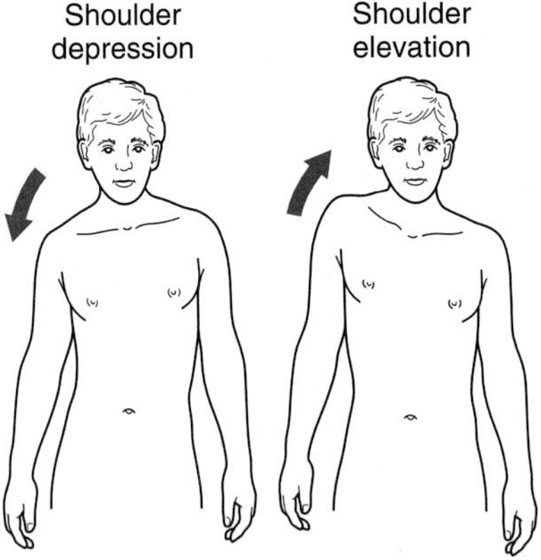

PROTRACTION is movement forward in the transverse or horizontal plane.

RETRACTION is movement backward or retrusion in the transverse or horizontal plane.

sistance (weight of body and/or an object) and effort (muscular contraction).

Levers are categorized into three classes, according to how the fulcrum, effort, and resistance are arranged (Fig. 6–6). Let's examine them briefly.

1. **Class 1 Lever.** Class 1 levers resemble a seesaw. The fulcrum is positioned between the effort and the resistance. The cranium sitting on top of the vertebrae is an example of a class 1 lever. This is the least common type of lever in the body.
2. **Class 2 Lever.** Class 2 levers function like a wheelbarrow. The fulcrum is at one end, the resistance is in the middle, and the effort is at the opposite end. One example of a class 2 lever is raising up on the toes.
3. **Class 3 Lever.** Class 3 levers are the most common. The fulcrum is at one end, the effort located in the central portion, and the resistance is at the opposite end. Flexing the leg or arm are examples of class 3 levers.

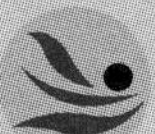

MINI•LAB

Flex your right elbow 90 degrees and affix your upper arm to your torso so it does not move. Place your left hand on your right ulna. Begin to pronate and supinate your right hand. Notice how your ulna never moves. Also notice how the thumb makes a 180-degree rotation. Pronation and supination results from the radius rotating over the distal end of the ulna. The hand follows the movement of the radius.

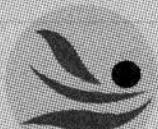

MINI•LAB

Perform the different joint movements like abduction of the arm and hip, rotation of the cervical region, flexion of the elbow and knee, and so on, until all joint movements have been experienced. Shout each movement as it is performed.

TYPES OF SYNOVIAL JOINTS

Synovial or diarthrotic joints are the largest classification of joints. There are six types of these joints, which allow different ranges of movement in one or all three known dimensions. They are ball-and-socket joints, hinge joints, pivot joints, ellipsoidal joints, saddle joints, and gliding joints (Fig. 6–7). All synovial joints contain a joint capsule and articular cartilage. They may also contain bursae and accessory ligaments. Let's look at each joint.

1. **Ball-and-socket** joint is also referred to as a spheroid or a triaxial joint. This type of joint permits all movements and offers the greatest range of motion, like the hip (iliofemoral joint) and shoulder (glenohumeral joint).
2. **Hinge** joint, also referred to as a ginglymus or a monaxial joint. The movements allowed in a hinge joint are limited to flexion and extension, like the knee, elbow, and interphalangeal joints.

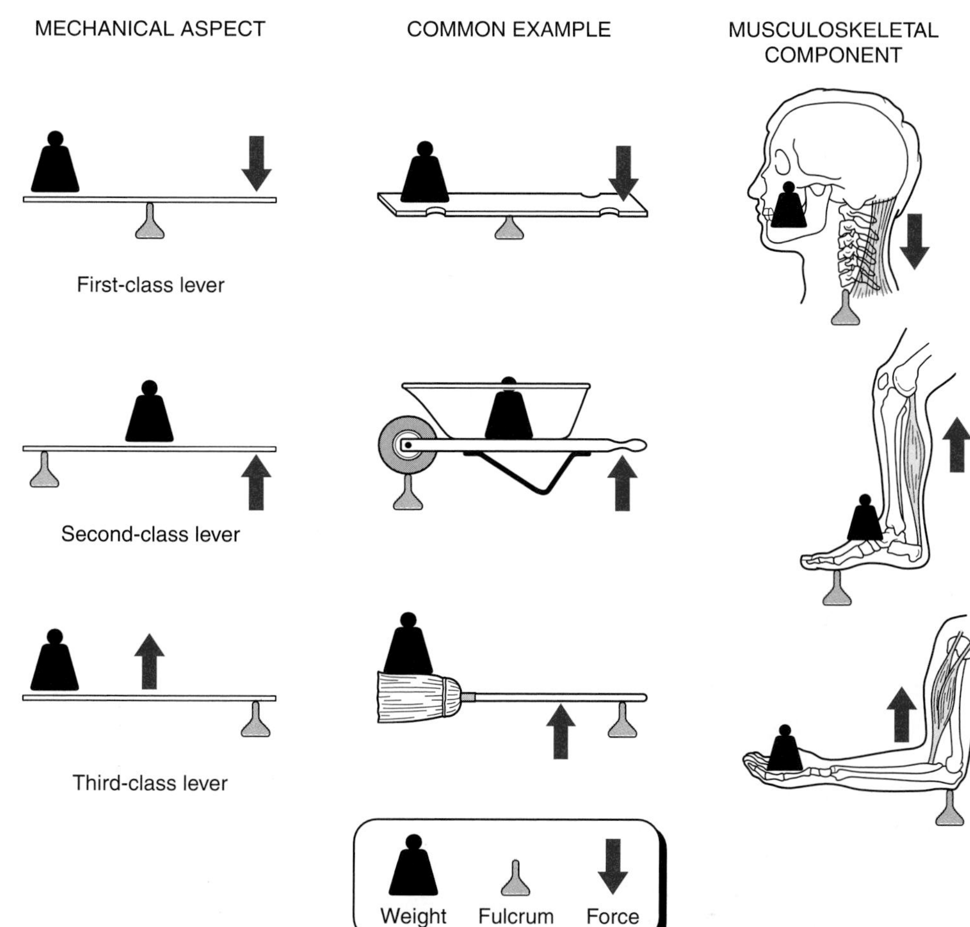

Figure 6•6 Three classes of levers.

3. **Pivot** joint, also known as a trochoid or a monaxial joint, allows movement that is limited to rotation, like the atlantoaxial or the proximal radioulnar joint.
4. **Ellipsoidal** joint is also referred to as a condyloid joint or a biaxial joint, and is essentially a reduced ball-and-socket joint. Ellipsoidal joints allow flexion, extension, abduction, and adduction, but rotation is not permitted. Examples of ellipsoidal joints are radiocarpal joints located in the wrist.
5. **Saddle** joints, also known as sellar or biaxial joints, allow all movements, but rotation is limited. An example of a saddle joint is the carpometacarpal of the thumb.
6. **Gliding** joints, also referred to as arthrodia or biaxial joints, permit movements limited to gliding in flexion, extension, abduction, and adduction; gliding is present in intercarpal and intertarsal joints.

SKELETAL CONDITIONS AND CLINICAL TERMS

1. **Dislocation.** A dislocation, also known as a luxation, occurs when bones are forced out of their normal position in the joint cavity. Associated ligaments, tendons, articular capsules, and blood vessels are torn in the process. An incomplete or partial dislocation is known as a subluxation.

   Local massage, especially range of motion, is contraindicated. However, once healing is complete, range of motion, deep specific friction, and cross-fiber friction can help increase mobility of the joint.
2. **Separation.** A separation is almost the same as a dislocation, but the joint structure is simply pulled and stretched; the bone is not displaced out of the joint capsule.
3. **Sprain.** Joint trauma that stretches or tears the ligamentous attachments is called a sprain. Sprains cause pain and possible temporary disability. Depending on the severity of the injury, it is not uncommon for a ligamentous sprain to take 6 months to a year to completely rehabilitate because ligaments have few blood vessels.

   Once a joint is sprained, use I-C-E (ice, compression, elevation) to bring down the swelling. Seventy-two hours after the initial injury, light effleurage and light friction are helpful massage techniques. Cross-fiber friction is an excellent rehabilitation technique. Do not begin the massage until the client receives medical clearance and DO NOT STRETCH the injured area.

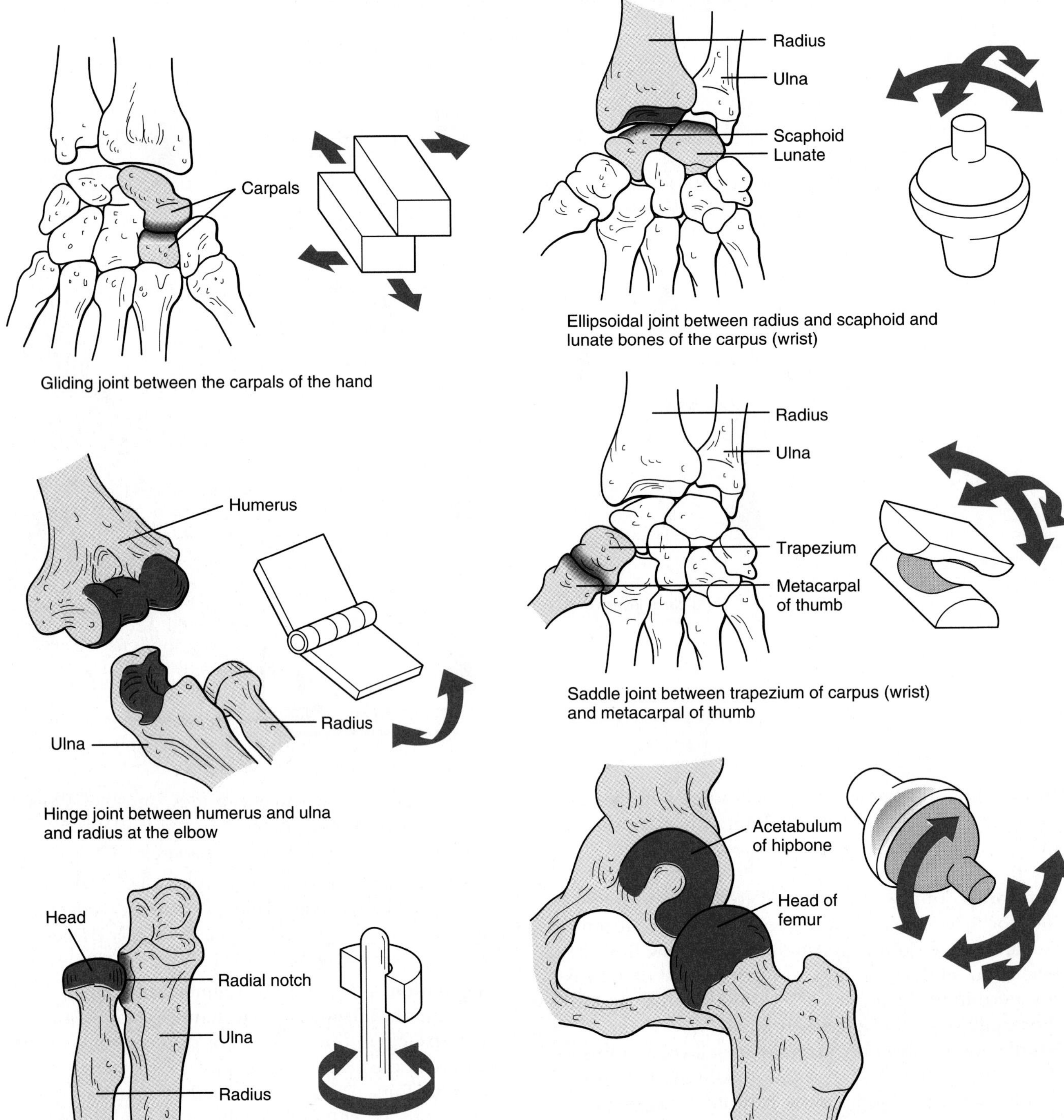

Figure 6•7 Types of synovial joints.

Acute ligament sprains can be classified into three grades or degrees of severity (Fig. 6–8). They are as follows:

First Degree. First degree is the stretching of the ligament without tearing or up to a 20 percent tearing of fibers with no palpable defects. The joint structures can maintain efficient motion and hold against resistance.

Second Degree. Between 20 and 75 percent tearing of a ligament with a defect felt in the structure is

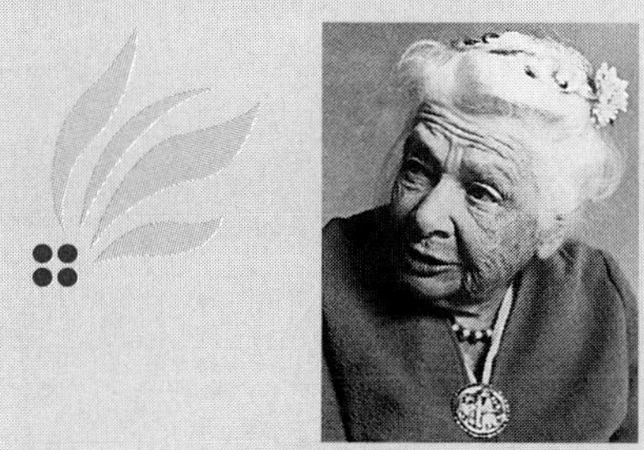

(Courtesy of the Rolf Institute, Boulder, CO; photo by David Kirk-Campbell.)

Ida Rolf

May 18, 1896–March 19, 1979

"God didn't come down and tell me; I had to find it out through many years of experience. The work came first; the inspiration came later."

It was the middle of WW II and most of America's men were far from home. Women began to fill roles they'd never dreamed would fall to them. One such young woman accepted a position with the Rockefeller Institute even though her father was dead set against it. War or peace, a proper lady stayed home where she belonged. After all, her family had money. She didn't need to earn her way.

But Ida Pauline Rolf had a mind of her own, and what a mind it was! Her doctorate was in biochemistry, but Rolf was just as passionate about philosophy and general semantics as she was about studying the science of the body. She explored homeopathy, was heavily influenced by osteopathy, and practiced yoga under the direction of a tantric yogi. And perhaps even more integral to her success than any other factor was that Rolf wasn't afraid to launch out in a new direction.

Her determination and boldness led her to drive across the country in order to study with Amy Cochran in a time when gas was being rationed. Cochran was an osteopath who claimed to have received her special abilities through a psychic encounter with Dr. Benjamin Rush, the physician who signed the Declaration of Independence.

When Rolf returned to New York she began work on a 45-year-old woman who had been crippled at age 8. In a couple of years the woman was up and walking.

Rolf believed that bodies are created balanced and comfortably supported by gravity, but injuries, overwork of one muscle group, or other postural dysfunctions result in fascia that are too tight here or too loose there. Thus, our bodies expend energy less efficiently and fight gravity rather than being supported by it. She also believed that anything that made individuals feel fear or guilt could manifest itself in bad physiology. For her, mental and physical health were two sides of the same coin.

Rolfing methodically restructures connective tissue through work on one body section at a time, gradually working deeper and deeper.

The massage that we know today as Rolfing was first called structural integration. When the container is aligned properly, the "stuff" inside functions as it should. Structural integration helps achieve homeostasis. But her vision went beyond physical change. Rolf believed that this tissue reorganization of the body was necessary to achieve spiritual growth.

Rosemary Feitis, Rolf's longtime secretary, writes: "IPR was not interested in curing symptoms; she was after a bigger game. She wanted nothing less than to create new, better human beings. The ills would cure themselves; the symptoms would melt as the organisms became balanced." (From Ida Rolf Talks About Rolfing and Physical Reality. Harper & Row, New York, New York.)

To achieve this Nirvana, Rolf used her arms, fingers, elbows, and forearms to loosen myofascial restrictions, moving tissue until it was "in the right place." Then she would proceed to the next problem area, asking for feedback as she went along. Eventually she developed a sequence of ten progressive sessions now referred to as the Basic Ten.

One of the most lasting impressions of Rolfing seems to be that sessions must be painful in order to be effective. This was never Rolf's goal, and because of the body's reactive mechanism to pain, too much force may have a negative effect on results. In fact, she was quoted in Feitis's book as saying: "Don't just go in there as though you were a locomotive charging in at a 100 miles an hour. In general, if there is trouble going on inside the body, fascia on the outside will be so tight it will tend to protect the area that's in trouble. So don't barge through fascia. If you are doing the right thing, and there isn't some deep pathology, the fascia will let go—let you in."

continued on page 120

Continued

Ida Rolf

Rolf tried to teach others what she'd discovered and at the same time preserve the integrity of her work, but her commitment was singular. Not everyone shared her enthusiasm, work ethic, or understanding of the body. According to Feitis, Rolf didn't want "mechanicalness." She taught who she could and cautioned them to wait until they were experienced before considering themselves "Rolfers."

Eventually, an invitation to present her work at Esalen, a California proving ground for new movements, landed Rolf in the midst of a new type of student. She began to teach her work to those with no preconceived notions and a variety of backgrounds. The world began to take notice of her work. Research established its effectiveness. Articles were published. The Rolf Institute, formerly the Guild for Structural Integration, was created in the early 1970s.

Today, Rolfing has undergone some change. Not all practitioners accept Rolf's notion of the perfect or ideal body. Others plan sessions according to clients' needs rather than sticking to the Basic Ten. It's hard to say what Rolf would think about this evolution.

second degree. The joint structures cannot hold against moderate resistance. Edema is typically found and the muscles surrounding the strain or sprain are splinted to restrict painful movement.

Third Degree. In a third-degree tear, 75 percent to a complete rupture of the structure (100 percent) is noted and a "snap" is often heard at the time of injury. A piece of the bone may be torn away as well (sprain fracture). A depression in the area of the torn muscle can be felt and is usually painful to touch. Function is greatly altered in third-degree tears.

4. **Fractures.** A fracture is a break, chip, crack, or rupture in a bone. Osseous tissue is highly vascularized, but healing sometimes takes months because sufficient calcium and phosphorus are deposited slowly in new bone. The three most common types of fractures are simple fractures, open fractures, and stress fractures (Fig. 6–9). Let's look at each briefly.

   Simple. Also known as closed fractures, the bone is broken, but does not protrude through the skin.

   Open. Also known as compound fractures, a broken end of the bone breaks through the skin and soft tissue.

   Stress. Stress fractures are accumulated microfractures (small cracks in a bone). These fractures are commonly a result of repeated activity, like running on a hard surface or high-impact aerobic dance. A common place for stress fractures are the metatarsal bones.

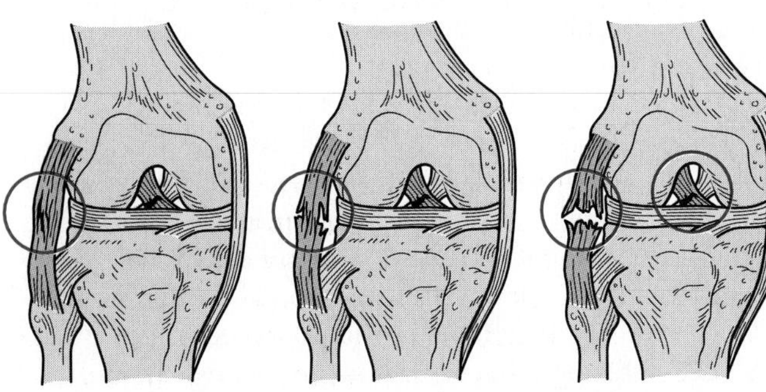

Figure 6•8 Three degrees of sprains.

While a bone is immobilized, massage can help maintain circulation, joint mobility, and muscle tone, and reduce edema. Elevate the affected limb to help with drainage. Massaging muscles close to the immobilized part can decrease spasms and reduce pain. A full-body, gentle massage can help reduce client stress.

Once healing is complete, massage and range of motion can help the client regain joint mobility and increase tone in muscles that have atrophied. Massage should begin slowly and gently, about a week after the

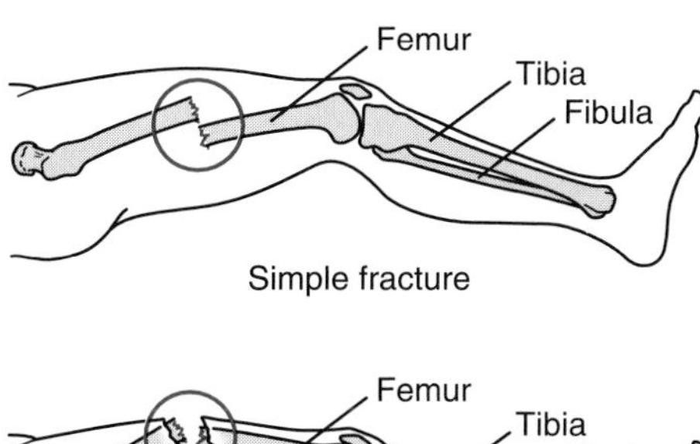

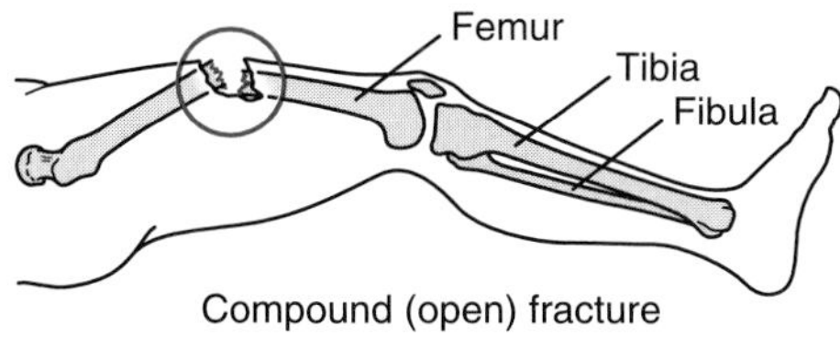

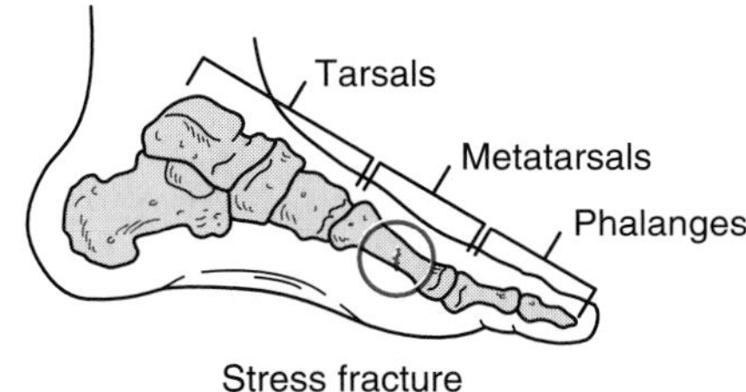

Figure 6•9 Three of the most common types of fractures.

cast has been removed. Gradually range of motion can increase, and massage can be deeper.

FYI FOR YOUR INFORMATION

The most commonly fractured bone in the body is the clavicle.

5. **Ankylosing Spondylitis.** This is an inflammatory disease leading to calcification and fusion of the joints between the vertebrae and the sacroiliac joint. It is more common in males between the ages of 20 and 40. There is pain and stiffness in the hips and lower back that can progress upward along the spine. Inflammation can lead to loss of movement of the joints (ankylosis) and kyphosis (hunchback). When the joints between the thoracic vertebrae and the ribs are involved, the person may have difficulty in expanding the rib cage for inhalation.

   Clients need to be positioned for their comfort. Clients who have kyphosis may need extra cushioning in the neck region. Massage treatments should retain joint mobility, strengthen weak muscles, and stretch tight ones. Ankylosed joints should not be forced into movement. The back and limbs should be massaged gently. Heat packs will help ease pain. Breathing exercises may help mobilize the thorax.

6. **Spondylolisthesis.** Spondylolisthesis is an anteriorly displaced vertebra, usually the fifth lumbar vertebra over the first sacral vertebra. This condition can range from mild to severe. Severe cases deform the spine.

   Gentle massage of the back is indicated. Tight muscles in the area can be stretched, but should not be forced.

7. **Crepitus.** A noisy discharge that may resemble a cracking sound and is produced by the body. Examples of crepitus are "popping" joints, rubbing of bone fragments, and flatulence. Can be the result of air present in subcutaneous tissue and can often be palpated.
8. **Bursitis.** Acute or chronic inflammation of the bursae is called bursitis. It is caused by infection, trauma, disease, excessive friction or pressure in the joint. The most common types of bursitis are subacromial bursitis, subcoracoid bursitis, subscapular bursitis, olecranon bursitis, trochanteric bursitis, ischial bursitis, prepatellar bursitis, and calcaneal bursitis.

   Cold packs can be applied to reduce swelling. Local massage is contraindicated until swelling has subsided. Friction can then be done, with ice packs applied afterward.

9. **Bunions.** Bunions are an abnormal medial tilting and enlargement of the joint between the first metatarsal of the great toe and the associated proximal phalanx. However, bunions can also be found on the lateral side of the foot. They are caused by chronic irritation and pressure from poorly fitted shoes, or inflammation of the plantar bursae.

   Local massage is contraindicated because of the pain, but general massage is all right.

10. **Osteoporosis.** Osteoporosis is characterized by decreased bone mass and increased susceptibility to fractures. As women and men age, they produce much smaller amounts of estrogen and testosterone, respectively. The decreased hormone levels result in osteoblasts becoming less active, so there is a decrease in bone mass. Bone mass becomes so depleted the skeleton can no longer withstand mechanical stress. Osteoporosis is responsible for hip fractures, shrinkage of the backbone, height loss, hunched backs, other bone fractures, and considerable pain.

    Gentle massage, avoiding undue pressure over bones, is indicated.

11. **Arthritis.** Arthritis refers to several chronic joint diseases characterized by inflammation, swelling, and pain in the joints. There are more than 100 types of arthritis and it usually affects the smaller joints first, like those found in the hands and feet. The three most common types of arthritis are rheumatoid arthritis, osteoarthritis, and gouty arthritis. Another type of arthritis is Lyme disease.

Rheumatoid Arthritis. Rheumatoid arthritis, or RA, is a systemic arthritis that destroys the synovial membranes of joints. These membranes are replaced by fibrous tissues that add to the joint stiffness already present. This process greatly reduces the person's range of motion. Usually there is bilateral involvement with a high incident of crippling deformity. The cause of RA is unknown, but it is believed to be an autoimmune disease. Persons who have RA experience flare-ups and remissions.

Massage is contraindicated when a client has a flare-up. When the client's RA is in remission, massage can be administered safely. Massage can help reduce stress, and gentle range of motion can help increase joint mobility. A shorter massage is indicated as the client may be on painkillers and/or anti-inflammatory drugs that may result in inadequate feedback.

Osteoarthritis. Osteoarthritis, or OA, is a chronic, progressive erosion of the articular cartilage due to chronic inflammation. The most common sites are weight-bearing joints, which may eventually become immovable. OA, which is more common than RA, is most common in the elderly population.

When applying massage techniques, do not use excessive pressure. Deep massage and range of motion are contraindicated because these movements may injure the client.

Gouty Arthritis. Gouty arthritis is characterized by an abnormal accumulation of uric acid in the body. Uric acid is produced when nucleic acids are metabolized; the uric acid is then converted to sodium urate crystals. In most cases, uric acid is eliminated in urine. Some individuals, usually males, either produce excessive amounts or are unable to excrete the uric acid, resulting in abnormally high levels of uric acid in the bloodstream. The sodium urate crystals eventually settle in the soft tissue around joints, typically the feet and toes, causing irritation, pain, and swelling.

Local massage is contraindicated.

Lyme Disease. Also called Lyme arthritis, Lyme disease is a recurrent form of arthritis caused by a bacterium *Borrelia burgdorferi,* which is transmitted by a tick bite. The condition was originally described in the community of Lyme, Connecticut, but has been reported throughout North America and in other countries. Large joints, such as the knee and hip, are most commonly involved, with local inflammation and swelling. Headaches, fever, and a scaly red skin eruption (erythematous), often precede the joint manifestations.

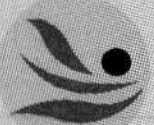

MINI•LAB

Imagine what you would look like if the ball-and-socket joints of the hip and shoulder were hinge joints. Or if the hinge joints of the elbow and knee were changed into ball-and-socket joints. Share with classmates new creatures that could be designed by joint alterations.

The Effects of Massage on the Skeletal System (Bone and Soft Tissue)

1. Massage increases the retention of nutrients such as nitrogen, sulfur, and phosphorus in bones, especially when performed locally on stable fractures. When a bone is fractured, the body forms a network of new blood vessels at the break site. Although the precise mechanism is not understood, it appears that local massage provides an increase in local circulation around the fracture, leading to increased deposition of callus to the bone scar.
2. Theoretically, massage flattens out adipose globules and makes the skin appear smoother. Cellulite, a type of adipose tissue, appears as groups of small dimples or depressions in the skin. This is caused by an uneven separation of fat globules below the skin's surface, which is displaced by manual manipulation. It does not reduce the amount of cellulite present below the skin; instead, it alters the shape or appearance of cellulite.
3. Massage can make the body more mobile by reducing hyperplasia (thickening) of connective tissue and freeing fascial restrictions.
4. Massage displaces adhesions and rearranges scar tissue. It can create an appropriate scar that is strong yet does not interfere with the muscle's ability to broaden as it contracts. This in turn helps to restore normal, pain-free motion of the affected joint.

Since the disease is chronic (lasting months or years), the massage needs to be tailored to the client's individual symptoms. Massage is contraindicated if the client is experiencing widespread inflammation. Generally, a gentle, full-body massage is indicated. Passive range of motion will retain joint mobility.

SUMMARY

The intricate structures of bone, cartilage, ligament, and joints are what comprise our skeletal system. The skeleton acts as a supportive framework for the rest of our body systems. It protects our delicate internal organs and acts as a storehouse for vital minerals.

Though we often associate bones with the dead, our bones are living tissue. They are strong, flexible, and relatively light. The bones of the human body number 206, or 210 if you count the sesamoid bones under each thumb and great toe.

The study of the skeletal system is not limited to bone alone. It includes the tissue of the bone itself, types of joints and articulations, movement, leverage, abnormal conditions, and the specific bony markings.

Finally, bones are the massage therapist's landmarks to muscle location. While the various soft tissues are at times indistinguishable from each other, bone is easily palpated. Since muscle attachment is fairly consistent from one person to the next, the bones act as reference points for locating muscles.

SELF-TEST

Multiple Choice • Write the letter of the best answer in the space provided.

_______ 1. The skeletal system is composed of bones, cartilage, joints, and

A. blood C. ligaments
B. tendons D. hormones

_______ 2. How many bones are in the human body?

A. 250 C. 206
B. 172 D. 197

_______ 3. Which of the following is *NOT* a function of the skeleton system?

A. produces melanocytes
B. protects the body's vital organs
C. supports the body
D. stores lipids and minerals

_______ 4. The fibrous membrane covering bone that is the bone's life support system is called

A. intraosteum C. diaphysis
B. periosteum D. Haversian canals

_______ 5. Cells located in bone that breaks down osseous tissue to maintain homeostasis is called

A. osteoclasts C. hemocyte
B. destructocyte D. periosteum

_______ 6. Bones are classified according to shape. Which of the following is *not* one of the four classifications?

A. long C. flat
B. short D. regular

_______ 7. The end of a long bone is known as the

A. intraosteum C. diaphysis
B. periosteum D. epiphysis

_______ 8. A hole or opening in a bone is called a

A. condyle C. process
B. foramen D. facet

_______ 9. The two regions of the skeleton are the axial skeleton and the

A. medial skeleton C. disarticulating skeleton
B. extremely skeleton D. appendicular skeleton

_______ 10. The bones of the skull, thorax, vertebral column, and the hyoid bone comprise the

A. axial skeleton C. disarticulating skeleton
B. central skeleton D. appendicular skeleton

_______ 11. When two or more bones come together, this is known as a/an

A. articulation or joint C. periosteum
B. axial skeleton D. structure

_______ 12. The three types of functional articulation are synarthrotic, amphiarthrotic, and

A. diarthrotic C. dysfibrous
B. osteoarthritic D. joint

_______ 13. The viscous lubricating fluid associated with articulations is called

A. serous fluid C. mucous
B. synovial fluid D. plasma

_______ 14. A saclike membrane that contains synovial fluid and is provided around joints to prevent friction is called

A. suture C. retinaculum
B. tendon D. bursae

_______ 15. Greatest range of movement is from

A. pivot joints C. ball-and-socket joints
B. hinge joints D. saddle joints

Matching • List the letter of the answer to the term or phrase that best describes it.

A. flexion
B. abduction
C. elevation
D. pronation
E. dorsiflexion
F. depression
G. retraction
H. extension
I. eversion
J. adduction
K. supination
L. inversion
M. circumduction
N. plantar flexion
O. protraction

_______ 1. movement where the sole of the foot is turned inward

_______ 2. circular movement; cone-shaped range of motion

_______ 3. movement away from the median axis

_______ 4. lateral rotation or outward rotation

_______ 5. movement backward, or retrusion

_______ 6. extension or planting the toes in the earth

_______ 7. bending or decreasing the angle of a joint

_______ 8. movement where the sole of the foot is turned outward

_______ 9. raising or elevating a body part

_______ 10. medial or inward rotation

_______ 11. foot hyperextension, as in walking on the heels

_______ 12. straightening or increasing the angle of a joint

_______ 13. movement forward

_______ 14. lowering or dropping a body part

_______ 15. movement toward the median axis

References

Applegate, Edith J., M.S. *The Anatomy and Physiology Learning System: Textbook.* Philadelphia: W. B. Saunders, 1995.

Dominguez, Richard and Robert Gajda. *Total Body Training.* New York: Warnerbooks, 1982.

Goldberg, Stephen, M.D. *Clinical Anatomy Made Ridiculously Simple.* Miami: Medmaster, Inc., 1984.

Haubrich, William S. *Medical Meanings, A Glossary of Word Origins.* New York: Harcourt Brace Jovanovich, 1984.

Kapandji, I. A. *The Physiology of the Joints.* New York: Churchill Livingstone, 1982.

Kordish, Mary and Sylvia Dickson. *Introduction to Basic Human Anatomy.* Lake Charles, LA: McNeese State University, Self-Published Manual. 1985.

Luttgens, Kathryn and Katharine Wells. *Kinesiology: Scientific Basis of Human Motion,* 7th ed. Philadelphia: Saunders College Publishing. 1982.

Marieb, Elaine N. *Essentials of Human Anatomy and Physiology,* 4th ed. New York: Benjamin/Cummings Publishing Company, Inc., 1994.

McAleer, Neil. *The Body Almanac.* Garden City, New York: Doubleday and Company, Inc., 1985.

McAtee, Robert. *Facilitated Stretching.* Colorado Springs, CO: Human Kinetics Publishing, 1993.

Moore, Keith L. *Clinically Oriented Anatomy,* 2nd ed. Baltimore: Williams & Wilkins, 1985.

Mosby's Medical, Nursing, and Allied Health Dictionary, 4th ed. St Louis: Mosby–Year Book, Inc., 1994.

Newton, Don. *Pathology for Massage Therapists,* 2nd ed. Portland: Simran Publications, 1995.

Premkumar, Kalyani, *Pathology A to Z—A Handbook for Massage Therapists.* Calgary, Canada: VanPub Books, 1996.

Southmayd, William and Marshall Hoffman. *SportsHealth: The Complete Book of Athletic Injuries.* New York and London: Quick Fox, 1981.

Tabers Cyclopedic Medical Dictionary, 13th ed. Philadelphia: F. A. Davis Company, 1977.

Tortora Gerald J. *Introduction to the Human Body: The Essentials of Anatomy and Physiology,* 3rd ed. New York: HarperCollins Publishers, 1994.

Education is not filling a bucket
but lighting a fire.
—William Butler Yeats

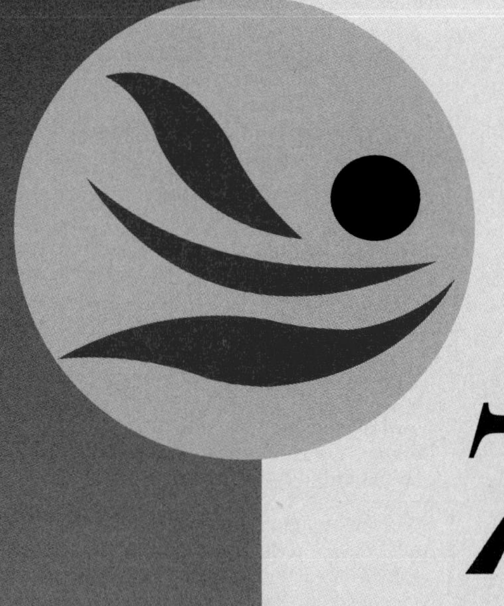

7
Skeletal Nomenclature

Student Objectives

After completing this chapter, the student should be able to:

- Describe the general locations of each bone listed in the chapter
- Explain the location of each bony marking listed in the chapter

INTRODUCTION

As a massage therapist, you will come to know the skeleton very well. Bones are landmarks for locating muscles and other soft tissues. Many of the terms we have learned in earlier chapters are repeated here. For example, the thigh bones are called the femurs because they are located in the femoral regions of the body. This information is a prerequisite to learning the muscular system, which is one of the main focuses for the study of massage therapy.

This chapter is divided into five lessons, and each lesson is divided into an anatomical region that includes the bones of that region (Fig. 7–1). Along with the bone names and locations, we will learn many bony markings and joints. Not all the bones and their surface markings or joints will be listed, just those that are the most important in the practice of massage

Terms and Word Roots Related to the Skeletal System

acetabulum – vinegar, saucer, or bowl; small
acromion – extremity; topmost; the shoulder
amphi – on both sides
arthric – joint
aspera – rough
atlas – to bear; as the giant of Greek mythology holding up the world
axis – an axis; an axle
bifid – cleaved or split in two; twice
bursa – a leather sac
carpus – wrist
calcaneus – heel
clavicle – little key
condyle – knuckle
coracoid – like a crow's beak
coronal – shaped like a corona or crown around the head
costa – rib
crepitus – a rattle
cribriform – sievelike
crista galli – cock's comb
cuneiform – wedge-shaped
diarthritic – two; joint
digit – resembling a finger or toe
dens – toothlike
epiphysis – epi upon, over; to grow
ethmoid – sievelike; shaped
fascia – strong central structural unit or band
femur – thigh
fontanel – a small fountain
gladiolus – small sword
glenoid – like a socket; shaped
hamate – to possess a small hook
Haversian – British physician and anatomist (1650–1702)
humerus – upper arm
hyoid – "U" shaped
ilium – flank
ischium – hip
kyphosis – humpbacked condition
lambdoidal – shaped like the Greek letter Λ
lamina – a thin plate
ligament – band
linea – line
lordosis – bent backward
malleolus – hammer or mallet; small
mandible – lower jawbone
manubrium – a handle
mastoid – breastlike; shaped
meatus – a passage
meniscus – moon; small
metacarpals – after or beyond; wrist
metatarsals – after or beyond; foot
navicular – a ship; small
obturator – to close, block up, or plug
odont – toothlike
olecranon – skull or head of the elbow
ossification – bone; to make
ossicle – small bone
osteo; osseo – bone
parietal – a wall or partition
patella – a little dish
pectoral – the breast or chest
pedicle – small foot
pelvis – a basin
periosteum – around, about; bone
phalanx – a battle line or a closely knit row
pisiform – pea-shaped
poples – ham
prominens – prominent or projecting
pterygoid – winglike; shaped
pubic – grownup
ramus – a branch
sacrum – sacred
sagittal – an arrow
scaphoid – boatlike; shaped
scoliosis – crooked condition
sella – a saddle or seat
sesamoid – sesame seed-like; shaped
sinus – a recess or cavity
skeleton – dried up
sphenoid – wedge-shaped; shaped
spine – spiny or thorny plant
stapes – a stirrup
styloid – a pillar; shaped
suture – to sew; a seam
symphysis – together with, joined; to grow
synarthritic – together; joint
talus – ankle
tarsals – broad, flat surface; foot
temporal – time
trochanter – a wheel or runner
tubercle – a hump, knob, or swelling; small
turcica – Turkish
ulna – elbow
vertebrae – turning joint
Volkmann's canals – named after a German physician (1800–1877)
xiphoid – swordlike; shaped
zygomatic – a yoke or bar

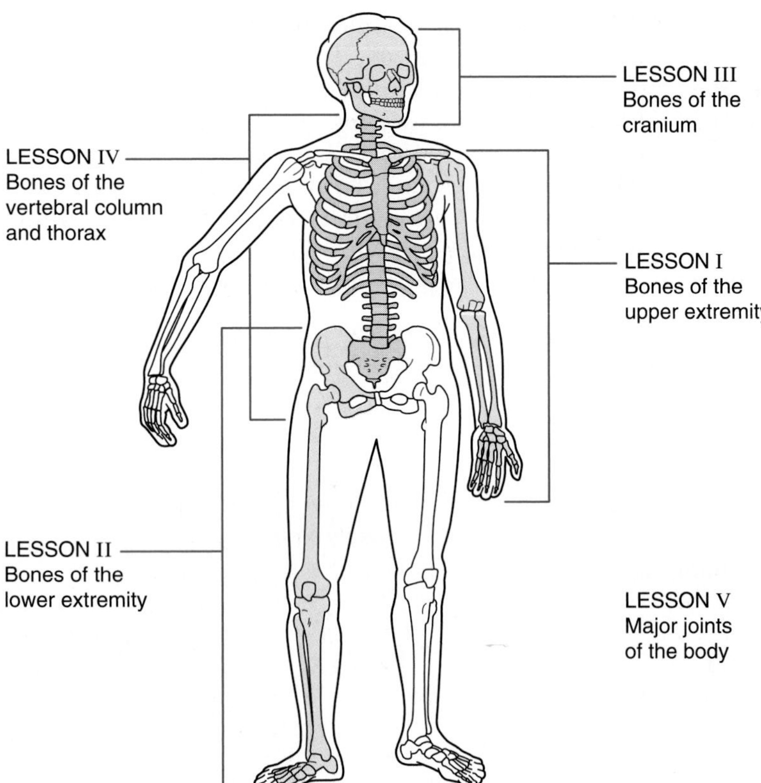

Figure 7•1 The relationship of the five lessons of this chapter to the human skeleton as a whole.

therapy. The best teacher is your own body and all the bodies you will be working with. Instead of saying, "I am massaging the arm," repeat to yourself the names "humerus, radius, and ulna." In this way, you will continually be reinforcing your new vocabulary. Try using scapula instead of shoulder blade or olecranon process instead of tip of the elbow. The sooner you begin to incorporate this new language into your massage work, the sooner you will have the confidence to progress into the world of muscles.

LESSON ONE—BONES OF THE UPPER EXTREMITY

There are eight bones in lesson one: the clavicle, scapula, humerus, ulna, radius, carpals (8 in number), metacarpals (5 in number), and phalanges (14 in number).

The upper limbs of most four-footed animals have evolved as crucial components of a running machine. Like their hind limbs, the forelimbs of a quadruped are made to bear weight and provide locomotion and quick acceleration. Dexterity is limited. When *Homo sapiens* went from being a quadruped (four footed) to a biped (two footed), our forelimbs or arms could be used for dexterity, articulation, and manipulation, rather than weight bearing, propulsion, and acceleration. Compared with the bones of the lower extremity, the bones of the upper extremity are light and less dense. The ball-and-socket joints of the shoulder are extremely shallow, thus achieving a large range of motion. The hip joint, by comparison, is a much deeper, more stable joint. It is made for weight bearing, but mobility is sacrificed. The joints of the hands, and particularly the opposable thumb, have evolved into a precision instrument capable of performing the most dexterous movements in the human body.

Shoulder or Pectoral Girdle. The bones of the shoulder or pectoral girdle are the clavicle and the scapula (Fig. 7–2). One of the reasons that we have such a wide range of motion in the upper extremity is because the shoulder girdle is attached to the axial skeleton at only one junction: the sternoclavicular joint. The sternal bone is associated with the axial skeleton and the clavicle bone is associated with the appendicular skeleton.

1. **Clavicle.** The clavicle acts as a brace to hold the arm away from the top of the thorax. If you know this bone as the "collar bone," remember C & C—the collar bone is the clavicle. When the clavicle is broken, the entire shoulder region caves in medially. This demonstrates how the clavicle functions as a brace. The clavicle has a sternal end, which is medial, and an acromial end, which is lateral.
2. **Scapula.** The scapula is a triangular-shaped bone located between the second and the seventh ribs. When the scapula is set in motion, it floats against the posterior aspect of the rib cage. If you already know the term "shoulder blade," then remember

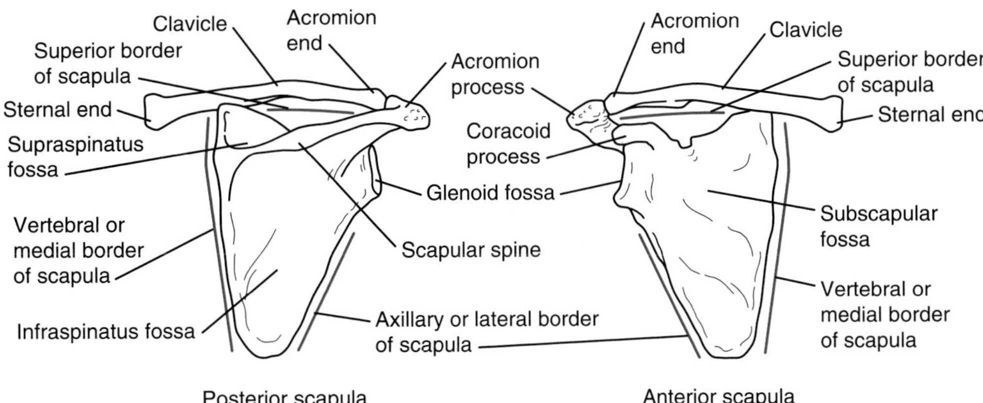

Figure 7•2 Scapula and the clavicle with surface markings.

S & S—shoulder blade is the scapula. The scapula has three borders: the superior, the medial or vertebral, and the lateral or axillary.

Scapular spine, also referred to as the spine of the scapula, can easily be palpated through the skin because muscles do not lie across this structure.

Acromion process is the enlarged lateral end of the scapular spine, which attaches to the clavicle. It is felt as the high point on the shoulder.

Coracoid process. This process protrudes anteriorly under the acromion for muscle attachment, namely the coracoid brachialis, the pectoralis minor, and the short head of the biceps brachii.

Glenoid fossa is the shallow socket on the lateral aspect of the scapula, which receives the head of the humerus to form the glenohumeral, or shoulder joint.

Subscapular fossa is the large depression in the anterior portion of the scapula and contains the subscapular muscle.

Supraspinatus fossa is a depression superior to the scapular spine and contains the supraspinatus muscle.

Infraspinatus fossa. This depression is inferior to the scapular spine and contains the infraspinatus muscle.

The Upper Extremity

3. **Humerus** The humerus is the upper arm bone (Fig. 7–3). It is also known as the "funny bone" or "crazy bone" because when you hit your elbow a certain way, it feels funny or "humorous." It's just a play on words. Actually, the sensation felt when you hit your funny bone is the ulnar nerve as it passes superficially over the medial epicondyle of the humerus. The proximal end of the humerus articulates with the scapula at the shoulder, and the distal end of the humerus articulates with the radius and the ulna at the elbow.

The **humeral head** is the part of the humerus that rests in the glenoid fossa of the scapula.

Surgical neck is located proximally to the section of the humerus where most fractures occur.

Greater tubercle is located on the proximal end of the humerus and on the lateral side of the bicipital groove.

Lesser tubercle is located on the proximal end of the humerus and on the medial side of the bicipital groove.

Intertubercular or bicipital groove lies between the lesser and greater tubercle of the humerus. The tendon of the long head of the biceps brachii lies in this groove.

Medial epicondyle is found at the medial distal end of the humerus and articulates with the ulna.

Lateral epicondyle is found on the lateral distal

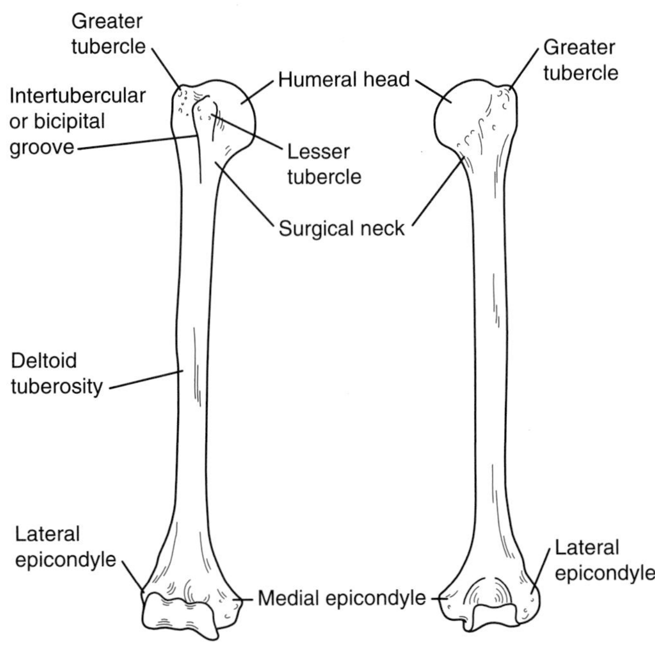

Figure 7•3 Humerus with surface markings.

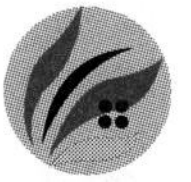

After graduation from massage school, I was ready to get a job to practice my new skill. Within 2 weeks, I was offered a job as the principal massage therapist at the Swedish Spa Resort. This was not a great feat because at that time I was the only massage therapist in town. It was an opportunity to massage a wide variety of people and learn a lot about the kind of injuries that occur in gyms.

Within a few short months I frequently noticed a "bump" on the midlateral upper arm on many of my clients. They seemed to be bilateral, so I ruled out injury, but what about pathology? "A little knowledge is a dangerous thing" were words of wisdom from my anatomy instructor.

The more clients I worked on, the more mysterious bumps I found. As luck would have it, one of my clients was an orthopedic surgeon. In desperation, I asked her what I was palpating on these clients. She began to laugh. I began to laugh, too, through embarrassment, when she told me that the bump that I was feeling on the upper arm was the deltoid tuberosity! ..

end of the humerus and articulates with the radius.

Deltoid tuberosity, also known as the deltoid tubercle, is the attachment site for the deltoid muscle.

4. **Ulna.** When looking at someone in the anatomical position, the ulna is the medial, or little finger, side of the arm (Fig. 7–4). The ulna articulates with the humerus (proximal end) and a carpal bone called the lunate (distal end).

Ulnar head. Located on the distal portion of the bone, the ulna is the only bone that stands on its head.

Olecranon process. This bony protrusion is located at the proximal end of the ulna and is the tip of the elbow. The olecranon process can also be referred to as the massage therapist's tool.

Styloid process is located at the distal end of the ulna and articulates with the lunate.

Trochlear or semilunar notch. The trochlear notch receives the posterior distal end of the humerus.

Coronoid process is located just below the trochlear notch, on the anterior side.

5. **Radius.** The radius is the lateral forearm bone, located on the thumb side of the arm. The easiest way to remember the radius from the ulna is to locate the radial pulse. You palpate the radial pulse by pressing it into the radial bone. Another way to remember the name of this bone is to remember that the *r*adius always *r*otates on the ulna. The radius articulates with the humerus (proximal end) and a carpal bone called the scaphoid (distal end).

Radial head. The radial head is located on the proximal end and articulates with the distal end of the humerus.

Radial or bicipital tuberosity. This is a small bony bump located near the proximal end of the radius.

Styloid process is located at the distal end of the radius and articulates with the scaphoid and the lunate.

An interosseous membrane weaves the ulna and the radius with bands of tough connective tissue. This anatomical arrangement gives the forearm lightness and mobility, while providing attachment sites for the many muscles of the hand. Imagine how heavy the arm would be if the ulna and radius were just one solid bone!

Hands. Each hand contains 27 bones: 8 carpals, 5 metacarpals, and 14 phalanges (Fig. 7–5). Our hands have evolved from mammalian paws and are a wondrous combination of balance, power, and dexterity. Dr. William Southmayd, author of *Sportshealth,* compares the hands to the eyes in the sense that both are extensions of the human brain and most skills require eye-hand coordination. It is our opposable thumb that makes the human hand vastly different from other mammals. The thumb is opposable and can be rotated

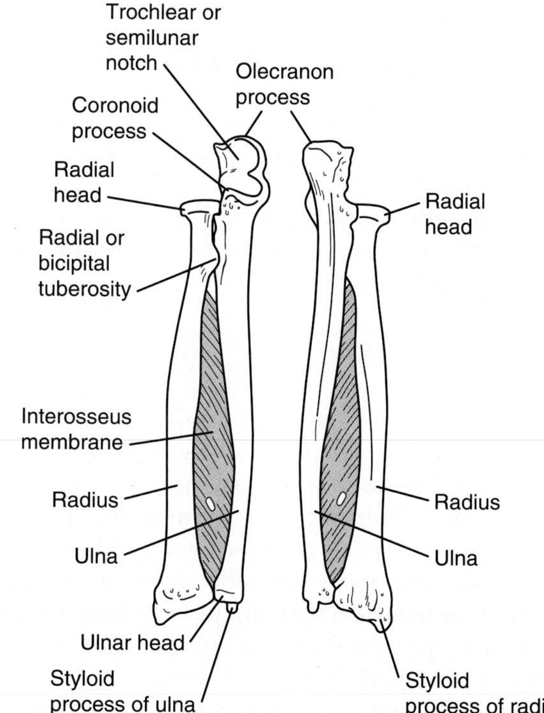

Figure 7•4 Ulna and radius with surface markings.

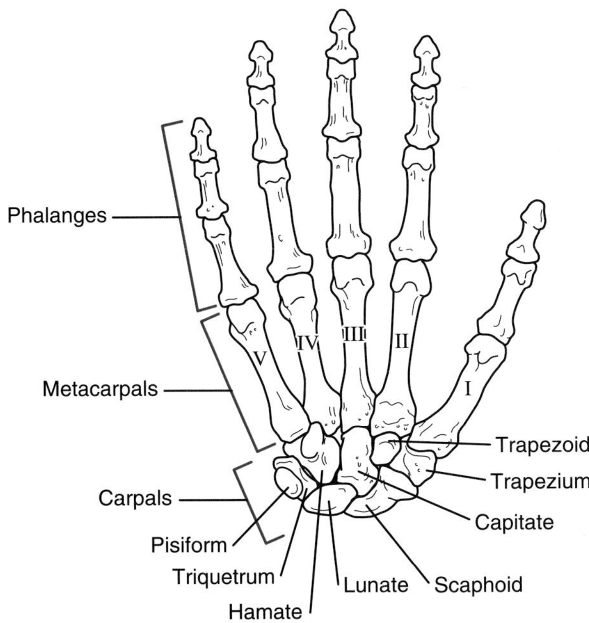

Figure 7•5 Carpals, metacarpals, and phalanges.

in front of the palm in the opposite direction of the other four digits. It is this flexibility that gives us the ability to create and use tools.

6. **Carpals.** The eight carpal bones of the wrist are arranged in two rows of four that are linked together by ligaments and bound in a joint capsule. The carpal bones function like eight ball bearings. For centuries, they were simply numbered one through eight. In the early 1800s, each bone was named individually. The names of the carpal bones are the scaphoid, lunate, triquetrum, pisiform, trapezium, trapezoid, capitate, and hamate.
7. **Metacarpals.** The metacarpals are also referred to as the hand bones. There are five in each hand, numbered I through V, starting from the thumb (I) to the little finger (V). When you clench your hand to make a fist, the heads of the distal ends of the metacarpals become obvious as the knuckles.
8. **Phalanges.** There are 14 phalanges in each hand. Three are located in each finger, and 2 are located in the thumb.

LESSON TWO—BONES OF THE LOWER EXTREMITY

Fourteen bones will be discussed in lesson two. Compared with the bones of the upper extremity, the leg bones are larger, heavier, and more dense. The individual bones of the lower extremity are the ilium, ischium, pubis, femur, patella, tibia, fibula, tarsals (7 in number), metatarsals (5 in number), and phalanges (14 in number).

Pelvic Girdle. The pelvic girdle is also known as the os coxa, the coxal bone, or the innominate bone. Each pelvic bone is made up of three fused embryonic bones: the ilium, ischium, and pubis. In contrast, the pelvis is formed by the two matched pelvic bones, anteriorly connected by the pubic bones at the symphysis pubis, and the sacrum, posteriorly connected by the ilium (Fig. 7–6). The sacrum is *not* part of the pelvic girdle, but it must be included when discussing the pelvis. The pelvis looks like a bowl of circles, holes, and arches. It holds the digestive, reproductive, and urinary organs and creates a passageway for birth and the elimination of wastes.

The pelvic girdle also provides a pathway for the nerves and vessels traveling from the trunk to the lower limbs. This bony unit serves as an attachment site for muscles, integrating the axial and lower appendicular skeleton. Over two dozen muscles attach on the pelvic girdle, including muscles of the spine, buttocks, abdominals, and several of the muscles of the anterior and posterior thigh. The pelvic girdle is a highly mobile structure, constantly responding to activity from above and below. Weight bearing is the most important function of the girdle because the total weight of the upper body sits on the pelvis.

1. **Ilium.** The ilium is the most superior pelvic bone in the pelvic girdle and looks like a broad expanding blade.

   Iliac crest. When you place your hands on your hips, they are resting on your iliac crests. This bony marking is easily palpable because no muscles or tendons lie across it.

   Anterior superior iliac spine. This is located on the anterior end of the iliac crest, and is a muscle attachment site for the sartorius muscle.

   Anterior inferior iliac spine is located on the anterior aspect of the ilium and is a muscle attachment site for the rectus femoris muscle.

   Greater sciatic notch. This is where the sciatic nerve traverses the ilium as it makes its way down the leg.

   Posterior superior iliac spine is the bony projection at the posterior end of the iliac crest. It can be located just below the "dimples" of the low back.

   Posterior inferior iliac spine is located below the posterior superior iliac spine, superior and medial to the greater sciatic notch.

   Superior, middle, inferior gluteal lines. These surface markings are located on the posterior aspect of the ilium. The large gluteal muscles attach in these bony lines.

2. **Ischium.** The ischium is the inferior and most posterior part of the pelvic girdle.

   Ischial tuberosity. This bony protrusion is also known as your sit bone. The ischial tuberosity receives the weight of the body when sitting and provides muscle attachments, namely the hamstrings and adductor magnus. Poor sitting

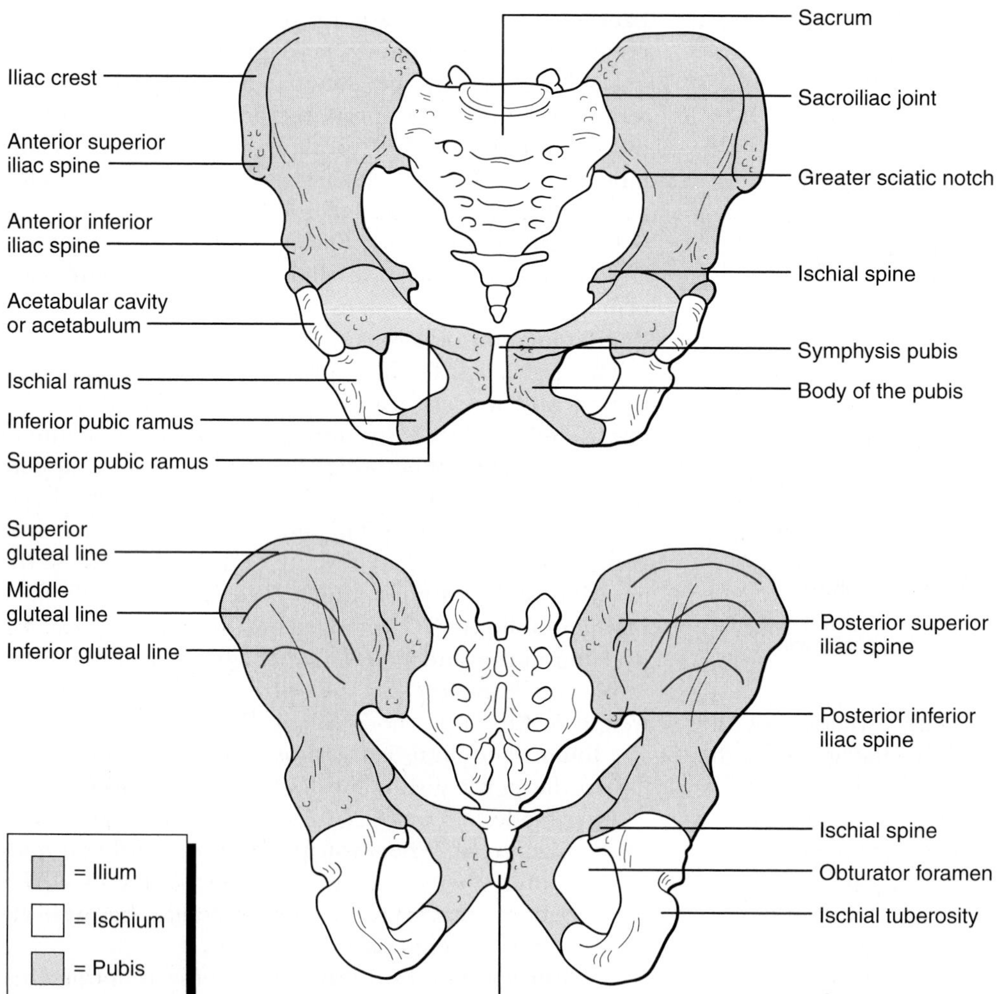

Figure 7•6 Pelvic girdle with surface markings.

posture can be the result of sitting on your sacral bone instead of the ischial tuberosity (Fig. 7–7).

Ischial spine. This structure varies in length from individual to individual and is a site for muscle attachment for some of the pelvic floor muscles and one of the hip rotators. It is also used as a landmark in pregnancy. In the final stages of pregnancy, the obstetrician will be able to locate the position of the fetal head by locating the ischial spine. If the head is at the level of the ischial spine, it is said to be at station zero. When the fetal head is superior to the ischial spine, it is in the negative station. If the head descends inferiorly from the ischial spine, it is in the positive station.

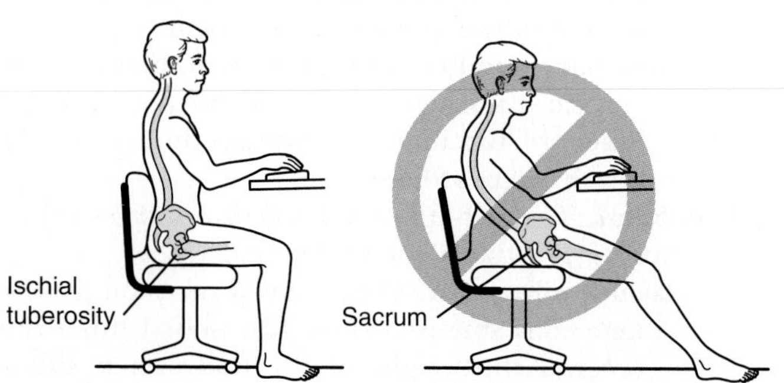

Figure 7•7 Sitting on your ischial tuberosity versus sitting on your sacrum.

Ischial ramus. This bony branch connects the ischial tuberosity with the pubis, forming the obturator foramen. It is also important for muscle attachments.

3. **Pubic bone or pubis.** In the most anterior portion of the pelvis, each of the two pubic bones resembles a wishbone, and they are collectively referred to as the pubis. These bones provide attachment sites for some of the abdominal muscles and fascia.

   Superior pubic ramus is the superior portion of the medial bony ring around the obturator foramen.

   Inferior pubic ramus is the inferior portion of the medial bony ring around the obturator foramen.

The **body of the pubis** forms the medial aspect of the pubis and the symphysis pubis. The symphysis pubis is the joint that superiorly connects the two pelvic bones.

Other Pelvic Structures

Acetabulum or Acetabular Cavity. Also known as the hip socket, the acetabulum receives the head of the femur. The ilium, ischium, and pubic bones all contribute to its makeup. Looking at the acetabulum laterally, it resembles a concave pie divided into roughly three equal pieces. Each piece is one of the three bones of the pelvic girdle. This allows equal force from all three dimensions to pass into the acetabulum.

Obturator Foramen. The obturator foramen is located inferior to the acetabulum. These bones are often referred as the "eyes" of the pelvis. The obturator membrane obstructs the foramen. This membrane provides attachment sites for the muscles of the hip.

Pelvic Inlet and Pelvic Outlet. The pelvic inlet is the superior opening of the pelvis and the pelvic outlet is the inferior opening of the pelvis. The digestive, urinary, and reproductive systems use this opening to empty their products externally.

The Lower Extremity

4. **Femur.** The femur is the longest, heaviest, and strongest bone in the body. It has a curved ball at the proximal end and two curved balls at the distal end (Fig. 7–8). The femur articulates proximally with the acetabulum, forming the hip joint and distally with the tibia, forming the knee joint. When looking at the femur, you will notice a distinct slant to the bone. The medial course of the femoral shaft (area between the two ends) is necessary to bring the hips back in line with the knee and lower leg bones. This medial direction of the femur is more noticeable in females because of their wider pelvis.

Femoral head. This is the "ball" part of the hip joint, located at the proximal end of the femur, which fits into the acetabulum, or hip socket. When turning the femur to the left or right, the femoral head is always pointed medially.

Femoral neck. This is the narrowed area of bone located between the femoral head and the femoral shaft. It is the most commonly fractured region of the femur, especially in postmenopausal women who have osteoporosis.

Greater trochanter. The large projection on the lateral side of the femur is known as the greater trochanter. This is what gets sore when you lie on your side on a hard floor.

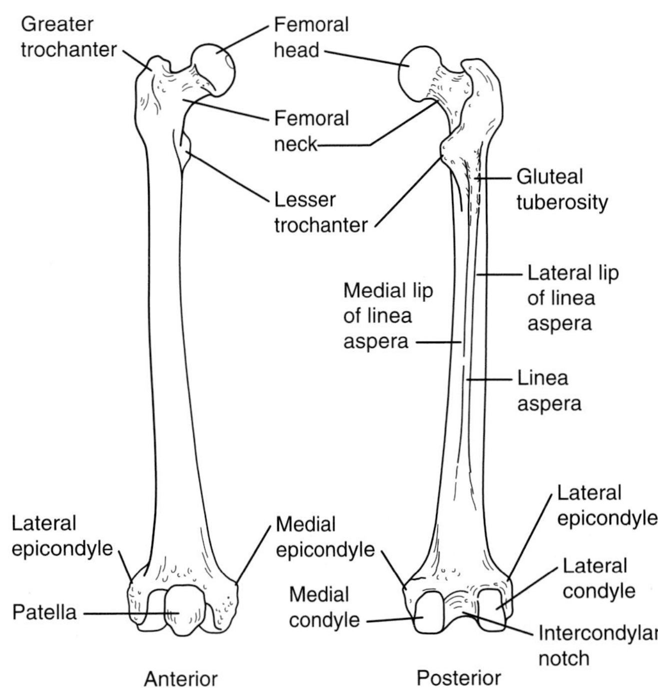

Figure 7•8 Femur and patella with surface markings.

Lesser trochanter is the superior medial bony marking for muscle attachment, namely the psoas major and the iliacus.

Medial condyle is the distal bony enlargement located on the medial aspect of the femur that articulates with the tibial plateau to form the knee joint.

Medial epicondyle is located on the distal aspect of the femur, superior to the medial condyle of the femur. The muscle that attaches here is the medial head of the gastrocnemius.

Lateral condyle is the distal bony enlargement located on the lateral aspect of the femur that articulates with the tibial plateau to form the knee joint.

Lateral epicondyle is located on the distal aspect of the femur, superior to the lateral condyle of the femur. The muscle that attaches here is the lateral head of the gastrocnemius.

Intercondylar notch. Also called the intercondylar fossa, this bony indentation is located between the medial and lateral condyles of the femur.

Linea aspera is the rough vertical ridge located on the posterior femoral shaft for muscle attachment, namely the hamstrings. Note that the linea aspera possesses a medial lip and a lateral lip.

Gluteal tuberosity. This is the roughened area located on the superior lateral lip of the linea aspera. The gluteus maximus muscle attaches here.

5. **Patella.** The patella, or kneecap, is the largest sesamoid bone in the body and is located anterior to the knee joint. It arises from the tendon of the quadriceps femoris muscle and can provide additional leverage for knee extension. However, the patella is not considered part of the knee joint. Its main function is to provide stabilization, cushion the hinge joints, and protect the knee by shielding it from impact.
6. **Tibia.** The tibia, or shin bone, is the stoutest and straightest bone in the body and is located below the femur on the medial side of the lower leg (Fig. 7–9). The distal aspect of the tibia articulates with the talus bone. The top of the tibia is relatively flat and the shaft has a triangular shape. It helps to transfer weight from the femur to the foot.

    Medial malleolus. This is the distal end of the tibia, forming the medial bulge of the ankle. The inferior surface of the medial malleolus articulates with the talus to help form the ankle joint.

    Tibial or patellar tuberosity. The tibial tuberosity is located on the proximal anterior side of the tibia. The large quadriceps femoris muscle attaches at this site via the patellar ligament.

    Tibial plateau. The superior ledge of the tibia that receives the condyles of the femur is known as the tibial plateau.

    Anterior crest. When you scrape your shin, you are actually striking the anterior crest of the tibia. It is the front point of the bony triangle.

    Medial condyle. The medial condyle of the tibia is located on the proximal end on the medial side, just below the tibial plateau.

    Lateral condyle. The lateral condyle of the tibia is located on the proximal end on the lateral side, just below the tibial plateau.

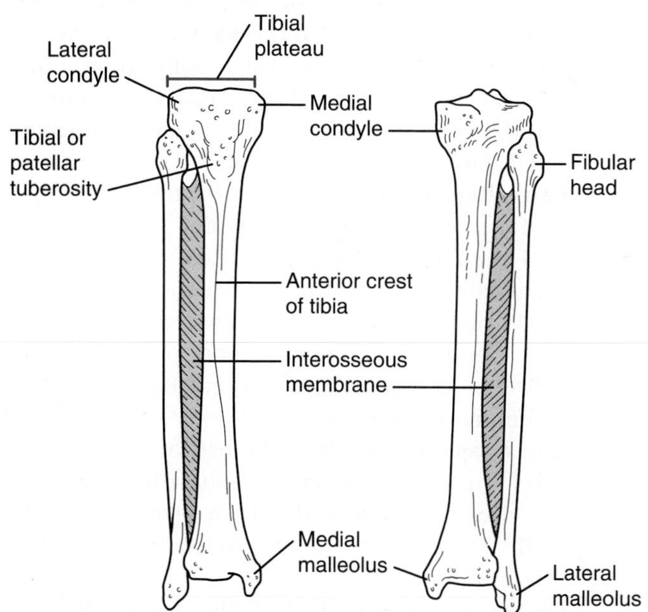

Figure 7•9 Tibia and fibula with surface markings.

7. **Fibula.** The fibula is located on the lateral side of the lower leg. Remember that a fib is a little white lie, so the *fib*ula is smaller than the tibia. The fibula attaches to the tibia below the tibial plateau and is not involved with the knee joint. The distal end of the fibula articulates with the talus bone. One can remove a section of the fibula for purposes of obtaining a bone graft without significant decrease in function of the lower extremity. Like the ulna and radius of the upper extremity, an interosseous membrane connects the tibia and the fibula.

    Fibular head. The head of the fibula is located at the proximal end of the fibula and articulates with the inferior surface of the lateral condyle of the tibia.

    Lateral malleolus. The distal end of the fibula, forming the lateral bulge of the ankle bone is known as the lateral malleolus. The inferior surface of the lateral malleolus articulates with the talus to help form the ankle joint.

Feet. During walking, running, jumping, or standing, our feet provide our base of support. Each foot contains 26 bones: 7 tarsals, 5 metatarsals, and 14 phalanges (Fig. 7–10). Each tarsal is an irregular bone that slides minutely over the next bone to collectively provide motion. This is similar to the way the spine creates movement. In massage therapy, range of motion exercises can help keep the tarsal bones mobile. If the tarsal bones become immobile or stuck, they will not be able to move properly or absorb shock.

8. **Talus.** The talus bone, or astragalus, is the main tarsal. It is also referred to as the ankle bone, but the ankle bones are usually thought of as the distal ends of the tibia and fibula. The talus articulates superiorly with the tibia and the fibula to form the ankle joint. To help you remember the location of this bone, the *t*alus, it is *t*allest of all the foot bones. The talus bears the weight of the entire body when standing or walking.
9. **Calcaneus.** The calcaneus is also known as the heel bone. It is the most inferior and posterior tarsal bone. It is also the largest and strongest bone of the foot. The longest foot ligament runs from the calcaneus to the metatarsal heads and is called the arch ligament or *plantar fascia.*
10. **Cuboid.** The cuboid bone is situated between the fourth and fifth metatarsals and the calcaneus bone.
11. **Cuneiform.** There are three cuneiform bones, numbered medially to laterally from I through III.

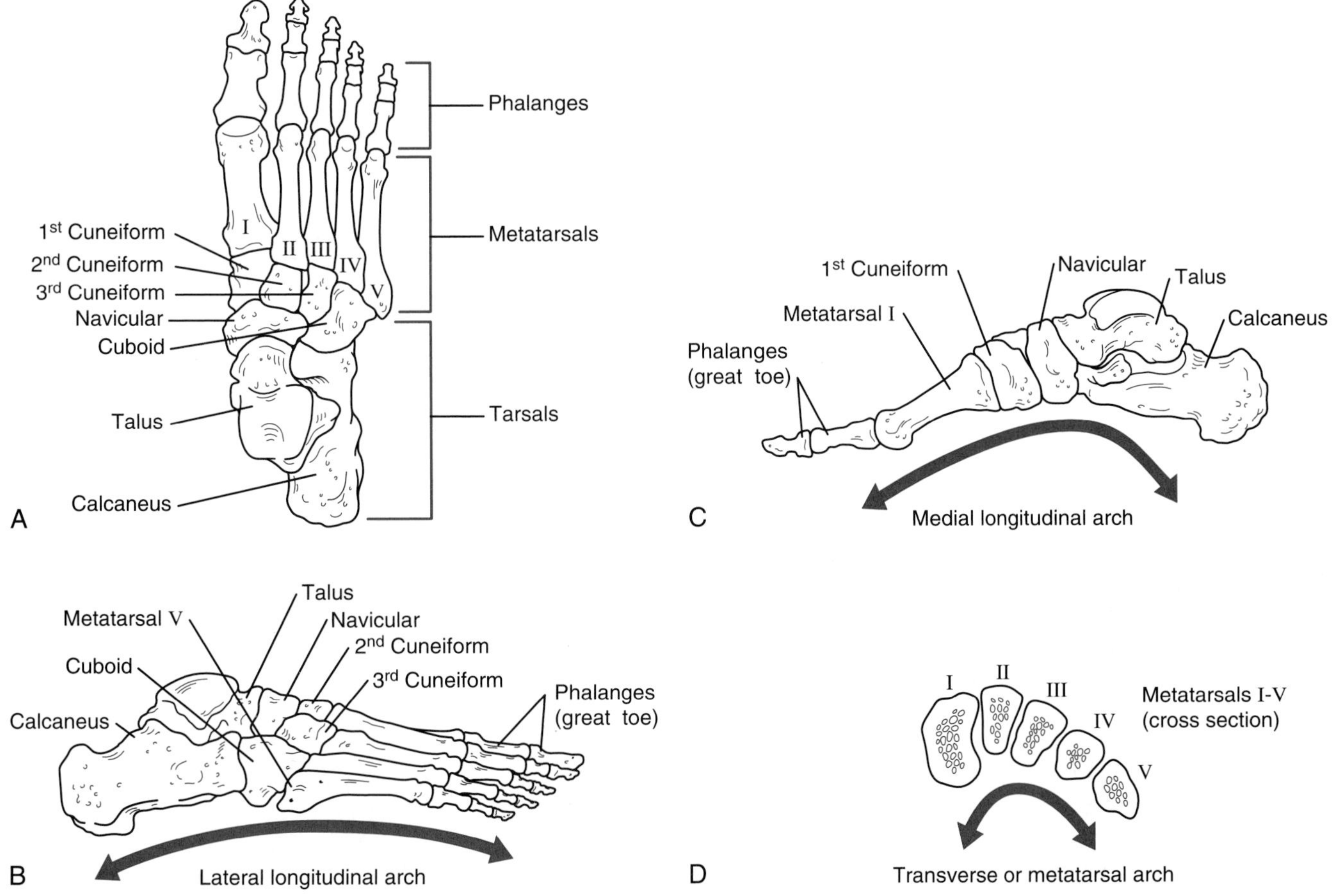

Figure 7•10 Tarsals, metatarsals, and the arches of the foot.

The most medial cuneiform is I, the middle cuneiform is II, and the most lateral cuneiform is III. All cuneiform bones are located between the navicular bone and the first three metatarsal bones.

12. **Navicular.** The navicular bone is located between the talus bone and the three cuneiforms.
13. **Metatarsals.** There are five metatarsals in each foot, numbered I through V. The length of your metatarsals determines if you wear a size six or a size ten shoe. When you flex your toes dorsally and look at your knuckles, you are actually looking at the distal ends of the metatarsals. The metatarsals articulate proximally with cuboid and cuneiforms and distally with the phalanges.
14. **Phalanges.** The phalanges are also known as the digits, or toes. There are 3 in each toe and 2 in the great toe for a total of 14 in each foot. As we walk, the first and second toe appears to be the fulcrum or pivot point for actions of the foot, like walking and jumping. The great toe is also referred to as the *hallux.*

The Plantar Vault or Foot Arch

In order for walking, running, and jumping to be springy, our feet must absorb shock. To help accomplish this, the foot uses a system of arches to prevent the plantar surface of the foot from becoming flat (see Fig. 7–10). These three strong arches look like a geodesic dome. Because the names of the arches are descriptive, they will be easy to learn. Weak arches are referred to as fallen arches or flat feet. To strengthen these arches and the intrinsic muscles of the foot, pick up marbles or rocks with your toes. The three arches are as follows:

1. Medial longitudinal arch
2. Lateral longitudinal arch
3. Transverse or metatarsal arch

LESSON THREE—BONES OF THE CRANIUM

There are ten bones in lesson three, which highlights the bones of the skull: the sinuses, ear bones, main sutures, and fontanels. The entire head contains 29 bones; 8 bones in the skull, 14 bones in the face, 6 ear ossicles, and 1 bone suspended from ligaments arising from the temporal bone. Except for one synovial joint located at the jaw, the temporomandibular joint, all skull bones and facial bones are joined by sutures. Note that all cranial bones are included in this lesson, but not all facial bones.

Cranial Vault. The cranial vault contains the frontal bone, two parietal bones, two temporal bones, the ethmoid bone, the sphenoid bone, and the occipital bone (Fig. 7–11). This bony region protects the brain and related nerves; it also provides a bony passageway for the organs of sight, taste, hearing, and olfaction.

1. **Frontal.** The frontal bone forms the forehead, and the roof of the eye sockets (eye orbits) and the anterior cranial floor.

    Supraorbital foramen or **supraorbital notch** is located along the superior ledge of the eye orbit on the lateral side where the supraorbital nerve and artery pass through this foramen. Some individuals have a foramen and others possess a notch. Surgeons often anesthetize the supraorbital nerve where it exits the supraorbital foramen prior to eye surgery.

2. **Parietal.** These two paired bones make up the majority of the sides and the roof of the cranium.
3. **Temporal.** The temporal bones form the inferior sides of the cranium as well as the lateral sides of the cranial floor.

    Styloid process is a short slender projection directed inferiorly and anteriorly located on the

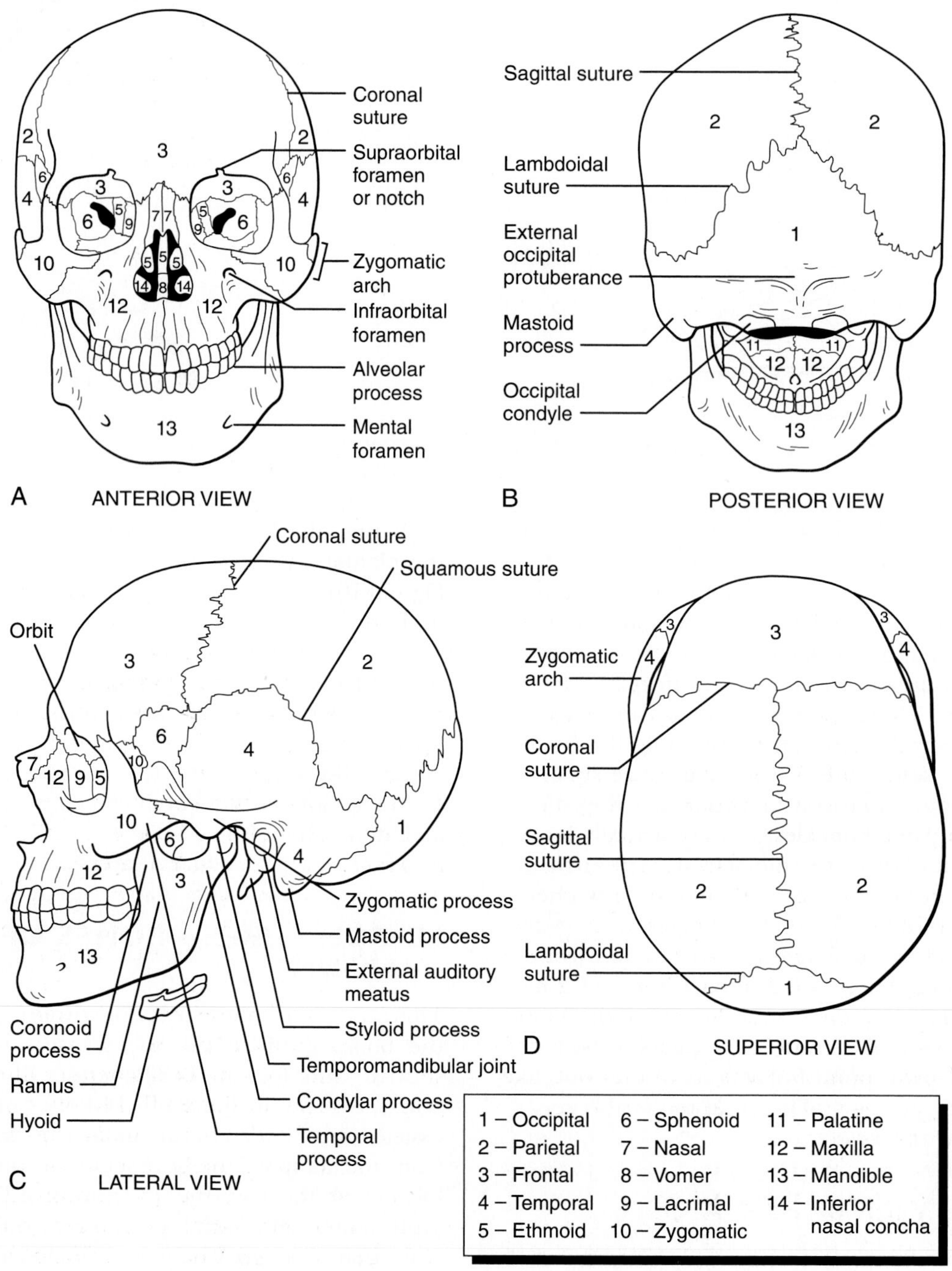

Figure 7•11 The cranial bones from different angles.

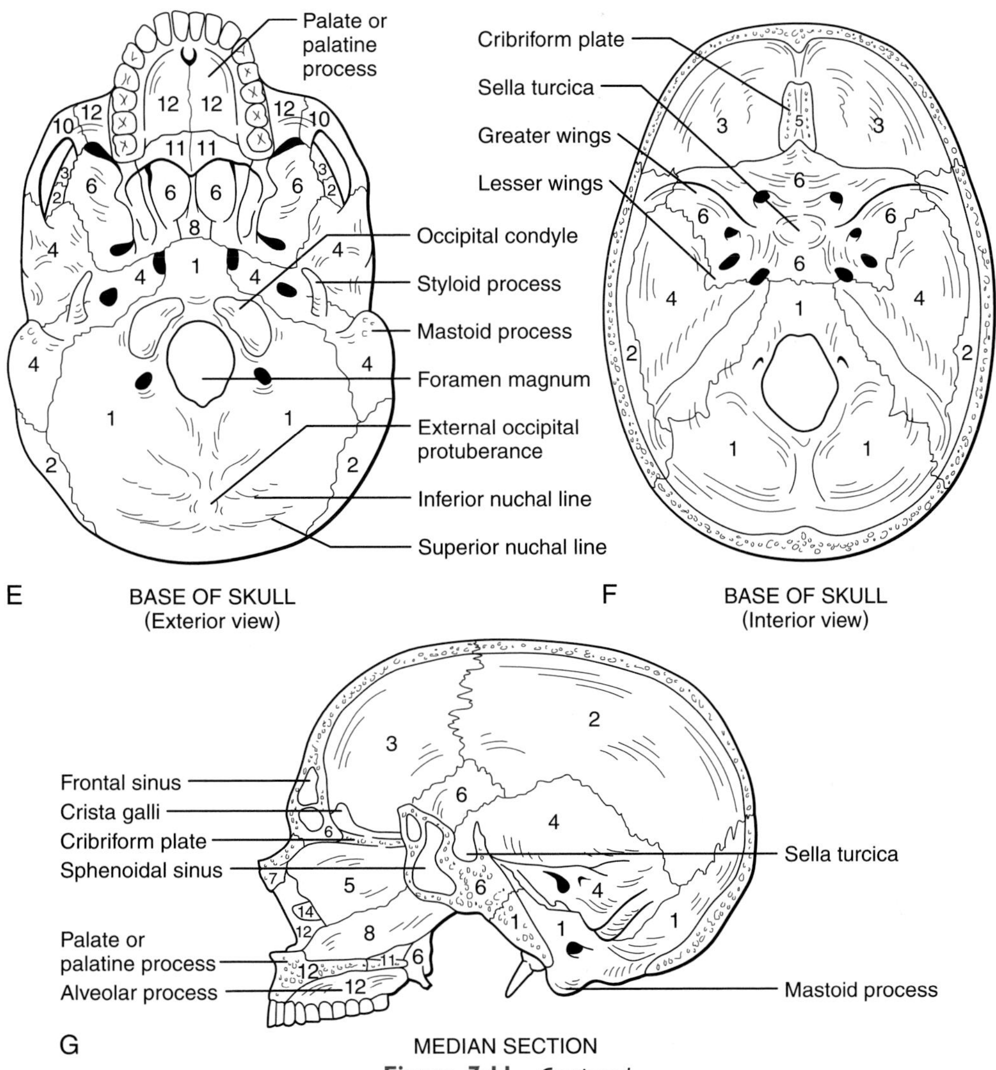

Figure 7•11 *Continued*

inferior surface of the temporal bone. Several neck muscles and the ligaments of the tongue attach on this bony marking. The styloid process of the temporal bone is an endangerment site for the massage therapist because it can be broken if direct pressure is applied on the site.

External auditory meatus. Also known as the ear canal, the external auditory meatus is the tubelike canal that leads to the middle and inner ear. The middle ear contains the six smallest bones in the body—the ear ossicles.

Ear ossicles. Each ear contains three tiny bones that vibrate with sound waves. These ear ossicles are the malleus, incus, and stapes. In the primary grades, they are known as the hammer, anvil, and stirrup.

Mastoid process. The large bony process inferior to the external auditory meatus is known as the mastoid process and is a site for neck muscle attachments.

Zygomatic process. The zygomatic process connects with the temporal process of the zygomatic bone anteriorly to form the zygomatic arch.

4. **Sphenoid.** This butterfly- or bat-shaped bone lies in the transverse plane, making a floor for the brain and a ceiling for the mouth. The sphenoid bone is known as the cornerstone of the cranial floor because it articulates with all other cranial bones.

Sella turcica. The sella turcica is the deep bony indentation that is located on the superior surface of the sphenoid bone, which receives the pituitary gland.

Greater wings. Located on either side of the sphenoid bone, these two processes extend laterally from the body, curving upward and outward. This bony marking is a site for muscle attachment and transmits blood vessels and nerves through numerous foramina.

Lesser wings. These two thin plates extend from the upper lateral surface of the body of the sphenoid bone. The lesser wing of the sphenoid forms the roof of the eye orbit and transmits several blood vessels and nerves and provides muscle attachment for several muscles of the eye.

5. **Ethmoid.** This bone forms part of the cranial floor, the medial border of the eye orbit, and the superior portion of the nasal septum.
   Cribriform plate, or the horizontal plate, forms part of the base of the skull and joins the frontal bones between the two orbital plates.
   Crista galli is a smooth, thick, triangular process that projects superiorly from the base of the cribriform plate. Its posterior border serves as an attachment for the falx cerebri (folds in the cranial meninges; see the nervous system chapter).
6. **Occipital.** The occipital bone makes up most of the posterior and inferior portion of the cranial base.
   Foramen magnum. This is the largest foramen in the skull. The medulla oblongata (part of the brain), the 11th cranial nerve, and spinal and vertebral arteries pass through this opening.
   Superior nuchal line is a linear elevation running transversely for muscle attachments located just above the inferior nuchal line.
   Inferior nuchal line is a linear elevation running transversely for muscle attachments located below the superior nuchal line.
   External occipital protuberance. This is a bony projection superior to the foramen magnum. This structure can be palpated just above the neck and feels like a bony bump in the middle of the back of the head.
   Occipital condyles. These bony markings have convex surfaces, positioned on either side of the foramen magnum, and articulate with the first cervical vertebra.
7. **Hyoid.** The hyoid bone is shaped like a miniature mandible (jawbone) with two incisor teeth. This bone does not articulate directly with any other bone. It is suspended from the styloid process of the temporal bone by ligaments and serves as a support for the tongue and provides muscle attachments for the tongue, neck, and pharynx. This bone is important in forensic medicine. When it is found broken, it usually means the victim was strangled or hanged.

Sutures. Sutures are located anywhere cranial bones join and are classified as synarthrotic joints. Very little movement exists in these sutural regions.

Sagittal Suture. The sagittal suture joins the two parietal bones.

Coronal Suture. This suture is shaped like a corona, or crown, around the head and separates the frontal bone from the parietal bones.

Lambdoidal Suture. The lambdoidal suture separates the parietal bones from the occipital bone.

Squamosal Suture. The parietal bones and the temporal bones are separated by this suture.

Author's Note

Dr. William Sutherland, a student of Dr. Andrew Still (father of osteopathy), became convinced through study and practice that the bones of the skull do not completely fuse, but rather retain a small, yet significant degree of motion relative to one another.

This idea was expounded on by Dr. John Upledger and was proven when he took pictures of sutural contents. Connective tissue and vascular tissue were discovered between the sutures!

From his finding, Dr. Upledger developed a system of nonintrusive diagnosis and treatment called craniosacral therapy.

Facial Bones. The face is the most expressive part of our body due to the many facial muscles. Our facial features are largely a result of our facial bone and cartilaginous structures. High cheekbones, a prominent nose, or a pointed chin are all representative of our facial bones. When recalling someone, we ordinarily don't instantly recall their legs or back, we remember the face.

The facial bones consist of the two nasal bones, the vomer bone, two zygomatic bones, two lacrimal bones, two palatine bones, two fused maxilla bones, two fused mandible bones, and two inferior nasal concha bones. Of the 14 bones of the face, only 3 will be featured.

8. **Zygomatic.** Also known as the cheekbone, the zygomatic bone connects the face to the cranium and forms the outer wall and base of the eye orbits.
   Temporal process. The temporal process of each zygomatic bone joins the zygomatic process of the temporal bone to form the zygomatic arch.
9. **Maxillae.** The two maxillary bones fuse to become one bone early in life, forming the upper jaw. All facial bones except the mandible join the maxillae. Most of the hard palate and the walls and base of the nasal cavity are formed by the maxillae.
   Infraorbital foramen. The infraorbital nerve and blood vessels exit the skull through the infraorbital foramen. Dentists and oral surgeons occasionally anesthetize the structures to deaden the upper jaw.
   Palatine process. The palatine process is the thick horizontal projection that makes up most of the base of the nostrils and about

three-quarters of the roof of the mouth (hard palate). If these processes from the two maxillary bones fail to unite completely during embryonic development, a condition called *cleft palate* occurs; which affects feeding and speech. Surgery and therapy usually can correct this problem.

Alveolar process is a bony depression that contains the sockets for the upper set of teeth. Each alveolar process varies in size according to the tooth it contains.

10. **Mandible.** The mandible, also referred to as the jawbone or chin, is the largest and heaviest bone in the skull. It is the only facial bone attached to the skull with a synovial joint; this is the only freely movable bone joint in the skull.

Mental foramen. The mental nerve passes through the mental foramen and is located inferior to the first molar. Dentists and oral surgeons occasionally anesthetize this nerve to deaden the lower jaw.

Ramus. The ramus is composed of two bony blades that connect the lower jaw to the joint region on either side of the jaw.

Coronoid process. The coronoid process is the superior and anterior portion of the ramus on each side. It serves as an attachment site for the temporalis muscle.

Condylar process. Also known as the condyloid process, the condylar process is located on the superior and posterior portion of the ramus and is a site for muscle attachment. These two processes articulate with both temporal bones to form the temporomandibular joints.

Alveolar process is a bony depression that contains the sockets for the lower set of teeth. Each alveolar process will vary in size according to the tooth it contains.

Paranasal Sinuses. The four pairs of paranasal sinuses, often referred to as the sinuses, are air-containing spaces in the skull and face that lighten the head, provide mucus, and act as resonance chambers for sound. These sinus cavities are named for the cranial bones or facial bones by which they are located. They are the frontal sinuses, the sphenoidal sinuses, the ethmoidal sinuses, and the maxillary sinuses, the last being the largest paranasal sinus (Fig. 7–12).

Other Cranial Structures. The fontanels are located in the fetal and neonatal cranium in the sutural regions. These membrane-filled spaces exist in the neonatal head to allow the head to be compressed during delivery and permit rapid growth of the brain. The anterior and posterior fontanels are also called soft spots. Obstetricians and midwives find these helpful in determining the position of babies during delivery. Although many fontanels exist in the newborn's head, these two are the most prevalent.

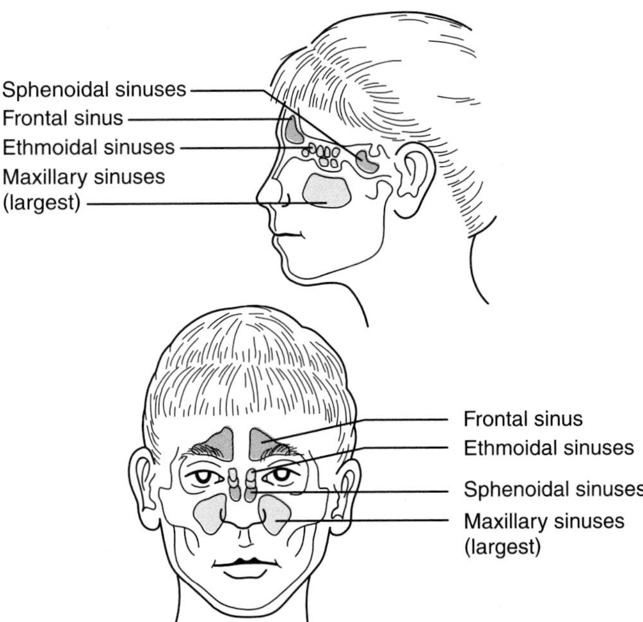

Figure 7•12 The paranasal sinuses.

The anterior fontanel is diamond-shaped and is the largest of all the fontanels. It is located where the coronal suture and sagittal sutures meet. The anterior fontanel completely ossifies by 18 to 24 months. You can often see a pulse under the membrane in this region of the head. One old wive's tale stated that if the anterior fontanel was depressed or concave-shaped, the infant was thirsty.

The posterior fontanel is located where the sagittal and lambdoidal sutures meet. It typically closes by the time the infant is 2 months old.

LESSON FOUR—BONES OF THE VERTEBRAL COLUMN AND THORAX

The vertebral column, or spinal column, consists of 26 individual bones in the adult and 33 to 35 in the embryo. These bones are divided into five regions: From superior to inferior they are the cervical, thoracic, lumbar, sacral, and coccyx regions. As we grow and develop, the last eight to ten vertebrae fuse into the last two vertebral regions; the sacral and the coccyx. The bones of the vertebral column are called the vertebrae. Each weight-bearing portion of the vertebra gradually increases in size, so that the larger lumbar vertebrae and sacral vertebrae form a stable base of support. This design spreads the weight of the body onto the pelvis. The vertebral column encloses the spinal cord and provides support for the spinal cord and the head, as well as an attachment site for the ribs and muscles of the back. The vertebral column allows us to bend forward and backward, lean sideways, and twist or rotate through the three planes of movement. All these spinal movements are a result of collective action. When the spine moves, it elicits a response from every other vertebra in the column, except for the axis, sacrum, and coccyx.

The spinal column of an infant is U-shaped, arching posteriorly. It soon becomes S-shaped when learning to walk on two feet. This S-shaped curve is required for a functional upright posture, providing better balance and better shock absorption qualities.

Thorax

The thorax, or chest cavity, consists of the 24 ribs, the sternum, and the 12 thoracic vertebrae. These bony structures support the body and protect the organs inside the thorax.

Sternum. The sternum, or breast bone, forms the anterior chest wall. In the adult, the sternum is a single bone made up of three fused bones (Fig. 7–13). These bones are the manubrium, the body of the sternum, and the xiphoid process. Not only does the sternum protect the chest organs, it also provides a place where the clavicle and the ribs attach.

Manubrium. The manubrium is located at the superior end of the sternum and articulates with the medial end of the clavicle and the medial end of the first rib.

Sternal notch. Also known as the suprasternal notch, or the jugular notch, the sternal notch is the depression located on the superior ledge of the manubrium.

Body or the gladiolus. This is the central portion of the sternum.

Xiphoid process. The xiphoid process is the distal end of the sternum and is an endangerment site for massage therapists because it can be broken off with excessive pressure. The xiphoid process is used as a landmark for applying cardiopulmonary resuscitation.

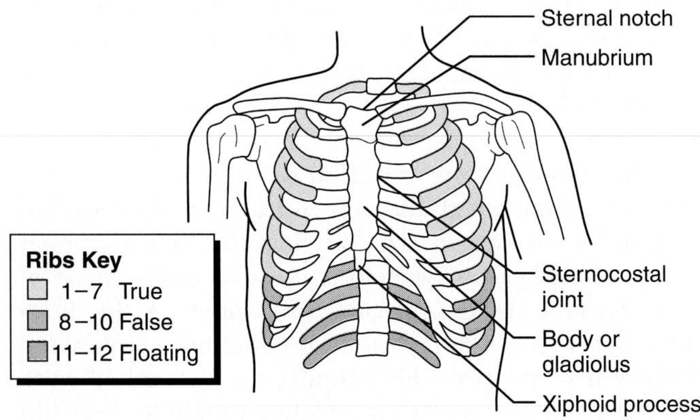

Figure 7•13 The sternum and ribs.

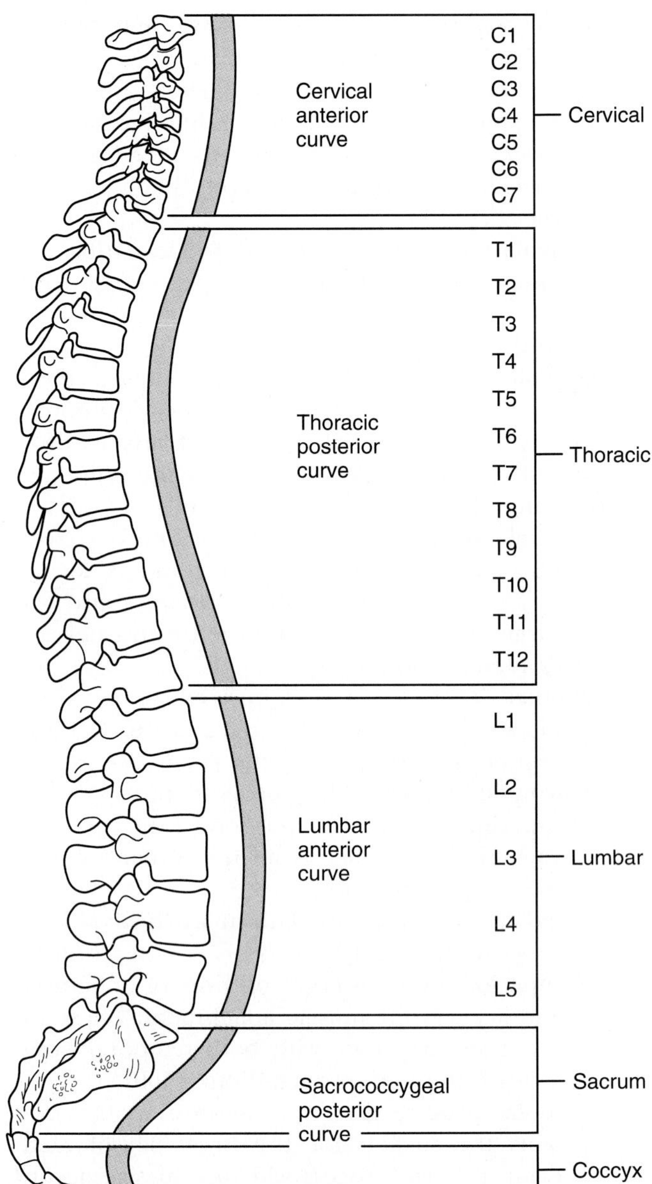

Figure 7•14 The vertebral column and its curves and divisions.

Ribs. The ribs are 24 individual or 12 pairs of long, slender, curved bones that articulate posteriorly with the thoracic vertebrae. Anteriorly, the first 7 pairs of ribs articulate directly with the sternum and are known as the *true ribs.* The next 3 pairs of ribs attach to the sternum through costal (hyaline) cartilage and are called the *false ribs.* The last 2 pairs of ribs do not attach to the sternum at all. These are known as the *floating ribs.* The first rib is short and thick, and the great vessels and main nerves run over it.

Divisions of the Vertebral Column

There are five regions or divisions of the vertebral column (Fig. 7–14). Each region has unique characteristics. As already stated, the vertebral column is

S-curved. This allows for a better balance and superior shock absorption. Let's look at the 5 regions.

- There are seven cervical vertebrae that make up the neck region of the spine. The cervical spine curves anteriorly.
- The 12 thoracic vertebrae are also known as the dorsal vertebrae. The thoracic region curves posteriorly.
- The five lumbar vertebrae are located in the low back region. The lumbar region of the spine curves anteriorly.
- There are five fused bones that make up the sacrum. This bone attaches to the pelvic girdle to form the pelvis. The sacrum region curves anteriorly.
- The coccyx bone consists of three to five fused bones and is the remnant of the tail other vertebrate animals possess. The coccyx also curves anteriorly.

Parts of a Vertebra

The typical vertebra of the spinal column has eight basic parts called the vertebral elements. These are the centrum or body, two pedicles, two transverse processes, two laminae, and the spinous process (Fig. 7–15). Each vertebra varies only in location, shape, and size. The circle of bone that extends out from the body of the vertebra is known as the vertebral arch, which is formed by the pedicles and the laminae on either side. Within the arch is the vertebral foramen, which encloses the spinal cord. The transverse process projects laterally from the arch and the spinous process projects posteriorly.

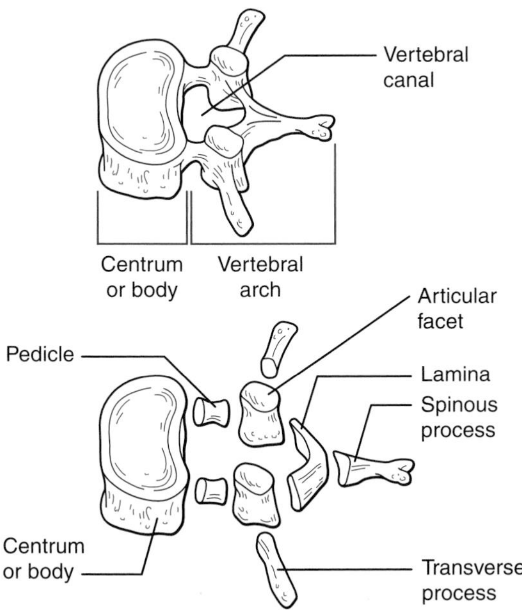

Figure 7•15 Parts of a typical vertebra.

Within each vertebra, from the first cervical vertebra to the last lumbar vertebra, are intervertebral disks, which attach to the body of the vertebra. These disks are composed of fibrocartilage. The functions of these disks are to maintain the joint spaces, assist with spinal movements, and absorb vertical shock. Within each disk is a soft, pulpy elastic middle called the *nucleus pulposus,* which can lose some of its elasticity with age; it can also become compressed and herniate. Just posterior to the intervertebral disk is a large central hole, or canal, for the spinal cord to pass. This opening in the vertebrae is known as the *vertebral foramen.* Each vertebra is attached to other vertebrae by two joints, called the facet joints.

Centrum or Body. The centrum is the thick anterior portion of the vertebrae. This is the weight-bearing part to which the intervertebral disks attach. Collectively, the vertebral bodies and their disks absorb shock and transfer the weight of the skull to the pelvis.

Pedicle. These two small, thick processes project back from the centrum to join the lamina posteriorly, forming the vertebral arch.

Lamina. The lamina is the flattened portion of the vertebral arch. The two laminae join posteriorly to form the posterior sides of the vertebral arch. Surgeons operating on the back occasionally remove the lamina in a surgical procedure called a laminectomy. This operation may be done to relieve pressure in the spinal canal.

Transverse Process. The transverse processes are the lateral projections from the point at which the pedical joins the lamina. Within the transverse process of the second through the sixth cervical vertebrae, a foramen exist which allows the vertebral artery, vein, and nerves to pass through the neck region. The lateral tip of the transverse process is an endangerment site for massage therapists because it is a bony projection. Massage therapists should avoid excessive pressure on osseous tissue.

Spinous Process. This bony structure projects posteriorly and is easily palpated over the skin of the back. The posterior end of the spinous process is an endangerment site for the massage therapist because it is a bony process.

Atypical Vertebrae

C1. The first cervical vertebra, also known as the atlas or C1, is shaped like a bony ring. The atlas possesses no centrum, pedicles, or laminae. The spinous process has been reduced to a posterior tubercle. Facets on the superior surface articulate with the occipital bone, permitting head nodding. On the inferior surface, facets articulate with the second cervical vertebrae.

C2. The second cervical vertebra is often referred to as the axis or C2. The axis has a spinous process that is thick and strongly bifurcated. The odontoid process, or dens, is a bony extension that projects superiorly through the ring of the atlas, permitting the rotation of the head (Fig. 7–16). It is speculated that the dens evolved from the old centrum of the atlas.

C7. The vertebral prominens, or C7, has a spinous process that is long and projects posteriorly. The vertebral prominens can be easily palpated at the base of the neck. This is the only cervical vertebra that does not possess a transverse foramen; the blood vessels pass directly over the transverse process.

T1–T12. Located on the centrum and transverse processes of all the thoracic vertebrae are demifacets for the posterior articulating ribs. Facets on the transverse process do not exist on the last two thoracic vertebrae.

L1–L5. The large lumbar vertebrae contain mammillary processes for the attachment of large ligaments of the low back. The spinous process and the transverse process of the lumbar vertebrae are short and thick.

Vertebral Structures

Supraspinous Ligament. This ligament connects and supports all of the spinous processes of the vertebral column. In American Indian culture, the supraspinous ligament of a deer was used for a bowstring.

Nuchal Ligament. The nuchal ligament is located in the posterior region of the neck. It attaches from the occipital bone to all the spinous processes of the cervical vertebrae and offers the neck some stability. To palpate this ligament, lean your head forward. The nuchal ligament will pop out as you drop your chin to your chest.

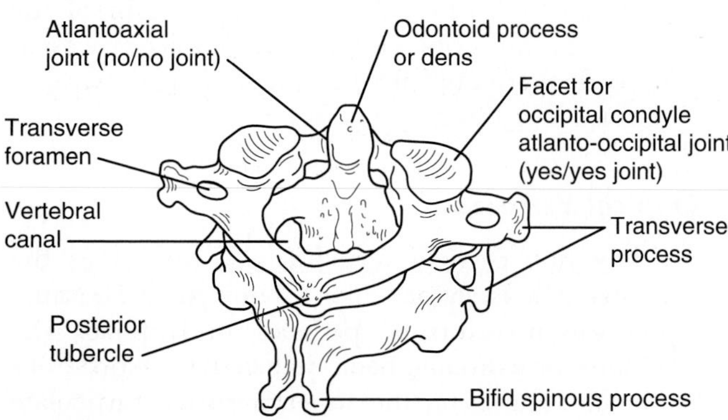

Figure 7•16 The atlas and axis—atlanto-occipital joint and atlantoaxial joint.

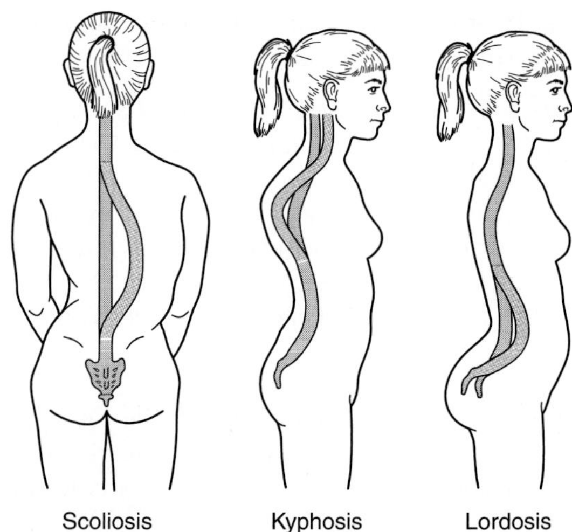

Figure 7•17 Scoliosis, kyphosis, and lordosis.

Abnormal Curvatures of the Spine

Scoliosis. Scoliosis is the lateral deviation or curvature in the normally straight vertical line of the vertebral column, usually in the thoracic region (Fig. 7–17). Distortion of the rib cage and unequal leg length are common. Causes of scoliosis include congenital malformations of the spine, poliomyelitis, paralysis, chronic spasticity of the iliopsoas muscle, and postural deviations such as poor posture and leg length discrepancy. Unequal position of the hips or shoulders may be one indication of this condition. Early detection, and intervention may prevent progression of the curvature. Treatment for scoliosis includes physical therapy, massage therapy, chiropractic, braces, casts, and corrective surgery. The vast majority of people who have scoliosis are female (80 percent). Refer to the chapter on adaptive massage to outline specific techniques for scoliosis.

Kyphosis. Also known as humpback, kyphosis is an exaggeration of the normal posterior thoracic curve. Typically, the chest appears caved in, the arms tend to hang in the front of the body, and the head moves forward. Kyphosis may be caused by rickets (vitamin D deficiency), degeneration of the intervertebral disks in the elderly, or tuberculosis of the spine. Mild to moderate back pain often accompanies this spinal condition. Conservative treatment of kyphosis consists of stretching the spine and modifications in sleep positions (sleeping without a pillow or with a board under the mattress). A modified brace may be used for severe kyphosis, and, rarely, spinal fusion may be required. Rounded shoulders and a dowager's hump are occasionally classified as a mild form of kyphosis.

Lordosis. Lordosis, or swayback, is an exaggeration of the anterior curvature of the lumbar concavity. A tightening of the back muscles followed by a weakening of the abdominal muscles are typical. Increased weight gain or pregnancy may cause or exacerbate this spinal condition. Because of the anterior tilt of the pelvis, hamstring problems are common.

LESSON FIVE—MAJOR JOINTS OF THE BODY

Articulations

Articulations, also known as joints, are the connections between the bones. Joints provide a space where one bone articulates with another for the transfer of weight and energy. Joints not only help us move, they also help us keep our skeletal system together.

The shape of a joint affects how it functions. As massage therapists, we often have problems in the joints of our hands because we expect them to function in ways for which they were not designed. For example, the wrist is not a weight-bearing structure. When a massage therapist spends too much time with the weight of his body on a flexed wrist, trouble is on its way. We will discuss this concept in greater detail in the body mechanics section of this text. Feet, on the other hand, are designed to bear the body's weight. The feet contain many joints for movement, for shock absorption, and for providing a stable base.

All the body's articulations have an inverse relationship regarding stability and mobility, where one function is sacrificed for the other. The more secure the joint, the more stable it is; however, it is less mobile. For example, the shoulder is the most flexible joint in the body. If you look at the joint structure, you will find a shallow socket and a greater incident of shoulder dislocations. The hip, on the other hand, has a deep socket. The hip joint does not have the flexibility that the shoulder possesses, but it is rarely dislocated. Often, the femur will fracture before the hip joint will be affected.

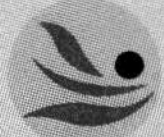

MINI•LAB

Proprioceptive awareness can be brought to our attention by focusing on the position of our joints and their relative positions in space. Close your right hand into a fist and place it behind your head. Now open any one finger of this closed fist. Which finger did you open? Can you see the finger? Then how do you know which one you opened? The answer is proprioception. It is proprioception that allows us to be aware of the position of each joint of our body.

Each joint contains nerve receptors that constantly give us proprioceptive information. These proprioceptive nerves detect stimuli originating from within the body regarding spatial position, muscular activity (motion and resistance), or activation of sensory receptors (see nervous system chapter). Two examples of proprioceptive nerves are muscle spindles and Golgi tendon organs.

We will examine 16 of the body's major joints in some detail. As you learn about each joint, touch and set into motion each joint while imagining the internal joint structures. This learning method will help you understand the mechanisms involved. If additional information is desired on these joints, or joints not listed, check the references at the end of the chapter.

1. **Temporomandibular Joint.** The temporomandibular joint (TMJ) is formed where the mandible articulates with the temporal bones (Fig. 7–18). Also known as the craniomandibular joint, the TMJ is classified as a ginglymoarthrodial joint, which is a combination hinge and gliding joint. Classified as an ellipsoidal joint, the movements permitted by this joint are not only depression and elevation but also protraction, retraction, adduction, and abduction.

Author's Note

Temporomandibular joint dysfunction is a common ailment afflicting either the jaw joint, its musculature, or both. Its chief symptoms are pain (at the jaws, toothache, headache, and earache), clicking of the joint and limited range of motion. Causes of TMJ dysfunction include trauma to the joint, chewing hard objects especially if only on one side of the mouth, biting fingernails, teeth clenching or grinding (bruxism) whether awake or asleep, and poor alignment (occlusion) of the upper and lower teeth.

TMJ dysfunction can be treated with massage. There are advanced techniques that require the donning of rubber gloves to enter the oral cavity and use ischemic compression to treat the muscles of the jaw. General massage techniques can benefit the TMJ sufferer because the majority of all TMJ dysfunction is associated with clenching or bruxism, which is often stress related. It is estimated that 60 percent of the population either clench or grind their teeth, but only 25 percent of these are aware of it.

2. **Atlanto-occipital Joint.** The atlanto-occipital joint allows you to nod your head in a yes/yes gesture and is classified as a gliding joint. The atlanto-occipital joint is an articulation involving the occipital condyles of the occiput and the condylar surface of the atlas or C1 vertebra (see Fig. 7–16).

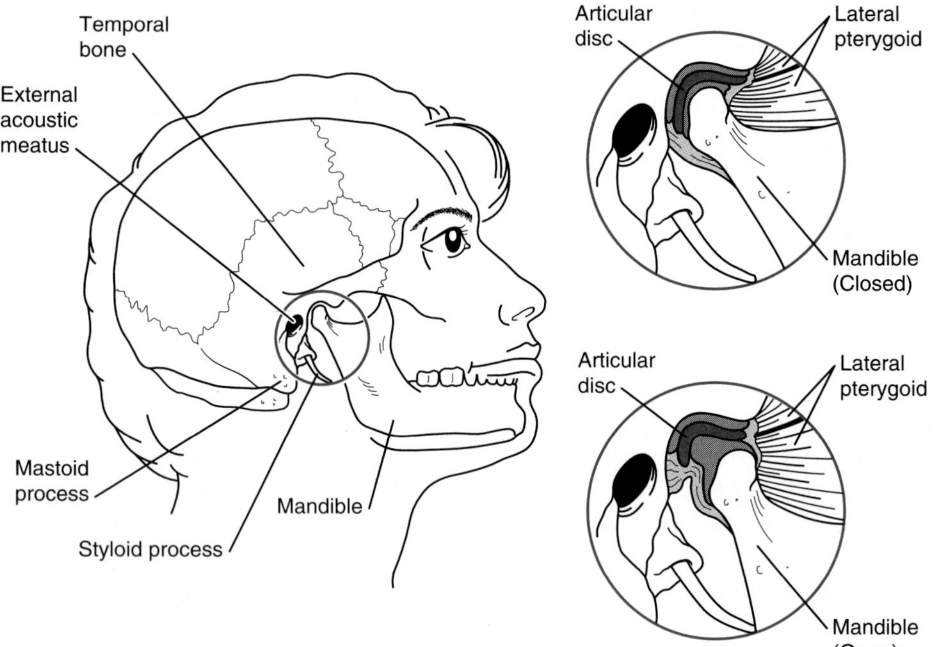

Figure 7•18 The temporomandibular joint.

3. **Atlantoaxial Joint.** The atlantoaxial joint allows you to shake your head, as in a no/no gesture and is considered a pivot joint. Think of this joint as Mother Nature's nut and bolt system of arrangement. This joint is the articulation between the C1 vertebra, or atlas, and the C2 vertebra, or axis (see Fig. 7–16). The specialized second cervical vertebra has a small, thick projection called the odontoid process, which protrudes superiorly from the anterior portion of the vertebra. This peg fits into a ring created by the anterior arch of the first cervical vertebra and is secured by a transverse ligament. The atlas then rotates around the pivot of the odontoid. Normal rotation is approximately 180 degrees.
4. **Glenohumeral Joint.** Other names for the glenohumeral joint are the scapulohumeral joint and the shoulder joint. The glenohumeral joint consists of the glenoid fossa of the scapula and the head of the humerus (Fig. 7–19). It is classified as a ball-and-socket joint, so all movements are permitted. The shoulder joint is poorly reinforced with ligaments, and the glenoid fossa of the scapula is too shallow to offer any real security for the head of the humerus. Thus stability is sacrificed in

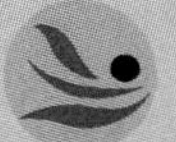

MINI•LAB

Nod your head slowly as if to say yes, then shake your head slowly as if to say no. Now repeat these movements while concentrating on the cervical-occipital area at the back of the neck. Which movement feels higher? Which one feels lower? Is the atlanto-occipital joint, also known as the yes/yes joint, more superior? Or is the atlantoaxial joint, also known as the no/no joint, more superior?

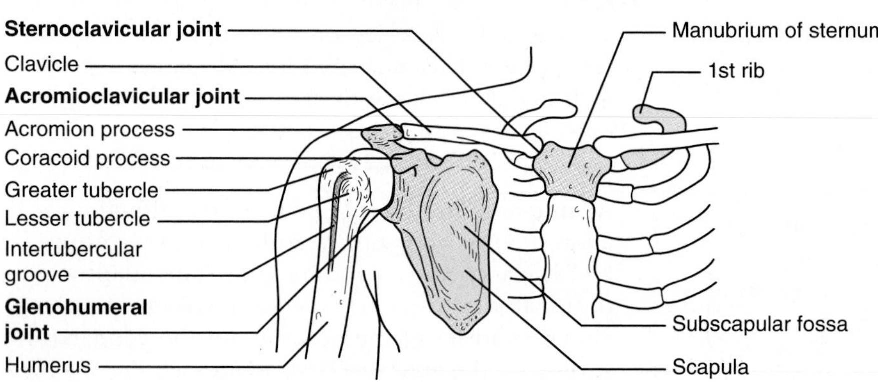

Figure 7•19 The glenohumeral joint and the acromioclavicular joint.

favor of mobility. The rotator cuff muscles function as ligaments to offer active support without sacrificing joint mobility.

5. **Acromioclavicular Joint.** Also known as the AC joint, the acromioclavicular joint is located on the lateral tip of the clavicle, where it articulates with the acromion process of the scapula (Fig. 7–19). The AC joint is classified as a gliding joint, which permits slight gliding movements in flexion, extension, abduction, and adduction. The AC joint can be injured due to direct blows and is commonly involved in shoulder separation and shoulder dislocation.
6. **Elbow Joint.** Also known as the humeroulnar joint and the elbow joint, is a three-bone articulation consisting of the humerus, ulna, and radius, held together by ligaments and a joint sleeve (Fig. 7–20). It is classified as a hinge joint and offers two-dimensional movements of flexion and extension in the given plane.
7. **Radioulnar Joint.** The radioulnar joint is located at the proximal end of the radius and ulna and is classified as a pivot joint (Fig. 7–20). This joint allows the hand to participate in pronation and supination.
8. **Radiocarpal Joint.** The radiocarpal joint, or wrist joint, is located on the distal end of the radius at the scaphoid and the lunate (Fig. 7–21). The radiocarpal joint is classified as an ellipsoidal joint. Movements that are permitted at the radiocarpal joint are flexion, extension, adduction, and abduction. True circumduction is not permitted.
9. **Intercarpal Joint.** The intercarpal joint is located in the area of the wrist (Fig. 7–21). The carpal bones glide across one another to create a limited sliding motion. The carpal bones are the trapezium, the trapezoid, the capitate, the hamate, the scaphoid, the lunate, the triquetrum, and the pisiform.

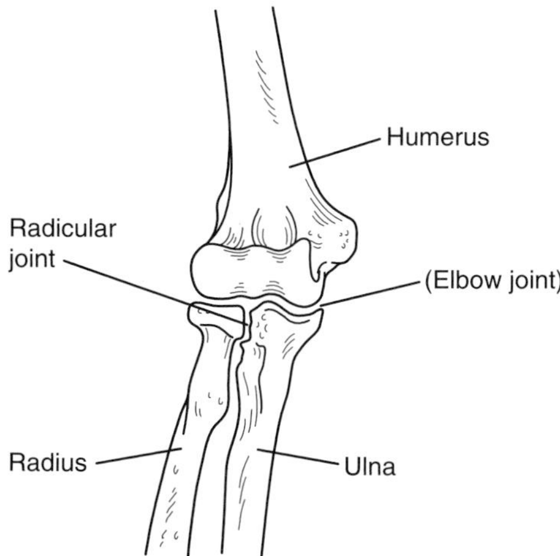

Figure 7•20 Close-up of the elbow joint and the radioulnar joint.

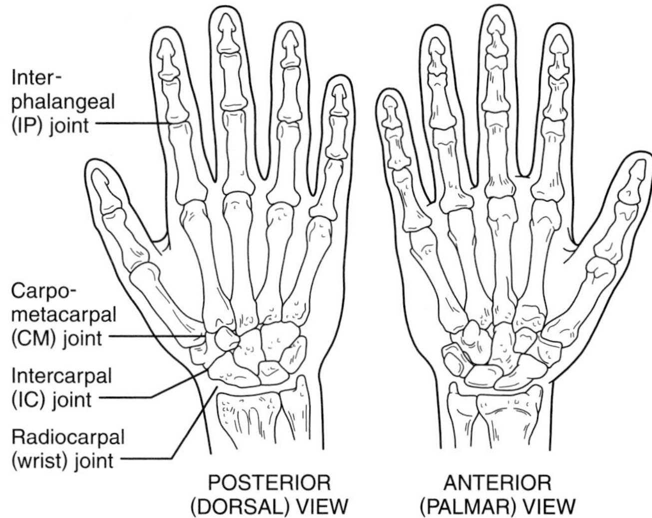

Figure 7•21 Close-up of the radiocarpal joint, the intercarpal joint, carpometacarpal joint of the thumb, and interphalangeal joints.

10. **Carpometacarpal of the Thumb.** This joint is classified as a saddle joint and is located between the trapezium (saddle portion of the joint) and the proximal metacarpal bone of the thumb (Fig. 7–21). A saddle joint permits two-dimensional movement in all planes, but does not support true rotation. It is the saddle joint that makes the thumb *opposable,* or able to pivot to face the fingers. It is this ability that allows humans to grasp and manipulate objects.
11. **Symphysis Pubis.** The symphysis pubis is often referred to as the pubic symphysis. This joint is located between the two pubic bones of the pelvic girdle (Fig. 7–22). Hormones secreted during pregnancy soften this synarthrotic joint to allow movement for expansion of the pelvis for fetal delivery.
12. **Sacroiliac Joint.** The sacroiliac joints, also known as the SI joints, are amphiarthrotic joints located

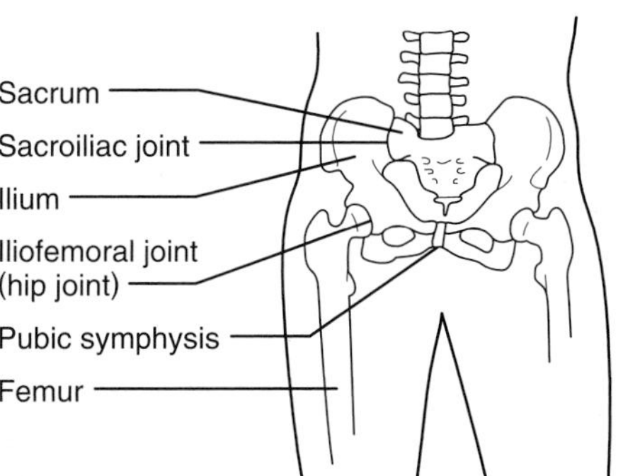

Figure 7•22 The three joints of the pelvis: the pubic symphysis, the sacroiliac joint, and the iliofemoral joint.

between the sacrum and the ilium on either side of the posterior pelvis (Fig. 7–22). This very stable joint allows limited motion of the pelvis. Within the space that separates these two bones are a synovial-like membrane, which suggests that the SI joints have characteristics of a diarthrotic joint.

13. **Iliofemoral Joint.** The iliofemoral joint is also known as the coxal joint or the hip joint. This two-bone articulation consists of the spherical femoral head and the acetabulum cavity (Fig. 7–22). The iliofemoral joint is a ball-and-socket joint that provides movement in all three dimensions. And yet, because the acetabulum cavity is a very deep socket and cups the ball of the femoral head firmly, mobility is sacrificed for stability. This extra stability is important because of the weight-bearing function of the hip joint. The iliofemoral ligament, also known as the Y ligament, is located within the hip joint and helps hold the femoral head in place. The iliofemoral ligament is the strongest ligament in the body and adds to the stability of the hip, making hip dislocation uncommon.
14. **Knee Joint.** The knee is the largest and most complex joint in the body (Fig. 7–23). It is actually three joints in one: two hinge joints and one gliding joint. The two hinge joints are the left and right *tibiofemoral joints,* which are composed of the medial and lateral femoral condyles and the superior ledge of the tibia (tibial plateau). The tibiofemoral joints allow movement in one plane as well as some limited medial and lateral rotation. Most individuals can flex the knee 150 degrees, but individuals who are hypermobile can touch their heels to their buttocks. In either motion of flexion and extension, weight does not pass through the patella, which is located anterior to the knee joint.

The gliding joint, the *patellofemoral joint,* is located in front of the knee. Here the patella articulates with the femur and actually protects, stabilizes, and cushions the hinge joints.

The knee has an internal and an external ligament system. The internal ligament system is composed of the anterior and posterior cruciate ligaments. The external ligament system is the medial (tibial) collateral ligament and the lateral (fibular) collateral ligament. The internal and external ligament systems are for static stabilization. Muscles and related tendons are dynamic stabilizers, supporting the knee joint in motion.

Because it is primarily a hinge joint, the normal movement of the knee is flexion and extension in the forward to backward plane. The knee does not hold up to repeated stress or blows in the lateral plane. Sports such as tennis and basketball with their quick lateral starts and stops, and sports like football with forceful contact can place high lateral stress on the knee joints. Damage is generally sustained to the menisci and/or the anterior cruciate ligament. Although there are many ligaments

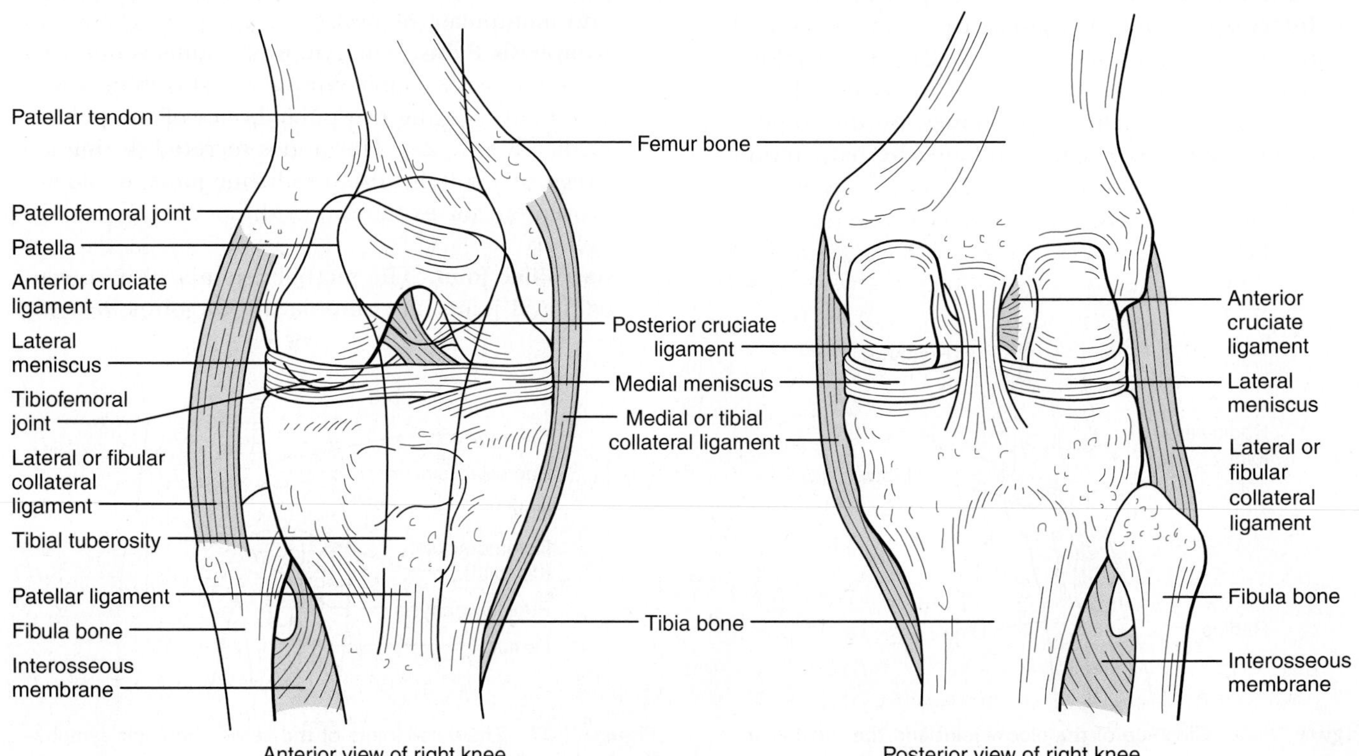

Figure 7•23 The knee joint with all its ligaments.

in the joint capsule of the knee, we will focus on the most important ones.

Patellar tendon. Also known as quadriceps tendon, this is the inferior tendon of the large quadriceps femoris muscle. This tendon attaches the quadriceps femoris muscle to the bone of the patella. The entire patella is actually embedded in this tendon, which continues to the tibia as the patellar ligament.

Patellar ligament. The patellar ligament is an extension of the quadriceps or patellar tendon. In the strictest sense, the section of the tendon between the patella and the tibia is referred to as the patellar ligament because it connects bone to bone.

Medial and lateral menisci. Each concave meniscus is composed of half-ringed fibroelastic cartilage that attaches on the tibial plateau. The two condyles of the femur are convex and articulate with the medial and lateral menisci during knee flexion and extension. The menisci absorb the shock of motion and locomotion.

Medial collateral ligament. Also known as the tibial collateral ligament, the medial collateral ligament connects the femur to the tibia. Damage to the medial collateral ligament may occur during lateral blows to the knee. The medial collateral ligament attaches to the medial meniscus, and they are commonly torn together.

Lateral collateral ligament. The lateral collateral ligament connects the femur to the fibula, hence the alternate term fibular collateral ligament. Because medial blows to the lateral collateral ligament are uncommon, this ligament is not often damaged. Both lateral and medial collateral ligaments provide external support and help prevent side-to-side movements.

Anterior cruciate ligament. Also known as the ACL, the anterior cruciate ligament crosses in front of the posterior cruciate ligament. The ACL anchors the superior surface of the tibia and prevents it from shifting forward during motion. The anterior cruciate ligament is often torn in knee injuries.

Posterior cruciate ligament. Both the anterior and posterior cruciate ligaments cross in the middle of the knee joint; they help to prevent anterior-to-posterior movement and provide an internal support system.

15. **Ankle Joint.** The ankle joint, or talocrural joint, is the articulation between the foot and the leg. The lower portion of the tibia and the fibula and the upper portion of the talus combine to form the ankle joint (Fig. 7–24). The talus swings forward and backward between the two lower leg bones, like a block of ice swinging between ice tongs.

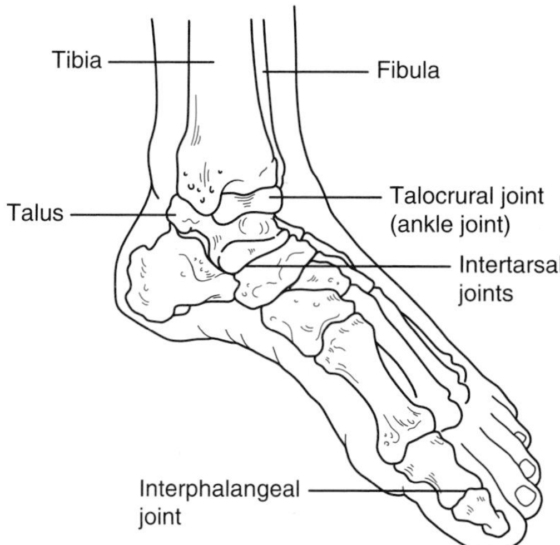

Figure 7•24 The ankle joint and the intertarsal joints.

This three-bone articulation classifies the ankle as a hinge joint. As you may recall from the previous chapter, the flexion and extension motions associated with this joint have been given specialized names; dorsiflexion and plantar flexion.

The ankle joint is stabilized on all sides by bands of ligaments. On the medial side of the ankle joint is the large deltoid ligament, which is the strongest ligament in the foot.

16. **Intertarsal Joints.** The intertarsal joints are located in the feet (Fig. 7–24). These bones glide across one another for collective but limited movement. This gliding effect allows the distribution of weight to be evenly transferred from one part of the foot to another. The most posterior tarsals contact the ground surface first as the heel strikes. The anterior tarsals glide into position forming an arch or bridge that distributes the weight onto the metatarsals as the ball of the foot contacts the ground. Finally, weight is transferred down to the phalanges as the foot toes off the ground for the next successive step. The gliding movements of the tarsals can produce a limited rotation effect, which is referred to as inversion and eversion.

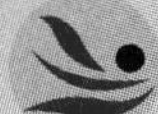

MINI•LAB

Obtain an articulated skeleton and a disarticulated skeleton. Most high-schools, colleges, or universities use them in their biology classes. Working in groups of two or three, locate all the bones, bony markings, and joints discussed in this chapter. Your instructor may add or delete particular structures to suit the needs of the class.

ARTHROMETRIC MODEL

The arthrometric model was developed by John Wilson of the University of Arizona. It describes the body's joint placement in radial symmetry. Radiating from the center of the circle are zones or perimeters that describe movement. The joints toward the center of this circle, or the central zone, are suited for directional movement. As we move out from the center toward the periphery, it is range, not direction, that is involved. For example, the hand may grasp the apple from the tree branch, but the shoulder must position the arm in space so that this task may be achieved. This model stimulates our imagination and the wisdom behind the articulate design of our skeleton. Let's look at Wilson's work (Fig. 7–25).

1. **Central Zone.** The function of the central zone is to position the body. Motion in all three dimensions is available, but motion from a single joint is limited.
2. **First Perimeter.** The first perimeter includes the ball-and-socket joints of the shoulder and hip, which are involved with directional movements.
3. **Second Perimeter.** The synovial joints of the elbow and knee are located in the second perimeter and allow movement in only one dimension. Note that the joints cannot change the direction of motion, but they allow for some fulfillment of the motion intended by the organism.
4. **Third Perimeter.** The third perimeter includes both ellipsoid and gliding joints. These are biaxial joints and allow movement in two dimensions. The joints in the third perimeter cannot change the direction of movement established by the central zone and the first perimeter, but can assist in the refinement of movement.
5. **Peripheral Zone.** The peripheral zone includes the most diverse arrangements of synovial joints. Hinge joints, ellipsoid joints, and saddle joints help the organism to express, manipulate, maneuver, and complete the motion that originated toward the center of the arthrometric model.

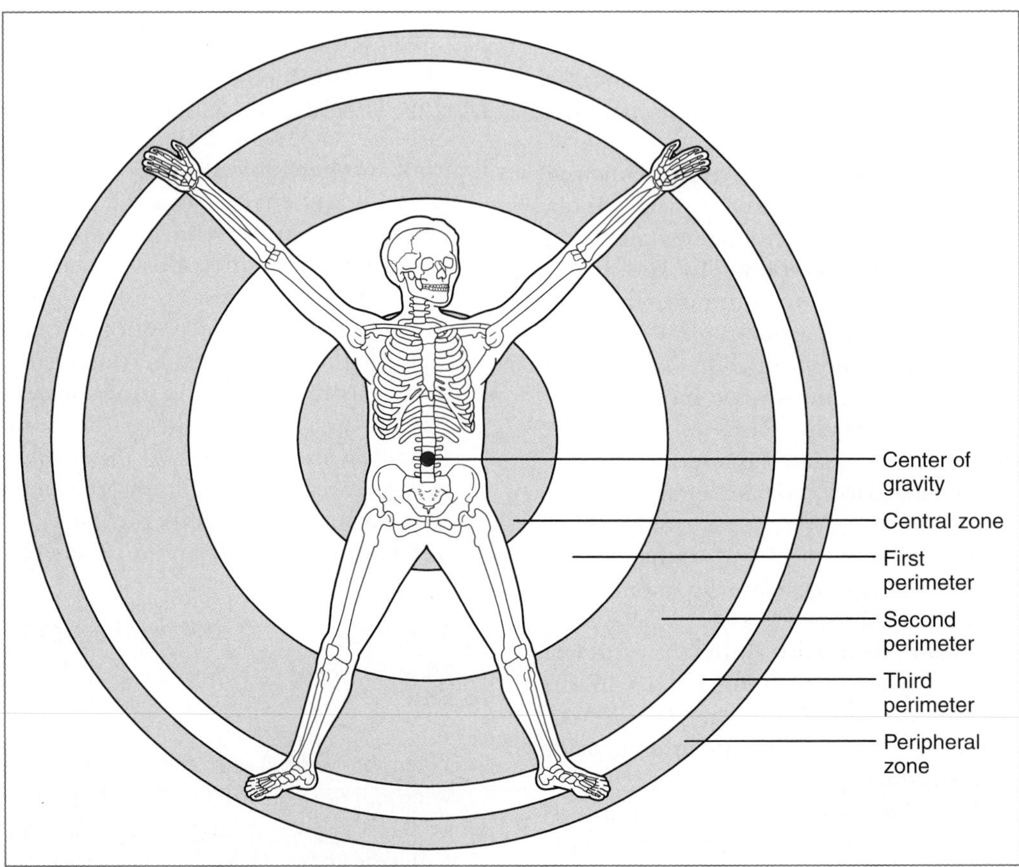

Figure 7•25 The arthrometric model.

SUMMARY

Skeletal nomenclature is the prerequisite to the muscular system and therefore fundamental to the study of massage. The bony skeleton provides a road map to the muscles, its signs being the bony markings that are the sites of tendon attachment. The 206 bones of the skeleton have been divided regionally: bones of the upper extremity, bones of the lower extremity, bones of the cranium, bones of the vertebral column and thorax, and major joints of the body. In each region, the specifics of each bone are detailed in regard to name, location, joint involvement, and important bony markings.

SELF-TEST

Matching I • List the letter of the bone to the bony marking or phrase that best describes it. Some terms will be used more than once.

A. scapula	E. radius
B. clavicle	F. carpals
C. humerus	G. metacarpals
D. ulna	H. phalanges

_______ 1. wrist bones that are arranged in two rows of four bones

_______ 2. olecranon process

_______ 3. acromion process

_______ 4. hand bones between carpal bones and phalanges

_______ 5. greater tubercle

_______ 6. deltoid tuberosity

_______ 7. most distal bones of each finger and thumb

_______ 8. collar bone; most frequently fractured bone

_______ 9. bicipital tuberosity

_______ 10. coracoid process

_______ 11. glenoid fossa

_______ 12. bicipital groove

Matching II • List the letter of the bone to the bony marking or phrase that best describes it. Some terms will be used more than once.

A. ilium	F. tibia
B. ischium	G. fibula
C. pubic bone	H. talus
D. femur	I. calcaneus
E. patella	J. metatarsals

_______ 1. ischial tuberosity

_______ 2. heel bone

_______ 3. iliac crest

_______ 4. linea aspera

_______ 5. knee cap; largest sesamoid bone in the body

_______ 6. anterior superior iliac spine

_______ 7. medial malleolus

_______ 8. greater trochanter

_______ 9. commonly called the ankle bone

_______ 10. greater sciatic notch

_______ 11. superior pubic ramus

_______ 12. gluteal tuberosity

_______ 13. lateral malleolus

_______ 14. bones between tarsel bones and phalanges

Matching III • List the letter of the bone or structure to the bony marking or phrase that best describes it. Some terms will be used more than once.

A. frontal bone	F. sagittal suture
B. temporal bone	G. zygomatic bone
C. sphenoid bone	H. maxilla
D. occipital bone	I. mandible
E. hyoid bone	J. maxillary sinus

_______ 1. mastoid process

_______ 2. infraorbital foramen

_______ 3. largest air-containing spaces in the skull; located in the jawbone

_______ 4. sella turcica

_______ 5. suspended from the styloid process of the temporal bone

_______ 6. superior nuchal line

_______ 7. separates the two parietal bones

_______ 8. supraorbital foramen

_______ 9. temporal process

_______ 10. mental foramen

_______ 11. foramen magnum

_______ 12. external auditory meatus

Matching IV • List the letter of the bone or condition to the bony marking or phrase that best describes it. Some terms will be used more than once.

A. sternum	G. C2
B. ribs	H. C7
C. centrum, or body	I. scoliosis
D. transverse process	J. kyphosis
E. lamina	K. lordosis
F. C1	L. scapula

_______ 1. also known as the atlas

_______ 2. the lateral projections from the lamina

_______ 3. manubrium

_______ 4. often referred to as the axis

_______ 5. an exaggeration of the normal posterior thoracic curve

_______ 6. xiphoid process

_______ 7. the weight-bearing part to which the intervertebral disks attach

_______ 8. an exaggeration of the normal anterior lumbar curve

_______ 9. long, slender, curved bones of the thoracic cavity

_______ 10. lateral curvature of the vertebral column in the thoracic region

_______ 11. the flattened portion of the vertebral arch

_______ 12. also known as the vertebral prominens

Matching V • List the letter of the joint to the phrase that best describes it.

A. atlanto-occipital joint
B. atlantoaxial joint
C. glenohumeral joint
D. acromioclavicular joint
E. elbow joint
F. radioulnar joint
G. radiocarpal joint
H. intercarpal joint
I. carpometacarpal joint of the thumb
J. sacroiliac joint
K. iliofemoral joint
L. knee joint

_______ 1. can be injured by direct blows and is commonly involved in shoulder separation and shoulder dislocation

_______ 2. allows pronation and supination of the hand

_______ 3. referred to as the yes/yes joint

_______ 4. also known as the coxal joint, or the hip joint, providing three-dimensional movement

_______ 5. also known as the scapulohumeral joint and the shoulder joint

_______ 6. referred to as the no/no joint

_______ 7. the largest and most complex joint in the body

_______ 8. this joint allows the wrist to flex, extend, adduct, and abduct, but true circumduction is not permitted

_______ 9. also known as the humeroulnar joint; a three-bone articulation

_______ 10. located between the sacrum and the ilium

_______ 11. these bones glide across one another to create a sliding motion

_______ 12. a saddle joint, permitting all movements except rotation

References

Brossman, A. B., D.D.S., M.S. *Some of the Finer Points About Temporomandibular Joint Anatomy and Physiology.* From a paper published on the internet located at home page: http://www.ovnet.com/userpages/rebross/tmjoints.html. Wheeling, WV, 1997.

Ardoin, Wes, D.D.S. From a lecture on temporomandibular joint dysfunction given at the Louisiana Institute of Massage Therapy, Lafayette, LA, 1994.

Goldberg, Stephen, MD. *Clinical Anatomy Made Ridiculously Simple.* Miami: Medmaster, Inc., 1984.

Gray, Henry, F.R.S., T. Pickering Pick. F.R.C.S., Robert Howden, M.A, M.B, C.M. *Gray's Anatomy,* 29th ed. Philadelphia: Running Press, 1974.

Guyton, Arthur, M.D. *Human Physiology and Mechanisms of Disease,* 3rd ed. Philadelphia: W. B. Saunders Company, 1982.

Haubrich, William S., M.D. *Medical Meanings, A Glossary of Word Origins.* New York: Harcourt Brace Jovanovich, Publishers, 1984.

Hoppenfeld, Stanley. *Physical Examination of the Spine and Extremities.* Norwalk, CT: Appleton-Century-Crofts, 1976.

Juhan, Deane. *Job's Body, A Handbook for Bodyworkers.* Barrington, NY: Station Hill Press, 1987.

Kapandji, I. A. *The Physiology of the Joints.* New York, NY: Churchill Livingstone, 1982.

Kordish, Mary and Sylvia Dickson. *Introduction to Basic Human Anatomy.* Lake Charles, LA: McNeese State University, Self-published manual, 1985.

Marieb, Elaine N. *Essentials of Human Anatomy and Physiology,* 4th ed. New York: Benjamin/Cummings Publishing Company, Inc., 1994.

McAleer, Neil. *The Body Almanac.* Garden City, New York: Doubleday and Company, Inc., 1985.

Moore, Keith L. *Clinically Oriented Anatomy,* 2nd ed. Baltimore: Williams & Wilkins, 1985.

Olsen, Andrea and Caryn McHose. *BodyStories: A Guide to Experiential Anatomy.* Barrytown, NY: Station Hill Press, 1991.

Tabers Cyclopedic Medical Dictionary, 13th ed. Philadelphia: F. A. Davis Company, 1977.

Tortora Gerald J. *Introduction to the Human Body: The Essentials of Anatomy and Physiology,* 3rd ed. New York: HarperCollins Publishers, 1994.

Wilson, John M. *A Natural Philosophy of Movement Styles for Theatre Performers.* Doctoral dissertation, University of Wisconsin–Madison, 1973.

Nothing happens until something moves.

—Albert Einstein

8 Muscular System

Student Objectives

After completing this chapter, the student should be able to:

- Recall six functions of the muscular system
- Identify three classifications of muscle tissue and the basic characteristics of each
- List the parts of a skeletal muscle
- Explain the sliding filament theory
- Identify how skeletal muscles interact to coordinate movement
- Demonstrate all types of skeletal muscle contraction
- Distinguish the difference between eccentric and concentric contractions

INTRODUCTION

At last, we get to the muscles, which is just what you've been waiting for! Everything you have learned until now was in preparation for learning and understanding your muscular system. This knowledge is essential for you as a massage therapist because the muscles and the related connective tissue (i.e., fascia) are the primary focus of Swedish massage.

When we think of ourselves as being alive, we generally think in terms of movement. Our heart beats, our muscles twitch, and our chest rises and falls with each breath. These visible signs of life are all created by muscle contraction.

In this chapter we will examine the muscular system. We will also study the internal mechanism of skeletal muscle contraction. The individual origin, insertion, and action of the muscles will be thoroughly explored later in the muscular nomenclature chapter.

In massage schools, the depth of knowledge regarding the muscular system exceeds that of many other health-care fields. Beyond a basic understanding of the anatomy and physiology of the muscles, it is necessary to consider a broad spectrum of information. These include the histology of muscle tissue; types of muscle tissue; connective tissue components; structures of skeletal muscles; the anatomy, neurology, and chemistry of muscular contraction; three types of skeletal muscle; muscle stretching and its barriers; types of skeletal muscle contractions; muscle fiber arrangement; parts of a skeletal muscle; how the body coordinates movement; and muscular conditions and terminology. This comprehensive study of muscles provides the therapist with a complex array of information that can be used to address muscular dysfunction due to stress, illness, or injury.

Author's Note

Muscle comes from the Latin word *musculus,* which means "a little mouse." How "little mouse" came to mean "muscle" seems to be explained by the appearance of movement of muscles under the skin to the scurrying of little mice. Dissected muscle may have looked like small rodents, and the tissue was named for this appearance. Anatomists of the pre-Galenic time had little knowledge of muscles. Plato and Aristotle, among other ancient authorities, regarded muscle tissue as part of the covering of the body, like skin.

FUNCTIONS

1. **External Mobility.** Skeletal muscles create movement we can see. This includes both motion and locomotion. *Motion* is defined as a change in position resulting from movement (e.g., manipulation); *locomotion* is movement from one place to another.
2. **Internal Mobility.** When we speak of internal mobility, we are referring to the movement resulting from the contraction of smooth muscles. An example of smooth movement is peristalsis of the colon. The special name given to the movement resulting from smooth muscle contractions is *motility.*
3. **Produce Heat.** All muscle contractions produce and release heat. This physiological mechanism is important to preserve correct body temperature. Additionally, when the body becomes chilled, skeletal muscles begin to rapidly contract and to produce heat. This is called *shivering.*
4. **Maintain Posture.** To maintain static positions, such as sitting and standing, the skeletal muscles contract to hold us in these postures. Muscles also contribute to joint stability.
5. **Move Lymph.** As skeletal muscles contract, lymph vessels are compressed and lymph fluid is displaced. Lymph flow can also be stimulated by peristaltic action of the gastrointestinal tract, by arterial pulsations, and by contraction of the diaphragm.

HISTOLOGY

The simplest unit of a muscle fiber is called a **myofibril.** Groups of these cells are organized into tissues. There are three types of muscle tissue in the body: smooth muscle, cardiac muscle, and skeletal muscle. We commonly refer to them by their features or characteristics. Smooth muscle is found in the viscera of the body and includes blood vessels and the organs of digestion, excretion (urinary), and reproduction. Cardiac muscle is found in the heart, and skeletal muscles generally attach to the bones of the skeleton either directly or indirectly. Each muscle tissue type will be discussed, but the skeletal muscles will be studied in detail. More information on cardiac muscle can be found in the circulatory chapter; and smooth muscle will receive additional coverage in the digestive, urinary, and circulatory chapters.

Smooth Muscle. Smooth muscle is also known as involuntary muscle or visceral muscle (mainly found in the viscera of the body). Smooth muscle forms the walls of hollow organs and tubes like the stomach, bladder, uterus, and blood vessels. These muscle fibers are adapted for long, sustained contraction, and consume very little energy. Imagine how dangerous it would be to the organism if the muscles of the internal organs fatigued quickly. When smooth muscles contract, they control the transport of materials, moving them along or restricting their flow. Properties and main characteristics of a smooth muscle are as follows (Fig. 8–1):

Word Roots and Terms Related to Muscles

antagonist – to struggle against
alba – white
aponeurosis – away from; nerve; condition
atrophy – lacking, without, not; to grow
brachi – arm
concentric – toward the middle
diaphragm – a fence or partition
eccentric – away from the middle
epicranius – upon; skull
fatigue – to tire
fasciculi – little bundle
flaccid – flabby
galea – helmet
gastro – belly
Golgi tendon organs – named for Italian histologist (1844–1926)
hypertrophy – over, above, excessive; to grow
intercalate – between; to put in place
isometric – same or equal measure
isotonic – same or equal tension
myo – muscle
myotatic – muscle; stretching
penniform – feather-shaped
peroneus – pin of the brooch; pertaining to the fibula
retinaculum – a halter
sarco – flesh
spasm – a convulsion
synergist – together, work
tendon – to stretch

1. The muscle cells are spindle-shaped and pointed at both ends
2. Each smooth muscle cell contains one centrally located, oval-shaped nucleus
3. Smooth muscles also exhibit a property of irritability: They will contract or relax in response to nerve impulses, stretching, or hormones but they are not under voluntary control.

Cardiac Muscle. The heart wall (i.e., myocardium) is made up of cardiac muscle, which is a type of involuntary striated muscle. The characteristics of cardiac muscle are (Fig. 8–2):

1. Each cardiac muscle cell is branched and shaped like the letter Y or H. This unique attribute allows the cells to fit together like clasped fingers and helps create the spherical shape of the heart. This branching and interlocking arrangement also allows for the rapid transmission of stimuli throughout an entire section of the heart, rather than in rows or bundles.
2. The nuclei of cardiac muscle cells are oval, centrally located, and are typically mononucleated (only one nucleus per cell), although cardiac muscle cells may be multinucleated.
3. Cardiac muscle is said to be "striated" because of its alternating light and dark bands, or striations, which are visible when this tissue is viewed under a microscope.
4. The contraction of the heart muscle is autorhythmic through a property called conduction. The stimulus to contract is transmitted from a specialized area of muscle in the heart called the sinoatrial (SA) node, which controls heart rate. Nerve impulses can speed up or slow down the heart rate, but the SA node initiates the heartbeat. Once the SA node produces a nerve impulse, it sends a message to the appropriate areas of the heart to stimulate rhythmic contractions generating the pumping action of the heart.
5. Between each cardiac muscle cell is a structure known as the intercalated disk. These disks function like the electrical synapses of the nervous system and assist the transmission of a stimulus from cell to cell. This transmission, along with the internal conduction system, allows the activity of the heart to be closely coordinated.

Skeletal Muscle. Skeletal muscle is both voluntary and striated muscle. There are over 600 skeletal mus-

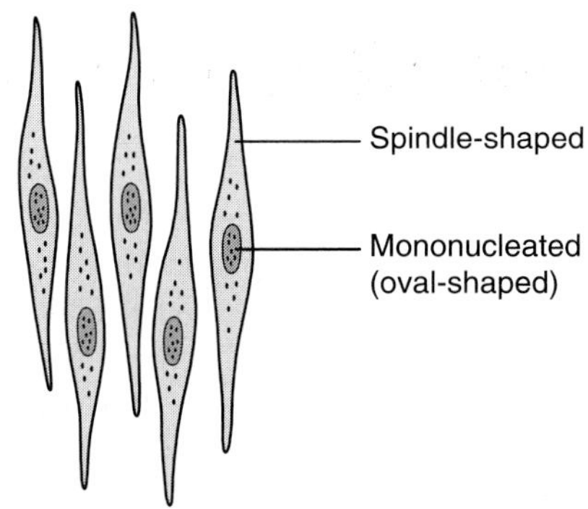

Figure 8•1 Smooth muscle characteristics.

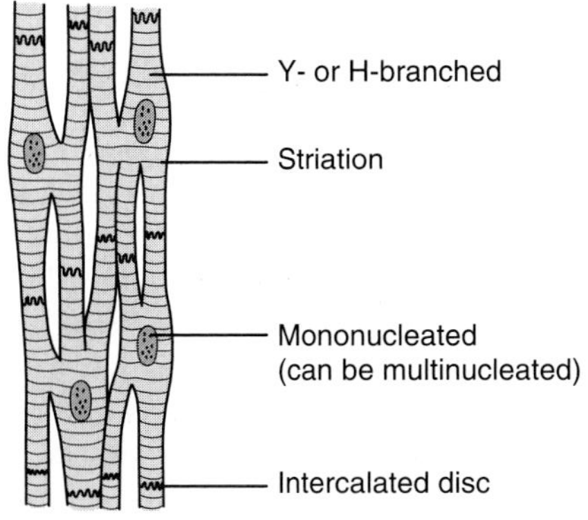

Figure 8•2 Cardiac muscle characteristics.

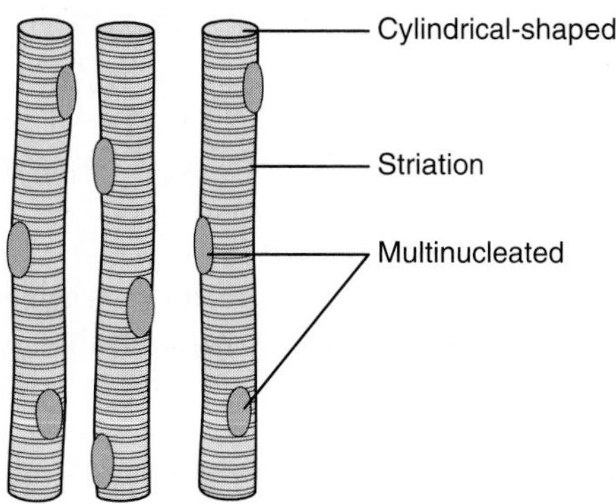

Figure 8•3 Skeletal muscle characteristics.

cles in the body. Skeletal muscles are those that attach to bones and their membranes, fascia, and other muscles. When we speak of the flesh of the body, we are referring to the muscles of the musculoskeletal system, which accounts for 40 to 50 percent of body weight. Skeletal muscles must be stimulated by a nerve impulse to contract. This may occur through voluntary control or through reflex action. The following are skeletal muscle cell characteristics (Fig. 8–3):

1. They are cylindrical or cigar-shaped.
2. Skeletal muscle fibers are multinucleated (more than one nucleus), and these nuclei are small, elongated, and located near the periphery.
3. Each muscle fiber of a skeletal muscle contains bands of red and white material, causing it to appear striped or striated under a microscope. Because of this characteristic, skeletal muscles are classified as striated muscles, making this characteristic common to both cardiac and skeletal muscles.

CONNECTIVE TISSUE COMPONENTS AND OTHER RELATED STRUCTURES OF SKELETAL MUSCLES

Muscle fibers are generally arranged in parallel rows. Some individual muscle fibers may be over 12 inches long. We think of muscles as being tough, but muscle fibers are quite fragile. Therefore, they are arranged and protected by a series of connective tissue wrappings, or fascia (Fig. 8–4).

Each muscle fiber is enclosed in a protective covering called the **endomysium.** Many of these muscle fibers are grouped into bundles of tissue known as **fasciculi,** and are bound together by another fascia layer known as the **perimysium.** These bundles are then wrapped together to form a single specific muscle by another layer of fascia, which then wraps around the entire muscle; it is called the **epimysium.** This particular covering is quite tough and thick. While the epimysium binds the fasciculi together, it also acts to separate one muscle from another. The epimysium reaches past the end of the muscle belly and encompasses the tendon as well.

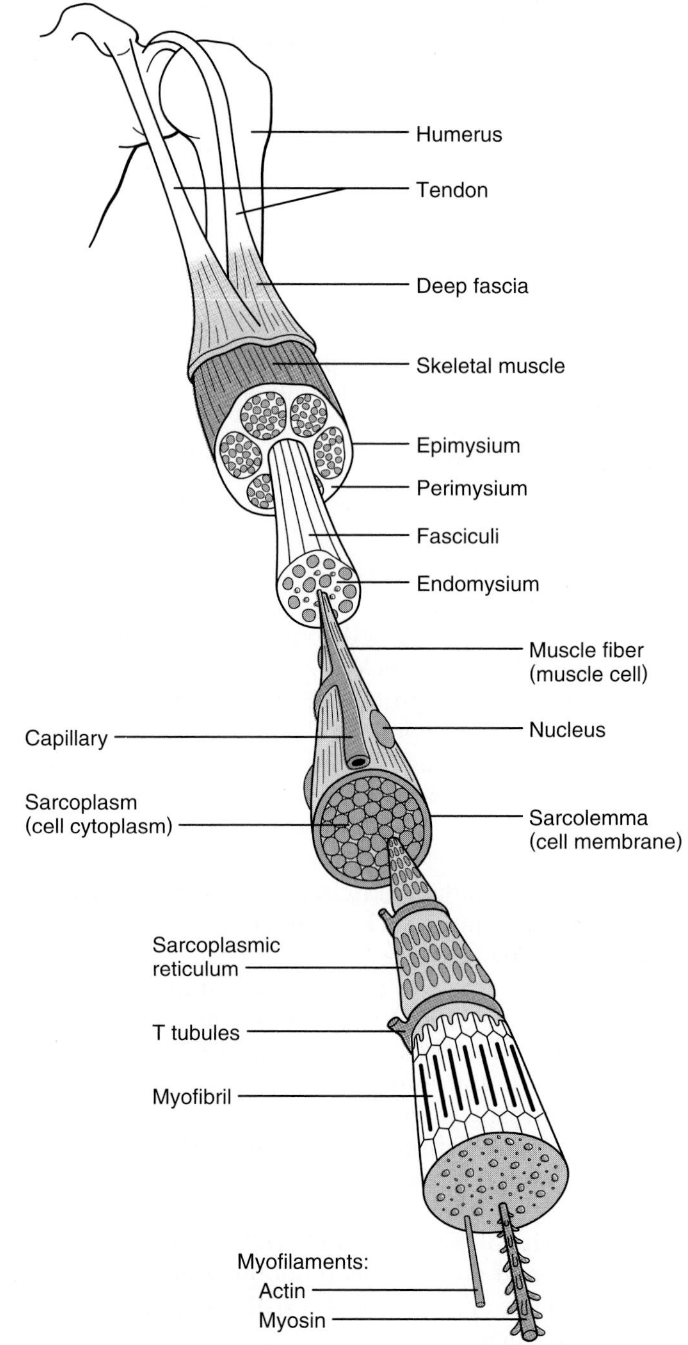

Figure 8•4 Connective tissue components of skeletal muscle.

A **tendon** is a cord of tough fibrous connective tissue that anchors the ends of muscle to bone, fascia, or other connective tissue structures. A broad, flat tendon is called an **aponeurosis,** and attaches skeletal muscle to bone, to another muscle, or to the skin. Both tendons and aponeuroses are tough, collagenous structures and differ only in shape; tendons are cords, whereas aponeuroses are sheetlike. When tendons cross multiple joints, as in the hands and feet, they are covered in **tendon sheaths.** These tubular-shaped structures look like "little sleeves" and are lined with synovial membrane. Synovial fluid reduces friction as the tendons glide back and forth within the sheath and also aids in protecting long tendons.

To keep tendons and tendon sheaths in place, **retinacula,** bandagelike retaining bands of connective tissue are found at the knees, ankles, and wrists. The retinaculum may also act as a pulley for the tendon at the joints of the wrist, ankle, and digits.

HOW DO MUSCLES CONTRACT?

Years ago, physiologists believed that skeletal muscles contracted by folding like an accordion or by changes in the diameter of each cell. Some hypothesized that muscles just grew or perhaps they moved like springs! To examine this "shortening," or contractile mechanism of the muscle, we must look within the muscle fibers themselves. Here, we will find the solution to this puzzle.

Sliding Filament Theory

In the 1950s, it was discovered that contraction does *not* occur by folding or "springing." The dimensional change of the overall size of a muscle is due to a change in the *relative positions of one muscle fiber to another.* Tiny divisions within muscle fibers, called filaments, slide past each other in order to create a change in the length of muscle fibers, resulting in a change in the muscle length. This was appropriately named the **sliding filament theory.**

Think of these filaments as parts of a sliding glass door. The sliding door has two sections that sit side by side in adjacent tracks. Usually one door is permanently secured and the other is movable. The entire glass door, when fully closed, represents a sarcomere (or muscle) at rest. The individual sections of the door represent muscle filaments. As the movable part of the door glides past the fixed door section, the length of the whole structure is shortened. As the door is pulled closed, the whole structure has greater length again. Muscle contractions are very similar. The lengths of the individual sections of filaments never change. Instead, they just slide over each other, changing the length of the sarcomere. Other examples of this concept is a telescoping car antenna or collapsible shower curtain rod. All these objects change their overall length by this sliding mechanism. Now let's examine the anatomy and neurology involved in muscle contraction.

THE ANATOMY OF MUSCULAR CONTRACTION

Each muscle fiber is enveloped by a cell membrane, or **sarcolemma** (Fig. 8–5). Contained in each skeletal muscle fiber is a cellular fluid called **sarcoplasm.** Within the sarcoplasm are sarcomeres; within sarcomeres are myofibrils. A fluid-filled system of cavities called the **sarcoplasmic reticulum** encircles each sarcomere. The sarcoplasmic reticulum plays a crucial role in muscular contraction by storing and releasing calcium ions. The sarcolemma is punctuated by extensions in the membrane called **transverse tubules,** or **T tubules.**

Myofibrils are composed of bundles of smaller structures called **myofilaments.** These myofilaments do not

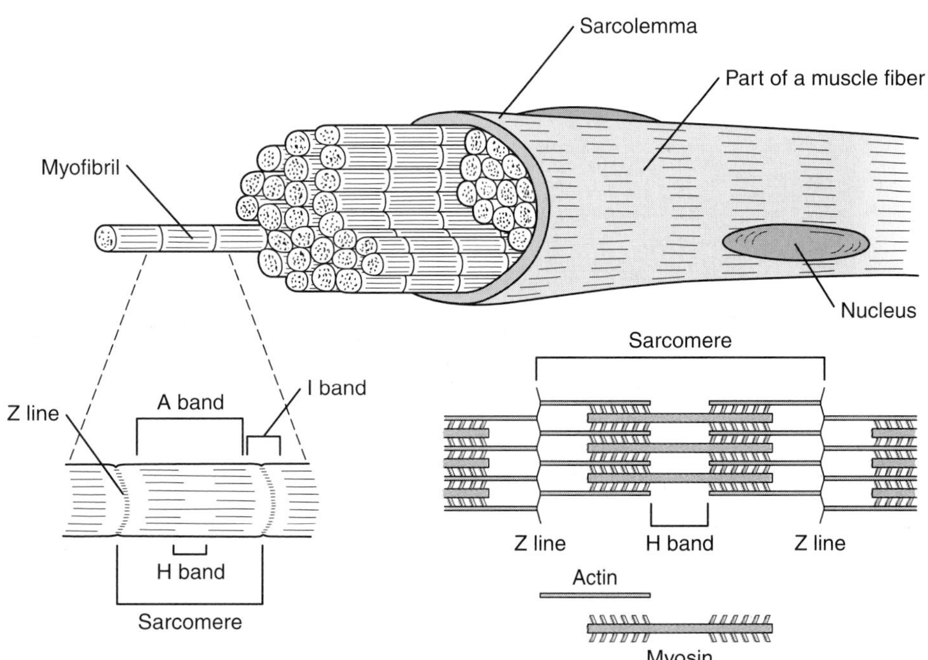

Figure 8•5 A myofibril with sarcomere and Z-lines. Sarcomere with actin and myosin.

run the entire length of the muscle. Rather, they are stacked end to end in a continuous chain of repeating compartments. The ends of the sarcomere are known as Z-lines, probably due to their jagged appearance. *The sarcomere is the basic contractile unit of the muscle* because it contains all the contractile elements. The sarcomere is made up of two types of myofilaments or protein threads. One is called **actin,** and the other is **myosin.** Actin is pulled over myosin filaments to produce the muscular contraction.

The stacked arrangement of the sarcomeres in long rows gives the muscle belly its striped appearance. Each sarcomere contains two bundles of actin strands and one bundle of myosin, and both actin and myosin bundles are connected to the Z-lines at the end of the sarcomere. Actin filaments are thinner than myosin filaments. The thin actin filaments do not run the entire length of the sarcomere. The central region of a resting sarcomere is devoid of actin filaments. This central portion of the sarcomere is known as the H-band.

Actin molecules are dotted with other protein molecules called **troponin** and **tropomyosin.** These protein molecules mark the sites of attachment of the myosin filament during contraction (Fig. 8–6).

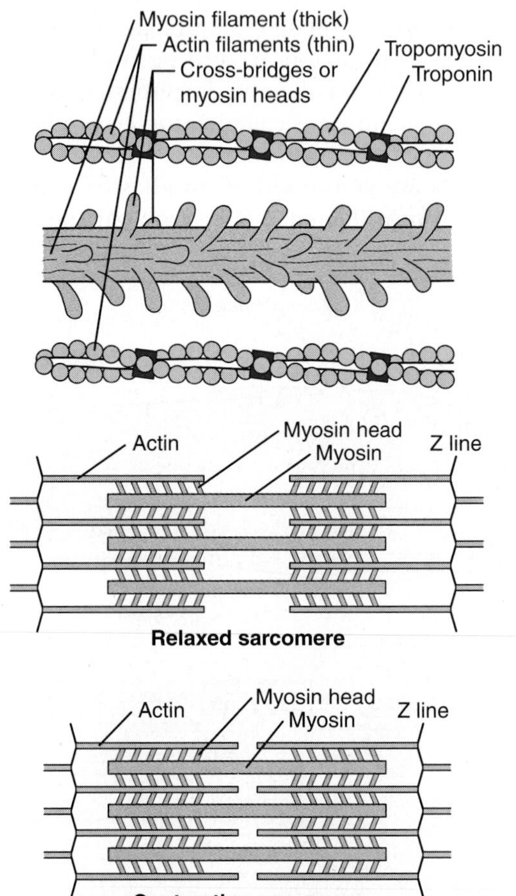

Figure 8•6 A drawing of the cross-bridge attachment process.

The myosin fibers are the thicker protein filaments and are easily recognizable under a microscope due to the presence of cross-bridges or **myosin heads.** The ends of the myosin filaments overlap the actin filaments located on either side. Actin and myosin filaments lie in parallel rows with interlocking ends in a honeycomb arrangement. The absence of myosin filament at either end of the sarcomere is known as the **I-band,** which has a light appearance.

The dark red area on either side of the H-band is known as the A-band. The A-band appears darker due to the presence of both actin and myosin. As the muscle contracts and the filaments slide, the white H- and I-bands become narrow.

THE NEUROLOGY OF MUSCLE CONTRACTION

The contraction of skeletal muscle begins with a nerve impulse that stimulates the conversion of chemical energy into mechanical energy. This nerve impulse may be initiated by either a reflex or a conscious desire to change the body's position. This stimulus travels down the **motor neurons** to the muscle. Motor neurons are responsible for carrying messages of contraction (or in some cases, inhibit contraction) *to* a muscle. One motor neuron may branch off and connect to 10 or 1,000 individual muscle fibers. A single motor neuron and all its associated skeletal muscle fibers are collectively known as a **motor unit.** A single muscle is composed of many motor units. The axons of the motor neurons terminate at the sarcolemma and form a **neuromuscular junction** (also known as a myoneural junction). This is a fluid-filled space between the nerve and the muscle fiber.

When a motor neuron delivers a stimulus, all the muscle fibers of the motor unit receive the signal to contract at the same time. If the stimulus lacks sufficient intensity (subthreshold stimulus), the motor neuron will not produce a response. Each individual muscle fiber, when sufficiently stimulated, will contract to its fullest extent. Likewise, in the absence of sufficient stimuli, each muscle fiber relaxes to its full resting length. With the individual fibers of motor units, there is no partial contraction. This is known as the **all-or-none response.**

Remember that this all-or-none response is true just for motor units, not the entire muscle. There may be thousands of motor units in a single muscle. The nervous system regulates the amount of muscular contraction by activating only the motor units that it needs to perform a given action. If more strength is required, then additional motor units will be stimulated and the muscle as a whole will further shorten. This process of motor unit activation based upon need is known as **recruitment.** More motor units are recruited to pick up a hammer than are required to pick up a nail.

THE CHEMISTRY OF MUSCLE CONTRACTION

When the nerve impulse travels through a motor neuron and enters the neuromuscular junction through the **axon terminal,** a chemical messenger is released (Fig. 8–7). This chemical is called **acetylcholine,** or ACh, and is stored in vesicles at the axon terminal located at the end of the motor neuron. The axon terminal is where the axon of the motor neuron ends. When ACh crosses the gap to the sarcolemma, it binds with receptor sites on the **motor end plate,** synapses with the muscle fibers, and chemically stimulates a muscle contraction impulse. This impulse travels across the surface of the sarcolemma and into the T tubules, causing calcium ions (Ca) to be released from storage in the sarcoplasmic reticulum. Calcium ions are the chemical driving force behind contraction.

These calcium ions bond with the troponin-tropomyosin complex located on the actin filaments. This bonding alters the troponin-tropomyosin complex, leaving an exposed site for the heads of the myosin filaments to attach. The connection between the myosin heads and the actin filaments creates a "cross-bridge" effect. The myosin heads are hinged at the base, and during a muscle contraction, toggle like a light switch. This ratchet effect of the myosin heads draws the actin filaments toward the center, or H-band. This process repeats itself; the actin and myosin filaments draw the Z-lines closer together, causing the entire sarcomere to shorten, the muscle fibers to shorten, and the muscle to contract.

These cross-bridges do not attach or toggle simultaneously, which would make motion jerky. The contraction process is relatively smooth. As the cross-bridge toggles, it is released from its bond with the actin filaments, recocks or toggles back the other way, and reattaches to the actin at a further binding site. This process repeats until the neural stimulation stops.

When the nerve stimulus stops, calcium ions are no longer released. A second chemical, **cholinesterase,** enters the sarcoplasmic reticulum, and neutralizes the effects of ACh. The troponin-tropomyosin complex reattaches to the actin filaments. The muscle is now at rest.

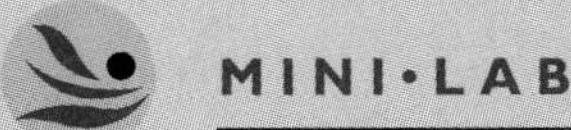

Hold your hands 18 inches from your face, palms facing you. Extend your thumbs up and interlace your fingers. Let your thumbs represent the Z-lines, and your fingers represent thick and thin myofilaments. Slide your fingers toward the middle. Notice how the space between your thumbs, or Z-lines, moves closer together. As the spaces between the thumbs shorten, do your fingers shorten? This illustrates how the sarcomere within a muscle creates movement by shortening.

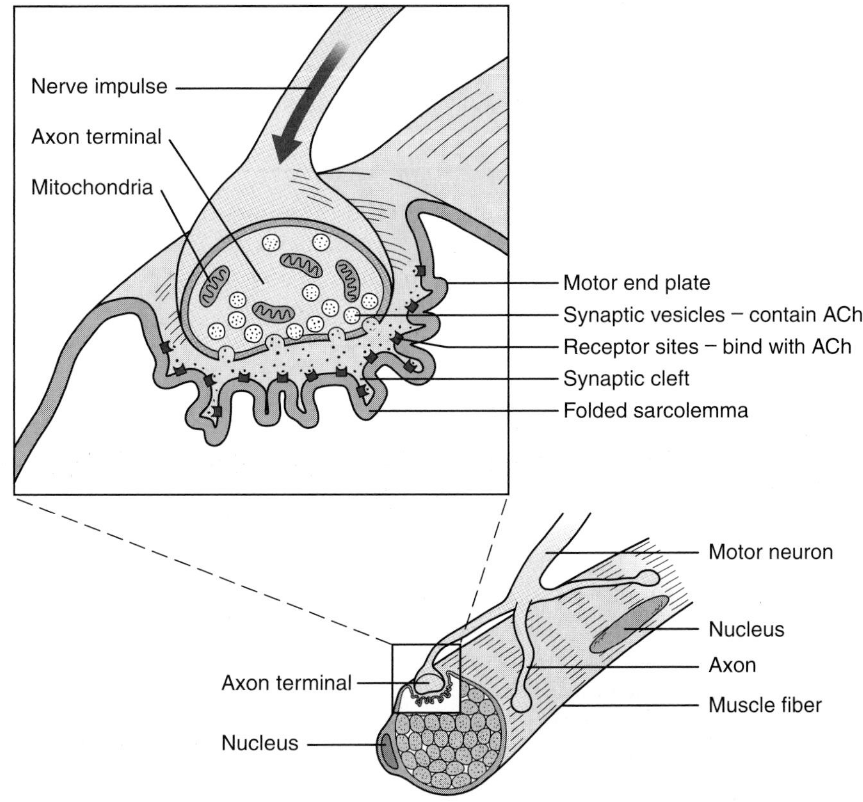

Figure 8•7 Motor end plate.

THREE TYPES OF SKELETAL MUSCLE FIBERS

There are three classifications of muscle fibers: **slow twitch, fast twitch A,** and **fast twitch B.** The ratio of slow twitch to fast twitch is unique to each individual. Some exercise physiologists believe that the ratio of slow twitch to fast twitch is genetically determined and therefore fixed. Others believe that with specialized training, the proportions of slow twitch to fast twitch can be changed. Let's look at the characteristics of each type of muscle tissue.

1. **Slow Twitch.** Also known as red muscle, slow twitch are fatigue-resistant fibers, are small in diameter, and have copious amounts of mitochondria and a red respiratory pigment called myoglobin. **Myoglobin,** or **myohemoglobin,** is chemically similar to the hemoglobin molecule present in red blood cells, which look red due to the presence of the myoglobin and many capillaries. Slow twitch fibers generate large amounts of ATP (adenosine triphosphate) aerobically, but break down the ATP slowly to reduce muscle contraction velocity so muscles are not easily fatigued. Most postural muscles are slow twitch muscles and include, for example, the trapezius, levator scapula, the scalene, and the gastrocnemius. A high ratio of slow twitch muscles is present in the legs of world-class long-distance runners.

Author's Note

The presence of myoglobin in skeletal muscles makes them appear darker. Notice that the dark meat of chickens are the legs and the thighs. Ducks, on the other hand, have dark breast meat. This is because, in general, chickens run around a chicken yard and ducks fly powered by their breast muscles.

2. **Fast Twitch A.** Fast twitch muscles are also fatigue-resistant fibers and are intermediate in diameter. They contain large amounts of myoglobin, many mitochondria, and numerous capillaries. These fibers are also red and generate copious amounts of ATP aerobically. However, they break down ATP quickly. Fast twitch A fibers are resistant to fatigue, but not as much as slow twitch fibers. Many world-class sprinters have a high ratio of fast twitch A muscles in their leg muscles such as the quadriceps and the gastrocnemius.
3. **Fast Twitch B.** Also known as white muscle, fast twitch B are rapidly fatiguable fibers. They possess the largest diameters, have the lowest amount of myoglobin, few mitochondria, and few capillaries, so they appear white. Fast twitch B fibers generate ATP anaerobically in short bursts, and these fibers fatigue quickly. However, their contractions are powerful and rapid. Muscles of the arm, such as the deltoid and biceps brachii, contain many fast twitch B fibers.

STRETCHING

The opposite of muscular contraction is stretching, or myotasis. While stretching is covered in "Classifying Swedish Massage Movements," it is important enough to warrant another brief mention here. When you stretch a muscle, you are extending it to its full length and elongating both muscle and connective tissue. How far you can stretch a muscle depends on several factors. Most factors are out of our control, like genetics and the movement capability of a joint. What we *can* change is the amount of tension in a muscle during a voluntary stretch.

Extensibility, the ability of muscles and other soft tissues to lengthen, can be improved by regular stretching. Stretching can also improve the range of movement of a joint because it influences the physiological characteristics of the muscle, tendons, ligaments, and other structures surrounding the joint. Hyperflexibility, or hypermobility, is flexibility beyond a joint's normal range of motion, and can affect joint stability.

Proprioceptors are sensory receptors located in muscles, tendons, and joints. They send information into the central nervous system about muscle length, muscle tension, and joint movements. One of the two proprioceptors that can be stimulated during a stretch are **muscle spindles** located within the muscle belly. If the muscle is stretched too rapidly (ballistic stretch), the muscle spindles detect the motion, and the central nervous system responds by reflexively contracting the muscle. This is a protective mechanism and is known as the **myotatic stretch reflex,** which is intended to protect the muscle from overstretching by causing the muscle to contract. This reflex is also important for maintaining posture, which is mediated by muscle spindles.

Other proprioceptors stimulated during a stretch are **Golgi tendon organs** or **tendon organs,** located in the musculotendinous junction. These receptors detect tension applied to the tendon during a slow, static stretch. The central nervous system responds by inhibiting muscle contraction, which allows the muscle to relax and stretch. This protective mechanism is known as the **inverse stretch reflex** or the **autogenic inhibition.** It works the exact opposite of stretch reflex and represses contraction to prevent tearing of a muscle or avulsion (separation by tearing) of the tendon from its attachment.

Massage therapists can use this information when applying or instructing clients in stretching. To enhance flexibility, apply only slow, static stretches. Movements that are perceived by the nervous system as "dangerous" will be met with resistance.

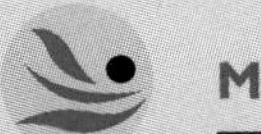

MINI•LAB

Hold a shoestring by the two coated ends with both of your hands. Slowly begin to pull the ends apart. Watch what happens to the individual strands in the string. Do the fibers spread apart or draw closer together? Imagine that this string is a muscle and the two ends are tendinous attachments. Within this muscle is a spasm. Pull the ends again. As the muscle is being stretched, is the spasm released? Note that separation in the muscle fibers does not occur when the muscle is stretched. This explains why stretching does not release local muscle spasms.

Reciprocal Inhibition

When the central nervous system sends a message for the agonist (muscle causing movement) to contract, the tension in the antagonist (muscle opposing movement) is inhibited by impulses from motor neurons, and thus must simultaneously relax. This neural phenomenon is called *reciprocal inhibition.*

This information can be used to ease the pain of an acute muscle spasm or cramp. Contract the muscle opposite (antagonist) of the muscle spasm and the muscle spasm will let go. This conscious contraction may have to be repeated several times, and the contraction must be isometrically resisted. It is as if the brain is turning off the message of contraction, and relaxation is the result. A further discussion can be found in the nervous system chapter.

TYPES OF SKELETAL MUSCLE CONTRACTIONS

1. **Isotonic Contractions.** During isotonic, or dynamic, contractions, the muscle changes length against resistance, and movement occurs. This is the most common type of muscle contraction. Isotonic contractions result from increased nerve activity and increased blood supply to the muscles being contracted.

   When a muscle is involved in dynamic contractions, it can shorten or lengthen. In fact, lengthening contractions are as much a part of coordinated motion as shortening contractions. Without the ability of a muscle to shorten and lengthen during contractions, we could not lower objects after we lifted them.
2. **Concentric (Positive) Contractions.** This type of isotonic contraction occurs as the muscle shortens and pulls on a bone to produce movement. When movement occurs as the muscle is shortening, it is called a concentric or shortening contraction. An example of a concentric contraction is the lifting phase of a biceps curl. The biceps brachii is flexing the elbow while you are holding a 5-pound barbell. Muscles involved in concentric contractions are also known as **accelerators** or **spurt** muscles. They may provide a forward acceleration in locomotion.
3. **Eccentric (Negative) Contractions.** Eccentric contractions, or lengthening contractions, occur when the muscle lengthens during a muscle contraction. For example, during the lowering phase of a biceps curl, the biceps brachii muscle will be eccentrically contracted as you extend the elbow. The biceps brachii is contracting, but it is getting longer. Repeated eccentric contraction causes more muscle damage and muscle soreness than concentric contraction, such as running downhill. These muscles are also known as **decelerators** or **shunt** muscles because they slow down the powerful concentric contractors. Unless the body compensates with some corrective braking action, we could tear tissue.
4. **Isometric Contractions.** Muscles do not always shorten or lengthen when they contract. If you attempt to pick up a weight that is too heavy, do the muscles still shorten? No. In isometric muscle contractions, the muscle increases in tension by contraction but does not change its length or angle of the joint. Isometric contractions are important because they stabilize some joints as others are moved. Isometric contraction can also be used clinically to reset tone on muscles weak from nonuse. It is often the first method of rehabilitation after surgery or injury, because isometric contractions are relatively painless and increase local blood circulation without stretching tissues.

   Isometrics are the therapy of choice when a client fears pain during movement or refuses to move an injured part. However they only strengthen muscles in the position of the actual contraction. Isometrics are great for building muscle bulk or increasing strength in certain positions, but these exercises do not increase the efficiency or endurance of skeletal muscles.

MUSCLE FIBER ARRANGEMENT

Muscle fibers are arranged mainly in one of two basic patterns: **longitudinal** and **penniform** (Fig. 8–8). The differences between them are the shape of the muscle and the resulting strength. Longitudinal muscles have greater range of motion, but are less powerful. The penniform shape allows more force in contraction but offers less range of motion.

Longitudinal muscles have fibers aligned in a parallel formation along a long axis. Types of longitudinal muscles are *quadrilateral* (e.g., rhomboids), *triangular* or fan-

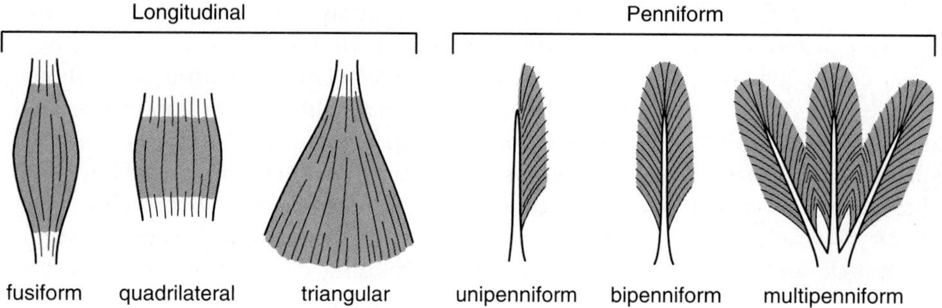

Figure 8•8 Longitudinal and penniform muscle fiber arrangement.

shaped (e.g., pectoralis major), and *fusiform* or spindle-shaped (e.g., coracobrachialis). Most of the muscles in the upper extremity are longitudinally arranged.

Penniform muscles are arranged with a central tendon and muscle fibers extending from the tendon diagonally, which gives the muscle a feather-like appearance. Types of penniform muscles are a *unipenniform, bipenniform,* and *multipenniform.* Occasionally these penniform muscles are referred to as unipennate, bipennate, and multipennate. In the unipenniform arrangement, the muscle fibers come off just one side of the tendon (e.g., tibialis posterior). When the muscle fibers are arranged on both sides of the central tendon, it is called a bipenniform (e.g., rectus femoris). Some muscles have several tendons within the belly, and muscle fibers run diagonally between them (e.g., subscapularis). These muscles are called a multipenniform. Most muscles in the lower extremity are of the penniform arrangement because of the added requirement of strength.

PARTS OF A SKELETAL MUSCLE

The gross structures of a skeletal muscle come in a range of shapes and sizes, but all possess a central portion of the muscle and at least two points of attachment. At the simplest level, a muscle shortens, one attachment moves toward the other, and movement occurs. Some schools call the two points of attachment proximal and distal attachments or the medial and lateral attachments. These attachment sites can also be referred to as the "origin" and "insertion," which are terms that indicate movement caused by muscle contraction. Generally, insertion moves toward origin; however, the roles can be reversed, and the origin can move toward the insertion (e.g., iliopsoas). Below are the parts of a muscle.

1. **Belly.** The belly of the muscle is also referred to as the gaster (Fig. 8–9). This central portion comprises the bulk of the muscle. The belly of the muscle produces movement of the joint by the shortening of its fleshy mass during contraction. This action pulls the tendons attaching the muscle to the bone closer together. Within the tissue of the muscle belly is the structure known as sarcomeres, which are the functional contractile unit of the muscle discussed earlier.
2. **Origin.** The tendinous attachment of the muscle that is relatively fixed and does not move when the body is in motion is called the origin. It is usually located on the medial or proximal end of the skeleton.
3. **Insertion.** The insertion, usually located lateral or distal, is the muscle attachment undergoing the greatest movement. When a muscular contraction occurs, the insertion commonly moves toward the origin.

As you learn individual skeletal muscles, the origins and insertions will help you to think about muscles causing a desired action. Once muscle actions are understood, you will be able to comprehend a series of actions, or dynamic motion. As we will see next, mus-

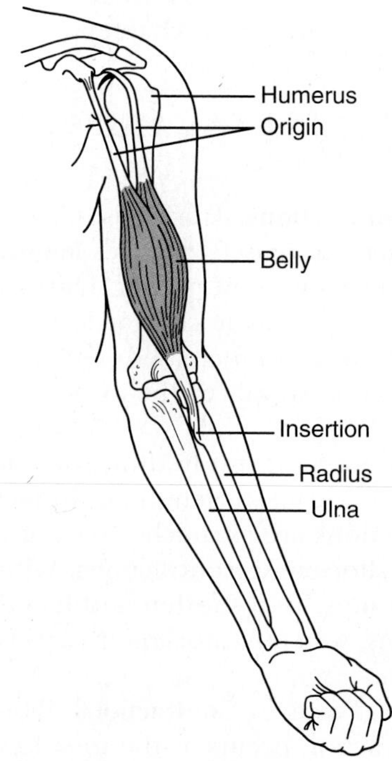

Figure 8•9 Parts of a skeletal muscle.

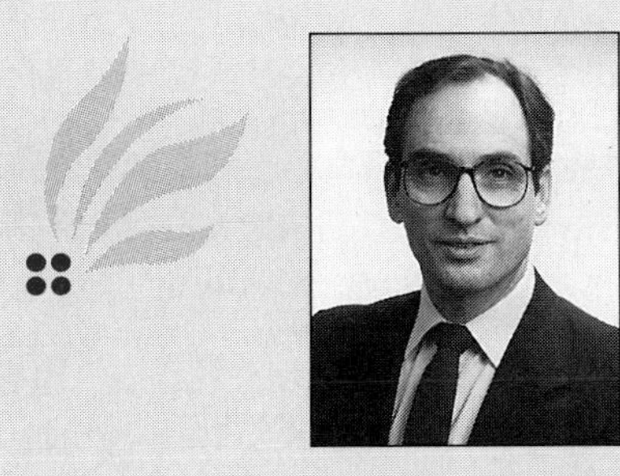

Jon Zahourek

Born: January 5, 1940

"The mind cannot forget what the hands have learned."

Artists dream of creating a work designed to last. Jon Zahourek is no exception. What makes him unique, however, is that his masterpiece could influence the way future generations learn how the body—especially the muscles—works.

It was a painful process for Zahourek, but not your typical artistic angst. For years Zahourek, a sculptor, artist, and Parson's School of Design instructor, was plagued with debilitating back pain. As a drawing teacher he taught a detailed anatomy class. "The names of some of the muscles scared me to death," he laughs. So, like a lot of teachers, he would gloss over these and go on. But a new way to teach anatomy led to a revelation for Zahourek, who began building clay muscles—layer by layer—on a model skeleton.

"It was like 'whoosh,' a wind rushed through me and suddenly everything that I had been trying to teach about how the muscles work became integrated within me. I spent all weekend trying to understand what happened," he says. "What most of us grasp about how our bodies work is either very childlike or dead wrong."

But he wasn't able to see this—or feel it in his own body—until he actually modeled each muscle in space. By building each muscle, one by one, and learning how it connected to bone and worked with or against other muscles, Zahourek moved from the ability to point to a muscle, name it, and tell his students which action it performed to a deeper level of knowing. Suddenly his body understood and felt how each muscle worked. "It set me free physically! My back problems of 20 years were gone. It wasn't the pain that was disabling me. It was the fear and lack of knowledge. I didn't understand what was causing the pain until I began to see the conflicts between the muscles."

If this could have such a liberating effect on him, it could also help others. So, what started as the perfect way to instruct art students became a creative work in itself. At first he intended to build clay muscles on a life-sized wooden skeletal model, then realizing the weight would be not only unwieldy but downright deadly if it toppled over on someone, he began to create scaled-down models. When these were perfected, Zahourek Systems, Inc. was born. A complete system package contains detailed videos, workbooks, clay, sculpting tools, and mannequins (skeletons of varying degrees of complexity and price ranges).

He began marketing his entire "learning process" package to anyone who could benefit from understanding how the body works, including physical therapists, college anatomy classes, even elementary-aged children, massage therapy schools, and of course, massage therapists.

For massage therapists, Zahourek's model and ideas have several implications. For massage schools who use the system, it's a guaranteed method to learn—really learn—the musculoskeletal system, not just about where a muscle is and its name and shape. It's hands-on, which benefits all massage students, especially those who are tactile learners, as many massage therapists are. Otherwise, a therapist may complete a degree program and merely work on a very surface level—literally, as well as figuratively—and often that's not enough for a client with a specific problem.

There's also the chance, that like Zahourek, the massage therapist will somehow have his or her own chance for the great "aha" to rush through his body, and experience the opportunity to travel from a conceptual understanding of how the muscles work to a deeper, cognitive level—to know the body from the inside out. Massage therapists lucky enough to have had this experience can often tell from the moment the client walks

continued on page 164

Continued

Jon Zahourek

into the office, what's happening with her body. The therapist doesn't just see it, he senses it or even feels it.

Massage therapists absolutely and unequivocally must understand their own bodies. Massage therapy can be such physically demanding work, many therapists don't last for more than 5 years. Not understanding their own bodies—and their hands in particular—is occupational suicide. As Zahourek says, "It's like working hard for a diploma and someone telling you, 'Congratulations, in 4 years you'd better find something else to do.'" Massage therapists need to understand how it all works. Zahourek offers the analogy: If you were a runner and you woke up one morning and your legs were sore, you wouldn't stop running, would you?

One way to stay strong? "Socrates was right," says Zahourek. "Know thyself." As massage therapists we must return again and again to the learning laboratory—our own minds and bodies, peeling layer from layer, then rebuilding layer upon layer until we get it right. Jon Zahourek, in his attempt to teach art students how to draw more lifelike figures, stumbled upon a new lease on life for himself and a model that allows massage therapists to learn how the body works in a way that will never be forgotten.

cles can play several roles in contributing to the body's dynamics.

HOW DOES THE BODY COORDINATE MOVEMENT?

Muscles do not simply contract simultaneously to achieve dynamic motion. Even the simplest movements would be impossible with all the muscles fully contracted. Instead, muscles assume different responsibilities to carry out a variety of movements. A muscle may function as agonist, antagonist, synergist, or fixator depending on its role in performing a particular task. Agonists are also called prime movers, and fixators are also referred to as stabilizers.

Most skeletal muscles are arranged in pairs. The muscle that is most responsible for causing desired joint action is the **agonist.** The opposing muscle, or **antagonist,** must resist, or yield to the joint motion initiated by the agonist. The antagonist usually lies on the opposite side of the joint and causes the opposite joint action. Imagine what movement would be like without the antagonist opposing the pull of the prime mover. The upper fibers of the trapezius muscle would contract, creating hyperextension of the head. When the movement task is fulfilled, your head would fall, uncontrolled, in response to the pull of gravity. The antagonist allows movements to be more controlled and refined.

To help things run smoothly, other muscles, called **synergists,** aid the prime movers by causing the same movement. For example, the peroneus longus and peroneus brevis are synergistic to the gastrocnemius and soleus when they are plantar flexing the ankle.

Fixators or **stabilizers** are specialized synergists. They stabilize the joint over which the prime mover exerts its action. This allows the prime mover to perform a motion more efficiently. For example, the postural muscles stabilize the vertebral column so the iliopsoas and the rectus femoris can flex the thigh (Fig. 8–10).

Strain between body segments alters patterns of movement. Tight muscles can affect movement partly because antagonists cannot fully elongate. Any given movement evokes response not only from the prime movers but also from the antagonists, synergists, and fixators. Imagine watching a baseball player throw a baseball. His foot goes forward, one hip swings back, then forward as his entire upper torso and arm are propelling the baseball. Full, powerful motion is a synchronized wave of smaller motions rather than a single movement.

Let's apply one of these concepts to a clinical setting. One rehabilitative approach for musculoskeletal problems is to strengthen the antagonist. This corrects positional and postural distortions by creating balanced motion on both sides of the joint. For example, if poor posture is due to hypercontracted back muscles, strengthening the abdominals can create a change in the resting length of these tight muscles. Don't be surprised if a client with a low back condition comes home from a doctor's appointment with a recommended daily routine of proper abdominal exercises.

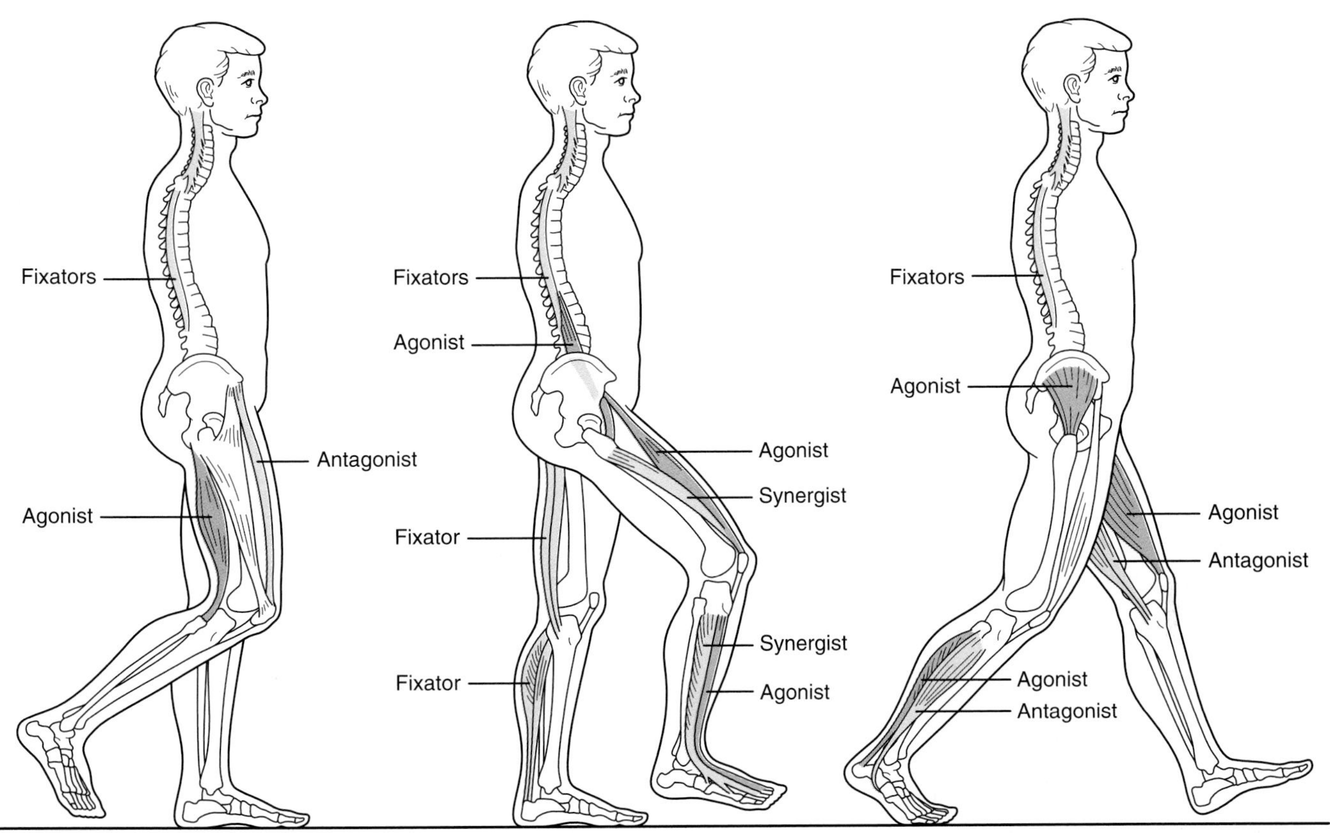

Figure 8•10 Man walking depicting agonist, antagonist, synergist, and fixators.

MUSCULAR CONDITIONS AND CLINICAL TERMS

1. **Contracture.** Also known as ischemic contracture, contracture is an abnormal, usually permanent condition of a joint in which the muscle is fixed in a flexed position. It may be the result of spasm, paralysis, or fibrotic tissue surrounding a joint. A contracture can be brought on by heat or medication.

   Use broad strokes to increase blood flow in the affected area. Friction, followed by the application of ice, can be used to reduce adhesions. The muscles should be kneaded thoroughly to stretch the fascia. Myofascial release would also be helpful. Slow and gentle stretches may help elongate the muscles.
2. **Muscle Spasm.** An increase in muscle tension with or without shortening, due to excessive motor nerve activity, may result in a rigid zone (i.e., knot, rope) in the muscle called a spasm. Muscle spasms cannot be alleviated by voluntary relaxation.
3. **Muscle Cramp.** An acute, painful contraction of a single muscle or group of muscles is a muscle cramp. They are often associated with mineral deficiency or muscle fatigue and are usually short-lived.
4. **Spasticity.** Spasticity is characterized by increased muscle tone and stiffness and is associated with an increase in tendon reflexes. A spastic muscle will resist stretching and typically involves the arm flexors and leg extenders and effects can range from mild to severe. In severe cases, movement patterns become uncoordinated or impossible and usually involve a neurological dysfunction.
5. **Tonus.** Also referred to as muscle tone or muscle tension, tonus is a state of continuous, partial contraction of muscles. This slight contraction firms up a muscle without causing movement and is necessary for maintaining posture.

Author's Note

The two worst things for your muscular system are overuse and no use. Somewhere in between is the right use.

6. **Flaccid.** Muscles lacking normal tone are loose and appear flattened rather than rounded. Flaccidity is often considered the first stage of muscular atrophy. Muscles will become flaccid if they are not used and exercised regularly.
7. **Muscular Atrophy.** A decrease in the size of muscle fibers or a wasting away of muscles from poor

nutrition, lack of use, motor unit dysfunction, or lack of motor nerve impulses is called muscular atrophy.

8. **Hypertrophy.** An increase in the size and diameter of muscle fibers without cell division is known as hypertrophy. Exercise and weight lifting may cause muscular hypertrophy, which increases the number of actin and myosin filaments in the sarcomere.
9. **Muscle Fatigue.** Muscle activity cannot be sustained indefinitely. The inability of a muscle to contract even though it is still being stimulated is called muscle fatigue. Insufficient oxygen, exhaustion of energy supply, or the accumulation of lactic acid can cause muscles to lose their ability to contract efficiently. A muscle may become fatigued if it generates wastes faster than the circulatory system can carry them away.

   Furthermore, muscles laden with lactic acid or lacking ample oxygen cannot relax as easily or quickly as they should. When muscle fatigue occurs, muscle strength and coordination decrease. Muscular performance drops off like that of a car with a fouled sparkplug.
10. **Tendinitis.** Inflammation of the tendon, accompanied by pain and swelling, is called tendinitis. When inflammation also involves the tendon sheath, it is referred to as *tenosynovitis.*
11. **Fibromyalgia.** Also known as fibrositis, fibromyositis, myofascial syndrome, or muscular rheumatism, fibromyalgia is a chronic inflammatory disease that affects muscle and related connective tissues. There is pain, joint stiffness, and the presence of "tender points" or "trigger points" as this disease progresses. This condition may develop after physical or emotional trauma, local or general infections, or even changes in climate. Like rheumatoid arthritis, fibromyalgia may go into remission, only to flare up at a later date.

Massage should be tailored to how the client is feeling at the time of the treatment because symptoms vary from day to day. Generally, a relaxing, full-body massage is indicated.

12. **Strain.** A strain, commonly called a pull, is an injury of a muscle or tendon due to a violent contraction, forced stretching, or synergistic failure. Most muscle strains occur on the antagonist, or the muscle that must resist the muscle creating the action. When the antagonist is tight or spasmed, it cannot stretch easily and may become injured.

    Acute muscle strains can be classified into three grades or degrees of severity (Fig. 8–11). *First-degree* strains involve up to 10 percent of stretching or a partial tear of fibers with no palpable defects. There is typically mild pain at the time of injury and there may be mild swelling and localized tenderness. The joint structures can maintain efficient motion and hold against resistance.

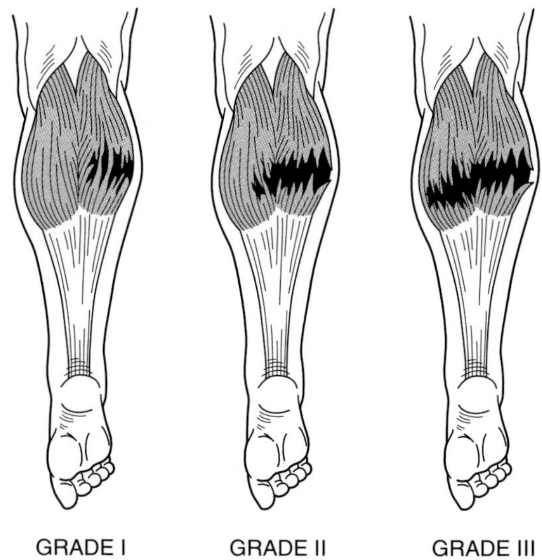

Figure 8•11 Three degrees of strain.

    When the muscle or tendon is torn between 10 and 50 percent, it is classified as a *second-degree* strain. A palpable defect is noted and the joint structures cannot hold against moderate resistance. Edema is typically found, and the muscles surrounding the strain or sprain splint to restrict painful movement.

    In *third-degree* tears, 100 percent of the fibers are torn and a "snap" is often heard at the time of injury. Third-degree tears may represent a complete rupture (avulsion) of the involved structures. A piece of the bone may be torn away as well (sprain fracture). A depression in the area of the torn muscle usually can be palpated and is usually painful to touch. Function is greatly altered in third-degree tears.
13. **Myasthenia Gravis.** Myasthenia gravis is a weakness in the muscles characterized by chronic fatigability. This condition is caused by a deficiency of acetylcholine, causing a malfunction at the myoneural junction. The onset of myasthenia gravis is gradual, with dropping of the upper eyelids, throat, and facial muscles. The weakness may extend to the respiratory muscles. Muscular exertion may exacerbate this condition and is not advised.

Massage may slow the muscle atrophy. Also, active and passive range of motion of the joints may be helpful.

14. **Muscular Dystrophy.** A collection of genetically transmitted diseases, muscular dystrophy is characterized by the progressive atrophy of skeletal muscles without any indication of neural degeneration or damage. All forms of muscular dystrophy involve a loss of muscular strength, disability, and deformity.

Massage may slow muscular atrophy. Also, active and passive range of motion of the joints may be helpful. Abdominal massage may help with constipation because this disorder affects involuntary muscles, including those of the large intestine.

15. **Hernia.** A hernia is a protrusion of an organ or part of an organ through its surrounding connective tissue membranes or cavity wall. This condition may be congenital, resulting from failure of structures to completely close after birth, or a hernia may be developmental due to obesity, chronic illness, or surgery. There are many types of hernias named for their location (i.e., hiatal or inguinal).

    Local massage is contraindicated. General massage is okay to do. If the client is experiencing pain in the area of the hernia, refer him immediately to his health-care professional.

The Effects of Massage on the Muscular System

1. Massage relieves muscular restrictions, tightness, stiffness, and spasms. These effects are achieved by direct pressure on the spasm by manipulating the tissue that sends messages of "length" to the central nervous system, and by the increase in circulation. Results are more flexible, supple, and resilient muscle tissues.
2. Massage enhances blood circulation, thus increasing the amount of oxygen and nutrients available to the muscles. Increased oxygen and nutrients reduce muscle fatigue and postexercise soreness. Due to increased circulation, massage improves muscular nutrition.
3. Massage promotes rapid disposal of waste products and replenishment of nutritive materials through increased circulation, further reducing muscle fatigue and soreness.
4. Massage interrupts the pain cycle by relieving muscular spasms, increasing circulation, and promoting rapid disposal of waste products.
5. Massage helps to maintain the muscle in the best possible state of nutrition, flexibility, and vitality, thus hastening muscle recovery and enabling muscles to function at maximum after recovery.

SUMMARY

The understanding of the structure and functions of muscle tissue and its related fascia is vital to the practice of massage therapy. Physiologically, muscles serve five basic functions; they provide external mobility and internal motility, produce heat, maintain posture and move lymph. It takes three different types of muscle tissue to perform these various functions: smooth, cardiac, and skeletal.

Each skeletal muscle is composed of bundles of muscle fibers known as fasciculi. These are bound together individually and collectively with layers of fascia, which is a tough, white, protective membrane. The main part of the muscle is the belly, which is attached to the bone by two or more tendons, which are known as the origin and insertion(s). The shortening of the muscle belly draws the tendons closer together to produce movement of the skeletal system. This shortening is produced by a change in the relative size of the basic contractile unit known as the sarcomere. An explanation of the cellular processes of muscular contraction is known as the sliding filament theory.

In the coordination of movement, muscles work in pairs or groups. Muscles involved in these groups are classified by function as agonists (prime movers), antagonists, synergists, and fixators (stabilizers). The muscle tissue can also be classified by its chemistry as slow twitch or fast twitch.

Biomechanically, muscles do one of two things: stretch or contract. Muscular contractions can be isometric or isotonic. Isotonic contractions may be further classified as either concentric or eccentric. The opposite of contracting is stretching, which extends the muscle. Overstretching is prevented by a mechanism known as the myotatic reflex.

With an understanding of the theory and actual mechanics of the muscular system, as well as the structure and location of the individual muscles, the application and effectiveness of the massage strokes can be greatly enhanced.

SELF-TEST

Multiple Choice • Write the letter of the best answer in the space provided.

_______ 1. Which of the following is *not* a function of the muscular system?

A. effecting external and internal mobility
B. maintaining posture
C. producing heat
D. exchanging of gases

_______ 2. The simplest unit of a muscle fiber is called

A. endomysium
B. agonist
C. myofibril
D. penniform

_______ 3. What layer of connective tissue wraps around the entire muscle?

A. endomysium
B. perimysium
C. ectomysium
D. epimysium

_______ 4. The fibrous cords of connective tissue that attaches muscle to bone are the

A. sarcomere
B. myofibril
C. tendon
D. fibrocord

_______ 5. The most stationary attachment of a muscle is the

A. agonist or prime mover
B. origin
C. antagonist
D. insertion

_______ 6. What is the moving attachment of a muscle called?

A. agonist or prime mover
B. origin
C. antagonist
D. insertion

_______ 7. The muscle fiber arrangement with a central tendon and muscle fibers extending from the tendon diagonally is

A. sarcomere
B. agonist
C. myofibril
D. penniform

_______ 8. The functional contractile unit in muscle fibers composed of actin and myosin filaments is the

A. sarcomere
B. agonist
C. myofibril
D. penniform

_______ 9. Which of the following is involved in skeletal muscle contraction?

A. acetylcholine
B. cross-bridge formation
C. actin and myosin
D. all of the above

_______ 10. The sarcoplasmic reticulum stores copious amounts of

A. sodium
B. protein
C. calcium
D. potassium

_______ 11. The motor neuron and its associated muscle fibers are called the

A. myoneural junction
B. motor unit
C. all-or-none response
D. intercalated disk

_______ 12. The muscle that is responsible for the resisting or opposing action is called the

A. agonist or prime mover
B. synergist
C. antagonist
D. insertion

_______ 13. A muscle that assists the agonist or prime mover is called the

A. agonist or prime mover
B. synergist
C. antagonist
D. insertion

_______ 14. The muscle causing the desired action is the

A. agonist or prime mover
B. retinaculum
C. antagonist
D. insertion

_______ 15. If an athlete has fast twitch A muscles, she is more suited for

A. sprints
B. long-distance running
C. walking
D. golf

_______ 16. Skeletal muscle contraction in which there is an increase in tension but no change in muscle length is called

A. isometric
B. eccentric
C. isotonic
D. concentric

_______ 17. A contraction of a muscle while it is in the process of lengthening is called

A. isometric
B. eccentric
C. isotonic
D. concentric

Matching • List the letter of the answer to the term or phrase that best describes it.

A. muscle tone
B. hypertrophy
C. muscular dystrophy
D. stretching
E. atrophy
F. muscle soreness
G. fibromyalgia
H. reciprocal inhibition

_______ 1. A chronic inflammatory disease that affects muscle and related connective tissues.

_______ 2. A decrease in the size of muscle cells or wasting away of muscles.

_______ 3. When a muscle is extended.

_______ 4. An increase in the size and diameter of muscle cells without cell division.

_______ 5. A buildup of lactic acid, minute tears as a result of overexertion, or stiffened connective tissue due to a lack of oxygen-rich blood.

_______ 6. When a muscle receives a message to contract and its antagonist receives a message to relax.

_______ 7. A collection of genetically transmitted diseases characterized by the progressive atrophy of skeletal muscles without any indication of neural degeneration or damage.

_______ 8. A state of continuous, partial contraction of muscles resulting from systematic stimulation of the nervous system.

References

Applegate, Edith J., M.S. *The Anatomy and Physiology Learning System: Textbook.* Philadelphia: W. B. Saunders, 1995.

Ardion, Christine. Certified manual lymphatic drainage practitioner, 1996.

Goldberg, Stephen, M.D. *Clinical Anatomy Made Ridiculously Simple.* Miami: Medmaster, Inc., 1984.

Guyton, Arthur, M.D. *Human Physiology and Mechanisms of Disease,* 3rd ed. Philadelphia: W. B. Saunders Company, 1982.

Haubrich, William S. *Medical Meanings, A Glossary of Word Origins.* New York: Harcourt Brace Jovanovich, 1984.

Kordish, Mary and Sylvia Dickson. *Introduction to Basic Human Anatomy.* Lake Charles, LA: McNeese State University, Self-Published Manual. 1985.

Marieb, Elaine N. *Essentials of Human Anatomy and Physiology,* 4th ed. New York: Benjamin/Cummings Publishing Company, Inc., 1994.

Mattes, Aaron. *Active Isolated Stretching.* Published by Aaron Mattes, 1995.

McAleer, Neil. *The Body Almanac.* Garden City, New York: Doubleday and Company, Inc., 1985.

Moore, Keith L. *Clinically Oriented Anatomy,* 2nd ed. Baltimore: Williams & Wilkins, 1985.

Mosby's Medical, Nursing, and Allied Health Dictionary, 4th ed. St Louis: Mosby–Year Book, Inc., 1994.

Newton, Don. *Pathology for Massage Therapists,* 2nd ed. Portland: Simran Publications, 1995.

Premkumar, Kalyani. *Pathology A to Z—A Handbook for Massage Therapists.* Calgary, Canada: VanPub Books, 1996.

Southmayd, William M. D. and Marshall Hoffman. *Sportshealth: The Complete Book of Athletic Injuries.* New York and London: Quickfox, 1981.

Tabers Cyclopedic Medical Dictionary, 13th ed. Philadelphia: F. A. Davis Company, 1977.

Tortora Gerald J. *Introduction to the Human Body: The Essentials of Anatomy and Physiology.* 3rd ed. New York: HarperCollins Publishers, 1994.

Travell, Janet G. M. D. and David G. Simons M. D. *Myofascial Pain and Dysfunction, The Trigger Point Manual.* Baltimore: Williams & Wilkins, 1983.

It takes seventeen muscles to smile and forty-three to frown. Humor is a great way to conserve energy. A smile has face value, and, if you grin, you get a double dose.
—Charles Linder

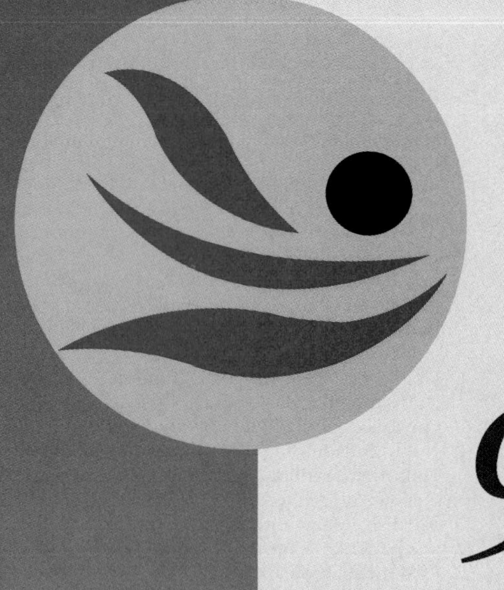

9

Skeletal Muscle Nomenclature

Student Objectives

After completing this chapter, the student should be able to:

- Describe the general locations of each muscle listed in the chapter
- Explain the location of each muscle listed in the chapter according to its muscle attachment site
- Demonstrate the actions of each muscle listed in the chapter

INTRODUCTION

This chapter will examine 116 of the major muscles of the body. To get the most out of this chapter, we must look at how it is organized. These muscles are divided into two units and nine lessons. The first unit is called Muscles of the Appendicular Skeleton and consists of six lessons: Muscles of Scapular Movement; Muscles of Shoulder Movement; Muscles of the Forearm, Wrist, and Hand; Muscles of Hip and Knee Movement; and Muscles of Foot Movement. The second unit is called Muscles of the Axial Skeleton and consists of three lessons: Muscles of the Head and Neck, Muscles of the Trunk and Vertebral Column, and Muscles of Respiration. It is recommended that the muscles be learned in the sequence presented, as these are generally the order in which muscles can be addressed during a massage. This system will support students of massage to gain a strong foundation of musculoskeletal anatomy and muscle nomenclature.

There are many ways to arrange and classify muscles into groups. They can be grouped regionally (e.g., arm, leg, abdomen), according to their attachment sites (i.e., clavicle, ribs, femur), or by how they move the joints (actions). Muscles in these units are grouped in regions, and the muscles of each lesson are grouped according to actions. You can look at each muscle individually, or you can look at them in the bigger context of motion.

One of the best approaches to learning the muscles is to reduce the task into bite-size pieces. Five learning phases are presented to assist you in this task. Understanding is a process, like learning a dance. First, you must hear the music, then you observe others, and then follow them with your body, until you are moving through space. This muscle-learning system uses the building-block approach to learning, in which a foundation is laid before something is built. However, feel free to design your own learning system and use this system as a starting point for further exploration.

Phase I. Decode muscle names and learn pronunciations.

Phase II. Learn general locations of muscles.

Phase III. Learn specific muscle locations using attachment sites.

Phase IV. Study muscle actions using a multisenory approach.

Phase V. Application of knowledge including palpation of muscle

In **Phase I,** spend time looking over all the muscles in this chapter and learn exactly how they were named. Do not be surprised if it feels like a history lesson. Try to imagine a small group of people dissecting a cadaver and having to name all the structures they find. All muscles are named using descriptive words. Read over the information in the box to familiarize yourself with six ways in which muscles are named. It may take you some time to read, pronounce, decode, and absorb each new word, but it will give you a solid foundation of understanding. It's also fun to try to look at these terms as a puzzle that you have to figure out.

Once you feel comfortable with the language of musculoskeletal anatomy, use a muscle chart and look at all muscle locations (Fig. 9–1.) Point to them and say their name. Locate them on your body and pronounce their name. **Phase II** gets you familiar with their general locations on the body.

Phase III adds a very important dimension to understanding muscle location for a massage therapist by focusing on attachment sites. Using an articulated skeleton, find each bony attachment site. Using a piece of colorful yarn or cording, touch both bony markings at once. This will give you a graphic idea of the muscles.

Most Muscles are Named by . . .

1. **Attachment Sites or Origin and Insertion.** An example of this is the sternocleidomastoid (sterno-cleido-mastoid) muscle, which is attached to the sternum, the clavicle, and the mastoid process of the temporal bone.
2. **Action or Function.** When muscles are named by function, the function is usually named first and the body part it is acted upon is usually named second. Examples are flexor pollicis (flexes the thumb), levator scapulae (elevates the scapula), and erector spinae (keeps the spine erect).
3. **Number of Origins.** When naming muscles by number of origins, the number of origins, or heads, is given first and the body part it is associated with is given second. For example, biceps femoris (two-headed muscle), triceps brachii (three-headed muscle), and quadriceps femoris (a group of four muscles).
4. **Relative Shape and Size.** Some muscles are named for their geometric shape or their gross size. Examples are gluteus maximus (largest), gluteus minimus (smallest), adductor longus (long), and deltoid (triangular).
5. **Location and Direction of Fibers.** Muscles can be named for where they are located or the direction of the majority of their fibers. Examples are temporalis (temporal bone), frontalis (frontal bone), rectus femoris (straight), internal abdominus oblique (slanted), and latissimus dorsi (dorsum or posterior).
6. **Combinations.** Many muscles are named using a combination of the aforementioned. For example, extensor digitorum longus (long muscle that extends the digits or fingers) and flexor digitorum profundus (deep muscle that flexes the fingers). ••

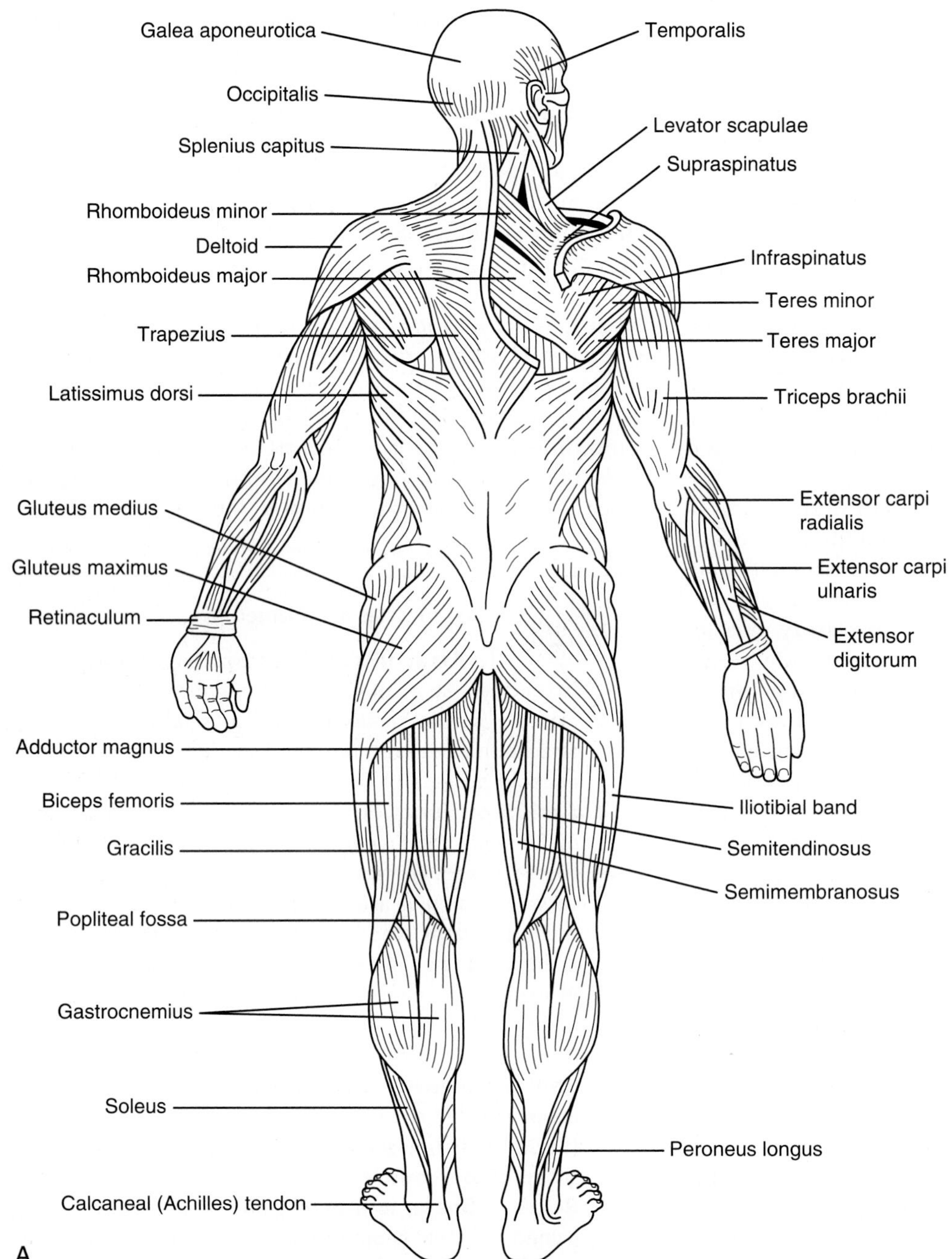

Figure 9•1 Muscles of the body.

A large picture of a skeleton may be used if a skeletal model is not available; use a color marker and draw in the muscle, going from origin to insertion. You can also practice this activity in pairs or groups.

Phase IV is to learn the action of muscles. Typically, the insertion or "I" moves toward the origin or "O." You can learn them by rote memory or by a multisensory approach. If you have chosen the latter, go back to the Phase III learning strategy, the yarn on the articulated skeleton, and shorten the string! This will produce the action of the muscle because muscles produce movement by contracting their fibers. Another useful technique is to say aloud the name of the muscle while you are doing the action with your own body. You can even touch the muscle, say the muscle name aloud, and perform the action. The muscle producing the action will feel harder and become shorter and thicker.

Phase V is to APPLY, APPLY, APPLY! With your instructor's help, learn how to palpate these muscles, if possible. Use all this anatomical information in massage class, and use the names of these muscles with your clients. Use the anatomical terminology as much as you can so it becomes part of *you.* As the names, locations, and actions of the muscles become more fixed in your brain, your confidence will grow.

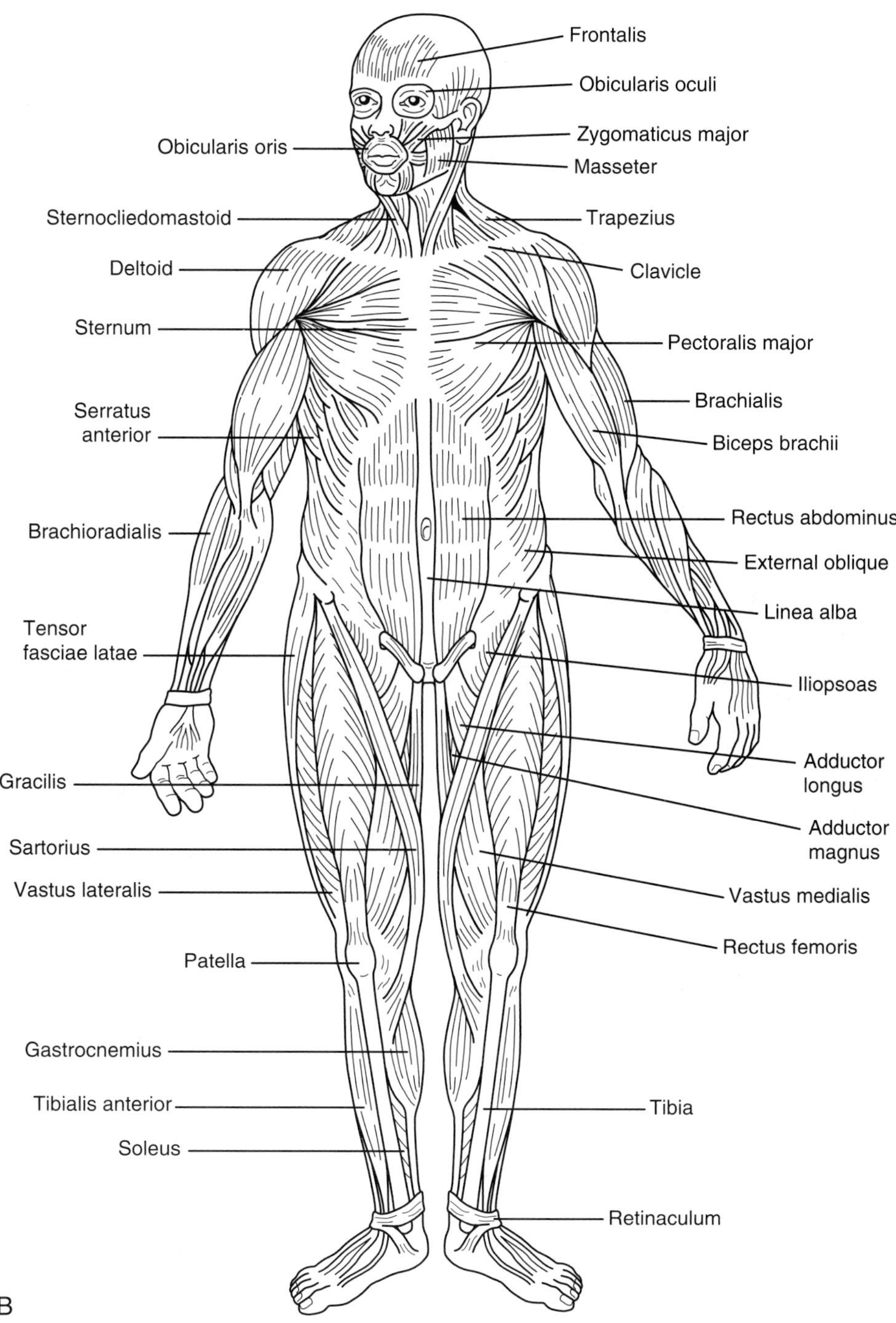

Figure 9•1 *Continued* B

Author's Note

In researching muscle origin, insertion, action, and nerve supply information, I discovered that there are numerous variations, inconsistencies, and disagreements on the subject of muscle nomenclature. Please realize this as you read and work with the information found in this chapter. It is helpful to collect the books mentioned in the reference section and many other books concerning this fascinating subject.

The muscles that have been featured in this chapter were determined by surveying teachers who taught this subject at massage schools and through the suggestions of numerous reviewers of this book.

You will notice some muscle names in a shaded box. These are words that are commonly used when discussing a group of muscles. An example of muscle groups are the hamstrings and the adductors.

Contract, relax, contract, relax—that's all muscles do. So relax your brain and enjoy this part of the book by learning through application. The retention of this knowledge will come with reinforcement.

Let's get started.

Other Tips for Learning Skeletal Muscles

Write each muscle on an index card, draw pictures, and write word roots. Study these at red lights, traffic jams, or while waiting for supper to cook.

Find new ways to group muscles together! Make one list of all muscles that have their origins on the occiput; make another list for clavicular origins, etc. You could also do this type of listing for insertions. You could even do this listing arrangement by actions.

Draw muscles on a real body! This body may be one of your classmates or recruit a body, *any* body. Use nontoxic, water-soluble markers.

Make paper cut-outs of muscles for a skeletal chart or build muscles with clay on a skeletal model.

UNIT ONE—MUSCLES OF THE APPENDICULAR SKELETON

LESSON ONE—MUSCLES OF SCAPULAR MOVEMENT

MUSCLE	ORIGIN	INSERTION	ACTION	NERVE
Trapezius	occipital protuberance, nuchal ligament, spinous process of C1–T12	lateral ⅓ of the clavicle, acromion process, and spine of the scapula	upper fibers: extend the head, elevate and laterally rotate the scapula; middle fibers: retract (adduct) the scapula; lower fibers: depress and laterally rotate the scapula; unilateral contraction: lateral flexion of the cervical spine, contralateral rotation of the head; bilateral contraction: extension of the head and cervical spine	accessory (cranial nerve XI), third and fourth cervical
Greek: trapezoeides—tablelike	**Notes:** Also known as the "coat hanger muscle" because clothes hang from the trapezius, like a coat hanger. The trapezius muscle behaves like three muscles in one. Covering more than half the back, the upper, middle, and lower fibers contract to perform three separate actions. The trapezius, or "traps," is to the neck and head what the erectors are to the back. Note that this muscle can be an antagonist to itself.			

LESSON ONE—MUSCLES OF SCAPULAR MOVEMENT *(continued)*

Levator Scapulae 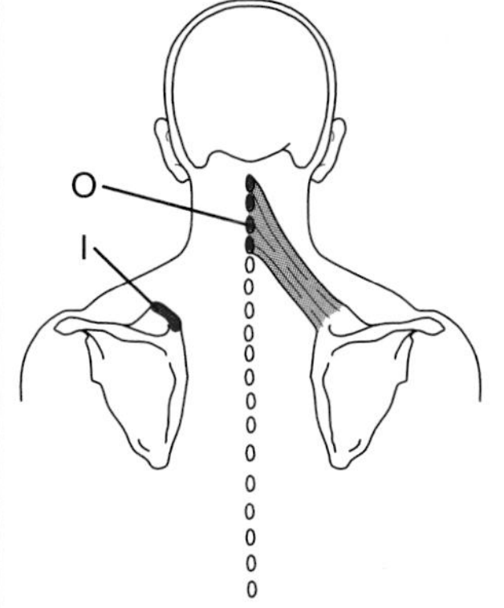 *Latin:* *levator—a lifter* *scapulae—shoulder blade*	transverse processes of C1–C4	vertebral border of the scapula from the superior angle to root of spine	elevates, retracts (adducts), and medially rotates the scapula	dorsal scapular nerve (C5), third and fourth cervical
Rhomboids	Rhomboids is the name given for the rhomboid major and the rhomboid minor. Both lie deep to the trapezius; the rhomboid minor is superior to the rhomboid major. They are also known as the "Christmas tree muscles" because the fiber direction is obliquely arranged, like Christmas tree branches.			
Rhomboid Major and Minor 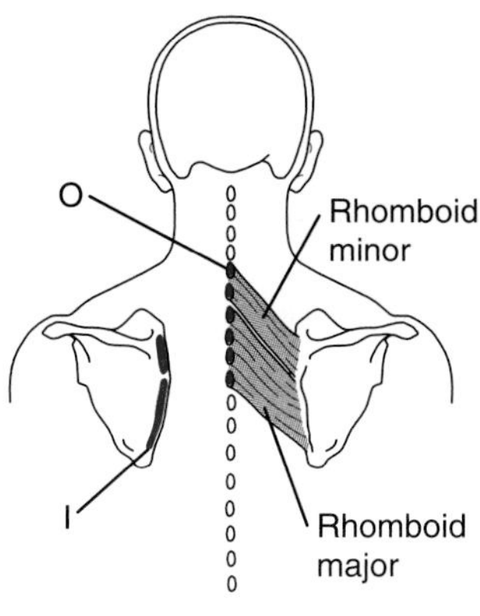 *Latin:* *rhombos—all sides even* *major—larger* *minor—smaller*	major: spinous process of T2–T5; minor: spinous process of C7–T1	vertebral border of the scapula from the root of the spine (minor) to the inferior angle (major)	elevates, retracts (adduction), and medially rotates the scapula	dorsal scapular nerve (C5)

continued on page 176

LESSON ONE—MUSCLES OF SCAPULAR MOVEMENT *(continued)*

MUSCLE	ORIGIN	INSERTION	ACTION	NERVE
Serratus Anterior	ribs 1–9, lateral to costal cartilage	anterior vertebral border and inferior angle of the scapula	protraction and lateral rotation of the scapula	long thoracic nerve (C5–C7)
Latin: *serratus—notched or jagged like a saw* *ante—before*	**Notes:** This, along with the triceps brachii, is called the "boxer's muscle" because the forward movement of the scapula enables a boxer to deliver a punch.			
Pectoralis Minor	ribs 3–5, lateral to costal cartilage	coracoid process of the scapula	depresses, protracts, and laterally rotates the scapula	medial pectoral nerve (C8 and T1)
Latin: *pectoralis—pertaining to the chest* *minor—smaller*	**Notes:** Pectoralis minor, along with the scalenes, is known as the "neurovascular entrappers." This is because the pectoralis minor forms a bridge over the axillary artery and the distal portion of the brachial plexus.			

Many of the figures in the charts in this chapter have been modified with permission from Bates A, Hanson N. *Aquatic Exercise Therapy*. Philadelphia, W. B. Saunders, 1996.

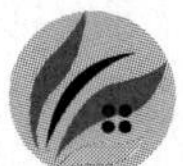

Tips on How to Palpate Muscles

- Locate the bony markings (origin and insertion) of the muscle you wish to palpate. It may be necessary to reposition your subject to allow neighboring muscles to relax.
- Ask your subject to perform the action of the muscle. The muscle contraction will probably be the muscle you are trying to locate. Apply resistance to the movement. Palpate the muscle in its contracted state. Ask your subject to relax and repeat the contraction.

LESSON TWO—MUSCLES OF SHOULDER MOVEMENT

MUSCLE	ORIGIN	INSERTION	ACTION	NERVE
Latissimus Dorsi	spinous process of T6–L5, lower four ribs, posterior iliac crest, sacrum	intertubercular or bicipital groove of the humerus	extends, medially rotates, and adducts the shoulder	thoracodorsal nerve (C6–C8)

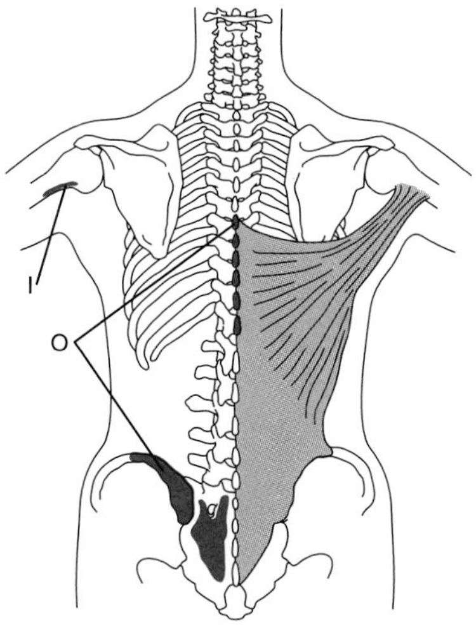

Latin:
latus—broad
dorsum—back

Notes: Also known as the "swimmer's muscle" because this muscle allows us to extend our arm and propel us in water. The latissimus dorsi is the widest muscle of the body and one of the major muscles involved with back pain. Because of its iliac attachments, improper lifting can cause trauma and tearing in the iliosacral region, resulting in low back pain.

MUSCLE	ORIGIN	INSERTION	ACTION	NERVE
Teres Major	inferior half of the lateral border of the scapula	medial lip of the bicipital groove of the humerus	extends, medially rotates, and adducts the shoulder	lower subscapular nerve (C5 and C6)

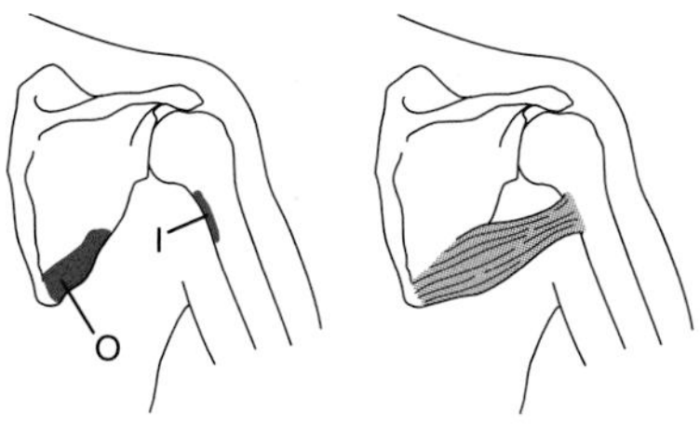

Latin:
teres—round
major—larger

Notes: The teres major muscle is a synergist to the latissimus dorsi muscle.

Rotator Cuff

Also known as the musculotendinous cuff, the rotator cuff is a group of muscles deep to the deltoids. They do a great deal for the stability of the glenohumeral joint and may function as ligaments. They are also called the "SITS muscles": *s*upraspinatus, *i*nfraspinatus, *t*eres minor, and *s*ubscapularis.

MUSCLE	ORIGIN	INSERTION	ACTION	NERVE
Supraspinatus	supraspinatus fossa of the scapula	greater tubercle of the humerus	assists deltoid in abducting and flexing the shoulder	subscapular nerve (C5 and C6)

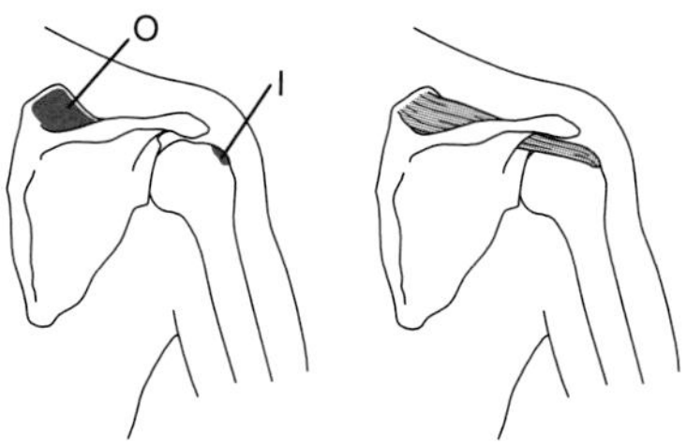

Latin:
supra—above
spinatus—spine

Notes: The supraspinatus muscle is the only muscle of the rotator cuff that does not rotate the humerus. The supraspinatus prevents downward dislocation of the humerus when carrying a heavy portable massage table!

continued on page 178

LESSON TWO—MUSCLES OF SHOULDER MOVEMENT *(continued)*

MUSCLE	ORIGIN	INSERTION	ACTION	NERVE
Infraspinatus 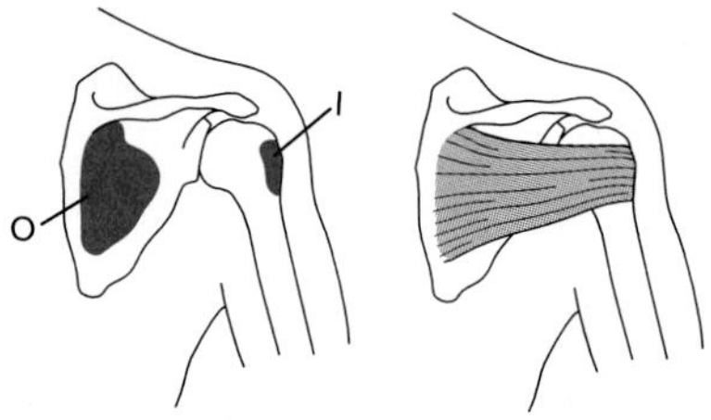 *Latin:* *infra—beneath* *spinatus—spine*	infraspinatus fossa of the scapula	greater tubercle of the humerus	extends and laterally rotates the shoulder	subscapular nerve (C5 and C6)
Teres Minor 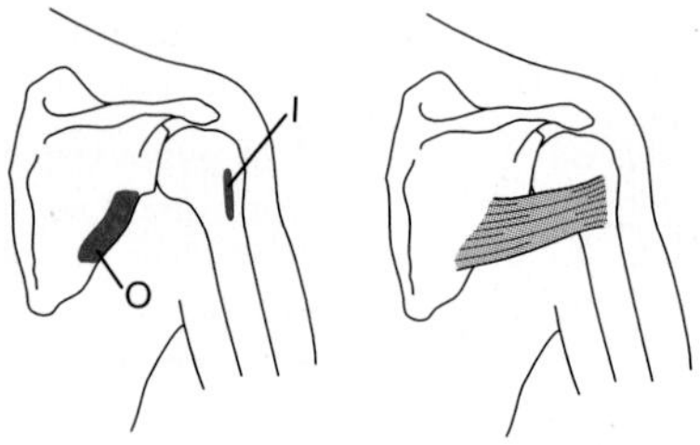 *Latin:* *teres—round* *minor—smaller*	superior lateral border of the scapula	greater tubercle of the humerus	abducts and medially rotates the shoulder	axillary nerve (C5 and C6)
	Notes: The teres minor muscle is the synergist to the infraspinatus muscle.			
Subscapularis 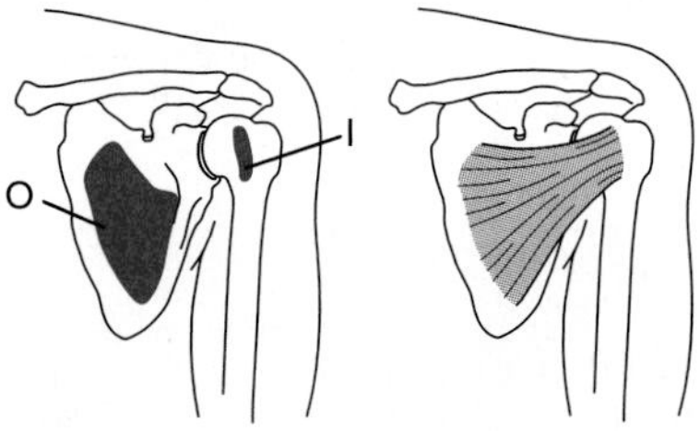 *Latin:* *sub—below* *scapulae—shoulder blade*	subscapular fossa of the scapula	lesser tubercle of the humerus	adducts and medially rotates the shoulder	upper and lower subscapular (C5 and C6) nerve
	Notes: Dr. Janet Travell, author of *Myofascial Pain and Dysfunction,* refers to the subscapularis muscle as the "frozen shoulder" muscle.			

LESSON TWO—MUSCLES OF SHOULDER MOVEMENT *(continued)*

MUSCLE	ORIGIN	INSERTION	ACTION	NERVE
Deltoid O O I *Greek:* *delta—triangular-shaped*	lateral ⅓ of the clavicle, acromion, and spine of the scapula	deltoid tuberosity of the humerus	anterior fibers: flex, medially rotate the shoulder; middle fibers: abduct the shoulder; posterior fibers: extend and laterally rotate the shoulder	axillary nerve (C5 and C6)
	Notes: Mary Kordish, a biology professor at McNeese State University, Lake Charles, LA, said that if the deltoids were discovered today, they would be considered three independent muscles. The anterior, middle, and posterior fibers of the deltoids function like three separate muscles. Structurally, they resemble the gluteals. To get a better understanding of this concept, get on your hands and knees and imagine yourself as a four-legged animal. Note that this muscle can be antagonist to itself.			
Pectoralis Major O I *Latin:* *pectoralis—pertaining to the chest* *major—larger*	medial half of the clavicle, edge of the sternum, costal cartilages of ribs 1–8	bicipital groove of the humerus	flexes, adducts, and rotates the arm medially; clavicular fibers only: shoulder flexion; sternal fibers only: shoulder extension	medial and lateral pectoral nerves (C5–T1)
	Notes: The pectoralis major muscle, or "pecs," forms the upper anterior chest wall and anterior axillary fold. Tightness in this muscle may cause constriction of chest and angina pectoralis-like pain or postural distortions such as rounded shoulders.			
Coracobrachialis O I *Greek:* *korax—crow's beak* *Latin:* *bracchium—arm*	coracoid process of the scapula	medial midshaft surface of the humerus	flexes, adducts, and medially rotates the shoulder	musculocutaneous nerve (C5–C7)

Claire was an avid weekend warrior. On Saturday and Sunday mornings she would run 6 miles. Then in the afternoons, Claire would ride her bike 15 miles. She was a long, lean, aerobic machine. By Monday morning, she would fall on my massage table, and I would try to soothe away her overworked muscles with massage.

On one of her weekend bike trips, she hit a train track at a wrong angle and fell off her bike. She felt okay, but by Monday morning she was having trouble breathing, and there was a feeling of constriction in her chest. After a visit to her physician, to make sure massage was appropriate, she scheduled a massage appointment.

Claire described to me how she landed when she fell off her bike. Apparently, she had thrown her arms out in front of her to protect herself from the rapidly approaching asphalt. This sudden force was absorbed by her scalenes and pecs, which went into spasms. Focusing on these two pairs of muscles seemed to reduce the tightness in her chest and restore her breathing. After a few visits, she felt terrific, and, by the following weekend, Claire was back in running shoes. ••

LESSON THREE—MUSCLES OF ELBOW MOVEMENT

MUSCLE	ORIGIN	INSERTION	ACTION	NERVE
Biceps Brachii	long head: supraglenoid tubercle of the scapula; short head: coracoid process of the scapula	radial tuberosity	flexes the elbow, supinates the forearm, flexes the shoulder	musculocutaneous nerve (C5–C6)
Latin: *bis—twice + caput—head* *bracchium—arm*	**Notes:** The biceps brachii muscle is called the "corkscrew muscle" because its two actions resemble how you uncork a wine bottle.			
Brachialis	distal half of the anterior surface of the humerus	ulnar tuberosity	flexes the elbow	musculocutaneous, radial, and median nerves (C5–C7)
Latin: *bracchium—arm*	**Notes:** The brachialis is the most effective arm flexor because of its mechanical advantage, lying deep to the biceps brachii.			

LESSON THREE—MUSCLES OF ELBOW MOVEMENT *(continued)*

MUSCLE	ORIGIN	INSERTION	ACTION	NERVE
Brachioradialis *Latin:* *bracchium—arm* *radialis—spoke of a wheel*	lateral supracondylar ridge of the humerus	styloid process of the radius	flexes the elbow	radial nerve (C5–C6)
Notes: The bulge you can palpate on the radial side of your forearm is the brachioradialis.				
Triceps Brachii *Greek:* *treis—three* *Latin:* *bracchium—arm*	long head: infraglenoid tubercle of the scapula; lateral head: posterior humerus above the spiral groove; deep or medial head: posterior humerus below the spiral groove	olecranon process of the ulna	extends the elbow and shoulder	radial nerve (C7–C8)
Notes: This, along with the serratus anterior, is called the "boxer's muscle," because it delivers a straight-arm knockout punch.				

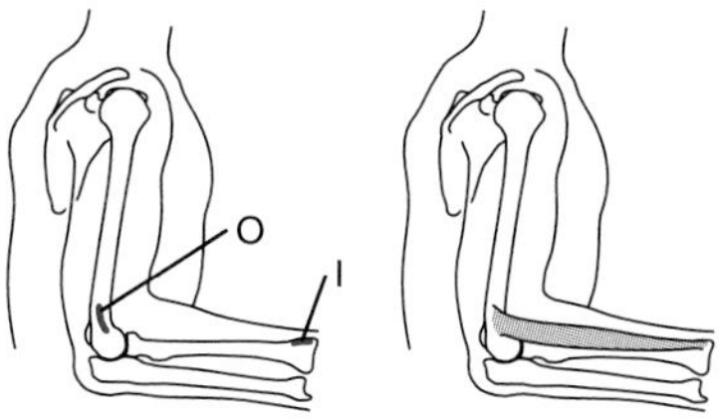

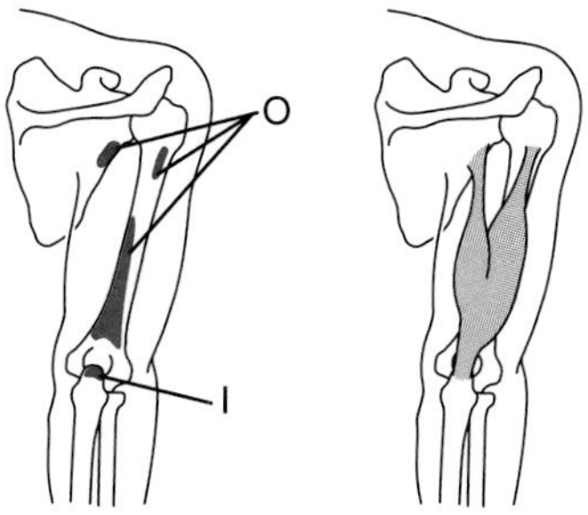

LESSON FOUR—MUSCLES OF THE FOREARM, WRIST, AND HAND

MUSCLE	ORIGIN	INSERTION	ACTION	NERVE
Pronator Teres *Latin:* *pronus—downward* *teres—round*	medial epicondyle of the humerus and coronoid process of the ulna	lateral surface of the proximal radial shaft	pronates the forearm and flexes the elbow	median nerve (C6–C7)

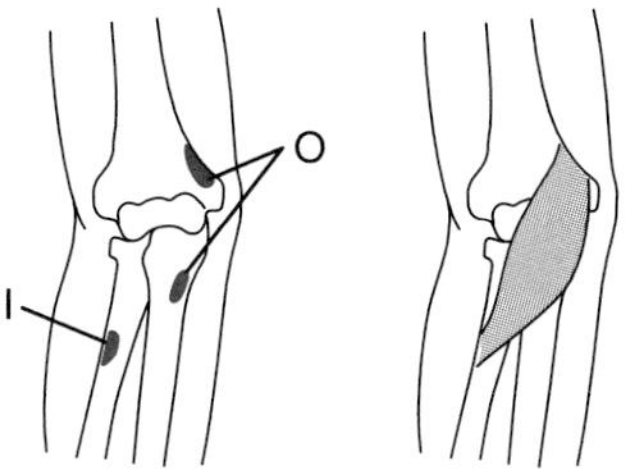

continued on page 182

LESSON FOUR—MUSCLES OF THE FOREARM, WRIST, AND HAND

MUSCLE	ORIGIN	INSERTION	ACTION	NERVE
Pronator Quadratus 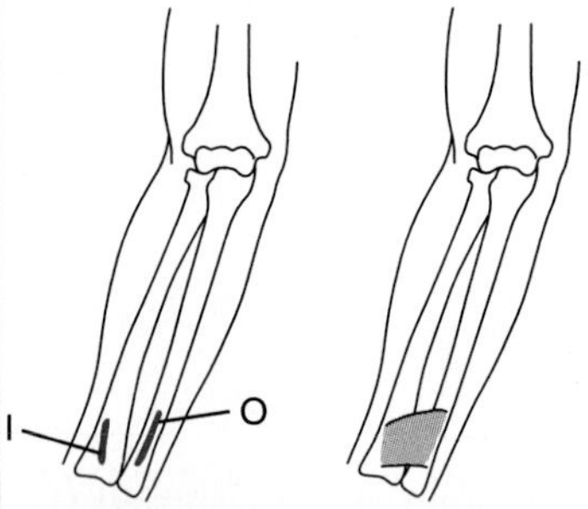 I O *Latin:* *pronus—downward* *quadratus—four sided*	distal ¼ of anterior ulna	distal ¼ of anterior radius	pronates the forearm	median nerve (C8–T1)
Supinator 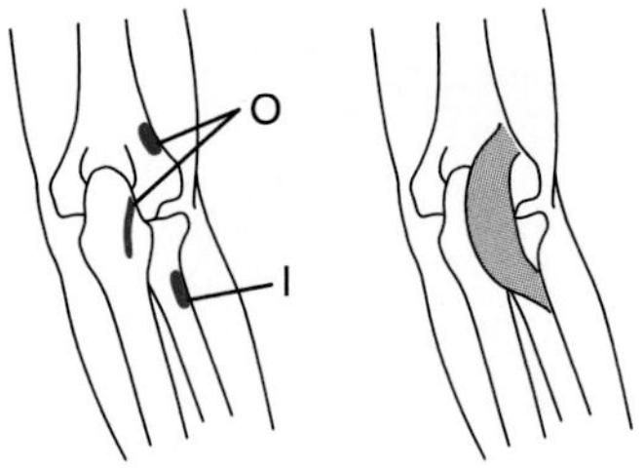 O I *Latin:* *supinatus—bent backward*	lateral epicondyle of the humerus, oblique line of the ulna, elbow joint	proximal lateral surface of the radius	supinates the forearm	radial nerve (C6)
Flexor Carpi Radialis 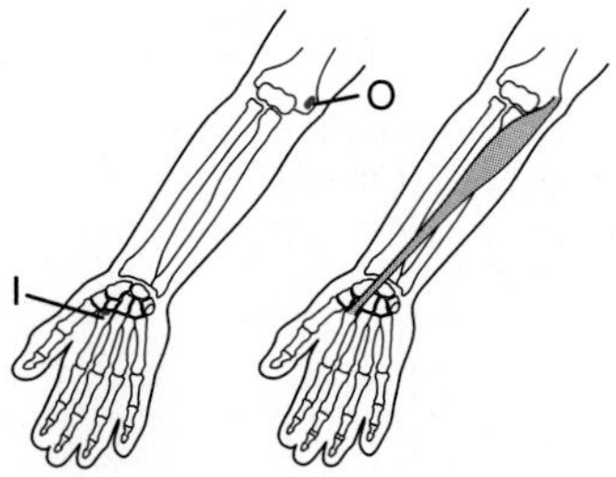 O I *Latin:* *flexus—bent* *karpos—wrist* *radialis—spoke of a wheel*	medial epicondyle of the humerus	bases of the second and third metacarpals	flexion of the wrist	median nerve (C6–C7)

LESSON FOUR—MUSCLES OF THE FOREARM, WRIST, AND HAND *(continued)*

MUSCLE	ORIGIN	INSERTION	ACTION	NERVE
Flexor Carpi Ulnaris 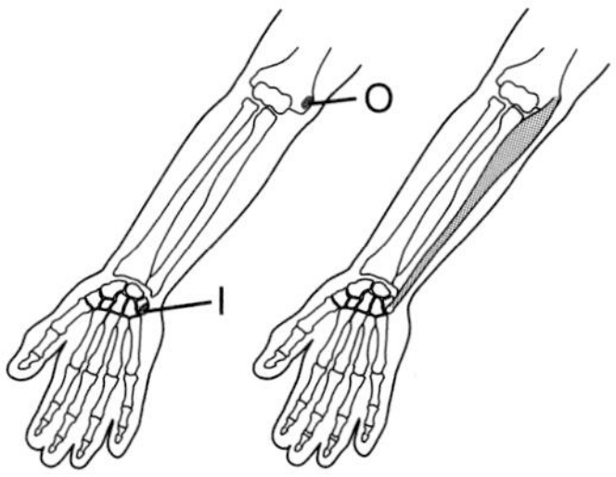 O I *Latin:* *flexus—bent* *karpos—wrist* *ulna—elbow*	medial epicondyle of the humerus	base of the fifth metacarpal	flexion of the wrist	ulnar nerve (C8–T1)
Extensor Carpi Radialis Longus and Brevis O O I I Extensor carpi Radialis longus Extensor carpi Radialis brevis 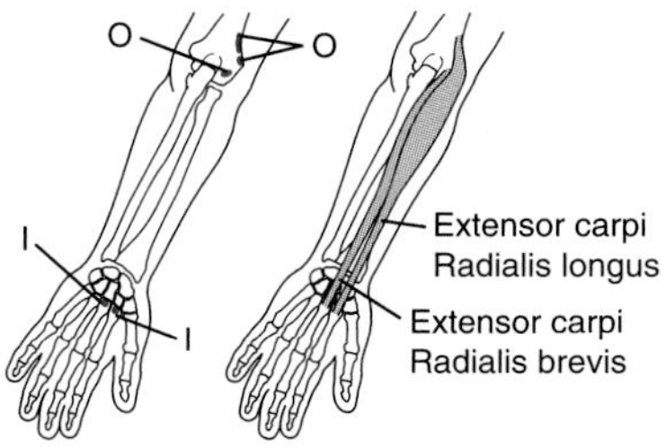 *Latin:* *extensio—to extend* *karpos—wrist* *radialis—spoke of a wheel* *longus—long* *brevis—brief*	lateral epicondyle of the humerus; supracondylar ridge of the humerus	base of the second and third metacarpals	extension of the wrist	radial nerve (C6–C7)
Extensor Carpi Ulnaris 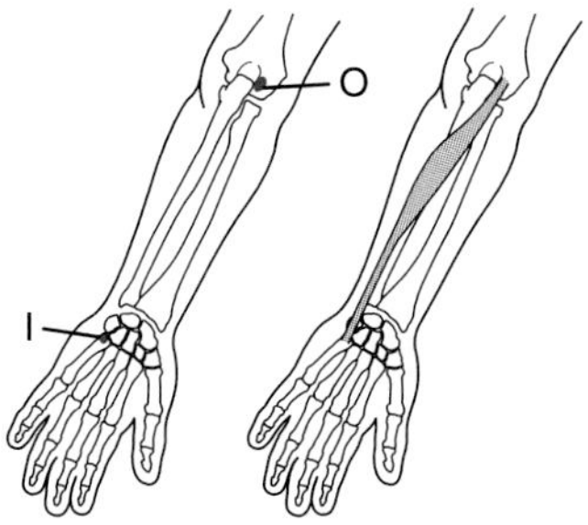 O I *Latin:* *extensio—to extend* *karpos—wrist* *ulna—elbow*	lateral epicondyle of the humerus	base of the fifth metacarpal	extension and adduction of the wrist	radial nerve (C6–C8)

continued on page 184

LESSON FOUR—MUSCLES OF THE FOREARM, WRIST, AND HAND *(continued)*

MUSCLE	ORIGIN	INSERTION	ACTION	NERVE
Palmaris Longus 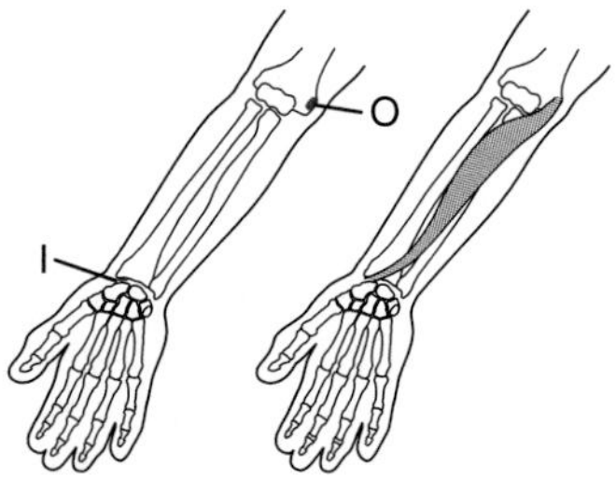 *Latin:* *palma—hand* *longus—long*	medial epicondyle of the humerus	transverse carpal ligament and palmar aponeurosis	flexes the wrist and cups or tenses the palm	median nerve (C6–C7)
Flexor Digitorum Superficialis 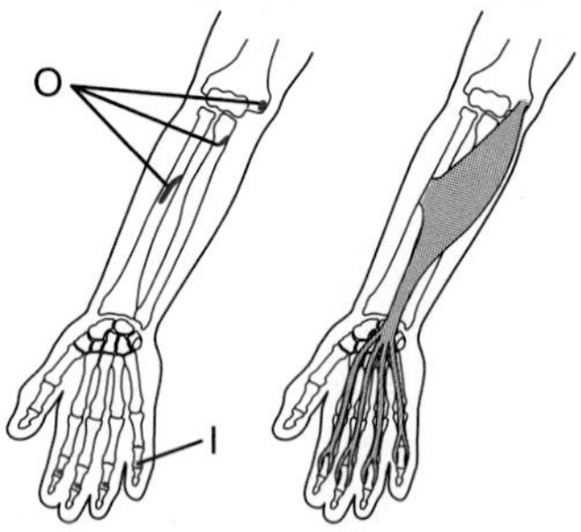 *Latin:* *flexus—bent* *digitus—finger* *superficialis—toward the surface*	medial epicondyle of the humerus, proximal radius, and proximal ulna	middle phalanx of each of fingers 2 through 5	flexes the wrist and proximal interphalangeal joints of the fingers	median nerve (C7–T1)
Flexor Digitorum Profundus 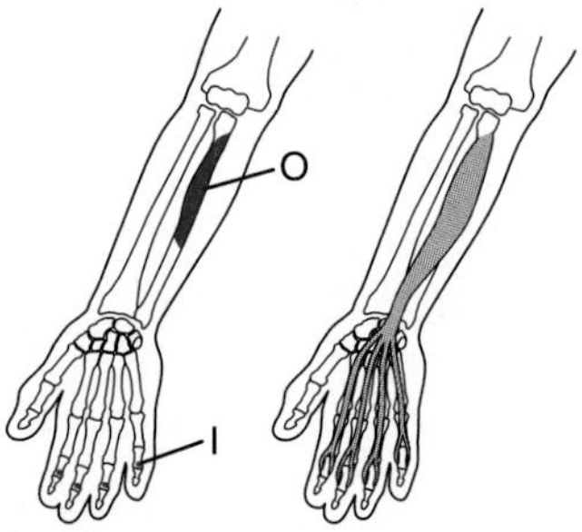 *Latin:* *flexus—bent* *digitus—finger* *profundus—deep*	anterior proximal ¾ of the ulnar shaft	distal phalanges of fingers 2 through 5	flexes all distal interphalangeal joints of the fingers	ulnar nerve (C8–T1), median nerve (C8–T1)

LESSON FOUR—MUSCLES OF THE FOREARM, WRIST, AND HAND *(continued)*

MUSCLE	ORIGIN	INSERTION	ACTION	NERVE
Flexor Pollicis Longus 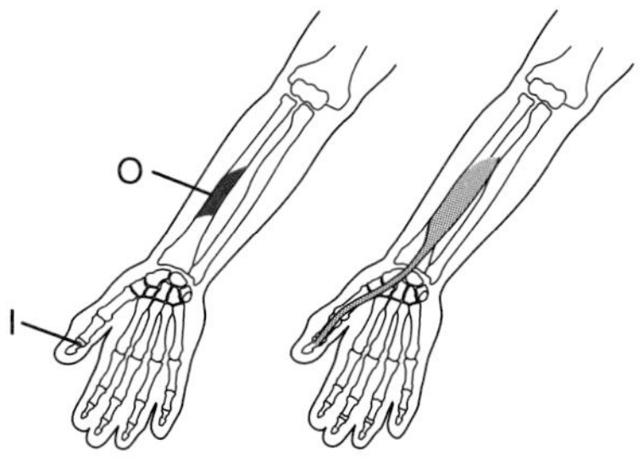 O I *Latin:* *flexus—bent* *pollex—thumb* *longus—long*	anterior surface of the radius	distal phalanx of the thumb	flexes the thumb	median nerve (C8–T1)
Extensor Digitorum 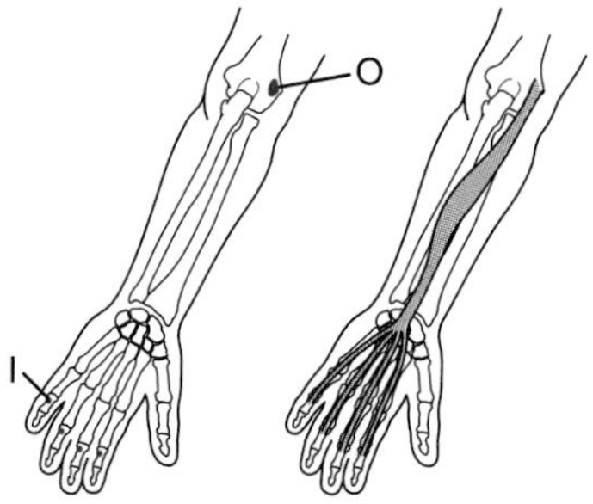 O I *Latin:* *extensio—to extend* *digitus—finger*	lateral epicondyle of the humerus	proximal, middle, and distal phalanges of each finger and thumb (posterior surface)	extends the fingers	radial nerve (C6–C8)
Extensor Digiti Minimi 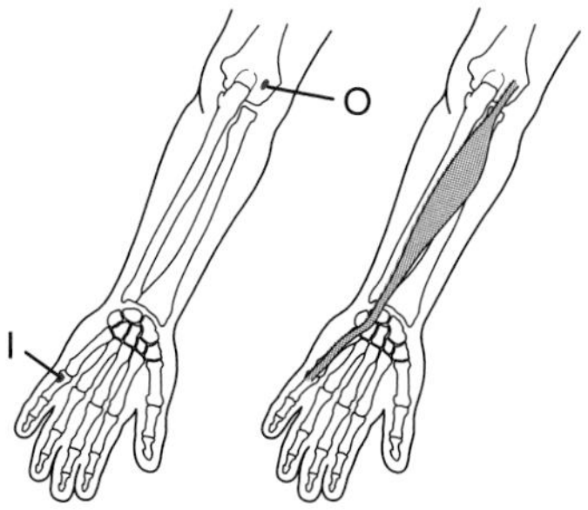 O I *Latin:* *extensio—to extend* *digitus—finger* *minimum—least*	lateral epicondyle of humerus	posterior surface of the proximal phalanx of the fifth (little) finger	extends the little finger at the proximal phalanx	radial nerve (C6–C8)

Notes: Also known as the "tea drinker's muscle," because it extends the little finger while you raise the tea cup to your lips.

continued on page 186

LESSON FOUR—MUSCLES OF THE FOREARM, WRIST, AND HAND *(continued)*

MUSCLE	ORIGIN	INSERTION	ACTION	NERVE
Extensor Indicis 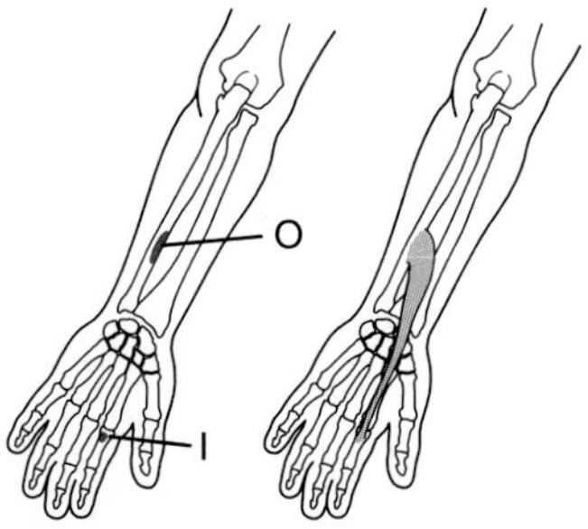 O I *Latin:* *extensio—to extend* *indices—forefinger*	posterior midsurface of the ulna and radius	base of the distal phalanx of the second (index) finger	extends the index finger	radial nerve (C6–C8)
Extensor Pollicis Longus 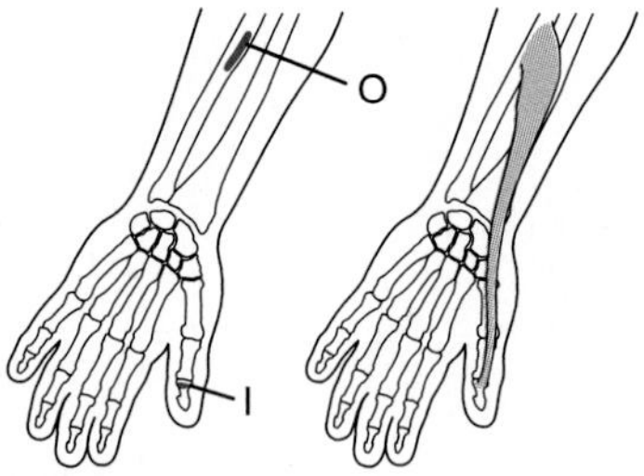 O I *Latin:* *extensio—to extend* *pollex—thumb* *longus—long*	midshaft dorsal surface of the ulna and radius	base of the distal phalanx of the thumb (posterior surface)	extends the distal phalanx of the thumb	radial nerve (C6–C8)
Extensor Pollicis Brevis 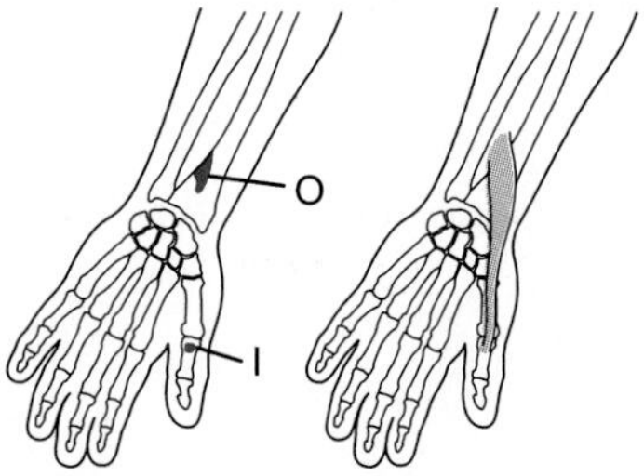 O I *Latin:* *extensio—to extend* *pollex—thumb* *brevis—brief*	midshaft dorsal surface of the radius and interosseous membrane	base of the proximal phalanx of the thumb (posterior surface)	adducts and flexes the metacarpophalangeal joint at the thumb	radial nerve (C6–C7)

LESSON FOUR—MUSCLES OF THE FOREARM, WRIST, AND HAND *(continued)*

Thenar Eminence

The thenar eminence is the thumb pad on the anterior surface of the hand. It is made up of three individual muscles called the opponens pollicis, abductor pollicis brevis, and the flexor pollicis brevis.

Greek:
thenar—palm of hand
minere—to hang on

MUSCLE	ORIGIN	INSERTION	ACTION	NERVE
Opponens Pollicis 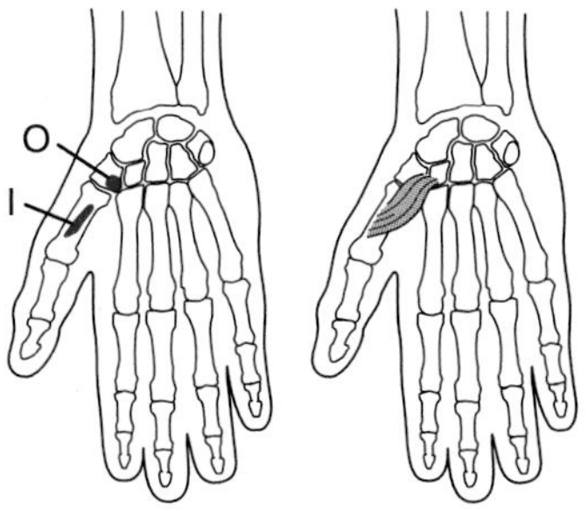 O I *Latin: opponens—opposing pollex—thumb*	trapezium and the transverse carpal ligament	first metacarpal (anterior surface)	flexes and adducts the thumb (rotates the thumb into opposition)	median nerve (C6–C7)
Abductor Pollicis Brevis 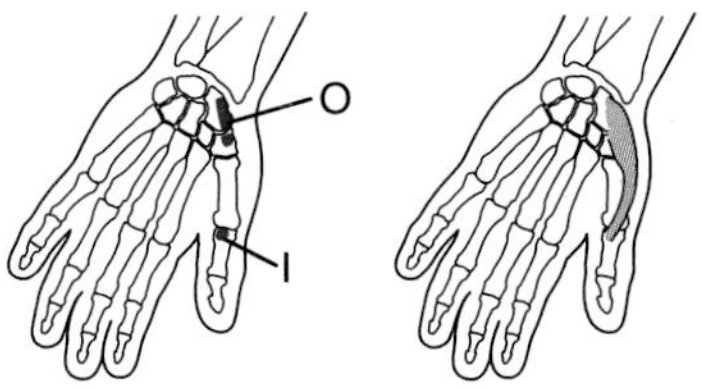 O I *Latin: abductus—led away pollex—thumb brevis—brief*	ridge of the trapezium and transverse carpal ligament	proximal lateral side of the first phalanx of the thumb	abducts the thumb	median nerve (C6–C7)
Flexor Pollicis Brevis 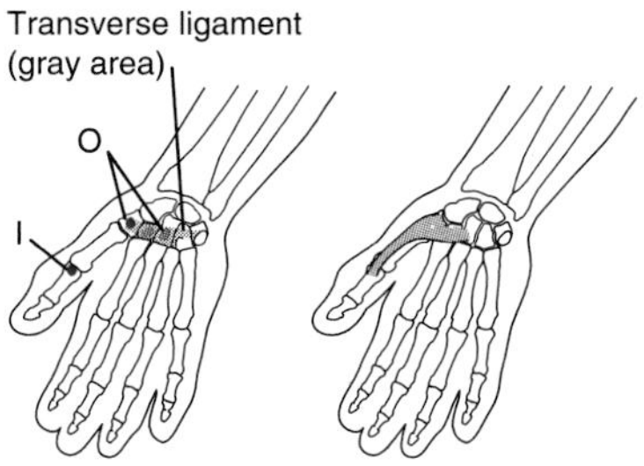 Transverse ligament (gray area) O I *Latin: flexus—bent pollex—thumb brevis—brief*	transverse carpal ligament	proximal first phalanx of the thumb	flexes the metacarpophalangeal joint of the thumb	median nerve (C6–C7), ulnar nerve (C8–T1)

continued on page 188

LESSON FOUR—MUSCLES OF THE FOREARM, WRIST, AND HAND *(continued)*

Hypothenar Eminence

The hypothenar eminence is the little finger pad on the anterior surface of the hand. It consists of three individual muscles called the opponens digiti minimi, flexor digit minimi brevis, and abductor digiti minimi.

Greek:
hypo—under
thenar—palm of hand
minere—to hang on

MUSCLE	ORIGIN	INSERTION	ACTION	NERVE
Opponens Digiti Minimi 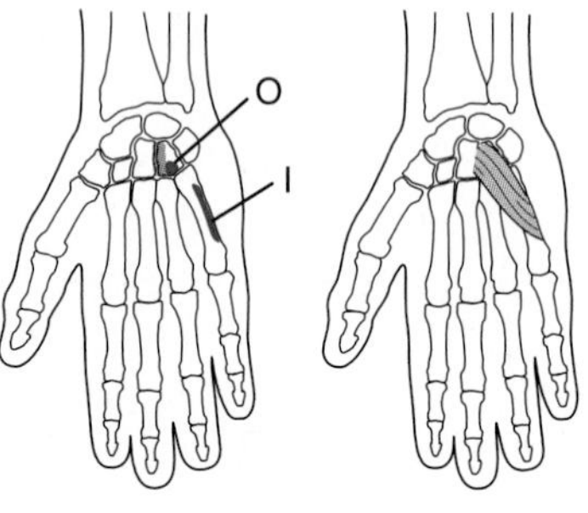 *Latin:* *opponens—opposing* *digitus—finger* *minimum—least*	transverse carpal ligament	fifth metacarpal	rotates the little finger into opposition	ulnar nerve (C8 and T1)
Flexor Digiti Minimi Brevis 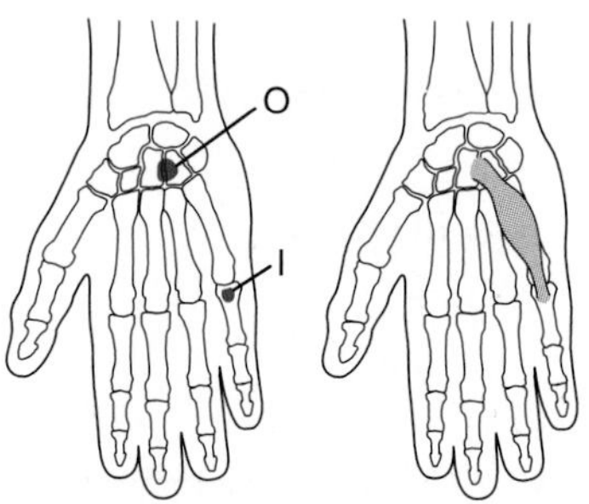 *Latin:* *flexus—bent* *digitus—finger* *minimum—least* *brevis—brief*	transverse carpal ligament	proximal phalanx of the fifth finger	flexion of the fifth (little) finger	ulnar nerve (C8–T1)

LESSON FOUR—MUSCLES OF THE FOREARM, WRIST AND HAND *(continued)*

MUSCLE	ORIGIN	INSERTION	ACTION	NERVE
Abductor Digiti Minimi Transverse ligament (gray area) O I *Latin:* *abductus—led away* *digitus—finger* *minimum—least*	transverse carpal ligament	proximal phalanx of the fifth finger	abduction of the fifth (little) finger	ulnar nerve (C8–T1)

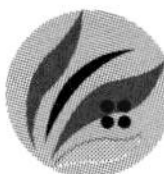

ANATOMICAL SNUFFBOX

If you hyperextend your fingers, a triangular "pocket" will appear on the posterior surface of your hand just distal to your wrist and proximal to your thumb. This depression is known as the "anatomical snuffbox" and is bound by the extensor pollicis longus and extensor pollicis brevis. At one time in history, European men and women would put snuff in this "box," hold it up to their nostrils, and inhale briefly.

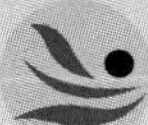

MINI•LAB

Gently grasp the posterior aspect of your right elbow with your left hand. Slowly flex and extend your wrist. Do this movement about six times, focusing on the muscular contractions near the elbow. Notice that the wrist flexors originate at the medial epicondyle of the humerus. In contrast, the wrist extensors originate at the lateral epicondyle of the humerus.

LESSON FIVE—MUSCLES OF HIP AND KNEE MOVEMENT

Iliopsoas

The psoas major, the psoas minor, and the iliacus are usually referred to as the iliopsoas. Because the psoas minor is absent in most cadavers, it will not be included for discussion. Tightness in the iliopsoas muscle can play a significant role in functional lordosis and scoliosis. When you eat a filet mignon, you are eating the iliopsoas muscle of a cow. The iliopsoas is the main flexor of the hip and is the muscle that initiates walking.

Latin:
ilium—flank
Greek:
psoa—muscle of the loin

continued on page 190

LESSON FIVE—MUSCLES OF HIP AND KNEE MOVEMENT *(continued)*

MUSCLE	ORIGIN	INSERTION	ACTION	NERVE
Psoas Major O I *Greek:* *psoa—muscle of the loin* *major—larger*	anterior transverse processes and vertebral bodies of T12–L5	lesser trochanter of the femur	bilateral contraction: flexes the hip by moving the lumbar spine; unilateral contraction: flexes the hip by moving the femur	lumbar nerve (L2–L3)
	Notes: The psoas major is the strongest hip flexor.			
Iliacus O I *Latin:* *iliacus—ilium*	iliac fossa, anterior inferior iliac spine	lesser trochanter of the femur	flexes and laterally rotates the femur	femoral nerve (L2–L4)

LESSON FIVE—MUSCLES OF HIP AND KNEE MOVEMENT *(continued)*

Deep Lateral or Outward Rotators

The six deep lateral rotators are located beneath the gluteals and correspond, to some degree, to the rotator cuff muscles of the shoulder joint. Because of a common action, each rotator is synergistic to the other. To help you learn the names of these muscles, from superior to inferior, use the mnemonic phrase "*p*ieced *g*oods *o*ften *g*o *o*n *q*uilts." *P*iriformis, *g*emellus superior, *o*bturator internus, *g*emellus inferior, *o*bturator externus, and *q*uadratus femoris are the six deep lateral rotators. The gemellus superior and inferior, along with the obturator internus, can be collectively referred to as the triceps coxae because of their common origins, insertions, and actions.

MUSCLE	ORIGIN	INSERTION	ACTION	NERVE
Piriformis O I *Latin:* *pirum—pear* *forma—shape*	anterior sacrum	greater trochanter of the femur	lateral rotation and abduction of the hip, assists in hip extension	sacral nerve (L4–S2)
	Notes: The piriformis is the largest of all the lateral rotators and the most likely to become chronically shortened. Fifteen percent of the population has all or part of the sciatic nerve running *through* this muscle. The piriformis may be in spasm if one or both feet are laterally rotated, in a ducklike position.			
Gemellus Superior O I *Latin:* *gemellus—twin* *superus—upper*	margin of the obturator foramen, spine of the ischium (passing over the ischium and through the lesser sciatic notch)	greater trochanter of the femur	laterally rotates the femur when the hip is flexed	sacral nerve (L4–S2)

continued on page 192

LESSON FIVE—MUSCLES OF HIP AND KNEE MOVEMENT *(continued)*

MUSCLE	ORIGIN	INSERTION	ACTION	NERVE
Obturator Internus 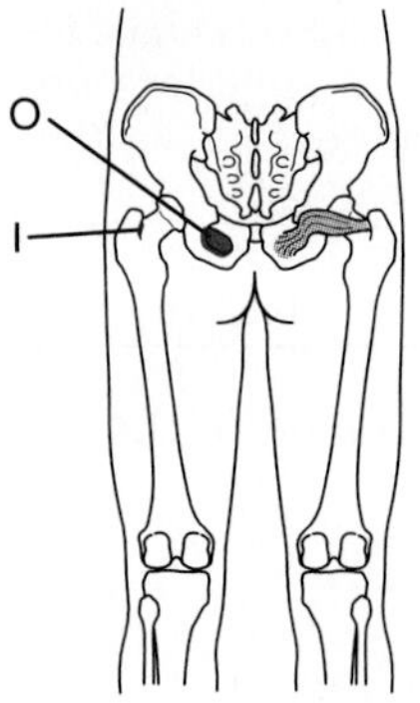 O I *Latin:* *obturare—obstruct* *internus—within*	margin of the obturator foramen, obturator membrane, spine of the ischium (passing over the ischium and through the lesser sciatic notch)	greater trochanter of the femur in front of the piriformis	laterally rotates the femur when the hip is flexed	sacral nerve (L4–S2)
Gemellus Inferior 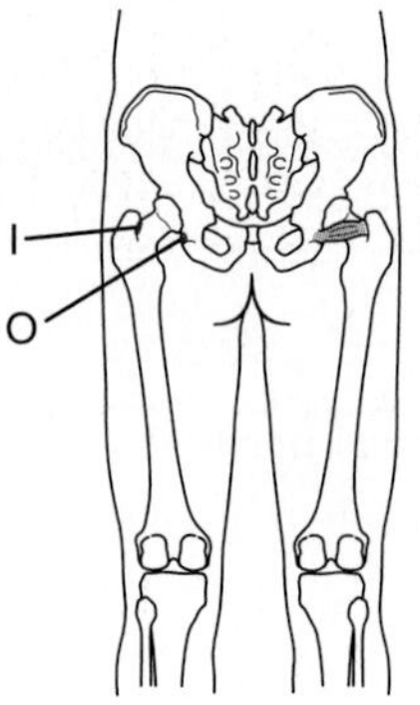 I O *Latin:* *gemellus—twin* *inferus—beneath*	margin of the obturator foramen, spine of the ischium (passing over the ischium and through the lesser sciatic notch)	greater trochanter of the femur	laterally rotates the femur when the hip is flexed	sacral nerve (L4–S2)
Obturator Externus 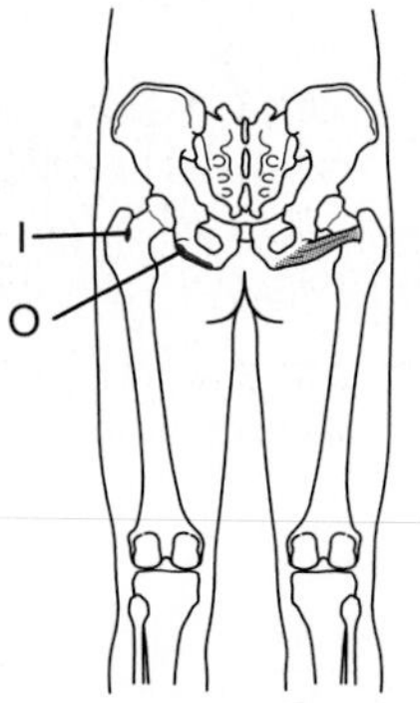 I O *Latin:* *obturare—obstruct* *externus—outside*	medial margin of the obturator foramen and obturator membrane	greater trochanter of the femur	adducts and laterally rotates the hip	obturator nerve (L3–L4)

LESSON FIVE—MUSCLES OF HIP AND KNEE MOVEMENT *(continued)*

MUSCLE	ORIGIN	INSERTION	ACTION	NERVE
Quadratus Femoris O I *Latin:* *quadratus—four-sided* *femoralis—pertaining to the femur*	medial margin of the obturator foramen and obturator membrane	greater trochanter of the femur	adducts and laterally rotates the hip	sacral nerve (L4–S2)
Gluteals	The gluteals, or "glutes," refer to a group of muscles: the gluteus maximus, the gluteus medius, and the gluteus minimus. Note that these muscles can be antagonists to themselves. Also known as the iliotibial tract, the iliotibial band (ITB) is a band of connective tissue stretching from the iliac crest to the tibia. The ITB is an insertion for the tensor fascia lata and the gluteus maximus, and helps to stabilize the knee.			
Gluteus Maximus O I *Greek:* *gloutos—buttock* *Latin:* *maximus—greatest*	posterior sacrum, coccyx, and iliac crest	gluteal tuberosity of the femur and iliotibial band	forceful extension, lateral rotation of the hip, abduction of the hip (by insertion of the ITB), and adduction of the hip (by insertion on the gluteal tuberosity)	gluteal nerve (L5–S2)

Notes: The gluteus maximus is the strongest hip extensor and one of the strongest muscles of the body; it is often more than 1 inch thick. This muscle is mainly used for power, as in climbing stairs, rising from a seated position, or running instead of walking.

continued on page 194

MUSCLE	ORIGIN	INSERTION	ACTION	NERVE
Gluteus Medius 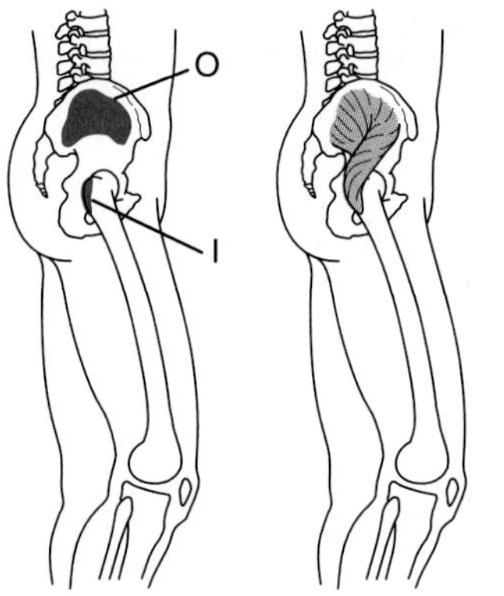 O I *Greek:* *gloutos—buttock* *Latin:* *medius—middle*	posterior lateral surface of the ilium	greater trochanter of the femur	anterior fibers: hip abduction, flexion, and medial rotation; posterior fibers: hip abduction, extension, and lateral rotation	gluteal nerve (L4–S1)
Gluteus Minimus 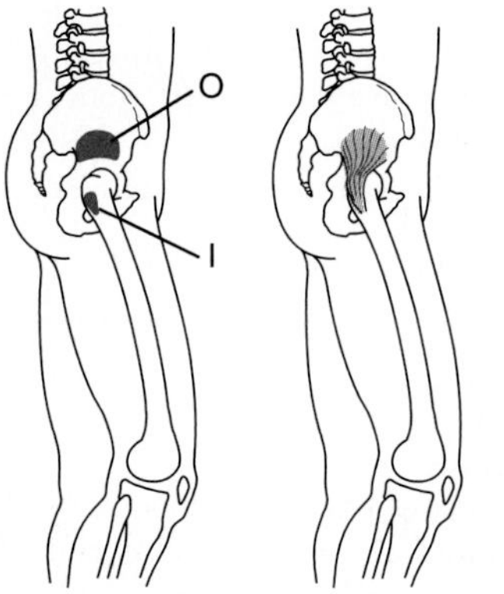 O I *Greek:* *gloutos—buttock* *Latin:* *minimum—least*	posterior lateral surface of the ilium	greater trochanter of the femur	same as the gluteus medius	gluteal nerve (L4–S1)
	Notes: The gluteus minimus is the synergist to the gluteus medius.			
Tensor Fascia Lata 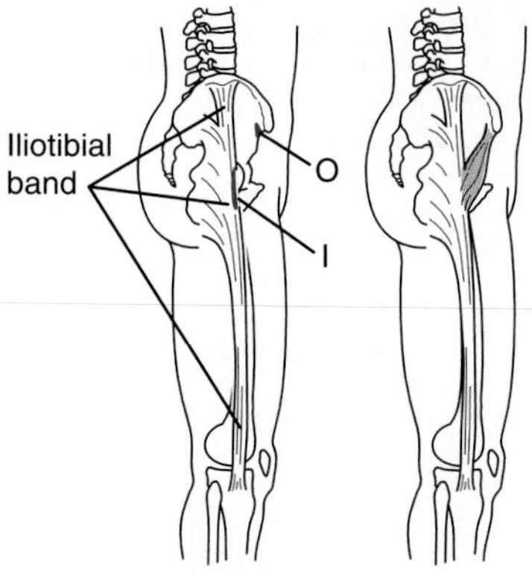 Iliotibial band O I *Latin:* *tensor—stretching* *fascia—band* *lata—broad*	anterior iliac crest, iliac spine	iliotibial band	same as anterior fibers of the gluteus medius and minimus: hip abduction, flexion, and medial rotation	gluteal nerve (L4–S1)

LESSON FIVE—MUSCLES OF HIP AND KNEE MOVEMENT *(continued)*

Quadriceps Femoris

The quadriceps femoris is a group of four muscles sharing a common attachment site on the tibia. The four muscle heads, which are frequently listed as four individual muscles, are the rectus femoris, vastus intermedius, vastus medialis, and vastus lateralis. Lengthening and softening of the quadriceps femoris may provide quick relief from knee problems because the quadriceps tendon crosses the knee joint. Conversely, overuse of quads may create knee problems.

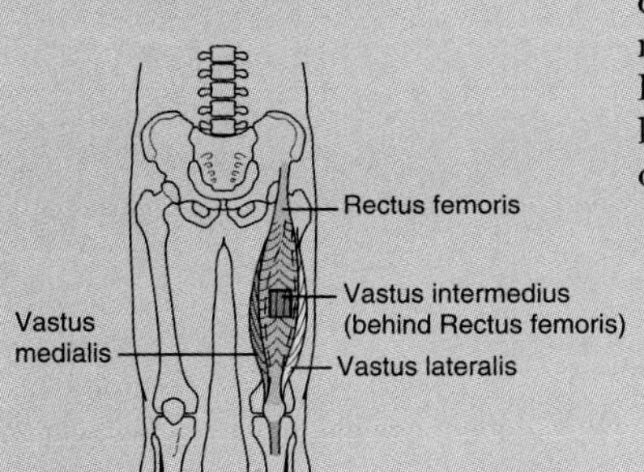

Latin:
quattuor—four
caput—head
femoralis—pertaining to the femur

MUSCLE	ORIGIN	INSERTION	ACTION	NERVE
Rectus Femoris	anterior inferior iliac spine	tibial tuberosity by way of the patellar tendon and patellar ligament	flexes the femur at the hip and extends the leg at the knee joint	femoral nerve (L2–L4)
Vastus Intermedius	anterior and lateral femoral shaft	same as the rectus femoris	extends the knee	femoral nerve (L2–L4)

Rectus Femoris — *Latin:*
rectus—straight
femoralis—pertaining to the femur

Notes: The rectus femoris overlies the vastus intermedius. It is the only muscle in the quadriceps femoris group that crosses two joints (hip and knee) and has two actions.

Vastus Intermedius — *Latin:*
vastus—immense
inter—internal
medius—middle

continued on page 196

LESSON FIVE—MUSCLES OF HIP AND KNEE MOVEMENT (continued)

MUSCLE	ORIGIN	INSERTION	ACTION	NERVE
Vastus Medialis 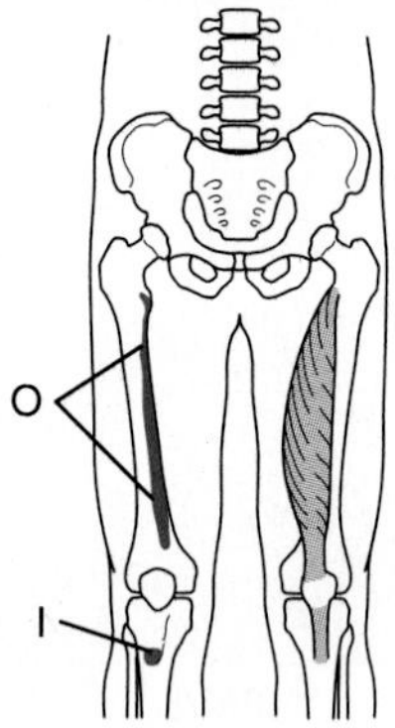 *Latin:* *vastus—immense* *medius—middle*	linea aspera of the femur	same as the rectus femoris	extends the knee	femoral nerve (L2–L4)
Vastus Lateralis 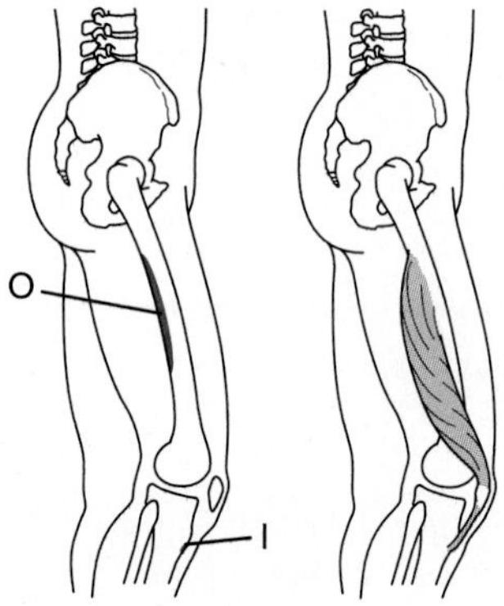 *Latin:* *vastus—immense* *lateralis—toward the side*	linea aspera, greater trochanter, gluteal tuberosity of the femur	same as the rectus femoris	extends the knee	femoral nerve (L2–L4)

Hamstrings

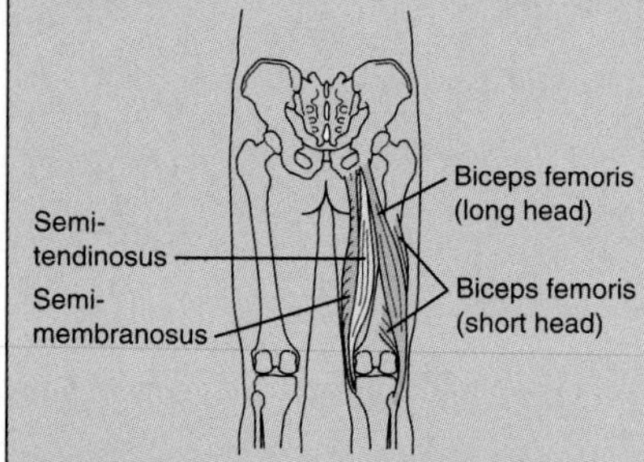

The name hamstrings comes from the fact that butchers use the tendons of the thighs and hips of pigs to hang "ham." Use the mnemonic BMT to indicate their location on the posterior thigh: *B* for *b*iceps femoris, *M* for semi*m*embranosus, *T* for semi*t*endinosus. Both semimembranosus and semitendinosus occupy the medial posterior thigh, with the biceps femoris occupying most of the lateral posterior thigh.

Anglo-Saxon:
haun—haunch

LESSON FIVE—MUSCLES OF HIP AND KNEE MOVEMENT *(continued)*

MUSCLE	ORIGIN	INSERTION	ACTION	NERVE
Semimembranosus O I *Latin:* *semis—half* *membrana—membrane*	ischial tuberosity	medial proximal tibia	hip extension and knee flexion	sciatic nerve—tibial and peroneal (L5–S3) nerves
	Notes: Use the mnemonic M&M to remember that the semi*m*embranosus is the most *m*edial hamstring muscle.			
Semitendinosus O I *Latin:* *semis—half* *tendinosus—tendinous*	ischial tuberosity	medial proximal tibia	hip extension and knee flexion	sciatic nerve—tibial and peroneal (L5–S3) nerves
	Notes: The semitendinosus is superficial to, or on *t*op of, the semimembranosus.			
Biceps Femoris O I *Latin:* *bi—twice* *caput—head* *femoralis—pertaining to the femur*	long head: ischial tuberosity; short head: linea aspera of the femur	head of the fibula	hip extension and knee flexion	sciatic nerve—tibial and peroneal (L5–S3) nerves
	Notes: The biceps femoris occupies both sides of the posterior thigh, crossing the midline from medial to lateral to reach the fibula. The short head of the biceps femoris does not cross the hip joint.			

continued on page 198

LESSON FIVE—MUSCLES OF HIP AND KNEE MOVEMENT *(continued)*

MUSCLE	ORIGIN	INSERTION	ACTION	NERVE
Sartorius	anterior superior iliac spine (ASIS)	medial proximal shaft of the tibia	laterally rotates and flexes the hip and knee (actions needed to sit cross-legged)	femoral nerve (L2–L4)

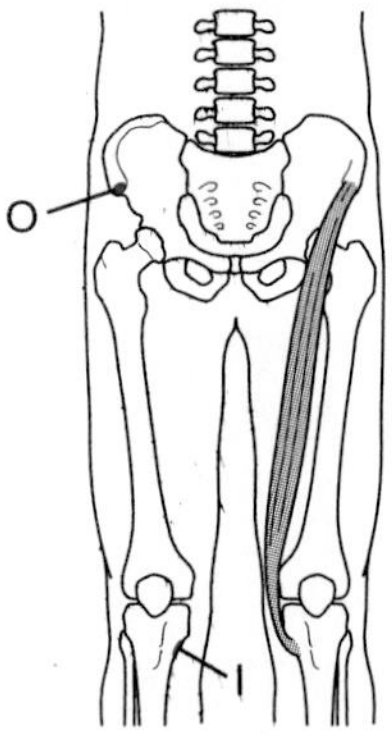

Latin: sartor—tailor

Notes: Also known as the "tailor's muscle" because in older times, tailors sat cross-legged while they sewed. The sartorius is the longest muscle in the body, crossing both the hip and knee joints, running superficially and obliquely across the quadriceps femoris muscle.

Adductors

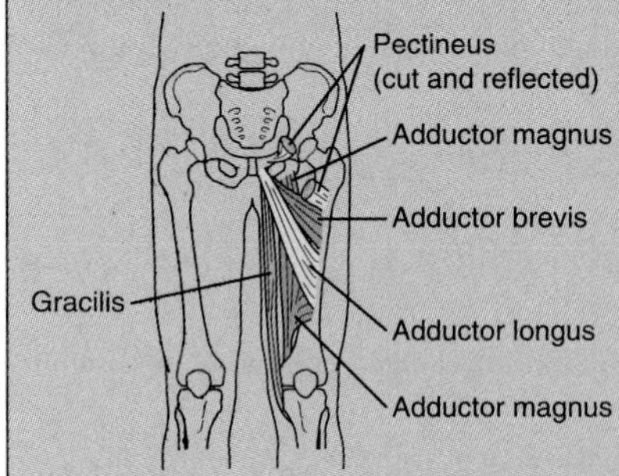

The adductors are a group of muscles forming the inner thigh. They are the *g*racilis, adductor *m*agnus, adductor *l*ongus, adductor *b*revis, and *p*ectineus. Use the mnemonic phrase "*G*irls *M*ostly *L*ike *B*ig *P*ecs" to learn the names of the adductors from medial to lateral to superior.

MUSCLE	ORIGIN	INSERTION	ACTION	NERVE
Gracilis	anterior pubic ramus	medial proximal tibia	hip adduction and knee flexion	obturator nerve (L2–L4)

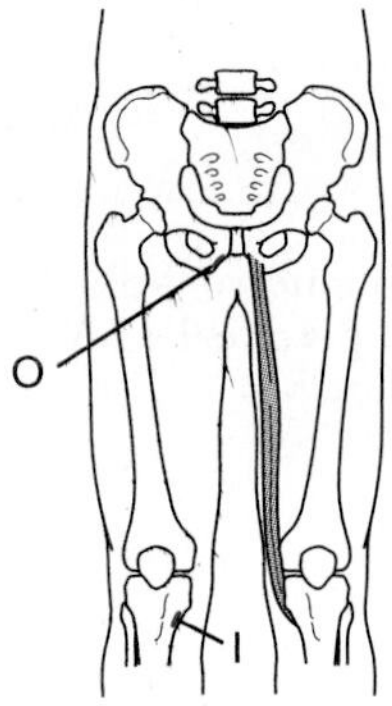

Latin: gracilis—slender

Notes: The femoral shaft and the gracilis form the letter "V."

LESSON FIVE—MUSCLES OF HIP AND KNEE MOVEMENT *(continued)*

MUSCLE	ORIGIN	INSERTION	ACTION	NERVE
Adductor Magnus 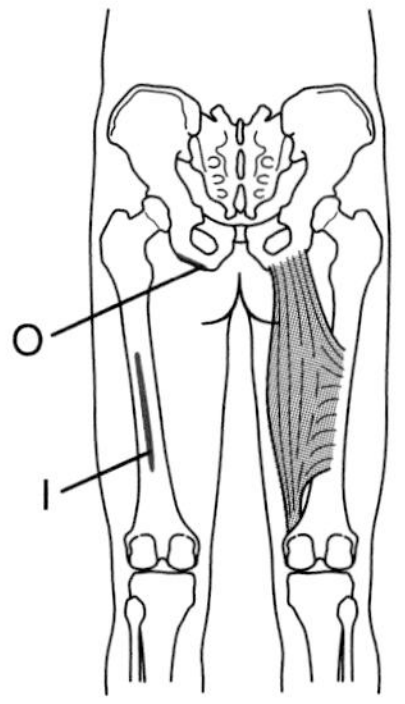 O I *Latin:* *adductus—brought toward* *magnum—large*	pubic and ischial rami, ischial tuberosity	linea aspera and medial epicondyle of the femur	adducts the hip, assists in flexion and medial rotation of the hip	obturator and sciatic nerve (L2–S3)
	Notes: The adductor magnus deep to the hamstrings.			
Adductor Longus 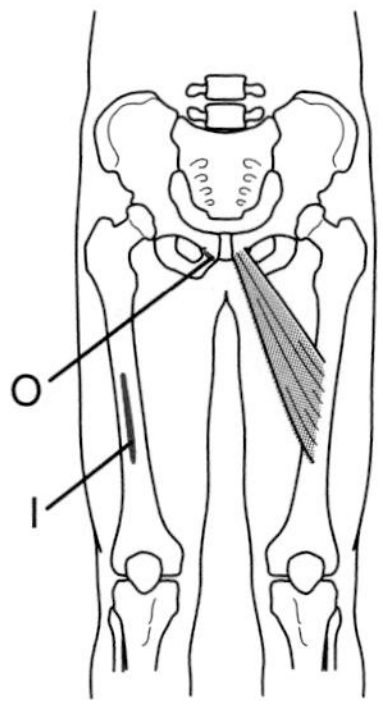 O I *Latin:* *adductus—brought toward* *longus—long*	anterior pubis near the pubic symphysis	linea aspera of the femur	adducts the hip and assists in flexion and medial rotation of the hip	obturator nerve (L3–L4)
Adductor Brevis 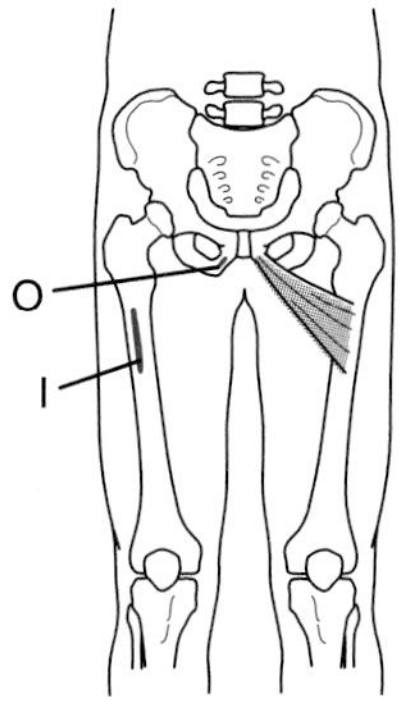 O I *Latin:* *adductus—brought toward* *brevis—brief*	anterior pubis	linea aspera of the femur	adducts the hip and assists in flexion and medial rotation of the hip	obturator nerve (L3–L4)

continued on page 200

LESSON FIVE—MUSCLES OF HIP AND KNEE MOVEMENT *(continued)*

MUSCLE	ORIGIN	INSERTION	ACTION	NERVE
Pectineus *Latin:* *pecten—comb*	anterior pubis	between the lesser trochanter and linea aspera of the femur	flexes the hip and assists hip adduction	femoral nerve (L2–L4)
	Notes: This muscle is medial to femoral artery and is often considered an extension of the iliopsoas muscle owing to its insertion and action.			
Pes Anserinus *Latin:* *pedes—footlike* *anserinus—goose*	The pes anserinus is the tendinous expansions of the *s*artorius, *g*racilis, and the semi*t*endinosus inserting at the medial border of the tibial tuberosity. Use the mnemonic phrase "*S*ay *G*race before *T*ea" to assist you in remembering the three muscles that contribute to this structure.			

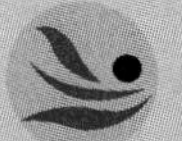

MINI•LAB

To better understand the gluteus maximus, place both hands on your buttocks and walk around the room. Notice how this muscle never fully contracts. Begin running or climbing stairs. Feel this muscle contract to extend the femur. Walking is great exercise, but leisurely walking does not activate this large muscle.

LESSON SIX—MUSCLES OF FOOT MOVEMENT

MUSCLE	ORIGIN	INSERTION	ACTION	NERVE
Tibialis Anterior 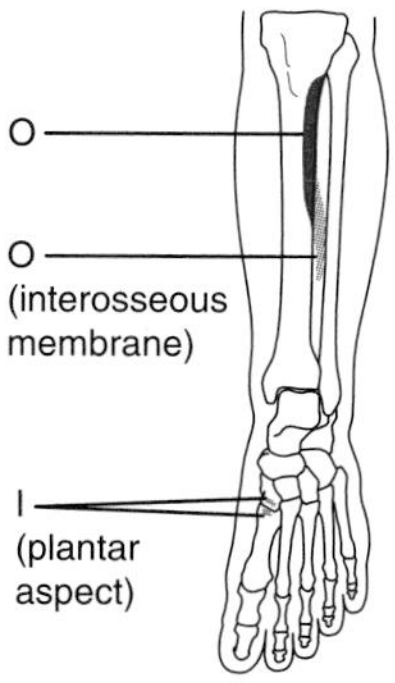 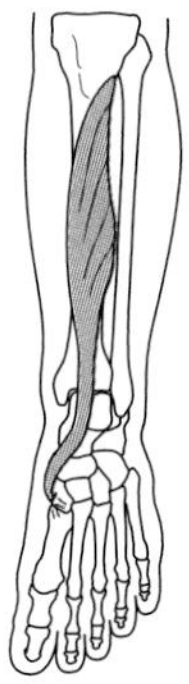 O O (interosseous membrane) I (plantar aspect) *Latin:* *tibialis—shinbone* *ante—before*	lateral shaft of the tibia and interosseous membrane	base of the first metatarsal and plantar aspect of the first (medial) cuneiform	dorsiflexes and inverts the foot	peroneal nerve (L4–S1)
	Notes: The tibialis muscle is strengthened after an inversion sprain is healed to aid in rehabilitation			
Extensor Digitorum Longus 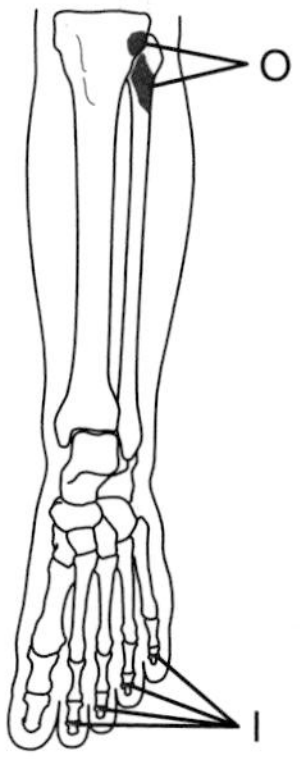 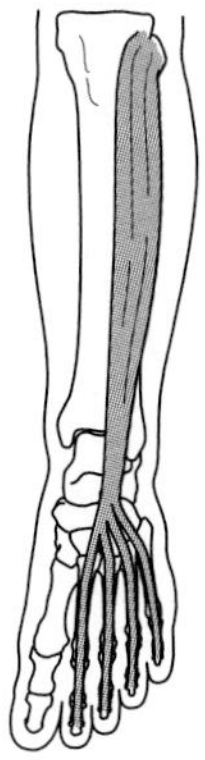 O I *Latin:* *extensio—to extend* *digitus—finger or toe* *longus—long*	head and superior ⅔ of fibula, lateral tibial condyle	dorsal surfaces of distal phalanges 2 through 5	extends digits 2 through 5 and assists dorsiflexion of the foot	peroneal nerve (L4–S1)

continued on page 202

LESSON SIX—MUSCLES OF FOOT MOVEMENT *(continued)*

MUSCLE	ORIGIN	INSERTION	ACTION	NERVE
Extensor Hallucis Longus 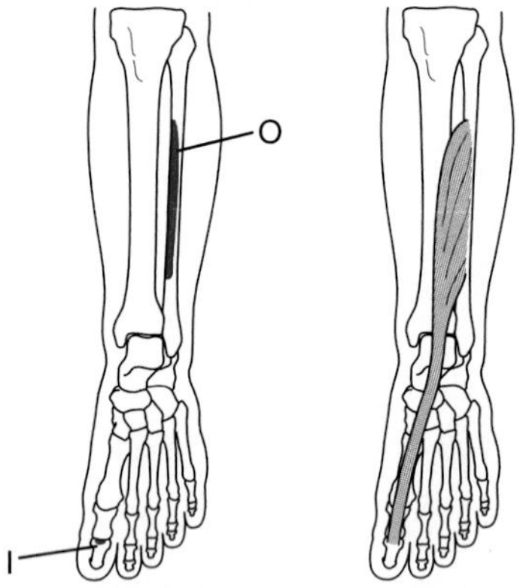 O I *Latin:* *extensio—to extend* *hallex—large toe* *longus—long*	middle half of medial fibula, interosseous membrane	dorsal surface of the distal phalanx of the great toe	extends the great toe and assists dorsiflexion of the foot	peroneal nerve (L4–S1)
Peroneus Longus 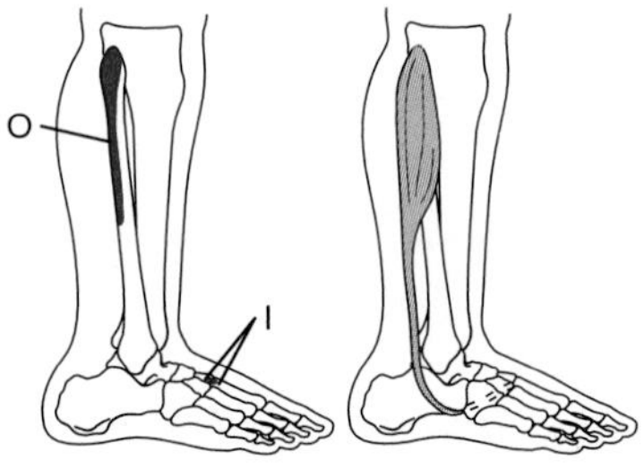 O I *Greek:* *perone—pin* *Latin:* *longus—long*	head and lateral shaft of the fibula (tendon passes behind the lateral malleolus)	base of the first metatarsal and plantar aspect of the first (medial) cuneiform	everts the foot and assists in plantar flexion	peroneal nerve (L4–S1)
	Notes: Peroneus longus is also known as fibularis longus.			
Peroneus Brevis 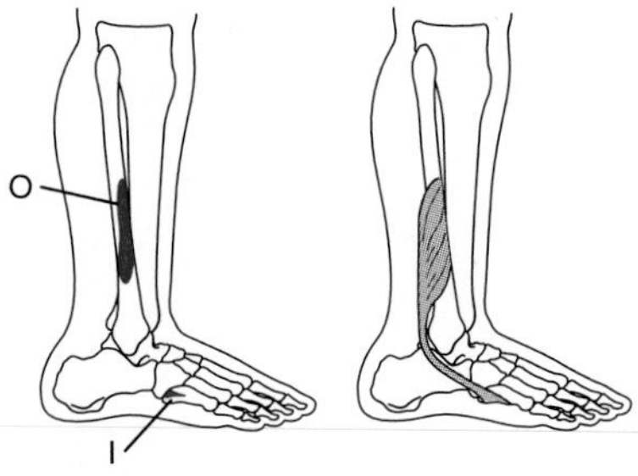 O I *Greek:* *perone—pin* *Latin:* *brevis—brief*	lower ⅔ of the lateral inferior fibula (tendon passes behind the lateral malleolus)	base of the fifth metatarsal	everts the foot and assists in plantar flexion	peroneal nerve (L4–S1)
	Notes: Peroneus brevis is also known as fibularis brevis.			

LESSON SIX—MUSCLES OF FOOT MOVEMENT *(continued)*

Triceps Surae

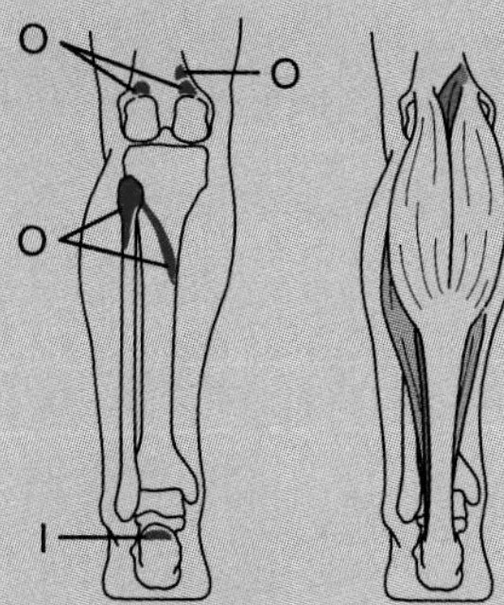

Greek:
treis—three
Latin:
sura—pertaining to the calf of the leg

The triceps surae is another name for the gastrocnemius, the soleus, and the plantaris muscles (some references include only the gastrocnemius and the soleus as the triceps surae). These three muscles share a common tendon and are viewed as the triceps brachii of the lower extremity. These muscles make up the superficial layer of the posterior lower leg.

MUSCLE	ORIGIN	INSERTION	ACTION	NERVE
Soleus	middle of the posterior tibia and superior ⅓ of the fibula	posterior calcaneus via Achilles tendon	plantar flexion of the foot	tibial nerve (S1–S2)
Latin: *solea—sole of the foot*	**Notes:** According to one story, the soleus was so named because it looks like a sole fish from the Mediterranean sea.			
Gastrocnemius	two heads, each superior to the medial and lateral epicondyles of the femur	posterior calcaneus via the Achilles tendon	plantar flexion of the foot, assists in knee flexion	tibial nerve (S1–S2)
Greek: *gaster—belly* *kneme—leg*	**Notes:** The gastrocnemius is also known as the "toe dancer's muscle" because it helps a ballerina stand on toe.			

continued on page 204

LESSON SIX—MUSCLES OF FOOT MOVEMENT *(continued)*

MUSCLE	ORIGIN	INSERTION	ACTION	NERVE
Plantaris 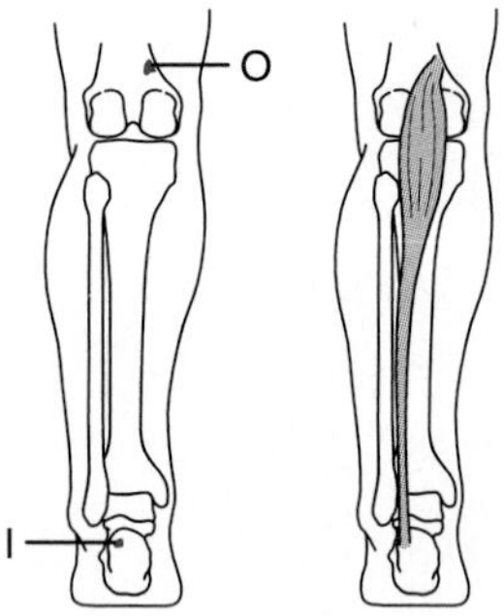 O I *Latin:* *planta—sole*	superior lateral femoral condyle	posterior calcaneus via the Achilles tendon	plantar flexion of the foot, assists in knee flexion	tibial nerve (L4–S1)
Notes: The plantaris is occasionally missing in cadavers.				
Tibialis Posterior 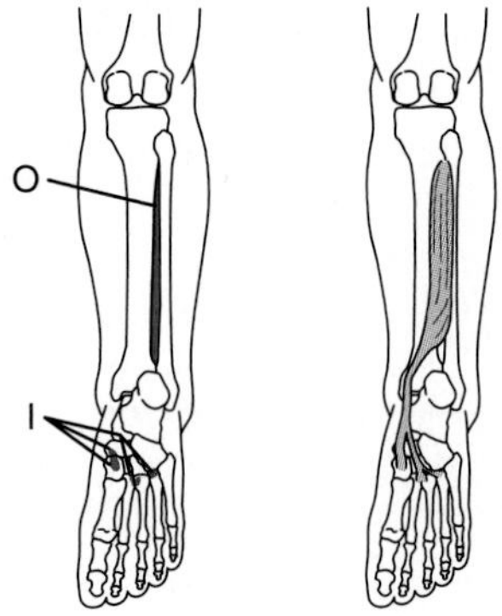 O I *Latin:* *tibialis—shinbone* *posterus—behind*	posterior tibia, fibula, and interosseous membrane	plantar aspect of the navicular bone, third cuneiform, and metatarsals II, III, and IV	assists in plantar flexion and inverts the foot	tibial nerve (L5–S1)
Flexor Digitorum Longus 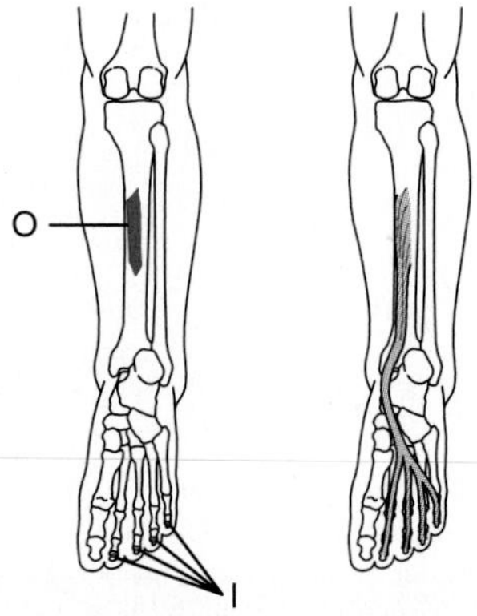 O I *Latin:* *flexus—bent* *digitus—finger or toe* *longus—long*	middle posterior tibia	plantar surfaces of distal phalanges 2–5	weighted: supports the longitudinal arch; unweighted: flexion of digits 2–5, plantar flexion and inversion of the foot	tibial nerve (L5–S1)

LESSON SIX—MUSCLES OF FOOT MOVEMENT *(continued)*

MUSCLE	ORIGIN	INSERTION	ACTION	NERVE
Flexor Hallucis Longus 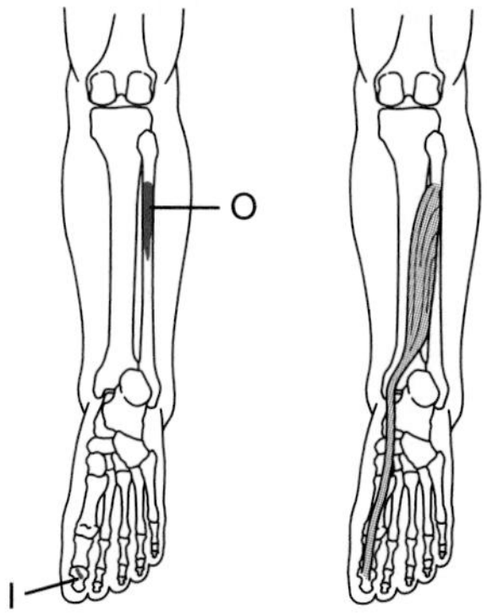 O I *Latin:* *flexus—bent* *hallex—large toe* *longus—long*	inferior posterior fibula, interosseous membrane	plantar surfaces of the distal phalanx of the great toe	weighted: supports the longitudinal arch; unweighted: flexion of the big toe, plantar flexion and inversion of the foot	tibial nerve (L5–S2)

UNIT TWO—MUSCLES OF THE AXIAL SKELETON

LESSON SEVEN—MUSCLES OF THE HEAD AND NECK

Occipitofrontalis

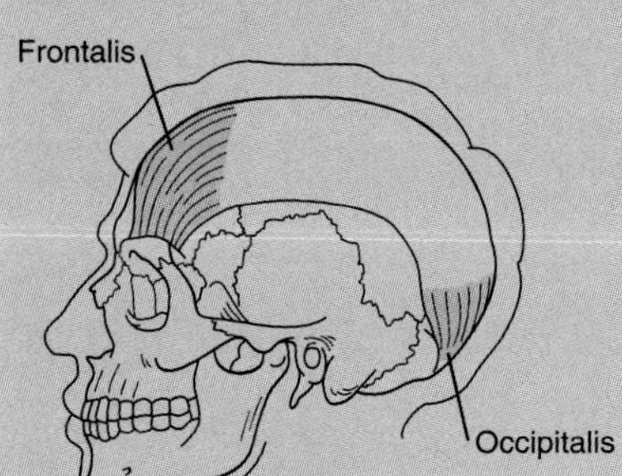

The occipitofrontalis, a two-bellied muscle containing the occipitalis and the frontalis, is connected by an extensive network of cranial fascia called the galea aponeurotica or the epicranius. The galea aponeurotica is firmly connected to the hypodermis and slides over the periosteum of the cranium.

MUSCLE	ORIGIN	INSERTION	ACTION	NERVE
Frontalis	galea aponeurotica	hypodermis of the eyebrows	allows you to raise your eyebrows as in surprise and wrinkle the skin on your forehead horizontally	facial nerve (cranial nerve VII)

Latin:
frons—brow or referring to the frontal bone

Notes: The frontalis muscle contributes to tension headaches.

LESSON SEVEN—MUSCLES OF THE HEAD AND NECK *(continued)*

MUSCLE	ORIGIN	INSERTION	ACTION	NERVE
Occipitalis 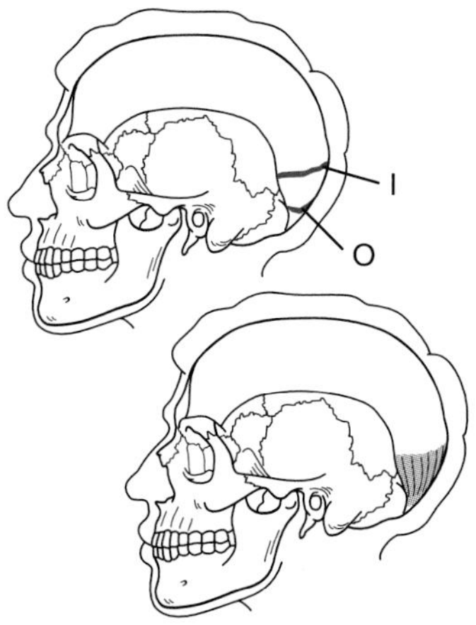 I O *Latin:* *occipitalis—pertaining to the back of the head*	lateral ⅔ of the superior nuchal line of the occipital bone	galea aponeurotica	allows you to move the scalp over the cranium	facial nerve (cranial nerve VII)
Orbicularis Oculi 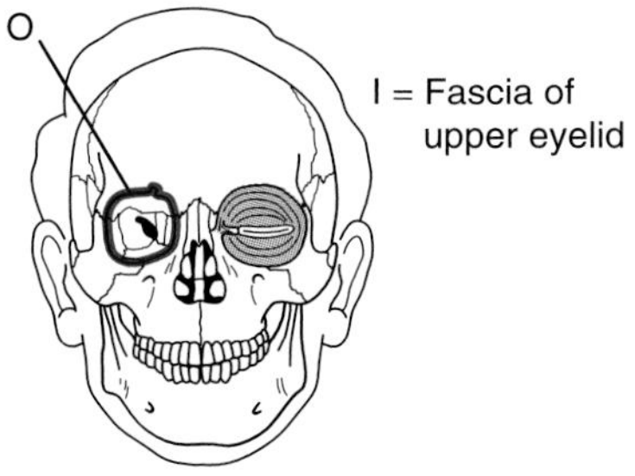 O I = Fascia of upper eyelid *Latin:* *little circle* *oculus—eye*	orbital margin	fascia of the upper eyelid	closes the eyelid, wrinkles the forehead vertically, squints, and blinks	facial nerve (cranial nerve VII)
	Notes: Also known as the "winking muscle" because it closes the eyelid in a wink.			
Orbicularis Oris 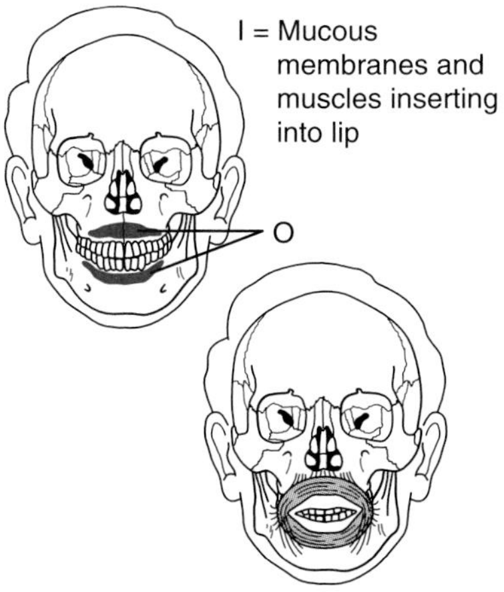 I = Mucous membranes and muscles inserting into lip O *Latin:* *little circle or mouth*	maxilla, mandible, lips, and buccinator	mucous membranes and muscles inserting into lip	closes the mouth, protrudes the lips, and allows dozens of activities such as eating, drinking, talking, and sucking	facial nerve (cranial nerve VII)
	Notes: Also known as the "kissing muscle" because it puckers the lips for a kiss.			

continued on page 208

LESSON SEVEN—MUSCLES OF THE HEAD AND NECK *(continued)*

MUSCLE	ORIGIN	INSERTION	ACTION	NERVE
Zygomaticus Major 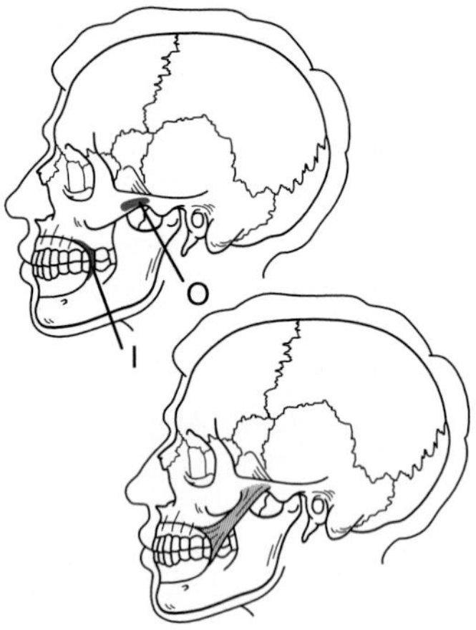 *Latin:* *zygotos—yoked or to connect* *major—larger*	zygomatic arch	lateral angle of the mouth	lifts corner of the mouth upward and outward into a smile or grin	facial nerve (cranial nerve VII)
Buccinator 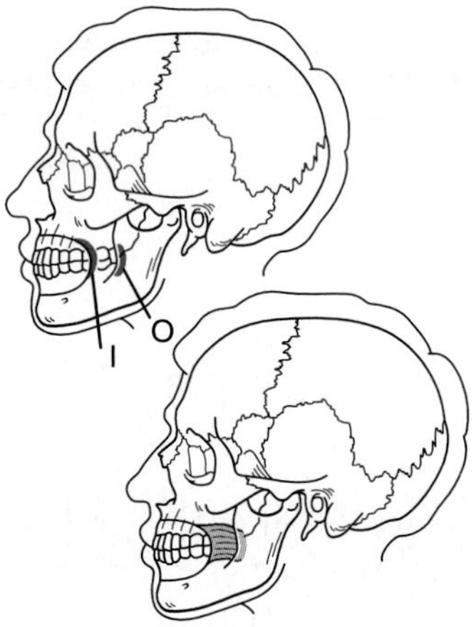 *Latin:* *buccinator—trumpeter*	maxilla and mandible	orbicularis oris	compresses the cheeks and retracts angles of the mouth (enabling air to be puffed out of cheeks as in whistling or blowing a trumpet)	facial nerve (cranial nerve VII)
Platysma 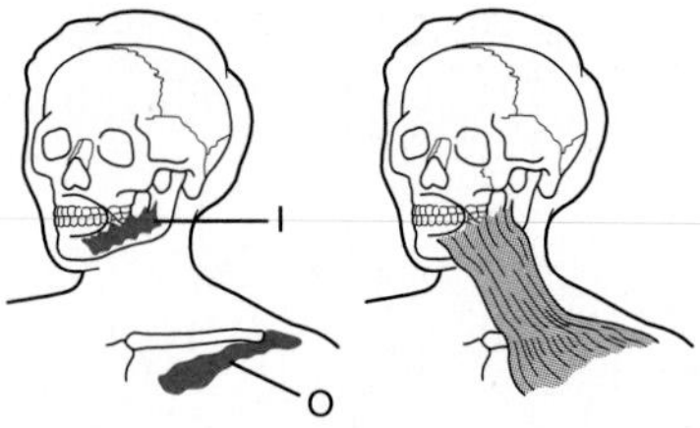 *Greek:* *platysma—plate*	fascia of both deltoid and pectoralis major	muscles around the angle of the mouth and hypodermis of the lower face	tenses the skin of the anterior neck (as in shaving), pulls the corner of the mouth down (as in pouting), and depresses the mandible	facial nerve (cranial nerve VII)

Notes: This is the most superficial muscle of the anterior neck.

LESSON SEVEN—MUSCLES OF THE HEAD AND NECK (continued)

Muscles of Mastication

MUSCLE	ORIGIN	INSERTION	ACTION	NERVE
Temporalis 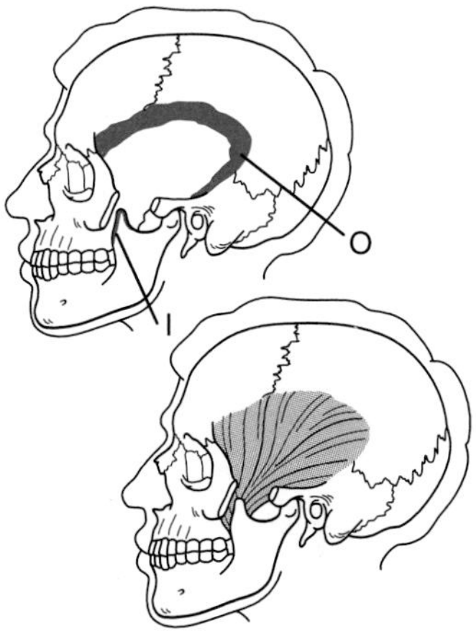 *Latin:* *temporalis—pertaining to the temporal bone*	lateral surface of the temporal fossa	coronoid process of the mandible	closes, elevates, and retracts the jaw	trigeminal nerve (cranial nerve V)
Masseter 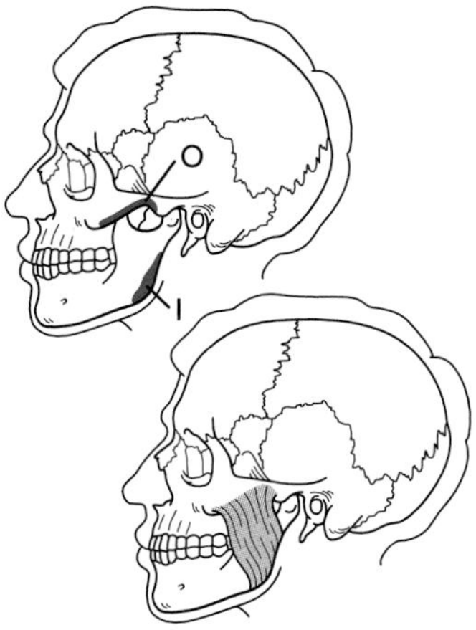 *Greek:* *masseter—chewer*	zygomatic arch	angle of the mandible	bilateral contraction: prime mover of jaw closure and assists in jaw protraction; unilateral contraction: assists in side-to-side grinding movements of the jaw	trigeminal nerve (cranial nerve V)

continued on page 210

LESSON SEVEN—MUSCLES OF THE HEAD AND NECK *(continued)*

MUSCLE	ORIGIN	INSERTION	ACTION	NERVE
Lateral Pterygoid 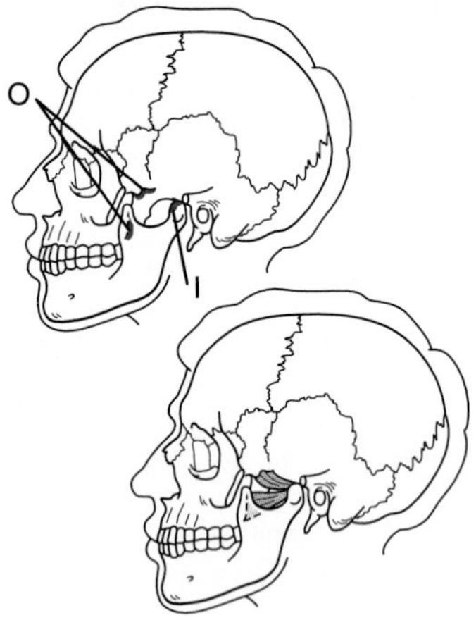 *Latin:* *lateralis—toward the side* *Greek:* *pterygodes—a wing*	lateral surface of the pterygoid plate and greater wing of the sphenoid bone	mandibular condyle and temporomandibular joint capsule	bilateral contraction: closes and protracts the jaw; unilateral contraction: assists in side-to-side grinding movements of the jaw	trigeminal nerve (cranial nerve V)
Medial Pterygoid 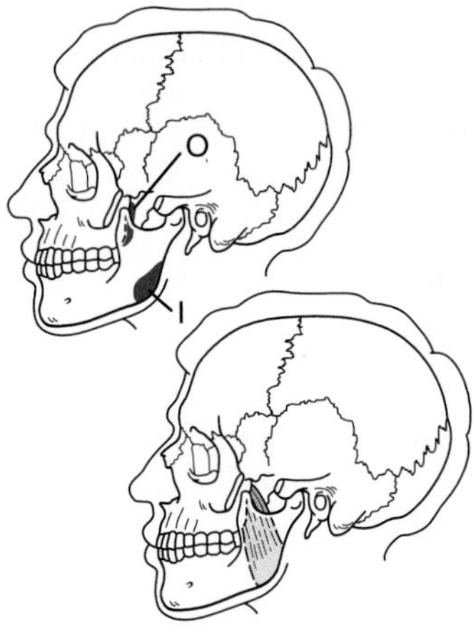 *Latin:* *medialis—toward the midline* *Greek:* *pterygodes—a wing*	medial surface of the pterygoid plate of the sphenoid bone	inner surface of the mandibular angle	bilateral contraction: closes and protracts the jaw; unilateral contraction: assists in side-to-side grinding movements of the jaw	trigeminal nerve (cranial nerve V)

LESSON SEVEN—MUSCLES OF THE HEAD AND NECK *(continued)*

Longus Colli

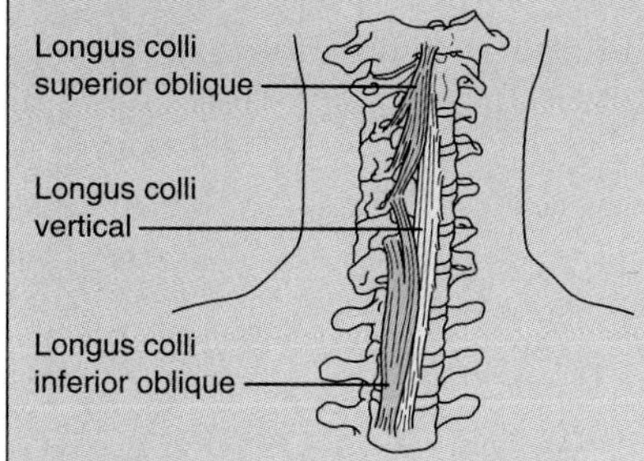

Longus colli superior oblique
Longus colli vertical
Longus colli inferior oblique

The longus colli, like the iliopsoas of the lower extremity, contains three different muscles: the longus colli superior oblique, the longus colli inferior oblique, and the longus colli vertical.

MUSCLE	ORIGIN	INSERTION	ACTION	NERVE
Longus Colli Superior Oblique 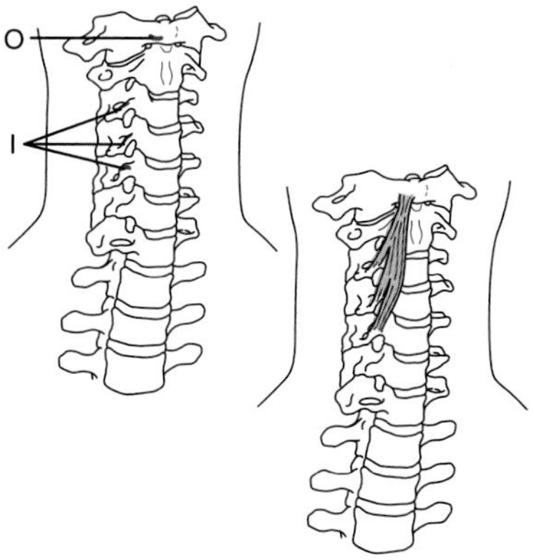 O I *Latin:* *longus—long* *colli—collar* *superus—upper* *obliquus—slant*	anterior transverse processes of C3–C5	anterior tubercle of the atlas	rotates C1 and laterally flexes the neck	anterior rami (C2–C4)
Longus Colli Inferior Oblique 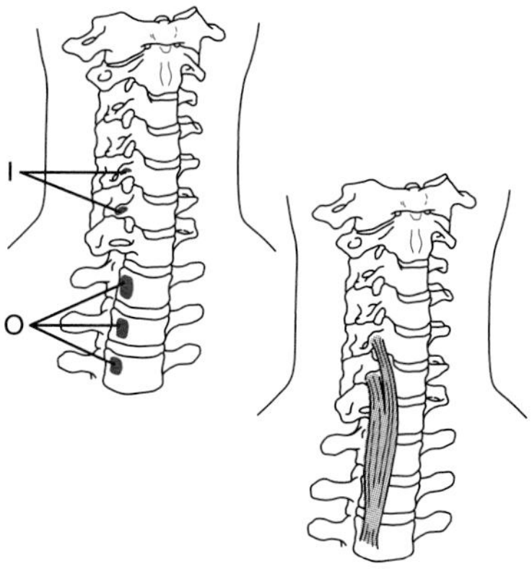 I O *Latin:* *longus—long* *colli—collar* *infra—beneath* *obliquus—slant*	bodies of T1–T3	anterior transverse processes C5–C6	rotates and flexes the neck	anterior rami (C2–C4)

continued on page 212

LESSON SEVEN—MUSCLES OF THE HEAD AND NECK *(continued)*

MUSCLE	ORIGIN	INSERTION	ACTION	NERVE
Longus Colli Vertical *Latin:* *longus—long* *colli—collar* *vertex—whirlwind or tornado*	bodies of C5–C7 and T1–T3	bodies C2–C4	rotates and flexes the neck	anterior rami (C2–C4)
Sternocleidomastoid 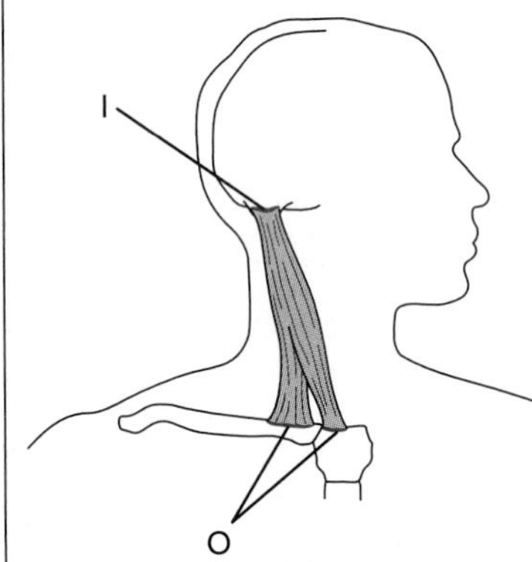 *Greek:* *sternon—sternum* *cleido—clavicle* *mastos—breastlike or the mastoid process of the temporal bone*	manubrium of the sternum and medial ⅓ clavicle	mastoid process of the temporal bone	bilateral contraction: flexes the cervical spine; unilateral contraction: lateral flexion of the cervical spine, contralateral rotation of the head	accessory nerve (cranial nerve XI)

Notes: The sternocleidomastoid (SCM) feels like a cable on both sides of the neck just lateral to the carotid artery. A condition called torticollis, or wryneck, involves spasms of the sternocleidomastoid muscle. Spasm in this muscle may also cause vertigo because of the many sensory and positional receptors located here. The SCM is the only muscle that moves the head but does not attach to any vertebrae.

LESSON SEVEN—MUSCLES OF THE HEAD AND NECK *(continued)*

Scalenes

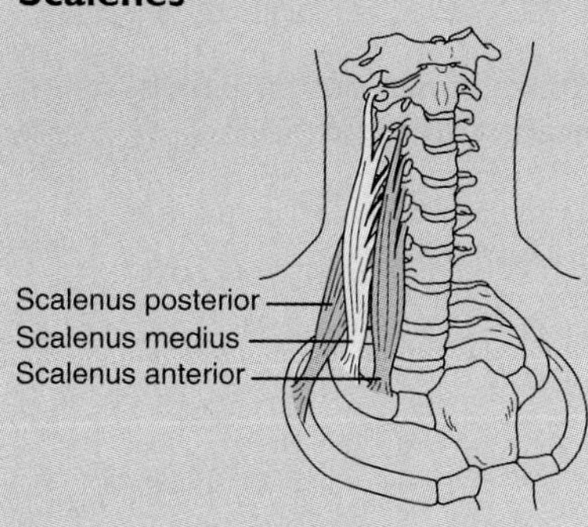

The scalenes are a group of muscles consisting of the scalenus anterior, the scalenus medius, and the scalenus posterior. These muscles, along with the pectoralis minor, are known as the "neurovascular entrappers" because the subclavian artery and the brachial plexus pass between the scalenus anterior and the scalenus medius. All scalene muscles are palpable in the triangular opening between the sternocleidomastoid and the trapezius. Place your hands in this triangle and take a deep breath. You should be able to feel these muscles shortening. Acting unilaterally, they mobilize the neck; acting bilaterally, they actively aid in respiration. Additionally, when the body is in motion, the scalenes stabilize the neck by preventing side swaying.

MUSCLE	ORIGIN	INSERTION	ACTION	NERVE
Scalenus Posterior 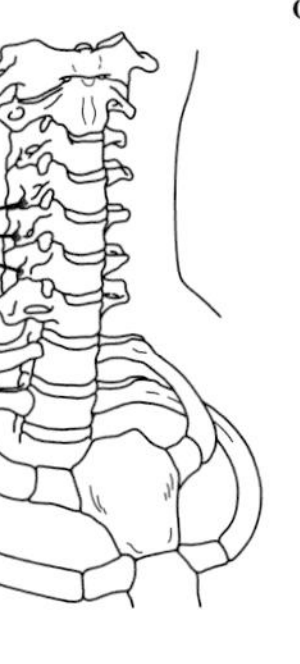 *Greek:* *skalenos—uneven* *Latin:* *posterus—behind*	transverse processes of C4–C6	lateral surface of the second rib	elevates the second rib and assists ipsilateral flexion of the neck	posterior rami of C3–C8
Scalenus Medius 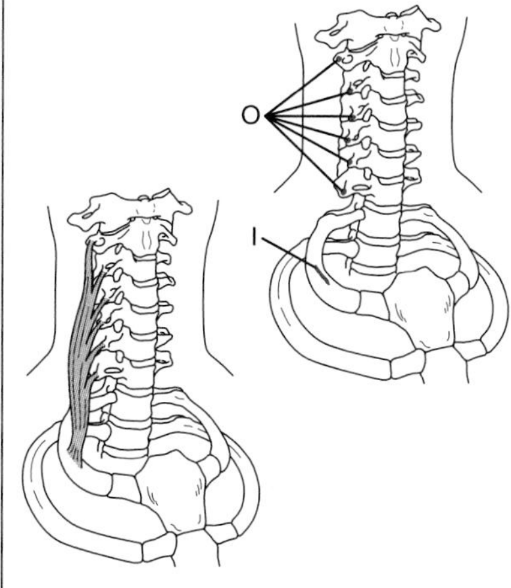 *Greek:* *skalenos—uneven* *Latin:* *medialis—toward the midline*	transverse processes of C2–C7	superior surface of the first rib	bilateral contraction: elevates the first rib; unilateral contraction: assists in rotation and lateral flexion and ipsilateral rotation of the cervical spine	posterior rami of C3–C8

continued on page 214

LESSON SEVEN—MUSCLES OF THE HEAD AND NECK *(continued)*

MUSCLE	ORIGIN	INSERTION	ACTION	NERVE
Scalenus Anterior 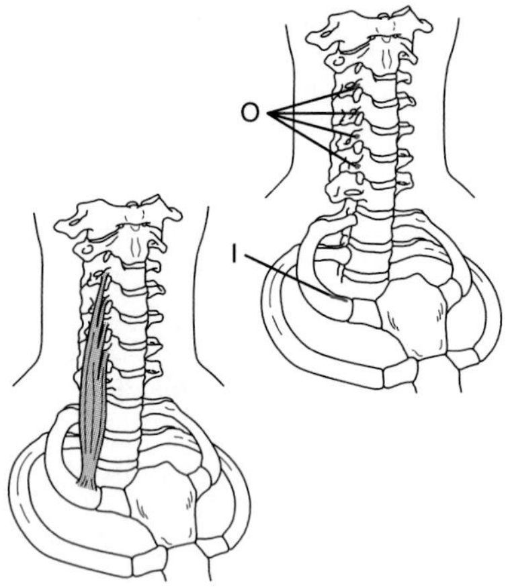 O I *Greek:* *skalenos—uneven* *Latin:* *ante—before*	transverse processes of C3–C6	superior surface of the first rib (anterior to scalenus medius)	bilateral contraction: elevates the first rib; unilateral contraction: assists in lateral flexion and ipsilateral rotation of the cervical spine	posterior rami of C3–C8
Suboccipitals 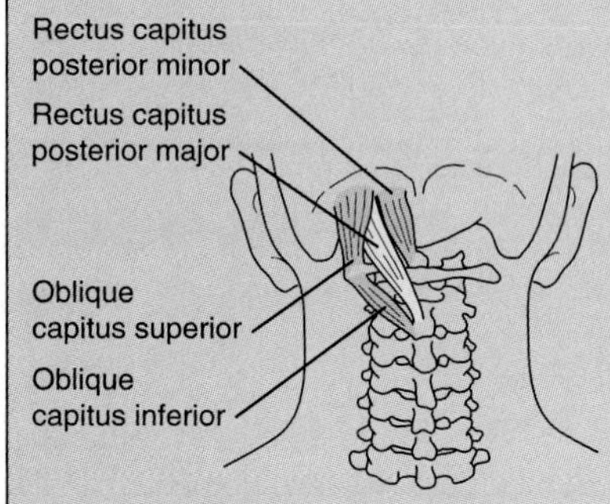 Rectus capitus posterior minor Rectus capitus posterior major Oblique capitus superior Oblique capitus inferior	The suboccipital muscles include the rectus capitus posterior major, the rectus capitus posterior minor, the oblique capitus inferior, and the oblique capitus superior. Dr. Janet Travell refers to the suboccipitals as the "ghost headache muscles," because the pain referred from these muscles seems to penetrate the skull and is difficult to locate. All suboccipitals attach on C1–C2 and are responsible for most of the head movements.			
Rectus Capitus Posterior Major 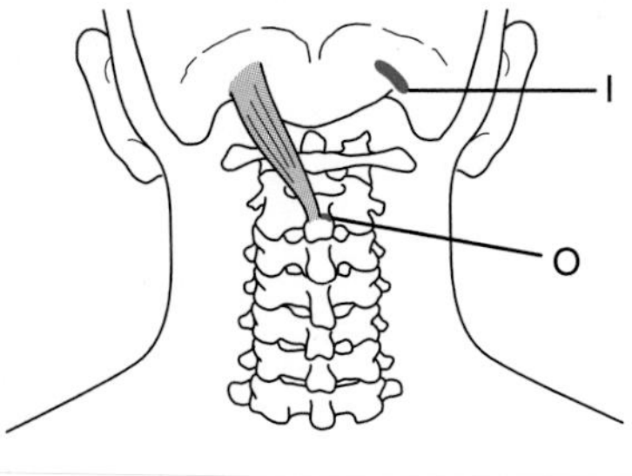 I O *Latin:* *rectus—straight* *caput—head* *posterus—behind* *major—larger*	below the spinous process of C2	occipital bone lateral to the inferior nuchal line	extension, lateral flexion and rotation of the head	posterior ramus of C1

LESSON SEVEN—MUSCLES OF THE HEAD AND NECK *(continued)*

MUSCLE	ORIGIN	INSERTION	ACTION	NERVE
Rectus Capitus Posterior Minor 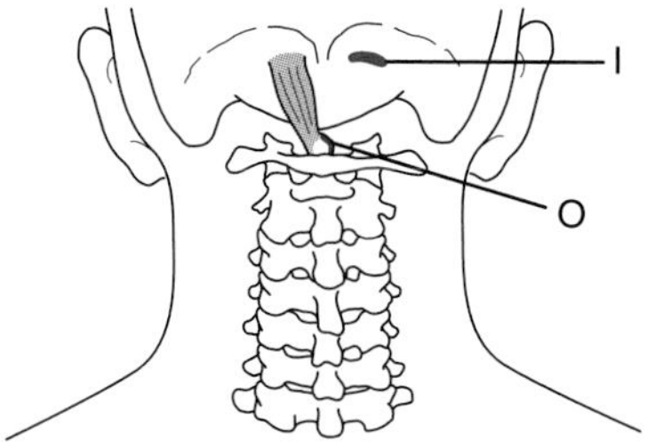 *Latin:* *rectus—straight* *caput—head* *posterus—behind* *minor—smaller*	posterior tubercle of C1	occipital bone lateral to the inferior nuchal line	extension and lateral flexion of the head	posterior ramus of C1
Oblique Capitus Inferior 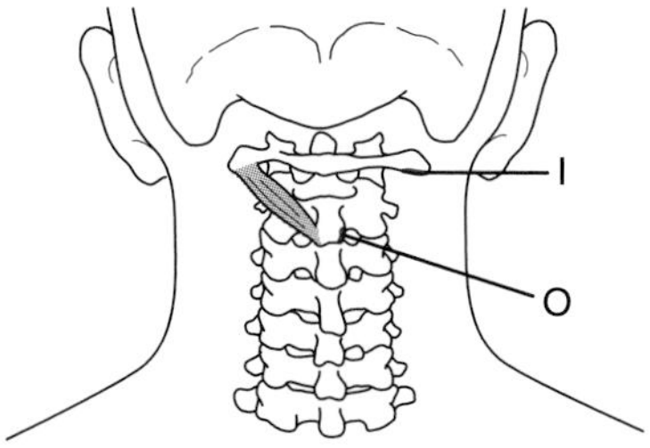 *Latin:* *obliquus—slant* *caput—head* *infra—beneath*	spinous process of C2	transverse process of C1	extension and lateral flexion of the head	posterior rami of C1 and C2
Oblique Capitus Superior 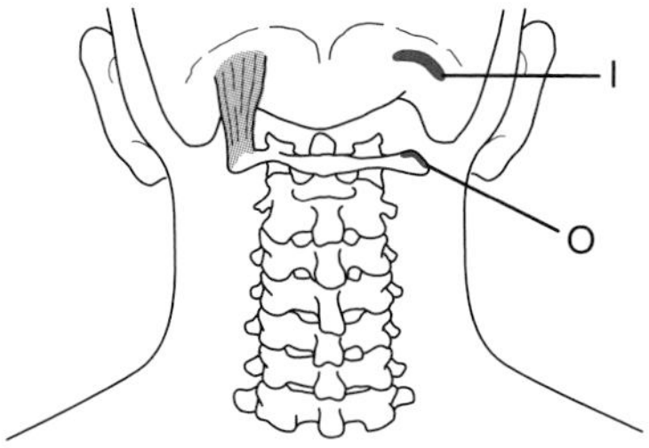 *Latin:* *obliquus—slant* *caput—head* *superus—upper*	transverse process of C1	occipital bone above the inferior nuchal line	extension and lateral rotation of the head	posterior ramus of C1

continued on page 216

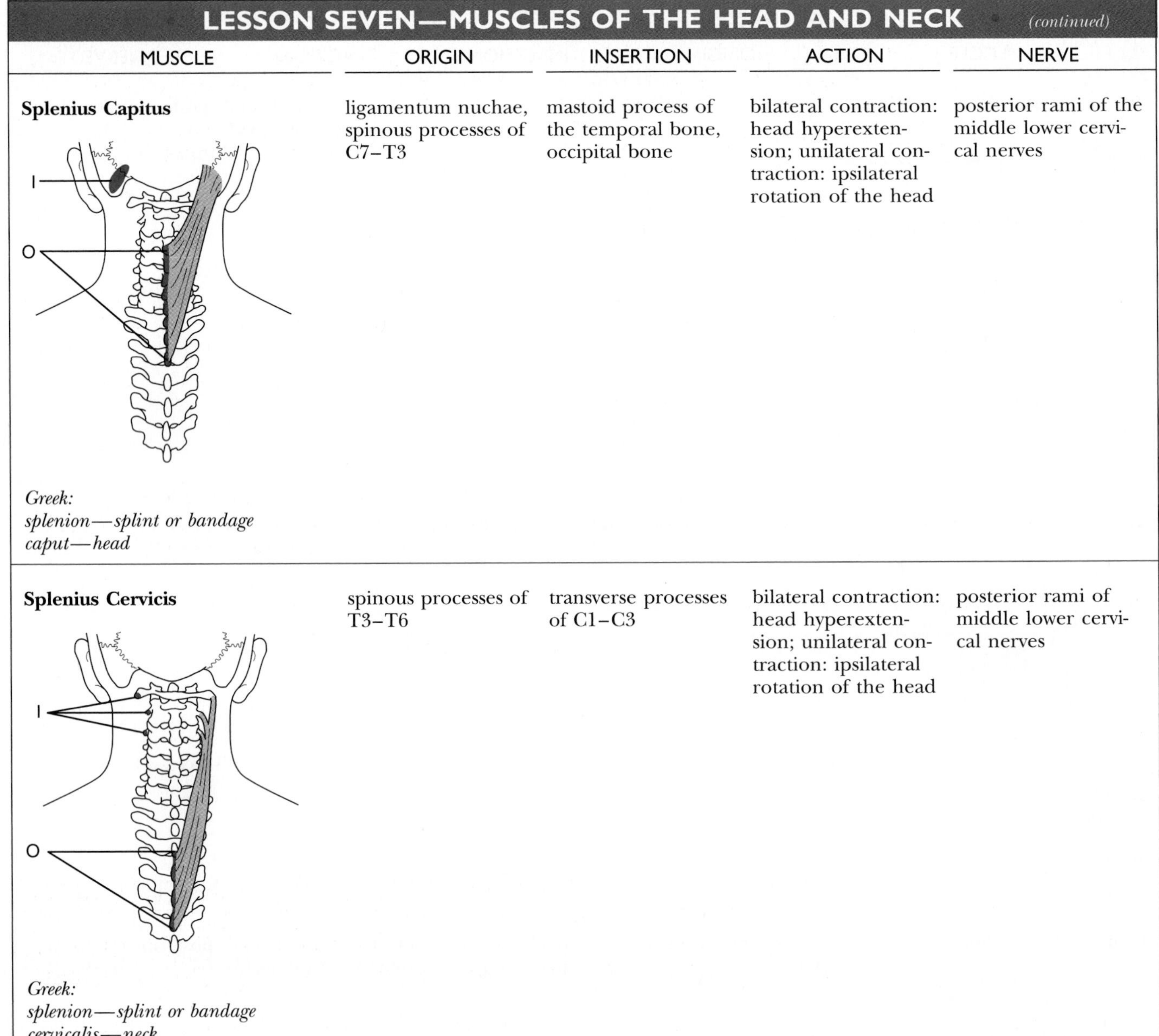

LESSON SEVEN—MUSCLES OF THE HEAD AND NECK *(continued)*

MUSCLE	ORIGIN	INSERTION	ACTION	NERVE
Splenius Capitus *Greek:* *splenion—splint or bandage* *caput—head*	ligamentum nuchae, spinous processes of C7–T3	mastoid process of the temporal bone, occipital bone	bilateral contraction: head hyperextension; unilateral contraction: ipsilateral rotation of the head	posterior rami of the middle lower cervical nerves
Splenius Cervicis *Greek:* *splenion—splint or bandage* *cervicalis—neck*	spinous processes of T3–T6	transverse processes of C1–C3	bilateral contraction: head hyperextension; unilateral contraction: ipsilateral rotation of the head	posterior rami of middle lower cervical nerves

Two other muscles of the head and neck are the ***levator scapulae*** and the ***trapezius*** (upper fibers). Both of these muscles are included in Muscles of Scapular Movement.

Author's Note

The two pterygoid muscles are named for their attachment on the pterygoid plate of the sphenoid bone. This can be felt as the bony lump in the back of the roof of the mouth.

LESSON EIGHT—MUSCLES OF THE TRUNK AND VERTEBRAL COLUMN

Abdominals

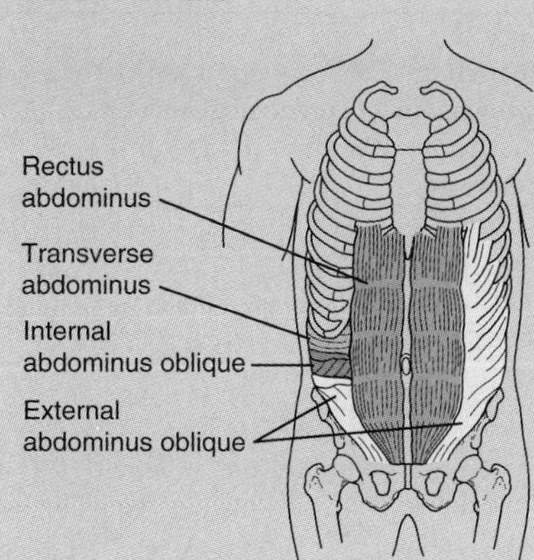

The abdominal muscles are the rectus abdominus, the external and internal abdominus oblique, and the transverse abdominus. The fiber arrangement of the abdominal muscles runs in four different directions and forms the shape of a six-pointed star. Think of this organization as the "plywood principle of anatomy," used for added strength to hold in internal abdominal organs. You can feel how these muscles compress the abdominal contents by placing your hands on your belly while you laugh, cough, defecate, or vomit (your choice).

MUSCLE	ORIGIN	INSERTION	ACTION	NERVE
Rectus Abdominus 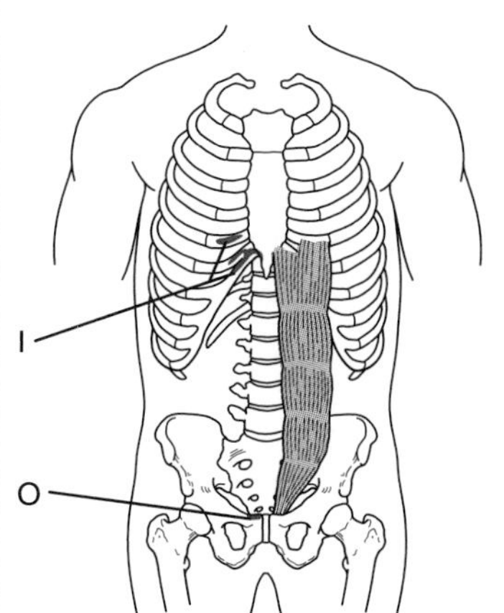 *Latin:* *rectus—straight* *abdomen—belly*	pubic symphysis	costal cartilage of ribs 5–7 and xiphoid process	bilateral contraction: trunk flexion, compression of the abdominal contents; unilateral contraction: lateral flexion of the vertebral column	anterior rami of intercostal nerves (T7–T12)
	Notes: The rectus abdominus goes a long distance without any skeletal attachment, so Mother Nature has provided a way of keeping its length constant by including a horizontal layer of connective tissue every few inches. This band of connective tissue is called a tendinous intersection.			
External Abdominus Oblique 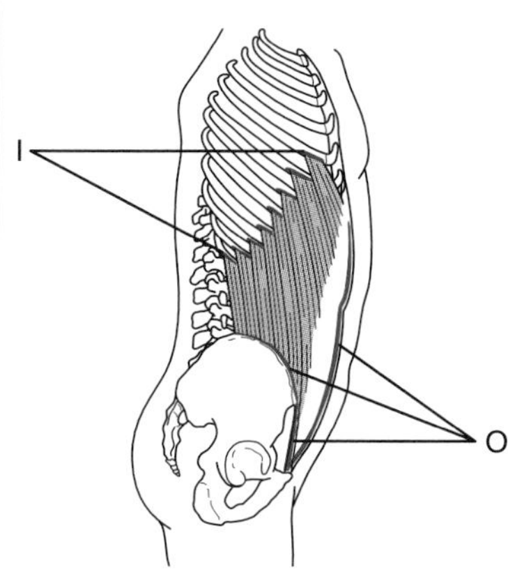 *Latin:* *externus—outside* *abdomen—belly* *obliquus—slant*	anterior lateral aspect of ribs 5–12	iliac crest, abdominal fascia, inguinal ligament, linea alba (via the rectus sheath)	bilateral contraction: trunk flexion and compresses the abdomen (as in sucking in the tummy); unilateral contraction: lateral flexion and contralateral rotation of the vertebral column	anterior rami of intercostal nerves (T7–T12)
	Notes: The fiber direction of this muscle is similar to the direction of your fingers when your hands are in the pockets of a jacket. The pockets of most jackets do not reach the midline. Likewise, the external abdominus obliques (external obliques) do not reach the midline. They insert into the sheath of the rectus abdominus instead.			

continued on page 218

LESSON EIGHT—MUSCLES OF THE TRUNK AND VERTEBRAL COLUMN *(cont.)*

MUSCLE	ORIGIN	INSERTION	ACTION	NERVE
Internal Abdominus Oblique *Latin:* *internus—within* *abdomen—belly* *obliquus—slant*	anterior iliac crest, thoracolumbar fascia, inguinal ligament	anterior lateral part of ribs 7–12, linea alba	bilateral contraction: trunk flexion, compression of the abdominal contents; unilateral contraction: lateral flexion of the vertebral column, ipsilateral rotation	anterior rami of intercostal nerves (T8–T12)
	Notes: The fiber direction of the internal abdominus oblique (internal obliques) is similar to the direction of your fingers when your hands are holding on to suspenders resting on your chest.			
Transverse Abdominus *Latin:* *transversus—lying across* *abdomen—belly*	anterior lateral aspect of ribs 7–12, iliac crest, thoracolumbar aponeurosis, inguinal ligament	abdominal aponeurosis, linea alba (via the rectus sheath), pubic bone	compression of the abdominal contents	anterior rami of intercostal nerves (T7–T12)
	Notes: The transverse abdominus is the deepest abdominal muscle and wraps around the internal organs like a cummerbund. The lower fibers of the rectus abdominus are enclosed by the transverse abdominus, probably for added strength.			
Quadratus Lumborum *Latin:* *quadratus—four-sided* *lumbus—loins*	posterior iliac crest	rib 12 and transverse process of L1–L4	bilateral contraction: tilts pelvis anteriorly and hyperextension of lumbar spine; unilateral contraction: lateral flexion of trunk or ipsilateral elevation of the hip	anterior rami (T12–L4)
	Notes: Also known as the "hip hiker muscle" because it hikes the hip up.			

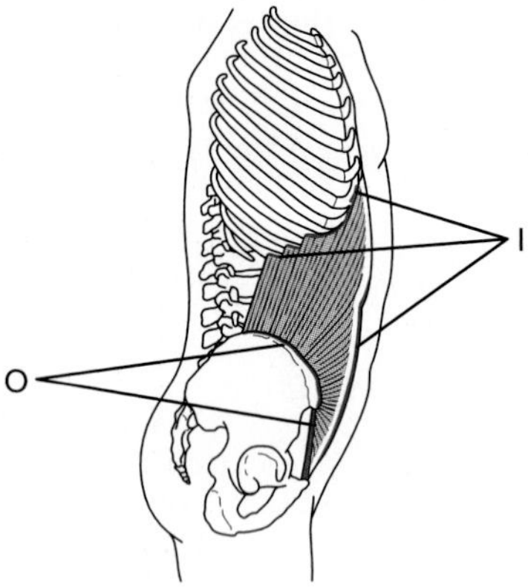

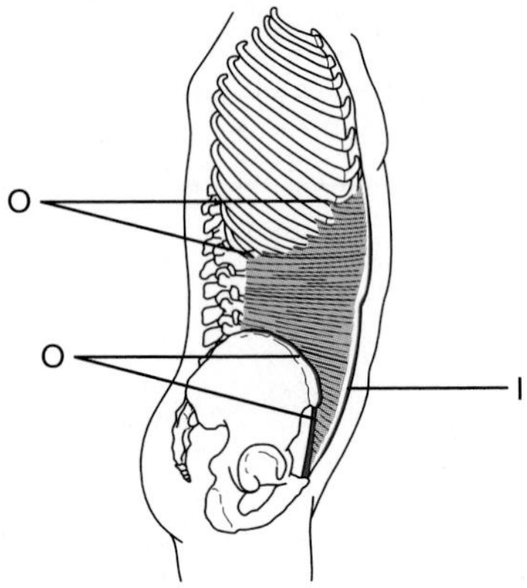

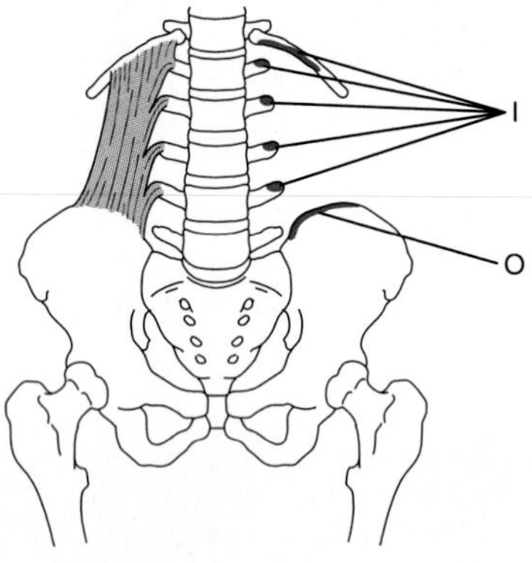

LESSON EIGHT—MUSCLES OF THE TRUNK AND VERTEBRAL COLUMN *(cont.)*

Paraspinals

The paraspinals are the collective term given to a group of back muscles composed of two groups, the transversospinalis and the erector spinae.

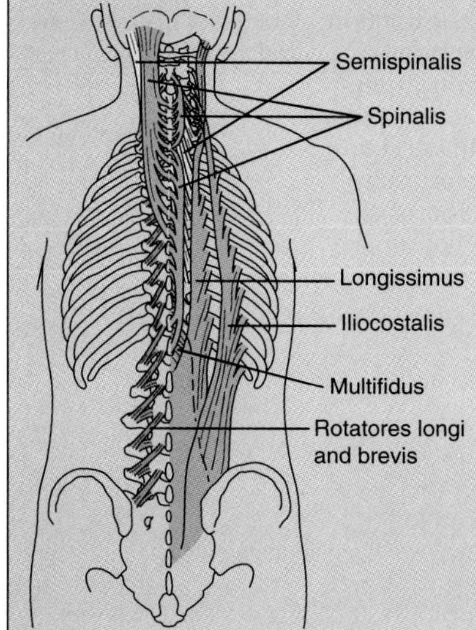

Greek:
para—beside
Latin:
spinatus—spine

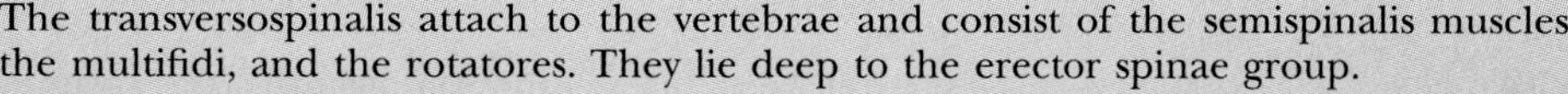

Transversospinalis

The transversospinalis attach to the vertebrae and consist of the semispinalis muscles, the multifidi, and the rotatores. They lie deep to the erector spinae group.

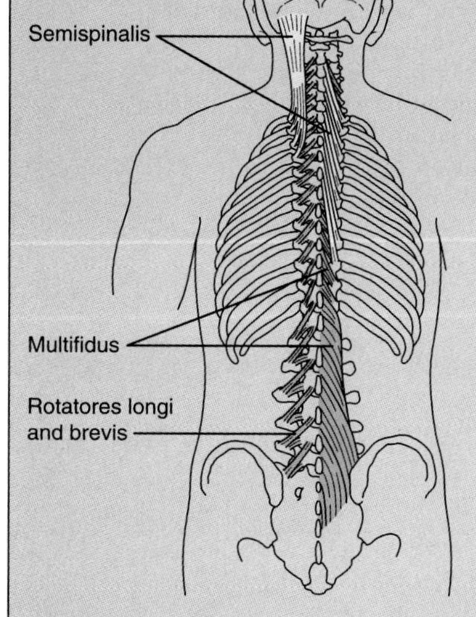

Latin:
transversus—lying across
spinatus—spine

continued on page 220

LESSON EIGHT—MUSCLES OF THE TRUNK AND VERTEBRAL COLUMN (cont.)

MUSCLE	ORIGIN	INSERTION	ACTION	NERVE
Rotatores Longi and Brevis 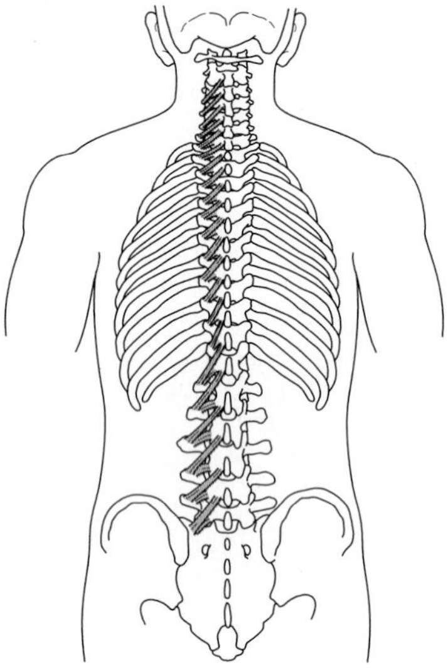 *Latin:* *rotare—to turn* *longus—long* *brevis—brief*	ORIGIN AND INSERTION: rotatores longi: transverse process of one vertebral segment to the spinous process of the second vertebral segment above; rotatores brevis: the transverse process of one vertebral segment to the spinous process of the vertebral segment above.		bilateral contraction: extends vertebral column (important in maintaining posture); unilateral contraction: contralateral rotation of the vertebral column	posterior rami of spinal nerves
	Notes: The rotatores longi is the deepest muscle of the transversospinalis group.			
Multifidus 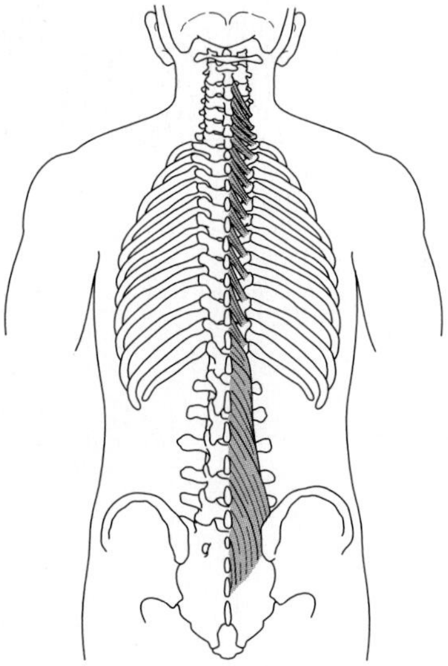 *Latin:* *multus—many* *fidus—to split*	the transverse process of one vertebral segment	the spinous processes of the second, third, and fourth vertebral segments above	bilateral contraction: extends the vertebral column (important in maintaining posture); unilateral contraction: contralateral rotation of the vertebral column	posterior rami of spinal nerves

LESSON EIGHT—MUSCLES OF THE TRUNK AND VERTEBRAL COLUMN *(cont.)*

MUSCLE	ORIGIN	INSERTION	ACTION	NERVE
Semispinalis	transverse process of one vertebral segment	spinous processes of the fifth, sixth, and seventh vertebral segments above	bilateral contraction: extends the vertebral column (important in maintaining posture); unilateral contraction: contralateral rotation of the vertebral column	posterior rami of spinal nerves
Latin: *semis—half* *spinatus—spine*	**Notes:** This group of muscles runs in only the thoracic and cervical regions of the vertebral column. This is the most superficial of the transversospinalis.			
Erector Spinae *Latin:* *erigere—to erect* *spinatus—spine*	Also known as the sacrospinalis muscle, the erector spinae runs parallel to the spine and erects it like a SILo. The word SILo can be used as a mnemonic phrase to recall the names of the erector spinae muscles: *s*pinalis, *i*liocostalis, *lo*ngissimus.			
Spinalis	spinous processes of C4–T12	spinous processes of C2–T8 and the occipital bone	bilateral contraction: extension of the vertebral column and head (important in maintaining posture); unilateral contraction; rotates and lateral ipsilateral flexion of the vertebral column	posterior rami of spinal nerves
Latin: *spinatus—spine*	**Notes:** The spinalis is the medial tract of the erector spinae and interconnects the upper 80 percent of the vertebral column with the skull. The *spin*alis hugs the *spine*.			

continued on page 222

LESSON EIGHT—MUSCLES OF THE TRUNK AND VERTEBRAL COLUMN *(cont.)*

MUSCLE	ORIGIN	INSERTION	ACTION	NERVE
Longissimus 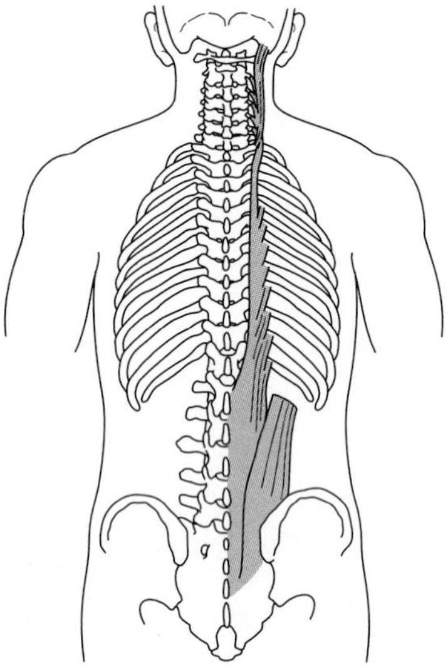	sacrum, spinous processes of T1–L5, transverse processes of C4–T12	mastoid process of the temporal bone, transverse processes of C2–T12	bilateral contraction: extension of the vertebral column and head (important in maintaining posture); unilateral contraction; rotates and lateral ipsilateral flexion of the vertebral column	posterior rami of spinal nerves
Latin: *longus—long*	**Notes:** The *long*issimus is the intermediate tract of the erector spinae and covers a *long* territory stretching from sacrum to skull.			
Iliocostalis 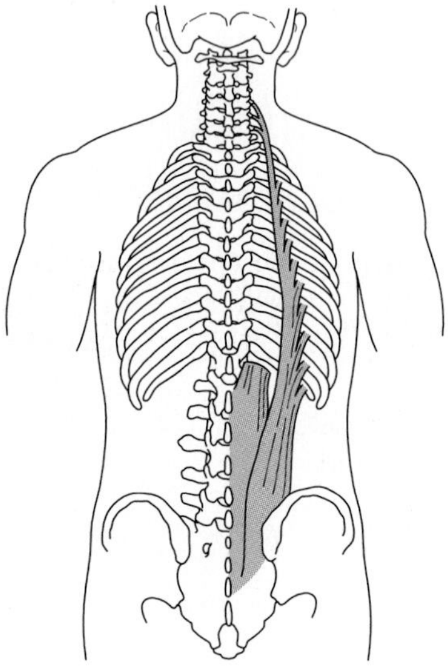	posterior iliac crest, sacrum, posterior surface of the ribs	posterior surface of ribs and transverse processes of C4–C6	bilateral contraction: extension of the vertebral column (important in maintaining posture); unilateral contraction; rotates and lateral ipsilateral flexion of the vertebral column	posterior rami of spinal nerves
Latin: *ilium—flank* *costae—rib*	**Notes:** The iliocostalis is the lateral tract of the erector spinae. The ilio*costal*is hugs the *costals* (ribs).			

LESSON NINE—MUSCLES OF RESPIRATION

MUSCLE	ORIGIN	INSERTION	ACTION	NERVE
Diaphragm	L1–L3, lower six costal cartilages, xiphoid process of the sternum	central tendon (a cloverleaf-shaped aponeurosis)	expands the thoracic cavity by pulling the belly of the diaphragm down via the central tendon	phrenic nerve (C3–C5)
Greek: *diaphragma—a partition*	**Notes:** The diaphragm divides the thoracic from the abdominal cavity and is the prime mover of inspiration.			
Internal Intercostals	superior border of the rib below	inferior border of the rib above	depress the rib cage, which helps to move air out of the lungs when exhaling, and maintain the intercostal spaces	intercostal nerves
Latin: *internus—within* *costae—rib*	**Notes:** The fiber direction of the internal intercostals is the same as the internal abdominus obliques.			
External Intercostals	inferior border of the rib above	superior border of the rib below	help to elevate the rib cage during inhalation and maintain the intercostal spaces	intercostal nerves
Latin: *externus—outside* *internus—within* *costae—rib*	**Notes:** As the name implies, the external intercostals are external, or superficial, to the internal intercostals and in between the ribs. The fiber direction of this muscle is the same as the external abdominus oblique.			

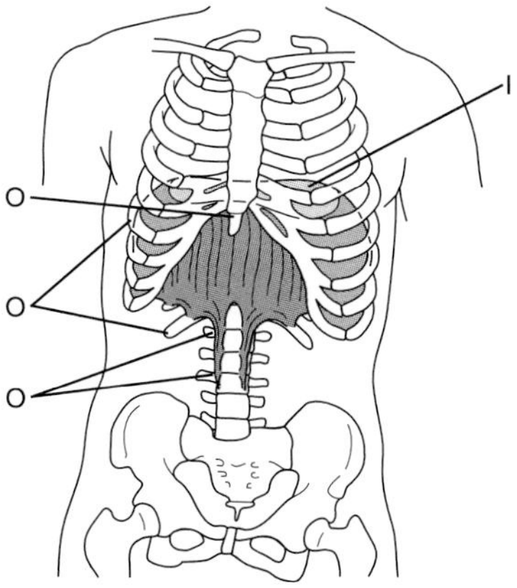

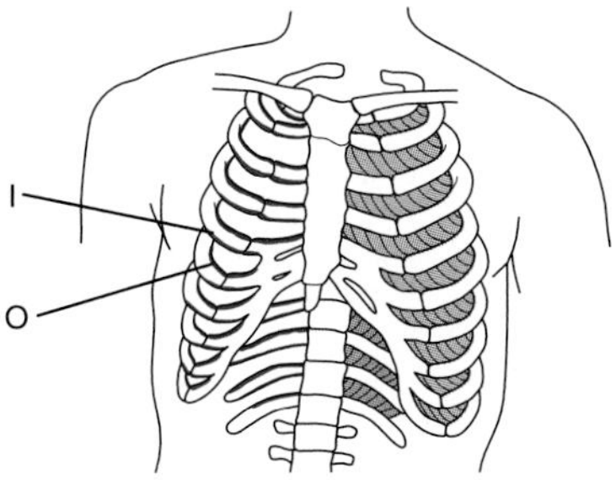

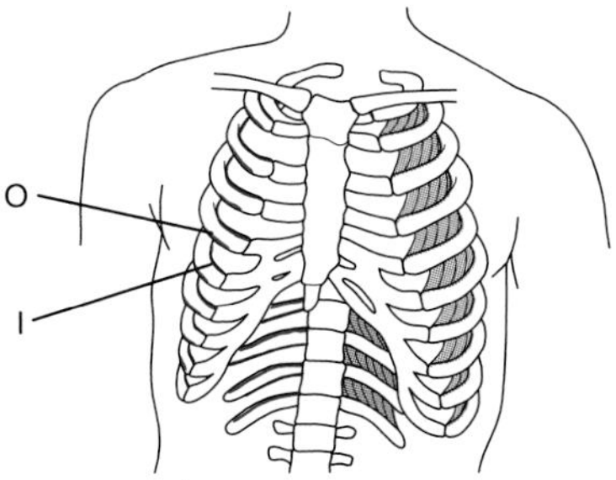

continued on page 224

LESSON NINE—MUSCLES OF RESPIRATION *(continued)*

MUSCLE	ORIGIN	INSERTION	ACTION	NERVE
Serratus Posterior Superior 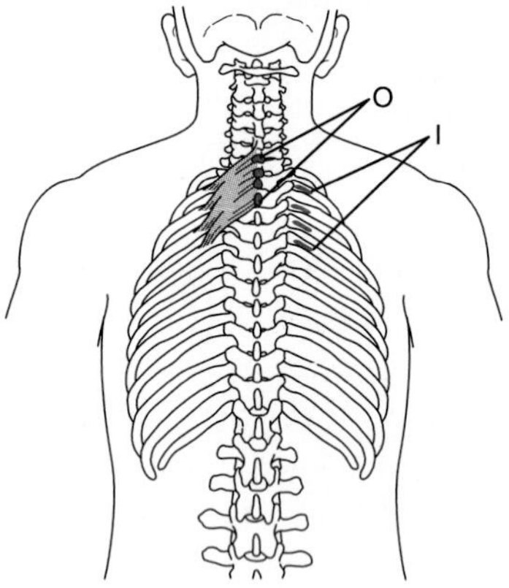 O I *Latin:* *serratus—notched or jagged like a saw* *posterus—behind* *superus—upper*	nuchal ligament and spinous process of C6–T2	posterior aspect of ribs 2–5	elevates ribs 2–5 during inspiration	intercostal nerves (T1–T4)
	Notes: These two muscles aid in the process of labored breathing; however, many notable anatomy texts, such as *Myofascial Pain and Dysfunction, The Trigger Point Manual,* by Janet Travell, M.D., and David Simons, M.D., do not consider these muscles as respiratory muscles, because they appear to remain passive during normal respiration.			
Serratus Posterior Inferior 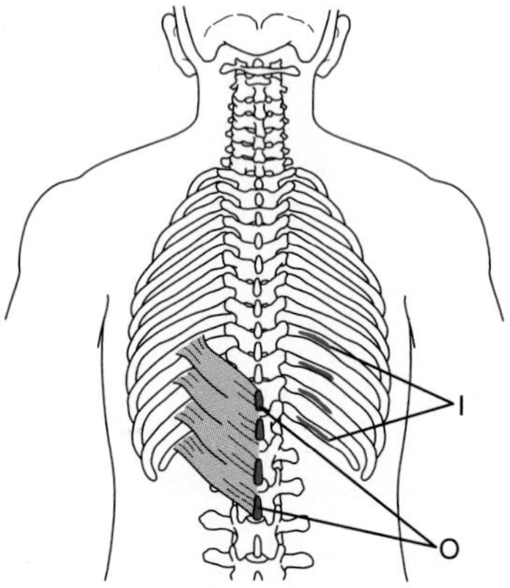 I O *Latin:* *serratus—notched or jagged like a saw* *posterus—behind* *infra—beneath*	spinous process of T11–L2	posterior aspect of ribs 9–12	depresses ribs 9–12 during exhalation, may contribute to lateral rotation of the vertebral column	intercostal nerves (T9–T12)

The three ***scalene muscles*** also contribute to the act of respiration. They are included in lesson seven, Muscles of the Head and Neck.

FYI FOR YOUR INFORMATION

The smallest muscle in the body: the stapedius muscle of the middle ear. Largest muscle in the body: Latissimus dorsi. The longest muscle: the sartorius. The thickest muscle: the gluteus maximus. The strongest muscle: some authorities say the masseter, some have claimed the tongue to be the strongest muscle, and still others say that it is the gluteus maximus.

SUMMARY

Muscular nomenclature deals with the names, locations, attachment points, actions, and nerve supply of individual skeletal muscles. The muscles of the appendicular skeleton are divided into the following groups: Muscles of Scapula Movement; Muscles of Shoulder Movement; Muscles of Elbow Movement; Muscles of the Forearm, Wrist, and Hand; Muscles of the Hip and Knee Movement; Muscles of Foot Movement. The muscles of the axial skeleton are broken down into the following groups: Muscles of the Head and Neck, Muscles of the Trunk and Vertebral Column, Muscles of Respiration.

For each muscle in these groups, the origin of its name is broken down, synonyms are listed, and specific actions, origins, and insertions are detailed.

SELF-TEST

Multiple Choice • Write the letter of the best answer in the space provided.

_______ 1. The four major abdominal muscles are the
- A. rectus torsalis, vastus lateralis, vastus medialis, vastus intermedius
- B. rectus abdominus, transverse abdominus, internal and external intercostals
- C. rectus abdominus, transverse abdominus, internal and external abdominus obliques
- D. transverse abdominus, biceps abdominus, semimembranosus, semitendinosus

_______ 2. Which muscle expands the chest cavity by pulling the belly of the muscle down via the central tendon?
- A. internal intercostals
- B. diaphragm
- C. multifidus
- D. levator scapulae

_______ 3. The paraspinals refer to the transversospinalis and the
- A. longus colli
- B. quadriceps femoris
- C. erector spinae
- D. triceps surae

_______ 4. The three tracts of the erector spinae group, from medial to lateral are
- A. iliocostalis, spinalis, longissimus
- B. longissimus, spinalis, iliocostalis
- C. spinalis, iliocostalis, longissimus
- D. spinalis, longissimus, iliocostalis

_______ 5. Which is the only muscle that moves the head but does *not* attach to any vertebrae?
- A. splenius capitus
- B. scalenes
- C. trapezius
- D. sternocleidomastoid

_______ 6. Torticollis affects which muscle?
- A. sternocleidomastoid
- B. pectoralis major
- C. trapezius
- D. rectus abdominus

_______ 7. The "neurovascular entrappers" are pectoralis minor and the
- A. splenius capitus
- B. scalenes
- C. trapezius
- D. sternocleidomastoid

_______ 8. The triceps brachii attaches on what bony marking?
- A. coracoid process of the scapula
- B. tibial tuberosity
- C. olecranon process of the ulna
- D. radial tuberosity

_______ 9. The four main muscles of mastication are
- A. orbicularis oris, temporalis, zygomaticus major, buccinator
- B. orbicularis oris, zygomaticus major, pterygoid medialis and lateralis
- C. masseter, temporalis, buccinator, pterygoid lateralis
- D. masseter, temporalis, pterygoid medialis and lateralis

_______ 10. What are the four rotator cuff muscles?
- A. supraspinatus, infraspinatus, serratus posterior, teres minor
- B. supraspinatus, pronator teres, subscapularis, deltoids
- C. supraspinatus, infraspinatus, teres minor, subscapularis
- D. brachialis, serratus posterior, teres minor, subscapularis

_______ 11. In general, where do the flexors of the wrist originate?
- A. lateral epicondyle of the humerus
- B. greater tubercle of the humerus
- C. medial epicondyle of the humerus
- D. lesser tubercle of the humerus

_______ 12. If Mrs. Brown's right shoulder is elevated, which muscle would you most likely find contracted?
- A. levator scapula
- B. pectoralis major
- C. serratus anterior
- D. subscapularis

_______ 13. What three muscles form the thenar eminence?
- A. opponens pollicis, abductor pollicis brevis, flexor pollicis brevis
- B. abductor pollicis brevis, flexor pollicis brevis, extensor pollicis

C. opponens pollicis, flexor pollicis brevis, extensor digiti minimi
D. abductor pollicis brevis, extensor digiti minimi, opponens digiti

_______ 14. Identify the three gluteal muscles.
A. gluteus maximus, gluteus intermedius, gluteus minimus
B. gluteus maximus, gluteus intermedius, gluteus lateralis
C. gluteus femoris, gluteus medius, gluteus minimus
D. gluteus maximus, gluteus medius, and gluteus minimus

_______ 15. There are six hip rotators; they are the
A. piriformis, obturator internus and externus, gemellus superior and inferior, quadratus femoris
B. piriformis, obturator superior and inferior, gemellus internus and externus, quadriceps lumborus
C. piriformis, rotator internus and externus, scalenus medius, anterior and posterior
D. piriformis, lumborum superior and inferior, femoris internus, externus, and medius

_______ 16. Which of the following are the three muscles of the iliopsoas?
A. iliacus, lumborum superior and inferior
B. psoas major and minor, iliacus
C. gluteus femoris, psoas medius, gluteus minimus
D. iliacus, rotator internus and externus

_______ 17. The five adductor muscles of the lower extremity are
A. adductor magnus, longus, and brevis, gracilis, pectineus
B. sartorius, adductor magnus, longus, and brevis, gracilis
C. semitendinosus, semimembranosus, gracilis, pectineus, adductor femoris
D. adductor magnus, longus, and brevis, semitendinosus, gracilis

_______ 18. Identify the four muscles of the quadriceps femoris.
A. sartorius, rectus femoris, vastus lateralis and intermedius
B. gracilis, sartorius, semimembranosus, pectineus
C. rectus femoris, vastus lateralis, intermedius, and medialis
D. rectus femoris, vastus lateralis and intermedius, sartorius

_______ 19. Which are the three hamstring muscles?
A. sartorius, semitendinosus, semimembranosus
B. quadriceps femoris, vastus medialis and intermedius
C. biceps femoris, adductor brevis and longus
D. semitendinosus, semimembranosus, biceps femoris

Don't forget to breathe!

_______ 20. Which of the rotator cuff muscles does not rotate the humerus?
A. supraspinatus
B. infraspinatus
C. subscapularis
D. teres minor

_______ 21. What is the muscle in the lower leg that spans two joints?
A. semitendinosus
B. pectineus
C. gracilis
D. soleus

Matching I • Choose one response and write the letter in the space provided.

A. orbicularis oris
B. buccinator
C. intercostals
D. gastrocnemius
E. tensor fascia latae
F. tibialis posterior
G. teres major
H. sartorius
I. platysma
J. zygomaticus major

_______ 1. located between the ribs; muscle of respiration

_______ 2. compresses cheeks as in whistling or blowing a trumpet

_______ 3. the "kissing muscle"

_______ 4. inserts on the calcaneus; two heads

_______ 5. longest muscle in the body; the "tailor's muscle"

_______ 6. posterior lower leg muscle; attaches on the tibia, fibula, and interosseous membrane

_______ 7. muscle that draws the corners of your mouth up into a smile or grin

_______ 8. inserts on the iliotibial band

_______ 9. a synergist to the latissimus dorsi

_______ 10. most superficial anterior neck muscle

Matching II • Choose one response and write the letter in the space provided.

A. deltoid
B. brachialis
C. extensor digiti minimi
D. latissimus dorsi
E. rhomboids
F. suboccipitals
G. trapezius
H. biceps brachii
I. orbicularis oculi
J. subscapularis
K. rotator cuff
L. triceps brachii

_______ 1. "Christmas tree muscle"; collective term

_______ 2. widest muscle in the body; "swimmer's muscle"

_______ 3. four shoulder muscles, collectively called the "SITS muscles"

_______ 4. three origins and one insertion; the "boxer's muscle"

_______ 5. because of its mechanical advantage, the most effective arm flexor

_______ 6. according to Dr. Travell, the "ghost headaches" muscles

_______ 7. resembles gluteals in structure; abducts, adducts, and elevates the shoulder

_______ 8. known as the "tea drinker's muscle"

_______ 9. "coat hanger muscle"

_______ 10. a muscle involved in frozen shoulder

_______ 11. the "winking muscle"

_______ 12. two origins and one insertion; upper arm

References

Applegate, Edith J., M.S. *The Anatomy and Physiology Learning System: Textbook.* Philadelphia: W. B. Saunders, 1995.

Goldberg, Stephen, M.D. *Clinical Anatomy Made Ridiculously Simple.* Miami: Medmaster, Inc., 1984.

Guyton, Arthur, M.D. *Human Physiology and Mechanisms of Disease,* 3rd ed. Philadelphia: W.B. Saunders Company, 1982.

Haubrich, William S., M.D. *Medical Meanings, A Glossary of Word Origins.* New York, NY: Harcourt Brace Jovanovich, Publishers, 1984.

Hoppenfeld, Stanley. *Physical Examination of the Spine and Extremities.* Norwalk, CT: Appleton-Century-Crofts, 1976.

Juhan, Deane. *Job's Body, A Handbook for Bodyworkers.* Barrington NY: Station Hill Press, 1987.

Kapit, Wynn, and Lawrence M. Elson. *The Anatomy Coloring Book,* 2nd ed. New York, N.Y: HarperCollins Publishers, 1993.

Kapit, Wynn, Robert Macey, and Esmail Meisami. *The Physiology Coloring Book.* New York, N.Y: HarperCollins Publishers, 1987.

Kendall, Florence P., and Elizabeth K. McCreary. *Muscles: Testing and Function,* 3rd ed. Baltimore: Williams & Wilkins, 1983.

Kordish, Mary, and Sylvia Dickson. *Introduction to Basic Human Anatomy.* Lake Charles, LA: McNeese State University, Self-published manual, 1985.

Lauderstein, David. *Putting the Soul Back in the Body: A Manual of Imaginative Anatomy for Massage Therapists.* Chicago, IL: Self-published manual, 1985.

Lowe, Whitney W. *Functional Assessment in Massage Therapy.* Corvallis, OR: Pacific Orthopedic Massage, 1995.

Marieb, Elaine N. *Essentials of Human Anatomy and Physiology,* 4th ed. New York: Benjamin/Cummings Publishing Company, Inc., 1994.

Mattes, Aaron. *Active Isolated Stretching.* Published by Aaron Mattes, 1995.

McAleer, Neil. *The Body Almanac.* Garden City, NY: Doubleday and Company, Inc., 1985.

McLaughlin, Craig. *The Bodyworker's Muscle Reference Guide.* Bellvue, CO: Bodyguide, 1996.

Moore, Keith L. *Clinically Oriented Anatomy,* 2nd ed. Baltimore: Williams & Wilkins, 1985.

Mosby's Medical, Nursing, and Allied Health Dictionary, 4th ed. St. Louis: Mosby–Year Book, Inc., 1994.

Olsen, Andrea, and Caryn McHose. *BodyStories: A Guide to Experiential Anatomy.* Barrytown, NY: Station Hill Press, 1991.

Rolf, Ida P., Ph.D. *Rolfing: The Integration of Human Structures.* New York: Harper and Row, Publishers, 1977.

Sieg, Kay, and Sandra Adams. *Illustrated Essentials of Musculoskeletal Anatomy,* 3rd ed. Gainesville, FL: Megabooks, 1996.

St. John, Paul. *St. John Neuromuscular Therapy Seminars Manual I.* Largo, FL, 1995.

Tabers Cyclopedic Medical Dictionary, 13th ed. Philadelphia: F. A. Davis Company, 1977.

Tortora, Gerald J. *Introduction to the Human Body: The Essentials of Anatomy and Physiology,* 3rd ed. New York: HarperCollins Publishers, 1994.

Travell, Janet, M.D., and David Simons, M.D. *Myofascial Pain and Dysfunction, The Trigger Point Manual.* Baltimore: Williams & Wilkins, 1983.

Warfel, John H. *The Extremities: Muscles and Motor Points,* 5th ed. Philadelphia: Lea and Febiger, 1985.

Warfel, John H. *The Head, Neck, and Trunk,* 5th ed. Philadelphia: Lea and Febiger, 1985.

The greatest undeveloped territory in the world lies under your hat.
—*Anonymous*

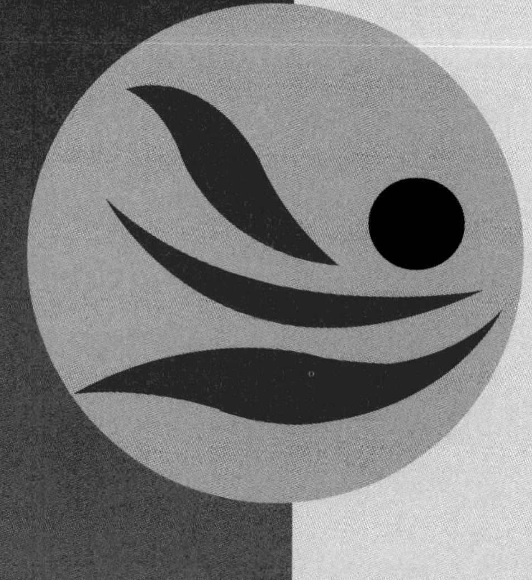

10

Nervous System

Student Objectives

After completing this chapter, the student should be able to:

- List the functions of the nervous system
- Discuss the basic organization of the nervous system
- Identify the types of nerve tissue
- Label the parts of a neuron
- Classify neurons according to their structure and function
- Describe how nerves initiate, receive, and transmit impulses
- Name the important neurotransmitters of the nervous system
- List the structures of the central nervous system, identifying the regions of the brain and spinal cord
- List the structures of the peripheral nervous system
- Explain the mechanisms involved in a reflex arc
- Name the cranial nerves
- Name and discuss the five basic types of sensory receptors
- List the physiological effects of the sympathetic nervous system and the parasympathetic nervous system
- Briefly discuss the senses (taste, smell, hearing, and vision)

INTRODUCTION

The human body has two specialized centers of control that make important adjustments to maintain homeostasis. The endocrine system, which will be discussed later, is the slower of these two centers. The faster control system is the nervous system, the most complex and most fascinating system of the body. It is the body's master controlling and communicating system; it even monitors and regulates the endocrine system. Every thought, action, and sensation reflect its activity. We are what our brain has experienced. If all past sensory input could be completely erased, we would be unable to walk, talk, or communicate; we would remember no pain and no pleasure.

The study of the functions and disorders of the nervous system is referred to as **neurology.** As we explore neurology, we will examine the structural and functional classifications of the nervous tissue. We will begin with an overview of nerves and with the chemistry behind nerve impulses and synaptic transmissions, then look at the two divisions of the nervous system itself: the central and the peripheral nervous systems. Finally, we will examine the specialized nerve receptors that give us our five senses and will review common clinical nervous conditions, some of which may affect the application of massage.

FUNCTIONS

1. **Sensory Input.** The sensory receptors of the body detect changes, such as pressure, temperature, and motion, both inside the body and out.
2. **Interpretive and Integrative Functions.** After registering these changes, the nervous system interprets the perceived information to provide a response. Integration occurs between the sensory input of information and the motor output.
3. **Motor Output.** Once the nervous system has received and interpreted the **stimuli** (any change in the internal or external environment), a motor response may be activated in the form of muscular contractions or glandular secretions.
4. **Higher Mental Functioning and Emotional Responsiveness.** The nervous system is also responsible for mental processes (cognition and memory) and emotional responses (anger and anxiety).

Word Parts and Terms Related to the Nervous System

arachnoid – spider; shaped
autonomic – self; law
axon – axis
baroreceptor – weight; to receive
Broca's area – named after the French surgeon (1824–80)
cauda equina – tail-like; horse
cerebellum – little brain
cerebrum – brain
chemoreceptors – chemical; to receive
cochlea – land snail
corpus callosum – body; hard or callused
cortex – bark or rind
cyton – cell
dendrites – treelike
diencephalon – two or second; brain
dura mater – hard or tough; mother
encephal – brain
filum terminale – threadlike; at the end
ganglion – knot
gyri – circle
incus – anvil
internuncial – between; together, midst; messenger
macula – spot
mechanoreceptors – machine; to receive
medulla oblongata – marrow or middle; long
meninges – membrane
myelin – marrow
neurilemma – nerve; husk
neuro – sinew; nerve
neuroglia (glial cells) – nerve; glue
neurotransmitters – nerve; a sending across
nociceptor – hurt; to receive
nodes of Ranvier – named after the French pathologist (1835–1922)
oligodendrocytes – little; tree; cell
otolith – ear; stone
papilla – nipple
parasympathetic – by the side of, sympathetic
photoreceptors – light; to receive
pia mater – tender, soft; mother
plexus – braid
proprioceptor – one's own; a receiver
pons – bridge
reciprocal inhibition – alternate; to restrain
reflex – bent back
retina – a net
Schwann cell – named after the German anatomist (1810–82)
soma – body
stapes – stirrup
stimuli – a goad (a pointed rod or spear); to urge on
sulci – groove
summation – adding
sympathetic – sympathy
synapse – point of contact
telodendron – end; a tree
thalamus – chamber
thermoreceptors – heat; to receive
tympanic – drum
vagus – wandering
vermis – wormlike
Wernicke's area – named after the German neurologist (1848–1905)

BASIC ORGANIZATION OF THE NERVOUS SYSTEM

Because of the complexity of the nervous system, it is often difficult to "swallow it whole." The central nervous system and the peripheral nervous system possess unique structural and functional characteristics.

The **central nervous system** (CNS) occupies a central or medial position in the body (dorsal body cavity). It is primarily concerned with interpreting incoming sensory information and with issuing instructions in the form of motor response. It is also the major control center for thoughts and emotional experiences. The major components of the CNS include the brain (cerebrum, cerebellum, diencephalon, and brain stem), meninges, cerebrospinal fluid, and spinal cord. These structures are surrounded by the bones of the spinal column or the skull. The nerve cells of the central nervous system are not capable of regeneration.

The **peripheral nervous system** (PNS) is composed of the nerves emerging from the central nervous system: the **cranial nerves,** which originate from the brain, and **spinal nerves,** which originate from the spinal cord. Both sets of nerves are involved with carrying impulses to and from their respective areas. Sensory nerves are said to be *afferent,* that is, they carry impulses from nerve receptors *to* the brain or spinal cord. Motor nerves are classified as *efferent,* which means that they carry messages *from* the brain or spinal cord. There are 43 pairs of nerves in the peripheral nervous system: 12 pairs of cranial nerves and 31 pairs of spinal nerves. It is best not to think of the peripheral nervous system as separate from the central nervous system; imagine that the PNS is the tentacles of the CNS. In this way, you can begin to see the intricate relationship between these two regions.

Within the PNS are several special divisions, the somatic and the autonomic nervous systems. The **somatic,** or voluntary, **nervous system** governs the impulses from the CNS to the skeletal muscles. The **autonomic nervous system** supplies impulses to smooth muscles, cardiac (heart) muscle, skin, special senses, some proprioceptors, organs, and glands. This system, also referred to as the involuntary nervous system, consists of a sympathetic and parasympathetic division, which possess complementary responses. For example, if the sympathetic nervous system speeds up the heart rate, the parasympathetic nervous system regulates normal heart rate. We will discuss the autonomic nervous system and its two divisions later in this chapter.

NERVE TISSUE

There are two types of nerve tissue: neuroglia and neurons.

Neuroglia, or **glial cells,** are connective tissue that supports, nourishes, protects, insulates, and organizes the delicate neurons. Glial cells are smaller and more numerous than neurons. Over 50 percent of the brain is made up of glial cells. These cells are unable to transmit impulses and never lose their ability to divide (mitosis). For this reason, most brain tumors are made up of glial cells. A type of neuroglial cell, *ependymocyte* (ependyma), line the cranial ventricles and probably assist in the circulation of cerebrospinal fluid.

Neurons (Fig. 10–1) are the basic impulse-conducting cells. They have two major properties: *excitability* (the ability to respond to a stimulus and convert it to a nerve impulse) and *conductability* (the ability to transmit the impulses to other neurons, muscle, and glands). Neurons act like tiny sense organs. A neuron at rest is negatively charged. Some neurons (CNS neurons) do not undergo mitosis.

Author's Note

Nerve tissue has the highest metabolic rate in the body, and lack of oxygen (even for a few minutes) leads to its destruction. Smoking decreases the amount of oxygen that can be carried in the blood, which has a negative effect on neurons. With this in mind, a smoking mother might be sentencing her infant to possible brain damage. In difficult deliveries, the temporary lack of oxygen often leads to cerebral palsy. Lack of oxygen to the brain is the largest single cause of crippling in children.

Parts of a Neuron

Even though neurons vary widely in shape and size to accommodate a number of neural connections, they all have three basic parts: a cell body and two or more cytoplasmic extensions (dendrite and axon). These extensions are often referred to as the nerve fibers.

The **cell body, cyton,** or **soma** contains the nucleus and other standard equipment (organelles) of the cell. The cell body of neurons lacks centrioles, which assist in cell division. The lack of centrioles is one of the reasons neurons cannot reproduce. Neural cell bodies are also the gray matter of the nervous system. In the brain, gray matter is found on the outer layer (cortex) and in the very deep part of the brain; in the spinal cord it is centrally located and forms regions called horns.

Dendrites, or **afferent processes,** are typically short, narrow, and highly branched extensions of the nerve cell. These neural extensions receive and transmit stimuli *toward* the cell body.

Axons, or **efferent processes,** are typically single cylindrical extensions of the cell. Their job is to transmit impulses *away* from the cell body. Axons can possess collateral extensions. As axons terminate, they branch

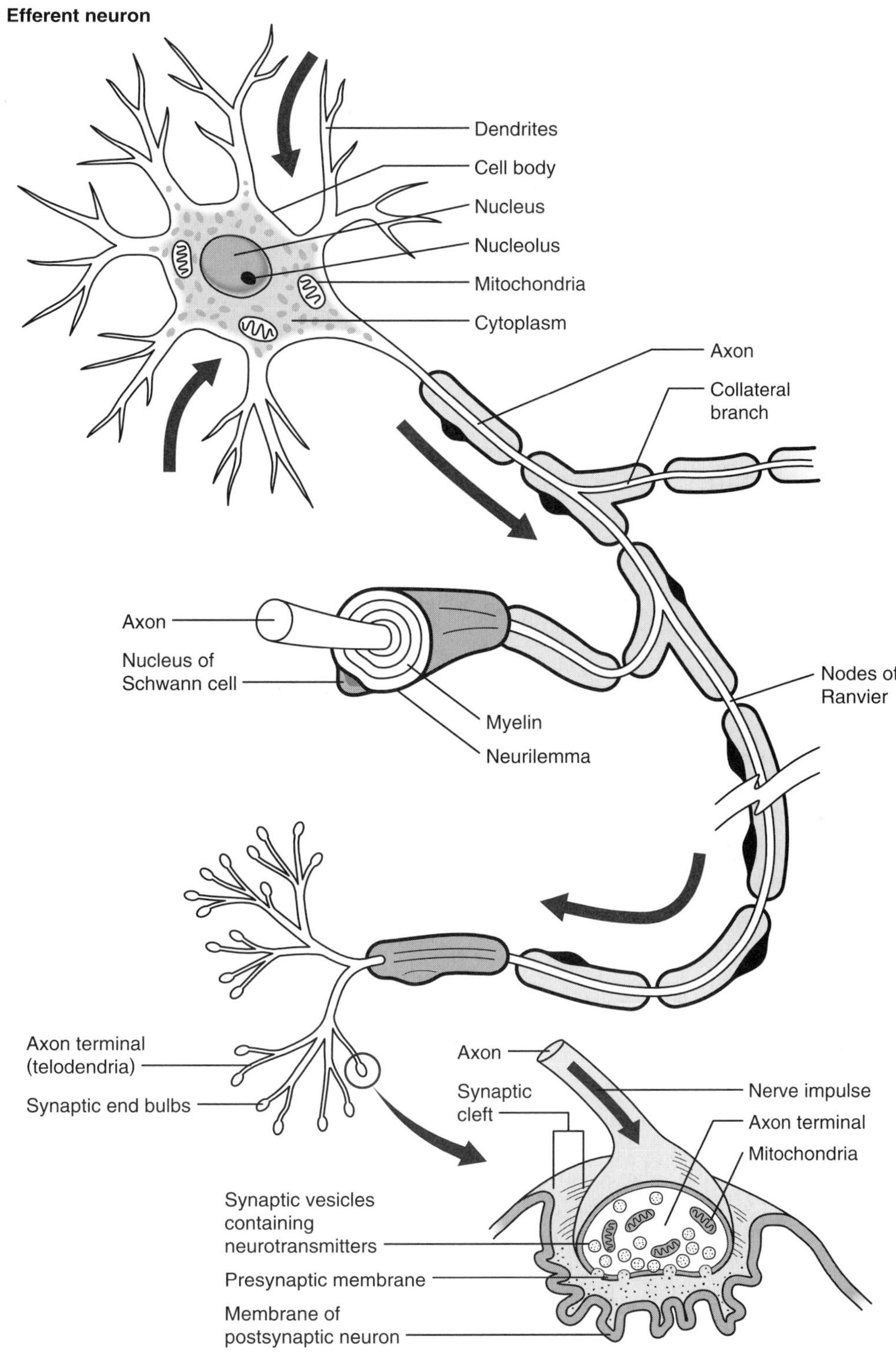

Figure 10•1 A neuron.

into many fine filaments called **axon terminals (telodendron).** The ends of axon terminals have **synaptic end bulbs** (terminal bulbs), bulblike structures that contain sacs called **synaptic vesicles.** These vesicles store **neurotransmitters,** chemicals that facilitate, arouse, or inhibit the transmission of nerve impulses between neurons across synapses.

Most axons are wrapped by a fatty insulating sheath called a **myelin sheath.** Myelin sheaths on axons located in the PNS are produced by one type of glial cell called a **Schwann's cell.** The myelin sheath is actually the cell membrane of a Schwann's cell, with a peripherally located nucleus. The Schwann's cell (a large, flat cell containing a nucleus and cytoplasm) wraps itself around the axon in a spiral fashion, layer after layer. The tighter-wrapped center layers are virtually devoid of cytoplasm, which is pushed along with the nucleus to the outermost spiral layer of the cell, hence the peripheral location. The myelinated axons are known as white matter. Myelin not only electrically insulates the neuron, but also increases the speed of nerve impulse conduction. A layer of one or more Schwann's cells enclosing the myelin sheath is called **neurilemma** (sheath of Schwann), which plays an important role in the regeneration of PNS nerve fibers. At certain intervals along an axon, the myelin sheath has gaps called **nodes of Ranvier.** During neural activity, impulses jump from one node to another, resulting in an increased rate of conduction.

In the CNS, the cells that produce myelin are **oligodendrocytes;** however, these nerve fibers are not enclosed by neurilemma. The lack of neurilemma in the CNS is why nerves within the CNS do not regenerate.

Author's Note

A mnemonic device to help you remember that axons carry neural impulses away from the cell body is both that axon and away begin with the letter A.

Classification of Neurons

Nerves can be classified as either structural (based on the number of cytoplasmic extensions from the cell body) or functional (based on the direction that the impulse is traveling in relation to the CNS).

Structural Classification

Nerves that are classified according to their structure are either unipolar, bipolar, or multipolar.

Unipolar. Associated with sense organs, unipolar neurons possess one extension from the cell body, split into two portions, one portion functioning as a dendrite and another as an axon.

Bipolar. Found in the retina of the eye, inner ear, and olfactory bulb of the nose, bipolar neurons possess one dendrite and one axon extending from the cell body.

Multipolar. The most common type of structural classification, multipolar neurons contain many dendrites and only one axon. These are found in the brain, spinal cord, and peripheral nerves.

Functional Classification

Nerves that are classified according to function are either sensory, association, or motor.

Sensory or **Afferent Neurons.** These nerve cells carry impulses from the internal and external environment toward the brain; sensory neurons are generally close to the surface of the skin. Some sensory receptors lie deep within the body (e.g., proprioceptors, nociceptors). A map of the distribution of afferent nerves is called a *dermatome map.* A dermatome is an area of skin that has sensory innervation originating from a given cord segment (C2–S5) or one of three branches of the fifth cranial (trigeminal) nerve. Dermatomes are roughly the same from person to person, although there is sometimes a significant overlap in innervation between adjacent dermatomes.

Association, Connecting, Interneuron, or **Internuncial.** These neurons connect sensory to motor neurons and vice versa. Association neurons play an important role in reflexes and are typically found in the center of the spinal cord as well as the brain.

Motor or **Efferent Neurons.** These neurons transmit impulses away from the CNS to activate (or inhibit) a muscle or gland.

Grouping of Nerve Tissue

A **nerve** is a group of impulse-carrying fibers connecting the brain and the spinal cord with other parts of the body. A bundle of nerve fibers running down the spinal cord in columns is called a **tract.** Afferent signals travel up the cord in *ascending tracts,* and efferent signals travel down the cord in *descending tracts.* A cluster of nerve cell bodies located in the PNS is called a **ganglion.**

A network of intersecting nerves is called a **plexus.** The body contains many plexuses, such as the cervical, the brachial, the cardiac, the solar, and the lumbosacral.

NERVE IMPULSES

Nerve impulses are the "messages" or "signals" of the nervous system that travel along the neuron(s) from dendrite to axon, and whose movement is accomplished by two characteristics of the neuron: excitability and conductivity. Nerve impulses are electrochemical in nature. *Ions* are electrically charged particles that pass through the ion channels of the neural cell membrane. Their movement is controlled by sets of protein molecules that open or close a gate in response to different stimuli to the neuron. *Neurotransmitters* are chemicals that initiate the change in the plasma membrane. Hormones can also begin a nerve impulse.

Nerves may become excitable due to a stimulus. Any alteration in the environment (internally or externally) can initiate a nerve impulse, such as pain, pressure, movement, heat, light, and the chemicals present in food and odors. The strength and frequency of the stimulus determine whether a nerve impulse is generated. When the stimulus is of sufficient intensity to generate a nerve impulse, **threshold stimulus** is the result. Any single stimulus that is below the threshold level will not result in the creation of a nerve impulse. However, if a **subthreshold stimulus** (one lower than the threshold) should be repeated in succession, the **summation** of these small stimuli may act cumulatively to create a nerve impulse.

Individual receptor thresholds vary. Some respond only to actual tissue damage such as lacerations. When chopping carrots, there is no impulse generated by the knife being near the fingers, yet if the blade slips and cuts the finger, the impulse is created by the tissue damage. Other receptors respond before actual damage has occurred such as in the case of exposure to a flame. Getting too close to a gas burner will create a nerve impulse that produces a rapid recoil from the heat, often without even sustaining a first-degree burn to the tissues.

The nerve impulse itself is always constant and does not vary with the type of stimulus. Nerve impulses created by summation of consecutive subthreshold stimuli have the same effect as nerve impulses created by a threshold stimulus. When a stimulus generates a nerve impulse, the impulse is conducted along the entire neuron at maximum capacity. This principle is referred to as the **all-or-none response.** For example, a firecracker with an 8-foot-long fuse can be lit by a match or by a torch. These are two vastly different stimuli in intensity, yet both methods result in the same rate of fuse burning (impulse) and in the same result or response, the firecracker's exploding. This is a system even simpler than Morse code—just dots, no dashes. The dots are all equal, and the only way to vary the intensity is to alter the frequency or the number of dots per second.

When such a stimulus is constant over time, **adaptation**—a decrease in sensitivity to a prolonged stimulus—may occur. Adaptation tends to be rapid regarding pressure, touch, and smell. We become accustomed to the weight of our clothes during the day and an odor that offended us when we first entered the room is no longer detected at the end of the day. It occurs more slowly with pain, position, and internal regulation. This is a protective mechanism that prevents us from "becoming used to severe pain" on a short-term basis or that allows us to "forget" that we are standing with our weight on our left foot rather than our right.

Now that we understand the relationship between the stimulus and the impulse, let's look at the dynamics of the nerve impulse itself. The nerve impulse is the body's quickest way of controlling and maintaining homeostasis. **Action potential** is a measurement of electrical difference between the charge inside the cell and the charge outside the neural cell membrane. The difference in voltage is created by the presence of ions or charged particles. The resting neuron is one that is *not* conducting a nerve impulse at a given time. The outside of the cell holds a positive charge and the inside of the cell is negatively charged.

As mentioned earlier, a system of gateways controls the flow of ions both into and out of the neuron through the cellular membrane. When a stimulus is applied, the cell responds by changing the membrane's level of ion permeability. The main ions related to nerve cells are the sodium ion (Na^+) and the potassium ion (K^+), both positively charged and existing inside and outside the membrane. The concentration of sodium ions is greater outside the membrane, and the concentration of potassium ions is greater inside the resting cellular membrane. Also inside the cell membrane are large, negatively charged proteins and organic phosphate particles. The membrane is polarized when the inside of the membrane bears a negative charge and the outside of the membrane bears a positive charge, and an action potential is generated.

When a stimulus is added to a neuron, the sodium ion channels open, permitting sodium ions to flow into the cell. Since there are more positively charged sodium ions going into the cell than leaving, the interior negative charge goes first to zero (neutral). This reduces the polarization of the cell membrane, a process known as depolarization.

As the large migration of sodium ions across the neural membrane continues, the polarity of the cell membrane *reverses* due to the increased presence of positive ions inside the cell. This is referred to as reverse polarization. The cell's interior is now positive due to the higher concentration of positive ions. This creates a differential in charge, which translates to a negative charge on the outside of the membrane.

Once this charge has occurred, the cellular membrane once again becomes impermeable to sodium ions. The potassium ion channels open and allow potassium to leave the cell. As the positive potassium ions leave the cell, the outside once again becomes positively charged, and the inside of the membrane resumes its negative charge. This is known as repolarization.

It is the reverse polarization in the initial section of the cell membrane that acts as the stimulus for the adjacent sections of the neuron. The initial stimulus has created a ripple or wave effect that travels down the cell as the depolarization–reverse polarization–repolarization or action potential or nerve impulse, process is repeated. Much like a line of dominoes, the ripple of current travels the length of the neuron until it reaches its destination. This is true for sensory neurons that may be bringing temperature information to the brain, for motor neurons that may be sending a message to the eyelids to blink, and for chains of neurons that stimulate adjacent neurons.

After the cell has returned to its normal polarized state during the repolarization process, the charge is

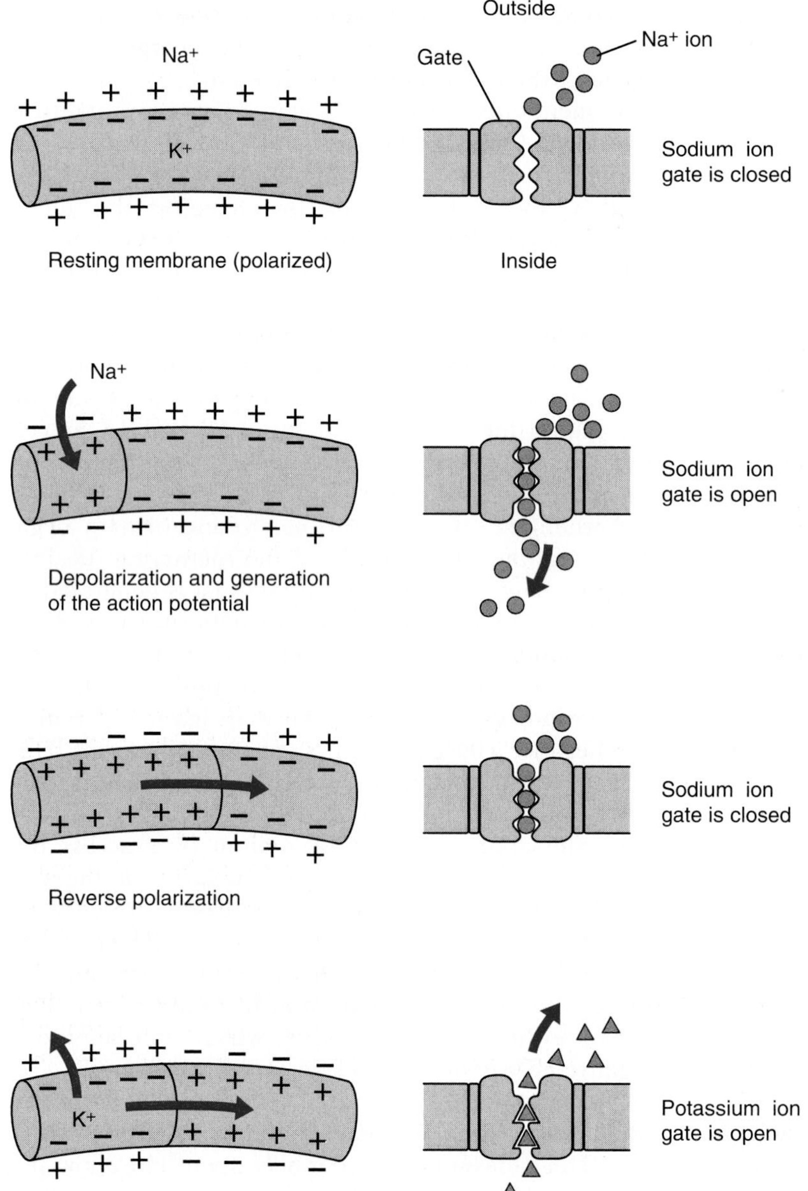

Figure 10•2 Neural membrane resting and action potential and/or sodium-potassium pump.

reinstated, but the distribution of sodium and potassium ions is often reversed. This distribution will be set back to normal by means of the sodium-potassium pump (Fig. 10–2).

The Sodium-Potassium Pump

The **sodium-potassium pump** is a function of the ion channels of the neurons. The pump, however, actively transports sodium and potassium, even when the cell is resting, in order to maintain cell membrane polarity. The sodium-potassium pump is easier to understand if it is pictured as a sprocket. The sodium and potassium ions attach between the spokes or teeth of the sprocket that will move them from one side of the cell membrane to the other, just as a revolving door moves people between the inside and outside of a building.

The sodium ions (Na^+) inside the cell membrane attach themselves to the spaces between the "teeth" of the pump, triggering the breakdown of adenosine triphosphate (ATP) into adenosine diphosphate and a free phosphate. The free phosphate attaches itself to the pump, and this action changes the shape of the pump in a way that moves the sodium ions to the outside of the cellular membrane. At this point, the potassium ions (K^+) outside the cellular membrane attach to the pump, releasing the phosphate. The pump reverts to its original shape, drawing the potassium ions into the cell where they are released, and the cycle perpetuates itself again.

Nerve Impulse Conduction

Nerve fibers with larger diameters conduct impulses faster than those with smaller diameters. Rapid reflexes require fast impulse conduction along nerves. However, if these axons were all large, they would be cumbersome and create a packaging problem. The problem is solved by keeping axon diameters small and by using another means, myelin sheaths, to achieve rapid conduction velocities. A myelin sheath is a lipid or fatty insulator surrounding sections of the axon. The myelin aids in conduction and insulation and prevents the "leaking" of microcurrent from one neuron to influence another.

Located along the axon are unmyelinated gaps called nodes of Ranvier. Since the myelinated segments of the axon are insulated, the action potential or depolarization process occurs only where there is an absence of myelin (at the nodes of Ranvier). The impulse then jumps across the myelinated section of the axon to the next node, and so on. This jumping effect enables the impulse to traverse a much longer distance in a much shorter time. It's basically like a game of checkers. You can move your checker across the board one square at a time, or you can jump the opposing pieces and make it across the board much quicker. In this way, myelinated fibers conduct impulses faster than unmyelinated.

SYNAPSE AND SYNAPTIC TRANSMISSION

The **synapse** is the junction between two neurons, or between a neuron and a muscle or gland, where they connect to transmit information. This junction is actually more of a fluid-filled separation or space than it is an actual connection. **Synaptic transmission** is the electrochemical method by which the nerve impulse from one neuron bridges the synaptic gap (or synaptic cleft) to convey the nerve impulse to the next neuron (Fig. 10–3). This is a one-way nerve impulse conduction from the axon of one cell to the dendrite of another.

The synapse is located between the end of the axon of one neuron and the dendrites of the subsequent neuron. The axon carries the nerve impulse away from the nerve cell body. At the distal end of each axon are clusters of short branches called telodendria. Each telodendrium terminates in a small bud known as a synaptic bulb or knob, which bulb contains synaptic vesicles that produce and store chemical neurotransmitters. These neurotransmitters are released into the fluid-filled gap and are absorbed by the dendrite, muscle, or gland cell terminal on the other side of the synaptic gap.

Neurotransmitters

Neurotransmitters is a collective term for a vast range of chemicals that facilitate, arouse, or inhibit the transmission of nerve impulses between synapses. These chemical messengers are stored in vesicles at the synaptic bulbs, and each vesicle may store as many as 10,000 different molecules. Neurotransmitters depart the synaptic knobs and cross the synaptic cleft, thereby bridging the gap between the neurons. The neurotransmitter then attaches itself to a receptor site on the postsynaptic neuron. The receptor sites are located adjacent to the ion channels. The action of chemical bonding at the receptor site acts as a stimulus on the adjacent neuron by affecting sodium and potassium movement across the neural membrane.

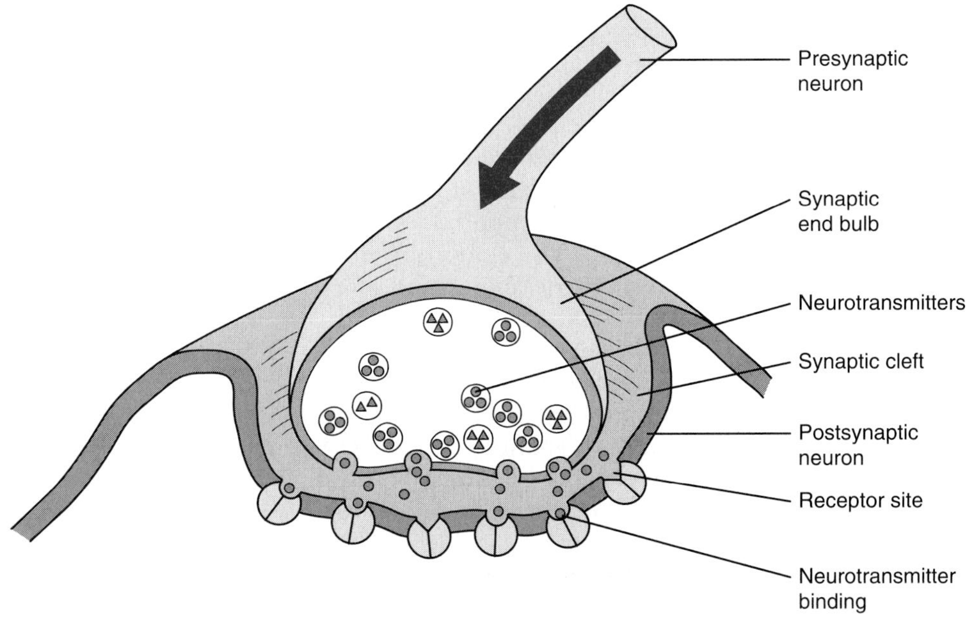

Figure 10•3 Synaptic cleft and neurotransmitter action.

Neurotransmitters can be either excitatory or inhibitory. Excitatory neurotransmitters decrease the negativity of postsynaptic membrane potentials, thereby increasing the impulse rate. Inhibitory neurotransmitters increase membrane potentials, which increases the threshold needed to create the nerve impulse.

The action of the neurotransmitter does not persist for a long time because it is continuously removed from the synaptic cleft by either enzymes or by reuptake (the drawing up of a substance) into nerve terminals. Ninety-nine percent of neural impulses are caused by chemicals; the other 1 percent is electrical and exists in intercalated disks of heart muscle (myocardium).

Types of Neurotransmitters

There are about 30 known or suspected neurotransmitters in the body. The following list contains some of the more important ones.

1. *Acetylcholine,* which is vital for stimulating muscle contraction, is made from choline, which is found in egg yolks, liver, soybeans, butter, peanuts, and other foods. This neurotransmitter stimulates vagus nerve and parasympathetic nervous system activity and is rapidly destroyed by the enzyme acetylcholinesterase.
2. *Catecholamines* are a chemical family containing norepinephrine, epinephrine, and dopamine. The major functions of catecholamines include the excitation and inhibition of certain muscles, cardiac excitation, metabolic action, and endocrine action. Catecholamines act directly on sympathetic effector cells to cause the desired action.

   Epinephrine is a hormone as well as a neurotransmitter secreted by the adrenal medulla, and this chemical simulates the functions of the sympathetic nervous system.

   Norepinephrine, like epinephrine, is both a hormone and a neurotransmitter secreted by the adrenal medulla; this chemical mediates several physiologic and metabolic responses that follow the stimulation of the sympathetic nerves. For example, norepinephrine acts to increase blood pressure by vasoconstriction but does not affect cardiac output. This neurotransmitter may be related to arousal, dreaming, and mood regulation.

   Dopamine is a neurotransmitter that is the precursor of norepinephrine and may have an inhibitory effect on movement. Dopamine is also implicated in attention and learning. A depletion of dopamine produces the symptoms of rigidity, tremors, and uncoordinated and slower than normal movement.
3. *Serotonin,* a naturally occurring derivative of tryptophan (an amino acid), acts as a potent vasoconstrictor. It is theorized to be important for sensory perception, mood regulation, and normal sleep.
4. *Gamma-aminobutyric acid* (GABA) is an amino acid with neurotransmitter activity; found in the brain, it has an inhibitory effect of nerve transmission.
5. *Histamine,* a compound found in all cells, causes dilation of capillaries, decreased blood pressure, and constriction of smooth muscles of the bronchi. The release of histamine is stimulated by allergic, inflammatory reactions.

Conditions That Affect Neurotransmitters

Synaptic transmission can be altered by drugs, disease, and direct pressure.

1. *Clostridium botulinum* (responsible for food poisoning) inhibits the neurotransmitter release of acetylcholine, thus inhibiting muscle contraction. The botulism toxin is a carefully controlled substance that can be used medically to correct chronic contractions of muscles caused by injuries such as brain lesions.
2. *Curare* is a toxin derived from plants and was often used by South American tribes to enhance the power of a blowgun. Modern synthetic forms of curare are used during surgery to produce muscle relaxation. Curare and its synthetic cousins compete for acetylcholine receptor sites, thus preventing muscular contraction.
3. The *"-caine"* drugs (procaine [Novocain], lidocaine, cocaine) are painkillers. They affect the neuron on the electrical level by attaching to the sodium gates, which prevents sodium from crossing the membrane, preventing a nerve impulse.
4. *Nicotine, caffeine,* and *benzedrine* mimic the neurostimulant effects of epinephrine. They lower the threshold for neural excitation, which enhances facilitation of the nerve impulse; however, there are no enzymes to neutralize them or to remove them from the synaptic cleft. The net effect is that action potential is prolonged, resulting in a general increase of nerve stimulation.
5. *Hypnotics, tranquilizers,* and *anesthetics,* the opposites of caffeine and nicotine, are groups of drugs that raise the threshold for neural excitation and inhibit the facilitation of nerve impulses.
6. *Neostigmine* (Sevin dust) and strychnine (rat poison) are poisons used for pest control (insecticides). They block acetylcholinesterase, which prolongs muscular contractions and may cause convulsions and death.
7. *Opiates* are a family of drugs that can permeate the blood-brain barrier (a very selective semipermeable membrane that controls which substances are allowed into the brain). Opiates are chemically similar to naturally produced enkephalins of the body,

which means opiates can attach to the same receptor sites. This similarity can fool the body into letting the opiates cross the blood-brain barrier. Opiates alter pain perception and tend to be analgesic. An example is morphine, which is chemically similar to endorphin (endogenous morphine).

8. *Sustained pressure* applied to a nerve can interrupt both sensory and motor function. A small amount of pressure sustained for a prolonged time, such as sitting with the legs crossed, may cause the tingling sensation experienced as "the leg is asleep." Trying to stand on the leg may prove unsuccessful due to impaired motor function.
9. *Myasthenia gravis* is a disease in which antibodies are produced that affect the acetylcholine receptors in the tissue of skeletal muscles, thereby disrupting muscular response.

CENTRAL NERVOUS SYSTEM

The central nervous system, surrounded and protected by the cranium and vertebral column, is located in the dorsal cavity. The CNS is further protected by a liquid called cerebrospinal fluid and a connective tissue membranous covering called the meninges.

Cerebrospinal Fluid

Circulating around the brain and spinal cord is a clear, colorless fluid called **cerebrospinal fluid** (CSF) that functions as a shock absorber and provides a medium for nutrient exchange and waste removal. CSF is produced in chambers called the choroid plexus within the ventricles of the brain and is similar in composition to blood, minus the red blood cells. The fluid is sensitive to glucose and electrolyte balance as well as to changes in the carbon dioxide content.

Meninges

The entire central nervous system (brain and spinal cord) is enveloped by special connective tissue membranes: the **meninges.** The innermost layer is called the **pia mater,** which is thin and vascular and hugs the brain; so tight is the covering that it is difficult to remove the pia mater without damaging the brain's surface (Fig. 10–4).

The middle layer is called the **arachnoid** which possesses many threadlike strands, giving it a webbed appearance.

The outermost layer, the thick and durable **dura mater,** lies up against the bone and contains a double layer of connective tissue (the outer layer representing periosteum). Within the two layers are thick venous channels called sinuses. The dura mater dips down between the cerebral hemispheres *(falx cerebri),* separates the cerebrum and the cerebellum *(tentorium cerebelli),* and divides the paired cerebellar hemispheres (*falx cerebelli*).

The *subdural space,* filled with circulating serous fluid, lies between the dura mater and the arachnoid. Between the pia mater and the arachnoid is the *subarachnoid space,* filled with CSF. The *epidural space* lies between the dura and the vertebral canal; this space,

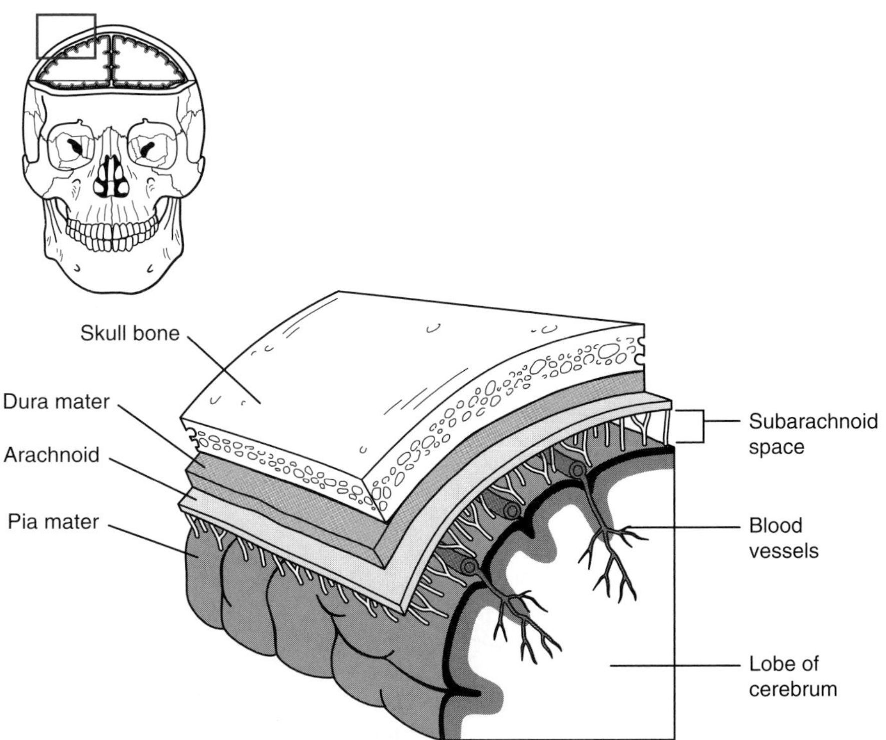

Figure 10•4 The meninges around the brain.

which is the safest place for injections such as saddle blocks, contains adipose tissue, connective tissue, and blood vessels.

Author's Note

A mnemonic device to recall the three layers of the meninges, from deep to superficial, is *PAD*. *P*, pia mater; *A*, arachnoid; *D*, dura mater.

BRAIN

One of the largest organs in the body, the **brain** contains an estimated 9 to 15 billion neurons. Brain cells can use glucose only as an energy source, and this glucose cannot be stored as glycogen, unlike the glucose stored by liver or muscle cells. Glucose only breaks down by aerobic respiration, so the brain needs a continuous supply of both glucose and oxygen. Although comprising only 2 percent of body weight, the brain utilizes about 20 percent of the body's oxygen intake. Oxygen deprivation kills brain cells quickly, in as little as 1 to 2 minutes.

The brain is where sensory information is fused into character and behavior. The brain's unimpressive appearance gives no hints of its remarkable abilities. In the embryo, the skull forms before the brain is finished; this results in the forebrain turning in on itself and mushrooming. Fissures (sulci) are grooves or depressions in the outer layer of the brain (cortex), and gyri are elevated ridges of tissue. Fissures divide the brain into hemispheres and lobes (Fig. 10–5).

The brain is divided into four major regions: cerebrum, diencephalon, cerebellum, and brain stem (stalk) (Fig. 10–6).

Cerebrum

Shaped like a boxing glove, the **cerebrum** is divided by the longitudinal fissure into two large (right and left) *cerebral hemispheres*. The cerebrum governs all higher

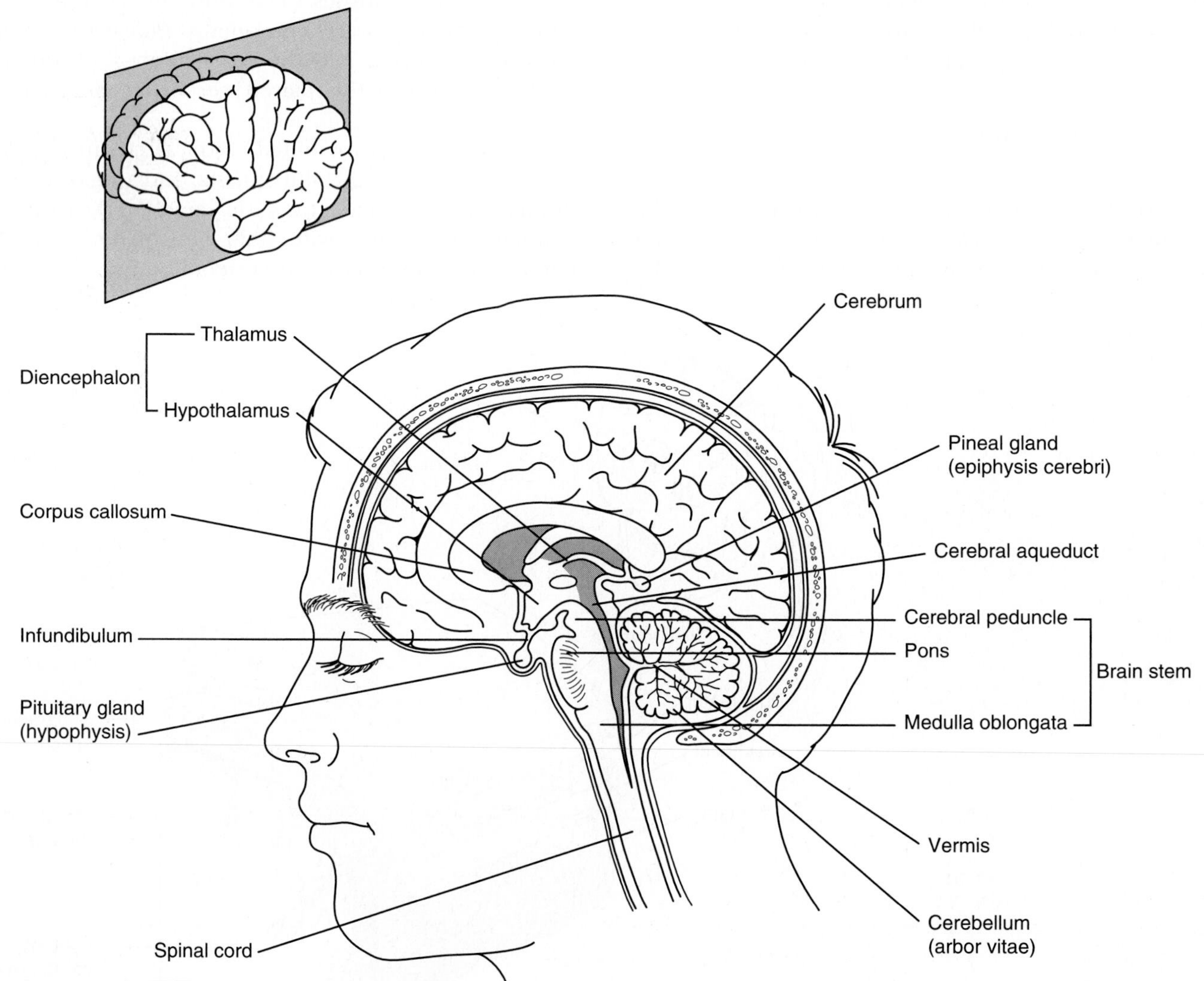

Figure 10•5 Sagittal slice of the brain.

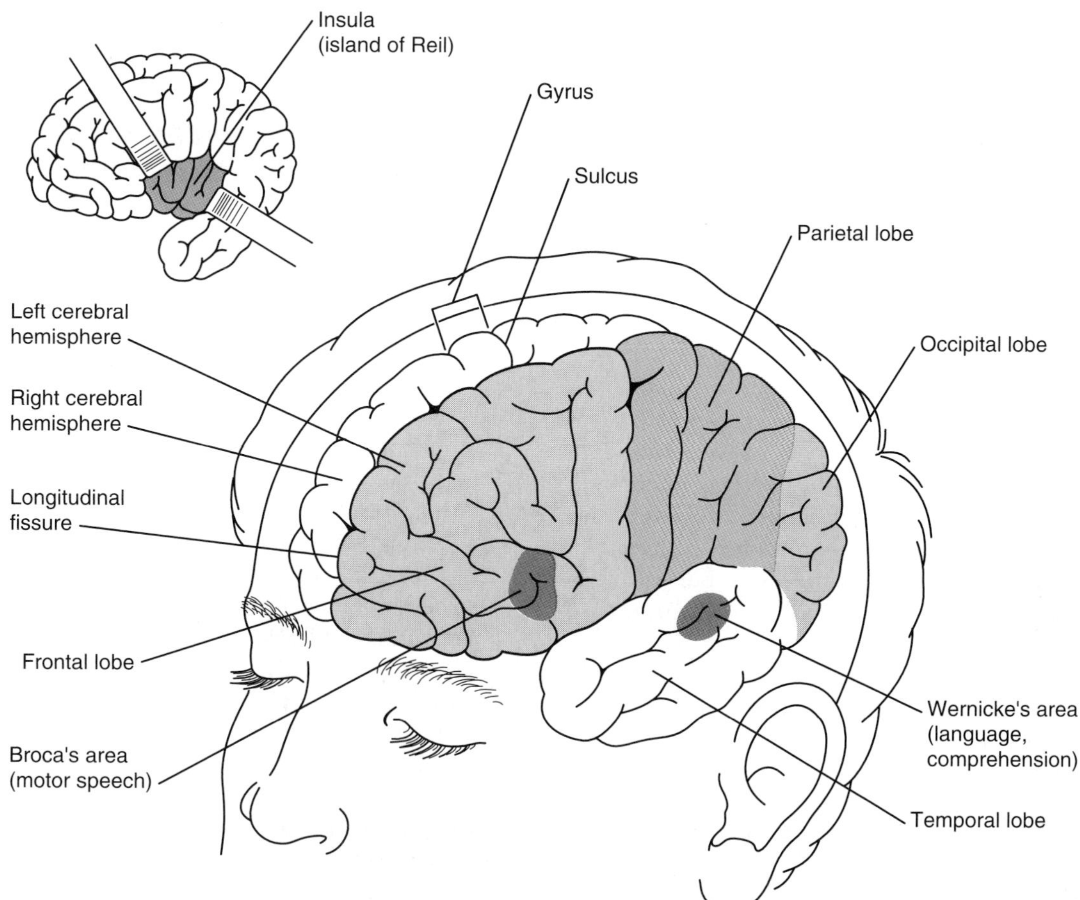

Figure 10•6 Cerebrum outlining lobes and insula.

functions (i.e., language, memory, reasoning, and some aspects of personality) and is the largest region of the brain. Connecting the two cerebral hemispheres are large fibrous bundles of transverse (arcuate) fibers, the **corpus callosum,** which provides a communicative pathway for impulses to move from one hemisphere to another (contralateral control).

The **cerebral cortex** is a thin gray layer covering the outer portion of the cerebrum. White matter, which constitutes most of the cerebrum, lies beneath the cerebral cortex. On the surface of the cerebrum are elevations called **gyri** and depressions called **sulci** (grooves).

Within each hemisphere of the cerebrum are **lobes,** which are named for the bone each lies beneath. The *frontal* lobe regulates motor output, cognition, and speech production (**Broca's area;** typically the left hemisphere only); the *parietal lobes* govern somatosensory input (namely the skin and muscles); the *temporal lobes* house an auditory and an olfactory area, as well as **Wernicke's area** (an area critical to language comprehension; typically the left hemisphere only); and the *occipital lobe* contains a center for visual input. Hidden by parts of the frontal, parietal, and temporal lobes is a structure called the *insula* (*island of Reil*), which is sometimes considered a fifth lobe of the cerebrum.

Diencephalon

Located in the center of the brain, the **diencephalon** houses two primary structures: the thalamus and hypothalamus.

The **thalamus,** which is nearly 80 percent of the diencephalon, is a relay station and interpretation center for all sensory impulses except olfaction.

Suspended by a slender stalk (*infundibulum*), the **hypothalamus** is a small structure that governs many important homeostatic functions: It regulates the autonomic nervous system and the endocrine system by governing the pituitary gland; and it controls hunger, thirst, temperature regulation, anger, aggression, hormones, sexual behavior, sleep patterns, and consciousness. A *Lancet* reader once asked, "Is there any pie in the vertebrate organism into which the hypothalamus does not dip its finger?"

The **pituitary gland** (*hypophysis*), which sits in the sella turcica of the sphenoid bone, is considered the "master gland" of the endocrine system because its hormones control and stimulate all other glands to produce their individual products. The **pineal gland** *(epiphysis cerebri)* is located below the corpus callosum. The pineal gland, or *epiphysis cerebri,* is a pinecone-shaped structure in the brain, attached to the roof of the third ventricle and inferior to the corpus callosum. Although its function is not clear, the pineal gland produces and secretes the hormone melatonin. Both of these glands are discussed in the endocrine chapter.

Cerebellum

The **cerebellum** is a cauliflower-shaped structure located posterior and inferior to the cerebrum. The cerebellum is the second largest part of the brain and consists of two cerebellar hemispheres connected by a middle section, the **vermis.** Like the cerebrum, the cerebellum consists of a **cerebellar cortex** (thin outer layer of gray matter). White matter lies beneath the cerebellar cortex and is structured as the *arbor vitae* (tree of life).

The cerebellum is concerned with muscle tone, coordinates skeletal muscles and balance (posture integration and equilibrium), and controls fine and gross motor movements.

Brain Stem

The **brain stem** contains three main structures: the midbrain, the pons, and the medulla oblongata.

The most superior structure of the brain stem, the **midbrain** (mesencephalon), contains two *cerebral peduncles* that house the voluntary motor tracts descending from the cerebral cortex to the spinal cord. The *cerebral aqueduct,* a narrow canal conveying CSF, is located in the midbrain.

The large rounded area below the midbrain is the **pons,** which relays messages from the cerebral cortex to the spinal cord and helps regulate breathing. The pons can be compared to the thalamus in the sense that both are relay stations. Four pairs of cranial nerves branch off the pons.

The most inferior portion of the brain stem is the **medulla oblongata,** which continues downward to form the spinal cord. The medulla oblongata contains much of the crossing-over fibers that cause the left cerebral hemisphere's association with the body's right side (*decussation*). Conversely, the right hemisphere is associated with the left side of the body.

The medulla, often considered the most vital part of the brain, contains the respiratory center, the cardiac center, and the vasomotor center. The medulla also controls gastric secretions and reflexes such as sweating, sneezing, swallowing, and, vomiting. Five pairs of cranial nerves branch from the medulla. Medullary disease or injury is often fatal.

Electrical Brain Wave States and States of Consciousness

Scientists have noted four different types of brain wave patterns and identified the sort of activity the brain is usually engaged in during these states of consciousness. Brain waves are rhythmic electric impulses produced in the cerebral cortex. Most patterns, identified by Greek letters, are similar for all normal people. These wave patterns are beta, alpha, theta, and delta.

Beta (13 to 30 Hz). Beta is associated with wakeful consciousness and being mentally active. Attention is focused on external surroundings, and activity is typified by rational thinking, some scattered thought patterns, and occasional distractions. High-intensity beta waves are associated with extreme stress. Dreaming while sleeping (rapid eye movement, or REM) appears as beta waves.

Alpha (8 to 12 Hz). The alpha state is regarded as awake but relaxed; there is focused awareness with synchronization between the right and left cerebral hemispheres. Alpha activity is related to inner consciousness and is associated with relaxation, self-healing, creativity, and meditation.

Theta (4 to 8 Hz). Theta is associated with deep relaxation, unfocused attention, dreamlike awareness, sleep, the collective subconscious, and out-of-body experiences. This state of consciousness is used to access deep-rooted memories.

Delta (0.5 to 4 Hz). Delta patterns are associated with deep sleep or comalike states.

Blood-Brain Barrier

The **blood-brain barrier** is a selective semipermeable wall of blood capillaries with a thick basement membrane and glial cells (oligodendrocytes) that prevent or slow down the passage of some drugs and other chemical compounds and that keep disease-causing organisms such as viruses from traveling from the blood into the central nervous system. Blood itself contains chemicals that can damage neurons; if blood comes into contact with neurons, they die.

Spinal Cord

The **spinal cord,** located in the vertebral canal of the vertebral column, is an extension of the brain stem from the foramen magnum to about the region of L2.

The spinal cord stops growing before the spinal column; hence, there is a difference in length. The functions of the spinal cord are to carry sensory impulses to the brain, to carry motor impulses from the brain, and to mediate the reflex response. Some texts consider the spinal cord to be part of the brain; others see the cord as a cable of nerves.

There are two enlargements located in the length of the spinal cord: one in the cervical region (cervical enlargement) and a second one in the lumbar region (lumbar enlargement). The lower end of the spinal cord is marked by the threadlike **filum terminale,** which is anchored to the coccyx. The ends of the cord fan out like a horse's tail, and form a structure appropriately called the **cauda equina.**

The spinal cord consists of 31 segments, each of which gives rise to a pair of spinal nerves. Beginning at the top of the cord, there are 8 cervical nerves, 12 thoracic nerves, 5 lumber nerves, 5 sacral nerves, and 1 coccygeal nerve (Fig. 10–7).

Each pair of spinal nerves joins the spinal column at two points, one on the left and another on the right. Each spinal nerve of each pair has an anterior and a posterior root. The *anterior,* or *ventral, root* contains motor neurons, and the *posterior,* or *dorsal, root* contains sensory neurons. The posterior root of the spinal nerve contains a swelling called the *posterior,* or *dorsal* (*sensory*), *root ganglion,* which is a collection of cell bodies of sensory neurons.

In cross-section of the spinal cord, white matter is on the outside and gray matter (H-shaped or butterfly-shaped) is on the inside of the cord. In the center of the spinal cord is the central canal, which runs the entire length of the spinal cord, containing CSF. The sides of the gray H are called horns, which are divided into the anterior, lateral, and posterior horns. White matter is organized into regions called columns (funiculi): the anterior, lateral, and posterior columns, within which are groups of myelinated axons called *nerve tracts.* Sensory impulses travel up the cord to the brain on ascending tracts, and motor impulses travel down and out the cord on descending tracts.

The spinal dura mater separates from the spinal cord and adheres to the spinal column. The space created by this separated dura filled with adipose and connective tissue is called the *epidural space.*

Reflexes

The farther an impulse has to travel, the longer it takes to reach its destination. When we see the light turn red, there is a brief delay of time before our foot goes for the brake pedal. Some situations require less of a time delay to prevent significant tissue damage (e.g., touching a hot skillet). For this reason, we have reflexes.

Although the neuron is a structural unit of the nervous system, a functional component of the nervous system is the **reflex arc.** The reflex arc consists of two or more neurons, at least one of which is sensory and one of which is a motor neuron innervating a muscle, gland, or organ. A **reflex** is an instantaneous, involuntary response to a stimulus originating from either inside or outside the body. Instead of the sensory impulse going all the way to the brain where it can be analyzed and a correct motor response selected, a reflex allows a shorter and quicker response.

The strong afferent stimuli coming into the posterior horn of the spinal cord excites an interneuron (also referred to as the *internuncial pool*), which synapses with a motor neuron to create a strong efferent motor response. We drop the hot skillet without thinking about it. Reflexes are essentially a protective shortcut or bypass around the brain and can be a reaction to stimuli such as pain, pressure, or even loud noises. The **flexor withdrawal reflex** is the one most commonly associated with pain. **Somatic reflexes** are those that are responsible for the contraction of skeletal muscle (*effector*) such as when the doctor taps your patellar tendon with the little rubber hammer (knee-jerk or patellar reflex). **Visceral,** or **autonomic, reflexes** maintain homeostasis through coughing, sneezing, blinking, and correcting the heart rate, respiratory rate, and blood pressure.

In the normal reflex arc, afferent impulses generate normal levels of efferent impulses resulting in muscular tonus, in proper skin function, in good joint movement, and in vascular function. In the specific case of pain stimulus, the resulting phenomenon is known as a **physiopathological reflex arc.** The increased afferent impulses (pain) cause a disturbance in the internuncial pool, which generates a spontaneous increase in efferent motor impulse, sending an awareness of the pain to the brain. The increased motor stimuli cause vasoconstriction, epidermal constriction, a decrease in visceral function, an increase in muscular tonus, and an increase in intrajoint pressure. This basic response is supported by **Hilton's law,** which states that the nerve trunk that supplies innervation to a joint in the body also supplies enervation to the muscle of that joint and to the skin and connective tissue surrounding the muscles (Fig.10–8).

Author's Note

Reciprocal inhibition is an involuntary reflex that occurs when a muscle receives a nerve impulse to contract and its antagonist simultaneously receives an impulse to relax. It would be difficult to move if all muscles contracted at the same time. Reciprocal inhibition ensures that when the prime mover (agonist) is creating movement, its antagonist cooperates by elon-

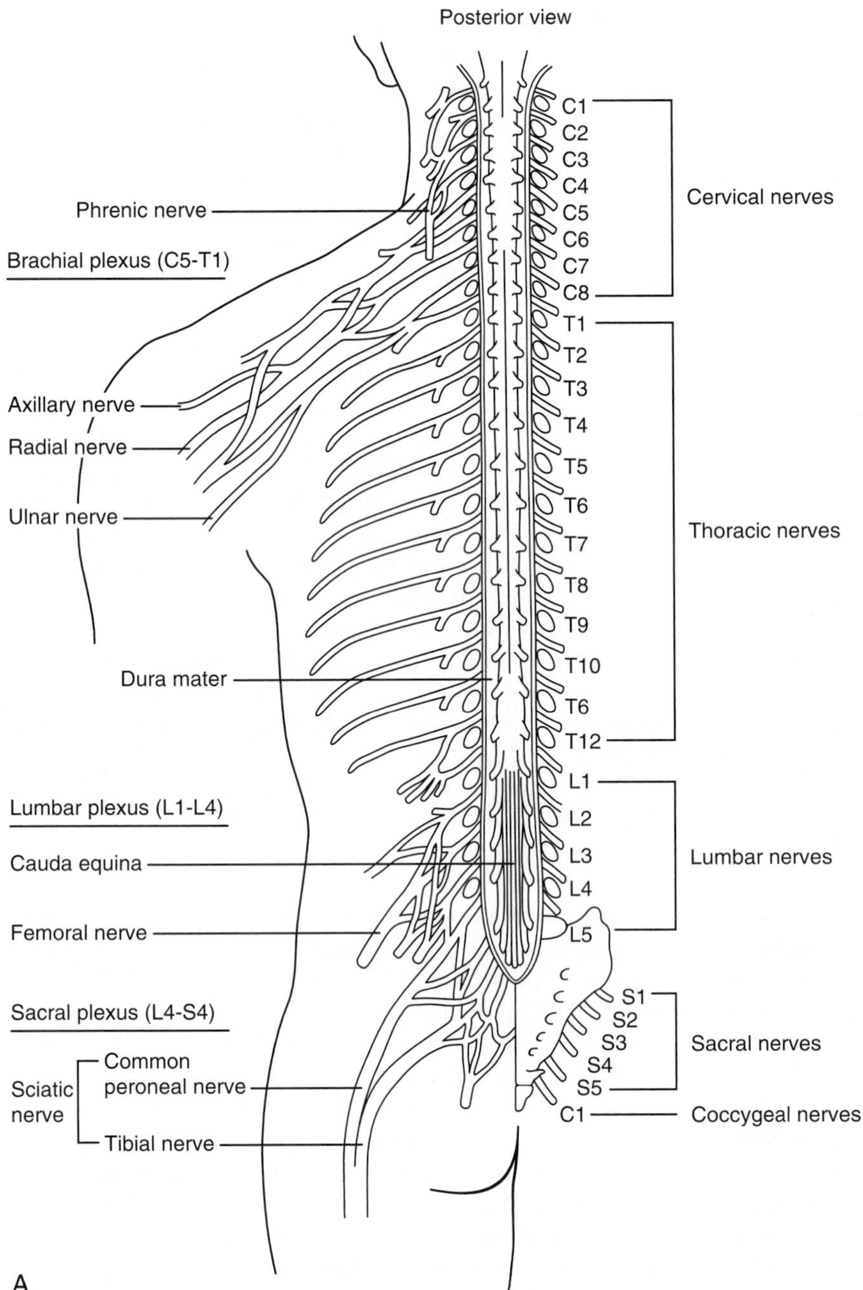

Figure 10•7 The spinal cord.

gating. In a subject with normal neurological function, these two impulses automatically occur simultaneously.

This principle can be used by massage therapists to turn off temporarily neural messages of contraction in acute muscle cramps. For example, when the soleus and gastrocnemius are experiencing a muscle cramp, the cramp could be relieved by forcibly contracting their antagonist, the tibialis anterior. This is best accomplished through isometric contraction (contraction against resistance). Instruct the supine client to dorsiflex her ankle while the massage therapist applies resistance. The therapist can accomplish this by interlacing her fingers around the top of the foot and leaning backward as the client tries to point her toes toward her chin. Maintain the contraction for 10 to 20 seconds, then release. Repeat three times.

The term "reciprocal inhibition" is also used in behavioral therapy. During an anxiety-producing event, an activity that decreases anxiety is intentionally performed. The introduction of the relaxing event diminishes anxiety; the stressful stimulus creates less anxiety. Examples of relaxing stimuli are deep abdominal breathing or systematically relaxing the facial muscles.

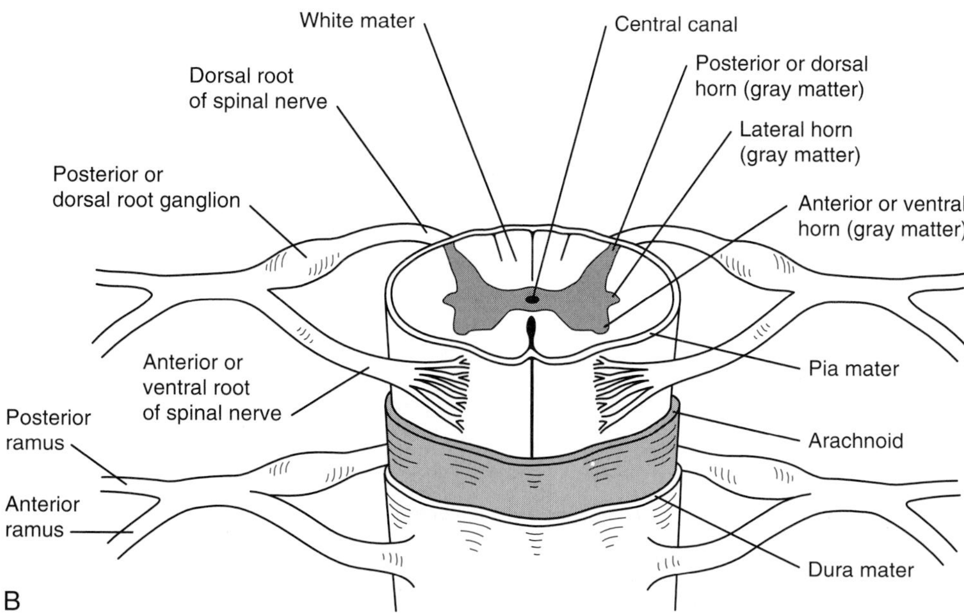

Figure 10•7 *Continued*

This is one of the principles in the Lamaze childbirth method (Fig. 10–9).

PERIPHERAL NERVOUS SYSTEM

The **peripheral nervous system** (PNS) contains all the nerves outside the central nervous system. The PNS can be subdivided into the somatic nervous system and the autonomic nervous system. The somatic nervous system contains the cranial nerves (those nerves originating from the cranium or brain) and spinal nerves (those originating from the spinal cord). The somatic nervous system will be discussed in this section; the autonomic nervous system will be discussed in the next section.

Cranial Nerves

There are 12 pair of cranial nerves. They emerge from the inferior surface of the brain and are named by roman numerals or the areas that the nerves supply.

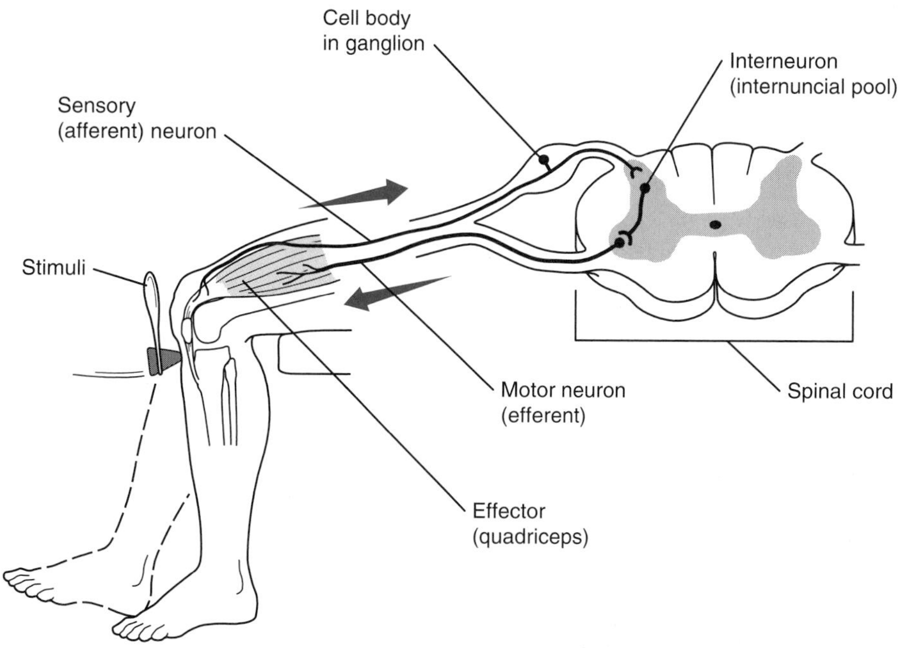

Figure 10•8 A reflex arc.

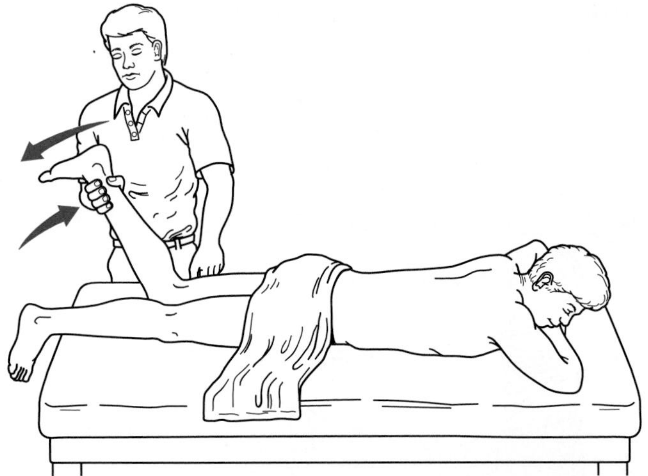

Figure 10•9 Demonstrating reciprocal inhibition.

Some cranial nerves are sensory, some motor, and some are both sensory and motor (Fig. 10–10). These cranial nerves are listed below:

I: *Olfactory*—smell
II: *Optic*—vision
III: *Oculomotor*—moves the eyeball and eyelid; constricts the pupil
IV: *Trochlear*—moves the eyeball
V: *Trigeminal* (*trifacial*) —the great sensory nerve of the face and head; contains three branches for chewing, pain, and temperature
VI: *Abducens*—moves the eyeball
VII: *Facial*—facial expression; saliva and tear production
VIII: *Vestibulocochlear* (*auditory* or *acoustic*) —two branches to the inner ear; conveys messages of equilibrium and hearing
IX: *Glossopharyngeal*—saliva production, taste, and swallowing
X: *Vagus*—receives sensations from the external ear and external auditory canal, and thoracic and abdominal organs; aids digestion; important in regulating heart activity
XI: *Accessory* (*spinal accessory*) —controls the tongue for speech and swallowing, innervates the trapezius and sternocleidomastoid
XII: *Hypoglossal*—moves the tongue for speech and swallowing

Author's Note

There is a mnemonic device to help you remember the names of the 12 cranial nerves: Oh, Oh, Oh! To Touch And Feel Very Green Vegetables, AH! (olfactory, optic, oculomotor, trochlear, trigeminal, abducens, facial, vestibulocochlear, glossopharyngeal, vagus, accessory, and hypoglossal)

OR

On Old Olympus's Towering Tops, A Finn And German Viewed Some Hops. (olfactory, optic, oculomotor, trochlear, trigeminal, abducens, facial, auditory, glossopharyngeal, vagus, spinal accessory, and hypoglossal)

Spinal Nerves

There are 31 pairs of spinal nerves, numbered according to the region from which they emerge and the level of spinal cord (example C7, T5, L4, S2). The first pair emerges between C1 and the occipital bone. When a spinal nerve exits the spinal cord, it divides into two branches: the **anterior (ventral) ramus** and the **posterior (dorsal) ramus.** The anterior ramus innervates the extremities, the lateral and anterior trunk, and the superficial muscles of the back; the posterior ramus innervates the skin and deep muscles of the back. All spinal nerves have sensory and motor components. When the nerves leave the spinal cord, they branch out to supply organs, muscles, and skin.

Types of Sensory Receptors

Special sensory receptors in the body detect sensory information. They are chemoreceptors, mechanoreceptors (proprioceptors), thermoreceptors, photoreceptors, and nociceptors. All initiate nerve impulses in sensory neuron membranes, and differ in the nature of the stimulus that initiates an impulse (e.g., chemical, pressure, light, heat, and pain).

Chemoreceptors

Located in the nose, tongue, within the walls of certain arteries, and within the brain, **chemoreceptors** are activated by chemical stimuli and detect smells, tastes, and chemistry changes in the blood. To create an action potential, certain molecules fit into certain receptor sites.

Chemoreceptors that are sensitive to changes in pH and carbon dioxide concentration are located in the aorta, the carotid arteries (carotid bodies), and the medulla oblongata. These receptors are occasionally sensitive to low oxygen levels in the blood (e.g., at high elevations). If oxygen is low or carbon dioxide is high, the chemoreceptors stimulate the respiratory center in the medulla oblongata to increase or decrease the respiration rate.

Mechanoreceptors

Mechanoreceptors are sensory receptors that respond to mechanical stimuli and are located in the skin (tactile), ears, muscles, tendons, joints, and fascia. They detect tactile sensations such as touch, pressure,

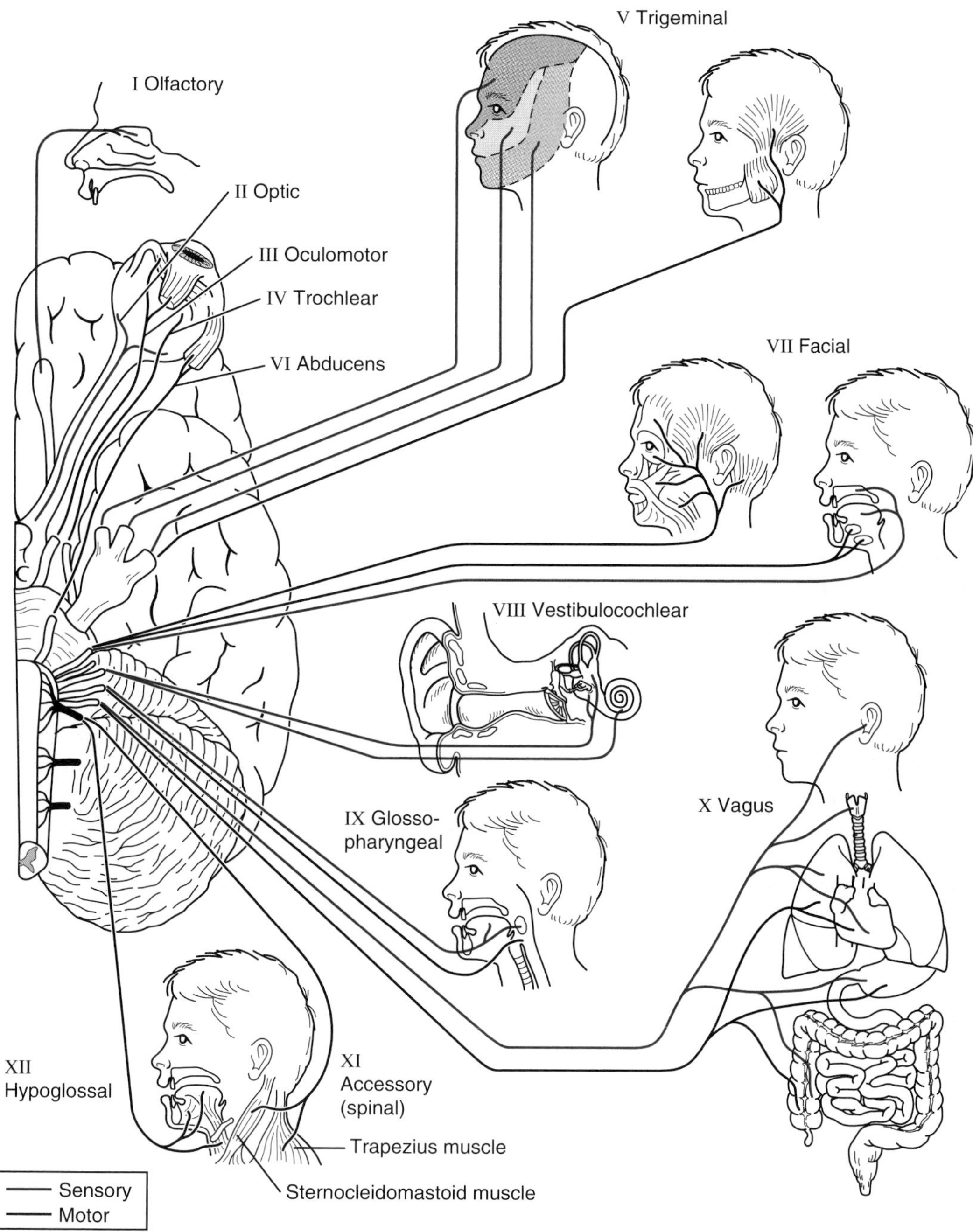

Figure 10•10 Cranial nerves.

vibration, stretching, muscular contraction, proprioception, sound, and equilibrium. Examples of mechanoreceptors are Pacini's (lamellated) corpuscles, Merkel's disks, Ruffini's end organs, hair follicle receptors, and proprioceptors. Mechanoreceptors detect mechanical forces on the cellular membrane and initiate action potentials. A discussion of many of these receptors can be found in the integumentary chapter.

A special type of mechanoreceptor detecting stimuli within the body is called a **proprioceptor.** Internal receptors are generally simpler than exterior receptors. Proprioceptors respond to changes in muscle length and tension, limb position, pain, and blood pressure; these receptors are located in muscles, joints, the walls of certain arteries, and the inner ear. This kinesthetic sense helps us consciously orient our body in space without the use of vision. Examples of proprioceptors are muscle spindles, Golgi tendon bodies, and baroreceptors.

Muscle spindles (neuromuscular spindles) are stretch-sensitive receptors wrapped around intrafusal muscle fibers (striated muscle fiber within a muscle spindle), which monitor changes in the length of a muscle and the rate of this change. When the muscle is stretched quickly (ballistic stretch), the muscle spindle elongates and conducts action potentials to the spinal cord. This causes motor neurons to produce action potentials, resulting in the muscle's contraction. This response is a protective reflex mechanism to defend against muscle damage by counteracting the sudden stretch with muscle contraction. This mechanism provides the basis for reflexes such as the knee-jerk reflex.

Receptors that are stimulated by both tension and excessive stretch are called **Golgi tendon organs** (GTOs, or Golgi tendon bodies). They are located at the musculotendinous boundary of skeletal muscles and activate a reflex response to inhibit the motor neuron if tension is too high. This protective mechanism helps ensure that muscles do not become excessively stretched or do not contract too strongly and damage their tendons. The stimulated GTOs cause relaxation (inhibit contraction) through the entire muscle.

Proprioceptors located in the carotid sinus (in the wall of the carotid arteries) and in the aortic arch are called **baroreceptors.** These pressure-sensitive receptor cells affect blood pressure by sending impulses to the cardiac center and to the vasomotor center in the medulla oblongata. Rates of neural firing are determined by the pressure exerted on the vessel walls. An increase in firing occurs with an increase in blood pressure, and a decrease in firing results from decreased blood pressure. The CNS responds by stimulating the autonomic nervous system; this action either increases or decreases the heart rate and vessel wall diameter.

To help us determine orientation with respect to gravity, the walls of our inner ear are lined with special receptors called maculae. Each **macula** contains a membrane with groups of modified hair cells, or *cilia,* that are attached to sensory nerves. Floating above the membrane is layer of calcium carbonate particles known as **otoliths.** As the body moves, the otoliths and the underlying otolithic membrane shift position, much like a pancake sliding back and forth across the bottom of a skillet as the frying pan is tilted. The weight of the otoliths responds to movement and changes in inertia. As they move, the cilia are disturbed, initiating a nerve impulse.

The three fluid-filled semicircular canals located within the inner ear help orient our position in different planes. Tips of cilia protrude in the gelatin-filled canals, and rotation of our head causes movement of fluid, which bends the cilia, creating action potentials. This process helps us maintain our body's position in space and aids in equilibrium.

Photoreceptors

Photoreceptors are nerve cells that are sensitive to light stimuli. There are two types of photoreceptors, rods and cones, which are located in the retina. The **retina** is a delicate nervous tissue membrane of the eye, which is continuous with the optic nerve. The cellular structures of both types of photoreceptors are similar. Each retina possesses over 100 million rods and 3 million cones.

Rods are thin cellular structures with slender rodlike projections that are very sensitive to dim light (night vision) and to shades of black, white, and gray. Notice how difficult it is to determine color and detail in dim light. Rods contain a substance called *rhodopsin* (a purplish tint) that is very sensitive to light. When light hits a rod photoreceptor, rhodopsin is broken down into two components (scotopsin and retinal). This process triggers an action potential, and neural messages are carried to the brain (occipital lobe).

Cones are needed for color vision; they are shorter and thicker than rods with short, blunt projections. Most cones are found in the fovea centralis (an area at the center of the retina), where very few rod cells are located. The fovea is designated for acute, detailed vision partly because blood vessels do not exist there, and thus color vision is not hindered.

Cones and rods function in a similar way. There are three different types of cones, each possessing a different color pigment (blue, red, and green). When colored light hits a cone cell, a nerve impulse is sent to the brain, and the color pigment of the cone cell is perceived. Different cone combinations create different colors. If all color pigments are activated, white is perceived; if no color pigments are activated, black is seen. To see color, more light is required; color vision is also known as daytime vision. Cones provide sharper images and finer detail than rods do.

Nociceptors

Receptors for detecting pain are **nociceptors.** These free nerve endings are actually bare dendrite endings and are located in almost every tissue of the body, especially near the surface. The brain lacks nociceptors; however, other tissues of the cranium, such as the meninges and blood vessels, have a large supply of them.

Nociceptors are the simplest sensory receptors and serve a protective function. They rarely adapt and may continue to fire once the painful stimulus is removed. Otherwise, pain would stop being sensed, and irreparable damage could result.

Nociceptors respond to stimuli that cause tissue damage, to irritants (e.g., ones released by injured cells), and to extreme stimuli (e.g., excessive heat, bright light, loud sound, and intense mechanical stimulation such as pressure). The painful sensation may cause reflexive withdrawal of the involved body segments if from an external source and stimulation of the sympathetic nervous system such as changes in heartbeat and blood pressure.

In most instances, pain is felt at the point of noci-

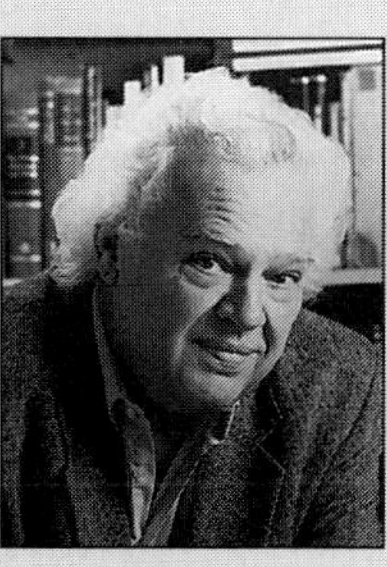

John Upledger

Born: February 10, 1932

"Trust the universe . . . accept its messages . . . and keep your motives clean. The client's body will tell you which way to go."

John Upledger, osteopathic physician, surgeon, and researcher, known by massage therapists as the man who observed a whole new physiological system and developed the form of massage called craniosacral therapy, grew up poor in an Italian neighborhood in Detroit. One of his strongest childhood memories is being held at gunpoint by the junior Mafia and threatened with execution. It turned out to be a BB gun, but from that moment on, he realized the role that fear can play in a person's life and vowed he'd never let it paralyze him again.

At 14 his father died. He hung out with gangs—with blacks during a time when segregation was the norm—played the piano in neighborhood bars, and thought one day he would become a very rich criminal lawyer.

Instead, he graduated with a psychology degree and joined the Coast Guard. Rowing a boat in the dead of winter off the coast of Long Island was less than rewarding. As the only enlisted man with a college education, he took a lot of ribbing. Then he went to Hospital Corpsman school, not because he was particularly interested in practicing medicine, but because medics seemed to have enough spare time to sit around and play cards. He'd played a few rounds with them during basic training.

While still a medic, he performed his first surgery, removing an appendix. But don't call him a healer. Upledger abhors the term, preferring to say that we are all facilitators of our own healing. "Everyone is born with healing abilities," says Upledger. "It's trained out of us by society as we grow to rely on external health care methods."

You might say that his observation of the craniosacral system was his most "moving" experience. While assisting a neurosurgeon during a very risky neurological membrane operation, Upledger's job was to hold the dura mater membrane perfectly still so that the surgeon could remove a spot of calcium plaque from its surface. A slip of the knife might injure the dura and open an avenue for infection.

> *It wouldn't hold still no matter what I did. It kept moving toward and away from us rather slowly but rhythmically and irresistibly. My pride was hurt. I was embarrassed at my own ineptitude. But I also became very curious. Wonder of wonders, I was experiencing the privilege of seeing first-hand the physiological performance of an as-yet-undiscovered bodily system. It would turn out to be another system just like the cardiovascular system, the digestive system, and the like.*
>
> —From: *Your Inner Physician and You,* by John Upledger, 1991

As early as the 1900s, Dr. William Sutherland had been studying the possibility of skull bone movement and developed cranial osteopathy. Using his experience in the operating room and Sutherland's work as a beginning point, Upledger forged on to document support of this physiological phenomenon. At Michigan State University he supervised a team of anatomists, physiologists, biophysicists, and bioengineers in the study of the craniosacral system for almost a decade.

The result of these endeavors is craniosacral therapy. The craniosacral system consists of the membranes and cerebrospinal fluid that surround and protect the brain and spinal cord. It extends from the bones of the skull, face, and mouth, which make up the cranium, down to the sacrum.

Upledger, who sounds more like a metaphysic guru than a scientist, has spent much of his life trying to demystify what happens during a craniosacral therapy session. Though it is much more complex, in *Craniosacral Therapy,* by John E. Upledger and Jon D. Vredevoogd, the authors describe

continued on page 250

Continued

John Upledger

the craniosacral system as a "semi-closed hydraulic system." It is the therapist's job to "feel" for restrictions in the motion of this system and facilitate their release. Craniosacral therapy practitioners assess the entire body to discover restrictions that may be caused by inflammation, adhesion, somatic dysfunction, and neuroreflexes. These restrictions keep our bodies from obtaining complete homeostasis or optimal health. The touch is extremely light, the pressure applied usually no heavier than the weight of a nickel.

Results have been phenomenal at times. Mentally retarded children have been mainstreamed. One child, spastic and paralyzed, walked into his fourth session. Craniosacral therapy has helped women through difficult labor, eased chronic pain, and helped an Olympic athlete recover from vertigo.

If, as a massage therapist, you feel as though your own results have been less than miraculous, Upledger urges you to remember that something as simple as "massage stimulates serotonin, the great tranquilizer." Asked how he likes to feel after a Swedish massage, Upledger replied: "Good . . . tingly . . . vibrant . . . mobile . . . warm . . . energized . . . as though everything is circulating."

Who practices craniosacral therapy? Through the Upledger Institute, Inc., the educational and clinical resource center in Palm Beach Gardens, Florida, osteopaths, medical doctors, psychiatrists, psychologists, dentists, physical therapists, occupational therapists, acupuncturists, doctors of chiropractic medicine, and of course, massage therapists have learned this valuable technique.

ceptor stimulation. However, visceral pain may be sensed in the cutaneous tissue that overlies the organ or can be projected to another cutaneous area of the body. This may be because the visceral organ and the distant pain are innervated by the same spinal segment. For example, the pain of angina may cause pain down the left arm due to a common spinal nerve connection. As pressure is applied to a hypersensitive area on a muscle, painful (noxious) stimuli may be felt in other regions of the body.

Thermoreceptors

Located immediately under the skin, **thermoreceptors** include two types of free nerve endings: one that detects cold and one that detects heat. Cold receptors are ten times more numerous than heat receptors and are stimulated by lowering temperatures. Heat receptors are stimulated by rising temperatures. Once temperature falls below 10°C (50°F) or rises above 45°C (113°F), nociceptors rather than thermoreceptors are activated.

The word crisis is written with two characters in Chinese. One symbol represents danger and the other stands for opportunity. ”

—Robert Cantor

AUTONOMIC NERVOUS SYSTEM

The **autonomic nervous system** (ANS), together with the endocrine (hormone) system, regulates the body's internal organs; the hypothalamus regulates the activity of the ANS. The ANS innervates smooth muscle, cardiac muscle, and glands, and it controls the circulation of blood, the activity of the gastrointestinal tract, body temperature, respiration rate, and many other functions. The ANS is regarded as a *visceral efferent system* because motor signals are sent to the visceral organs. Most of these motor activities are not under conscious control and thus are involuntary.

Within the ANS, there are two divisions (branches)—the **sympathetic nervous system** and **the parasympathetic nervous system.** Their effects on the visceral organs are complementary (one system excites while the other system inhibits) because nerves from both divisions supply the same organs (dual intervention), with one exception (the adrenals). This complementary relationships controls the body's internal organs in a way to maintain homeostasis. In extreme fear, both systems may act simultaneously, producing involuntary emptying of the bladder and rectum, along with a generalized sympathetic response (Fig. 10–11).

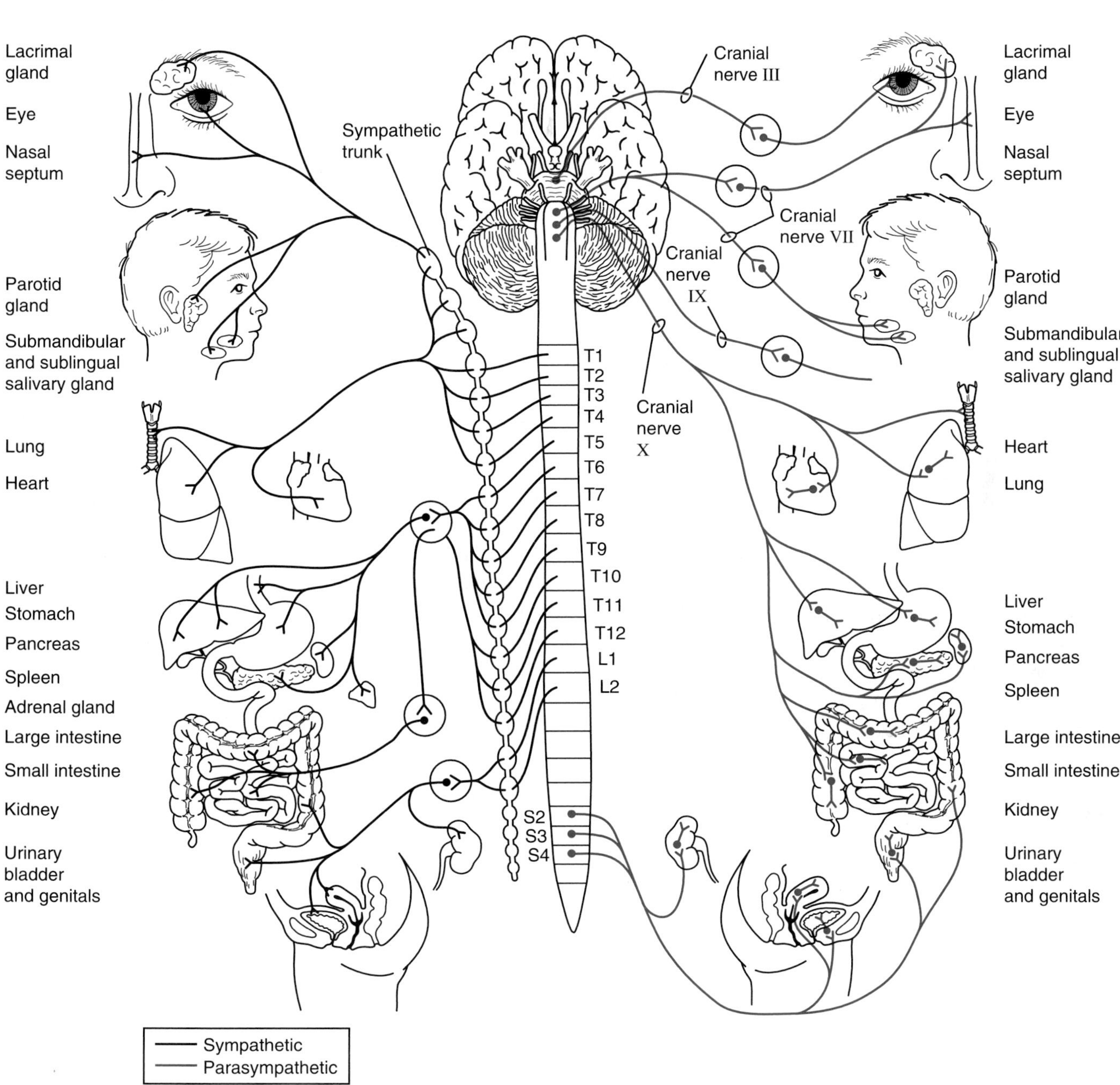

Figure 10•11 The autonomic nervous system: sympathetic and parasympathetic branches.

Author's Note

During stressful situations, the sympathetic nervous system narrows the perceptual field; during times of rest and relaxation, the parasympathetic nervous system broadens the perceptual field. One gift of parasympathetic response during a massage is the client's relaxation; he suddenly can contemplate more options. These added options may help to solve troublesome situations in the client's life.

Sympathetic Nervous System

The sympathetic nervous system (SNS), as a whole, is a catabolic system and is involved with spending body resources and with preparing the body for emergency situations. However, the SNS is activated anytime you experience an alarm reaction (anger, fright, anxiety, or any other type of emotional upset—real or imagined). The sympathetic division is also stimulated in situations where you are physically stressed.

The SNS inhibits most visceral activities momentarily

during emergency situations. All reactions of the sympathetic division occur quickly. The nerves of this system cause the adrenal gland to secrete epinephrine, which sustains the actions of the SNS through the endocrine system.

Most of the cell bodies of the sympathetic system lie outside the spinal cord at the level of T1 to L2. These fibers terminate almost immediately in the *paravertebral ganglia*. For this reason, the sympathetic nervous system is often called **thoracolumbar outflow.**

Effects of Sympathetic Activity

- Increased heart rate
- Increased respiratory rate
- Bronchiolar dilation
- Glucose released from liver
- Increased blood pressure
- Pupillary dilation
- Increased perspiration and oil gland activity in the skin
- Inhibited salivation
- Vasoconstriction
- Decreased gastrointestinal motility (inhibits digestion)
- Inhibited elimination
- Stimulation of adrenal glands to release epinephrine and norepinephrine

Author's Note

Studies show that simply posing the facial muscles in a smile, even if we are not actually thinking happy thoughts, can trigger the same nervous system effects that occur when we are actually feeling happy (parasympathetic arousal). Wearing a negative face, on the other hand, will produce heart rate and skin temperature changes associated with negative emotions (sympathetic arousal). So smile!

Parasympathetic Nervous System

The parasympathetic system (PSNS), in general, is an anabolic system, conserving the body's resources energy. Representing a body calmness, the PSNS's actions are complementary to the sympathetic system. Because the PSNS is most active under relaxed conditions and stimulates visceral organs for normal functions and maintains homeostasis, it is referred to as the "housekeeping system."

The fibers of the parasympathetic nervous system terminate near or within the visceral organ called the *terminal ganglion*. The cell bodies of the PSNS occupy spaces at the spinal cord level S2 to S4 and cranial nerves 3, 7, 9, and 10. For this reason, the parasympathetic nervous system is often called craniosacral outflow.

Effects of Parasympathetic Activity

- Resting heart rate
- Resting respiratory rate
- Resting blood pressure
- Increased gastrointestinal motility—stimulated digestion and elimination
- Pupillary constriction
- Bronchiolar constriction
- Stimulated tearing
- Stimulated salivation
- Increased pancreatic secretions
- Dilated coronary arteries

SPECIAL SENSES

All sense receptors arise from ectoderm (the cellular layer from which the brain and spinal cord come). Receptors for general senses (e.g., pain, pressure, temperature, proprioception) are distributed throughout the body. They are part of the nervous system and are made up of special sensory neurons that receive stimuli from the outside environment, such as vibration, light, and chemicals.

In this section, the special senses (taste, olfaction, vision, hearing, and equilibrium) will be briefly discussed. Information on the touch sense is located in the integumentary chapter because it is often considered a general sense.

Taste

Mediated by taste buds (gustatory organs), taste is a collection of chemosensitive receptors concentrated on projections on the tongue (called **papillae**). Within each papilla are taste (gustatory) hairs extending from taste pores. These hairs are attached to a gustatory receptor that supports a chemoreceptor), which becomes aroused when a molecule of a particular size and shape enters a receptor site (like a lock and key mechanism). Controversy exists whether these receptors detect four primary tastes (salty, sweet, bitter, and sour) or if there is a continuum of many tastes. Most textbooks assert that these four primary tastes are localized in specific regions on the tongue, but new research indicates that there are more taste receptors than the four primaries. Our perception of taste is a combination of impulses from many taste receptors. The input from one receptor means little without the combined information from other receptors, just as the letter K is relatively meaningless without surrounding letters to form a word.

Taste is strongly influenced by our sense of smell. It is difficult to taste food without scent molecules rising

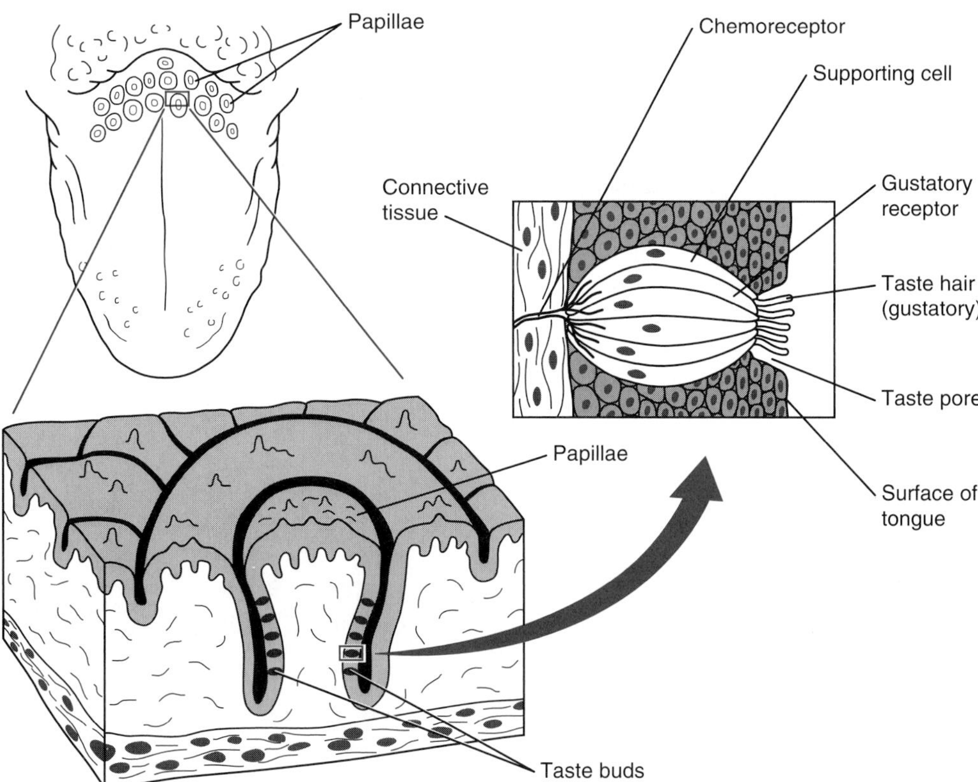

Figure 10•12 Taste buds on the tongue.

up to our nostrils (cold food does not have as much taste as hot food). When we have a condition, such as a cold, that interferes with our sense of smell, taste is inhibited. Cigarette smoking inhibits our detection of sweet and salty tastes. Monosodium glutamate increases flavor by making the gustatory organs more sensitive to sour and bitter taste (Fig. 10–12).

Author's Note

In fish, taste buds are located all over the body and are used to locate food.

Olfaction

Olfaction (sense of smell) utilizes chemoreceptors to detect smells. The cell bodies of olfactory receptors are found in the olfactory mucosa, and dendritic extensions or cilia (hair cells) are located in the mucous layer. The act of inhalation forces airborne molecules up to the mucous layer where they dissolve and come into contact with the chemosensitive receptors. Once certain gaseous chemical molecules fit into the correct receptor site, action potentials are created, and impulses of odor are sent to the olfactory bulb and to the temporal lobe of the cerebrum. It has been suggested by scientists that there are between 7 and 32 primary odors (e.g., ether, camphor, musk, floral, mint, pungent, putrid) and, therefore, a large number of chemoreceptor sites that detect odors. Regarded as the most primitive of all senses, smell plays an important role in sexual behavior for most mammals (Fig. 10–13).

Vision

Vision uses photoreceptors that are located in the eye. Light enters the eye through the *pupil* (the opening in the center of the iris) and strikes the *retina,* which is essentially a membranous screen composed of delicate nervous tissue at the rear of the eye.

There are two types of photoreceptors located on the retina; rods and cones. Rods receive shades of black, white, and gray; cones receive color images. There are only three different types of cones, and each one is sensitive to a different wavelength of light (blue, red, and green). Combinations of these three colors give us an entire color spectrum. Color (cone) perception is based on the differences in the wavelength of light. The shortest visible light wavelength is perceived as violet; as the wavelengths become longer, we perceive different colors (Fig. 10–14).

The photoreceptors on the retina convert light energy into action potentials, which are transmitted to the brain via the optic nerve for visual interpretation. There is a blind spot where the optic nerve exits the retina, but this does not affect our vision because we have two eyes, and the blind spots do not coincide with each other.

Olfactory bulb
Olfactory tract
Nasal cavity
Cribriform plate of ethmoid bone
Afferent nerve fibers (olfactory nerve)
Supporting cell
Olfactory receptor cell (chemoreceptor)
Cilia receptor cell
Olfactory mucosa
Mucus layer

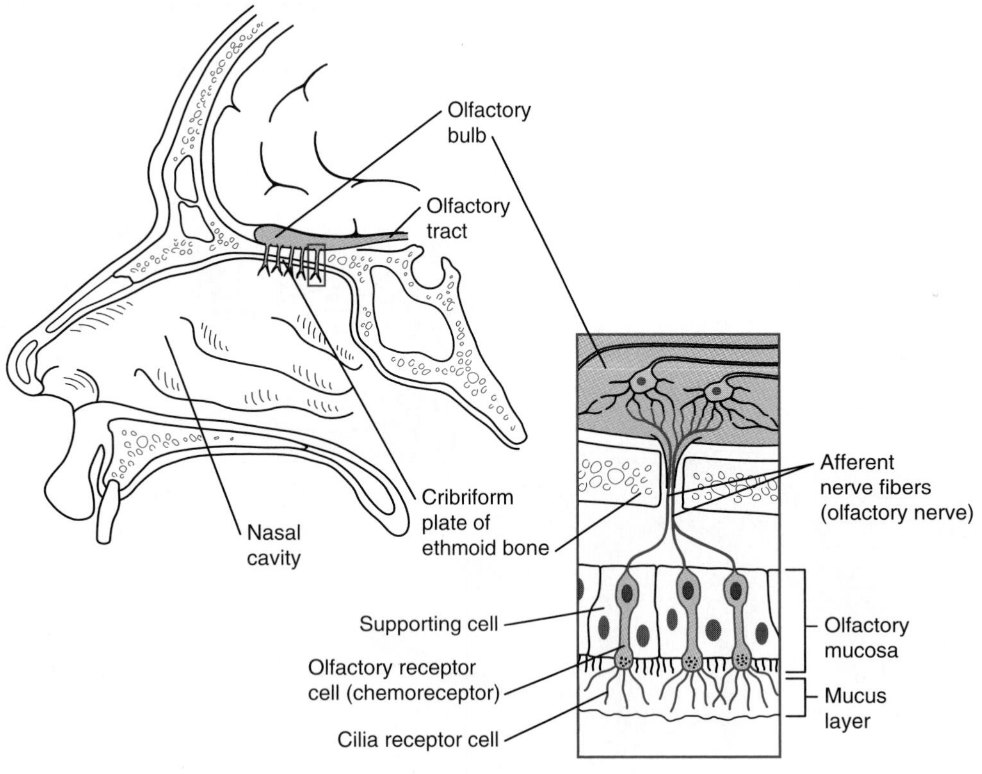

Figure 10•13 Nasal cavity and the olfactory bulb.

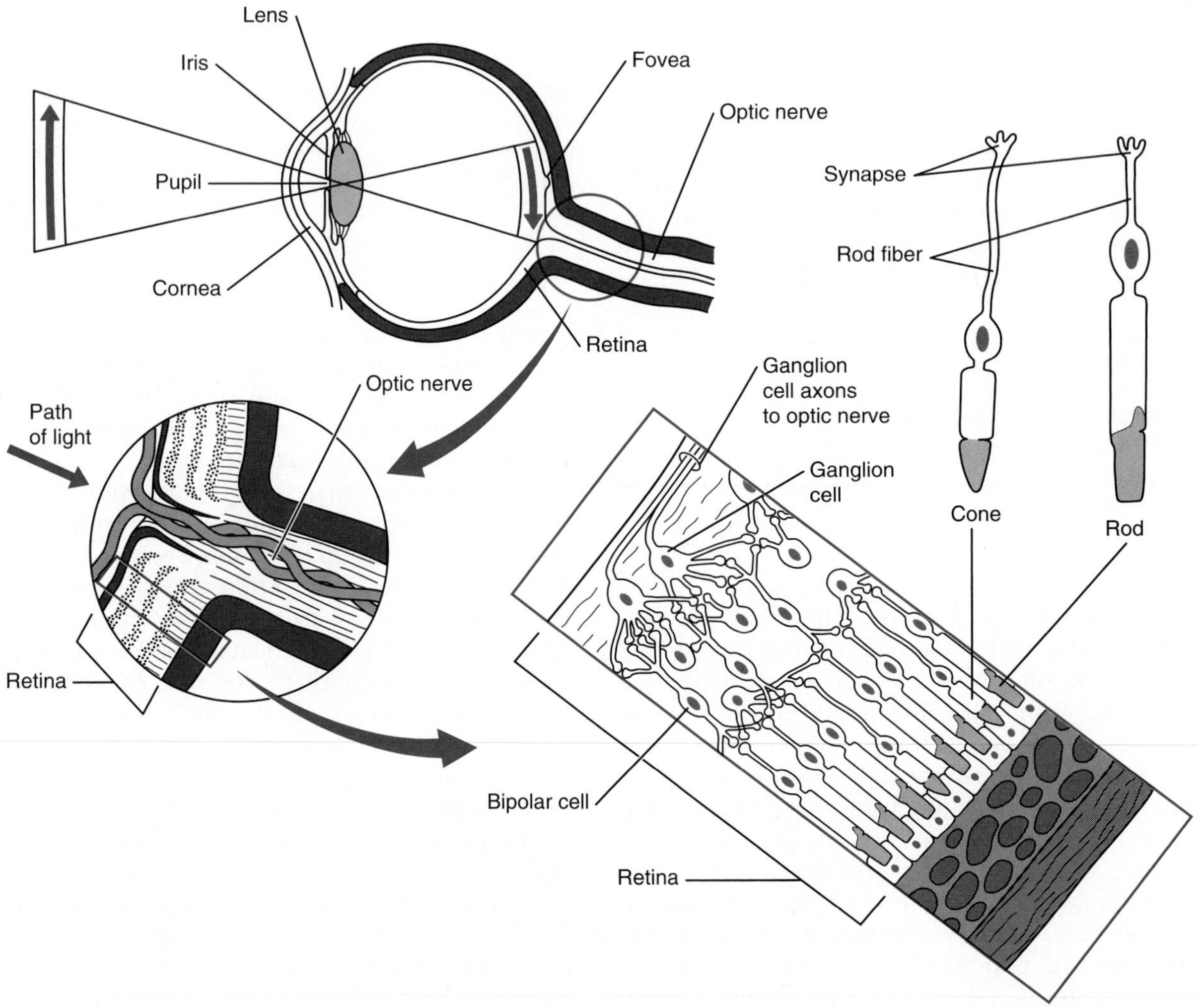

Lens
Iris
Fovea
Optic nerve
Pupil
Cornea
Retina
Synapse
Rod fiber
Path of light
Optic nerve
Retina
Ganglion cell axons to optic nerve
Ganglion cell
Cone
Rod
Bipolar cell
Retina

Figure 10•14 Rods and cones in the retina.

Hearing

Hearing responds to air vibrations that are detected by mechanoreceptors. Air vibrations, or sound waves, are transmitted into neural messages in an indirect, roundabout process.

Sound waves hit the **tympanic membrane** (eardrum) at the back of the auditory canal. The membrane, which separates the outer ear from the middle ear, vibrates like a drum at the same frequency as the sound waves that strike the membrane. These waves are transmitted through three small bones (ossicles) in the middle ear: the malleus (hammer), incus (anvil), and stapes (stirrup). The vibration of these three small bones causes a domino effect to relay this auditory information to the oval window.

The **oval window** is a membrane that covers the opening to a coiled, fluid-filled cavity (**cochlea**) of the inner ear. It then transfers the sound vibrations to the fluid of the cochlea (endolymph). Within the cochlea are three fluid-filled canals, one of which contains a **basilar membrane** (sensory cells are located on top of this basilar membrane where hair cells attach to the auditory nerve). Bending of the hair cells sends action potential through the auditory nerve to the cerebral cortex (temporal lobe) and it is interpreted as sound. It's as though the moving fluid "plucks" the hair cells in the lining, producing the impulses for sound (Fig. 10–15).

Two aspects of sound are pitch and volume. **Pitch** is the quality of a tone or sound, which is dependent on the relative rapidity of the vibrations (slow vibrations produce deep sounds, and fast vibrations produce high sounds). Hearing high-pitched sounds declines with age. **Volume** is the loudness of sound; volume can change without altering pitch.

Skin (Touch)

Most all regions of the skin are sensitive to different sensations. Tactile sensations include touch, pressure,

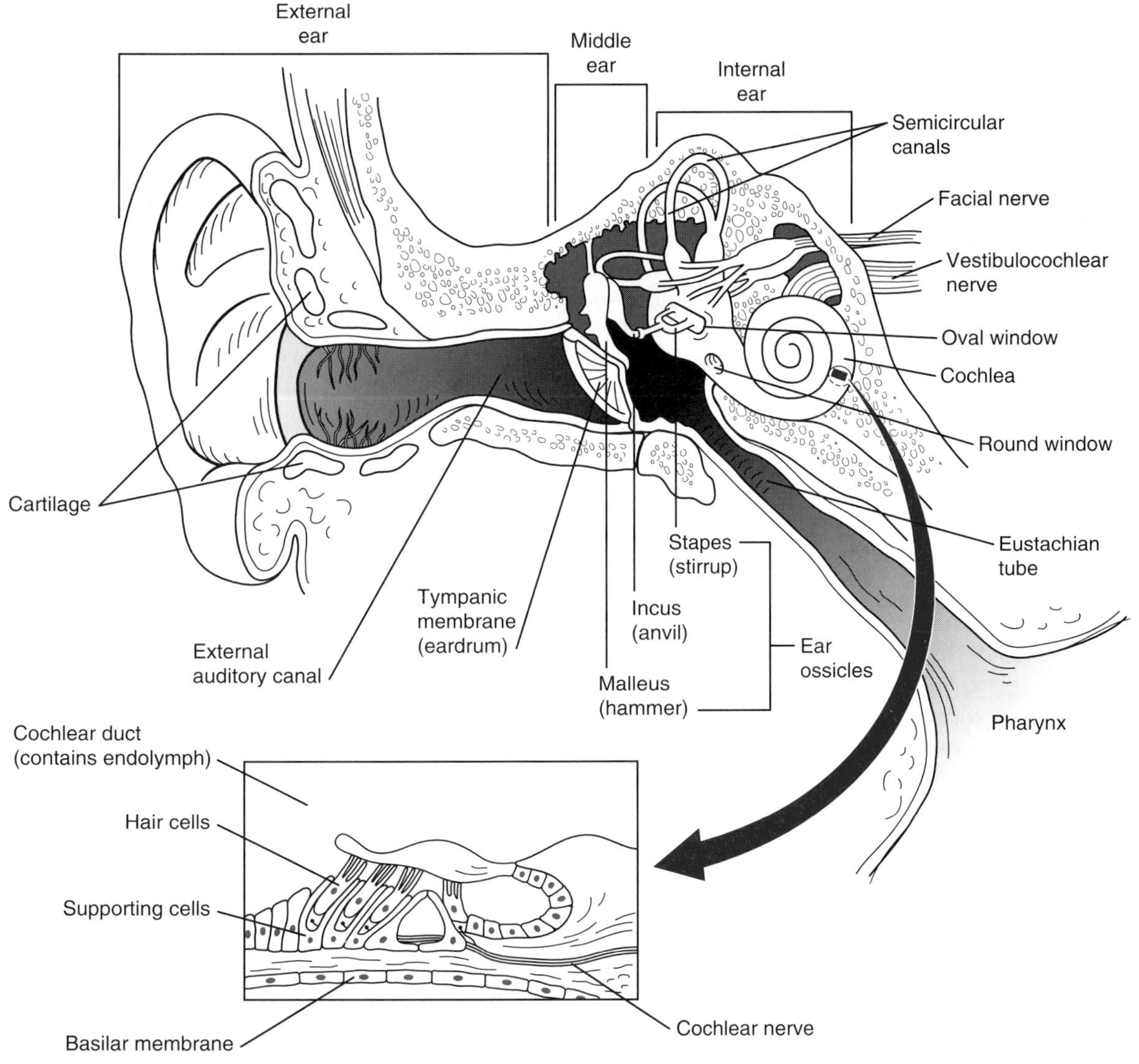

Figure 10•15 Tympanic membrane, oval window, ear ossicles, cochlea, and mechanoreceptors.

and vibration. Thermoreceptors are receptive to heat or to the absence of heat (cold).

NERVOUS CONDITIONS AND CLINICAL TERMS

1. **Pinched Nerve.** Pinched nerve can refer to a broad spectrum of nervous conditions: sciatica; thoracic outlet syndrome; Bell's palsy; ruptured disks; slipped disks; vertebral subluxations; carpal tunnel syndrome; paresthesia; symptoms of radiating pain, numbness, or weakness in the extremities; and a host of other symptoms. It is most commonly used when referring to conditions such as nerve compressions or nerve entrapments.
2. **Nerve Entrapment.** Nerve entrapments are also known as entrapped nerves or entrapment neuropathy, a dysfunction of a nerve as a result of pressure against it by adjacent soft tissues such as muscle, tendon, fascia, and ligaments. The entrapment can be caused by muscle tightness and shortening due to injury or overuse. These tight soft tissues can affect the nerve two ways. They may press an underlying nerve against hard tissues such as bone, disrupting normal nerve function (e.g., thoracic outlet syndrome caused by either the scalene or pectoralis minor muscles pressing the brachial plexus against the ribcage). The other type of entrapment occurs when a nerve actually passes through the belly of a muscle and is constricted by the tightening muscle, much like a rubber band stretched between two fingers (e.g., triceps brachii entrapment of the radial nerve or piriformis entrapment of the sciatic nerve). Both types of entrapment may have symptoms of sharp radiating pain (especially in the extremities), burning, numbness, pins and needles, or weakness in the affected muscles.

   The main goal of the massage treatment is the release of the muscles involved. Most clients will already have a medical diagnosis that may be used to locate, along with trigger point books and charts, the muscles involved. Work deeply, but briefly, to release the tissues responsible for the entrapment; overworking the affected area will further traumatize it.

3. **Nerve Compression.** Nerve compression is also known as nerve impingement. A nerve compression is similar to a nerve entrapment except that the pressure against the nerve is due to contact with hard tissues such as bone or cartilage. Common nerve compressions are found when vertebral disks "slip" from between the bodies of adjacent vertebrae and migrate into the nerve root branching from the spinal cord. The symptoms of nerve compressions are almost identical to those of nerve entrapments (i.e., sharp radiating pain, burning, numbness, tingling, and weakness) except that they may be more severe or occasionally result in loss of all strength or dexterity.

   While deep pressure should not be applied to vertebral disks and bony surfaces, massage may be indicated for the muscles in the area of the compression or muscles which are ennervated by the nerve being compressed. However, a physician's clearance is needed, especially in the spine area.

4. **Carpal Tunnel Syndrome.** Carpal tunnel syndrome is a painful repetitive strain injury (RSI) of the hand and wrist caused by compression of the median nerve. Tendinous sheaths may become swollen and irritated through an improper arm-to-wrist angle and overuse. As these tendons become irritated, extra synovial fluid is secreted, and extra interstitial fluid causes edema. The sheath is inelastic and cannot expand to accommodate the extra fluid. The accumulated fluid compresses the median nerve. Chronic inflammation causes the tendon sheath to thicken, compounding the problem.

   Because this is an occupational hazard for massage therapists, take preventive measures like keeping your wrists neutral while you work, massaging your forearms and hands regularly, and stretching and doing range of motion exercises for your hands, shoulders, and neck. To prevent RSIs, strengthen your forearm and hand muscles using isometric and isotonic contractions; also, use a variety of strokes, rest your hands by spacing your clients, stretch between sessions, and adjust the height of the massage table.

   For clients with this syndrome, local massage over the wrist is contraindicated if there is acute inflammation. In chronic conditions, edema can be reduced by elevating the limb and using lymphatic drainage techniques. Penetrating moist heat can help soften and allow stretch of fibrous adhesions. Cross-fiber friction loosens scar tissue. Passive movement of the elbow, wrist, and finger joints maintains range of motion. It is also essential to massage the neck, shoulders, and arms.

   Massage therapists should help the client identify and avoid risk factors. Also, remedial exercises such as passive stretching of the wrist flexors and extensors will help clients.

5. **Spina Bifida.** Spina bifida is a congenital defect characterized by a lack of osseous development in the lamina (posterior vertebral arch). This condition may be mild (only a small deformed lamina with a gap) or it may be associated with the complete absence of laminae surrounding a large area (usually the lumbar spine). In the more severe cases, the meninges and spinal cord protrude, producing a saclike appearance in the region. The severe forms cause weakness or paralysis of the legs.

In the less severe forms, massage in the lumbosacral area is contraindicated. The more severe forms have neurological problems. The aim is to prevent contractures, prevent pressure ulcers, and reduce spasticity. Passive range of motion helps prevents contractures; force should not be used to stretch muscles that are in spasm. These clients may be prone to pressure ulcers and edema in the legs or sacral region. Avoid massaging the ulcer area, and bring it to the notice of the client's caregiver.

6. **Cerebrovascular Accident.** See this section in Chapter 12.
7. **Transient Ischemic Attack.** Transient ischemic attack, or TIA, is an event of temporary cerebral dysfunction caused by ischemia or reduced blood circulation. TIAs are characterized by abnormal vision in one or both eyes, vertigo, shortness of breath, general loss of sensation, or unconsciousness. Common causes are occlusion by embolus, thrombus, or atherosclerotic plaque. The attack is typically sudden and brief (lasting only a few minutes), leaving no long-term neurological damage.
8. **Shingles.** Shingles is an acute infection of the peripheral nervous system caused by the reactivation of the latent herpes zoster (chickenpox) virus. Affecting mainly adults, shingles presents itself as painful, blisterlike eruptions in a striplike pattern along the affected nerves. The distribution of the blisters is usually unilateral, although both sides of the body may be involved. The skin in the area of the blisters is hypersensitive.

   Local massage is contraindicated. General massage, if the client feels up to it, is fine.
9. **Meningitis.** Meningitis is an infection or inflammation of the meninges, often characterized by a sudden severe headache, vertigo, stiffness of the neck, and severe irritability. As the condition progresses, individuals experience nausea, vomiting, and mental disorientation. An elevated body temperature, pulse rate, and respiration rate are often noted. Meningitis can be life threatening.

   Massage is contraindicated.
10. **Encephalitis.** Inflammation of the brain, or encephalitis, is an infectious disease typically transmitted by the bite of an infected mosquito. Encephalitis may be the result of hemorrhage, lead or other type of poisoning, or as a secondary complication of another condition. This condition is characterized by headaches, fever, vertigo, nausea, and vomiting. In severe cases, encephalitis causes seizures, paralysis, and coma.

    Massage is contraindicated.
11. **Sciatica.** Inflammation of the sciatic nerve, or sciatica, is a type of neuritis often experienced as a dull pain and tenderness in the buttock region with sharper radiating pain or numbness down the leg. The pain is felt along the path of the of the sciatic nerve. As inflammation increases, motor function may be affected, with the knee becoming "rubbery" or unstable. Frequently, sciatica results in muscle flaccidity of the lower leg due to lack of use. The branches of the sciatic nerve may also be affected. Sciatica may be unilateral or bilateral, and can be brought on by injury, overuse, or excessive emotional stress.

    It is a good idea to assess the motor and sensory function and keep a record of it. Treatment needs to be modified according to the cause. For example, if the sciatica is due to a herniated disk, massage in the area of the disk is contraindicated. However, treatment of quadratus lumborum and psoas major may be helpful. If the sciatic is due to a tight piriformis muscle, deep specific work in the area is indicated. Deep work right over the sciatic nerve is contraindicated. The aim is to relax muscles, reduce atrophy, prevent spasms, and reduce edema.
12. **Poliomyelitis.** Poliomyelitis, or polio, is an infectious disease transmitted through fecal contamination or nasal secretions. It is caused by one of the three polioviruses and can range in severity from relatively asymptomatic to severe paralysis. Factors that influence the susceptibility to the viruses are gender, stress, and age. In spinal poliomyelitis, the virus replicates in the anterior horn cells of the spinal cord, causing inflammation and eventual destruction of the spinal neurons.

    Massage therapists are most likely to encounter adults in the chronic noninfective stage. A lighter massage is indicated because the skin may be dry and fragile. Massage treatments should increase joint mobility and prevent contractures. The paralysis of one group of muscles causes antagonist muscles to increase in tone. The increased tone results in excessive stretch and adhesions of the affected muscle group. Passive range of motion helps with joint mobility. Cross-fiber friction over joints and atrophied muscle helps loosen adhesions. It is important to remember that the loss of motor function is irreversible. There may be pressure sores in clients who wear braces or use crutches. Avoid massaging the ulcer area and bring it to the attention of the client.
13. **Parkinson's Disease.** Parkinson's disease is a progressive, degenerative, neurological disorder marked by the destruction of certain areas of the brain (specifically, dopamine-producing neurons) and depletion of the neurotransmitter dopamine, which causes unnecessary skeletal muscle movements that often interfere with voluntary movements. Muscles may alternately contract and relax, causing tremors while other muscles contract con-

tinuously, causing rigidity in the involved part. Injections of dopamine are useless because the blood-brain barrier does not permit passage of this neurotransmitter. Levodopa, a dopamine precursor that does cross the blood-brain barrier, is often used to treat this disease.

The goal of massage treatments is to reduce rigidity. Gentle, slow massages of shorter duration are indicated. Passive movements of joints after the massage are also indicated, but force should not be used. Symptoms will be reduced, though temporarily.

14. **Multiple Sclerosis.** Multiple sclerosis, or MS, is the progressive destruction of myelin sheaths in the central nervous system. Plaque formation in the cerebellum interferes with the ability of nerves to transmit impulses, producing a lack of coordination. The symptoms depend on what areas of the central nervous system are most laden with plaque. As the disease progresses, even handwriting becomes strained and irregular. It usually begins slowly in young adulthood, worsening throughout life with periods of exacerbation and remission. The interims between remissions grow shorter and shorter as the disease advances.

    Massage is contraindicated during flare-ups. Clients should be assessed thoroughly at every visit because symptoms may change from day to day. The goal of massage treatments is to shorten exacerbations, relax the client, decrease tone in rigid muscles, and prevent stiffness and contractures. Heat and cold therapies are contraindicated because temperature extremes can make symptoms worse. Treatments should be slow and gentle and of shorter duration because clients may tire easily.

15. **Epilepsy.** Epilepsy is the presence of abnormal and irregular discharges of cerebral electrical activity; billions of neurons in the brain fire at once. During these episodes, the individual may experience sensory disturbances, seizures, abnormal behavior, and loss of consciousness. The causes of most epileptic cases are unknown, but it has been linked to cerebral trauma, brain tumors, cerebrovascular disturbances, or chemical imbalances. It is viewed as a "lightning storm in the brain."

    Massage is fine for clients who have a history of epilepsy. However, it is important to have the address and phone number of a contact person in case a seizure occurs during a massage treatment. Certain types of epilepsy can be triggered by specific smells, so aromatherapy can serve as a trigger, and is therefore contraindicated.

16. **Rabies.** Rabies is an acute infection that most often is fatal. This condition is caused by the rabies virus often transmitted by animals (dogs, cats, bats, raccoons, and skunks) to people by infected blood, tissue, or, most commonly, saliva. The incubation period for individuals infected with the rabiesvirus is between 10 days and 1 year. Early symptoms are headaches, fever, and loss of sensation. Within several days, the individual develops encephalitis, painful muscle spasms, seizures, paralysis, and coma. Death usually follows these symptoms. Early diagnosis of the disease allows treatment by injection that can prevent death.

17. **Cerebral Palsy.** This is a group of motor disorders resulting in muscular coordination and loss of muscle control. It is caused by damage to the brain's motor areas during fetal life, birth, or infancy. Causes include rubella infection, toxemia, or malnutrition during pregnancy or damage during birth in which oxygen to the baby is reduced. Cerebral palsy is not progressive, meaning it does not worsen as time goes on; however, the damage is irreversible. Intelligence is usually not affected, but speech is impaired. The muscles may be spastic and hyperexcitable. Even small movements, touch, muscle stretch, pain, or emotional stress can increase spasticity.

    Relaxing massage treatments with light pressure help reduce spasms and involuntary movements. Passive movements and range of motion prevent muscle contractures. Force should not be used to stretch muscles in spasm. Pressure sores may form in clients who use wheelchairs. Avoid massaging ulcer areas and bring them to the attention of the client's caregiver.

18. **Glaucoma.** Glaucoma is a condition of elevated pressure within an eye due to an obstructed outflow of aqueous humor. The two most common types of glaucoma are chronic and acute, chronic being the most common. Acute glaucoma is characterized by severe ocular pain, blurred vision, and dilated pupils. If left undiagnosed or untreated, acute glaucoma results in permanent blindness within 2 to 5 days. Chronic glaucoma usually produces no symptoms except for a gradual loss of peripheral vision; this type of glaucoma is genetically determined.

19. **Paralysis.** Paralysis is the loss of muscle function and/or the loss of sensation. This condition can be caused by trauma during an automobile or motorcycle accident, sporting incidents, or gunshot wounds, as well as from disease and poisoning. Paralysis of the lower extremities and trunk is called *paraplegia,* whereas paralysis of the arms and legs is called *quadriplegia.* When the paralysis is restricted to one side of the body, it is called *hemiplegia.*

    Massage is fine for clients with paralysis. Because these clients cannot give feedback about their affected limbs, a lighter pressure is indicated. They may also be prone to pressure sores. Avoid massaging the ulcer area and bring it to the notice of the client's caregiver.

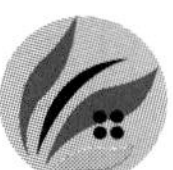

Effects of Massage on the Nervous System

1. Massage activates sensory receptors and can stimulate or soothe the nervous system. Results will depend on the massage stroke you choose and on the pressure applied. Slow, light, and rhythmic movements are soothing to the nerves because such movements produce a low level of excitement to the nervous system. Vigorous movements applied in short duration stimulate the nervous system due to their high level of excitation. The stimulatory massage movements are deep petrissage, friction, vibration, and tapotement. Sedative massage movements are light effleurage, light petrissage, light friction, and light vibration.
2. Massage decreases pain. One of the ways this occurs is by the release of endorphins (endogenous morphine), enkephalins, and other pain-reducing neurochemicals. General relaxation brought on by massage therapy has a diminishing effect on pain.
3. Massage inhibits pain by interfering with nociceptive (pain) information, which enters the spinal cord through stimulation of cutaneous thermo- and mechanoreceptors.
4. Massage relieves pain caused from hypersensitive trigger points or referred pain, presumably by increasing circulation to the tissue (reactive hyperemia), thereby reducing ischemia-related pain.
5. Massage mechanically stretches and broadens tissue. These changes are detected by mechanoreceptors (Golgi tendon organs) and reflexively alter the contraction signal.
6. Muscle spindle activity is increased during abrupt massage strokes, such as tapotement and some forms of vibration. These strokes create minute muscle contractions to help tone weak muscles.
7. Massage increases delta wave activity and decreases alpha and beta wave activity (EEG determined).
8. Massage stimulates the parasympathetic nervous system, thus promoting relaxation and decreasing insomnia.
9. Massage has been proven to reduce norepinephrine and cortisol (stress hormones) levels by activation of the relaxation response.
10. Massaged individuals possess an increase in dopamine and serotonin levels. This suggests a decrease in stress levels and depression.

20. **Reflex Sympathetic Dystrophy.** Reflex sympathetic dystrophy (RSD) is a complex disorder or group of disorders affecting the limbs that may develop as a result of trauma (accident, repetitive motion, or surgery). It is characterized by pain, sensory and motor dysfunction, localized abnormal blood flow, and the inability of the body to control pain messages to the brain.

    Massage treatments need to be tailored to the client's specific needs, depending on the extent of the disorder. If the client is experiencing acute symptoms, massage is contraindicated. With less severe symptoms, a gentle massage is indicated, with passive range of motion to increase joint mobility.

SUMMARY

A study of the nervous system includes the details of the anatomy and physiology of individual nerve fibers and nerve transmission and a look at the system as a whole.

The neurons are the functional unit of the nervous system and can be classified according to structure (unipolar, bipolar, and multipolar). Functionally, nerves are classified as sensory (or afferent), association (or connecting, internuncial), or motor (or efferent) neurons. The connecting neurons are found in the brain and spinal cord where they connect the sensory and motor neurons, which generally run as a pair between somewhere in the body back to the spinal cord. The sensory nerve of the pair runs from a remote nerve receptor and enters the posterior horn of the spine. The motor neuron originates at the anterior horn of the same spinal segment and runs back inside the sheath alongside the sensory nerve, until the motor neuron reaches its target muscle or gland.

The nerve impulse generated when the receptor senses input is an electrochemical reaction to stimuli. This happens when the stimulus exceeds the limit of the neuron, and an action potential or nerve impulse is created. This all-or-none response is fueled by a process in which the polarized membrane of the nerve cell becomes depolarized, reverse polarized, and then repolarized. This is accomplished by a complex exchange of sodium and potassium ions across the cellular membrane, which is driven by a mechanism known as the sodium-potassium pump. Action potentials, or nerve impulses, are affected by neurotransmitters. The neurotransmitters may facilitate, arouse, or inhibit nerve impulse transmission.

The nervous system as a whole is divided into two units: the central nervous system and the peripheral nervous system. The CNS is composed of the brain, spinal cord, cerebrospinal fluid, and meninges. Nervous control of the body is regulated by chemicals that can cross the blood-brain barrier. Protective body reflexes are found within the spinal cord itself.

The peripheral nervous system consists of the intricate network of many millions of branching nerve fibers that leave and return to the brain and spinal cord, some of which are sensory and some of which are motor. Nerves leaving directly from the brain are referred to as cranial nerves; spinal nerves are those originating from and terminating at the spine. The types of sensory nerves include chemoreceptors, mechanoreceptors, photoreceptors, nociceptors, and thermoreceptors; these give us our specialized senses of taste, olfaction, vision, hearing, and touch.

A subdivision of the peripheral nervous system is the autonomic nervous system, which in turn is divided into two parts: the sympathetic nervous system and the parasympathetic nervous system.

SELF-TEST

Multiple Choice • Write the letter of the best answer in the space provided.

_______ 1. Which of the following is *not* a function of the nervous system?

A. nutrient transport
B. sensory input and motor output
C. interpretation and integration
D. emotional responsiveness

_______ 2. The nervous system is divided into two major divisions, the

A. epi nervous system and endo nervous system
B. axial nervous system and appendicular nervous system
C. central nervous system and peripheral nervous system
D. central nervous system and superficial nervous system

_______ 3. The central nervous system includes the

A. mesoderm, endoderm, and ectoderm
B. brain, meninges, cerebrospinal fluid, and spinal cord
C. brain, cranium, spinal cord, and vertebral column
D. cranial nerves and spinal nerves

_______ 4. The peripheral nervous system consists of

A. mesoderm, endoderm, and ectoderm
B. brain, meninges, cerebrospinal fluid, and spinal cord
C. brain, cranium, spinal cord, and vertebral column
D. cranial nerves and spinal nerves

_______ 5. Within the peripheral nervous system, there are two special divisions that supply impulses to smooth muscles, cardiac muscles, skin, special senses, some proprioceptors, organs, and glands. They are also referred to as the involuntary nervous system. These two divisions are the

A. somatic nervous system and autonomic nervous system
B. brain and spinal cord
C. sympathetic and parasympathetic divisions
D. cranial nerves and spinal nerves

_______ 6. The autonomic nervous system is further divided into the

A. somatic nervous system and autogenic nervous system
B. brain and spinal cord
C. sympathetic and parasympathetic divisions
D. cranial nerves and spinal nerves

_______ 7. Which of the following connective tissue cells support, nourish, protect, and organize the delicate neurons?

A. osteocyte
B. neuroglia
C. dendrites
D. cartilage

_______ 8. The basic impulse-conducting cells that act like tiny sense organs are the

A. neurons
B. plexus
C. ganglions
D. glial cells

_______ 9. A typically short, narrow, and highly branched extension of the nerve cell that receives stimuli from other neurons and that moves it toward the cell body is the

A. cyton
B. synaptic end bulb
C. axon
D. dendrite

_______ 10. The nerve fiber that is a single cylindrical extension of the cell and carries impulses away from the cell body is the

A. cyton
B. synaptic end bulb
C. axon
D. dendrite

_______ 11. Chemicals that facilitate, arouse, or inhibit the transmission of nerve impulses across synapses are

A. hormones
B. histamines
C. steroids
D. neurotransmitters

_______ 12. A group of impulse-carrying fibers connecting the brain or the spinal cord with other parts of the body is a

A. neuron
B. nerve
C. plasma
D. synapse

_______ 13. A network of intersecting nerves is referred to as a

A. neuron
B. plexus
C. ganglion
D. glial cell

_______ 14. Nerve impulses are accomplished by two characteristics of neurons:

A. contractility and extensibility
B. digestion and elimination
C. active transport and osmosis
D. excitability and conductivity

_______ 15. When the stimulus is of sufficient intensity to generate a nerve impulse, it is referred to as a

A. threshold stimulus
B. all-or-none response
C. subthreshold stimulus
D. subliminal message

_______ 16. When a stimulus generates a nerve impulse, it is conducted along the entire neuron at its maximum capacity. This principle is the

A. threshold stimulus
B. all-or-none response
C. subthreshold stimulus
D. subliminal message

_______ 17. The junction between two neurons, or between a neuron and a muscle or gland where information is transmitted, is a(n)

A. synapse
B. neural space
C. neural gap
D. axon cleft

_______ 18. The neural structure where neurotransmitters are produced and stored is the

A. transmitter pocket
B. synaptic bulb or knob
C. neural bladder
D. bulb of Ranvier

_______ 19. A collective term for a vast range of chemicals that facilitate, arouse, or inhibit the transmission of nerve impulses between synapses is

A. transmitter chemicals
B. neural activation substances
C. axon secretions
D. neurotransmitters

_______ 20. Which of the following is a neurotransmitter?

A. acetylcholine
B. dopamine
C. serotonin
D. all of the above

_______ 21. The connective tissue membranes that envelop the central nervous system are the

A. cerebrospinal membranes
B. meninges
C. myelin sheaths
D. neural coverings

_______ 22. The regions of the brain are the

A. pia mater, arachnoid, and dura mater
B. cerebrum, midbrain, and hindbrain
C. cerebrum, diencephalon, cerebellum, and brain stem
D. cerebellum, corpus callosum, midbrain, and hindbrain

_______ 23. The largest region of the brain that governs all higher functions (language, memory, reasoning, and some aspects of personality) is the

A. cerebellum
B. cerebrum
C. medulla oblongata
D. diencephalon

_______ 24. Within the cerebrum are regions named for the bones they lie beneath. These regions are called

A. neural spaces
B. cranial zones
C. lobes
D. cerebral tracts

_______ 25. The lobe that contains a center for visual input is the

A. frontal lobe
B. parietal lobe
C. temporal lobe
D. occipital lobe

_______ 26. The part of the brain that houses the thalamus and hypothalamus is the

A. cerebrum
B. cerebellum
C. diencephalon
D. brain stem

_______ 27. Which region of the brain concerns muscle tone, coordinates skeletal muscles and balance (posture integration and equilibrium), and controls fine and gross motor movements?

A. cerebrum
B. cerebellum
C. diencephalon
D. brain stem

_______ 28. The brain stem contains the

A. midbrain
B. pons
C. medulla oblongata
D. all of the above

_______ 29. Often considered the most vital part of the brain, which of the following structures contains the respiratory center, the cardiac center, and the vasomotor center, and which also controls gastric secretions and reflexes such as sweating, sneezing, swallowing, and vomiting?
A. cerebellum C. medulla oblongata
B. hypothalamus D. meninges

_______ 30. A semipermeable wall of blood capillaries and glial cells that prevents or slows down the passage of some drugs, other chemical compounds, and disease-causing organisms (such as viruses) from the blood into the central nervous system is the
A. cerebrospinal boundary
B. neurotransmitter block
C. blood-brain barrier
D. neurocranial barrier

_______ 31. Which structure consists of two or more neurons, at least one of which is sensory and at least one of which is a motor, innervating a muscle, gland, or organ?
A. interconnecting neuron
B. reflex arc
C. ascending tract
D. communicating system

_______ 32. An instantaneous, involuntary response to a stimulus originating from either inside or outside the body is a
A. synapse
B. sodium potassium response
C. action potential
D. reflex

_______ 33. Which of the following is *not* one of the 12 cranial nerves?
A. sciatic C. trigeminal
B. optic D. facial

_______ 34. Sensory receptors stimulated by both tension and excessive stretch and activate an inhibitory responses in the motor neuron are called
A. muscle spindles C. nociceptors
B. Golgi tendon organs D. baroreceptors

_______ 35. Pressure-sensitive receptors located in the carotid sinus and in the aortic arch are called
A. muscle spindles C. nociceptors
B. Golgi tendon organs D. baroreceptors

_______ 36. Sensory receptors that are sensitive to light stimuli are called
A. mechanoreceptors C. photoreceptors
B. chemoreceptors D. light receptors

_______ 37. Photoreceptors that are very sensitive to dim light (night vision) and shades of black, white, and gray are
A. dim light receptors C. cones
B. rods D. spindles

_______ 38. Photoreceptors that are used for color vision are
A. dim light receptors C. cones
B. rods D. spindles

_______ 39. Located in almost every tissue of the body, the receptor for detecting pain is a
A. mechanoreceptor C. photoreceptor
B. chemoreceptor D. nociceptor

_______ 40. Sensory receptors that are sensitive to temperature changes are
A. chemoreceptors C. nociceptors
B. thermoreceptors D. photoreceptors

_______ 41. Taste and smell are interpreted by which sensory receptor?
A. chemoreceptor C. nociceptor
B. thermoreceptor D. photoreceptor

_______ 42. Color perception is based on the differences in the
A. amount of light entering the eye
B. number of cones stimulated
C. number of inhibited rods
D. wave length of light

_______ 43. Receptors responding to air vibrations or sound waves that are transmitted into neural messages are
A. mechanoreceptors C. photoreceptors
B. chemoreceptors D. nociceptors

_______ 44. The loudness of sound is called

A. symphonic quality
B. pitch
C. volume
D. orchestral intensity

_______ 45. Which of the following is involved with spending body resources and preparing the body for emergency situations?

A. central nervous system
B. somatic nervous system
C. sympathetic nervous system
D. parasympathetic nervous system

_______ 46. The sympathetic division of the autonomic nervous system is also called

A. relaxation response
B. thoracolumbar outflow
C. housekeeping system
D. somatic division

_______ 47. Which of the following are effects of the sympathetic nervous system?

A. increased heart rate
B. increased respiratory rate
C. inhibited salivation and digestion
D. all of the above

_______ 48. Which division of the nervous system conserves body resources and represents a body calmness?

A. central nervous system
B. somatic nervous system
C. sympathetic nervous system
D. parasympathetic nervous system

_______ 49. The parasympathetic division of the autonomic nervous system is also called

A. alarm response
B. thoracolumbar outflow
C. craniosacral outflow
D. somatic division

_______ 50. Which of the following is *not* an effect of the parasympathetic nervous system?

A. decreased blood pressure
B. decreased heart rate
C. increased respiration rate
D. increased gastrointestinal motility

References

Applegate, Edith J. *The Anatomy and Physiology Learning System: Textbook.* Philadelphia: W. B. Saunders, 1995.

Crooks, Robert, and Jean Stein. *Psychology: Science, Behavior, and Life.* New York: Holt, Rinehart, & Winston, Inc., 1988.

Damjanov, Ivan. *Pathology for the Health-Related Professions.* Philadelphia: W. B. Saunders, 1996.

Gould, Barbara E. *Pathophysiology for the Health-Related Professions.* Philadelphia: W. B. Saunders, 1997.

Gray, Henry, et al. *Gray's Anatomy,* 29th ed. Philadelphia: Running Press, 1974.

Haubrich, William S. *Medical Meanings, A Glossary of Word Origins.* New York: Harcourt Brace Jovanovich, 1984.

Juhan, Deane. *Job's Body, A Handbook for Bodyworkers.* Barrington, NY: Station Hill Press, 1987.

Kalat, James W. *Biological Psychology,* 2nd ed. Belmont, CA: Wadsworth Publishing Company, 1984.

Kapit, Wynn, and Lawrence M. Elson. *The Anatomy Coloring Book,* 2nd ed. New York: HarperCollins Publishers, 1993.

Kordish, Mary, and Sylvia Dickson. *Introduction to Basic Human Anatomy.* Lake Charles, LA: McNeese State University. Self-published manual, 1985.

Marieb, Elaine N. *Essentials of Human Anatomy and Physiology,* 4th ed. New York: Benjamin/Cummings Publishing Company, Inc., 1994.

McAleer, Neil. *The Body Almanac.* Garden City, NY: Doubleday & Company, Inc., 1985.

McAtee, Robert. *Facilitated Stretching.* Champaign, IL: Human Kinetics Publishing, 1993.

Mosby's Medical, Nursing, and Allied Health Dictionary, 4th ed. St. Louis: Mosby–Year Book, Inc., 1994.

Newton, Don. *Pathology for Massage Therapists,* 2nd ed. Portland: Simran Publications, 1995.

Premkumar, Kalyani. *Pathology A to Z—A Handbook for Massage Therapists.* Calgary, Canada: VanPub Books, 1996.

St. John, Paul. *St. John Neuromuscular Therapy Seminars.* Largo, FL: self-published manual, *Manual I.* 1995.

Tabers Cyclopedic Medical Dictionary, 13th ed. Philadelphia: F. A. Davis Company, 1977.

Tortora, Gerald J. *Introduction to the Human Body: The Essentials of Anatomy and Physiology,* 3rd ed. New York: HarperCollins Publishers, 1994.

Travell, Janet G., and David Simons. *Myofascial Pain and Dysfunction, The Trigger Point Manual.* Baltimore: Williams & Wilkins, 1983.

Voss, Dorothy E., Marjorie K. Ionta, and Beverly J. Myers. *Proprioceptive Neuromuscular Facilitation.* Philadelphia: Harper & Row, 1985.

The intellect is powerless to express thought without the aid of the heart, liver and every member.
—Wordsworth

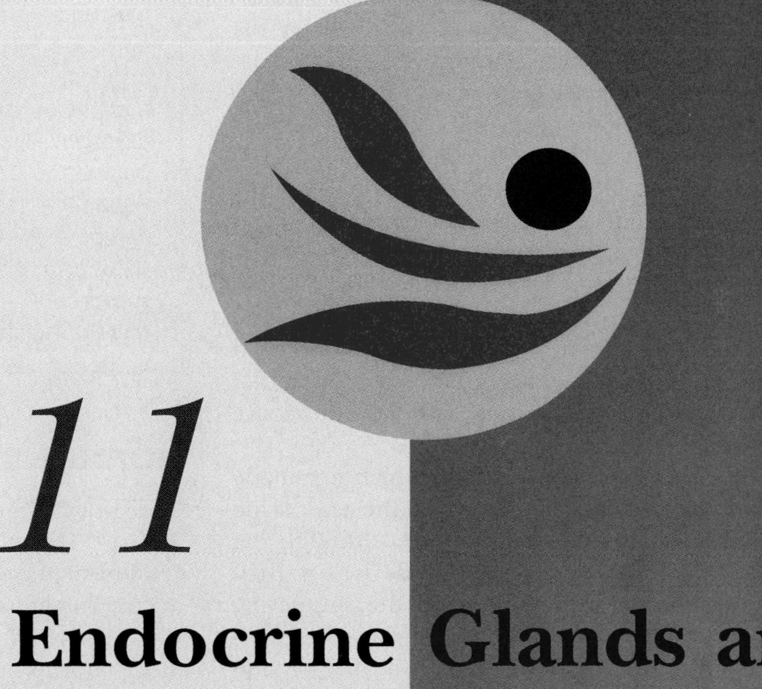

11

Endocrine Glands and Hormones

Student Objectives

After completing this chapter, the student should be able to:

- Identify the four functions of the endocrine system.
- Describe the types of hormones
- Explain the hormonal control systems
- Classify glands as either endocrine or exocrine
- Identify specific endocrine glands
- Name the hormones produced and secreted by each endocrine gland
- Discuss the function of each glandular hormone

INTRODUCTION

The body has two types of glands: exocrine and endocrine. **Exocrine glands** contain cells that produce glandular secretions and use ducts to transport their products to the site of action. Examples of exocrine glands are sudoriferous glands, sebaceous glands, and salivary glands. **Endocrine glands** have cells that produce glandular secretions called hormones that diffuse directly into the bloodstream. Also known as "ductless glands," endocrine glands empty their products directly in the blood, which carries the hormones to the sites of action.

Some glands, such as the pancreas and the ovaries, are endocrine *and* exocrine glands.

The endocrine system is the second major controlling and communicating system of the body. The first major system is the nervous system and its activity is relatively fast. The nervous system and the endocrine work together to integrate body activities. In comparing the endocrine system to the nervous system, one could say that the nervous system is built for speed and that the endocrine system regulates processes that go on for relatively long periods, and its effects are more widespread.

Compared with other body systems, which are made up of fairly large organs, the glands of the endocrine system may seem small and unimportant. Although the total weight of all the endocrine glands is less than half a pound, normal functioning of the endocrine system is vital to our body's physiology, which becomes apparent when hormone levels are too low or too high. Drastic changes in our body's metabolism occur when hormonal levels are out of balance.

The endocrine system consists of the endocrine glands and glandular secretions called hormones, which are surrounded by rich capillary networks. The purpose of the vascularity of the endocrine glands is to assist the delivery of hormones to their sites of action. Hormones are carried by the blood, so it is vital for endocrine glands to have good blood supply.

FUNCTIONS

The functions of the endocrine system are to:

1. produce and secrete hormones;
2. regulate body activities, such as growth, development, metabolism, and fluid, mineral, and electrolyte balance;
3. help the body to adapt during times of stress, such as infection, trauma, dehydration, emotional stress, and starvation; and
4. contribute to the reproductive process.

Each hormone has its own specific role to play in regulating body activities. Each of the endocrine glands and the functions of their hormones will be discussed in the section, Endocrine Glands, but first let's get a better understanding of hormones.

Terms and Word Roots Related to the Endocrine System

adenohypophysis – gland; below; to grow
adrenal – kidney
antidiuretic – against; urine; production
diabetes – overflow; passing through
endocrine – within; to separate
exocrine – away from; to separate
hormone – to excite, arouse, or urge on
insipidus – not; tasty
mellitus – sugar; honey
oxytocin – swift; childbirth
pancreas – all flesh
peptide – to digest
pineal – pine cone
polydipsia – much or many; thirst
suprarenal – above; kidney
thyroid – shield; shaped

HORMONES

The word "hormone" means to set in motion or to arouse. **Hormones** are internal secretions that are "chemical messengers" of the endocrine system. They act as catalysts in biochemical reactions and regulate the physiological activity of other cells in the body. Since hormones circulate freely in the blood, they have the potential of coming into contact with every type of cell in the body. But hormones *do not affect* every cell they may encounter. Each type of hormone is specifically programmed to seek out a corresponding type of cell, which are called **target cells.** The target cells contain *receptor sites,* which are chemically compatible with their corresponding hormone. When the hormone comes into contact with the receptor site of the target cell, they lock together like puzzle pieces, and the resulting chemical change produces the desired effect on the cell. This arousal of the target cell is usually an increase or decrease in the rate of its primary metabolic function.

Types of Hormones

Hormones may be grouped according to their chemical makeup. The four most common types of hormones are steroids, peptides, biogenic amines, and eicosanoids.

1. **Steroid Hormones.** Steroid hormones are derived from cholesterol and alter the cell's activity by turning genes on or off. Hormones of the adrenal cortex and gonads are steroid hormones, which are fat soluble (can be stored in body fat).
2. **Peptide Hormones.** Peptide or protein hormones

are derivatives of amino acid chains. These hormones are water soluble. They attach to the cell membrane and introduce a series of chemical reactions to alter the cell's metabolism. These reactions can last from several minutes to several hours. Hormones of the pituitary gland, parathyroid glands, and some of the hormones of the thyroid glands are peptides.

3. **Biogenic Amines.** These are the simplest hormone molecules and are derived from amino acids, like peptide hormones. These hormones also act as neurotransmitters. Hormones of the adrenal medulla and thyroid gland are biogenic amines as well as the catecholamines: histamine, serotonin, and dopamine. These substances regulate blood pressure, waste elimination, body temperature, and many other functions.
4. **Eicosanoids.** Also called local or tissue hormones, eicosanoids are produced by almost every cell in the body. Derived from fatty acids found in cell membranes, eicosanoids work on the cells that produce them or on nearby cells. They are inactivated quickly and have actions such as altering smooth muscle contractions, blood flow, nerve impulse transmission, and immune responses.

Hormonal Control Systems

The body uses three mechanisms to control the amount of hormones secreted by the endocrine glands. These are the negative feedback system, the hormonal control system, and the neural control system.

If these control systems do not function properly, physiological disorders may result. Great strides have been made in understanding the complex control mechanisms of the body. New ideas about endocrine system regulation are being formulated as more research is conducted. Let's take a brief look at what we know about each system of control.

The Negative Feedback System. Most hormone levels in the body are regulated by a negative feedback system. Information about blood hormone levels is relayed back to the endocrine gland, and the gland responds by secreting more or less hormones. This process is known as the *negative* feedback system because the stimulus triggers the negative, or opposite, response; this process may or may not involve the nervous system. For example, when the negative feedback system senses a low level of calcium ions in the bloodstream, it triggers an increase of parathyroid hormone, which causes an increase in blood calcium ions. This increase continues until the level of calcium ions exceeds the target value or becomes high; the parathyroid then responds negatively by decreasing production. This principle may be confusing unless we apply it to something that we use every day.

A more familiar example would be a home's central-air unit that controls the climate by using a negative feedback system. When the temperature rises above a set point or target value, the air-conditioning unit is activated and cold air blows through vents to cool the dwelling. When the room temperature drops below the set point, the cooling system is shut down. Conversely, the central heat unit will work in the opposite direction; it will warm the house when the temperature drops too low. In comparing the two, remember that the direction of change is not important; the effect is always opposite the stimulus. The temperature is thus controlled in a narrow range by responding negatively to the input.

In summary, a high stimulus is a deviation from the set point or target value, such as the desired level of hormone in the bloodstream. A deviation on the high side results in reduced hormone production. A deviation below the set point or target range, results in an increase of hormone production.

Hormonal Control System. Hormones themselves can trigger the release of other hormones in the endocrine system. For example, thyroid-stimulating hormone, released by the anterior lobe of the pituitary, activates the thyroid gland to secrete thyroxine and triiodothyronine. One hormone can stimulate or inhibit the release of another through the hormonal control system.

Neural Control System. Some hormones are secreted as a result of direct nerve stimulation, the most classic example being the release of epinephrine and norepinephrine from the adrenal medulla. Sympathetic arousal, also known as the stress response, releases epinephrine and norepinephrine into the bloodstream to maintain the fight-or-flight response. The neural control system has a much faster response time than the negative feedback or the hormonal control systems.

INDIVIDUAL ENDOCRINE GLANDS

There are nine individual endocrine glands. These are the pituitary gland, pineal gland, thyroid gland, parathyroid glands, thymus gland, adrenal glands, pancreas, and the female ovaries and male testes (Fig. 11–1). The posterior lobe of the pituitary and the adrenal medulla are not technically endocrine glands because they contain neurosecretory cells (specialized nervous tissue that secrete hormones). The placenta and some cells of the digestive tract also serve an endocrine function but will not be discussed here because they are usually included in discussion of the reproductive and digestive systems.

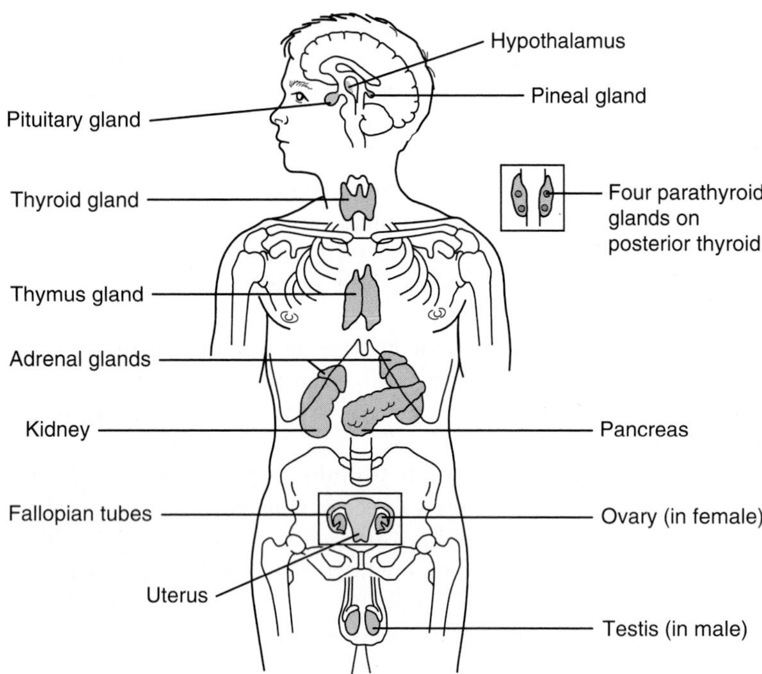

Figure 11•1 Location of all endocrine glands.

Pituitary Gland. The bilobed pituitary gland, or hypophysis, is located in the sella turcica of the sphenoid bone and extends from the hypothalamus by a stalk-like structure known as the *infundibulum.* Approximately the size of a small grape, the pituitary gland is protected on all sides by osseous tissue and is considered the "most protected gland in the body." The pituitary gland is also known as the "master gland" because its hormones control and stimulate other glands to produce their individual products (Fig. 11–2). The pituitary itself also has a master—the hypothalamus, which sends hormones and nerve impulses to control secretions of the pituitary gland.

Most hormones of the pituitary gland, except for human growth hormone, are *tropic hormones;* these regulate the growth and secretory activity of other endocrine glands.

The pituitary gland consists of two parts: an anterior lobe and a posterior lobe.

1. **Anterior Lobe.** Also known as the *adenohypophysis,* the anterior lobe of the pituitary constitutes about 75 percent of the total weight of the entire gland. Of the nine hormones secreted by the pituitary gland, seven are produced by the anterior lobe. The anterior lobe and the hypothalamus are interconnected by a rich vascular network. Hormones from the hypothalamus travel this network to stimulate or inhibit the release of hormones from the anterior lobe.

    Adrenocorticotropic hormone, or ACTH, regulates the endocrine activity of the adrenal cortex, especially cortisol secretion.

    Human growth hormone, hGH, GH, somatotropin, or somatogrowth hormone, stimulates protein synthesis for muscle and bone growth and maintenance. It also plays a role in metabolism.

    Thyroid-stimulating hormone, or TSH, stimulates the thyroid gland to produce and secrete triiodothyronine (T_3) and thyroxine (T_4).

    Follicle-stimulating hormone, or FSH, stimulates oogenesis or egg development in the ovaries. It also stimulates estrogen production by the ovaries. In men, FSH stimulates sperm production, or spermatogenesis, in the testes.

    Luteinizing hormone, or LH, stimulates ovulation in women. It also stimulates the production of estrogen and progesterone by the ovaries. In men LH stimulates testosterone secretion by the testes.

    Prolactin, PRL or lactogenic hormone, along with many other hormones, stimulates the mammary glands to create milk production in women. Prolactin's role in men is not known.

    Melanocyte-stimulating hormone, or MSH, seems to stimulate the distribution of melanin granules, therefore increasing skin pigmentation.

Author's Note

To memorize the hormones of the anterior pituitary, use the mnemonic phrase "*FLAT* *M*iles *P*er *G*allon," *f*ollicle-stimulating hormone, *l*uteinizing hormone, *a*drenocorticotropic hormone, *t*hyroid stimulating hormone, *m*elanocyte-stimulating hormone, *p*rolactin, and *h*uman growth hormone.

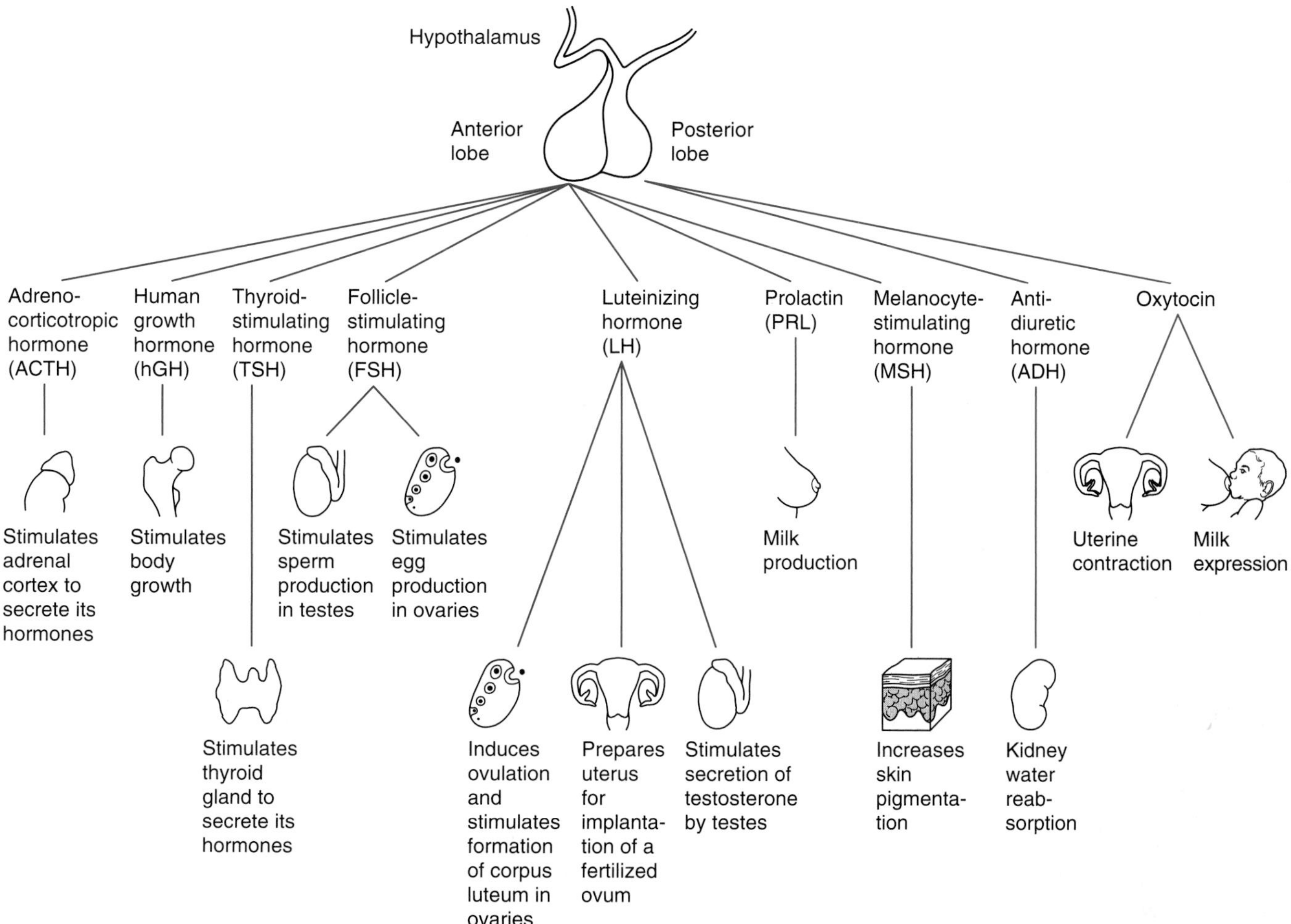

Figure 11•2 The pituitary gland with all hormones.

2. **Posterior Lobe.** Also known as *neurohypophysis,* the posterior lobe of the pituitary is not technically an endocrine gland because it does not produce the hormones it releases. It stores and releases hormones produced by the hypothalamus. The cellular makeup of the posterior lobe is similar to the neuroglia cells of the nervous system and are called neurosecretory cells. The cells in the hypothalamus produce two hormones.

   Antidiuretic hormone, ADH or vasopressin, decreases urine output by stimulating the kidneys to reabsorb water to prevent dehydration. ADH also raises blood pressure by constricting arterioles, and, during severe blood loss, the amount of ADH in the blood increases. Alcohol consumption inhibits secretion of ADH and increases urine production.

   Oxytocin is involved in milk expression from the mammary glands and in uterine muscular contraction. A synthetic version of oxytocin, Pitocin, is used to stimulate labor in pregnant women. Oxytocin's function in men is unknown.

Pineal Gland. The pineal gland, or *epiphysis cerebri,* is a pine cone–shaped structure in the brain, attached to the roof of the third ventricle and inferior to the corpus callosum. Although its function is not clear, the pineal gland produces and secretes the hormone melatonin.

Melatonin is a controversial hormone that may be involved in the control of circadian rhythm or diurnal cycles (occurring daily, such as sleeping and eating) and in the growth and development of sexual organs. When injected into the body, melatonin produces drowsiness. It also appears to inhibit the secretion of luteinizing hormone.

Thyroid Gland. Located at the base of the neck, posterior and inferior to the larynx, is the butterfly-shaped thyroid gland (Fig. 11–3). The thyroid gland is a bilobed gland connected in the center by a mass of tissue known as the *isthmus.*

1. **Triiodothyronine (T_3)** and **thyroxine (T_4).** Both triiodothyronine and thyroxine regulate growth and development as well as influence mental, physical, and metabolic activities. These hormones consist of

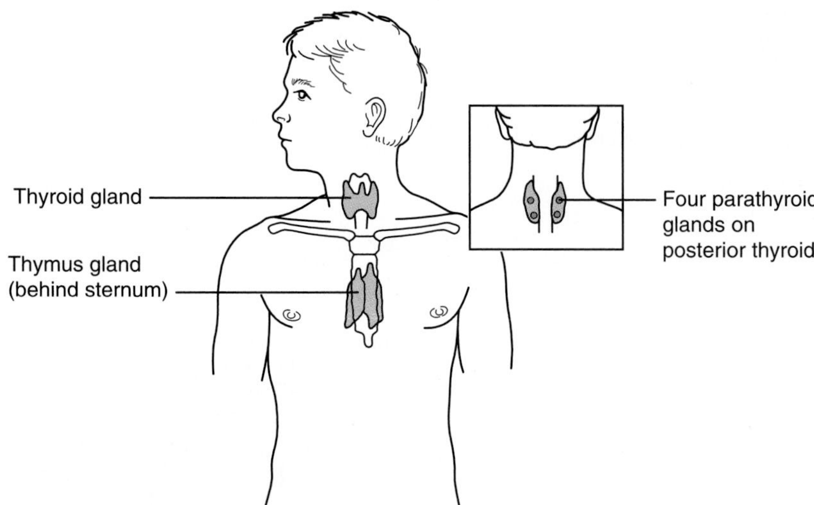

Figure 11•3 The thyroid, parathyroid, and thymus glands.

a small peptide molecule bound to iodine; therefore, they cannot be made without iodine. Some good sources of iodine are iodized salt and seafood.

2. **Calcitonin,** or CT, decreases blood calcium and phosphorus by stimulating osteoblasts (bone-forming cells) to make bone matrix. This causes calcium and phosphorus to be deposited in the bones. Low calcitonin production contributes to insufficient calcium in the body. It is believed that calcitonin production decreases in elderly adults, which may explain why many elderly people experience an increase in the decalcification of bones.

Parathyroid Glands. Usually four in number, the tiny parathyroid glands are located on the posterolateral surface of the thyroid lobes (see Fig. 11–3).

Parathyroid hormone, or PTH, increases blood calcium levels by stimulating osteoclast (bone-destroying cells) activity and breaks down bone tissue. The liberated calcium is released in the bloodstream, and blood calcium levels increase. PTH also increases calcium reabsorption from urine and the intestines back into the blood.

Thymus Gland. The thymus gland is a bilobed gland posterior to the sternum (see Fig. 11–3). It is large in infants, reaches its maximum size at puberty, then atrophies and is replaced by adipose tissue in adults. The thymus secretes a number of hormones, such as thymosin and thymopoietin.

Thymosin and **thymopoietin** are immunologic hormones that play a role in the body's growth and development, in sexual maturation, and in the growth and maturation of antibodies, namely T cells. T cells are a type of white blood cell that destroys foreign invaders like bacteria and viruses; therefore, the thymus gland plays an important role in the body's immunological response. Thymosin appears to be present in copious amounts in young children and decreases throughout life.

Adrenal Glands. The adrenal glands, or suprarenals, are located superior to each kidney and are among the most vascular organs in the body. These important glands are divided into two regions and, like the pituitary gland, possess two types of tissue, each producing a different hormone (Fig. 11–4).

1. **Adrenal cortex** is the outer region and makes up most of the gland. It arises from embryonic tissue, endoderm, which is similar to that of the kidneys. The hormones of the adrenal cortex are steroid hormones.
   Aldosterone stimulates the reabsorption of sodium and water in kidney filtration, helping to maintain proper mineral balance and monitoring blood volume.
   Cortisol affects carbohydrate, protein, and fat metabolism, and when needed, produces an anti-

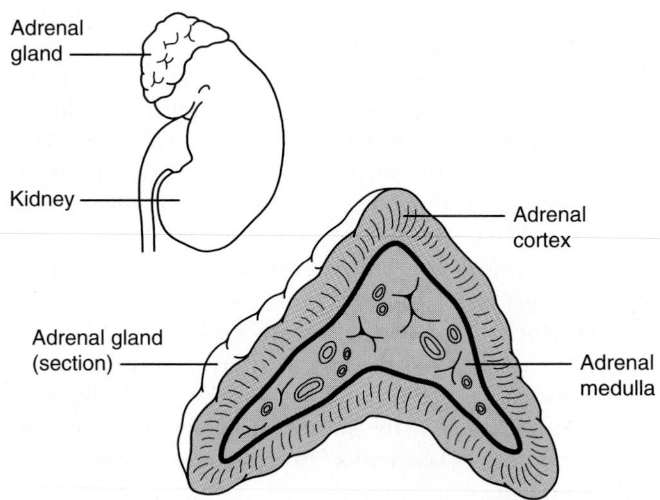

Figure 11•4 The adrenal cortex and medulla.

inflammatory response. A synthetic version, hydrocortisone, is used as an anti-inflammatory agent.

Androgens are hormones that maintain male sexual characteristics.

2. **Adrenal medulla** is the inner region of the adrenals, which arises from ectoderm. The hormones of the adrenal medulla, also called neurohormones, mimic the effects of the sympathetic nervous system and account for the sudden emergency energy required for the stress response.

Epinephrine, or adrenaline, is an adrenal hormone that increases blood pressure by stimulating vasoconstriction, rather than by affecting cardiac output. This occurs in response to stress.

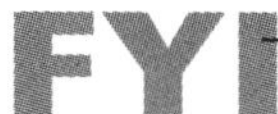

FOR YOUR INFORMATION

Even though it is commonly used, the term "adrenalin" is a registered trademark for epinephrine held by the Parke-Davis company.

Norepinephrine, or noradrenaline, helps the body to maintain the stress response. When you are threatened physically or emotionally, your sympathetic nervous system brings about the fight-or-flight response to help you cope with the stressful situation. The effects of norepinephrine are increased heart rate, blood pressure, and blood glucose levels, and dilatation of the small passageways of the lungs. This results in more oxygen and glucose in the blood and a faster circulation of blood to the body organs—most importantly, to the brain, muscles, and heart. Epinephrine and norepinephrine are broken down slowly, so the effects on the sympathetic nervous system are long lasting.

When you are having dental work done, it's very hard to have a conversation with your dentist or dental hygienist. Somehow, I manage to ask a lot of questions about anatomy and physiology. One day, after my dentist administered a local anesthetic, within minutes, my heart began to race, and my breathing accelerated. It alarmed me, because I was not anxious in the least. It must be the drug he injected in my mouth.

I asked my dentist what could be causing this reaction. He told me that a small amount of epinephrine was added to the drug to hasten the effect of the drug.

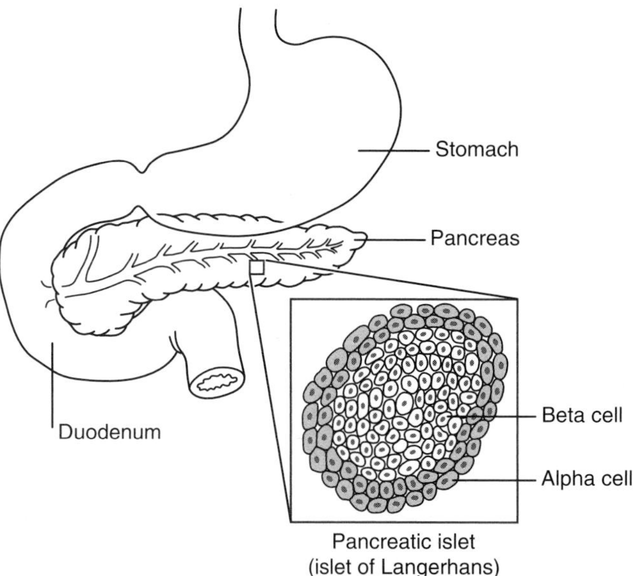

Figure 11•5 Beta cells of alpha cells of the islets of Langerhans.

Pancreas. The pancreas, or pancreatic gland, is located inferior to the stomach and is both endocrine and exocrine. Within the pancreas are islands of specialized cells called the **islets of Langerhans** or **pancreatic islets.** The pancreas contains over a million islets, each consisting of *alpha* and *beta cells* (Fig. 11–5) that function like an organ within an organ. Both hormones of the pancreas help regulate carbohydrate metabolism.

1. **Insulin,** secreted by beta cells, decreases blood glucose levels by enhancing the uptake of glucose into the cells. Its effects are said to be hypoglycemic. Insulin is the only hormone that decreases blood glucose levels and is absolutely necessary for metabolism. Because this hormone is deactivated by digestive enzymes, it cannot be administered by mouth. If an individual requires insulin, it must be given by injection.
2. **Glucagon** is secreted by the alpha cells of the pancreatic islets, which increase blood glucose levels and produce hyperglycemic effects. This hormone release is stimulated by low blood levels of glucose. It causes the liver and the skeletal muscles to break down stored glycogen into glucose, thus increasing blood glucose levels.

Ovaries and Testes. The ovaries and testes, or gonads, are the reproductive glands. They function both as endocrine and exocrine glands. The testes are located in the male scrotum, and the ovaries are located in the abdominopelvic region of the female body. The hormones of both glands stimulate the growth and development of primary sex organs and the secondary sex characteristics and play a very important role in reproduction (Fig. 11–6).

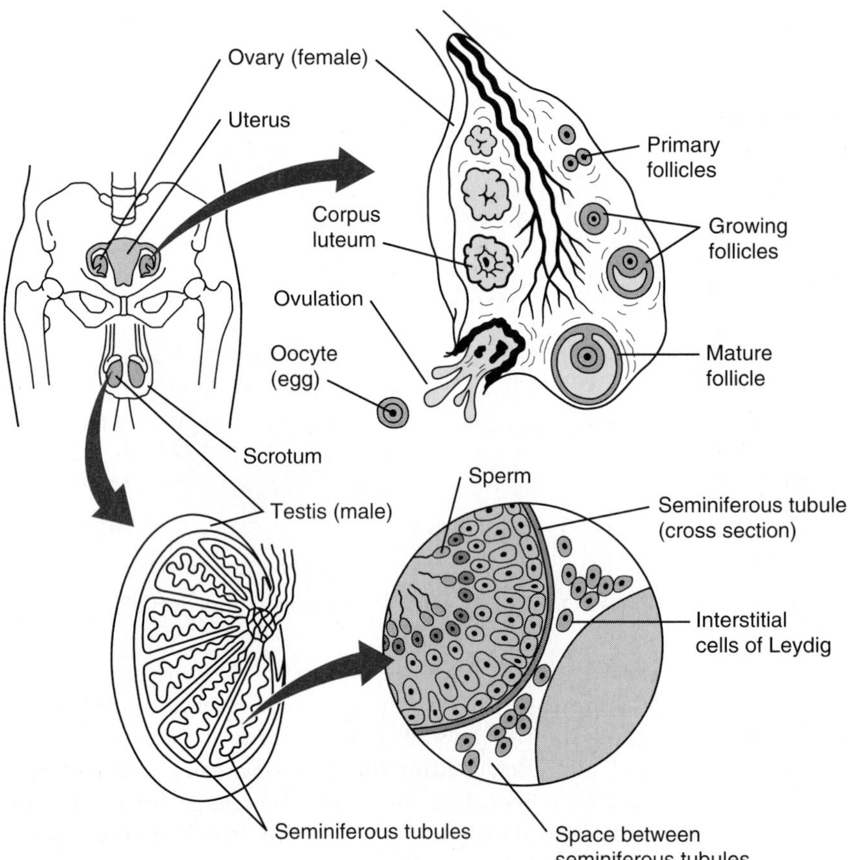

Figure 11•6 The gonads and hormonal function of each.

1. **Ovaries.** Within the ovaries, a structure called the corpus luteum produces the hormones estrogen, progesterone, and relaxin.

   Estrogen is also known as the "feminizing" hormone, because it is responsible for female secondary sex characteristics. During the menstrual cycle, estrogen triggers the preparation of the female genital tract for fertilization and implantation of the early embryo. Estrogen is also produced in the testes and placenta.

   Progesterone prepares the endometrium for pregnancy and helps to maintain the corpus luteum once conception and implantation occur. If this does not occur, the uterine lining is sloughed off. One cause of spontaneous abortion (miscarriage) is a drop in progesterone levels.

   Relaxin softens the connective tissue in the body of a pregnant woman, especially the pelvic ligaments, for fetal delivery. It also helps to dilate the cervix during labor and delivery.

Author's Note

Because relaxin loosens connective tissue during pregnancy, all range of motion and stretching modalities must be kept to a minimum and must be performed with caution.

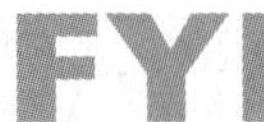
FOR YOUR INFORMATION

The first oral contraceptive, Enovid, was approved by the Food and Drug Administration (FDA) in 1960. It was manufactured and distributed that same year. Over 9 million women in the United States and Europe use oral contraceptives (birth control pills) every year.

2. **Testes.** Within the testes are groups of specialized cells called the interstitial cells of Leydig. These cells produce and secrete androgens, namely testosterone.

   Testosterone is an androgenic hormone that promotes secondary male sex characteristics, as well as libido (sex drive) and sperm production.

ENDOCRINE CONDITIONS AND CLINICAL TERMS

1. **Diabetes.** Diabetes refers to a family of metabolic disorders that alter the fluid balance of the body. There are four main types of diabetes.

   Diabetes Mellitus. This is a group of disorders that lead to elevated blood glucose levels (hyperglycemia). Glucose appears in the urine and is accompanied by polyuria (excessive excretion of urine), polydipsia (excessive thirst), and excessive eating (polyphagia). In Type I diabetes, there is a deficiency of insulin and regular injections of insulin are needed. It is thought to be an autoimmune disease because the beta cells of the pancreas, which produce insulin, are destroyed. Type II diabetes represents more than 90 percent of all cases. It usually occurs later in life, and symptoms are mild. This type of diabetes can usually be controlled by diet, exercise, and weight loss.

Relaxing and gentle massage is indicated for clients with diabetes mellitus. Sometimes clients cannot give accurate feedback about pressure due to accompanying neuropathy, so lighter pressure is indicated. It is important that clients have their necessary medications (e.g., insulin, ADH) with them when they come for treatment, in the event of a diabetes related emergency.

Diabetes insipidus. This is caused by a posterior pituitary gland dysfunction that results in deficient production of ADH. Diabetes insipidus has absolutely nothing to do with insulin production or pancreatic dysfunction, but like diabetes mellitus, it results in polyuria, thus reducing fluid volume in the body, and increasing thirst.

A massage of shorter duration is indicated. It is important that clients have their necessary medications (e.g., insulin, ADH) with them when they come for treatment, in the event of a diabetes-related emergency.

Nephrogenic diabetes insipidus. This is much the same as diabetes insipidus, except that the cause is due to kidney dysfunction, often as a result of disease or damage, rather than pituitary gland dysfunction. Blood levels of ADH are normal, but the kidneys do not respond to it. Instead of concentrating impurities into a small amount of urine, the kidneys filter large amounts of water with impurities, resulting in very dilute urine and excessive fluid loss.

A massage of shorter duration is indicated. It is important that clients have their necessary medications (e.g., insulin, ADH) with them when they come for treatment, in the event of a diabetes-related emergency.

Gestational diabetes mellitus. This usually occurs in women in the second and third trimesters of pregnancy. Hormones secreted by the placenta disturb the function of insulin, causing expectant mothers to become glucose intolerant. This condition is temporary, usually diminishing after the baby is born.

A relaxing and gentle massage is indicated.

2. **Hypoglycemia.** Hypoglycemia is almost the opposite of diabetes, although it too can be related to pancreatic dysfunction. Hypoglycemia refers to an excessive loss in blood glucose levels that can result in a variety of symptoms including weakness, light-headedness, headaches, excessive hunger, visual disturbances, anxiety, and sudden changes in personality. If left untreated, the result may be delirium, coma, and death. Causes of hypoglycemia can be an overdose of prescribed insulin, an excessive level of insulin production by the pancreas, or extreme dietary deficiencies.

   Massage is fine for clients with hypoglycemia. However, they may experience light-headedness when getting up from the massage table, so they may need assistance.

3. **Goiter.** An enlarged thyroid gland, or goiter, is associated with hyperthyroidism, hypothyroidism, inflammation, infection, or lack of iodine in the diet. Goiters are more prevalent in countries where dietary iodine intake is inadequate. Iodized salt reduces the occurrence of goiters.

   Massage is fine for clients who have goiters. However, the neck region should be avoided.

4. **Addison's Disease.** Addison's disease is caused by failure of adrenal functions, often resulting from an autoimmune disease, local or general infection, or adrenal hemorrhage. The disease is characterized by general weakness, reduced endurance, and an increase in pigmentation of the skin and mucous membranes (called bronzing). Loss of appetite, anxiety, lethargy, depression, and other emotional disturbances often accompany this disease.

   A gentle, relaxing full body massage of shorter duration is indicated.

5. **Cushing's Disease.** Classified as a metabolic disorder, Cushing's disease is caused by an overproduction of adrenocortical steroids. An overabundance of these hormones causes an accumulation of fluids and fat on the face, neck, and upper back. Other conditions that may develop are muscle weakness, purplish streaks on the skin, acne, osteoporosis, and diabetes mellitus. The person bruises easily and wound healing is poor.

   A very gentle massage is indicated.

6. **Graves' Disease.** Graves' disease is caused by hyperthyroidism and is characterized by related anxiety, fatigue, tremors of the hands, loss of appetite, and increased metabolic rate. An enlarged thyroid gland (goiter) and enlarged lymph nodes often accompany this condition as well as an unusual protrusion of the eyeballs. This disease is thought to be an autoimmune disorder.

   A gentle full-body massage is indicated. Massage over the anterior neck and any enlarged lymph nodes is contraindicated.

7. **Acromegaly.** Acromegaly, or acromegalia, is caused by the overproduction of growth hormone. It is characterized by elongation and enlargement of the bones of the extremities, face, and jaw. The condition mainly affects middle-aged and older persons.
8. **Cretinism.** A congenital deficiency in the secretion of the thyroid hormones, cretinism is characterized by a lack of physical and mental development. This condition is typical in countries where the diet is deficient in iodine and where goiters are common. The addition of iodized salt reduces the occurrence of cretinism.

   A relaxing gentle massage is indicated, avoiding the neck region.

SUMMARY

The endocrine glands and the hormones they secrete make up the endocrine system. The endocrine glands are ductless and discharge directly into the bloodstream via their surrounding network of capillaries. The functions of the endocrine system are to regulate growth, development, metabolism, and fluid balance, to maintain homeostasis, and to contribute to the reproductive process.

Hormones are the chemical messengers and act as catalytic agents that affect the physiological activity of other cells in the body. The most common types of hormones are steroids, peptides, biogenic amines, and eicosanoids. The amount of hormone secreted into the bloodstream is governed by negative feedback systems, other hormones, and the nervous system.

Hormones are produced by the following glands: pituitary, pineal, thyroid, parathyroids, thymus, adrenals, pancreas, ovaries, and testes. Abnormal hormone production may result in diseases such as diabetes, hypoglycemia, and obesity.

SELF-TEST

Multiple Choice • Write the letter of the best answer in the space provided.

_______ 1. The endocrine system consists of the endocrine glands and their glandular secretions called

A. capillaries
B. hormones
C. sebum
D. insulin

_______ 2. Endocrine glands

A. use ducts to transport their products to the site of action
B. include sudoriferous glands, sebaceous glands, and salivary glands
C. produce secretions that diffuse directly into the bloodstream
D. A and B

_______ 3. Hormones act as catalysts in biochemical reactions and

A. aid in increasing the oxygen content of the blood
B. provide a protective covering to the outside environment
C. regulate the physiological activity of body cells
D. eliminate waste products

_______ 4. The four most common types of hormones are

A. steroid, peptide, biogenic amines, and eicosanoids
B. pituitary, pancreas, thymus, and pineal gland
C. erythrocytes, leukocytes, thrombocytes, and platelets
D. cortex, medulla, alpha, and beta

_______ 5. The mechanism regulating the amount of hormones secreted by endocrine glands by stimulating the opposite response is the

A. positive feedback system
B. negative feedback system
C. hormonal control system
D. neural control system

_______ 6. Hormones that regulate the growth and secretory activity of other endocrine glands are called

A. dominant hormones
B. tropic hormones
C. climatized hormones
D. eicosanoids

_______ 7. A metabolic disorder characterized by excessive thirst and urination and caused by a deficiency in antidiuretic hormone is

A. carbohydrate diabetes
B. diabetes mellitus
C. diabetes insipidus
D. urinal diabetes

_______ 8. A metabolic disorder that is the result of a deficiency of the hormone insulin is called

A. carbohydrate diabetes
B. diabetes mellitus
C. diabetes insipidus
D. urinal diabetes

Matching • List the letter of the answer to the term or phrase that best describes it. Some will be used more than once.

A. adrenal gland (cortex)
B. adrenal gland (medulla)
C. pituitary (anterior lobe)
D. pituitary (posterior lobe)
E. ovaries
F. thyroid gland
G. pancreas
H. parathyroid gland

_______ 1. prolactin

_______ 2. aldosterone

_______ 3. insulin

_______ 4. thyroxin and triiodothyronine

_______ 5. estrogen and progesterone

_______ 6. cortisol

_______ 7. calcitonin

_______ 8. parathyroid hormone

_______ 9. ACTH

_______ 10. glucagon

_______ 11. oxytocin

_______ 12. epinephrine

_______ 13. human growth hormone

_______ 14. antidiuretic hormone

References

Applegate, Edith J., M.S. *The Anatomy and Physiology Learning System: Textbook*. Philadelphia: W. B. Saunders, 1995.

Guyton, Arthur, M.D. *Human Physiology and Mechanisms of Disease,* 3rd ed. Philadelphia: W. B. Saunders Company, 1982.

Haubrich, William S. *Medical Meanings, A Glossary of Word Origins.* New York: Harcourt Brace Jovanovich, 1984.

Kalat, James W. *Biological Psychology,* 2nd ed. Belmont, CA: Wadsworth Publishing Company, 1984.

Kordish, Mary and Sylvia Dickson. *Introduction to Basic Human Anatomy.* Lake Charles, LA: McNeese State University, Self-published manual. 1985.

Marieb, Elaine N. *Essentials of Human Anatomy and Physiology,* 4th ed. New York, NY: Benjamin/Cummings Publishing Company, Inc., 1994.

McAleer, Neil. *The Body Almanac.* Garden City, NY: Doubleday and Company, Inc., 1985.

Mosby's Medical, Nursing, and Allied Health Dictionary, 4th ed. St Louis: Mosby–Year Book, Inc., 1994.

Newton, Don. *Pathology for Massage Therapists,* 2nd ed. Portland: Simran Publications, 1995.

Premkumar, Kalyani, *Pathology A to Z—A Handbook for Massage Therapists.* Calgary, Canada: VanPub Books, 1996.

Tabers Cyclopedic Medical Dictionary, 13th ed. Philadelphia: F. A. Davis Company, 1977.

Tortora Gerald J. *Introduction to the Human Body: The Essentials of Anatomy and Physiology,* 3rd ed. New York: HarperCollins Publishers. 1994.

A man is only as old as his arteries.

—Pierre Cabanis, French physician

12 Circulatory System

Student Objectives

After completing this chapter, the student should be able to:

- List the functions of the circulatory system (cardiovascular and lymphatic)
- Describe blood's characteristics and physical composition (formed elements and plasma)
- Identify how oxygen is transported in the blood
- Explain three blood-clotting mechanisms
- Identify and discuss two types of commonly used blood type groupings
- Trace blood through the heart, and identify each chamber and valve
- Discuss the heart's conduction system
- List the three main types of blood vessels, and identify characteristics of each
- Name all the major arterial pulse points of the body
- Discuss blood pressure and factors that can influence both blood pressure and heart rate
- Within the systemic circuit, name and locate all the major arteries and veins of the body
- Name the lymphatic organs and vessels of the body
- Discuss the flow of lymph from the lymphatic capillaries to the major lymphatic ducts

INTRODUCTION

The circulatory system consists of two different subsystems: the cardiovascular system and the lymphvascular system, both regarded as "pick-up and delivery" systems because their primary function is transportation. We will discuss the cardiovascular system in the first section of this chapter; the lymphatic system will be discussed later.

CARDIOVASCULAR SYSTEM

The cardiovascular system consists of the blood, the heart, and blood vessels—a sustaining "river of life." We will examine the characteristics of blood: its formed elements and plasma, its clotting function, blood typing, and its main function of transport. Blood is the primary transport medium for a variety of substances that travel through the body. Blood makes its way through the body in a circular direction due to the pumping action of the heart. We will learn, in detail, about the heart's various structures, chambers, valves, and heart rate. Circulation is accomplished by a vast network of vessels, and each vessel plays a different role in the circulatory process.

FUNCTIONS OF THE CARDIOVASCULAR SYSTEM

1. Transportation and distribution of respiratory gases such as oxygen and carbon dioxide, of nutrients from the digestive tract, of antibodies, of waste materials, and of hormones from endocrine glands.
2. Protection of the body through disease-fighting white blood cells and the removal of impurities such as pathogens and poisons.
3. Prevention of hemorrhage through clotting mechanisms; prevention of loss of body fluids from damaged vessels.
4. Regulation of body temperature by moving heat to and from active muscles to the skin where the heat can be dissipated through the mechanisms of perspiration and vasodilation.

BLOOD

Blood is classified as a liquid connective tissue that is essential for human life because the body's tissues can get oxygen and nutrients only from its blood supply. Blood is composed of a pale fluid called plasma, in which living cells possessing different functions are suspended. Under normal circumstances, a blood cell makes a round trip through the circulatory system every 60 seconds.

Terms and Word Roots Related to the Circulatory System

aorta – a strap; to suspend
atrium – corridor
bicuspid – two; pointed
brady – slow
capillary – hairlike
cardio, cardia – heart
chordae tendineae – cordlike; tendon
cisterna chyli – a reservoir or cavity; juice
coagulation – to curdle
coronary – shaped like a crown or circle
cyanosis – dark blue; condition
diastole – to expand
edema – swelling
erythrocyte – red cell
fibrinogen – fiber; to produce
hemo – blood
hemocytopoiesis/hemocytogenesis – blood; cell; formation or birth
hemoglobin – blood; globe
hemorrhage – blood; to burst forth
hemostasis – blood; stopping
intima – innermost
ischemia – to hold; blood
leukocytes – white; cell
lumen – light
mediastinum – standing in the middle
mitral – headdress
phagocytosis – to eat; cell; condition
phleb – vein
pinocytosis – to drink; cell; condition
plasma – a thing formed
platelet – flat
Purkinje fibers – named after the Bohemian anatomist (1787–1869)
saphenous – the hidden
semilunar – half; moon
sphygmomanometer – pulse; thin; measure
systole – contraction
tachy – rapid, fast, or swift
thrombocytes – clot; cell
tricuspid – three; pointed
tunica – a sheath
vascular – a vessel or duct
vasoconstriction – vessel; a binder
vasodilation – vessel; to widen
vena cava – vein; cavity
ventricle – little belly

Characteristics of Blood

1. Blood is a viscous fluid that is thicker and more adhesive than water.
2. Its pH is slightly alkaline.
3. Blood constitutes about 8 percent of the total body weight.
4. Blood volume in the average-size male is approximately 5 to 6 liters (6 quarts or 12 pints).
5. The color varies from bright scarlet red to dull maroon, depending on oxygen content.

Components of Blood

Blood consists of formed elements and plasma.

Formed Elements

Also referred to as blood corpuscles, the three formed elements—the erythrocytes, the leukocytes, and the thrombocytes—comprise approximately 45 percent of blood. Each element performs a different function.

Blood cells are formed by a process called **hemocytopoiesis** or **hemocytogenesis.** After birth, blood forms primarily in the red bone marrow of long, flat, and irregular bones. Some blood cells (white) are formed in lymphoid tissue. A matrix blood cell is called a **hemocytoblast.** Almost all types of blood cells are formed from this single cell (Fig. 12–1).

Erythrocytes. Erythrocytes, red blood cells or red corpuscles, are the most numerous components of blood, outnumbering white blood cells by about 1,000 to 1. Erythrocytes are the major factor contributing to blood viscosity. These cells do not have a nucleus, which keeps them from reproducing or carrying out extensive metabolic activities. The primary function of erythrocytes is to transport oxygen and a small amount of carbon dioxide in the blood. Each functional erythrocyte is biconcave to allow greater surface area for more efficient diffusion of gas molecules and for ease of movement through tiny capillaries (minute blood vessels). Erythrocytes are occupied by a red respiratory pigment called **hemoglobin,** which constitutes about 33

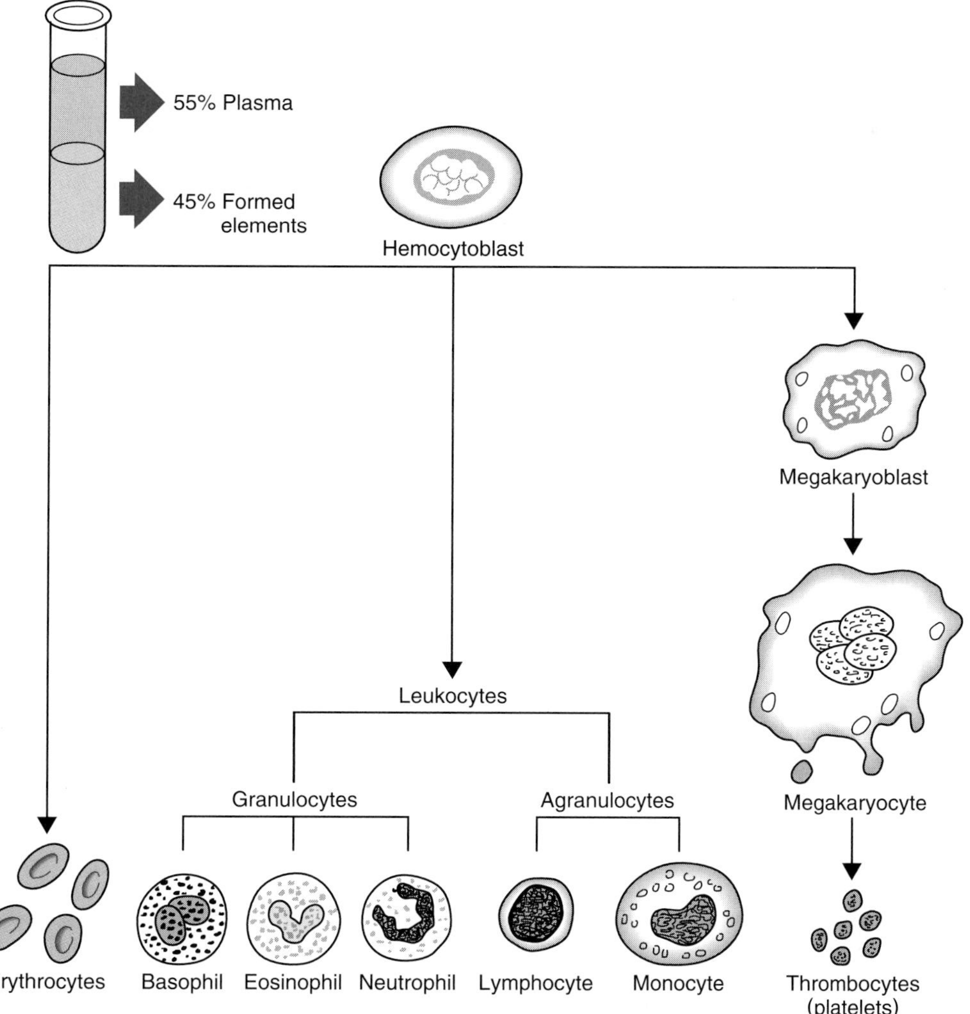

Figure 12•1 Different kinds of blood cells.

percent of a cell's weight. This red pigment is what gives blood its characteristically red color. Hemoglobin consists of a protein called globin and a pigment called heme (containing iron). This molecule combines with oxygen so that the gas can be transported through this liquid medium to body tissues. Because oxygen has a low solubility in water, hemoglobin requires the heme molecule to carry oxygen.

The life span of an erythrocyte is between 100 to 120 days, after which it begins to fragment, and the remains are eliminated by the spleen, liver, and other body tissues. Hemoglobin is also recycled. Globin broken down into amino acids is reused in protein synthesis, and heme is broken down into iron and biliverdin. The iron component is sent to bone marrow for reuse in hemoglobin synthesis, and biliverdin (green pigment) is converted into bilirubin (yellow) and is sent to the liver for excretion in bile.

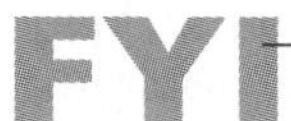

FOR YOUR INFORMATION

Cigarette smoking damages about 20 percent of the smoker's hemoglobin due to the presence (and crowding) of carbon monoxide.

Leukocytes. Leukocytes, white blood cells or white corpuscles, serve as part of the body's immune system by protecting the body from invading wastes, debris, bacteria, viruses, and tumor cells. Think of these cells as the blood's defensive "mobile army." Leukocytes begin to mobilize and destroy the invader in processes known as phagocytosis and pinocytosis. Phagocytosis is the process by which specialized cells engulf and digest harmful microorganisms and cellular debris. When a pathogen is absorbed rather than "eaten" by leukocytes, this is known as pinocytosis. In this process, the cell develops a saccular indention, engulfing the pathogen.

Some leukocytes combat irritants that cause inflammation, as well as irritants that produce allergies by producing **histamine** (a compound found in all cells that is released in allergic, inflammatory reactions, causing dilatation of capillaries, decreased blood pressure, and constriction of smooth muscles of the bronchi) and **antigens** (substances, usually proteins, that stimulate production of antibodies).

Whenever leukocytes mobilize for action, the body doubles their production within a few hours. Leukocytes are able to squeeze through intracellular spaces and migrate to their sites of action. Their life span lasts from a few hours to a few days.

There are two major types of leukocytes: granular (possessing grains in the cytoplasm) and agranular (possessing very few grains or devoid of grains in the cytoplasm). Granular leukocytes include neutrophils, eosinophils, and basophils. Monocytes and lymphocytes make up a type of agranular leukocyte.

Thrombocytes. Also known as **platelets, thrombocytes** are not complete cells but are fragmented parts of larger blood cells called megakaryoblast/megakaryocytes. Thrombocytes help to repair leaks in the blood vessels through various clotting mechanisms. A thrombocyte life span is from 5 to 9 days. **Hemostasis** is the term used to indicate the cessation of vascular bleeding by either mechanical (i.e., pressure), chemical (vitamin K) means, or by the coagulation process of the body.

Plasma

Plasma is a straw-colored liquid that remains when the formed elements are removed from the blood. Approximately 55 percent of blood volume is plasma, but plasma itself is 90 percent water and 10 percent **solutes** (substances dissolved in a solution). One of the solutes is **fibrinogen,** which functions in blood clotting. When necessary, fibrinogen is converted to an insoluble fibrin, forming the foundations of a blood clot.

BLOOD CLOTTING

The ability for the blood to clot is vital for the repair of damaged blood vessels. Vitamin K is required for the blood-clotting process. The three main mechanisms for blood clotting are a platelet plug, vascular spasm, and coagulation.

1. **Platelet Plug.** When platelets come into contact with a damaged blood vessel, their physical characteristics change drastically. They enlarge, become sticky, and clump together, forming a plug that helps to seal the damaged vessel. The mass of platelets closing off (or attempting to close off) a break in a vessel is called a platelet plug.
2. **Vascular Spasm.** The smooth muscle in the broken blood vessel begins to spasm, reducing the blood flow for up to 30 minutes.
3. **Coagulation.** Coagulation, or clot formation, is the process of transforming liquid blood into a viscous ball or clot. Because coagulated blood flows at a slower rate than liquid blood, blood loss is reduced. The coagulation process involves a chemical reaction that forms fibrin (the threadlike components of a clot). Once a clot is formed, it goes through a process of retraction (tightening of the clot) that draws the injured vessel walls closer together for repair. At the time a clot is formed, an enzyme called plasmin is also formed, which has the ability to slowly dissolve the clot over time.

BLOOD TYPES

Currently, there are at least 14 blood group systems (ways to classify blood types). The most popular system is the ABO system, which uses antigens to classify blood groups. The surfaces of erythrocytes may contain genetically determined proteins called antigens. Common antigens and antibodies are chemically reactive to each other; this is part of the body's defense system. The body does not normally produce antibodies for naturally occurring antigens. When a foreign antigen is introduced to the body, its corresponding antibody recognizes the foreigner as an intruder and attacks it.

The two known blood antigens are antigen A and antigen B. People with antigen A are type A, and those with antigen B are type B. Those with both antigens are type AB, and those with neither antigen are type O.

Correspondingly, the blood *plasma* has an antibody that is associated with the antigen on the erythrocyte. Type A blood has a type B antibody, type B blood has a type A antibody, type AB blood has neither antibody, and type O blood has both A and B antibodies. If a type A individual is given type B or type AB blood, the recipient's body will recognize the type B antigens as a foreign protein. The type B antibodies present in the recipient's type A blood will attack the type B antigen in the donor blood, causing erythrocytes to clump. These clumps can block smaller blood vessels and may lead to tissue damage, organ blockage, and death.

Since type AB has no antibodies, it can receive all other blood types and is referred to as a **universal recipient.** Type O has no antigens and will not react to any other blood types and hence is referred to as a **universal donor.** Blood transfusions must be made with compatible blood types because mismatching can cause severe medical problems or death.

The Rh blood group system depends on the presence or absence of the Rh protein on the erythrocyte membrane. **Rh factor** is so named because the theory was refined in the blood of rhesus monkeys. Rh-positive (about 85 percent of the population) describes the presence of the Rh protein and is not a health problem. Rh-negative (about 15 percent of the population) indicates the absence of the Rh protein and can become a problem during pregnancy. If the pregnant mother is Rh-negative and the fetus is Rh-positive, blood incompatibility may occur if the blood interacts, such as through a ruptured vessel. Due to medical advances, this situation is rarely life threatening for the fetus.

THE HEART

The heart is located in the mediastinum region of the thoracic cavity and rests on the respiratory diaphragm. About the size of a clenched fist, the heart possesses four hollow chambers: two atria and two ventricles. A septum separates the ventricles and extends between the atria (interatrial septum) (Fig. 12–2). These hollow chambers function as a double pump; the right-hand pump forces oxygen-depleted blood to the lungs, while the left-hand pump squeezes oxygen-rich blood out to the rest of the body and back. The primary function of the heart is to pump blood through the body. When the heart or cardiac muscle contracts, it squeezes the hollow cavities, forcing blood out while valves open and shut to keep it on its course. The heart pumps blood intermittently, on the average of 70 beats per minute in a resting person.

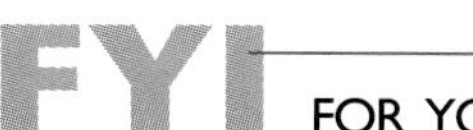

FOR YOUR INFORMATION

The heart beats an average of more than 100,000 times a day. The blood is pumped through 60,000 miles of blood vessels, or roughly two and a half times around the world at the equator.

Heart Coverings and Heart Wall

Surrounding the heart is a structure called the **pericardium,** or the **pericardial sac** (see Fig. 12–2). The outer layer of the pericardial sac is the *fibrous pericardium,* a dense, fibrous connective tissue layer that anchors the heart into the middle of the chest and to the diaphragm. Within the fibrous pericardium is a double-layered serous membrane. One layer is the *parietal pericardium,* which lies close to the surface of the heart; the second layer, which actually touches the heart, is the *visceral pericardium* (epicardium). The space created by the visceral and the parietal pericardiums is called the *pericardial cavity.* The serous fluid produced by these membranes fills the pericardial cavity to reduce friction between the membranes as the heart contracts and expands.

The heart wall itself possesses three layers: the epicardium, the myocardium, and the endocardium (see Fig. 12–2). The **epicardium,** which is the same membrane as the visceral pericardium, is the thin outer layer of serous membrane. This protective layer possesses adipose tissue and the blood vessels that nourish the heart. The **myocardium** is the thick muscular layer that makes up the bulk of the heart wall. Contraction of the myocardium forces blood out of the cardiac chambers. For a discussion of cardiac muscle tissue, refer to the insert from the muscular system chapter. The **endocardium** comprises the thin, inner lining of the heart and is continuous with the endothelial lining of the heart chambers and blood vessels, as well as with the valves of the heart.

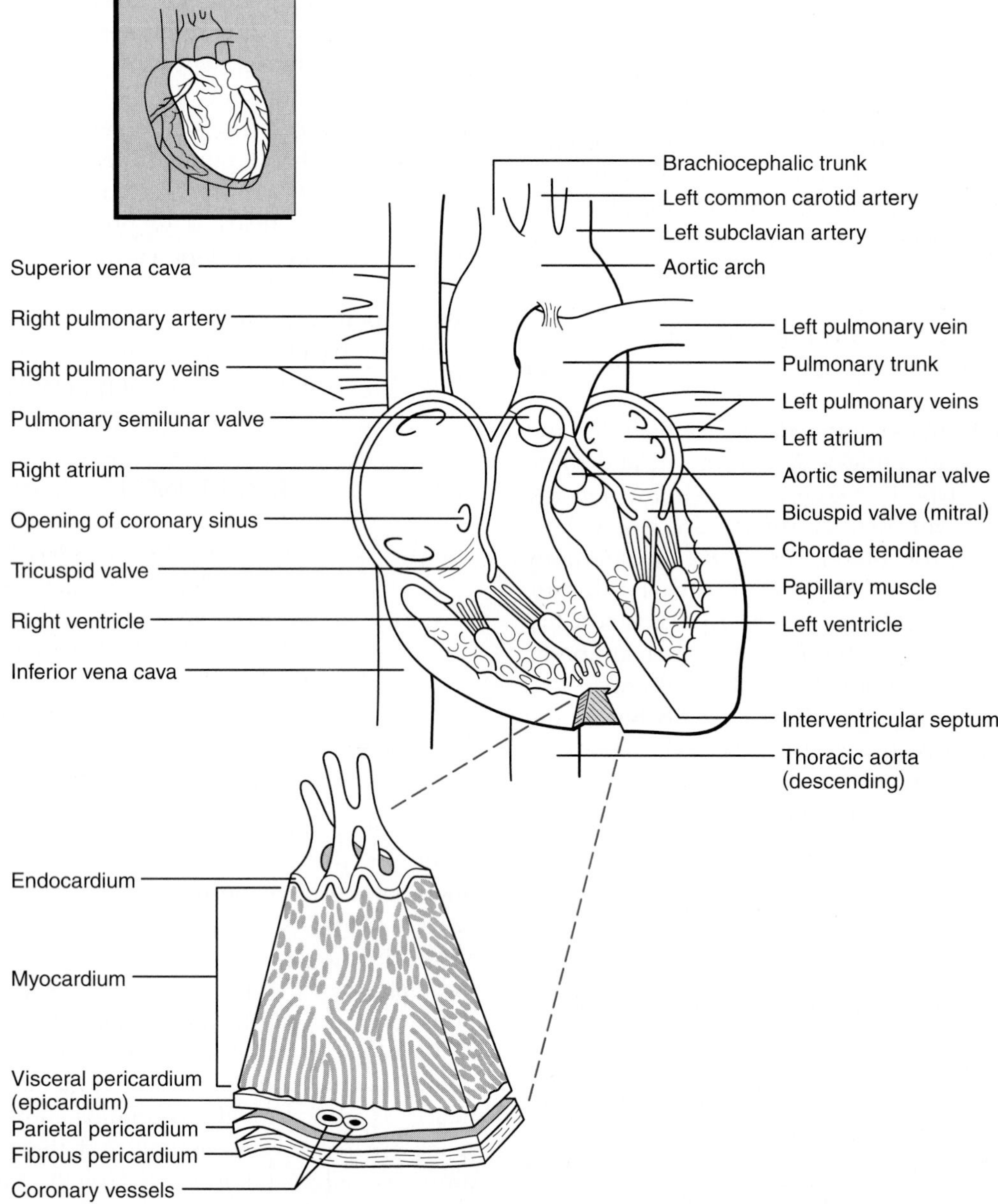

Figure 12•2 The heart, its wall, and the valves.

Flashback

From the Muscular System Chapter . . .
The heart wall is made up of cardiac muscle, which is a type of involuntary striated muscle.

1. Each cardiac muscle cell is branched and shaped like the letter Y or H. This unique attribute allows the cells to fit together like clasped fingers and helps create the spherical shape of the heart. This branching and interlocking arrangement also allows the transmission of stimuli throughout an entire section of the heart, rather than in rows or bundles.
2. The nuclei of cardiac muscle cells are centrally located and are typically mononucleated (only one nucleus per cell), although they may be multinucleated.
3. Cardiac muscle is said to be striated because of its alternating light and dark bands, or striations, which are visible when this tissue is viewed under a microscope.
4. The contraction of the heart muscle is autorhythmic through a property called conduction. When the heart is stimulated to contract, this stimulus is transmitted from a specialized area of muscle in the heart called the sinoatrial node (SA node), which controls heart rate. Nerve impulses can speed up or slow down heart rate, but the SA node initiates the heartbeat. Once the SA node produces an impulse, it sends a message to the appropriate areas of the heart to stimulate rhythmic contraction, generating the pumping action of the heart.

5. Between each cardiac muscle cell is a structure known as the intercalated disk, which functions like the electrical synapses of the nervous system and assists the transmission of a stimulus from cell to cell. This transmission, along with the internal conduction system, allows the activity of the heart to be closely coordinated.

Heart Chambers

The hollow heart is subdivided into four chambers that receive and pump blood. The superior chambers are called the atria and take in blood from the body through large veins, then pump it to the inferior chambers. The lower chambers, or ventricles, pump blood to the body's organs and tissues. The septum separating the right and left atria is called the *interatrial septum,* and the septum separating the right and left ventricles is called the *interventricular septum.* Let's examine the heart chambers more closely (the vessels will be discussed later in the chapter).

Right Atrium. Atria, in general, are thin walled because they only need enough cardiac muscle to deliver the blood into the ventricles. The right atrium receives blood from all parts of the body except the lungs. Blood is received from the superior and the inferior vena cavae and the coronary sinus. Blood from the right atrium is delivered into the right ventricle beneath it.

Right Ventricle. The right ventricle receives blood from the right atrium and pumps blood through the pulmonary trunk and into the right and left pulmonary arteries. Blood is routed to the lungs to release carbon dioxide and to pick up oxygen. The oxygenated blood is returned to the heart via the pulmonary veins.

Left Atrium. The oxygen-rich blood from the pulmonary veins enters the left atrium. During an atrial contraction, blood passes from the left atrium to the left ventricle.

Left Ventricle. The left ventricle receives blood from the left atrium. This ventricular structure has the thickest heart wall because it must pump blood using high pressure through literally thousands of miles of vessels throughout the body. The amount of blood ejected from the left ventricle during each contraction is called **stroke volume.**

In review, the blood travels through the heart as follows (Fig. 12–3): Blood from the body enters the heart through the inferior and superior vena cavae

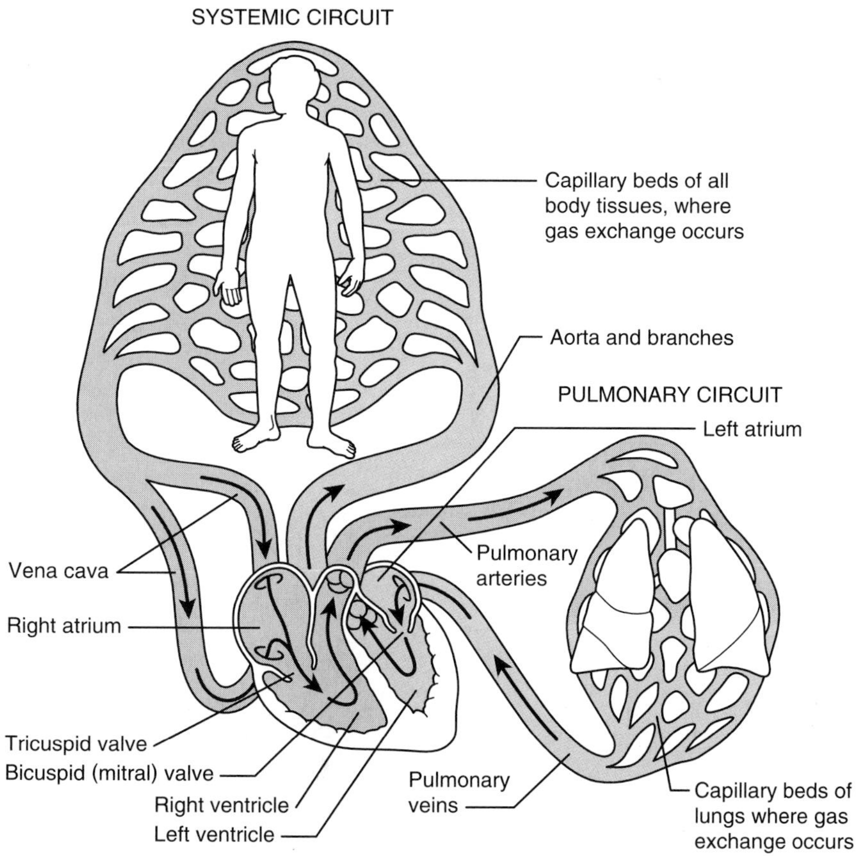

Figure 12•3 Blood moving through the heart.

and the coronary sinus into the right atrium. The superior vena cava returns blood from the chest area, the arm, and the head. The inferior vena cava returns blood from the abdominal area and the legs. The coronary sinus (veins) returns blood from the heart itself. Once blood from these vessels enters the right atrium, it is delivered into the right ventricle and then to the pulmonary trunk. This vessel becomes the right and left pulmonary arteries and transports blood to the lungs for the release of carbon dioxide and to obtain oxygen.

The oxygenated blood returns to the heart through the right and left pulmonary veins and enters the left atrium. The left atrium moves the blood into the left ventricle, and from here the blood moves into the aorta to all parts of the body via the arteries.

Heart Valves

The heart valves are little flaps of endothelium located between the chambers of the heart (atria and ventricles) and between the ventricles and some of the great vessels. These valves work to keep blood flowing in one direction as the pressure exerted on the blood changes as the heart pumps. These valves include the **atrioventricular (AV) valves** and the **semilunar (SL) valves.**

The AV valves separate the atria from the ventricles; their names indicate their anatomical position. The right AV valve has three flaps or cusps and is called the **tricuspid valve;** the left AV valve has two flaps or cusps and is called the **bicuspid valve** or **mitral valve.** These valves are held in place by tendonlike cords called chordae tendineae, which are attached to the ventricular walls through cardiac muscle projections called papillary muscles.

Between both ventricles and their adjacent arteries are the semilunar valves. Each valve consists of three half moon–shaped cusps that allow blood to flow in only one direction. They are named for the vessels they lead to: the **pulmonary semilunar valve** and the **aortic semilunar valve.** The pulmonary semilunar valve lies between the right ventricle and the pulmonary trunk; the aortic semilunar valve is between the left ventricle and the aorta.

Conduction System of the Heart

The heart's rate of contraction is controlled by a system of modified cardiac cells that *conduct* impulses through the muscle tissue of the heart. The purpose of this conduction system is to coordinate and synchronize the heart's activity. The cardiac tissues of the heart are autorhythmic (capable of self-excitation). Thus, the heart has the ability to generate its own regular series of action potentials that cause each section to contract independently without neural input. Each structure in the conduction system is a mass of specialized conducting cells. The main parts of this system are the **sinoatrial node** (SA node) and the **atrioventricular node** (AV node), the **atrioventricular bundle** (AV bundle), and the **conducting myofibers (Purkinje fibers)** (Fig. 12–4).

The SA node lies within the right atrium and initiates the cardiac impulse, stimulating both the right and left atria to contract. The purpose of the SA node is to initiate the heartbeat cycle. While this is accomplished without the input of the nervous system, the

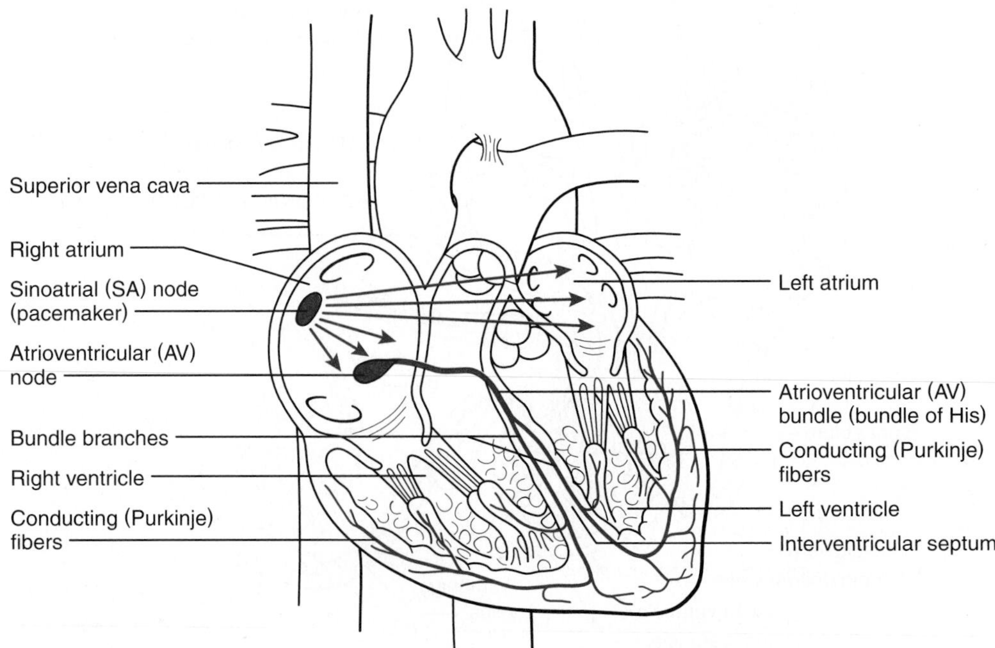

Figure 12•4 The heart's conduction system.

rate at which the contractions are generated can be influenced by nervous system input. Firing on the average of about 72 times per minute, the SA node sets the pace of the heart; this is why it is called the "pacemaker."

The firing of the SA node is much like pushing the first in a row of dominos standing on end. It is the first impulse or push that initiates a sequence of events. Each domino causes another to fall until the cycle is complete. Compare this concept with the heart's conduction system. The SA node fires, causing the atria to contract; blood in these chambers is then pushed by the atrial contraction into the ventricles; and the impulses from the SA node immediately arrive at the AV node in the interventricular septum.

The AV node is designed to work at a slower rate than the SA node in order to give the atria plenty of time to empty themselves of blood. It is this brief delay that causes the slight pause between two sounds of the heart (lubb, dubb). The AV node relays the impulses to the AV bundle **(bundle of His).** The AV bundle branches into right and left bundles which run in the interventricular septum to the right and left ventricles. These bundles branch out to form conduction myofibers (Purkinje fibers), the function of which is to spread the impulse throughout the myocardium. This second stimulation through the myocardium causes the ventricles to simultaneously contract, expelling the blood from the ventricles to the arteries.

The cycle of events occurring with each alternating contraction and relaxation of the heart muscle, coordinated by the conducting system, is called the **cardiac cycle.** The firing action of the cardiac cycle remains constant when the SA node acts alone; however, other factors can regulate the cardiac cycle to increase or decrease the output of the heart to meet the demands of the body.

Author's Note

Dr. Janet Travell documents a myofascial trigger point in the right pectoralis major muscle whose pain referral zone refers noxious impulses into the sinoatrial node. This trigger point is related to cardiac arrhythmia (any deviation from a normal heartbeat). Releasing the trigger point with massage techniques can often end symptoms of tachycardia or "runaway" heartbeat. It is important to note that this procedure is only performed while the client is asymptomatic (or without symptoms at the time of treatment). A client experiencing tachycardia while in your office should be referred *immediately* to a physician.

The majority of heart rate changes are controlled by a specialized portion of the medulla oblongata known as the cardiac center of the brain. The autonomic nervous system can control the heart's activity and it responds like "spurs" or "reins" to alter the heart rate depending on which division of the nervous system is activated (sympathetic or parasympathetic). Heart rate and cardiac output are generally increased by impulses from the sympathetic nervous system, while stimuli from the parasympathetic nervous system decrease heart rate.

Oxygen demand and carbon dioxide levels in the bloodstream are constantly monitored by the body through chemoreceptors (receptors activated by chemical stimuli). Signals are sent to the cardiac center to increase cardiac output whenever oxygen is needed or when carbon dioxide levels are too high. Exercise, emotional stress, and altitude changes can create this need for oxygen or increase carbon dioxide levels.

Other factors that can increase or decrease heart rate are blood hormone levels, blood pH, ion and mineral balance of the blood, temperature (elevated temperatures will increase heart rates whereas colder temperatures decrease heart rate), age (younger people require a higher cardiac rhythm to operate efficiently), and general health or vitality. For further discussion, refer to the section in this chapter on blood pressure.

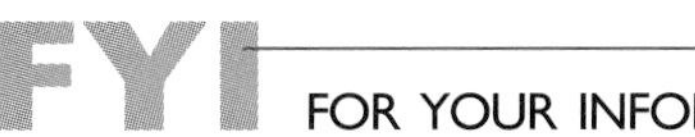

FYI FOR YOUR INFORMATION

An electrocardiogram (ECG or EKG) records the electrical changes in the heartbeat as the impulse travels through the heart.

Sound of Heartbeat

When you listen to a beating heart—lubb, dubb; lubb, dubb—the sounds *by a beating heart* are due to the closing of the heart's valves. The "lubb" sound is the closing of the AV (tricuspid and bicuspid) valves when the atria contract, and the "dubb" sound is the closing of the pulmonary and aortic semilunar valves after the ventricles contract. *The pulse rate is the number of ventricular contractions per minute.*

BLOOD VESSELS

Blood vessels are a closed network of tubular structures connected to the heart that transport blood to all the cells of the body. These blood vessels are divided into three main groups based on their structure and function: arteries, veins, and capillaries. The walls of both arteries and veins possess three layers (tunics). The innermost layer is called the **tunica intima** (or **tunica interna**), which is endothelial tissue fused with a small quantity of connective tissue. The middle layer is the **tunica media,** which contains quantities of both connective tissue and smooth muscle. The outer layer,

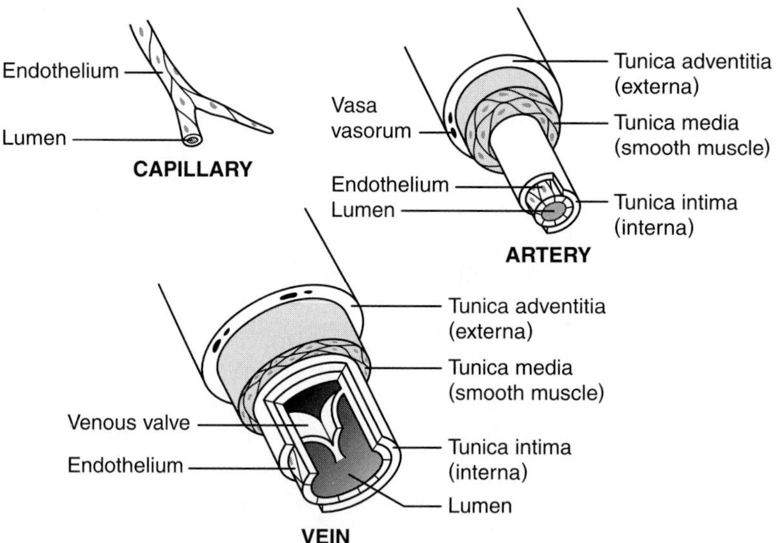

Figure 12•5 Comparing arteries and veins—layers or tunics of blood vessels.

possessing mostly dense connective tissue, is the **tunica adventitia** (or **tunica externa**) (Fig. 12–5).

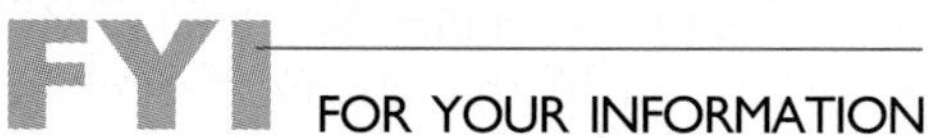

FOR YOUR INFORMATION

Blood vessels have their own blood supply called the vasa-vasorum, which are often referred to as the "vessels of the vessels." They are typically located in the tunica externa layer of the vessels.

The walls of arteries and veins possess two specific properties: elasticity and contractility. The levels of these properties differ greatly between the arteries and the veins; arterial walls are more elastic and have a thicker muscular (middle) layer than veins.

The muscular layer of the arteries and veins can dilate and contract to change the diameter of the vessel. The open space within the blood vessel is known as the **lumen.** When the diameter of the vascular lumen enlarges, the process is called **vasodilation;** when the diameter becomes narrower, it is called **vasoconstriction.**

Vasodilation and vasoconstriction may be initiated by two sources. One source is by direct nerve stimulus from the vasomotor center located in the medulla oblongata of the brain; this may be a systemic response to raise or lower blood pressure. The other source is by a local reflex response to a stimulus such as pressure (i.e., massage) or temperature (i.e., heat or cold application).

Arteries

Arteries, by definition, are vessels that move blood away from the heart. In general, blood within the arteries is oxygenated. The only artery that contains deoxygenated blood is the pulmonary artery, moving blood from the right ventricle of the heart to the lungs; conversely, the pulmonary vein carries oxygenated blood. Since arteries are closer to the pumping action of the heart, their vascular walls are considerably thicker and stronger in order to withstand higher blood pressure, compared with veins. Arteries continue to branch off into smaller and thinner vessels, becoming **arterioles,** then lose the two outer layers. When the vessels are one layer thick, they are called capillaries (discussed later).

Because arteries deliver oxygenated blood to the body's tissues, pressure applied on these vessels could interfere with blood delivery and could damage tissues. Thus, there are several important arteries that must be avoided by the massage therapist (i.e., endangerment sites). Please refer to the massage physiology chapter for a complete list of vascular endangerment sites.

Author's Note

A mnemonic device to help you remember that arteries carry blood away from the heart is both that *a*rteries and *a*way begin with the letter A.

Arterial Pulse. The word "pulse" refers to the expansion effect that occurs when the left ventricle contracts, producing a wave of blood that surges through and expands the arterial walls. This pulse can be felt in the arteries that are located close to the surface of the body or where they lie over bone or other firm tissue. Avoid using your thumb or index finger when taking someone's pulse because you may register your own pulse instead. Each pulse point is named for the region of the body in which it is located. The common pulse points are listed in Figure 12–6.

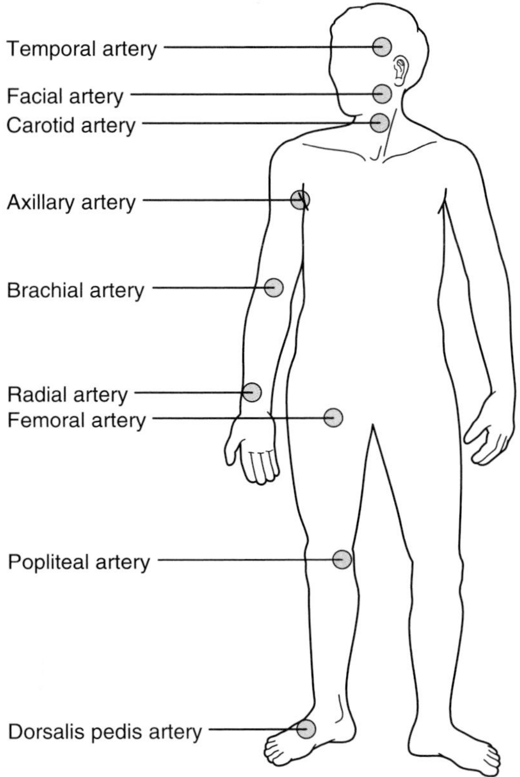

Figure 12•6 Map of pulse points.

1. **Carotid artery**—sides of the neck
2. **Temporal artery**—anterior to the ear; temple region
3. **Facial artery**—inferior to the corner of the mouth
4. **Axillary artery**—in the armpit region
5. **Brachial artery**—the midbiceps brachii
6. **Radial artery**—lateral aspect of the wrist
7. **Femoral artery**—inferior groin area to the upper medial thigh
8. **Popliteal artery**—the posterior knee
9. **Dorsalis pedis artery**—the anterior medial foot

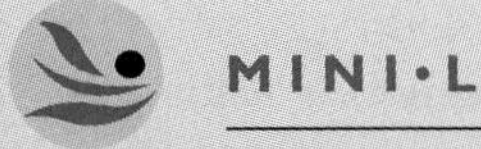

MINI•LAB

Using the map of pulse points, locate these areas on a partner or on yourself. Note that pressure must be used to feel the pulse, but too much pressure prevents blood from flowing in the vessel.

Capillaries

When the arterioles lose their two outer layers, leaving only endothelium, they become the capillaries, which possess a thin, permeable membrane for efficient gas exchange. Erythrocytes carry oxygen in the blood on the hemoglobin molecule; these blood cells must move in a single file to squeeze through each capillary. The movement of blood in capillaries is the slowest of all the vessels, and its flow is intermittent, providing ample opportunity for an exchange to occur. The process by which nutrients and oxygen are provided to the tissues and waste from cells is removed from interstitial fluid is called **capillary exchange.** The exchange of gases is referred to as *internal* or *tissue respiration.* Capillary exchange is the main function of the capillaries and is achieved by diffusion. Tissues and organs that have extensive capillary networks are the muscles, the liver, the spleen, and the kidneys. Connective tissue has a sparse capillary network. Areas of the body that are devoid of capillaries are the epidermis of the skin and its derivatives (i.e., hair and nails) and the lens and cornea of the eye.

Veins

Veins begin at the capillary level and gradually become larger; small veins are called **venules.** Veins drain the tissues and organs and return blood, which is now low in oxygen, back to the heart and lungs. Unlike arteries, no pulse is felt in veins, and they are considerably less elastic, possess thinner walls, and are easily collapsed. By the time blood leaves the capillaries and moves into the veins, it has lost a great deal of pressure. The blood pressure in veins is usually too low to force the blood back to the heart (and venous return is often flowing against gravity).

To assist venous flow, the lumens in veins are larger, and small and medium-sized veins have numerous valves formed by folds in the endothelium, which open in the direction of the heart. This one-way valve system to prevent backflow, together with the pumping action of muscular contraction in the limbs, is called the **venous pump.** Veins also depend on pressure changes in the thorax and abdomen during breathing (**respiratory pump**) to push blood back to the heart.

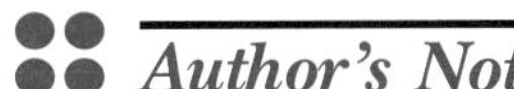

Author's Note

Arterial circulation is called *deep circulation,* and venous circulation is called *superficial circulation.* During massage therapy, the pressure strokes are applied centripetally (toward the heart or thorax). This is because massage therapy directly assists venous circulation or the circulation that is near the surface of the skin, whereas arterial blood flow is affected indirectly by massage.

BLOOD PRESSURE

To understand blood pressure, it is helpful to review some of the basics of simple physics. A basic law of physics is that pressure of a liquid in a closed system is distributed equally in all directions to the confines of the container. Hence, blood pressure is generally consistent in different areas of the body at a given time. In order to distribute itself equally, a liquid will always flow from a higher pressure to a lower pressure area. When a liquid such as blood flows into the heart, it does so because the empty chamber expands, creating a lower pressure or suction effect. Once the blood has filled the chamber, the contraction places force on the blood, and pressure builds. When the pressure inside the chamber of the heart overcomes the combination of the pressure outside the heart and the resistance of the valve, blood begins flowing out of the heart. Blood continues to move forward by the one-way action of the valves of the heart.

Blood pressure (BP) is the pressure exerted by blood on an arterial wall during the contraction of the left ventricle. Blood pressure is most often measured in the brachial artery using a **sphygmomanometer,** or blood pressure cuff. The reading gathered during the blood pressure measurement looks like a fraction or ratio. The top number (**systole**) represents the pressure exerted on the arterial wall during active ventricular contraction. The bottom number (**diastole**) represents the static pressure against the arterial wall during the rest or pause between contractions. Blood pressure is measured in millimeters of mercury, abbreviated mmHg. This is the pressure required to lift a column of mercury into the gauge to a given height (millimeters). A reading of 120/80 mmHg is considered to be normal blood pressure for adults. Borderline high blood pressure is above 140/90 mmHg. Readings over 160/95 mmHg are considered high, requiring medical attention. The diastolic reading is considered to be the most critical in health considerations. The heart is designed for periodic exertion; it will work harder to supply the body with blood during times of high demands, but cannot keep up a high rate for an extended period of time without resting. A high diastolic reading may indicate that the heart is working too hard even during its resting phase.

Blood flow, the amount of blood passing through a vessel in a given amount of time, depends on two factors: blood pressure and the resistance of friction between the blood cells and the vessel wall. When blood pressure rises, the friction resistance rises slightly due to the greater amount of blood being forced through the vessels. The main factor influencing blood flow is the blood pressure. The greater the difference between systolic and diastolic pressures, the higher the flow rate will be. For example, a blood pressure of 120/80 mmHg has a pressure difference of 40 mmHg during the cardiac cycle. If the blood pressure is increased to 140/90 mmHg due to physical exertion, the pressure difference has increased to 50 mmHg. A greater quantity of blood will be pushed through the vessel with the higher pressure drop or greater difference in pressures. However, the rate of blood flow through vessels does not significantly increase with hypertension because of the notable increase in vascular resistance.

We have seen that blood flow is directly influenced by blood pressure. Let's now look at the factors that influence blood pressure itself: resistance, cardiac output, blood volume, homeostatic regulation, and diseases or pathologies.

1. **Resistance.** This represents the effects of friction between the blood and the vessel walls. Resistance is directly influenced by the viscosity or composition of the blood, the length of the blood vessel, and the diameter of the blood vessel.

   Viscosity. As stated, blood thickness (viscosity) can influence blood pressure by increasing blood resistance. Dehydration may result in a reduction of blood plasma, causing blood volume to decrease and the blood to thicken. An increase in erythrocyte count can also cause a rise in viscosity. The thicker the blood, the more friction that is created. The higher the rate of friction resistance, the higher the blood pressure. Blood-thinning medication, such as aspirin, which depletes erythrocytes, can decrease blood viscosity and blood pressure.

   Length of the blood vessels. The longer the distance traveled through the vessel, the greater the contact between the blood cells and the vessel wall. This results in an increase in friction or resistance.

   Diameter of the blood vessels. The smaller the diameter of the blood vessel (lumen), the more resistance it offers the blood. The resistance in the arteries and veins is negligible due to their larger diameter. It is the smaller vessels, namely the arterioles, capillaries, and venules, that act as the bottleneck of the circulatory system, causing an increase in resistance and hence blood pressure. A discussion of how the arterioles are used to control blood pressure can be found in the section on vasomotor activity.

2. **Cardiac Output.** Cardiac output represents the blood volume expelled by the ventricles of the heart, multiplied by the heart rate (number of beats) per minute. The ventricles of the heart in a resting adult pump a volume of blood varying from about 4 to 8 liters of blood per minute. Blood pressure is directly proportional to cardiac output when all other factors stay the same. Cardiac output is influenced by the cardiovascular center of the brain as well as certain blood chemicals, physical characteristics, and genetic characteristics of the subject.

3. **Blood Volume.** Blood pressure is also directly proportional to blood volume. The greater the volume

of blood in the body, which might be due to a condition such as pregnancy, the higher the blood pressure. As blood volume decreases, perhaps due to blood loss by hemorrhage, blood pressure decreases.

4. **Homeostatic Regulation.** The body seeks to maintain homeostasis by regulating chemical and physical activities in the body. In regard to blood pressure, it is essential that the systolic and diastolic pressures be kept within normal ranges, which prevents cellular malnutrition and oxygen deprivation caused by low blood pressure, or physical damage to major organs such as the heart, brain, and kidneys caused by high blood pressure. Maintaining normal blood pressure is accomplished by regulating vasomotor activity due to chemoreceptor input, baroreceptor input, and the presence of hormones.

   Vasomotor activity. The vasomotor center located in the medulla oblongata of the brain helps to control blood pressure. By varying the number of sympathetic nervous system impulses to the vessels, the diameter of the arterioles can be dilated or constricted. Increased sympathetic impulses boost vasoconstriction, and the blood pressure elevates in response. Conversely, when impulses are decreased, vessel diameter dilates, and blood pressure falls. Vasomotor control is influenced by input from chemoreceptors, baroreceptors, and hormones. The body uses this information to determine the demand for bodily resources and then regulates the various body activities to supply these demands. Stimuli such as pressure, temperature, pain, or strong emotions can create a temporary increase in blood pressure, whereas a condition such as emotional depression may lower blood pressure.

   Chemoreceptors. These receptors measure pH, carbon dioxide, and some oxygen concentration of the blood. If oxygen is low or carbon dioxide is high, the chemoreceptors located in the aorta, carotid, and medulla stimulate the vasomotor system to constrict arterial flow until the blood pressure begins to rise.

   Baroreceptors. These pressure-sensitive receptor cells affect blood pressure in two ways. First, they communicate information about the blood pressure in the aorta and in the internal carotid arteries to the cardiac center in the medulla oblongata, which responds by increasing or decreasing cardiac output. Second, they transmit blood pressure information to the vasomotor center, also located in the medulla oblongata, which results in vasoconstriction or vasodilation.

   Hormones. Several hormones affect blood pressure. Epinephrine and norepinephrine produced by the adrenal medulla increase cardiac output and cause vasoconstriction to bring about a rise in blood pressure. Antidiuretic hormone (ADH) produced by the hypothalamus of the brain causes vasoconstriction during blood loss (hemorrhage).

5. **Diseases or Pathologies.** Deposits of plaque on the vessel walls may result in an increase of resistance due to friction, and/or a diameter restriction, causing an increase in blood pressure. Conditions such as edema may cause extravascular pressure against the vessels, particularly the veins, causing the heart to work harder to achieve circulation. Vascular diseases such as arteriosclerosis may raise systolic blood pressure due to the loss of elasticity in the arterial wall.

PATHS OF BLOOD CIRCULATION

As you may recall, the primary function of the circulatory system is transportation. Within the cardiovascular system, there are two circuits based on the areas of the body that are served: the pulmonary and the systemic. The **pulmonary circuit** brings deoxygenated blood from the right ventricle to the alveoli of the lungs to release carbon dioxide and to regain oxygen. Oxygenated blood returns to the left atrium of the heart and moves into the systemic circuit with the contraction of the left ventricle.

The **systemic circuit** brings the oxygenated blood from the left ventricle through numerous arteries into the capillaries. From here, blood moves back through the veins and returns the now deoxygenated blood to the right atrium to enter the pulmonary circuit.

Not all circulation routes begin with arteries and end with veins. There are several other circulatory networks for transporting blood within the body systems. Located within the systemic circuit are venous portal systems. As the name suggests, the venous portal systems of the body both start and end with veins that are used to transport materials such as hormones and nutrients. The main venous portal system is the **hepatic portal system,** which collects blood from the digestive organs (stomach, intestines, gallbladder, spleen, and pancreas) and delivers this blood to the liver for processing. Since the liver is a key organ involved in maintaining the proper glucose, fat, and protein concentrations in the blood, the hepatic portal system allows the blood from the digestive organs to "take a detour" through the liver to process these substances before they enter the systemic circulation (Fig. 12–7). The other venous portal system is located between the hypothalamus and the posterior pituitary of the brain.

Pulmonary Circuit

The pulmonary circuit is the circulatory system's contribution to respiration. The purpose of the pulmo-

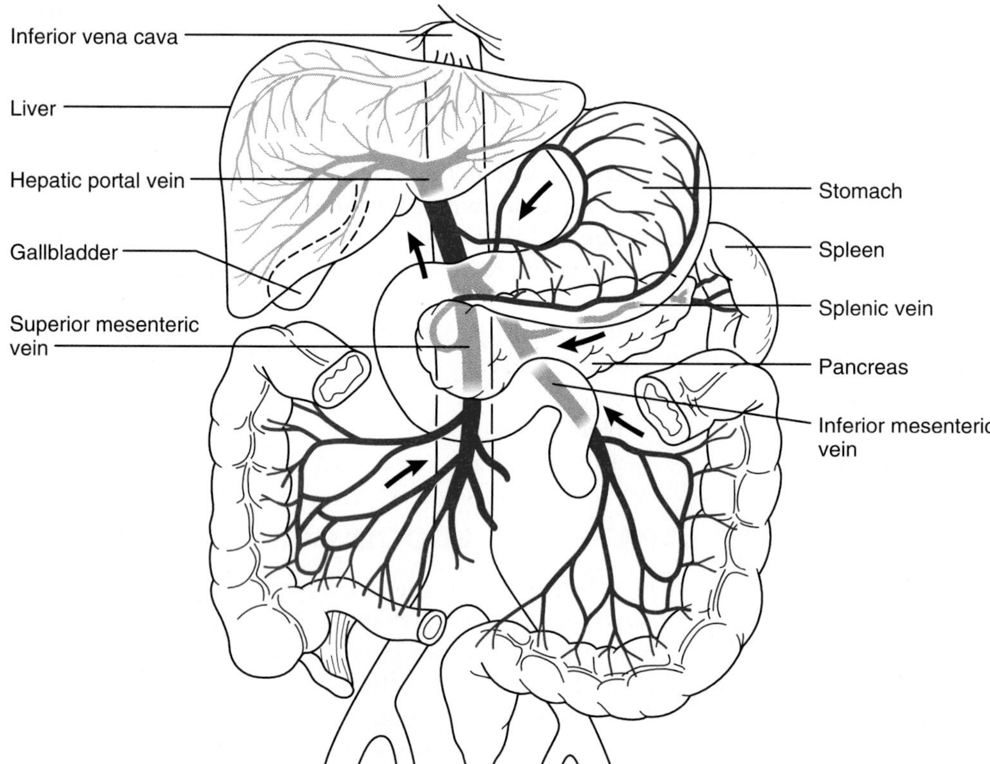

Figure 12•7 Venous portal system.

nary circuit is to replenish the oxygen supply of the blood and to eliminate gaseous waste products. The pulmonary circuit pumps blood to the lungs (pulmonary organ), where at each moment over 900 milliliters of blood are exposed to air by the rich capillary network in the alveoli. Here, gas exchange takes place by diffusion across the cellular membrane. The oxygen-depleted blood attracts the oxygen molecules from the lungs while releasing the waste gases such as carbon dioxide, which is exhaled. (For more information, see Internal and External Respiration in Chapter 13.) When the pulmonary arteries carry blood away from the heart and the pulmonary veins carry blood back to the heart, the oxygen content of the blood is reversed, that is, the pulmonary arteries carry deoxygenated blood (away from the heart to the lungs) and pulmonary veins carry oxygenated blood (back from the lungs to the heart).

Systemic Circuit

The systemic circuit is the body's highway system (its routes are hollow streets that consist of all other arteries, capillaries, and veins). The function of this circuit is to bring nutrients and oxygen to all systems of the body and to carry waste materials from the tissues for elimination.

Major Systemic Arteries. Arteries are named for their locations; they generally lie deep and are well shielded within tissues and muscles. Following is a list of the major systemic arteries (use Figure 12–8 to assist you in learning their locations in the body).

- temporal
- facial
- aorta (aortic arch, ascending, descending, thoracic, and abdominal)
- coronary
- brachiocephalic
- common carotid
- subclavian
- vertebral
- internal carotid
- external carotid
- axillary
- brachial
- radial
- ulnar
- celiac
- hepatic
- gastric
- splenic
- superior and inferior mesenteric
- renal
- gonadal (testicular and ovarian)
- common iliac
- internal and external iliac
- femoral
- popliteal
- anterior and posterior tibial

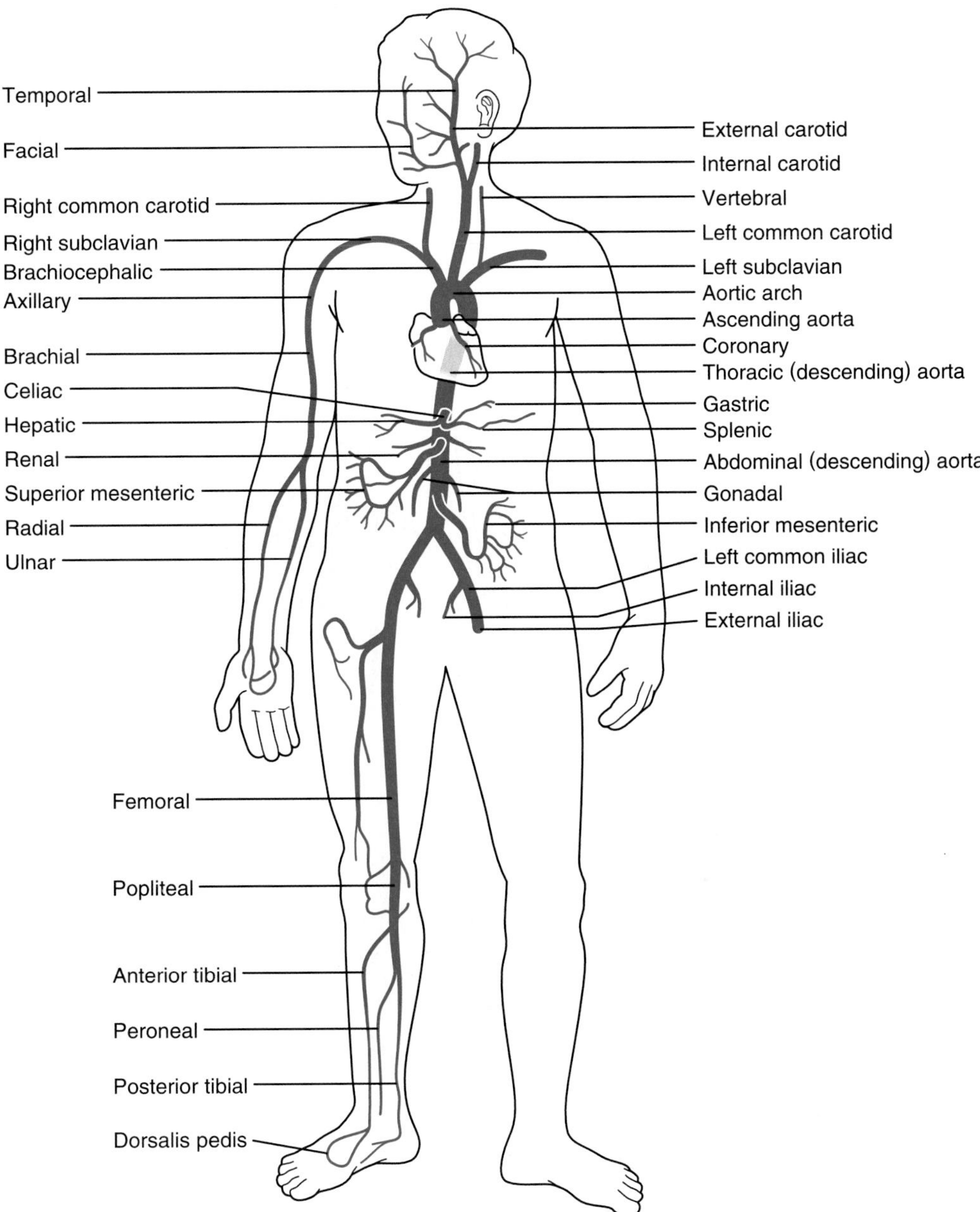

Figure 12•8 All major arteries of the body.

- peroneal
- dorsalis pedis

Major Systemic Veins. Veins, like arteries, are also named for their locations. Following is a list of the major systemic veins found in the body. Use Figure 12–9 to assist you in learning their locations.

- superior and inferior vena cava
- brachiocephalic
- internal and external jugular
- subclavian
- vertebral
- axillary
- cephalic
- brachial
- median cubital
- ulnar
- radial
- basilic
- hepatic
- hepatic portal
- superior and inferior mesenteric
- splenic
- renal
- gonadal (testicular and ovarian)
- common iliac
- internal and external iliac
- femoral
- great saphenous
- small (lesser) saphenous
- popliteal
- posterior and anterior tibial
- peroneal

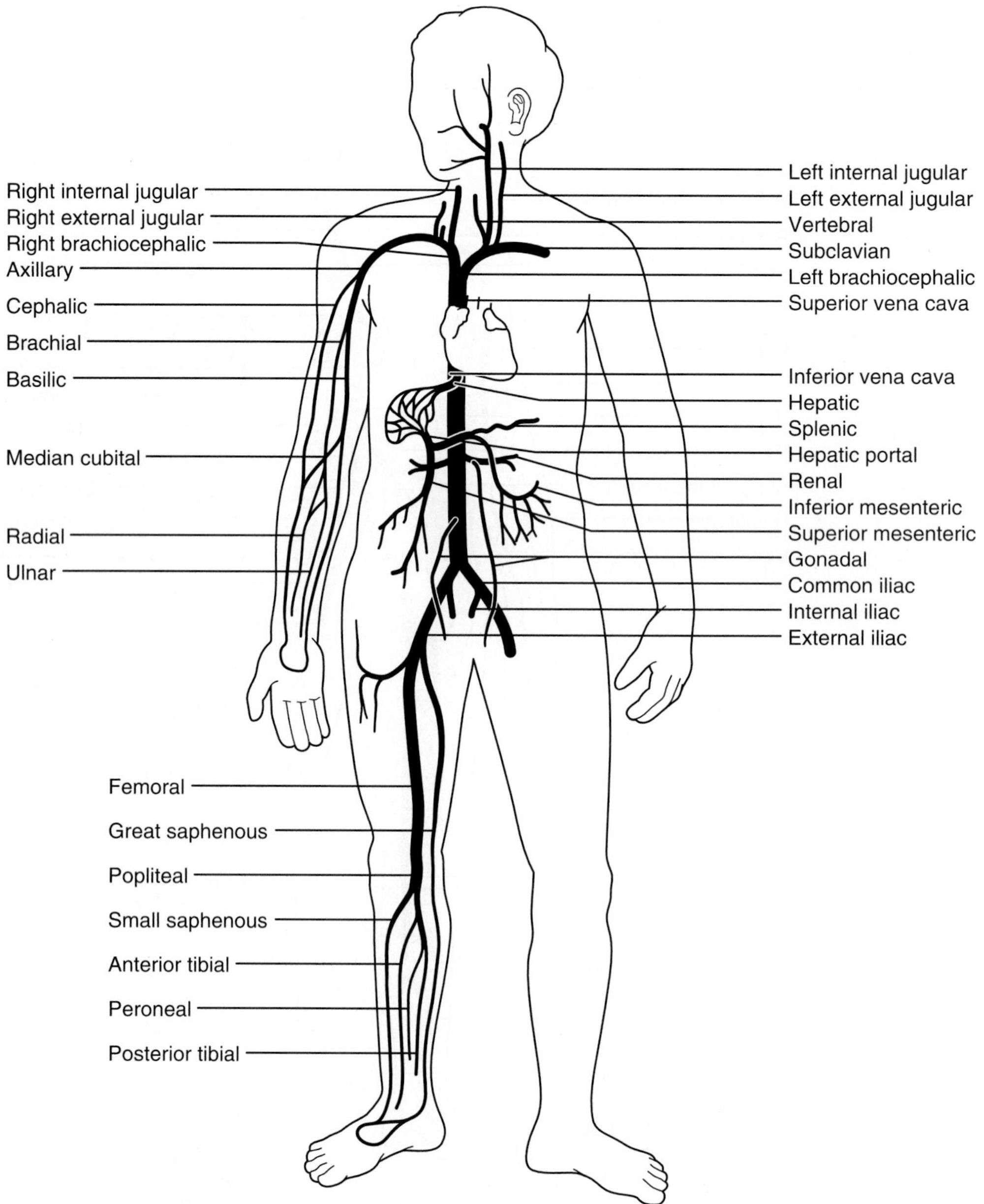

Figure 12•9 Major veins.

LYMPHATIC SYSTEM

The lymphatic system is a one-way system for drainage of excess fluid from the body's tissues, and is a complementary system for the circulatory system. Like the circulatory system, the lymphatic system has disease-fighting functions. The lymphatic system is composed of lymph fluid, lymph vessels, and specialized organs such as lymph nodes, tonsils, Peyer's patches, appendix, thymus, and the spleen. Lymph, the fluid of the lymphatic system, is transported through progressively larger and larger vessels until it is returned to the venous system through one of two large ducts in the thoracic region. In this section, we will explore the structures, functions, and pathways of the lymphatic system.

FUNCTIONS OF THE LYMPHATIC SYSTEM

1. After draining the tissues of excess interstitial fluid, the lymphatic system returns this fluid to the cardiovascular system. This helps maintain blood volume and blood pressure and prevent edema.
2. The lymphatic system transports fats and some vita-

mins from the digestive tract to the blood. As you may recall from the chapter on the digestive system, these specialized lymphatic vessels are called lacteals. The lymphatic system also returns proteins and cellular debris that have escaped from the blood back to the general circulation.
3. Through the filtering action of lymph nodes and organs, the lymphatic system provides immunity against disease. Many pathogens and other impurities are removed from the lymph and destroyed by disease-fighting lymphocytes and antibodies.

LYMPH

Lymph is similar in composition to both interstitial fluid and blood plasma with a few minor differences. The main difference between lymph and interstitial fluid is location. Once this fluid leaves the cells and tissues and enters the lymphatic system, it is referred to as lymphatic fluid or lymph. Lymph contains fewer proteins than blood plasma.

Unlike the cardiovascular system, the lymphatic system is an open system that moves in only one direction, toward the subclavian veins. Without a pump to assist flow, lymph moves only through pressure gradients from external sources. Transportation of lymph depends entirely on smooth muscle contraction within the vessel walls, on the milking action of skeletal muscle contractions, and on the pressure changes in the thorax and abdomen during breathing. Lymph moves slowly when compared with blood circulation.

LYMPH VESSELS

Lymphatic vessels (lymphatics) include lymph capillaries, lymph vessels, lymphatic trunks, and two main collecting ducts.

Lymph capillaries have the same structures as blood capillaries, but they are larger, more irregular, and more permeable. They start blindly in the tissues and exist in all parts of the body except bone marrow, the epidermis, the central nervous system (brain and spinal cord), and the eyes. Lymph nodes are located throughout lymphatic tributaries to filter the lymph moving through the system.

Lymph capillaries become larger vessels called lymph vessels. Compared with veins, lymphatic vessels have thin walls and more valves that open up in only one direction. These merge along similar pathways to form **lymphatic trunks,** which join to form one of two lymphatic ducts: the right and the thoracic. The **right lymphatic duct** drains lymph from the right arm and the right side of the head and the right half of the thorax into the right subclavian vein. The thoracic duct drains lymph from all remaining parts of the body into the left subclavian vein. The **thoracic duct** begins as an enlarged lymphatic trunk in front of L2 called the cisterna chyli. The **cisterna chyli,** inferior to the thoracic duct, is a large collecting chamber, gathering drained fluids from the lower extremities and from the digestive organs.

Author's Note

If one of your objectives in massage is to reduce swelling in a limb, elevate the limb during the massage session. Elevation will promote dependent drainage (lymph drainage assisted by gravity). Massage proximal to the edematous area first, then the edematous area; this will encourage blood and lymph flow proximal to the swollen area. Otherwise, you will be moving lymph into areas that have not been massaged and do not yet have increased blood and lymph circulation.

LYMPH ORGANS

Lymphatic organs include the lymph nodes, tonsils, Peyer's patches, vermiform appendix, thymus, and spleen. Because the bone marrow produces lymphocytes, it is sometimes considered a lymphatic organ.

1. **Tonsils** are a group of large specialized lymph tissues embedded in the mucous membranes around the throat. They include the adenoids or pharyngeal tonsils, the palatine tonsils, and the lingual tonsils. The function of the tonsils is to protect the body from airborne pathogens or other harmful substances that might enter through the nose or mouth. The lymphatic tissues use lymphocytes and macrophages to combat hostile intruders. (See Chapter 14, the Digestive System, for more information on tonsils.)
2. **Intestinal tonsils** or **Peyer's patches** are groups of lymphatic nodules found in the mucous membrane of the small intestine, usually in the ileum and the jejunum. These lymphatic cells constitute another member of the body's defense mechanisms by combating pathogens we ingest.
3. **Vermiform appendix.** Located inferior to the cecum, this wormlike appendix varies from 3 to 6 inches in length. Like other members of the lymphatic system, the appendix helps to fight pathogens and other bodily intruders.
4. **Lymph nodes** are bean-shaped structures located along lymph vessels that collect and filter lymph. These are powerful defense stations that help to protect the body from unwanted invaders. Within these nodes are white blood cells that destroy bacteria, viruses, and other foreign substances in the lymph before it is returned to the blood. Lymph nodes also produce white blood cells called lymphocytes, which help to battle pathogens. When the

body is experiencing a local infection, the regional lymph nodes enlarge.

Afferent lymphatic vessels bring lymph into the lymph node to be filtered and cleaned. Lymph nodes are the only place where lymph is filtered in the lymphatic system. **Efferent lymphatic vessels,** located at the **hilus** (a depression in an organ where vessels and nerves enter), take lymph out of the node. There are more afferent lymphatic vessels entering the node than there are efferent vessels leaving the node, an imbalance that creates a pressure differential that slows down the flow of lymph for filtering to occur.

Although lymph nodes are located along all lymphatic vessels, nodes collect superficially in three areas on each side of the body and are palpated on routine physical examinations. They are named for their location: **cervical nodes, axillary nodes,** and **inguinal nodes.**

5. **Thymus.** The thymus gland is a bilobed organ anterior to the ascending aorta and posterior to the sternum in the mediastinal region of the thorax. Large in infants, the thymus reaches its maximum size at puberty, then atrophies and is replaced by adipose tissue in adults. The thymus aids in the maturation process of T lymphocytes or T cells. These mature T cells are introduced into the bloodstream and are carried to other lymphatic organs where they can be used to fight disease.
6. **Spleen.** The largest lymphatic organ, the spleen lies within the left lateral rib cage (between ribs 9 and 11) just posterior to the stomach. This dark purple organ varies in shape between individuals and within the same individual at different times. The functions of the spleen appear to be destroying bacteria (defense), hemocytopoiesis, destroying red blood cells and platelets, storing these destroyed and worn-out blood cells, and returning these blood cells to the liver for bile production. Macrophages located in the lining of the splenic sinuses destroy microorganisms by phagocytosis. The spleen also produces leukocytes and lymphocytes.

PATHS OF LYMPH CIRCULATION

All lymph moves back toward the cardiovascular system. Lymph, which starts out as interstitial fluid, is collected by lymph capillaries and moves into lymph vessels, which become successively larger and larger. Periodically along its one-way path, lymph flows into lymph nodes through afferent vessels and leaves through efferent vessels. Ultimately, lymph converges into either the right lymphatic duct or the thoracic duct and then enters the bloodstream through the right and left subclavian veins. The thoracic duct enters only the left venous circulation. In fact, most of the body's lymph empties on the left side. Only the right side of the head and neck, the right upper extremity, and right half of the upper trunk empty into the right lymphatic duct (Fig. 12–10).

In general, lymph flows in this pathway: it starts out as tissue fluid ⇒ collected by the lymphatic capillaries ⇒ lymphatic vessels ⇒ lymph nodes ⇒ larger lymph vessels ⇒ lymph trunks (either thoracic duct or right lymphatic duct) ⇒ subclavian veins.

The deeper structures of the thorax, abdomen, pelvis, and perineum drain directly into the larger lymph vessels rather than passing through lymph capillaries.

CIRCULATORY CONDITIONS AND CLINICAL TERMS

1. **Hemorrhage.** Hemorrhaging is excessive bleeding, either internally (from blood vessels into tissues) or externally (from blood vessels directly to the surface of the body). The blood spillage may come from arteries, veins, or capillaries.
2. **Ischemia.** Ischemia is a localized, usually temporary deficiency of blood flow due to an obstruction of circulation. Ischemia can cause tissue necrosis (death).
3. **Anemia.** Anemia is a condition in which the oxygen-carrying capacity of the blood is decreased due to a decrease in red blood cells or in the amount of functional hemoglobin in the blood. It is a sign of other disorders instead of a diagnosis. Characteristics of anemia include fatigue, vertigo, headaches, insomnia, paleness, and intolerance to cold.

   There are many types of anemia. The most common is iron-deficiency anemia due to lack of iron, and pernicious anemia in which not enough vitamin B_{12} is absorbed from the digestive tract into the blood.

   Massage can help rest and oxygenate an anemic client. However, if the anemia is due to a bleeding disorder, lighter pressure should be used since the client may bruise easily and bleeding could occur under the skin.

4. **Sickle cell anemia.** An inherited type of severe, chronic anemia, sickle cell anemia is a condition in which red blood cells are "sickled." This shape greatly reduces the amount of oxygen that can be supplied to the tissues, eventually causing extensive tissue damage. Sickle cell anemia is characterized by lethargy, fatigue, pain in the joints, thrombosis, and headaches.

   Sickle cell genes are found mainly among populations or descendants of populations that live in the malaria belt around the world. These include parts of Mediterranean Europe, sub-Saharan Africa, and tropical Asia. Treatments include analgesics to relieve pain, antibiotics to counter infections, and blood transfusions.

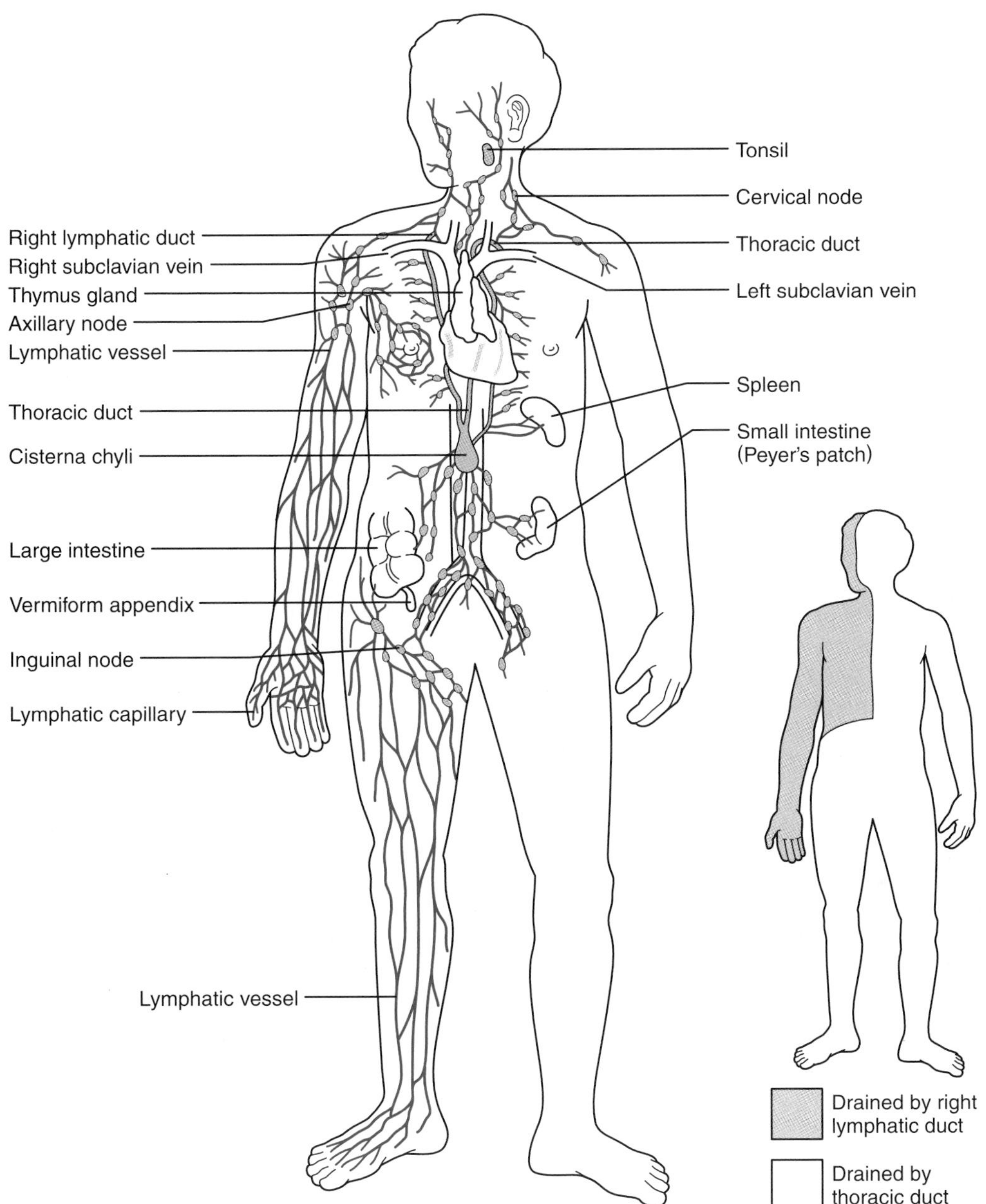

Figure 12•10 Lymph ducts and node clusters—lymph drainage on right and left sides of the body.

Clients with this disorder have periods of remission and flare-ups. Massage is contraindicated during flare-ups because the client will be in pain and debilitated. During periods of remission, a lighter massage, paying close attention to the client's vitality, is indicated.

5. **Hemophilia.** There are three types of hemophilia and each is genetically determined. In each case, only one clotting factor is missing, making it difficult or impossible for the blood to clot. Large hematomas can develop in the muscle or under the skin with mild trauma. There may be bleeding into the joints causing pain, swelling, and permanent joint stiffness. Often referred to as "free bleeders," people with hemophilia receive transfusions of their missing clotting factor.

   Massage is contraindicated for people with severe hemophilia. In milder forms light massage is indicated.

6. **Angina pectoris.** Often felt as chest pain, angina pectoris is frequently caused by constriction of coronary arteries and myocardial anoxia (lack of oxygen in the heart muscle). However, there is no lasting tissue damage. The pain originates from the chest then radiates down the inner side of the left arm. Angina pectoris is often associated with physical overexertion, emotional stress, and exposure to intense cold.

   Massage can help clients by reducing stress. Massage also decreases the effects of the sympathetic nervous system, which is partially responsible for coronary artery vasoconstriction. Since sudden exposure to extreme

cold or heat can bring on an attack, keep the client warm and avoid using heat or cold packs. If a client has an attack during a massage treatment, bring him to a sitting or standing position to decrease the load on the heart, and call for help. It is important that clients have with them their necessary medications (e.g., beta-blocker, nitroglycerin) when they come for treatment, in the event of a medical emergency.

7. **Hypertension.** Hypertension is a common (more common in men than in women), often asymptomatic disorder of elevated blood pressure: 140/90 mmHg is regarded as the threshold of hypertension, and 160/95 is classified as serious hypertension. With sustained hypertension, arterial walls become inelastic and resistant to blood flow, and as a result the left ventricle becomes enlarged in order to maintain normal circulation. Risk factors for hypertension are cigarette smoking, obesity, lack of exercise, diabetes, and genetic predisposition.

   People having hypertension that is not under control by diet, exercise, or medication should not have massage.

   For clients who do have their hypertension under control, massage helps keep blood pressure lowered by reducing stress and the activity of the sympathetic nervous system. Clients on antihypertensives may be prone to postural hypotension (a low blood pressure from the massage treatment). These clients will feel lightheaded, and need to get up slowly from the massage table, perhaps needing assistance.

8. **Cyanosis.** The presentation of bluish or dark purplish skin due to reduced blood flow, oxygen deficiency, and an increase in carbon dioxide is referred to as cyanosis.
9. **Aneurysm.** An aneurysm is a weakness and dilation of a blood vessel wall. The most common causes are atherosclerosis, hypertension, and trauma, but it can also be due to a congenital vascular weakness. The most common areas for aneurysms are the aorta and the circle of Willis, but they can occur in the extremities. Aneurysms may burst, causing hemorrhage, thrombi, and possibly death.

   If a client has a history of hypertension or atherosclerosis, the massage therapist should consult the client's physician before performing deep massage. If a client has been diagnosed with an abdominal aortic aneurysm, abdominal massage is contraindicated.

10. **Phlebitis.** Phlebitis, or thrombophlebitis, is an inflammation of the veins, frequently accompanied by a thrombus (blood clot). Phlebitis usually occurs after acute or chronic infection, surgery or childbirth, or prolonged sitting, standing, or immobilization. The affected area is hypersensitive to pressure and swollen and can be either hot or cold to the touch. It generally affects the arms or the calf area.

    Local massage is contraindicated. A lighter, general massage would be all right.

11. **Coronary artery disease.** In coronary artery disease (CAD), the coronary arteries are narrowed so that there is a reduced blood flow to the heart. CAD is the leading cause of death in the United States, with symptoms ranging from mild angina to a full-scale heart attack. Usually symptoms start when about 75 percent of the coronary artery is blocked. The three main causes are atherosclerosis, coronary artery spasm, and blood clots.
12. **Myocardial infarction.** This is a heart attack. Death (necrosis) of myocardial tissue is due to an interrupted coronary blood supply. Blood clots, atherosclerosis, and vascular spasms could lead to a myocardial infarction. Preceding symptoms are a viselike pain in the chest, which may radiate down the left arm, neck, or sternal region.

    Massage considerations are the same as for angina pectoris.

13. **Cardiac arrest.** A cardiac arrest is the sudden and complete cessation of the heartbeat, stopping all cardiac output, including pulmonary and systemic circulation. Once a cardiac arrest occurs, vascular delivery of oxygen and nutrients, as well as removal of carbon dioxide and waste products, is interrupted. Anaerobic metabolism begins and, if measures are not taken to stimulate the pumping action of the heart, damage to the brain, kidneys, heart, and lungs, or death can occur.
14. **Cerebrovascular accident.** Also known as a stroke, a cerebrovascular accident (CVA) is an occlusion of cerebral blood vessels by an embolus or thrombus, or cerebrovascular hemorrhage. Muscular weakness or paralysis, an increase or decrease in sensation, speech abnormalities, or death may occur. Subsequent damage due to the CVA depends on the location and extent of neurological damage.
15. **Congestive heart failure.** In congestive heart failure (CHF), the heart is a failing pump. Causes include coronary artery disease, long-term hypertension, and myocardial infarcts (areas of dead heart tissue from previous heart attacks). If the left ventricle fails first, blood backs up in the lungs and can result in pulmonary edema. If the right ventricle fails first, blood backs up in peripheral blood vessels and can result in edema in the extremities, most noticeably the feet and ankles.

    Massage should only be performed after obtaining clearance from the client's physician. A light massage of shorter duration is indicated because vigorous massage may tax an already debilitated heart.

16. **Tachycardia.** Rapid heart rate (more than 100 beats per minute) is called tachycardia. This condition may be due to fever, strenuous exercise, or emotions such as anxiety. Tachycardia is the body's response to an increased demand for oxygen by the tissues. Any deviation from a normal heart rate pattern is termed *arrhythmia.*
17. **Bradycardia.** Slow heart rate (under 50–60 beats per minute) is called bradycardia. The condition may be the result of disease; however, it is often normal for people who are physically fit.
18. **Pericarditis.** Pericarditis is an inflammation of the parietal pericardium and may be due to trauma or infectious disease.
19. **Atherosclerosis.** An arterial disorder, atherosclerosis is associated with a build-up of plaque (made of lipids) in the blood vessels. It is a form of arteriosclerosis. The inner vessel walls become dense and fibrotic as the lumen, or hollow center of the blood vessel, narrows. This reduces blood flow and typically raises blood pressure. Atherosclerosis is often associated with obesity, hypertension, and diabetes.

    If a client has atherosclerosis, she may be prone to thrombosis (blood clot) formation. Deep strokes may dislodge the thrombus that could float as an embolus and lodge in smaller blood vessels in the lungs, heart, or brain leading to difficulty breathing, heart attack, or stroke. Massage should be given only after consulting the client's physician. A lighter massage is indicated.

20. **Arteriosclerosis.** This is the narrowing of arteries due to the accumulation of hard lipid plaques in their walls. The narrowed arteries reduce blood flow, especially to the heart and brain. Because the plaque has a rough surface, platelets can snag on it, then form clots, which can also impede blood flow. Treatments include angioplasty, which is the insertion of a small balloon that, when inflated, squashes the plaque against the arterial walls to enlarge the hollow center of the artery. Lasers are also used to evaporate plaque. Catheter arthrectomy is a procedure that shaves the plaque off arterial walls. Clot-dissolving agents can be injected to remove thrombi.

    Deep massage may dislodge a clot. If the client has a history of previous strokes, hypertension, or thrombus formation, massage should only be given after consulting her physician. Gentle massage is indicated for all clients with arteriosclerosis.

21. **Raynaud's phenomenon.** Raynaud's phenomenon (Raynaud's disease) is periodic attacks of vasospasm of blood vessels in the body's extremities, especially the most distal parts, such as the toes, fingers, ears, and nose. It is most frequently caused by exposure to cold or by emotional stress. This condition can lead to ischemia, tissue necrosis, and nerve damage.

    Massage helps increase local circulation. By reducing stress, massage helps reduce sympathetic stimulation and so relaxes the smooth muscle of blood vessels. Heat and ice packs are contraindicated.

22. **Occlusion.** Any clogged vessel or passage of the body is referred to as an occlusion.
23. **Thrombosis.** This is an abnormal vascular condition characterized by thrombus (blood clot) formation in an unbroken blood vessel. It may lead to tissue damage due to an interruption in blood supply.

    Local massage is contraindicated. A lighter, general massage would be all right.

24. **Embolus.** A blood clot, bubble of air, or any piece of debris transported by the bloodstream is an embolus. When an embolus becomes lodged in a vessel and cuts off circulation, it is then called an embolism.
25. **Mononucleosis.** Mononucleosis is an acute viral infection that results from the Epstein-Barr virus (EBV). Symptoms are a slight to high fever, sore throat, red throat and soft palate, stiff neck, enlarged lymph nodes, and coughing. It is highly contagious, transmitted by droplets that contain the virus. There is no cure; treatment is letting it run its course and treating any complications.

    Massage is contraindicated until the client has recovered. Lighter abdominal massage is indicated after the client has recovered because the spleen may be enlarged. Gentle massage with heat packs may help relieve persistent body ache.

26. **Leukemia.** Also called "cancer of the blood," leukemia is a cancer of white blood cells. There are many types of leukemia. Generally, there are two main categories: acute and chronic. Acute leukemia is a malignant disease of blood-forming tissues resulting in uncontrolled production and accumulation of immature leukocytes. Chronic leukemia results in an accumulation of mature leukocytes that do not die at the end of their life span. Complications include anemia and bleeding problems because the immature white blood cells crowd out platelet production in red bone marrow. There can also be uncontrolled infection due to lack of mature or normal leukocytes.

    Clearance from the client's physician is essential before performing massage. A gentle, relaxing massage is indicated because the client may bruise easily and have a tendency to bleed. Because there may be enlargement of the spleen or liver, abdominal massage is contraindicated.

27. **Hodgkin's disease.** Hodgkin's disease is a cancer of the lymph nodes, evidenced by painless, pro-

gressive enlargement of lymph nodes that may spread to other areas. Other symptoms include fever, night sweats, weight loss, fatigue, itching, and anemia. It is more common in young women between the ages of 15 and 35.

Clearance from the client's physician is necessary before performing massage. Massage is contraindicated if the client is debilitated. Otherwise, a gentle, relaxing massage is indicated.

28. **Lymphedema.** Accumulation of interstitial fluid (swelling) in the soft tissues is referred to as lymphedema. It is due to local or general inflammation, obstruction, or removal of lymph vessels. Lymphedema may be congenital or as a result of injury or surgery.

    Massage can help lymphatic drainage by moving excess fluid into lymphatic vessels. The client's edematous limb should be supported and elevated. Proximal areas should be worked first to clear the path for lymph from distal areas.

29. **Varicose veins.** Varicose veins are dilated veins possessing incompetent valves. In veins with weak valves, gravity prevents large amounts of blood from flowing upward. The back-pressure overloads the vein and pushes its walls outward. The veins lose elasticity and become stretched and flabby. Thromboses may form in the varicose veins. They are typically caused by a congenital defect or by repeated stress from overloading, such as pregnancy and obesity.

    Because clients with varicose veins may be prone to thromboses, clearance from their physician may be necessary. Massage should be geared to reduce edema and prevent venous and lymphatic stasis. These clients' legs should be raised above the heart during treatment.

30. **Allergies.** Allergies are a hypersensitivity and overreaction to otherwise harmless agents (most are environmental or dietary).

    The massage therapist should make sure that the massage products and treatment room do not contain items to which the client is allergic.

31. **Autoimmune diseases.** Autoimmune diseases are part of a large group of diseases characterized by an alteration of immune functions. These disorders result from an attack by the body's own immune system. The body makes a "mistake" in identifying one or more tissues as invading organisms and attacks that tissue. Examples of autoimmune diseases are rheumatoid arthritis, lupus, and MS.

    Massage is contraindicated during flare-ups. Massage for autoimmune diseases in remission depends on the individual disorder. Communication with the client and her healthcare provider on the client's vitality is essential for planning the massage treatment.

32. **Acquired immunodeficiency syndrome.** Acquired immunodeficiency syndrome (AIDS) is a disease caused by human immunodeficiency virus (HIV). Transmission of the virus occurs through body fluids such as blood, semen, vaginal secretions, and mother's milk. The average time between exposure to the virus and diagnosis is 8 to 10 years, but the incubation time may be longer or shorter. Generally, there may be enlarged lymph nodes, weight loss, fatigue, night sweats, and fever. An AIDS diagnosis is made when a person has three or more opportunistic infections (e.g., tuberculosis, pneumonia, fungi) and/or a T-cell count below 200. A normal T-cell count is 1,200.

    It is unlikely that massage therapists will come in contact with client blood or body fluids. However, if a massage therapist has an open wound on her hands, she should not treat any client. Massage treatment for a client with AIDS needs to be tailored to that client's vitality, but a gentle massage is indicated. Care needs to be taken so that any infectious disorders of the client are not spread to the therapist, and vice versa.

Effects of Massage on the Cardiovascular System

1. Deep stroking improves circulation by mechanically assisting venous blood flow back to the heart. Massage also stimulates tissue release of histamines and acetylcholine.
2. Because blood circulation is enhanced (venous blood flow directly and arterial blood flow indirectly), the delivery and removal of products in the blood (i.e., nutrients, oxygen, and metabolic wastes) are improved.
3. Blood pressure is temporarily decreased by dilation of the capillaries, affecting the permeability of capillary walls.
4. Massage temporarily increases systolic stroke volume.
5. Massage decreases heart rate through decreased stimulation of the sympathetic nervous system,
6. The number of functional red blood cells, and their oxygen carrying capacity, is increased by the application of massage.
7. The presence of white blood cells in the capillaries increases following massage.
8. Gentle but firm massage strokes also increase the number of thrombocytes (platelets) in the blood.
9. Massage reduces ischemia.

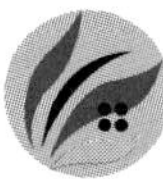

Effects of Massage on the Lymphatic System

1. Massage reduces lymphedema by improving circulation to the lymphatic system, thereby helping remove waste and bacteria from the system more effectively than passive range of motion or electrical muscle stimulation.
2. The presence of natural killer cells and their activity increase with massage, suggesting that massage may strengthen the immune system.

Author's Note

A central venous catheter is a flexible tube that is inserted into a large vein (usually the subclavian vein in the upper chest) and left in place for a long time. This type of catheter is used to keep a vein open for dialysis, blood withdrawal, chemotherapy, and frequent administration of medications, which must be taken regularly or cannot be taken orally. Common types of central venous catheters are Hickman's catheter and Quinton's catheter. Use bolsters, pillows, and positional modifications for the client's comfort. During the massage, the massage therapist should take precautions not to dislodge the catheter, which is sutured to fascia and muscle, by exerting tension or excessive movement on nearby skin tissues. Do not allow the massage lubricant to come into contact with the catheter dressing or sutures. If a catheter is placed in the arm, do not massage the area below the catheter. Massage work above the catheter in these extremities should be gentle.

Another consideration is the client with an artificial pacemaker. This device sends out a small electrical current to stimulate the heartbeat. Artificial pacemakers are inserted near the pectoralis major muscle with wires going directly to the heart. The newer ones are activity-adjusted; they automatically speed up the heartbeat during exercise. The primary concern is to make sure the incision from the surgery has completely healed before applying gentle effleurage over the area. Avoid vigorous massage on the pectoral region. While the client is prone, offer a soft pillow to be placed under the chest. This will provide added comfort for the client during the massage.

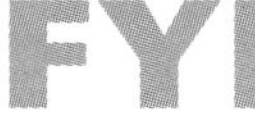

FOR YOUR INFORMATION

If you recall, hemoglobin is what gives blood its color. Lacking hemoglobin, most insect blood has a yellow or greenish tint.

SUMMARY

The cardiovascular and lymphatic systems are the main transport mechanisms of the body for various fluids, gases, nutrients, wastes, antibodies, and hormones. These two systems also play an important role in the body's defense system by fighting a variety of invaders. The clotting mechanism of the blood enables the body to make repairs to breaches of its tissues. The circulatory system also plays a part in the regulation of temperature, water balance, and chemical balance of the body. The main components of the cardiovascular system are the blood, the heart, and the vast network of arteries, capillaries, and veins that make up the circulatory vessels. There are two main circuits of the cardiovascular system: the pulmonary and the systemic.

Although the cardiovascular system provides the liquid nourishment to the body's tissues, it is the lymphvascular system that collects and "recycles" that fluid back into circulation. Along with fluid conservation, the lymph system also transports fats, vitamins, lost proteins, and cellular debris, in addition to filtering the lymph and combating diseases with its own immune functions. The lymphatic system's major structures include the lymphatic fluid or lymph, the tonsils of the throat, intestinal tonsils (Peyer's patches), the vermiform appendix, a vast network of lymphatic vessels and lymph nodes, the thymus, and the spleen. The lymphatic vessels route the collected fluids from all areas of the body and direct it to two main vessels, which return it into the cardiovascular system.

SELF-TEST

Multiple Choice • Write the letter of the best answer in the space provided.

_______ 1. Which of the following is *not* one of the functions of the cardiovascular system?

A. transportation and distribution of respiratory gases, nutrients, antibodies, and hormones
B. protection of the body through disease-fighting white blood cells
C. synthesizes vitamins A, E, and D
D. protection of the body through clotting mechanisms

_______ 2. Blood cells are formed by a process called

A. hemocytopoiesis
B. hemobirthocytosis
C. hemocytogenesis
D. A and C

_______ 3. Which of the following is *not* a characteristic of blood?

A. viscous fluid that is thicker and more adhesive than water
B. slightly alkaline pH
C. constitutes about 8 percent of the total body weight; blood volume in the average-size male is approximately 5 to 6 liters
D. is red in arteries and blue in veins

_______ 4. The most numerous blood cell, the primary function of _______ is to transport oxygen and a small amount of carbon dioxide in the blood.

A. hemoglobin
B. erythrocytes
C. thrombocytes/platelets
D. leukocytes

_______ 5. Which of the following are fragmented parts of megakaryoblast/megakaryocytes and help to repair leaks in the blood vessels through clotting mechanisms?

A. hemoglobin
B. erythrocytes
C. thrombocytes/platelets
D. leukocytes

_______ 6. When a pathogen is absorbed rather than "eaten" by these cells, this process is known as

A. pinocytosis
B. vascular spasm
C. platelet plug
D. fibrinogen

_______ 7. Which of the following are mechanisms for blood clotting?

A. platelet plug
B. coagulation
C. vascular spasm
D. all of the above

_______ 8. The "universal donor" is which type of ABO blood group?

A. type A
B. type B
C. type AB
D. type O

_______ 9. The sac surrounding the heart is called the

A. synovial sac
B. pericardium
C. pericardial sac
D. B and C

_______ 10. Which of the following best describes the path of blood through the heart?

A. blood flows into the right atrium, then into the right ventricle, then on to the pulmonary trunk; the blood returns from the lungs and enters the left atrium, then flows into the left ventricle and into the aorta to all parts of the body
B. blood flows from the capillaries, to the veins, to the arteries, then to the aorta
C. blood flows into the SA node, then to the right ventricle, the aorta, and the coronary sinus
D. blood flows from the brachial artery, to the left ventricle, the pulmonary trunk, and on to the right atrium

_______ 11. Another name for the bicuspid valve is the

A. tricuspid valve
B. mitral valve
C. sinoatrial valve
D. semilunar valve

_______ 12. The valves located between both ventricles and their adjacent arteries are the

A. tricuspid valves
B. mitral valves
C. sinoatrial valves
D. semilunar valves

_______ 13. The main part of the heart's conducting system is the

A. sinoatrial node (SA node)
B. the atrioventricular bundle (AV bundle)
C. atrioventricular node (AV node)
D. all are important parts of the conducting system of the heart

_______ 14. The majority of heart rate changes are controlled by the cardiac center located in a specialized portion of the brain called the

A. hypothalamus C. medulla oblongata
B. occipital lobe D. prefrontal lobotomy

_______ 15. The sounds created by a beating heart are due to the

A. contraction of the ventricles
B. closing of the heart's valves
C. blood moving from one heart chamber to another
D. compression from the respiring lungs

_______ 16. The three layers of both arteries and veins are

A. tunica intima, media, and adventitia
B. pia mater, arachnoid mater, and dura mater
C. epicardium, myocardium, and endocardium
D. epilayer, myodivision, and endosurface

_______ 17. When the diameter of the vascular lumen enlarges, it is called

A. vasoconstriction C. vasodilation
B. vasoelongation D. vasoamplify

_______ 18. Vessels that carry blood away from the heart and have thick muscular walls are called

A. afferent vessels C. veins
B. arteries D. capillaries

_______ 19. Vessels that return blood to the heart and possess valves are the

A. afferent vessels C. veins
B. arteries D. capillaries

_______ 20. The expansion effect that occurs in arteries when blood is pushed forward due to contraction of the left ventricle (and that can be felt when arteries are located close to the surface) is called

A. cardiac cycle C. fibrillation
B. vital capacity D. pulse

_______ 21. The pressure exerted by blood on an arterial wall during the contraction of the left ventricle is called

A. vascular pressure C. arterial pressure
B. blood pressure D. all of the above

_______ 22. In which artery is blood pressure most frequently taken?

A. brachial C. femoral
B. carotid D. peroneal

_______ 23. In a blood pressure reading, the top number, which represents the pressure exerted on the arterial wall during active ventricular contraction, is called

A. cerebral C. systole
B. diastole D. arterstole

_______ 24. A normal pressure reading is considered

A. 120/80 C. 140/95
B. 139/94 D. 80/120

_______ 25. Factors that influence blood pressure and blood flow are

A. diameter of the blood vessels, resistance, and blood viscosity
B. cardiac output and blood volume
C. feedback from chemoreceptors and baroreceptors
D. all of the above

_______ 26. Within the cardiovascular system, the two circuits based on the areas of the body they serve are the

A. right and the left
B. pulmonary and the systemic
C. cerebral and the systemic
D. pulmonary and the somatic

_______ 27. The main venous portal system, which collects blood from the digestive organs and delivers this blood to the liver for processing, is called the

A. digestive portal system
B. intestinal portal system
C. gastric portal system
D. hepatic portal system

_______ 28. The lymphatic system consists of

A. blood, blood vessels, and the heart
B. brain and spinal cord
C. lymph, lymph vessels, and lymph organs
D. lymph, blood vessels, and lymph organs

_______ 29. Which one of the following is *not* one of the functions of the lymphatic system?

A. mechanically and chemically converts blood into a usable state
B. drains tissues of excess interstitial fluid; the lymphatic system returns this fluid to the cardiovascular system
C. transports fats and some vitamins from the digestive tract to the blood
D. provides immunity against disease

_______ 30. Lymph flow depends entirely on the

A. milking action of the skeletal muscles
B. pressure changes in the thorax during breathing
C. ventricular contraction
D. A and B

_______ 31. The two main lymphatic ducts are the

A. right and left subclavian
B. thoracic and the left subclavian
C. thoracic and the right lymphatic
D. right and left lymphatic

_______ 32. Which large collecting chamber is located inferior to the thoracic duct?

A. corpus callosum C. lingual lymph nodes
B. cisterna chyli D. inguinal lymph nodes

_______ 33. Lymphatic organs include the

A. liver and gallbladder
B. hypothalamus and pituitary
C. small and large intestines
D. none of these

_______ 34. Usually located in the ileum and jejunum of the small intestines, these groups of lymphatic nodes combat pathogens

A. palatine tonsils C. thymus
B. Peyer's patches D. spleen

_______ 35. Which of the following are bean-shaped structures that collect and filter lymph?

A. lymph nodes C. tonsils
B. Peyer's patches D. spleen

_______ 36. Although lymph nodes are located along all lymphatic vessels, they collect superficially in three areas on each side of the body and are the

A. nodica intima, media, and adventitia
B. pia mater, arachnoid mater, and dura mater
C. epicardial, myocardial, and endocardial nodes
D. cervical nodes, axillary nodes, and inguinal nodes

_______ 37. The organ that aids in the maturation process of T lymphocytes or T cells is the

A. tonsils C. thymus
B. Peyer's patches D. spleen

_______ 38. The largest lymphatic organ that filters blood and destroys bacteria is the

A. palatine tonsils C. thymus
B. Peyer's patches D. spleen

_______ 39. Which duct collects the majority of lymph?

A. thoracic duct C. left lymphatic duct
B. right lymphatic duct D. cisterna chyli

References

Applegate, Edith J. *The Anatomy and Physiology Learning System: Textbook.* Philadelphia: W. B. Saunders, 1995.

Damjanov, Ivan. *Pathophysiology for the Health-Related Professions.* Philadelphia: W. B. Saunders, 1996.

Gould, Barbara E. *Pathophysiology for the Health-Related Professionals.* Philadelphia: W. B. Saunders, 1997.

Gray, Henry, F.R.S., T. Pickering Pick. F.R.C.S., Robert Howden, M.A., M.B., C.M. *Gray's Anatomy,* 29th ed. Philadelphia: Running Press, 1974.

Haubrich, William S. *Medical Meanings, A Glossary of Word Origins.* New York, NY: Harcourt Brace Jovanovich, Publishers, 1984.

Kapit, Wynn and Lawrence M. Elson. *The Anatomy Coloring Book,* 2nd ed. New York, NY: HarperCollins Publishers, 1993.

Marieb, Elaine N. *Essentials of Human Anatomy and Physiology,* 4th ed. New York: Benjamin/Cummings Publishing Company, Inc., 1994.

McAleer, Neil. *The Body Almanac.* Garden City, NY: Doubleday and Company, Inc., 1985.

Mosby's Medical, Nursing, and Allied Health Dictionary, 4th ed. St Louis: Mosby–Year Book, Inc., 1994.

Newton, Don. *Pathology for Massage Therapists,* 2nd ed. Portland: Simran Publications, 1995.

Premkumar, Kalyani. *Pathology A to Z—A Handbook for Massage Therapists.* Calgary, Canada: VanPub Books, 1996.

Tabers Cyclopedic Medical Dictionary, 13th ed. Philadelphia: F. A. Davis Company, 1977.

Tortora, Gerald J. *Introduction to the Human Body: The Essentials of Anatomy and Physiology,* 3rd ed. New York: HarperCollins Publishers, 1994.

Travell, Janet G., M.D. and David G. Simons, M.D. *Myofascial Pain and Dysfunction, The Trigger Point Manual.* Baltimore: Williams & Wilkins, 1983.

When you breathe, you inspire.
When you don't, you expire.
—Popular Science *quote*

13 Respiratory System

Student Objectives

After completing this chapter, the student should be able to:

- List the functions of the respiratory system
- Identify and discuss each respiratory structure
- Describe the mechanisms of breathing
- Name the six modified respiratory air movements
- Discuss olfaction as it relates to the use of aromatherapy

INTRODUCTION

Breathing has long been the inspiration of poets and philosophers. Books have been filled with references to "his dying breath," "her breast rose and fell," "his breath quickened," and "he breathed life into them." Breath and the breathing process are synonymous with life itself. Breathing is the most easily observable of the body's vital signs. It is through respiration that we take in new air, extract oxygen from it, and expel carbon dioxide, other waste gases, and stale air. Oxygen is needed by every cell of the body, and delivery is accomplished by way of the bloodstream. Therefore, the respiratory and the circulatory systems both participate in the respiratory process. Failure of either system has the same effect on the body, namely disruption of homeostasis and rapid cell death from oxygen starvation.

We will examine the various life-sustaining mechanisms of the respiratory system, as well as some of its modified respiratory functions. Included in this chapter discussion will be the following: basic anatomy of the respiratory system, the respiratory system's role in the senses of smell and speech, the mechanisms of breathing, internal and external respiration, and how breathing can aid massage (Fig. 13–1).

FUNCTIONS

1. **Exchange of Gases.** Oxygen and carbon dioxide exchange is the primary function of the respiratory system. A constant intake of oxygen is essential for maintaining life. Without oxygen intake and the elimination of carbon dioxide (a toxic gas), the body's cells would start to perish within 5 minutes. This gas exchange occurs in the lungs.

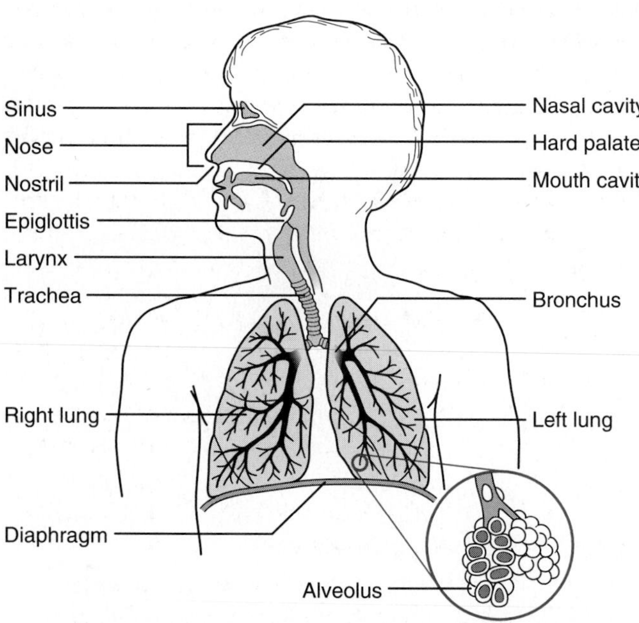

Figure 13•1 General respiratory structures.

2. **Olfaction.** Olfaction refers to the sense of smell. Through the act of inhalation, scent molecules enter the nose and are forced against the olfactory epithelium, in the nasal cavity. Nerve endings from the olfactory nerve are embedded in the olfactory epithelium, and send impulses for the sense of smell to the brain.
3. **Speech.** The production of speech is a complex coordination of muscles and nerves. Sound is produced by air moving over the vocal folds. Words are formed by movements of the facial muscles and tongue.
4. **Homeostasis.** The respiratory system helps to maintain oxygen levels in the blood. It also helps maintain homeostasis through the elimination of wastes (i.e., carbon dioxide and heat). Excess carbon dioxide in the blood can lead to an acidic condition. When carbon dioxide is expelled through exhalation, the respiratory system helps to regulate pH.

Terms and Word Roots Related to the Respiratory System

allergy – other; work
apnea – not; breathing
auditory – to hear
bronchus – windpipe
cilia – hairlike
eustachian – named for Italian anatomist (1524–1574)
exudate – to sweat out
glottis – back of the tongue
meatus – passage
olfaction – to smell
phrenic – diaphragm
pleura – rib-side
pneumo, pneum – air; lungs
pulmo – lung
trachea – rough
ventilation – to air
volitional – will

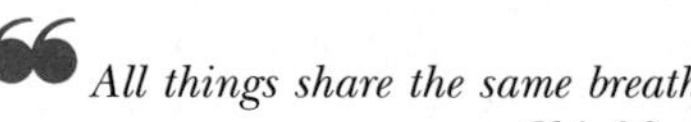

"*All things share the same breath.*"
—Chief Sealth, Duwamish tribe, 1885

ANATOMY AND PHYSIOLOGY

1. **Nose.** The nose is formed by several cranial and facial bones and hyaline cartilage. The paired nasal bones and process of the maxillae bone form the central region of the nose. The bridge of the nose consists of the nasal bones and the frontal bone.
2. **Nasal cavity.** Posterior to the nose is the nasal cav-

ity. The nasal septum, formed by the vomer and the ethmoid bones and hyaline cartilage, divides the nasal cavity into right and left sides. The nasal cavity leads to the **nasal conchae.** The superior, middle, and inferior nasal conchae are the ridges that extend out of each lateral wall of the nasal cavity (Fig. 13–2). The three conchae subdivide further into the creaselike passageways called **meatuses.** The nasal conchae terminate at the throat or pharynx. The mucosal lining of the nasal cavity contains blood capillaries, cells with cilia, and goblet cells. **Cilia** are projections on the outer surfaces of certain cells that can produce movement of particles or fluids. The sweeping effect of cilia not only moves particles but also determines the direction of mucus. Mucus can move down toward the throat (swallowing) or up for expectoration (spitting). **Goblet cells** produce mucus that moistens the air and traps incoming foreign particles. As air enters the nasal cavities, it becomes warm and moist. Because of all of these functions, the nasal cavities are called the "air-conditioning" chambers.

3. The **pharynx,** or throat, is a muscular tube approximately 5 inches long that is shared by the respiratory and the digestive systems. The pharynx, which extends from behind the nasal cavity (nasopharynx) to the back of the oral cavity (oropharynx), and down to the larynx (laryngopharynx), is located in front of the cervical vertebrae. It contains the pharyngeal tonsils, the palatine tonsils, and the lingual tonsils, which help our immune system by protecting against inhaled or ingested pathogens.

   The eustachian tube (auditory canal) opens into the pharynx. Because of this close structure, respiratory infections can easily create middle ear infections and vice versa.

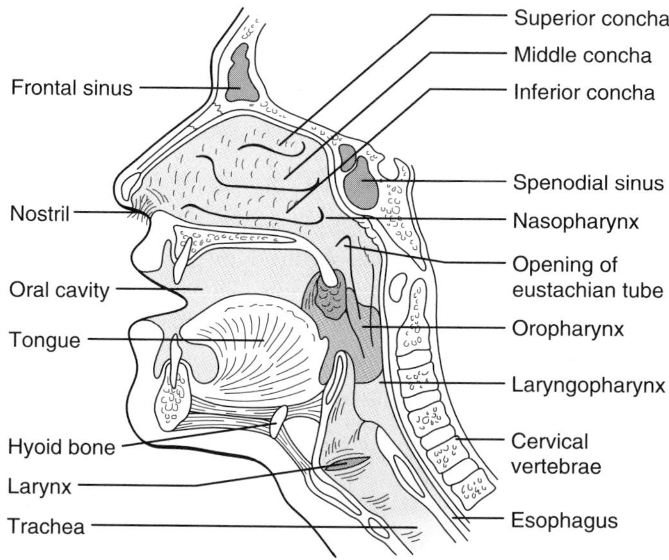

Figure 13•2 Upper respiratory anatomy.

4. The **larynx,** or voice box, is formed by three single and three paired pieces of cartilage. The single cartilages are the epiglottis, the cricoid, and the thyroid (laryngeal prominence or Adam's apple), which is the largest, especially in men because it is enlarged by the male hormone testosterone. The three paired cartilages — the arytenoid, corniculate, and cuneiform — attach to and support the vocal folds.

   There are two sets of **vocal folds:** a superior pair called the ventricular folds or false vocal cords and an inferior pair called vocal folds or true vocal cords. The vocal folds are used for normal voice production; however, a person can train the ventricular folds, as is shown in ventriloquism or singers who have two ranges.

   The vocal folds are bands of elastic ligaments that are attached to the rigid cartilage of the larynx by skeletal muscle. There is a space between the folds and when air passes over them, they vibrate and produce sound. The tighter the skeletal muscles pull the vocal folds, the higher the pitch of the voice.

   One of the single laryngeal cartilages, the **epiglottis,** closes the trachea (windpipe) during swallowing (deglutition), preventing food from entering the inferior passageways. Because of this function, the epiglottis is sometimes referred to as the "guardian of the airways."

5. The **trachea,** or windpipe, is a tube from the larynx to the upper chest. Located anterior to the esophagus, it measures about 5 inches long and consists of 16 to 20 half-ring hyaline cartilages. These half-ring cartilages serve a dual purpose. The incomplete sections of the ring allow the esophagus to expand into the trachea when a food bolus is swallowed. The rings also keep the tracheal wall from collapsing in spite of pressure changes that occur during breathing. At the base of the trachea, it bifurcates into the right and left primary bronchi.

6. The right and left **bronchi** are the large air-conduction passageways leading to each lung. Each tube-like structure is reinforced with hyaline cartilage to keep it open. The right primary bronchus is slightly wider and has a slightly steeper downward angle than the left, and because of this, foreign bodies more frequently lodge on the right side. The right and left primary bronchi branch out like roots of a tree into the secondary (lobar) bronchi, then into tertiary (segmental) bronchi. The tertiary bronchi branch out even more into smaller divisions called **bronchioles.** As the airways branch out, they become smaller and smaller, with less cartilage and more smooth muscle.

7. **Alveoli** are tiny sacs attached to the bronchioles. They are made of a single layer of epithelial tissue blended with elastic tissue. The walls are so thin

that it is hard to imagine their thinness, but a sheet of notepaper is much thicker. **Alveolar sacs** are two or more alveoli that share a common opening. The lungs contain 300 million alveoli, providing an immense surface area of about 1,000 square feet, roughly the area of a handball court. Superficial to the alveoli are numerous capillaries, so many that 900 milliliters of blood are able to participate in gas exchange at any given time. Alveolar macrophages remove duct particles and other debris of the alveoli.

The lungs continue to grow and mature throughout childhood, and more alveoli are formed until young adulthood.

Surfactants are phospholipids that assist in the exchange of gas in the alveoli, reduce surface tension, and contribute to the elasticity of pulmonary tissue. Lungs are the last organ to develop in utero. Infants born prematurely (before 28 gestational weeks) may not have produced enough surfactants to allow their lungs to expand with air. This infant respiratory distress syndrome (RDS) affects over 65,000 premature babies in the United States each year and accounts for over 20,000 neonatal deaths. The death rate from RDS of the newborns has decreased due to commercially prepared surfactants.

8. **Lungs** are the highly elastic, paired organs of respiration. Although the lungs fill most of the thoracic cavity, they weigh less than 1 pound each. The inferior surface of the lungs is broad and concave to match the shape of the superior surface of the respiratory diaphragm. The right lung has three lobes; the left lung has two lobes because the heart is more localized on the left side. This depression in the left lung to accommodate the heart is called the cardiac notch (Fig. 13–3). The external surfaces of the lungs are lined by a serous membrane, and both lungs are encased by a pleural membrane. The inside of this double-walled pleural cavity is lined with a pleural membrane that secretes a thin, serous fluid, which fills the pleural cavity. This fluid prevents friction between the lungs and the surrounding tissues, allowing the lungs to move easily during respiration.
9. The **respiratory diaphragm,** or the thoracoabdominal diaphragm, is a dome-shaped muscular partition that separates the thoracic cavity from the abdominal cavity. It is the main muscle of respiration. The diaphragm consists of both contractile muscular fibers and resistant, tendinous connective tissues, which serve to increase extensibility and help keep its firm shape. Passing through the transverse plane with an airtight seal and inserting into its central tendon, the diaphragm attaches around the circumference of the lower six ribs, connecting the spine, ribs, and xiphoid process. The descending aorta, inferior vena cava, and the esophagus pass through the diaphragm. During contraction, the diaphragm is pulled down, creating a vacuum in the chest cavity, which sucks air into the lungs. Relaxation of the diaphragm causes it to rise, allowing the lungs to deflate, and pushes out air as a result.

Because the respiratory diaphragm never stops contracting, the potential for trigger point development is tremendous. Tightening of the diaphragm's fibers can cause torquing of the rib cage around the spine and central tendon, thus limiting the efficiency of inhalation. There are some rib cage mobilizations and deep-tissue diaphragm releases that can actually increase the volume of air capacity within the lungs and the thoracic cavity.

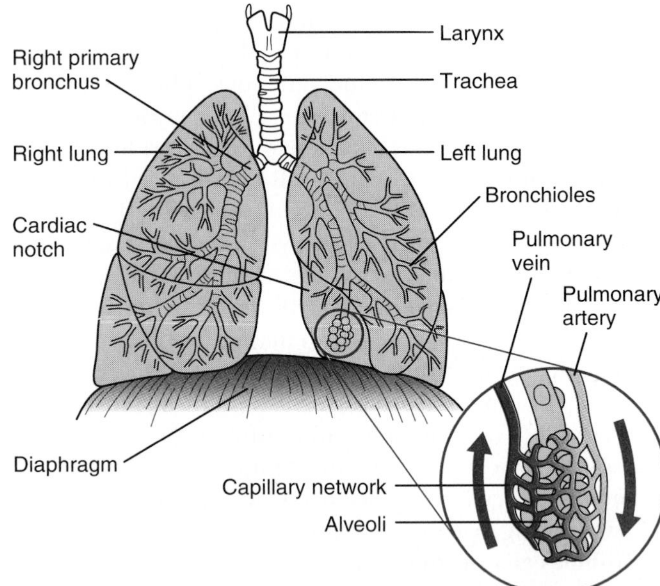

Figure 13•3 Lower respiratory anatomy.

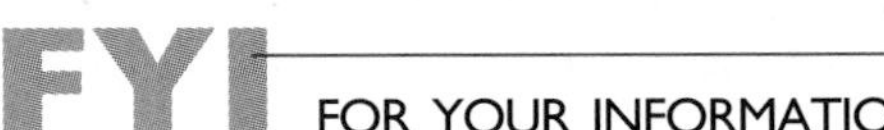

FOR YOUR INFORMATION

If an individual lives to be 72 years old, he or she will have taken more than 530 million breaths of air.

THE MECHANISMS OF BREATHING

There are three processes required to get oxygen from the atmosphere to the body's cells. They are pulmonary ventilation, external respiration, and internal respiration.

Pulmonary Ventilation

Pulmonary ventilation, or breathing, is primarily a mechanical process because muscular contraction and relaxation are required to move air in and out of the lungs. There are two phases in pulmonary ventilation: inspiration and expiration.

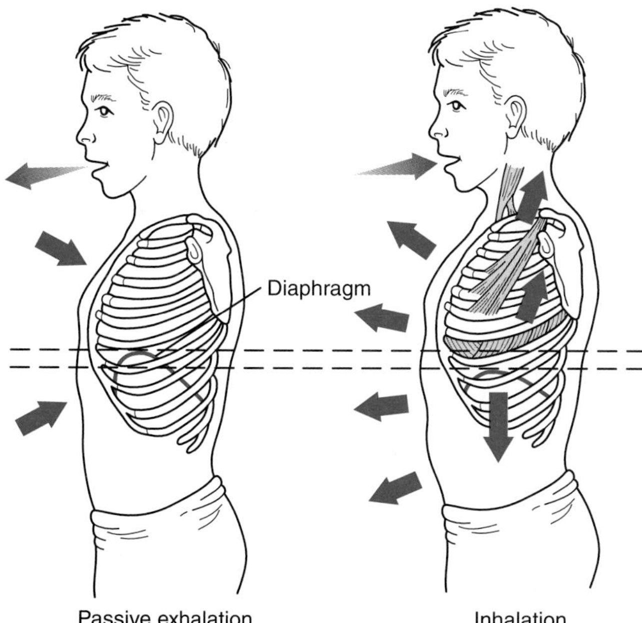

Figure 13•4 Air moving in and out of the lungs.

Inspiration, or **inhalation,** is the process that is responsible for drawing air into the lungs and can be divided into normal and forced inspiration. Normal inspiration occurs when the diaphragm contracts and descends into the abdominal cavity, and when the external intercostal muscles simultaneously contract to raise the ribs. Forced or labored inspiration requires additional muscular contraction by the sternocleidomastoid, scalenes, and pectoralis major. These muscles are considered accessory muscles of respiration.

Expiration, or **exhalation,** is the process that is responsible for expelling air from the lungs back to the atmosphere. Expiration can be classified as normal or forced. During normal exhalation the diaphragm relaxes and ascends back up toward the thoracic cavity. Air is forced out of the lungs due to elastic recoil of the alveoli (Fig. 13–4). Forced or labored expiration is an active process, utilizing voluntary muscular contractions of the internal intercostals and the abdominal muscles.

At rest, adults respire about 12 to 14 times a minute; children breathe twice as fast. Exercise can increase oxygen need up to 30 times. Respiration rates increase to match the oxygen needs of cells.

The respiratory center in the brain stem that controls the basic rhythm of breathing is influenced by the amount of carbon dioxide in the blood. It operates without conscious control and works by sending nerve impulses down the phrenic nerve to the diaphragm. These impulses are also sent to the other muscles of respiration.

Several other factors help regulate the respiratory center, for example, the cerebral cortex can modify our breathing patterns (i.e., laughing or crying) and can initiate volitional breathing. Volitional, or voluntary breathing, allows us to "hold our breath" during swimming under water and to "take a deep breath" and project our voice during public speaking. However, if you control your breath by rapid breathing (hyperventilation) or by holding your breath (hypoventilation) too long, you will become unconscious. How long the breath is held is limited by carbon dioxide buildup in the blood.

An increase in body temperature (i.e., fever, exercise) increases respiration whereas a decrease in body temperature (i.e., hypothermia, jumping into cool water) decreases respiration. Emotions such as anger or fear can change respiration rates, too. A sudden, severe pain can temporarily stop breathing (apnea), and stretching the anal sphincter muscle increases the respiration rate (this technique is sometimes employed to stimulate respiration during medical emergencies).

Author's Note

A relaxed muscle is more receptive to pressure than a contracted muscle. Because passive exhalation is basically the result of muscular relaxation, apply pressure to muscles as the client is exhaling.

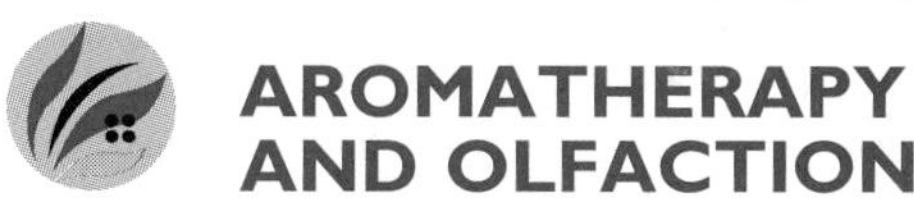

AROMATHERAPY AND OLFACTION

We don't smell with our noses; we smell with our *brains.* Aromatherapy can be used to enhance relaxation or stimulate the nervous system. The olfactory bulb is part of the limbic system, which is regarded as the neurological seat of the emotions. Other parts of the limbic system are the hypothalamus, the hippocampus, the amygdala, parts of the thalamus, and sections of the cerebral cortex. Scientists believe that these structures work as a system to regulate emotional behaviors.

In 1937, J. W. Papez identified these structures and stated that the structures of the limbic system responded to smell, taste, sound, sight, and painful stimuli, all of which elicit emotional responses. When these structures are damaged, emotional experience decreases significantly. When these neurological structures are stimulated electrically, individuals experience emotions, such as aggression, fear, and happiness.

The easiest way to stimulate the limbic system is through the sense of smell. Massage therapists can use aromatherapy in conjunction with massage therapy to enhance therapeutic benefits. A list of essential oils and their effects is found in the chapter Tools of the Trade. Enjoy!

Robert Tisserand

Born: November 11, 1948

"Love what you do. Enjoy listening to people. It can be hard work, but the potential for helping people is tremendous."

Robert Tisserand, author and aromatherapist, was born in London to a father who made baskets and a mother who "did a little of this and that, but mostly raised three kids." Luckily for his "mum," the two girls weren't quite as inquisitive as Tisserand, who shares his first "taste" of the aromatherapy experience.

"Curiously, I did actually drink a bottle of perfume when I was about 2 years old. My father bought it for my mother in a flea market in Paris in 1945, so the perfume would have been about 5 years old at the time. It was called Creme de Zofali. I survived, but the bottle has not."

Considering that it is often the smell and not the taste of foods that makes them appealing, it's easy to understand why a little boy wouldn't think twice before turning up a bottle of slightly aged perfume. However, aromas affect more than our appetites. Odors of certain plants have been used to dedicate newborns, banish evil spirits, guide dearly departed souls to the other side, and heal all manner of ills in between. Long before frankincense and myrrh were offered to the Christ child, Egyptian physicians were using it in their practices. Greek mythology includes stories regarding the healing properties of aromatic plants, and Romans enjoyed massage with wonderfully scented, unbelievably expensive oils.

What has become a popular trend in the past few years was an academic area of study as far back as the Middle Ages. During this time, essential oils were classified according to the four elements or humors, the degree of "hotness" or "coldness" and also by the shape or color of the plant from which it was derived. For example, lungwort looks like lungs, so it was used for the respiratory system. Blue is a calming color, so plants with blue flowers were considered to have sedative properties. This way of cataloging plant essences was called the *doctrine of signatures.* Astronomy also helped play a role in organizing certain scents. Late in the 16th century, Nicholas Culpepper, an astrological physician, associated oils with planetary characteristics. For instance, ylang-ylang is identified as having "Venus" properties because it has a strong, sweet odor and a slightly yellow tint and is considered an aphrodisiac.

The first people to dispense aromatics were the priests. They were the first perfumers, or what we would call an aromatherapist today. Physicians picked up the practice soon thereafter.

Although aromatherapy (the use of essential oils distilled from plants for certain conditions) has been widely used in England for some time, only recently did its climb in popularity start in the United States. Lately, massage therapists are learning more about how aromatherapy can benefit their practices. At the very least, aromatherapy adds another sensory-pleasing dimension to the pleasure of receiving a massage. However, due to the strong tie between our sense of smell and mood, it can add other benefits as well. For instance, lavender is thought to be calming. On the other end of the spectrum, mints and citrus oils have an energizing effect. Mixed with oil or lotion, essential essences are considered by many to work magic on myriad maladies, from clogged sinuses to diarrhea. Aromatherapy can also be ingested (by trained aromatherapists) for treatment of some ailments.

When asked which five essential oils are most important for massage therapists to always have on hand, Tisserand hesitates, pointing out that ideally there should not be a limit. However, if it is necessary to choose only five, he recommends eucalyptus, lavender, rosemary, geranium, and ylang-ylang. He also advises therapists to practice the craft in as professional a manner as possible, experiment, and attend some type of training in aromatherapy. The Tisserand School of Aromatherapy requires 6

Continued

months' full-time attendance or 2 years' part-time attendance. Massage therapists should also be aware that some oils do have contraindications. For example, a popular essential oil for muscular aches and pains, bergamot, can cause photosensitivity.

Tisserand's "taste" for aromatherapy piqued around 1967 when he attended a lecture on the subject along with his mother. She bought a book and had it signed by the speaker, Dr. Valnet (he was 19 at the time).

A couple of years later, Tisserand became interested in bodywork and did some training in that area. Soon he made a conscious decision to pursue a career in aromatherapy. "Not for the money," he laughs, "or I would have given up a long time ago. Basically I starved for 20 years."

Today he teaches others the art of aromatherapy. He has also developed and distributes Tisserand essential oil products all over the world. His works include the quintessential *The Art of Aromatherapy,* published by Inner Traditions; *Aromatherapy to Heal and Tend the Body,* published by Lotus Light; and *Essential Oil Safety,* Churchill Livingstone.

Tisserand still has his mother's signed copy of Valnet's French aromatherapy book. And after 30 years of hard work, audiences flock to his seminars, buy his books, seek his advice, and ask for his signature. The little boy who couldn't resist his mother's bottle of flea market perfume is finally able to sit back and enjoy the sweet smell of success.

External and Internal Respiration

Respiration takes place by *diffusion,* the tendency of molecules to move from a region of higher concentration to an area of lower concentration. The main functions of the respiratory process are to supply the body with oxygen and to dispose of carbon dioxide. Every cell needs oxygen to sustain life. Respiration occurs through two distinct processes: external respiration and internal respiration.

External, or pulmonary respiration, is gas exchange in the lungs, between blood and air in the alveoli that came from the external environment. Oxygen diffuses from the air inside the alveoli across the alveolar walls into the blood capillaries. The oxygen binds to the hemoglobin inside erythrocytes and is then transported to cells throughout the body. Carbon dioxide is transported by the blood from the cells of the body to the capillaries attached to the alveoli. The carbon dioxide then diffuses from the blood across the alveolar walls into the air inside the alveoli, which will then be exhaled. Oxygen and carbon dioxide exchange across the wall of the alveoli at the same time.

Internal respiration, or **tissue respiration,** is the gas exchange between blood and tissues throughout the body. Oxygen diffuses from the blood into the cells, and carbon dioxide diffuses from the cells into the bloodstream. Each cell participates in absorption of oxygen and removal of waste materials in connection with this process.

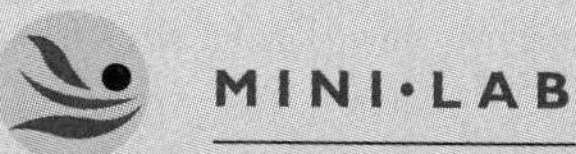

Using a tape measure, note the change in the circumference as you measure the rib cage during inspiration and expiration. Measure parts of the body such as the upper and lower ribs and abdomen.

MODIFIED RESPIRATORY AIR MOVEMENTS

Yawn. A yawn is a very deep breath, initiated by opening the mouth wide and by movements of the upper torso to expand the chest. Some believe that yawning is triggered by the need to increase the oxygen content and decrease carbon dioxide in the blood or as a result of drowsiness, boredom, or depression, but the precise cause is unknown.

Sneezing is a forceful involuntary expulsion of air through the nose and mouth to clear the upper respiratory passageways. Most sneezes occur due to irritation of the respiratory lining or to foreign particles such as dust or pollen.

Coughing is a sudden expulsion of air to clear the lungs and lower respiratory passageways of irritants or foreign materials. Coughing is a protec-

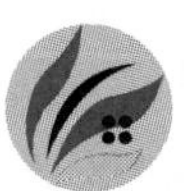

BREATHING AND MASSAGE THERAPY

Breathing not only reflects our physiological and psychological states, it also creates them. Actors have known this for many years. Whenever a particular scene requires them to appear anxious, they take shallow, rapid breaths before the scene. Conversely, when a scene requires that they look calm and relaxed, they use slow, deep breaths to bring them to a state of relaxation. Massage therapists use breathing techniques themselves while they are giving a massage and often teach these techniques to their clients.

The most effective type of breathing to produce relaxation is deep, slow abdominal or diaphragmatic breathing. During deep breathing, the muscles of the abdominal wall expand when the diaphragm moves inferiorly during inhalation. As we breathe, the abdominal contents get a massage as they are compressed and released.

When we breathe deeply, it is a total body experience. The nurturing air enters the nostrils and communicates internal and external movement. Deep breathing can ease pain, relax tension, or introduce much-needed energy into the body. Shallow breathing does not encourage relaxation and can create tension in the neck and shoulders.

Breathing creates and reflects our emotional sphere, so deep, full breaths will positively affect the free expression of our feelings. Restrictive breathing tends to constrict our expressions and wall off our feelings; we feel disconnected from the world around us.

The rhythm of breathing can give us an indication of how we feel about our environment. If we observe a slight pause before inhalation, this may announce a fear of new experiences. People inevitably stop breathing in an attempt to prevent something from happening. Clients will hold their breath during a massage when the pressure is uncomfortable. A slight pause before exhalation may indicate a fear of their own personal expression. Breath moves out of the lungs when we are trying to communicate. The most efficient breathing rhythm is a steady stream of inhalation and exhalation.

Imagine that the air around you has a fluid quality. As you inhale, the bottom portion of your lungs fills up first (like a glass of water). This filling causes a depression of the diaphragm and an expansion of the abdomen. As air fills the upper lungs, the rib cage expands and elevates on all sides. The spine also moves to accommodate the thoracoabdominal expansion. To complete your inhalation, puff out your cheeks and tightly close your lips. Allow your breath to burst out of your lips and exhale through your mouth, nose, or both. Although exhalation is typically a passive event, you may force air out of your lungs by contracting your abdominal muscles and "kissing your belly button to your spine." As you breathe, you should feel your body (especially your spine, ribs, and abdomen) move. Subtle movements may be felt in the extremities.

Children and most animals breathe with their bellies. Observe a sleeping cat or a toddler running around in a diaper. Her belly moves in a wave as she breathes. On mornings when you can wake up naturally (without an alarm), notice how you are breathing; you will probably be doing abdominal breathing. Encourage your body to breathe this way throughout the day.

To encourage your client to breathe properly, ask him to focus on his breathing by placing your hand just below his navel while he is lying supine. Ask him to take a deep breath and to allow his belly to elevate your hand. Occasionally, a simple goal like using the breath to move the therapist's hand will help the client understand the abdominal changes that occur while breathing.

While your client is prone, place your hand on the small of her back and ask her to take a deep breath, elevating your hand during inhalation. After instructing your client how to breathe for relaxation, teach her to use this simple technique when she feels stress or fatigue. These types of client/therapist interactions help to teach clients how to relax and to be aware of their bodies. Remember the old saying: "*If you give a man a fish, he eats for a day; if you teach a man to fish, he eats for a lifetime.*"

tive reflex, but can be voluntarily induced or inhibited. The act of coughing occurs after a brief inspiration. The abdominal muscles contract, forcing air out of the lungs. Productive coughing helps to clear the respiratory tract.

Crying is a response to emotions, such as grief, pain, fear, or joy. A common breath pattern while crying involves a sudden inspiration followed by the release of air in short breaths.

Laughing involves the same modified respiratory patterns as crying and is usually a response to happiness or being tickled. During laughter, the mouth is typically open in a grin. Laughing and crying can be so similar in sound that we typically have to look at a person's face to tell which emotion is being expressed.

Snoring is audible breathing during sleep due to vibration of the uvula and soft palate. Snoring can be accompanied by harsh sounds and is common among individuals who sleep with their mouths open. When a snorer sleeps on her back, the mouth opens due to gravity, and the tongue may rest in the back of the throat, partly blocking the air passage. In most cases, closing the mouth or simply rolling the snoring individual over will stop the snoring.

Hiccups, or hiccough, are spasmodic contractions of the diaphragm followed by a spasmodic closure of the vocal folds. The sound occurs when inspired air hits the closed vocal folds. Hiccups have a variety of causes that appear to be linked to irritation of gastrointestinal sensory nerve endings.

Author's Note

Cigarette smoking eventually destroys alveoli and negatively affects gas exchange in the lungs. Smoking also destroys respiratory cilia which remove particles in the nasal cavity and respiratory tract. As cilia die and the respiratory lining becomes irritated, the body produces excess mucus to trap the foreign particles in the cigarette smoke and to protect these delicate membranes and related tissues.

Smoking can also inhibit the macrophage cells, which increases the likelihood of respiratory infections. A recent medical discovery found that when smoking begins during early teen years, complete maturation of the lungs never occurs and those additional alveoli are lost forever.

As a result, individuals who smoke one pack of cigarettes a day will statistically take 7 years off their life expectancy.

RESPIRATORY CONDITIONS AND CLINICAL TERMS

1. **Hypoxia.** Hypoxia is a decrease in the amount of oxygen in the blood, often characterized by rapid heart rate, excessive carbon dioxide levels in the blood, cyanosis, vertigo, and mental confusion. Mild hypoxia increases respiration; severe hypoxia can lead to heart failure and death. The organs most effected by hypoxia are the brain, the heart, and the liver.
2. **Apnea** is a temporary cessation (usually lasting 15 seconds) or absence of spontaneous respiration. There are three types of apnea: central, obstructive, and mixed. During central apnea, there is an absence of a neurological drive to breathe, a lack of diaphragmatic movement, and no detectable air conduction. Central apnea is often seen in premature infants. Obstructive apnea airflow is created by a misformed or abnormal anatomical structure, the most common cause being a deviated septum. Mixed apnea is a combination of central and obstructive apnea.
3. **Minimal air.** When an infant takes its first breath, the alveoli are filled with air that is never expelled. This is known as minimal air. You actually have part of your first breath in your body right now. If an infant is found dead, lung tissue is often used to determine if the child was stillborn. If the lung tissue floats, the baby took his first breath. If the lung tissue sinks, the alveoli never filled with air and the baby was probably stillborn.
4. **Vital capacity.** The total amount that can be forcibly inspired and expired from the lungs in one breath is called vital capacity. This represents the greatest respiratory volume of an individual. Vital capacity is affected by age, gender, physical fitness, and disease. Average values range from 4,000 to 5,000 milliliters.
5. **Pleurisy** is inflammation and/or adhesion of the pleural membranes characterized by stabbing pain during breathing. The painful breathing is caused by friction created as the swollen pleural membranes rub against each other as they move. Chronic pleurisy may result in permanent pleural adhesions.

   Massage is contraindicated if the pleurisy is due to bacterial infection. If it is due to other causes, a full-body massage can be done, to the client's tolerance. Attention should be paid to the accessory muscles of respiration.
6. **Pulmonary edema** is a condition involving an excessive amount of blood and interstitial fluid in the lungs. Common causes of pulmonary edema are near drowning, congestive heart failure, infection (i.e., pneumonia, tuberculosis), renal failure, and cerebrovascular accidents.

   If the symptoms are severe, massage is contraindicated because the increased circulation can make the edema in the lungs worse. If the symptoms are less severe, a light, relaxing massage may be helpful as long as it has been approved by the client's physician.
7. **Laryngitis** is inflammation of the larynx that often results in loss of voice. Laryngitis is caused by respiratory infections or irritants such as cigarette smoke. Most long-term smokers acquire a permanent hoarseness from the damage created by chronic irritation and inflammation. Edema of the vocal fold often accompanies this disorder, as well as coughing and a scratchy throat.
8. **Bronchitis** is inflammation of the bronchial mucosa that causes the bronchial tubes to swell and extra mucus to be produced. The two types of bronchitis are acute and chronic. Acute bronchitis, caused by an upper respiratory tract infection, results in a productive cough and high fever. Chronic bronchitis involves copious secretions of mucus with a productive cough that typically lasts 3 full months of the year for 2 successive years. Cigarette smoking remains the most frequent cause of chronic bronchitis, followed by chronic

respiratory infections and anatomical abnormalities of the bronchi that interfere with normal respiratory drainage.

Postural drainage is very helpful in clearing the respiratory tract of mucus. Position the client so her head is lower than the rest of her body. This can be done by putting pillows under the client's abdomen or by making the head of the massage table lower than the back of the table. A full-body relaxing massage is helpful, with tapotement and vibration on the back for 10 to 20 minutes. Be sure to massage the accessory muscles of respiration.

9. **Asthma** is a chronic, inflammatory disorder in which the smooth muscles in the walls of the smaller bronchi and bronchioles spasm to close or partially close the respiratory passageways, causing labored breathing. Asthma usually is preceded by emotional stress, respiratory infections, strenuous exercise, or inhalation of allergens (substances that promote allergic reactions). Exercise-induced asthma produces asthmatic symptoms after vigorous exercise; this type usually occurs in people who already have asthma, allergies, or hypersensitivity respiratory reactions.

   Make sure from the client's intake form and premassage interview that there are no allergens in the massage office that would trigger an attack. Side-lying position may be the most comfortable for the client. A full-body, relaxing massage is helpful. Focus on the accessory muscles of respiration and the postural muscles because many clients with chronic asthma develop kyphosis. Vibration over the chest may help loosen mucus.

10. **Pneumonia** is an infection or inflammation of the alveoli caused by the bacterium *Streptococcus pneumoniae,* but other infectious agents, such as bacteria, protozoans, viruses, and fungi, may be responsible. During pneumonia, the alveoli fill with fluid and exudates such as dead white blood cells and pus. Exudates are substances that have been slowly discharged from cells or blood vessels as waste products. Pneumonia is the most common infectious cause of death in the United States, affecting, in particular, the elderly, infants, immunocompromised individuals, and cigarette smokers.

    Massage is contraindicated during the acute phase because it is infectious. Once a client has recovered, massage can be beneficial. Tapotement and vibration on the chest can help drain secretions. Range of motion and massage on the extremities can help prevent muscle atrophy from prolonged bed rest.

11. **Emphysema** involves destruction of the alveoli, producing abnormally large air spaces that remain filled with air during expiration. With the loss of the elasticity of the alveoli, a person can inhale easily but has to labor to exhale. The added exertion increases the size of the rib cage, resulting in a barrel chest. Emphysema is caused by a long-term irritation such as cigarette smoking, air pollution, and exposure to industrial dust.

    The client may need to be propped in a semireclining position for ease of breathing. The accessory muscles of respiration will be especially tight, so focus massage on them. In particular, the sternocleidomastoid, scalenes, and pectoralis minor need to be addressed.

12. **Tuberculosis,** the "white plague" or "consumption," is a chronic lung infection caused by the bacterium *Mycobacterium tuberculosis.* It is typically transmitted by the inhalation and exhalation (or consumption) of infected droplets. Even though the lungs are the disease's primary target, the liver, bone marrow, and spleen may be involved as well. During tuberculosis, lung tissue is destroyed by bacteria and is replaced by fibrous connective tissue, limiting gas exchange. Tuberculosis bacteria can withstand exposure to disinfectants but die quickly in sunlight.

    Generally, tuberculosis is not infectious from 2 to 4 weeks after the start of treatment with antitubercular medications. Massage is contraindicated unless the client is no longer infective. Check with the client's physician to be sure.

13. **Bronchogenic carcinoma,** or lung cancer, is caused by a long-term irritant such as air pollution, cigarette smoke, asbestos, or coal dust. Initially, there are usually no symptoms and it isn't detected until the late stages when symptoms include chronic cough, difficulty breathing, chest pain, coughing up blood, weight loss, and weakness.

    Massage can be beneficial in reducing stress for the client. However, it is essential to consult with the client's physician before performing any massage. It is also very important to consider the client's vitality because a long and vigorous massage may in fact make the client feel worse.

14. **Cystic fibrosis.** This is a genetic disorder involving the pancreas and the respiratory system. The bronchi secretes thick mucus, which causes obstruction and narrowing of the lumen. The prognosis is poor and there is no known cure.

    Postural drainage is very helpful. Position the client so his head is lower than his feet. Tapotement and vibration can help loosen phlegm. Massage of the accessory muscles of respiration is also very helpful.

15. **Respiratory distress syndrome**, also known as RDS or hyaline membrane disease, is an acute infantile lung disease characterized by inelastic lungs, respiration rate of more than 60 per minute, and nasal flaring. The condition occurs most often in premature babies due to inadequate pulmonary surfactants. Adult respiratory distress syndrome, or ARDS, is characterized by hypoxia and is often the

result of foreign objects (e.g., asbestos) aspirated into the lungs, cardiopulmonary bypass surgery, or pneumonia.

16. **Carbon monoxide poisoning** is a toxic, often lethal condition that is caused by the absorption of carbon monoxide through inhalation. Carbon monoxide binds at the same receptor sites as oxygen on the hemoglobin molecule, preventing oxygen from being carried by the hemoglobin. Carbon monoxide poisoning leads to oxygen starvation of cells. Its most common causes are automobile exhaust fumes and improperly functioning furnaces.
17. **Decompression sickness (the bends).** When people work in a high-pressure region, such as below sea level, the blood and body tissues can absorb unusual amounts of nitrogen, carbon dioxide, and oxygen. This condition is harmless as long as the pressures inside and outside the body are equal. If divers or aviators move too quickly between areas of high pressure or low pressure, a painful, often fatal syndrome called the bends, may occur. When pressure is reduced too quickly, nitrogen can not move from the tissues to the lungs fast enough for it to be dispelled through expiration. Nitrogen accumulates in the body and impairs normal tissue oxygenation. Symptoms include joint pain, dizziness, shortness of breath, extreme fatigue, paralysis, and unconsciousness. The name "the bends" comes from the fact that victims of decompression sickness double over from the extreme pain caused by the expansion of gases in the bloodstream. Gradual decompression is the safest way to normalize the gaseous condition.

Effects of Massage for the Respiratory System

1. Massage slows down the rate of respiration via reduced stimulation of the parasympathetic nervous system.
2. The mechanical loosening and discharge of phlegm in the respiratory tract increase with rhythmic alternating pressures. Tapotement (cupping) and vibration on the rib cage are often used to enhance this effect. Phlegm loosening and discharge are further enhanced when combined with postural drainage (promoting fluid drainage of the respiratory tract through certain body positions) and when the client is encouraged to cough.
3. By freeing tight respiratory muscles and fascia, massage can be used to increase vital capacity and pulmonary function.

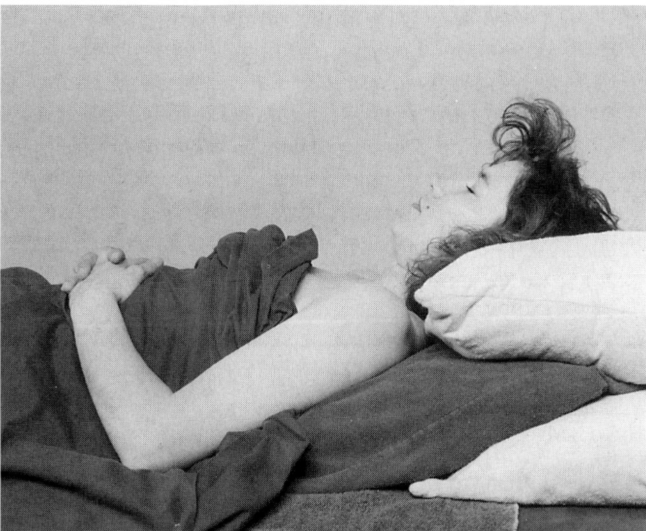

Figure 13•5 Client in the supine position supported by pillows.

Author's Note

Because of gravity a client receiving a massage in a recumbent position, when she is experiencing respiratory congestion, compounds the problem. There are a few things you can do to make the client more comfortable.

1. When the client is in the supine position, elevate the upper body to assist drainage. Dr. Keith De Sonnier; an ear, nose, and throat physician, recommends a 30-degree incline to assist sinus drainage (Fig. 13–5).

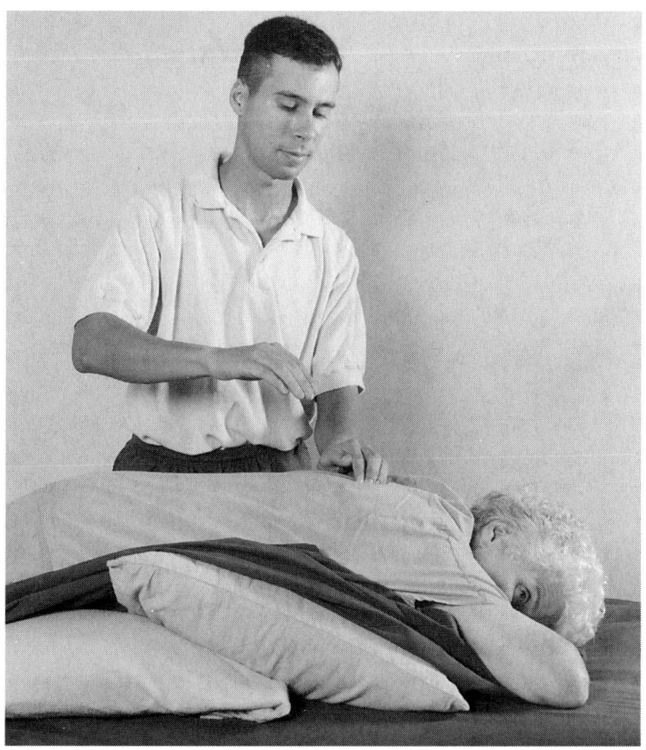

Figure 13•6 Client receiving percussion to loosen phlegm.

2. After massaging in the prone position, lower the upper body by placing pillows or other supportive cushions under the hips and abdomen. Use cupping percussion delivered to the posterior thoracic region to loosen phlegm. Expect the client to cough as a natural reflex (Fig. 13–6). Have tissues handy for client use.
3. You may elect *not* to massage the client in the prone position and choose a side-lying position instead.

SUMMARY

The respiratory system is physiologically and poetically associated with the very concept of life itself. The main functions of this system include the exchange of gases, homeostasis, olfaction, and the production of speech. This method of air movement and chemical exchange is accomplished by the anatomical structures of the respiratory system, including the nasal cavities, the pharynx, the larynx, the trachea, bronchi, alveoli, the lungs, and the respiratory diaphragm. Pulmonary ventilation, external respiration, and internal respiration are the processes necessary to get oxygen to cells and to eliminate gaseous wastes. The main mechanisms of air movement involved in the breathing process are inspiration and expiration. There are also several modified respiratory air movements, which include yawning, sneezing, coughing, crying, laughing, snoring, and hiccuping. The main purpose of air movement is to take in oxygen, which is vital to sustain life and to expel carbon dioxide, a waste product. Aromatherapy and massage therapy complement each other and benefit the client greatly.

SELF-TEST

Multiple Choice • Write the letter of the best answer in the space provided.

_______ 1. Which of the following is a function of the respiratory system?
- A. receptors for taste
- B. exchange of gases
- C. homeostasis of blood glucose levels
- D. protection against blood loss

_______ 2. The pitch of the voice is produced when air passes over the
- A. trachea
- B. epiglottis
- C. vocal folds
- D. nasal conchae

_______ 3. External and internal respiration takes place by which mechanism?
- A. active transport
- B. pinocytosis
- C. osmosis
- D. diffusion

_______ 4. Gas exchange between the blood and the tissues is called
- A. environmental respiration
- B. external/pulmonary respiration
- C. internal/tissue respiration
- D. diffusion of gases

_______ 5. Another name for the throat is the
- A. pharynx
- B. larynx
- C. epiglottis
- D. trachea

_______ 6. The "windpipe" is a common name for the
- A. pharynx
- B. larynx
- C. epiglottis
- D. trachea

_______ 7. Which structure covers the trachea during swallowing?
- A. pharynx
- B. larynx
- C. epiglottis
- D. trachea

_______ 8. Within the larynx, three paired cartilages attach to and support the
- A. thyroid cartilage
- B. Adam's apple
- C. epiglottis
- D. vocal folds

_______ 9. The incomplete sections of the tracheal rings allow the esophagus to
- A. expand into the trachea when swallowing a food bolus
- B. compress the trachea during vomiting
- C. close over the trachea, keeping food from entering the lungs
- D. there are no incomplete sections of tracheal rings

_______ 10. Because the right primary bronchus is slightly wider and has a slightly steeper downward angle than the left,
- A. respiratory infections are more frequent on the right side
- B. alveoli in the right lung are larger
- C. foreign bodies more frequently lodge on the right side
- D. foreign bodies more frequently lodge on the left side

_______ 11. The bronchi divide into smaller branches called
- A. tracheals
- B. bronchioles
- C. epiglottis
- D. surfactants

_______ 12. The balloonlike sacs made of epithelium are the
- A. bronchioles
- B. surfactants
- C. respiratory diaphragm
- D. alveoli

_______ 13. Phospholipids reducing surface tension and contributing to elasticity of pulmonary tissue is/are
- A. bronchioles
- B. surfactants
- C. the respiratory diaphragm
- D. pleurisy

_______ 14. The paired organs of respiration are the
- A. diaphragm
- B. adrenals
- C. lungs
- D. pharynx

_______ 15. The main muscles of respiration is/are the

A. scalenes
B. sternocleidomastoid
C. respiratory diaphragm
D. abdominal muscles

_______ 16. The respiratory center is located in the

A. lungs
B. cerebral cortex
C. limbic system
D. brain stem

_______ 17. At rest, respiration cycles occur in adults about

A. 20 to 30 times a minute
B. 12 to 14 times a minute
C. 20 times a minute
D. 72 times a minute

_______ 18. Some factors that affect respiration are

A. a sudden, severe pain
B. an increase in body temperature
C. an increase in carbon dioxide levels
D. all of the above

_______ 19. Breathing has two mechanical phases called

A. inhalation/exhalation
B. internal/tissue respiration
C. pulmonary/tissue respiration
D. all of the above

_______ 20. Contraction and descending of the diaphragm causes

A. inhalation
B. exhalation
C. pulmonary apnea
D. tissue respiration

_______ 21. During this phase of pulmonary ventilation, air moves out of the lungs due to elastic recoil of the alveoli.

A. inhalation
B. exhalation
C. pulmonary apnea
D. tissue respiration

Matching • List the letter of the modified respiratory air movement to its description.

A. cough
B. cry
C. hiccup
D. laugh
E. sneeze
F. yawn

_______ 1. A voluntary or involuntary response to emotions such as grief, pain, fear, or joy, involving a sudden inspiration followed by the release of air in short breaths

_______ 2. A very deep breath, initiated by opening the mouth wide and movements of the upper torso to expand the chest

_______ 3. A protective reflex involving a sudden expulsion of air to clear the lungs and lower respiratory passageways of irritants or foreign materials

_______ 4. A spasm of the diaphragm followed by a spasmodic closure of the vocal folds

_______ 5. Forceful involuntary expulsion of air to clear the upper respiratory passageways through both the nose and the mouth, due to irritation of the respiratory lining or foreign particles such as dust or pollen

_______ 6. A response to happiness or while being tickled, very much like crying, but the mouth is open in a grin

References

Applegate, Edith J., M.S. *The Anatomy and Physiology Learning System: Textbook.* Philadelphia: W. B. Saunders, 1995.

Damjanov, Ivan. *Pathophysiology for the Health-Related Professions.* Philadelphia: W. B. Saunders, 1996.

Ford, Clyde W. *Where Healing Waters Meet: Touching Mind and Emotions through the Body.* Barrytown, NY: Station Hill Press, Inc. 1992.

Gray, Henry, F.R.S., T. Pickering Pick, F.R.C.S., Robert Howden, M.A., M.B., C.M. *Gray's Anatomy,* 29th ed. Philadelphia: Running Press, 1974.

Haubrich, William S. *Medical Meanings, A Glossary of Word Origins.* New York: Harcourt Brace Jovanovich, 1984.

Kalat, James W. *Biological Psychology,* 2nd ed. Belmont, CA: Wadsworth Publishing Company, 1984.

Kordish, Mary and Sylvia Dickson. *Introduction to Basic Human Anatomy.* Lake Charles, LA: McNeese State University, Self-published manual. 1985.

Marieb, Elaine N. *Essentials of Human Anatomy and Physiology,* 4th ed. New York: Benjamin/Cummings Publishing Company, Inc., 1994.

McAleer, Neil. *The Body Almanac.* Garden City, NY: Doubleday and Company, Inc., 1985.

Mosby's Medical, Nursing, and Allied Health Dictionary, 4th ed. St Louis: Mosby–Year Book, Inc., 1994.

Newton, Don. *Pathology for Massage Therapists,* 2nd ed. Portland: Simran Publications, 1995.

Premkumar, Kalyani. *Pathology A to Z—A Handbook for Massage Therapists.* Calgary, Canada: VanPub Books, 1996.

Tabers Cyclopedic Medical Dictionary, 13th ed. Philadelphia: F. A. Davis Company, 1977.

Tortora, Gerald J. *Introduction to the Human Body: The Essentials of Anatomy and Physiology,* 3rd ed. New York: HarperCollins Publishers, 1994.

Make your words sweet, because one day you may have to eat them!
—Colombian proverb

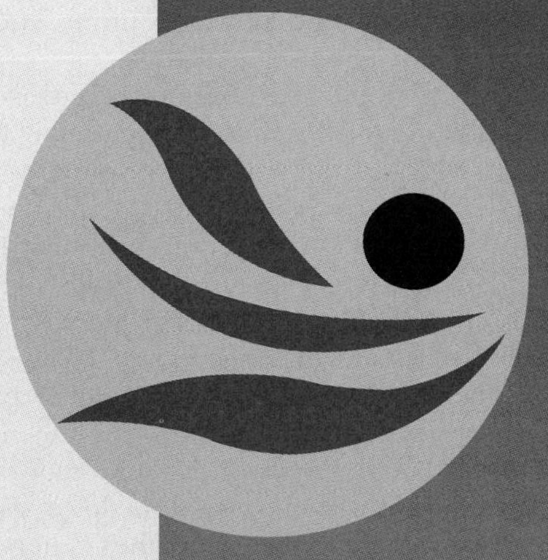

14

Digestive System

Student Objectives

After completing this chapter, the student should be able to:

- Explain the four functions of the digestive system
- Discuss the basic anatomical structures of the digestive system
- Identify the specific divisions of the alimentary canal
- Describe what happens to food when it enters the alimentary canal
- Trace the path food takes from the time it enters the mouth to the time wastes are eliminated
- Identify where the products of the salivary glands, liver, gallbladder, and pancreas enter the intestinal tube
- Describe the disassembly of foods in the body

INTRODUCTION

We each consume over 40 tons of food in an average lifetime. The digestive system provides processes by which molecules such as proteins, carbohydrates, and fats are broken down into a state more easily assimilated into the body. Essentially, the digestive process is a "disassembly line." These digestive processes themselves consume a tremendous amount of bodily resources, but fortunately they produce more energy than they use.

As we learned in Chapter 10, there are two divisions of the autonomic nervous system: sympathetic and parasympathetic. Digestive functions are initiated by the parasympathetic nervous system during periods of low stress. Because digestion requires a tremendous expenditure of energy, it occurs during times of low activity. The body can then reallocate energy that would normally be spent on muscular activity and route it to the digestive system. Activation of the parasympathetic nervous system is also known as the *relaxation response* or *rest and digest.* Stress and emotions such as anger, fear, and anxiety may slow down digestion because they stimulate the sympathetic nervous system, or the *stress response.* People in high-stress jobs or high responsibility positions are more likely to have problems with ulcers, heartburn, colitis, irritable bowel syndrome, and constipation due to frequent disruption of the digestive process.

The digestive system may be viewed as the refinery of the body. A refinery takes a product such as raw crude from the ground and fractionates or disassembles it into useful components such as gasoline, butane, and diesel. Likewise, the digestive system takes in the raw materials of food and drink and converts them both physically and chemically into highly refined fuel. Just as fuel oil or natural gas is transported to our homes by pipes, digested materials are delivered to our body's cells through the vessels of the circulatory system. Many unneeded resources can be stored for future metabolism.

As we study the anatomy of the digestive system, we will see that it is primarily composed of a tube, which is linked to the outside world. In this chapter, each tube section and organ will be identified and described by structure and function. Included are the various digestive secretions and the food types upon which they act.

FUNCTIONS

1. **Ingestion** is the process of orally taking materials into the body. This term applies to taking in food, liquids, and oral medications.
2. **Digestion** is the mechanical and chemical processes that occur as food is mixed with digestive enzymes and converted into an absorbable state. Mechanical digestion includes chewing in the oral cavity, churning in the stomach, and the mixing movements of the intestinal tube (peristalsis). After digestion, food is capable of being taken into the bloodstream. Digestion occurs through **hydrolysis,** or the chemical breakdown in the presence of water.
3. **Absorption** is the process by which the products of digestion move into the bloodstream or lymph vessels and then into the body's cells.
4. **Defecation** is the process of eliminating indigestible or unabsorbed material from the body.

Terms and Word Parts Related to the Digestive System

amylase – starch; enzyme
bolus – a lump
Brunner's glands – named after the Swiss anatomist (1653–1727)
bucca – cheek
cecum – blindness
chol – bile
chyme – juice
deglutition – to swallow
dens, dent, odont – toothlike
duodenum – 12
enzyme – leaven
fundus – base
gingiva – gums
gustatory – to taste
haustra – to draw, drink
hepato – liver
ileum – twisted
jejunum – empty
Kupffer's cells – Named after the German anatomist (1829–1902)
lacteal – of milk
mastication – to chew
mesentery – middle; intestine
omentum – a covering or apron
peristaltic – around; contraction
plicae circulares – a fold; a little ring
pylorus – gatekeeper
rectum – straight
rugae – a crease or fold
sacchar – sugar
sigmoid – the Greek letter "sigma" meaning "s"-shaped
sphincter – a binder
sphincter of Oddi – named after a 19th century Italian physician
taenia coli – tape; colon
tonsils – almond
vermiform appendix – wormlike; hanger-on
villi – tuft of hair

GENERAL DIGESTIVE ANATOMY AND RELATED PHYSIOLOGY

1. **Alimentary canal.** The alimentary canal, also referred to as the intestinal tube, the digestive tube, or the gastrointestinal (GI) tract, is the mostly coiled, muscular passageway leading from the mouth to the anus. The alimentary canal is approximately 30 feet long and includes the oral cavity, pharynx, esophagus, stomach, small intestine, and large intestine (Fig. 14–1). The tube itself has four layers, or **tunics.** From superficial to deep, the layers are the mucosa, the submucosa, the muscularis, and the serosa, all of which are host to blood vessels, lymphatic vessels, and glands that produce and secrete digestive enzymes. The alimentary canal is primarily smooth muscle and this muscle tissue is responsible for most of the movement and mixing action of the digestive tube. Skeletal muscle is present only in parts of the pharynx, the esophagus, and in the anus.

   Within the muscular layer (muscularis) of the alimentary canal, there are two types of contractions: tonic and rhythmic. **Tonic contractions** are sustained contractions that occur in sphincter muscles. A **sphincter** is a ring of muscle fibers that regulate movement of materials from one compartment of the gastrointestinal tract to another. **Rhythmic** or **peristaltic contractions** are the most common muscular contraction of the digestive system. These wavelike contractions mix and propel materials farther into the GI tract. Also known as *peristalsis,* the propelling motion of the tube occurs as a contraction just behind a **bolus** (a ball-like, masticated lump of food once swallowed). As the bolus approaches, the sphincter relaxes and then opens to allow passage. During mixing movements, peristaltic contractions occur as a rhythmic, sequential contraction of smooth muscle, moving the intestinal materials back and forth until they are thoroughly mixed.

2. **Peritoneum.** The peritoneum, which envelops the entire abdominal wall, is the largest serous membrane in the body. The free surface of the peritoneum is lubricated with a serous fluid, permitting the visceral contents to glide easily against the abdominal wall without friction. Within the peritoneum are blood vessels, lymph vessels, and nerves. Sections of the peritoneum include the mesenteries, the parietal and visceral peritoneum, and the greater and lesser omentum.

   Another part of the peritoneum, the **mesentery,** is a large, fan-shaped section connecting the small intestine to the posterior abdominal wall. Also referred to as the "fatty apron," the **greater omentum** is a double-layered structure that attaches from the greater curvature of the stomach and the duodenum, draping down over the coils of the small intestine, then attaches to the transverse colon. The **lesser omentum** is a fatty, membranous extension of the peritoneum and attaches from the right side of stomach and first section of the duodenum to the liver (Fig. 14–2).

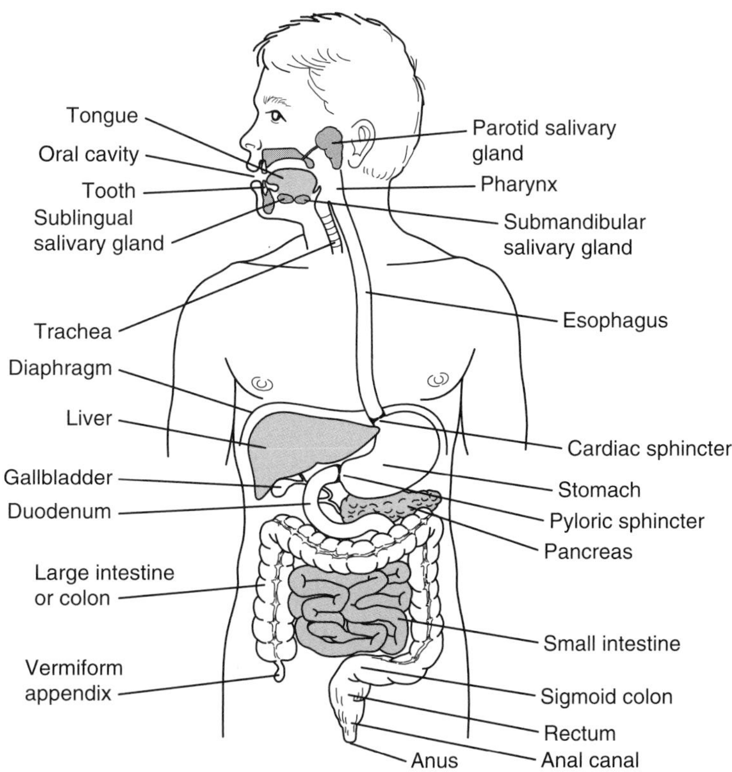

Figure 14•1 The digestive system and accessory organs.

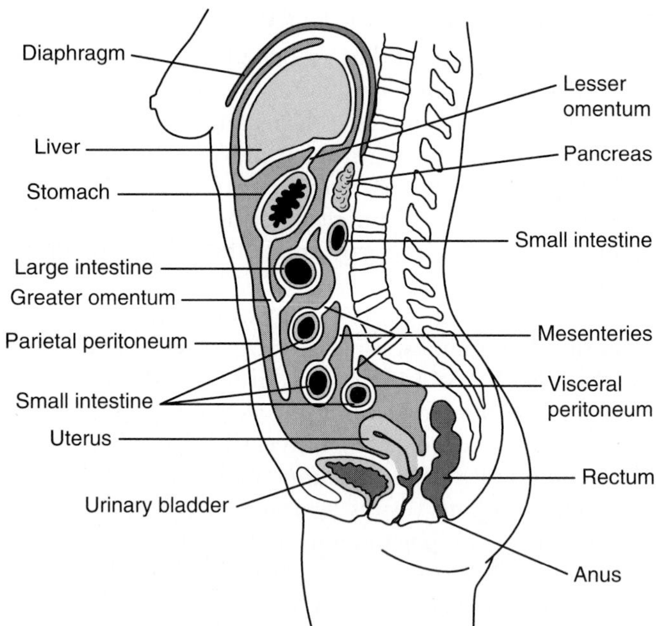

Figure 14•2 Lateral view of the peritoneum.

DIVISIONS OF THE ALIMENTARY CANAL

1. **Oral cavity.** Also known as the buccal cavity or mouth, the oral cavity contains the tongue, teeth, gums, and openings from the salivary ducts. Digestion begins in the oral cavity. **Mastication** (chewing) is aided by the tongue; digestive enzymes (an **enzyme** is a catalyst that accelerates chemical reactions) present in salvia break down food. **Saliva,** containing water, mucus, organic salts, and digestive enzymes, is a clear, nondigestible, viscous fluid secreted by the salivary and mucous glands in the mouth. The functions of saliva are to act as a lubricant and an adhesive by causing food to stick together and forming a bolus for **deglutition** (swallowing). Saliva stimulates the taste buds and protects the mucosa by acting as a buffer. With the exception of several medications, such as nitroglycerin, no absorption takes place in the oral cavity.

   Saliva also serves to initiate the digestion of starches and fats through salivary amylase and lingual lipase. Salivary amylase, or ptyalin, begins the digestion of carbohydrates. Lingual lipase, secreted by glands located in the tongue, breaks lipids down into glycerol and fatty acids.

   Saliva is produced in one of the three pairs of salivary glands. They are the submandibular glands (located inside the mandibular arch), the sublingual glands (located in the roof of the mouth under the tongue), and the large parotid glands (located superficial to the masseter muscle).

   The tongue aids in deglutition (by directing the bolus toward the back of the throat). Nestled in spheric pockets on the superior and lateral surfaces of the tongue are the **gustatory organs** (taste buds), chemoreceptors that detect the primary tastes of sweet, sour, bitter, and salty. However, taste is a response of many neurons, not just a signal from a single gustatory nerve. Even though the tongue is considered the primary organ of taste, the nose and the temperature of food play a significant role in how food tastes. Hot food tastes better than cold food because heat causes the aroma of the food to rise and enter our nose. Food does not taste as good when we have a condition that affects our sense of smell.

   Within the adult oral cavity are 32 secondary or permanent teeth. Children possess only 20 primary or deciduous teeth, that are usually shed between the ages of 6 and 12 years. Enamel, which is the hardest substance in the body, covers each tooth. Teeth are classified according to shape and function: the incisors; cuspids (canines); bicuspids (premolars); and the multicuspids (molars). The third molars are also called wisdom teeth because they evidently erupt when a person is old enough to be wise (usually between the ages of 17 and 25; however, many people reportedly do not begin to feel wise until later in life.

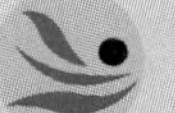

MINI•LAB

Most individuals can recall a biology experiment in elementary school in which different substances were placed on the tongue to grasp a better understanding of how different parts of the tongue detected tastes.

Gather a small container of sugar, a small container of salt, and a sliced lemon. Apply these foods on different areas of your tongue and notice the areas that clearly detect the tastes. Can you taste the lemon or the salt on the tip of your tongue? After wetting your finger, apply the sugar on the backside of the tongue. Can you taste the sweetness?

2. **Pharynx.** Also called the throat, the pharynx is the tube structure that transports food, liquid, and air to their respective destinations. In the digestive system, the pharynx takes food from the oral cavity to the esophagus during deglutition.
3. **Esophagus.** The esophagus (gullet) is the muscular tube that connects the pharynx to the stomach. The esophageal lining secretes mucus to aid in the transport of food. Bypassing the thoracic organs, the esophagus transports food to the stomach. The narrowest part of the gullet is where it traverses the diaphragm through the esophageal hiatus.

4. **Stomach.** The stomach is a J-shaped organ that is essentially an enlargement of the gastrointestinal tract bound at both ends by sphincters. The superior sphincter, found at the junction between the esophagus and the stomach, is the **cardiac** or **cardioesophageal sphincter.** The **pyloric sphincter** is located between the stomach and the small intestine. The stomach is situated directly under the diaphragm in the left upper quadrant of the abdomen and is divided into four main regions: the *cardia* (surrounding the superior opening to the stomach), the *fundus* (superior rounded section), the *body* (large central region), and the *pylorus* (distal portion). Exteriorly, the shape of the stomach reveals a greater curvature and a lesser curvature (Fig. 14–3).

   The stomach receives partially digested food and drink from the esophagus. When empty, the stomach is about the size of a large sausage! Depending on body size, the stomach, when full, can hold up to 1 gallon of food. This expansion is permitted by the longitudinal folds, or **gastric rugae.**

   The muscular tunic of the stomach has three layers of muscle: the oblique, the circular, and the longitudinal. It is the oblique layer that adds a new dimension to the churning action of the stomach, giving it an extraordinary ability to mix food. Entering the stomach, food mixes with gastric enzymes to initiate protein digestion. As food is further blended and digested, a bolus of food is reduced to a thin viscous fluid called **chyme.**

   The pyloric sphincter opens periodically to allow chyme to enter into the small intestine. The process of moving chyme into the small intestine may take up to 4 hours; therefore, the stomach also serves as a storage tank as well as a digestive chamber. Because of this slow release of chyme into the small intestines, it is possible for us to maintain our energy needs with only two or three meals a day, instead of requiring a steady supply of food like grazing animals.

   The gastric mucosa possesses both endocrine and exocrine cells. The endocrine glands are called **G cells** and secrete the hormone *gastrin,* which initiates the production and secretion of gastric juice and stimulates bile and pancreatic enzyme emission into the small intestines. The stomach produces about 2 to 3 quarts of gastric juice per day. The only substances that are absorbed by the lining of the stomach are water, some minerals, alcohol, and some medications such as aspirin.

   Two types of exocrine cells in the stomach are the parietal cells and the chief cells. The **parietal cells** produce intrinsic factor, a substance required for the absorption of vitamin B_{12} from the small intestine to the bloodstream. They also produce hydrochloric acid, a component of gastric juice, which breaks down protein and activates many gastric enzymes. Hydrochloric acid (HCl), which kills bacteria and other pathogens, is so powerful an acid that it can eat through wood! The gastric lining is protected from this strong acid by a thick layer of alkaline mucus produced by mucous cells in the gastric lining. **Chief cells** produce the gastric enzyme pepsinogen, which is a precursor to pepsin. Pepsin is secreted in an inactive form to prevent the gastric lining from eroding from pepsin's protein digestion. Pepsinogen converts to pepsin when it comes into contact with HCl and begins the chemical digestion of proteins by converting them into peptides.

   Rennin, an enzyme found in the gastric juices of infants, is used to aid in milk curdling and is used commercially to produce cheese.

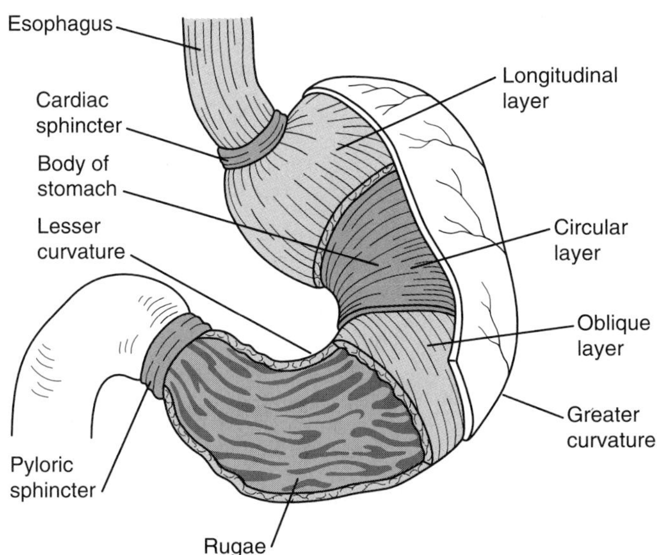

Figure 14•3 The stomach and its structures.

Author's Note

What causes hunger? Is it the need for food and energy? Heredity? There are several theories of why we get hungry. One theory is stomach contractions or stomach "growling," which may increase when the stomach is empty. Another idea is that our body detects a low level of blood sugar or a combined reduction of all available digestible foods. Additionally, the hypothalamus appears to regulate the sensation of hunger as well as the feeling of satiety (fullness). Many individuals eat when they are lonely, depressed, or bored. Other reasons besides hunger are often indicated when people are asked why they eat. Hunger is most likely a combination of several physiological and psychological events.

5. **Small intestine.** The small intestine is actually the longest section of the alimentary canal and is situ-

ated in the central abdomen, framed by the large intestine. This muscular tube is bound at both ends by the pyloric sphincter (at the stomach) and the **ileocecal sphincter** (at the large intestine). The lumen of the small intestine possesses circular folds called **plicae circulares** (Fig. 14–4). The lining of the small intestines contains numerous **villi,** finger-like projections that house blood and lymph capillaries. The lymph capillaries in the villi are called **lacteals,** which assist in the absorption of fat. The plicae circulares and the villi increase the surface area of the small intestine for more efficient absorption.

FYI FOR YOUR INFORMATION

The word "jejunum" is derived from the Latin adjective *jejunus,* "fasting or hungry," meaning being empty or devoid of food. The ancient Greeks, during the practice of necropsy (examination of a dead body), found that the lumen of the middle small intestine was always empty.

The three divisions of the small intestines, from beginning to end, are the duodenum, jejunum, and ileum. The **duodenum** is between 10 and 12 inches long and contains the sphincter of Oddi and the major duodenal papilla. The **sphincter of Oddi** regulates the flow of secretions from the pancreas, liver, and gallbladder; the **major duodenal papilla** is the site of entry for these secretions. The major duodenal papilla is a dilation that is formed by the juncture of the pancreatic and bile ducts as they open into the small intestines.

The intermediate portion of the small intestine, the **jejunum,** joins the duodenum with the ileum and is approximately 6 feet in length. The walls of the jejunum are slightly thicker than those of the ileum, and the jejunum possesses a smaller lumen. The villi are larger in this section, presumably to increase absorption.

The final division of the small intestine—the **ileum**—is approximately 9 feet long and terminates at the ileocecal sphincter which connects the ileum of the small intestine to the cecum of the large intestine. This section of the small intestine contains numerous clusters of lacteals to enhance fat absorption.

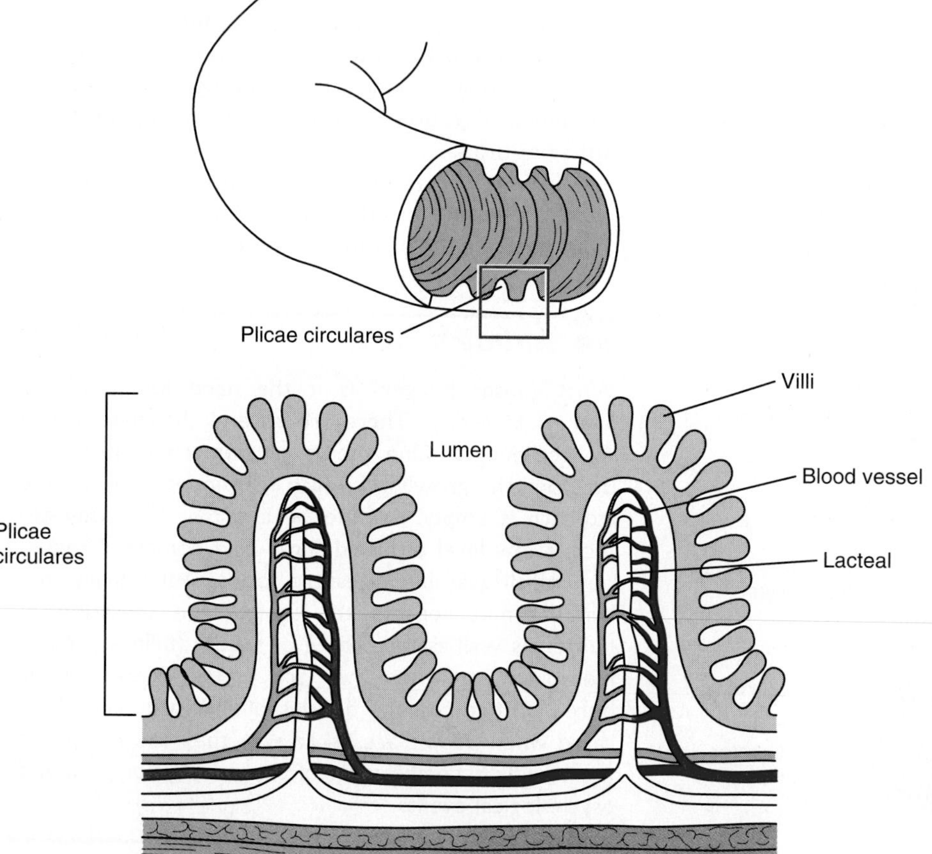

Figure 14•4 Cutaway of the small intestine exposing the plicae circulares and the villi and a close-up of a lacteal.

Ninety percent of all absorption takes place throughout the length of the small intestine (the other 10 percent occurs in the stomach and large intestine). Digested foodstuffs, absorbed through the intestinal walls, are transported by the blood (i.e., sugars and proteins) and lymph (i.e., fats) to be used by the body. If more food nutrients (i.e., fat, fat-soluble vitamins) are absorbed than the body requires, the extra is stored until needed.

Brunner's glands (duodenal glands) secrete alkaline mucus. Other intestinal glands secrete intestinal juice containing digestive enzymes such as *erepsin, enterokinase, peptidases, maltase, sucrase,* and *lactase.* These enzymes promote the digestion of proteins and carbohydrates. Hormones secreted by the intestinal mucosa are *enterocrinin, cholecystokinin,* and *secretin.* Enterocrinin stimulates the flow of intestinal juice, and cholecystokinin stimulates contraction of the gallbladder and pancreatic enzyme secretion. Secretin stimulates the pancreas to secrete an alkaline liquid that neutralizes the acid chyme facilitating the action of the intestinal enzymes.

6. **Large intestine.** The large intestine, or colon, is the final stretch that undigested and unabsorbed food takes before it is eliminated by the body. The lining of the large intestine does not produce digestive enzymes; instead it produces mucus that allows the developing fecal matter to move down more easily. With the exception of water, vitamins, and minerals, few substances are absorbed by the colon lining.

The large intestine is characterized by two structures: haustrum and taenia coli. Located in the muscularis tunic of the large intestine are thick, longitudinal bands called the **taenia coli,** which resemble a thread gathering fabric. The "gathers" or "tucks" along the length of the colon make a series of pouches, called **haustra.** Once filled, these pouches contract to push this contents to the next haustrum.

The divisions of the large intestine are the cecum, the colon proper, the rectum, the anal canal, and the anus. The colon proper is further divided into the ascending, transverse, descending, and sigmoid colons. Flexures exist where the colon turns in its upside U shape (Fig. 14–5).

The first section of the colon, the **cecum,** is a small saclike structure located in the right lower quadrant of the abdomen. The cecum is attached to the ileocecal sphincter. Suspended from and opening into the inferior portion of the cecum is a lymph gland called the **vermiform appendix.** The wormlike appendix varies from 3 to 6 inches in length.

The next segment of the colon is the ascending colon, continuing from the cecum up the lower right abdomen, turning from the hepatic or the right colic flexure. After the hepatic flexure, the colon moves horizontally from right to left, draping to form the transverse colon. The colon proper takes a downward turn at the splenic or left colic flexure, providing the path for the descending colon. At the level of the iliac crest, the descending colon turns back toward the right at the sigmoid flexure to become the sigmoid colon. Then, with a final S-shaped downward curve, the colon reaches

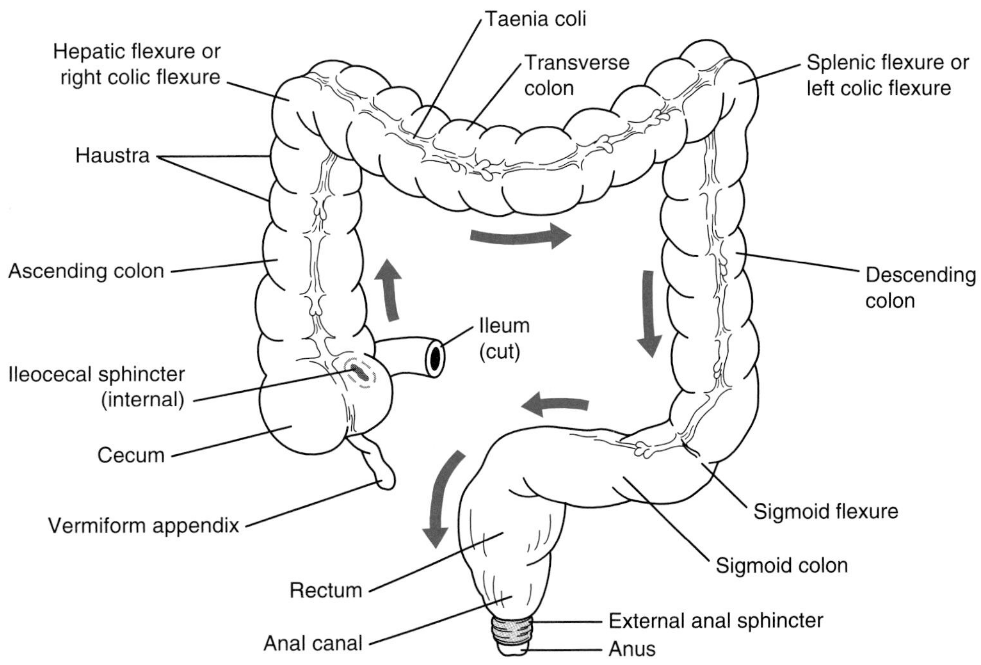

Figure 14•5 The large intestine.

the **rectum** and terminates at the **anal canal,** opening to the outside at the **anus.**

The rectum usually contains three circular folds that overlap when empty and grow in size as the rectum fills with "ready to excrete" wastes. The main function of the rectum and anal canal is storage.

The anal canal possesses two sphincters: an internal sphincter, containing visceral muscle; and an external sphincter, containing skeletal muscle. As the rectal contents move into the anal canal, the internal anal sphincter muscle distends, stimulating pressure-sensitive receptors and initiating the defecation reflex. If this urge is suppressed, it may dissipate, and it may be hours before the desire to defecate returns. If the urge to defecate is chronically suppressed, copious amounts of water are absorbed from the colon and constipation may result.

During defecation, the levator ani muscle raises the anus to eliminate fecal matter. Feces, or stool, is excrement from the GI tract formed in the intestine and released through the anus. Feces consists of indigestible foodstuffs, water, bacteria, and cells sloughed off the walls of the rectum and the anal canal.

ACCESSORY DIGESTIVE ORGANS

The accessory digestive organs produce substances such as enzymes that assist digestion and enter the small intestines. They are the liver, gallbladder, and pancreas (Fig. 14–6). The digestive enzymes produced and secreted by these organs continue the chemical digestion of food.

1. **Liver.** The largest organ of the body, the liver, weighs about 3 pounds. It is located in the upper right quadrant of the abdominal cavity. This reddish brown organ consists of *hepatocytes* (liver cells) that are arranged around thousands of specialized venous channels called **sinusoids,** which are larger than ordinary capillaries. Lining the sinusoids of the liver are phagocytic cells called **Kupffer's cells,** which filter bacteria and other foreign material out of the blood before sending it through the hepatic vein. Blood flowing through the sinusoids originates from the stomach and the intestines via the hepatic portal system (the hepatic portal system is discussed in the circulatory chapter). Due to the vascularity of this organ, the liver holds approximately 1 pint of blood at any given moment.

   One of the most complex organs of the body, the liver has more than 500 functions! One of its digestive functions is the production of bile—approximately 1 quart of bile per day. **Bile,** produced by the hepatocytes of the liver, enters the left and right hepatic ducts, which join to form the common bile duct that leads to the duodenum of the small intestine. Produced from the hemoglobin in worn-out red blood cells, bile is not an enzyme but an *emulsifier.* It physically breaks apart large fat globules in the GI tract into smaller ones and provides a larger surface area for the fat-digesting enzymes to work. Bile gives urine and the stool their characteristic color, as well as offering deodorizing properties to the intestines.

   Some other liver functions are the production, storage, and breakdown of glucose and hemoglobin. The liver produces amino acids, blood plasma proteins, fibrinogens (blood-clotting substances), and antibodies. It also stores vitamins A, D, E, K, minerals, iron, and copper and other compounds used by the body.

   The liver detoxifies numerous toxic substances, such as alcohol, nicotine, and other poisons, into nontoxic materials. Toxic substances that cannot be broken down and excreted are stored. One such substance is DDT (dichlorodiphenyltrichlorethane), which was banned in the United States in 1971.
2. **Gallbladder.** The gallbladder, which stores bile manufactured by the liver, is a pear-shaped sac located in a depression on the inferior surface of the liver. The sphincter of Oddi controls the release of bile into the duodenum. When the sphincter is closed, bile backs up into the gallbladder, where it is stored until needed. During digestion, the intestinal mucosa secretes a hormone, cholecystokinin, which stimulates the release of bile from the gallbladder.
3. **Pancreas.** Both an endocrine and an exocrine gland, the pancreas is a carrot-shaped organ located inferior and posterior to the greater curvature of the stomach. The pancreas is the most important digestive gland because it secretes enzymes that break down all categories of digestible foods: pro-

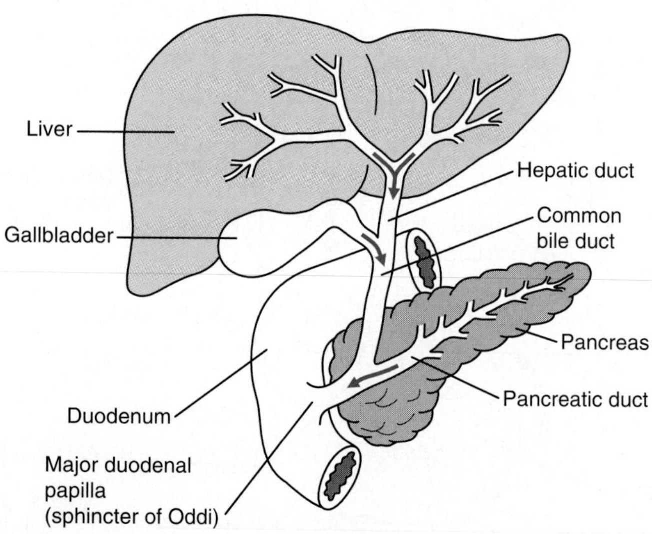

Figure 14•6 Liver, pancreas, and gallbladder in relationship to the duodenum.

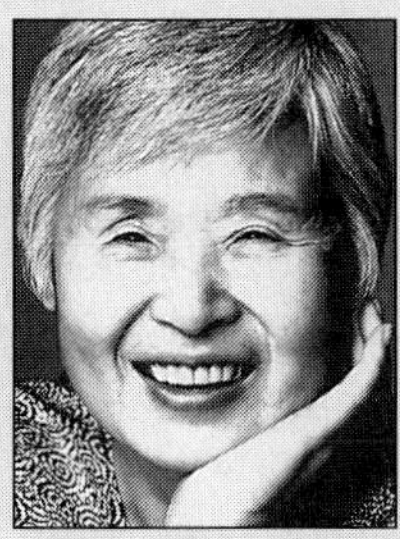

Shizuko Yamamoto

Born: June 1, 1924

"Carefully observe your activities of thinking, breathing, movement, diet, sex, and sleep, for these are the six fundamentals of health. Within this realm lies success or failure in your physical health and emotional happiness."

Shizuko Yamamoto is a bodyworker, author, and founder of the International Macrobiotic Shiatsu Society. What she believes, teaches, and practices is at once simple and sublime. In a nutshell, she advises us to return to nature as a means to promote health and well-being. Of course this isn't a new idea. Around 400 b.c. Hippocrates taught that violating nature's laws brought disharmony in the form of physical or emotional sickness. The cure was to re-create balance, so that the patient could cure herself.

Centuries after Hippocrates, Chinese medicine made its way to Japan and with it came the art of massage. But unlike the full spectrum of treatment practiced in Chinese medicine, massage soon became viewed as a pleasurable indulgence for the wealthy—much like the way we have viewed massage for generations. But there were those practitioners who stuck to the old, more holistic ways of healing. A segment of this group branched out and named their form of massage shiatsu.

Shiatsu is finger, forearm, elbow, or foot pressure and stimulation to certain points on the body, and includes rotation and stretching of joints. This pressure frees any blockage in what is the normal route of energy as it moves from organ to organ throughout the body and balances the *ki*, which means life force in Japanese.

Macrobiotic is an ancient term that describes healthy people who live a long life. Macrobiotic shiatsu is a blend of hand and barefoot shiatsu, diet, exercise, breathing, stretching, postural rebalancing, and use of medicinal plant foods to create balance, thus health, in individuals. Basic macrobiotic principles are as follows:

1. Health is the natural condition of human beings. It is our birthright.
2. Illness and unhappiness are unnatural conditions.
3. Health or sickness is not an accident or something inexplicable.
4. Sickness arises from how we live as a result of our own actions and thoughts.
5. Food is one of the very important factors in determining sickness.
6. We should eat seasonal foods that grow in our own environment.

One of the most enlightening gems you can receive from learning more about macrobiotic shiatsu makes you feel like the scene in the *Wizard of Oz* when Toto revealed that the great wizard was nothing but a mere man. Illness is not so much shrouded in mystery as it is a function of how you think, breath, move and sleep, your diet, and your relationship with others. To a certain degree you can influence your own health, even though it may not be as easy as clicking your heels together three times.

Shizuko Yamamoto was born in Tokyo, the youngest of three brothers and one sister. Her father had his own company; her mother was a homemaker. After WW II a generous cousin made it possible for her to be trained in yoga, shiatsu, aikido, and Chinese acupuncture. But it was a bout with ill health that changed her life. She had leukemia, lost her eyesight, and had absolutely no energy. She was counseled to eat only fresh, organic foods and whole grains. No animal foods. No sugar. She began walking for exercise and doing corrective breathing exercises. One month later she felt much better, something that 12 operations hadn't done. Now she shares her experience and expertise with others the world over.

"We are nature's creation. Our bodies should be organic. We need clean water and a good environment. We are not just existing as ourselves; we are part of the planet, otherwise we cannot survive."

Survive she has. With gusto. She travels all over the world, teaches and counsels at a pace that might be grueling for someone half her age. She's

continued on page 326

Continued

Shizuko Yamamoto

sturdy and exudes energy and warmth. But at a mere 5 feet 3 inches, she worked on many people who were much larger than she when she started her practice in the states. Her clients weren't just bigger, they were also less flexible, which she attributes to a higher consumption of animal fats and protein. She worked on so many people for so many years, her hands would get to the point that they couldn't move. To compensate for her size difference and to continue a strong practice for years to come, she developed barefoot shiatsu, a simple yet effective routine wherein the client lies on the floor and the practitioner stands and uses primarily her feet to deliver the treatment.

Yamamoto outlines her advice to beginning massage therapists: "I don't think about money. I concentrate on how I can help." She also recommends being sensitive to clients' needs, maintaining good health, and using good judgment. Increase your knowledge of your craft, then practice, practice, practice. And naturally her last bit of advice is, "Maintain a healthy balance in your life."

teins, carbohydrates, and fats. The main duct of the pancreas runs the length of the organ, draining the smaller ducts and emptying the pancreatic enzymes into the duodenum. Pancreatic enzymes are secreted in an alkaline fluid to neutralize the acid chyme from the stomach. The hormone produced by the intestinal mucosa, secretin, stimulates the production and secretion of pancreatic enzymes.

The pancreas produces about 1 to 1½ quarts of digestive enzymes per day; *trypsinogen, chymotrypsin, carboxypeptidase, pancreatic amylase,* and *pancreatic lipase.* Trypsinogen, a protein-splitting enzyme, is converted to trypsin when it enters the duodenum. Trypsin, activated by the intestinal enzyme enterokinase, breaks protein into smaller chains of amino acids called peptides. Chymotrypsin and carboxypeptidase also assist in the breakdown of proteins. Pancreatic lipase converts triglycerides into monoglycerides and fatty acids. Pancreatic amylase converts polysaccharides into disaccharides (maltose, sucrose, and lactose).

DISASSEMBLY OF FOODS

The major purpose of eating is to feed our body. This sounds simple enough, but the process is not quite so simple. Ultimately, feeding needs to take place at the cellular level. We have just examined the how-to part of getting food broken down. Next we will explore what food becomes and how these products are used by our cells.

To be beneficial on the cellular level, food must be disassembled into its component parts—proteins, carbohydrates, fats, vitamins, minerals, and water. Two functions of the digestive system are to disassemble these nutrients and to eliminate the unused matter. Nutrients such as vitamins, minerals, and water do not have to be digested before they are used in the body, but proteins, carbohydrates, and fats need to be mechanically and chemically broken down.

Proteins. Proteins are naturally occurring organic compounds that contain large combinations of amino acids. There are 20 identified amino acids vital for proper growth, development, and health maintenance. Ten of the 20 amino acids are classified as nonessential, meaning that they can be synthesized by the body. The remaining ten amino acids are essential amino acids, and these must be obtained from dietary sources. Sources rich in protein are meat, poultry, seafood, eggs, soy products, and milk products (including yogurt and cheese).

Amino acids are the building blocks of protein. Amino acids are the major components for building muscles, blood, skin and its appendages (hair and nails), and visceral organs. Protein is also essential for the formation of hormones, enzymes, and antibodies and is used by the body to repair and rebuild tissues because the body is in a constant state of tearing down and rebuilding.

Carbohydrates. Also known as starches and sugars, **carbohydrates** are classified according to molecular structure as mono-, di-, tri-, and polysaccharides. Monosaccharides, or simple sugars, are glucose (blood sugar), fructose (fruit sugar), and galactose (a milk sugar). Disaccharides, which are the union of two monosaccharides, are sucrose (table sugar), lactose (milk sugar), and maltose (malt sugar). Polysaccharides, carbohydrates containing three or more simple sugar molecules, are dextrins, glycogen, cellulose, and gums.

Carbohydrates are the body's preferred source of energy, particularly used for brain functions, and are required for the metabolism of other nutrients, such as proteins and fats. Ingested carbohydrates, mediated by the hormone insulin, are absorbed immediately by the cells of the body or stored as glycogen (stored glucose). Some dietary sources of carbohydrates are grains, cereals, vegetables, fruits, potatoes, and legumes.

Fats. Fats are composed of lipids or fatty acids and can range in consistency from a solid to a liquid. Stored fat (adipose tissue) helps to cushion and insulate visceral organs. Fats are classified as saturated or unsaturated, depending on whether they are solid (saturated) or liquid (unsaturated) at room temperature. Our body requires fats; they are needed for cell membranes, and steroid hormones, just to name a few examples.

Of all the nutrients, fats are probably the least understood of all. There are good fats and bad fats, and everyone talks about fat as if there were only one. The "bad" fats are in the categories of saturated fats and the "good" fats are unsaturated fats.

The following are good fats (oils): olive oil, peanut oil, flax seed oil, hemp oil, evening primrose oil, borage oil, sesame oil, and canola oil, to name a few. Bad fats include lard (animal fats), processed oils (hydrogenated or partially hydrogenated oils), and oils that have been used numerous times (many restaurant oils).

Vitamins. Vitamins are organic compounds that are essential for normal physiologic and metabolic functioning of the body. Many vitamins act as coenzymes. Most vitamins cannot be synthesized by the body and must be obtained from a healthy diet or vitamin supplements. Vitamins are either fat soluble or water soluble. Fat-soluble vitamins can be stored by the body, whereas water-soluble vitamins must be ingested regularly. Fat-soluble vitamins are A, D, E, and K; water-soluble vitamins are the B vitamins and C.

Vitamins have various functions: Vitamin E is an antioxidant (a substance that inhibits or retards oxidation), as is C and beta carotene; vitamin D functions as a hormone; and vitamin A enhances the immune system. Vitamins are necessary micronutrients for the body, and the U.S. government has recognized the importance of vitamins by establishing minimum daily requirements.

Minerals. Minerals are essential nonorganic compounds found in nature that are used by the body. Minerals are needed in trace amounts and are used to build bone (calcium, magnesium, boron, etc.), to work muscles (calcium and magnesium), to support various organs such as the pancreas (manganese, chromium, and vanadium), and to transport oxygen and carbon dioxide (iron). Minerals also play a vital role in regulating many body functions; many also function as coenzymes.

A mineral is usually referred to by the name of a metal, nonmetal, radical, or phosphate rather than by the name of the compound (i.e., sodium chloride or table salt).

Water. Although we do not usually think of water as food, water is an essential nutrient needed by every part of the body. Water-based fluids surround every cell in the body (except the outer layer in the skin) and all nutrients and wastes travel through fluids (blood and lymph). These fluids require a continuous supply of fresh water for proper body pH, for nutrient transport, for lymphatic transport, and for elimination. A key point to remember is that the nutrient is *water*—not coffee, cola beverages, tea, alcohol, or sports drinks! WATER.

DIGESTIVE CONDITIONS AND CLINICAL TERMS

1. **Nausea.** Nausea is a sensation that often leads to vomiting. Some common causes of nausea are motion sickness, severe pain, food poisoning, infection, first-trimester pregnancy (due to hormonal changes), and irritants such as spicy foods, toxins, bacteria, and certain medications.
2. **Vomiting.** Vomiting is "reverse peristalsis" of the upper gastrointestinal tract and is accomplished by contraction of the abdominal muscles squeezing the stomach against the diaphragm. As contraction of these muscles occurs, the stomach is forcibly emptied of its contents through the mouth.
3. **Heartburn.** If the lower esophageal sphincter fails to close normally after food has entered the stomach, hydrochloric acid from the stomach can enter the inferior portion of the esophagus. The hydrochloric acid irritates the esophageal wall and causes a burning sensation. It is called heartburn because the sensation is near the heart, not because of cardiac problems. Antacids neutralize the hydrochloric acid and decrease the burning sensation. If food is eaten in smaller amounts and the person does not lie down right after a meal, symptoms are less likely to occur.

   If a client is prone to heartburn, urge him to not eat a large meal right before the massage treatment.
4. **Achalasia.** This occurs when the lower esophageal sphincter does not relax normally to allow food to enter the stomach. A whole meal may stack up in the esophagus and enter the stomach slowly.

There may be chest pain that feels like pain from heartburn.

5. **Diarrhea.** The frequent passing of unformed, loose, watery stools is called diarrhea. Factors that cause diarrhea are stress, diet, infection, medication side effects, or inflammation. The stool may also contain blood, pus, or mucus. Other symptoms are abdominal pain, cramping, and intestinal crepitus. Diarrhea may also lead to dehydration.

   Clients who have an acute onset of diarrhea should not be massaged until all symptoms are gone because this is often due to infection. If a client has chronic diarrhea (lasting more than 3 weeks), it is usually due to conditions such as inflammatory bowel disease. In these cases, abdominal massage is contraindicated, but general massage would be all right.

6. **Constipation.** Constipation is infrequent or difficult passing of stools. Common causes of constipation are insufficient intake of fluid or dietary fiber, lack of physical activity, emotional disturbance, diverticulitis, pregnancy, enema abuse, and painful defecation.

   Abdominal massage can help relieve constipation by stimulating the forward movement of intestinal contents.

7. **Hemorrhoids or piles.** Hemorrhoids are varicosities of the rectal veins. The veins in the rectal area do not have valves, which makes them particularly susceptible to vascular congestion. Prolonged sitting, pregnancy, obesity, constipation, and straining to defecate can contribute to hemorrhoid development.
8. **Anorexia nervosa.** Classified as an eating disorder and emotional disorder, anorexia nervosa is the prolonged avoidance of eating. Lack of nutrients results in emaciation, amenorrhea (cessation of menstruation), decreased sleep, and psychological disturbance. When people with anorexia nervosa do eat, they often prefer foods low in calories. Although cases among young males are on the rise, most anorexia nervosa cases are young Caucasian females. Treatment consists of increasing dietary intake and psychological counseling.

   Massage therapy can be a very helpful adjunct to psychological counseling. Massage may help improve the client's self-image and may decrease anxiety.

9. **Bulimia.** Bulimia is characterized by overeating (bingeing) and self-induced vomiting (purging). Like anorexia nervosa, bulimia is classified as an eating and an emotional disorder, treated by psychological counseling.

   Massage considerations for a client with bulimia are the same as for a client with anorexia nervosa.

10. **Obesity.** Obesity is characterized by an abnormal increase in subcutaneous fat tissue, primarily in visceral regions of the body. Generally, an individual is regarded as obese if his body weight is 30 percent above desired body weight for his age, height, frame size, and sex. Normal (nonathlete) body fat is 18 percent in men and 25 percent in women.

    See Chapter 21 for considerations of clients who are obese.

11. **Mumps.** Mumps is an acute viral disease caused by a *paramyxovirus* (an airborne member of the herpes family). Symptoms are enlargement of the parotid salivary glands, fever, and extreme pain during swallowing. Transmitted by contact with infectious droplets, mumps is most likely to be contracted by children between 5 to 15 years old, but the disease may occur in adults.

    Massage is contraindicated because this is an infectious disease.

12. **Ulcer.** An ulcer is a lesion in a membrane. A peptic ulcer can develop in parts of the digestive tract exposed to acidic gastric juice. Those that occur in the first part of the duodenum are called duodenal ulcers. Some occur in the body of the stomach and are called gastric ulcers. Symptoms of ulcers are a nonradiating pain in the upper abdominal region, dark fecal stools, and bleeding that could lead to anemia.

    There are three main causes of ulcers. (1) Use of nonsteroidal anti-inflammatory drugs (NSAIDs), like aspirin; (2) hypersecretion of hydrochloric acid caused by a tumor of the pancreas; and (3) the bacterium *Heliobacter pylori*. Cigarette smoking, alcohol, caffeine, aspirin, and stress can exacerbate ulcers.

    Massage is beneficial for clients with peptic ulcers because massage is an effective stress management tool. Abdominal massage is contraindicated.

Author's Note

It is generally accepted that ulcers are attributed to stress. But the cause of ulcers is an overproduction of gastric enzymes, which is actually a parasympathetic response. And stress does the opposite; it stimulates a sympathetic nervous system response and reduces gastric secretions. So it's as if the condition of ulcers is an oxymoron.

Using monkeys as subjects, several experiments were conducted to study ulcers in 1971 and again in 1979. Situations were set up in which shocks were administered to monkeys at a predictive rate. One monkey, called the executive monkey, could, by using a lever, control whether or not the shock was administered. Another monkey, called the passive monkey, did not have the same control over the shock. If the executive monkey received a shock, both monkeys were shocked. Likewise, both were spared the shock if the executive monkey pressed the lever at the appropriate time.

So which monkey do you think got the ulcers? The executive monkey was full of ulcers, but the passive monkey had none. Although this was not a perfect experiment, it appears that ulcers may develop after periods of emotional strain, excessive responsibility, and worrying. But since gastric enzymes do not freely flow during periods of stress, ulcers seem to form during periods of rest or parasympathetic activity. It's as if the body is trying to play 'catch-up' after frequent and prolonged stress.

13. **Hepatitis.** Hepatitis is an inflammation of the liver that can be caused by alcohol, drugs, toxins and, infection by the hepatitis virus, of which there are several types. Symptoms include muscle and joint pain, fatigue, loss of appetite, nausea, vomiting, diarrhea or constipation, abdominal discomfort, tea-colored urine, white stools, and jaundice. Severity ranges from mild and brief to chronic and life threatening.

    Massage is contraindicated during the acute phases because it is infectious. If a client has chronic hepatitis (lasting more than 6 months) massage should be performed only after receiving a physician's clearance to make sure the client is not infectious and that the debilitated liver will not be stressed by massage. If clearance is given, abdominal massage is contraindicated.

14. **Cirrhosis of the liver.** Cirrhosis of the liver is a chronic degenerative disease in which the hepatic cells are destroyed and replaced with fibrous connective tissue, giving the liver a yellow-orange color. Liver functions deteriorate as hepatic cells are destroyed. As the disease progresses, gastrointestinal hemorrhage and kidney failure may also occur. Cirrhosis is usually the result of chronic alcohol abuse or severe hepatitis. The symptoms of cirrhosis are nausea, fatigue, and loss of appetite.

    If the cirrhosis is caused by viral hepatitis, massage is contraindicated because of the risk of infection. Otherwise, a gentle full body massage is indicated. Reducing the edema in the legs is not recommended because the return of the lymph to the blood may stress the liver and its filtering capacity.

15. **Korsakoff's syndrome.** Korsakoff's syndrome, also known as Korsakoff's psychosis, is caused by thiamine and other B vitamin deficiencies. Characterized by anterograde and retrograde amnesia, apathy, confusion, and the inability to learn new skills, Korsakoff's syndrome is commonly found in "career" alcoholics who neglect solid food for liquor over extended periods. If treated early, the syndrome can be arrested. Severe cases result in complete debilitation and confinement.

16. **Gallstones.** Gallstones result from the fusion of cholesterol crystals in bile. They gradually grow in size and number and may cause minimal to total obstruction of bile flow into the duodenum.

    Massage is contraindicated during a gallbladder attack. Otherwise, general massage is all right, with abdominal massage contraindicated.

Author's Note

A colostomy is an incision in the colon for the purpose of making an opening between the bowel and the abdominal wall. A bag is attached outside the body to gather fecal material that passes through the opening. Colostomies are sometimes temporary bypass methods, which are used in conjunction with surgeries.

An ileostomy is similar to a colostomy except the ileostomy connects the small intestine to the external abdominal wall. Clients who have lower colostomies can regulate their bowels. The bowel material of upper colostomies and ileostomies will be too loose to afford the client the ability to control bowel movements.

When clients who have a colostomy or ileostomy make an appointment for a massage, recommend that they not eat 2 hours before they arrive. This 2-hour delay will decrease the motility in the bowels. Because of the anterior abdominal opening, these clients may not be able to receive massage in the prone position. Accommodate these special individuals by using a side-lying position.

Suggest to a client that he empty his bag before the massage begins. A bag can burst or become unclipped during the session, spilling it's contents. Should this occur, do your best to calm the client and reassure him that accidents like this do happen. Ask him if he would prefer to clean himself up or if he would like your assistance. If he has a spinal injury, he may *require* your assistance. Treat the contents of the bag as a biohazard if tainted with blood.

Do not apply lubricant on or near the bag opening. Oily substances interfere with the ability of the adhesive or cement to anchor the bag to the skin.

17. **Pancreatitis.** An inflammation of the pancreas, pancreatitis is usually the result of trauma, alcohol

abuse, infection, or certain medications that damage the pancreas. In many cases, instead of inactive trypsinogen, the pancreas secretes active trypsin that digests the pancreatic cells and blood vessels. Early symptoms may be severe abdominal pain that refers to the back, fever, lack of appetite, nausea, and vomiting. Most of these symptoms are caused by a decrease in the production and secretion of pancreatic enzymes.

Acute pancreatitis needs medical attention. Abdominal massage is contraindicated in clients with chronic pancreatitis, but general massage would be okay.

18. **Appendicitis.** An inflammation of the vermiform appendix, appendicitis is often detected by acute pain in the lower right quadrant of the abdomen, vomiting, fever, and elevated white blood cell count. Appendicitis is typically caused by intestinal disease, intestinal obstruction or adhesions, or parasites. The most common treatment is an appendectomy.

    Massage is contraindicated for appendicitis. Immediate medical attention is needed.

19. **Colitis.** Colitis is an inflammation of the mucosa of the large intestine and rectum and is characterized by weight loss, intestinal ulcerations, diarrhea, and bleeding of the colon wall. The origins of colitis are not known, although it is thought to be an autoimmune disease. Some treatment recommendations are increased fluid intake, dietary alterations, and antibiotics.

    General massage is beneficial to the client, although the abdomen should be avoided.

20. **Crohn's disease.** A disease of unknown origin, Crohn's is a progressive inflammatory disease of the colon and/or ileum. Early symptoms are severe abdominal pain, diarrhea, fever, nausea, and loss of appetite. Typically, diseased colon segments are separated by normal colon segments. Crohn's disease is often confused with colitis.

    General massage is beneficial to the client, although the abdomen should be avoided.

21. **Irritable bowel syndrome.** Also known as spastic colon, irritable bowel syndrome is a condition of the large intestine characterized by abnormal muscular contraction and excessive mucus in stools. It is generally associated with young adults under extreme emotional stress. Early symptoms are diarrhea and pain in the lower abdomen. Because there is no disease present, there is no cure, but many individuals benefit from adding roughage to their diets. Other positive steps to take in reducing irritable bowel syndrome are counseling, stress reduction, change in dietary habits, and antispasmodic medications.

    General massage is beneficial to the client, although the abdomen should be avoided.

22. **Diverticulosis.** Diverticula are pouchlike herniations of the colon wall where the muscle has become weak. This condition is most likely to be found in individuals over 50 years old who have a low-fiber diet. Even though people who have diverticulosis have no symptoms, 15 percent will develop diverticulitis (inflammation of the diverticula).

    General massage is beneficial to the client, although the abdomen should be avoided.

23. **Peritonitis.** An acute inflammation of the peritoneum, peritonitis is produced by bacteria or irritating substances that gain access into the abdominal cavity. These substances are introduced into the cavity by a ruptured organ, a penetrating wound, perforation of the gastrointestinal or urogenital tract (e.g., ectopic pregnancy), or a ruptured appendix.

    Usually the client is too sick to be massaged. However, massage may be administered in the hospital to reduce stress and pain, but only after obtaining the physician's clearance. The massage should be gentle and soothing, avoiding the abdomen.

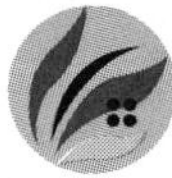

EFFECTS OF MASSAGE FOR THE DIGESTIVE SYSTEM

1. Massage promotes excitation of peristaltic activity in the large intestine, helping to relieve colic and intestinal gas.
2. Massage can promote evacuation of the colon, thus relieving constipation, provided that the direction of massage follows the normal intestinal flow (clockwise).
3. Massage also promotes stimulation of the parasympathetic nervous system, which stimulates digestion.

SUMMARY

The digestive system consists of a series of structures that are designed to break down complex food and liquids into usable body fuel by the processes of ingestion, digestion, absorption and defecation. In order to carry out these processes, the digestive system makes use of a series of specialized, interrelated organs known collectively as the alimentary canal. These organs include the oral cavity, pharynx, esophagus, stomach, small intestines, and large intestines. The alimentary canal makes use of a set of accessory organs that aid in the digestive processes. These accessory organs include the liver, gallbladder, and pancreas. There are six types of nutrients: proteins, carbohydrates, fats, vitamins, minerals, and water.

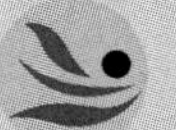

MINI•LAB

Calculate your total caloric intake over a 24-hour period by using a simple caloric guide obtainable in any drugstore. Look at the distribution of the basic food groups, and write a list of what improvements could be (and should be) made in your eating habits.

SELF-TEST

Multiple Choice • Write the letter of the best answer in the space provided.

_______ 1. The functions of the digestive system are
A. inhalation, digestion, absorption, and homeostasis
B. speech production, taste, digestion, and absorption
C. ingestion, digestion, absorption, and defecation
D. ingestion, digestion, movement, and storage

_______ 2. The process of orally taking materials into the body is called
A. ingestion C. homeostasis
B. digestion D. absorption

_______ 3. What is the mechanical and chemical process that occurs as food is converted into an absorbable state?
A. ingestion C. homeostasis
B. digestion D. absorption

_______ 4. The term used to denote the hollow muscular tube from the oral cavity to the anus includes all of the following *except*
A. alimentary canal C. absorption lumen
B. intestinal tube D. gastrointestinal tract

_______ 5. The major type of muscle of the GI tract is the
A. cardiac C. skeletal
B. voluntary D. smooth

_______ 6. The type of muscular contractions that occur in most sphincters are
A. rhythmic C. tonic
B. peristaltic D. voluntary

_______ 7. A ring of muscle fibers that regulates movement of materials from one compartment of the gastrointestinal tract to another is called
A. bolus C. mastication
B. sphincter D. enzyme

_______ 8. Which of the following is responsible for the chemical reactions of digestion?
A. bolus C. mastication
B. sphincters D. enzymes

_______ 9. A ball-like, masticated lump of food is a
A. bolus C. mastication
B. sphincter D. enzyme

_______ 10. The largest serous membrane of the body is the
A. perineum C. abdominal membrane
B. peritoneum D. lesser omentum

_______ 11. Contents of the oral cavity include the
A. tongue, pharynx, and esophagus
B. tongue, teeth, gums, and salivary ducts
C. duodenum, jejunum, and ileum
D. tongue, teeth, and nose

_______ 12. A clear, nondigestible, viscous fluid secreted by the salivary and mucous glands in the oral cavity is called
A. salivary juice C. serous fluid
B. saliva D. chyme

_______ 13. Nestled in spheric pockets on the superior and lateral surfaces of the tongue are
A. salivary glands C. sphincter of Oddi
B. deciduous teeth D. gustatory organs

_______ 14. Which of the following is *not* one of the three salivary glands?
A. submandibular glands
B. submaxillary glands
C. sublingual glands
D. parotid glands

_______ 15. Which division(s) of the alimentary canal transport food to the stomach?
A. duodenum C. esophagus
B. rectum D. A and B

_______ 16. Which of the following is first initiated in the stomach?

A. carbohydrate digestion
B. fat digestion
C. vitamin and mineral digestion
D. protein digestion

_______ 17. A viscous semifluid blended in the stomach is called

A. chyme
B. gastrin
C. enzymes
D. mucus

_______ 18. The parietal cells in the stomach produce

A. intrinsic factor and hydrochloric acid
B. gastrin
C. pepsinogen
D. gastric amylase

_______ 19. Chief cells produce

A. intrinsic factor and hydrochloric acid
B. gastrin
C. pepsinogen
D. gastric amylase

_______ 20. The three divisions of the small intestines, from beginning to end, are the

A. duodenum, ileum, and jejunum
B. ascending, transverse, and descending
C. jejunum, ileum, and duodenum
D. duodenum, jejunum, and ileum

_______ 21. Which structure contains the sphincter of Oddi and the major duodenal papilla?

A. oral cavity
B. stomach
C. sigmoid colon
D. duodenum

_______ 22. Most of digestion and absorption takes place in the

A. small intestine
B. oral cavity
C. cecum
D. esophagus

_______ 23. Which of the following is *NOT* a hormone secreted by the intestinal lining?

A. enterocrinin
B. intestin
C. cholecystokinin
D. secretin

_______ 24. Which of the following hormone stimulates the contraction of the gallbladder and pancreatic enzyme secretion?

A. enterocrinin
B. histamine
C. cholecystokinin
D. secretin

_______ 25. The colon lining primarily absorbs which substance?

A. proteins/peptides
B. carbohydrates/starches
C. water, vitamins, and minerals
D. fats and lipids

_______ 26. Along the length of the large intestine there are a series of pouches called

A. taenia coli
B. villi
C. haustra
D. ceca

_______ 27. Suspended from the inferior portion of the cecum is/are

A. taenia coli
B. vermiform appendix
C. sinusoids
D. Kupffer's cells

_______ 28. The phagocytic cells in the liver that eat bacteria and other foreign material out of the blood before sending it through the hepatic vein is called

A. taenia coli
B. vermiform appendix
C. sinusoids
D. Kupffer's cells

_______ 29. Which of the following describe(s) bile?

A. processed by using worn-out red blood cells
B. an emulsifier that also offers deodorizing properties
C. gives urine and the stool their characteristic color
D. all of the above

_______ 30. Functions of the liver include

A. production, storage, and breakdown of glucose and hemoglobin and production of bile
B. production of amino acids, blood plasma proteins, fibrinogens (blood-clotting substance), and antibodies, storage of vitamins A, D, E, K, iron and copper, and other compounds used by the body
C. produces gastrin, salivary amylase, pepsin, trypsin, and glucose
D. A and B

_______ 31. The pear-shaped sac located on the inferior surface of the liver that stores bile is called the

A. salivary gland
B. bursa
C. gallbladder
D. pancreas

_______ 32. Because it breaks down all categories of digestible foods, the most important digestive gland is the

A. salivary gland
B. liver
C. gallbladder
D. pancreas

_______ 33. Food is disassembled into six components; they are

A. amino acids, triglycerides, water, vitamin C, iron, and calcium
B. amino acids, water, vitamin A, magnesium, calcium, and folic acid
C. protein, carbohydrates, fats, vitamins, minerals, and water
D. protein, carbohydrates, lipids, iron, phosphorus, and zinc

_______ 34. What are the building blocks for protein?

A. cells
B. oxygen
C. lipids
D. amino acids

_______ 35. Of the 20 known amino acids, how many are called essential amino acids?

A. 14
B. 10
C. 12
D. 20

_______ 36. Carbohydrates are classified as

A. solid or liquid
B. mono-, di-, tri-, and polysaccharides
C. water soluble or fat soluble
D. saturated or unsaturated

_______ 37. Fats are classified as

A. solid or liquid
B. saturated or unsaturated
C. water soluble or fat soluble
D. A and B

_______ 38. Fat-soluble vitamins are

A. A, D, E, and K
B. iron and copper
C. B vitamins and C
D. mono- and disaccharides

_______ 39. Water-soluble vitamins are

A. A, D, E, and K
B. iron and copper
C. B vitamins and C
D. mono- and disaccharides

References

Applegate, Edith J., M.S. *The Anatomy and Physiology Learning System: Textbook*. Philadelphia: W. B. Saunders, 1995.

Crooks, Robert and Jean Stein. *Psychology: Science, Behavior, and Life*. New York, NY: Holt, Rinehart, and Winston, Inc., 1988.

Damjanov, Ivan. *Pathophysiology for the Health-Related Professions*. Philadelphia: W. B. Saunders, 1996.

Goldberg, Stephen, M.D. *Clinical Anatomy Made Ridiculously Simple*. Miami: Medmaster, Inc., 1984.

Gould, Barbara E. *Pathophysiology for the Health-Related Professionals*. Philadelphia: W. B. Saunders, 1997.

Haubrich, William S. *Medical Meanings, A Glossary of Word Origins*. New York: Harcourt Brace Jovanovich, 1984.

Kalat, James W. *Biological Psychology*, 2nd ed. Belmont, CA: Wadsworth Publishing Company, 1984.

Kordish, Mary and Sylvia Dickson. *Introduction to Basic Human Anatomy*. Lake Charles, LA: McNeese State University, Self-published manual, 1985.

Marieb, Elaine N. *Essentials of Human Anatomy and Physiology*, 4th ed. New York, NY: Benjamin/Cummings Publishing Company, Inc., 1994.

McAleer, Neil. *The Body Almanac*. Garden City, NY: Doubleday and Company, Inc., 1985.

Mosby's Medical, Nursing, and Allied Health Dictionary, 4th ed. St Louis: Mosby–Year Book, Inc., 1994.

Newton, Don. *Pathology for Massage Therapists*, 2nd ed. Portland: Simran Publications, 1995.

Premkumar, Kalyani. *Pathology A to Z—A Handbook for Massage Therapists*. Calgary, Canada: VanPub Books, 1996.

Tabers Cyclopedic Medical Dictionary, 13th ed. Philadelphia: F. A. Davis Company, 1977.

Tortora, Gerald J. *Introduction to the Human Body: The Essentials of Anatomy and Physiology*, 3rd ed. New York: HarperCollins Publishers, 1994.

One doesn't discover new lands without consenting to lose sight of the shore for a very long time.
—Andre Gide

15 Urinary System

Student Objectives

After completing this chapter, the student should be able to:

- Describe the five functions of the urinary system
- Identify the four basic structures of the urinary system, and explain their function
- Name the parts of the kidney and the nephron
- Trace blood flow through a kidney; include filtration and reabsorption
- Explain urine production
- Discuss how the antidiuretic hormones renin and aldosterone aid in regulating blood pressure, water balance, and blood volume

INTRODUCTION

The human body is a complex machine, and as such it does not perform properly if residues from fuel combustion and other processes are not removed. The cells of the body machine metabolize nutrients and produce wastes such as carbon dioxide, water, and heat. The breakdown of proteins produces the nitrogen wastes such as ammonia and urea, which are toxic to the system. Sodium chloride, sodium sulfate, phosphate, and hydrogen molecules and ions also build up in excess quantities due to metabolic activities. All of these waste materials must be excreted from the body for homeostasis to be maintained and for metabolism to function well.

Excretion of waste products is such a large task that no single body system can handle it alone. Several systems contribute to the job of waste elimination.

1. *The Respiratory System.* Waste elimination includes carbon dioxide, heat, and water through expiration.
2. *The Integumentary System.* Sudoriferous glands excrete sweat, a waste product, which is a solution of 98 percent water and 2 percent solids (salt ions, lactic acid, and other metabolic wastes). By contrast, urine is 96 percent water and 4 percent solids.
3. *The Digestive System.* It eliminates solid wastes and heat through excretion.
4. *The Urinary System.* Wastes, water, and heat are excreted through urination.

Terms and Word Roots Related to the Urinary System

antidiuretic – against or opposed; urine flow
Bowman's capsule – named after an English physician (1816–92)
calyx – cup
diuretic – urine flow
ducts of Bellini – named after an Italian anatomist (1643–1704)
glomerulus – little ball
hilus or hilum – a trifle
juxtapose – close by, adjacent, side by side
loop of Henle – named after a German anatomist (1809–85)
macula densa – spot; thick
nephro or nephra – kidney
peritubular – around, about; like a tube
renal – kidney
renin – kidney
retroperitoneal – retro–backward; the peritoneum
trigone – three-cornered figure

FUNCTIONS

1. **Eliminate Metabolic Waste.** Cellular metabolism produces waste products that are released in the urine. These waste products include excess potassium ions, carbon dioxide, ammonia, heat, and urea.
2. **Regulate Blood pH and Its Chemical Composition.** The kidneys possess specialized cells that monitor the acid–base balance of the blood. Metabolic wastes are laundered from the blood, and substances such as glucose, sodium, vitamins, and minerals are reabsorbed into the blood to adjust its chemical composition. Hydrogen ions are secreted from the blood into the urine as needed to maintain the blood's pH balance.
3. **Regulate Blood Volume and Fluid Balance.** The kidneys control the amount of water reabsorbed into the circulatory system in order to regulate blood volume. In this way, both the blood volume and body's water balance are altered. If fluid levels are not regulated, excess fluids collect in the tissues, producing edema of the hands, feet, face, heart, and other body areas.
4. **Regulate Blood Pressure.** The kidneys continuously monitor blood pressure and help maintain a normal range by secreting enzymes that stimulate vasoconstriction. Blood pressure is also kept in balance by the regulation of blood volume. Blood pressure is maintained by interaction of the circulatory, endocrine, and nervous systems.
5. **Maintain Homeostasis.** With the removal of metabolic wastes, the body maintains homeostasis by regulating the chemical composition of the blood, by regulating blood volume, and by maintaining fluid balance and blood pressure. Because of these many functions, the kidneys are the major homeostatic organs of the body. Malfunction of the kidneys causes dangerous changes in blood composition, which often lead to death.

ANATOMY AND RELATED PHYSIOLOGY

The urinary system contains four basic parts: the kidneys, the ureters, the urinary bladder, and the urethra (Fig. 15–1). The kidneys launder the blood and direct the filtered waste products to the ureters, which transfer the urine to the urinary bladder for storage. The bladder is then emptied through the urethra to the outside of the body. The filtered blood is routed back to general circulation.

Kidneys

The **kidneys** are a pair of organs located bilaterally in the upper lumbar region of the spine. They are bean-

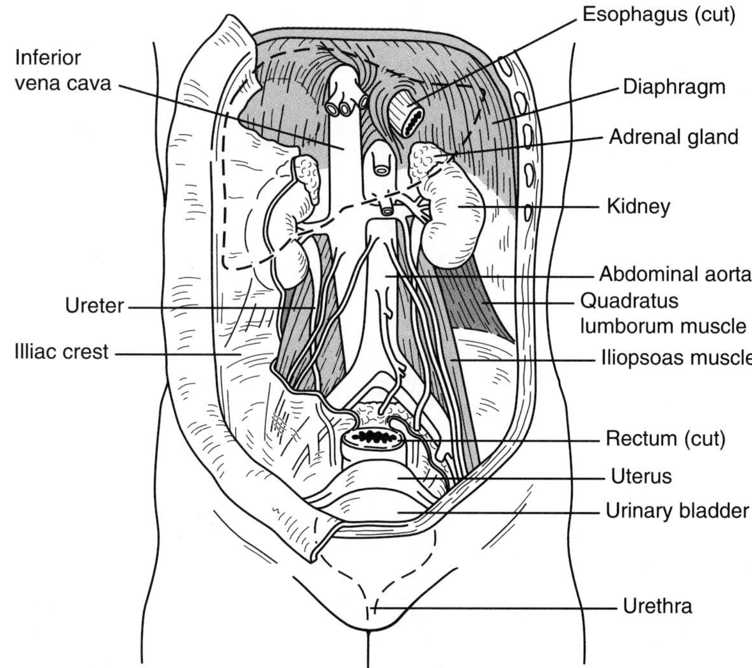

Figure 15•1 General urinary system.

shaped (convex laterally and concave medially, like a kidney bean) and are slightly smaller than a fist. The **retroperitoneal** kidneys (behind the abdominal peritoneum) are surrounded by a fibrous renal capsule and are imbedded in adipose tissue called perirenal fat; this fat serves as a barrier against trauma and the spread of infection. Due to the presence of the liver, the kidney on the right side of the body is slightly lower than the one on the left.

The **renal hilus/hilum,** or **renal sinus,** is the indentation located in the medially concave region of the kidney; here is where the renal arteries, renal veins, and the ureters attach. The interior compartment of the renal hilus houses the **renal pelvis,** which is the funnel-shaped origin of the ureters. Each kidney is divided into two major regions: the cortex and the medulla (Fig. 15–2).

The cortex is the soft, outer region of the kidney and is composed of millions of minute structures known as **nephrons,** the basic filtering units of the kidney that are responsible for filtering waste products from the blood, which are later excreted. It is possible to lose many nephrons, or even an entire kidney, and maintain good health. The filtration process is accomplished in the nephrons by a vast and intricate network made up of two different routing vessels: one channels blood through the nephron and the other collects urine from the nephron and routes it to the renal pelvis. The process begins in the section of the nephron known as the **glomerular capsule** or **Bow-**

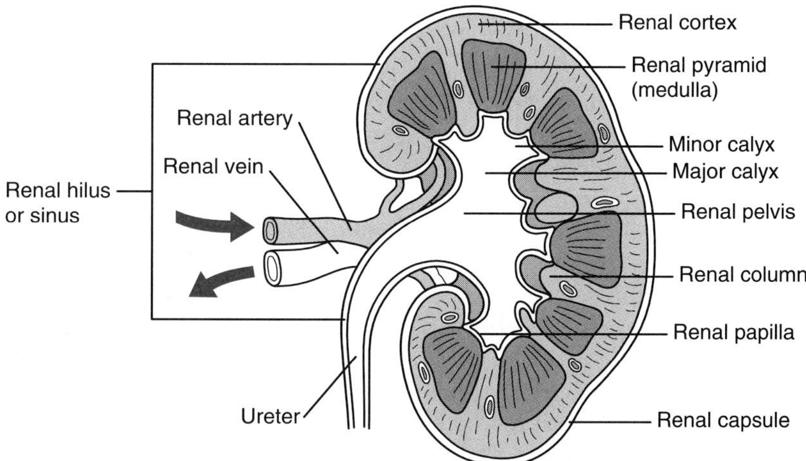

Figure 15•2 The kidney.

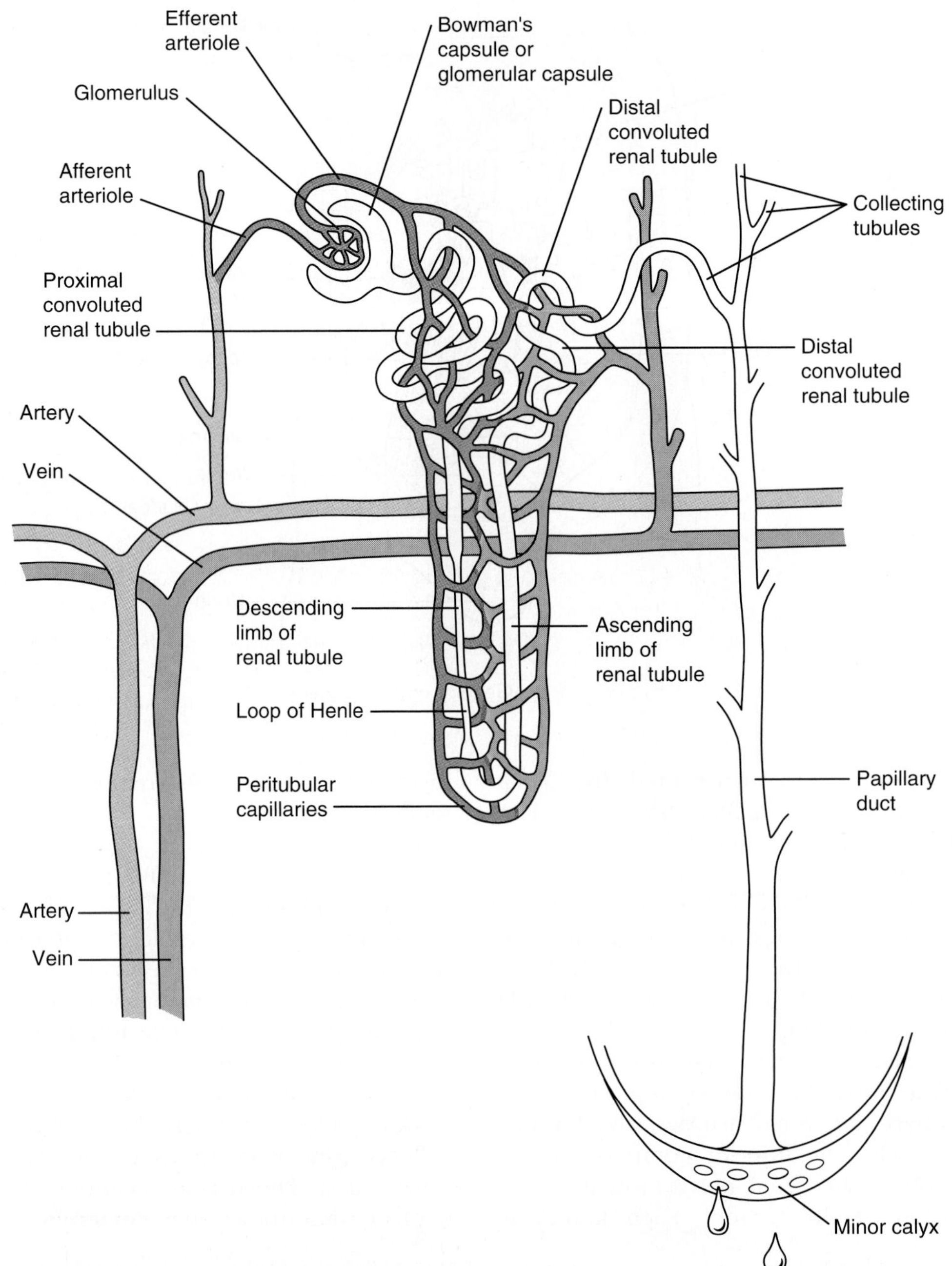

Figure 15•3 Cutaway view of the nephron.

man's capsule (Fig. 15–3). The glomerular capsule is where urine formation originates; the glomerular capsule then becomes the **renal tubule,** which is a urine routing vessel. Contained within the glomerular capsule are loops of minute blood vessels called **glomeruli.** It is here in the glomerulus that fluids from the blood cross the membrane to the glomerular capsule in the first stage of the blood filtration–urine formation process.

A second network of blood vessels branches off before the glomerulus: the **peritubular capillaries,** which are interwoven with corresponding renal tubules. These two structures are interlaced, providing a larger surface area for waste product exchange and water reabsorption. The renal tubules move the urine through the internal portion of the kidney, or the medulla to the ureters. Bundles of renal tubules in the medulla are called **renal** or **medullary pyramids.** Each kidney, composed of 8 to 18 renal pyramids, contains many straight collecting tubules, which gives each pyramid a striated appearance.

The filtration process depends on blood pressure being higher in the glomeruli than in the renal tubules so that fluid can easily move across the cellular membrane. This process is clearly understood if we trace the path of the blood throughout the kidneys.

Blood Vessels and Blood Flow in the Kidneys

Oxygen-rich blood enters the kidneys by the renal artery where it branches off the abdominal aorta (Fig. 15–4). As the renal artery enters the renal hilus, the artery becomes smaller, subdividing and looping through the kidney in two paths; one path consists of the afferent arterioles and the other consists of the peritubular capillaries. The afferent arterioles are high-pressure vessels that feed the glomerular capillaries. It is here in the glomeruli that blood plasma, with its dissolved solids, crosses over into the renal tubules. From the glomerular capillaries, the blood flows into the efferent arterioles. This is one of the few places in the body that arterial flow moves through a capillary network and into another artery instead of into a vein.

The second, smaller vascular path feeds directly into the peritubular capillaries, bypassing the glomeruli. The peritubular capillaries surround the renal tubule, where most reabsorption of water occurs. The blood from the efferent arterioles then joins with the flow from the peritubular capillaries, and together they stream into the venous system. The venous structures grow larger and larger and return the blood directly to the inferior vena cava.

Urine Production

Urine production begins in the renal cortex as the watery portion of the blood plasma exits the glomerulus, then enters the first section of the renal tubule, the glomerular capsule (Fig. 15–5). The glomerular capsule is a funnel-shaped pouch that surrounds the glomerulus. Once it crosses from the glomerulus into the glomerular capsule, the filtered fluids are referred to as **filtrate.** This filtrate first flows into the proximal convoluted tubule, the walls of which are lined with microvilli; they create a larger surface area for more efficient fluid exchange. The convoluted tubule feeds into the loop of Henle, which is a hairpin-shaped structure divided into a descending loop and an ascending loop. From here, the filtrate flows into the distal convoluted tubule and then into collecting tubules located in the medulla of the kidney.

The medulla is basically the urine-collecting facility. These straight collecting tubules route the urine produced in the cortex into larger papillary ducts, the

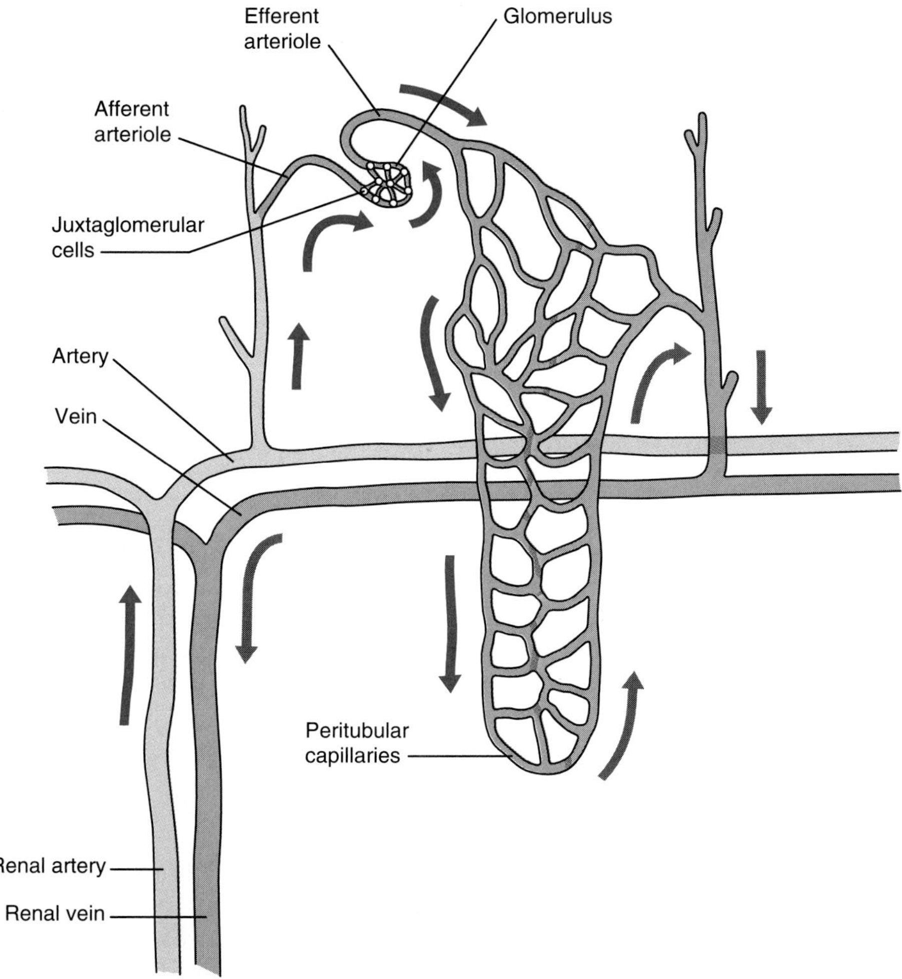

Figure 15•4 Close-up of the renal tubule focusing on the urine pathway.

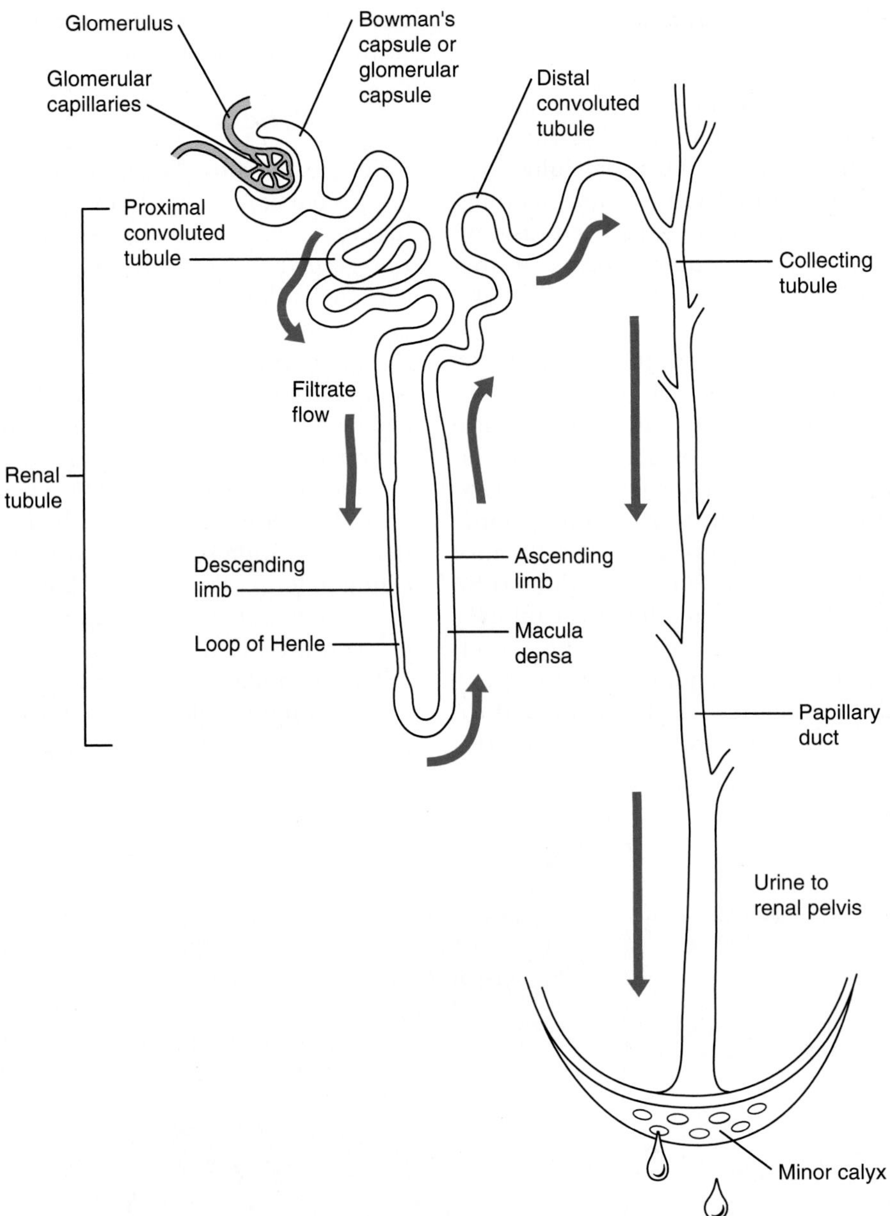

Figure 15•5 Close-up of the blood supply to and from the renal tubule.

ducts of Bellini. At the apex of the renal pyramid, a small expanded duct, the minor calyx (plural, calyces), encloses one or more papillae. There are 4 to 13 minor **calyces** in the renal sinus of each kidney. Several minor calyces unite to form a major calyx. There are only two or three major calyces in each kidney. The major calyces join to form the renal pelvis, which is the upper region of the ureter located at the renal hilus. When the concentrated filtrate of the kidney reaches the calyces, it is then called urine.

Author's Note

Because the kidneys do not have the extra protection of the abdominal peritoneal lining or the rib cage, massage tapotement (percussion) is contraindicated over the kidney area in the dorsum of the body. It may be helpful to draw the kidneys on a fellow student with a washable, nontoxic marker to identify the location of these structures.

The Filtration Process

Filtration of the blood and the formation of urine is a three-step process. First, the watery blood plasma is *filtered* in the glomeruli; second, water, nutrients, and ions are *reabsorbed* into the bloodstream from the renal tubules; and third, *tubular secretions* of unwanted elements are discharged back into the filtrate or urine. The filtrate descends down the collecting ducts into the renal pelvis.

Pressure in the kidneys is necessary for filtration to occur. The pressure in the glomeruli must be higher than in the renal tubule. The afferent arteriole feeding the glomerular vessels has a large diameter, which results in a slight reduction of pressure. The lumen (singular, lumina) of the efferent arterioles are narrower than the lumina of the afferent arteriole, which causes an additional increase in pressure. This difference creates a positive pressure of approximately 60 mmHg in the glomerulus as compared with only 18 mmHg in the renal tubule (pressure is measured in millimeters of mercury).

The entire blood supply of the body passes through the kidneys every 3 minutes, during which only about $\frac{1}{100}$ of the blood plasma crosses the glomeruli for waste removal processing by the kidneys. It takes about 5 hours to process all the blood plasma in the human body. As water from the plasma portion of the blood permeates the membranes between the glomeruli and the renal tubules, waste products pass into the filtrate. Proteins and formed elements of the blood that are too large to cross the membrane are retained by the bloodstream. Toxins and unessential substances such as urea, uric acid, ammonia, drug residue, excess water-soluble vitamins and minerals (especially B vitamins; this is why your urine turns bright yellow when taking these supplements), and excess free ions are collected in the renal tubules and are allowed to leave the body in the **urine,** which is a solution of water and dissolved waste. The filtration process is so efficient that about 45 gallons (180 liters) of filtrate are produced in a 24-hour day! Not all of this water is excreted as urine. Most of it is reabsorbed into the blood.

 *Author's Note*

The key to the filtration process is hydrostatic pressure. Hydrostatic pressure refers to the fluid movements that are dependent upon pressure differences on each side of the cell membrane. With hydrostatic movement, fluids always flow from a high pressure to a low pressure.

Reabsorption

Approximately 99 percent of the fluids removed from the blood are reabsorbed. The reabsorption process occurs when water from the renal tubule crosses back over the semipermeable cell membrane, returning into the peritubular capillary system. How can this happen when we already know that the hydrostatic pressure is greater in the blood vessels than in the renal tubules?

The answer is found in the mechanism of *osmosis.* Unlike hydrostatic pressure, osmotic movement of fluids does *not* depend upon pressure at all. Osmosis depends upon the concentration of the dissolved elements that lie in the solutions on each side of the membrane. Osmotic movement of water is always from the lowest (most dilute) to the highest concentration of solution (least dilute). Since most of the water has moved across to the renal tubule, the filtrate is very diluted, and the blood and plasma in the peritubular capillary network are highly saturated with solutes. Osmosis causes the reabsorption of water into the bloodstream and continues until the concentrations of the solutions on both sides of the membrane equalize. The majority of the body's water, along with much needed substances such as glucose and amino acids, are retained and returned to the blood plasma through the process of reabsorption.

Tubular Secretion

In the reabsorption phase, water and necessary nutrients are recovered from the filtrate by crossing back from the renal tubules to the bloodstream. The final phase of the filtration process is essentially moving toxins in the opposite direction. Toxins are transported from the blood plasma in the peritubular capillaries into the renal tubule by a process known as *tubular secretion.*

The purposes of tubular secretion are to rid the body of toxic elements and to control blood pH. Toxins are secreted back across the cell membrane from the blood to the filtrate. These toxins may include organic compounds, such as creatinine and histamine, that are naturally occurring within the body; they may also be residues from drugs, such as penicillin or marijuana, that are introduced to the body. Other potentially harmful substances that are secreted are ions. Hydrogen ion secretion is especially important because it is the major regulator of blood pH. Potassium ion secretion prevents a buildup of ions that would affect heart rhythm.

Ureters

The **ureters** are two slender hollow tubes that transport urine formed by the kidneys to the urinary bladder. Like the kidneys, the ureters are located bilaterally; there is one ureter for each kidney. Between 10 and 12 inches in length, each ureter originates at the renal hilus. Urine is drained by peristaltic activity from the major and minor calyces, and from the renal pelvis in the kidneys to the urinary bladder. This peristaltic activity continues until urine reaches the urinary bladder. Each ureter enters the urinary bladder through a specialized valve, which prevents backflow of urine as the bladder contracts and empties. When the bladder is empty, the ureters are spaced about 2 cm apart. However, when the bladder expands, the ureters move about 5 cm apart.

Urinary Bladder

Located in the pelvis behind the symphysis pubis, the muscular **urinary bladder** provides a temporary storage reservoir for urine. Within the urinary bladder is a small triangular region, the *trigone.* The three corners of the trigone are marked at the top by the left and right ureter ducts and at the bottom by the internal urethral orifice. The urinary bladder is frequently filled with and emptied of urine. Two types of structures allow expansion of the urinary bladder: folds within the interior lining, or rugae, that allow the urinary bladder to distend and transitional epithelium, which changes shape as pressure is exerted on the epithelial lining. This tissue expansion puts pressure on pressure-sensitive receptors located in the muscular wall, which causes the internal urethral orifice to relax and results in the conscious desire to void. Upon demand, the cerebral cortex of the brain sends impulses to the external urethral orifice muscle to relax, and urination takes place.

Urethra

The **urethra** is a small tubular structure that transports urine from the urinary bladder out of the body during micturition (urination). The proximal end of the urethra is closed by the internal sphincter muscle, whereas the external sphincter muscles are located in the wall of the urogenital diaphragm. The internal urethral sphincter contains visceral muscle, and the external urethral sphincter contains skeletal muscle and is typically under voluntary control after the age of 15 months.

The length of the urethra differs in males and females. In females, the path of the urethra is located anterior to the vagina and exits between the vaginal opening and clitoris. The female urethra is relatively short (about 1½ inches). This, as well as the fact that the female urinary orifice is close to the anal opening, may account for the much higher incidence of bladder infections in women.

Opening at the distal end, or the glans penis, the male urethra extends from the center of the prostate and passes through the length of the penis (about 8 inches, depending on penile length). Both semen from the testes and urine from the urinary bladder may be transported by the male urethra.

FYI FOR YOUR INFORMATION

If water loss exceeds 5 to 10 percent of total body weight, serious dehydration results. A 20 percent loss of water is often fatal. Common causes of water loss are infection, fever, severe burns, and diarrhea.

CONTROLLING THE WATER BALANCE OF THE BODY

The bloodstream is responsible for water transfer to and from all the cells of the body, as well as for oxygen and nutrient exchange. The key to the water balance of the entire body is regulating the fluid balance of the blood. The control of water balance of the body is regulated by the secretion of antidiuretic hormone (ADH). If the bloodstream becomes concentrated due to a loss of water through sweat or urination, the posterior pituitary gland releases ADH, which stimulates the kidneys to reabsorb more water. If the blood is too dilute, the pituitary reduces the production of ADH, and the kidneys begin to produce more urine. Along with the water, important substances such as glucose are reabsorbed into the bloodstream.

THE KIDNEYS, BLOOD PRESSURE, AND BLOOD VOLUME

Blood pressure is directly proportional to blood volume. As blood volume increases, blood pressure increases accordingly. The kidneys depend upon blood pressure to function properly. As long as systemic blood pressure is sufficient, the kidneys filter the blood and produce urine. However, if arterial blood pressure drops too low, renal pressure becomes inadequate to force substances out of the blood into the tubules, and filtrate formation stops. It makes sense that the mechanism that controls blood pressure and blood volume is located in the kidney.

The mechanism monitoring the blood pressure is known as the **juxtaglomerular apparatus.** It consists of two specialized groups of cells known as the **macula densa** and **juxtaglomerular cells.** The macula densa is located in the ascending limb of Henle loop. The juxtaglomerular cells are located in the afferent arteriole. The macula densa and the juxtaglomerular cells lie next to each other where the renal tubule touches the afferent arteriole. The juxtaglomerular cells monitor changes in blood pressure in the afferent arteriole, and the macula densa monitors the concentration of the filtrate.

When blood pressure drops or the chloride ion concentration of the filtrate drops, the juxtaglomerular apparatus responds by secreting the enzyme **renin** into the bloodstream. Renin reacts with the blood, producing a substance called **angiotensin II,** a powerful stimulant that has two major effects. First, it works directly on the blood vessels by causing vasoconstriction, which raises the blood pressure; second, it stimulates the adrenal cortex to release **aldosterone.** Aldosterone, produced by the adrenal cortex, causes the kidneys to retain sodium, which stimulates the reabsorption of more water back into the blood plasma. The plasma volume of the blood increases, and blood pressure rises correspondingly. When blood pressure becomes too high, the renin secretions are decreased, and blood pressure falls.

URINE

Urine is concentrated filtrate from the kidneys that is 96 percent water and 4 percent dissolved wastes (urea, creatinine, uric acid, sodium chloride, potassium, sulfates, phosphates, and drug residue). Urine tends to be slightly acidic, and the normal amber color is due to the presence of urochrome, a pigment resulting from protein digestion. The more concentrated the urine, the darker its color. Abnormal constituents in urine may include albumin, glucose, red blood cells, white blood cells, bilirubin, kidney stones, and bacteria.

When passing from the body, urine is odorless. Once out of the body, the urea in the urine quickly decomposes to form ammonia, which gives urine its characteristic odor. If urine is allowed to remain on the skin, as in the case of wet diapers or bedwetting, the skin becomes irritated and a rash may develop.

The average adult produces anywhere from 1 to 2 quarts (1,000 to 2,000 ml) of urine per day. Chemical, nervous, and even physical factors can affect the amount of urine produced and excreted by the body. An example of a chemical factor is the consumption of coffee, tea, and many carbonated beverages. Stimulating the production of urine, these drinks have a **diuretic** effect on the urinary system. A diuretic (substance promoting the formation and excretion of urine) can increase urine production by increasing the amount of blood fluid crossing the glomerulus or it can decrease the amount of water reabsorbed from the renal tubule; both increase urine production. Anxiety often suppresses the body's urge to void. During periods of physical activity, the heart beats more rapidly, moving the blood through the kidney faster and increasing urine production.

Author's Note

Cryotherapy has a diuretic effect on the body. General cold applications cause vasoconstriction of the superficial vessels of the skin, which results in a temporary increase in blood pressure. The raised blood pressure increases the amount of glomerular output and therefore urine production.

URINARY CONDITIONS AND CLINICAL TERMS

1. **Urinalysis.** Urinalysis is the examination of urine using microscopic, chemical, or physical means. Prior to examination, a urine specimen is frequently placed in a centrifuge to separate materials. Chemicals may be added to the urine specimen to identify abnormal amounts of substances, such as blood, white blood cells, glucose, and protein.
2. **Micturition or Voiding.** Also known as urination, micturition is the act of emptying the bladder by passing urine out of the body through the urethra.
3. **Urinary Incontinence.** The inability to control micturition is referred to as urinary incontinence. This condition may be the result of an infection or damage to the central or peripheral nervous system, or of injury to the urinary sphincter or perineal structures, which can occur during childbirth. Urinary incontinence is frequently precipitated by laughing, coughing and sneezing, late stages of pregnancy, or straining while lifting heavy objects.
4. **Gout.** Gout is a condition characterized by high levels of uric acid in the blood due to the inability of the kidneys to excrete this substance. High levels of uric acid in the blood are converted to sodium urate crystals, which are frequently deposited in joints, the kidneys, and other tissues. Gout is more common in men than in women. The great toe is a common site for the accumulation of sodium urate crystals, causing painful swelling. When gout settles in the joints, it is frequently called gouty arthritis.

Massage and passive range of motion are contraindicated during an acute phase of gout because of the inflammation and pain. However, cold packs could be beneficial. If the client is not having a flare-up, light massage can be done on the surrounding areas. Range of motion and local massage, though, are contraindicated.

5. **Glomerulonephritis.** Also known as Bright's disease, glomerulonephritis is an inflammation of the glomeruli. This disease frequently follows other infections and is characterized by blood in the urine, edema, and hypertension.
6. **Uremia.** Often seen in renal failure and glomerulonephritis, uremia denotes a toxic level of urea and other nitrogenous waste products in the blood. Uremia is due to a renal insufficiency and abnormal retention of these waste products normally removed by the kidneys.
7. **Cystitis.** Cystitis is an inflammation of the urinary bladder and/or ureters. This condition is frequently caused by a bacterial infection from neighboring organs such as the kidney, prostate, or urethra. Cystitis is often characterized by pain, blood in the urine, and by urgency and frequency of urination.
8. **Urinary Tract Infection.** Urinary tract infection, or UTI, is an infection of one or more structures of the urinary system. Most UTIs are caused by bacte-

ria and are more common in women than in men. Bacteria from feces can be transported to the urethra as a result of improper toilet habits (i.e., wiping from back to front rather than from front to back). The most common symptoms of UTIs are increased urination, burning and pain during urination, and, if the infection is severe, blood and pus in the urine.

Encourage your client to take the full treatment of antibiotics. Also encourage her to drink at least eight glasses of water each day to flush out microbes. Massage will depend on how the client is feeling. If the symptoms are severe, massage may be the last thing the person wants. If the symptoms are less severe, abdominal massage should be avoided, but a general massage would be okay. Keep in mind the client may need to take frequent trips to the bathroom.

9. **Renal Dialysis.** Renal dialysis is a process of using a mechanical kidney to remove substances from the blood in an attempt to restore its electrolyte and acid–base balance. This process is accomplished by diffusing previously unfiltered blood across a semipermeable membrane. Substances such as uric acid, creatinine, and drugs are ordinarily removed.
10. **Renal Failure.** Renal failure is the inability of the kidneys to perform their essential functions (i.e., filtering the blood, collecting and secreting wastes, retaining essential elements). This condition is caused by an impediment to renal blood flow, such as hemorrhage, trauma, obstruction of the urinary tract, toxic substances (i.e., mercury), or renal disease (i.e., glomerulonephritis). If someone has progressive renal failure, he may be on hemodialysis, a procedure in which the blood is filtered through an external source. It is usually done three times a week and lasts several hours at a time.

Someone who is undergoing hemodialysis may not be a good candidate for massage. Permission from the client's physician is a must. He may be taking anticoagulants that make the skin fragile and tear easily. A light massage of short duration is best.

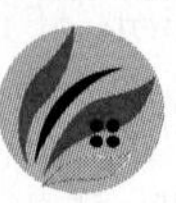

EFFECTS OF MASSAGE FOR THE URINARY SYSTEM

1. Massage, especially abdominal massage, increases urine output by activating dormant capillary beds and recovering lymphatic fluids for filtration.
2. Massage promotes the excretion of nitrogen, inorganic phosphorus, and sodium chloride. The levels of these metabolic wastes are elevated in urine after massage.
3. Massage promotes autonomic nervous system functioning, promoting general homeostasis, thus increasing urine output.

SUMMARY

The urinary system maintains homeostasis in the body by accomplishing several functions. This system eliminates metabolic waste, regulates the pH and chemical composition of the blood, and regulates blood volume, fluid volume, and blood pressure. This small system accomplishes these varied functions with only four types of organs: a pair of kidneys, a pair of ureters, a urinary bladder, and a urethra.

The kidney is a highly complex bean-shaped organ located bilaterally in the upper lumbar area. Kidneys have three main divisions—the cortex, the medulla, and the renal hilus—that are covered with a tough renal capsule. The renal hilus is the point where the artery and vein connect to permit blood circulation through the kidney, and is the origin of the ureters. The cortex carries out the process of blood filtration, and the medulla houses the urine collecting apparatus. The chief structural and functional unit of the kidney is the nephron, which is responsible for the filtration process. This is accomplished by two interlaced networks of vessels, one carrying blood and the other carrying filtrate or urine. The blood is carried through some specialized vessels known as glomeruli and peritubular capillaries. In the glomeruli, the liquid portion of the plasma filters across into the renal tubules, which are urine transport structures. Excess water and certain needed elements are reabsorbed from the renal tubules back into the bloodstream in the peritubular capillaries. The product remaining in the renal tubule is known as filtrate. Other toxins are secreted into this filtrate, which is collected and becomes urine.

The urine flows out of the kidneys through a pair of ureters and into the urinary bladder, where the liquid is stored until it can be excreted from the body. When full, the bladder is emptied through a tube to the outside known as the urethra. Analysis of urine is often useful for determining adverse conditions and diseases of the body.

SELF-TEST

Multiple Choice • Write the letter of the best answer in the space provided.

_______ 1. Which one of the following systems is *not* involved in waste elimination?

A. the muscular system
B. the integumentary system
C. the respiratory system
D. the digestive system

_______ 2. All of the following are functions of the urinary system except

A. elimination of metabolic waste
B. regulation of blood volume and blood pressure
C. regulation of chemical composition of the blood
D. movement and support

_______ 3. The kidneys are positioned behind the abdominal peritoneum. This position can also be referred to as

A. anterior
B. subperitoneal
C. infraperitoneal
D. retroperitoneal

_______ 4. The indentation in the medial aspect of the kidney, where the renal arteries, veins, and the ureters attach, is called the

A. renal hilus/hilum or renal sinus
B. renal cortex
C. renal pelvis
D. renal medulla

_______ 5. The internal portion of the kidney containing the renal tubules and the renal pyramids is called the

A. renal hilus or renal sinus
B. renal cortex
C. renal pelvis
D. renal medulla

_______ 6. The soft, outer region of the kidney is called the

A. renal hilus or renal sinus
B. renal cortex
C. renal pelvis
D. renal medulla

_______ 7. In which section of the kidneys are the nephrons located?

A. renal hilus or renal sinus
B. renal cortex
C. renal pelvis
D. renal medulla

_______ 8. The vast, intricate network of minute vessels in the nephron is referred to as the

A. capillaries
B. villi
C. nephrons
D. glomeruli

_______ 9. High-pressure vessels from the renal artery that feed the glomerular capillaries are the

A. afferent arterioles
B. renal tubules
C. efferent arterioles
D. peritubular capillaries

_______ 10. Where does water reabsorption occur?

A. afferent arterioles
B. glomerulus
C. efferent arterioles
D. peritubular capillaries

_______ 11. The funnel-shaped pouch surrounding the glomerulus is called the

A. renal capsule
B. glomerular capsule
C. Bowman's capsule
D. B and C

_______ 12. Fluids that cross from the glomerulus into the glomerular capsule are referred to as

A. lymph
B. filtrate
C. plasma
D. synovia

_______ 13. As urine is formed, it is collected in tubules and routed into larger papillary ducts called the

A. renal ducts
B. ducts of Bellini
C. urinary ducts
D. islets of Langerhans

_______ 14. At the apex of the renal pyramid, there is a small expanded duct called the

A. renal duct
B. major calyx
C. minor calyx
D. urinal duct

_______ 15. Filtration of the blood and the formation of urine is a three-step process. Which of the following is the correct procedural order?

A. filtration, reabsorption, and tubular secretions
B. digestion, absorption, and excretion

C. absorption, filtration, and reabsorption
D. absorption, reabsorption, and excretion

_______ 16. Proteins and formed elements of the blood are too large to cross the membrane and are ___ by the bloodstream.
A. absorbed C. retained
B. destroyed D. emulsified

_______ 17. The reabsorption of water that occurs in the renal tubule, returning into the peritubular capillary system, takes place by what mechanism?
A. active transport C. mastication
B. diffusion D. osmosis

_______ 18. Which of the following is retained by the body and returned to blood plasma?
A. urea and ammonia
B. creatinine, oxygen, and salts
C. glucose, vitamins, and amino acids
D. urea and glucose

_______ 19. The storage reservoir for urine is the
A. kidney C. ureter
B. urethra D. urinary bladder

_______ 20. The two urinary bladder structures that allow for expansion are the
A. villi and expansion joints
B. rugae and transitional epithelium
C. villi and cilia
D. haustra and rugae

_______ 21. Which small tubular structure transports urine from the urinary bladder out of the body during micturition?
A. kidney C. ureter
B. urethra D. urinary bladder

_______ 22. The control of the water balance of the body is regulated by the secretion of
A. antidiuretic hormone C. estrogen
B. melatonin D. glucagon

_______ 23. The juxtaglomerular apparatus consists of the
A. macula densa and the juxtaglomerular cells
B. internal and external urethral orifices
C. ureters and the urethra
D. renin and aldosterone

_______ 24. Which structure, located in the afferent arterioles, monitors changes in blood pressure?
A. juxtaglomerular cells C. macula densa
B. loop of Henle D. islets of Langerhans

_______ 25. Which of the following structures monitors the concentration of the filtrate?
A. juxtaglomerular cells C. macula densa
B. loop of Henle D. islets of Langerhans

_______ 26. When blood pressure drops or the chloride ion concentration of the filtrate drops, the juxtaglomerular apparatus responds by secreting
A. prostaglandin C. cellular fluid
B. renin D. fibrinogens

_______ 27. Angiotensin II has what effect on the urinary system?
A. raises the blood pressure through vasoconstriction
B. stimulates the release of aldosterone, causing sodium retention and the reabsorption of more water into the blood plasma
C. angiotensin II has no effect on the urinary system
D. A and B

_______ 28. Characteristics of normal urine are
A. slightly acidic C. odorless
B. amber color D. all of the above

_______ 29. Factors that can affect the amount of urine produced and excreted by the body are
A. chemical (consumption of coffee, tea, and carbonated beverages)
B. physical (physical activity)
C. nervous (anxious and other sympathetic nervous system reactions)
D. all of the above

References

Applegate, Edith J. *The Anatomy and Physiology Learning System: Textbook.* Philadelphia: W. B. Saunders, 1995.
Damjanov, Ivan. *Pathophysiology for the Health-Related Professions.* Philadelphia: W. B. Saunders, 1996.
Gould, Barbara E. *Pathophysiology for the Health-Related Professionals.* Philadelphia: W. B. Saunders, 1997.

Gray, Henry, F.R.S., T. Pickering Pick., Robert Howden, C.M. *Gray's Anatomy,* 29th ed. Philadelphia: Running Press, 1974.

Haubrich, William S. *Medical Meanings, A Glossary of Word Origins.* New York: Harcourt Brace Jovanovich, 1984.

Kalat, James W. *Biological Psychology,* 2nd ed. California: Wadsworth Publishing Company, 1984.

Kordish, Mary and Sylvia Dickson. *Introduction to Basic Human Anatomy.* McNeese State University, Lake Charles, LA: Self-published manual, 1985.

Marieb, Elaine N. *Essentials of Human Anatomy and Physiology,* 4th ed. New York: Benjamin/Cummings Publishing Company, Inc., 1994.

McAleer, Neil. *The Body Almanac.* Garden City, New York: Doubleday and Co., Inc., 1985.

Moore, Keith L. *Clinically Oriented Anatomy,* 2nd ed. Baltimore: Williams & Wilkins, 1985.

Mosby's Medical, Nursing, and Allied Health Dictionary, 4th ed. St Louis: Mosby–Year Book, Inc., 1994.

Newton, Don. *Pathology for Massage Therapists,* 2nd ed. Portland: Simran Publications, 1995.

Premkumar, Kalyani. *Pathology A to Z—A Handbook for Massage Therapists.* Calgary, Canada: VanPub Books, 1996.

Taber's Cyclopedic Medical Dictionary, 13th ed. Philadelphia: F. A. Davis Co., 1977.

Tortora, Gerald J. *Introduction to the Human Body: The Essentials of Anatomy and Physiology,* 3rd ed. New York: HarperCollins Publishers, 1994.

UNIT THREE

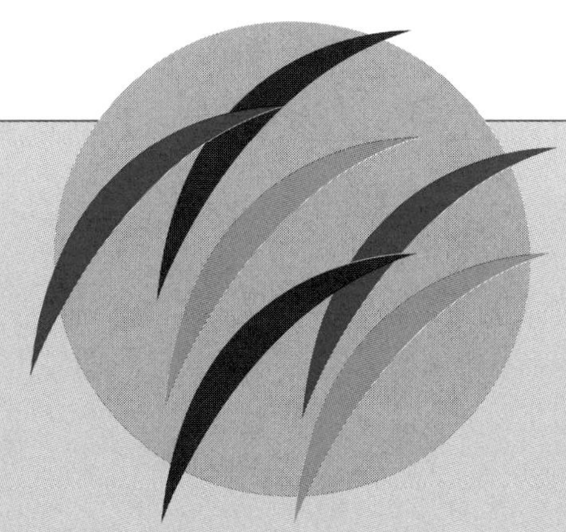

Benefits, Contraindications, Screening, Technique, and Special Considerations for the Massage Practitioner

If I felt any better, I'd be scared of myself.

—*Jack Johnson*

16

Health, Hygiene, Sanitation, and Safety Standards

Student Objectives

After completing this chapter, the student should be able to:

- List and give examples of infectious agents
- Explain the basic rules and procedures of sanitation and how they are used to control transmission of pathogens
- Discuss universal precautions and how they are applicable to the practice of massage therapy
- Determine when vinyl gloves are needed for massage therapy
- Demonstrate proper handwashing techniques
- List five hygiene tips
- Recommend three health tips to your clients and colleagues
- Design a massage facility using basic rules of safety and accessibility

INTRODUCTION

Massage therapy is probably one of the safest, least intrusive, and yet most effective treatment modalities in the healthcare field today. However, there are areas of our practice in which the client is susceptible to harm. These areas may often be obscure, such as incidental exposure to a possible disease-causing agent or an accidental injury. Hippocrates, the father of medicine, declared that physicians should "do no harm." Likewise, as healthcare professionals ourselves, we must protect our clients and ourselves through personal and professional habits and studio modifications that minimize disease transmission and prevent accidents.

In this chapter, we will examine safe procedures as well as why these procedures are necessary, including the following elements: basic pathophysiology as it relates to disease transmission, proper hygiene and sanitation, and safety standards for your massage facility. Familiarity with these facets of health will support you in providing the best environment possible for your clients. The pathophysiology section will include the causative agents and their related diseases, how to reduce the transmission of disease-causing microorganisms, and the handling of biohazardous material (blood and other body fluids). Health and hygiene will cover basic sanitation procedures and techniques for handwashing and gloving up, as well as health tips for therapists and clients. The safety module will provide standards for the physical facility and information on client safety. These standards for health, hygiene, sanitation, and safety are becoming a part of professional massage conduct across the country.

PATHOPHYSIOLOGY

In order to build a better understanding of disease and its transmission, let's begin with a fundamental overview of pathophysiology, the study of biological and physical manifestation of disease. A **pathogen** or **pathogenic agent** is a living biological agent that is capable of causing disease. Pathogen comes from the Greek words, "pathos," meaning "disease" and "gennan," meaning "to produce." One way to develop a disease is to be exposed to a pathogen. Effective exposure occurs due to many factors (time duration, concentration of pathogens, weakness of the subject's defenses, and other unidentified reasons). Effective exposure results in contamination.

Contamination occurs when an infectious, or causative, agent resides in or on an organism (e.g., airborne, fluid-borne, or direct contact). Once the organism is contaminated, the next phase is infection. Inanimate objects, or **fomites,** can also become contaminated. In the next section, we will look at causative agents in more detail. Once the agent is understood, ways to control its transmission become apparent.

The Host/Parasite Relationship

When a pathogen first penetrates a target organism, a relationship between the parasite and the host is initiated. The host's body will react to fight the disease, and the parasite will try to overcome the host's reactions. The outcome of health or disease is dependent upon which side of the relationship is stronger. As the parasite or causative agent enters the body, the immune system is put on alert and a complex series of reactions begins. This includes the secretion of chemicals, such as enzymes and acids of the gastrointestinal tract. Reflexes like coughing and vomiting may occur in a physical attempt to remove the infectious agent. Leukocytes (or white blood cells which are part of the body's immune system, protecting the body from damage of bacteria, viruses, and other invaders) begin to mobilize and destroy the invader in a process known as phagocytosis and pinocytosis. *Phagocytosis* is the process by which specialized cells engulf harmful microorganisms and cellular debris. When the pathogen is absorbed rather than "eaten" by these cells, this is known as *pinocytosis.* In this process, the cell develops a saccular indention, engulfing the pathogen.

The susceptibility of the host to infection is dependent on factors such as age, genetics, nutrition, state of health, immune response, and factors we have not identified. The success of the parasite depends on various factors including the portion or number of organisms that gain access, which areas are attacked, the parasite's ability to spread and replicate itself, and its resistance to host defenses. Thus, a weak host with a strong parasite results in disease, whereas a strong host with a weak parasite will overcome the introduction of disease.

However, if the immune system is depressed by chronic stress, malnutrition, radiation, some medications, or a preexisting illness, such as HIV or AIDS, the organism is then more susceptible to diseases caused by pathogens. It is for this reason that the HIV virus is so deadly; it hurts the host by crippling the host's immune response so that a second infection, which would normally be dormant or suppressed by the immune system, becomes fatal.

Types of Diseases

To understand how to reduce the likelihood of transmitting disease, we must look at disease itself. This section will explore the types of diseases, both pathogenic and nonpathogenic. *It is the pathogenic, infectious disease that most concerns the massage therapist.* As you may recall, the presence of a causative agent does not ensure that a disease will develop. Often the body's immune system declares biological war on the causative agent and destroys it before disease can manifest itself. Some symptoms that may lead us to believe that the organism is trying to defeat a pathogen are fever, mild nausea, altered metabolism, cardiovascular changes, anemia, leukocytosis, and a general feeling of despondency. The types of diseases are as follows:

1. **Infectious diseases** are caused by a biological agent, like a virus or a bacterium, and are highly contagious. Examples of infectious disease are pneumonia, measles, and tuberculosis.
2. **Deficiency diseases,** caused by a lack of an essential vitamin or nutrient, typically interfere with the body's growth and development or help to establish metabolic diseases. Types of deficiency diseases are scurvy (deficiency of ascorbic acid or vitamin C), rickets (deficiency of vitamin D), and beriberi (deficiency of thiamine or B_1). Deficiency diseases are not contagious.
3. **Metabolic diseases** involve abnormal activities of cells and/or tissues like Cushing's disease, diabetes, cardiovascular conditions, and jaundice. Metabolic diseases are not contagious but may have originated from a contagious disease, such as hepatitis, which can lead to jaundice or vice versa.
4. **Genetic diseases** are caused by an imperfect genetic code located in the chromosomes. Chromosomes are structures found in the nucleus of every cell of the body. Examples of genetic diseases are Down's syndrome, cystic fibrosis, sickle cell anemia, and hemophilia. These genetic disorders are not contagious, but may be genetically passed from generation to generation.
5. **Cancerous diseases** are characterized by the uncontrollable growth of abnormal cells that invade surrounding tissue and **metastasis** (process of cancerous cells spread to distant parts of the body, usually through the bloodstream or the lymphatic circulation). Cancerous diseases cause **malignant** (a condition that worsens and causes death) cancerous tumors, which often cause death if they are not treated. Conversely, **benign** refers to conditions that are not cancerous or life threatening. The definite cause of cancer is undetermined, but many potential causes are recognized. More than 80 percent of cancer cases are attributed to exposure to carcinogenic (cancer-causing) chemicals, tobacco, ionizing radiation, and ultraviolet rays. Stress tends to promote cancer growth. Cancer is not contagious, but it can spread internally.

Agents of Disease

There are six basic causative agents that promote disease in the body: bacteria, fungi, metazoa, protozoa, rickettsia, and viruses.

1. **Bacteria.** Most bacteria are not pathogenic and do not require living tissue for survival. Some bacteria are important for plant growth, such as nitrogen-fixing bacteria in the soil. Others are used for processing certain foods such as bread, cheese, yogurt, and wine. "Good" bacteria also occur as natural flora in the body (mouth, intestines) and aid the digestive processes. Harmful bacteria are transmitted directly from person to person or from a fomite. Bacteria may enter the body through ingestion and lead to diseases like botulism and salmonella. Improper food handling, such as chopping vegetables or fruits after handling raw meat, or chopping on unclean surfaces, can contaminate food. Another frequent method of obtaining bacteria is by not washing your hands after using the toilet then touching your nose or mouth. Some diseases that are caused by bacteria are boils (staph), tuberculosis, strep throat, and tetanus.
2. **Fungi.** Fungal agents include molds and yeast, and their growth is promoted by warm, moist environments. Only a few fungal varieties are pathogenic. When an individual has a fungal infection, it is typically superficial, tenacious, and difficult to eradicate. Generally, fungal spores are transmitted by a fomite; for example, athlete's foot fungus may be picked up off the locker room floor. However, some fungal infections can infect the body internally such as thrush, which is a yeast infection of the tissues of the mouth. In hosts with severely suppressed immune function, fungal causative agents can become systemic and may be life threatening. Fungi can be transmitted directly from person to person. *Candida albicans* normally grows in the mucous membranes of the mouth and vagina, can be found in the axilla and under the breast, and can be transmitted to a new host through touch. Another fungal infestation is ringworm.
3. **Metazoa.** These are parasites (organisms obtaining nourishment from other living organisms) that can produce diseases in the bodies of their living hosts. Parasite contamination may come from ingesting undercooked meats, drinking contaminated water, or bodily entry through an open wound (usually in the feet). Common parasites are hookworms, pinworms, and trichina worms.
4. **Protozoa.** These single-celled organisms are considered the lowest form of animal life; pathogenic protozoa can only survive in a living subject and are commonly transmitted through contaminated food, water, and feces. Protozoa are responsible for diseases such as trichomoniasis, amebic dysentery, African sleeping sickness, and malaria.
5. **Rickettsia.** Rickettsia are intracellular parasites that share characteristics of both bacteria and viruses. They are similar to viruses in that they require living cells for growth and replication, yet are also similar to bacteria in susceptibility to antibiotics.

Rickettsia diseases are usually transmitted from infected rodents to individuals by their bites or the bites of lice, fleas, mites, or ticks. Chlamydia is one of the most common sexually transmitted diseases and frequently causes sterility or pneumonia. Except for chlamydia, most diseases caused by rickettsia pathogens are uncommon in areas where rodents and vermin are controlled. Examples of rickettsia diseases are typhus, Rocky Mountain spotted fever, and Lyme disease.

6. **Viruses.** Viruses are considered to be nonliving entities because they do not carry out independent metabolic activities. They can only replicate themselves within the cell nucleus of a living plant or animal host. Because viruses easily mutate, antibiotics are relatively ineffective. Viruses are usually transmitted from person to person or animal to person. Viral diseases include the common cold, influenza, AIDS, measles, mumps, rabies, herpes simplex, viral hepatitis, and Ebola.

Premassage consultations should query the client regarding illness. In general, massage therapists are exposed to no more viruses and bacteria than the average person, with one major difference: We are touching an unclothed person. Massage therapists who are hospital-based or who work with hospice or nursing homes may be at a higher risk of infection. The pathogen that the massage therapist is most likely to contact is fungi and yeast. Massage therapists may not only contract the fungi, but the fungi also can be spread to other parts of their client's body. Contamination can occur in both directions: from therapist to client and from client to therapist. Clients with HIV or any condition where the immune system is compromised may require stricter sanitation standards, perhaps routine disinfection and mandatory glove use.

Paths of Infection

For infection to pass successfully from an infected agent (often referred to as a *reservoir,* which can be living or inanimate) to a living organism (or new host), a mode of transmission is required. By understanding the various modes of transmission, this information can be used to protect ourselves and our clients from disease.

1. **Pathogen Transmission by Direct Contact of Mucous Membranes.** This includes the touching of an infected mucous membrane to an uninfected mucous membrane (i.e., nose, mouth, and genitals) and the exchange of bodily fluids and secretions by oral, genital, or rectal sexual activity (also known as sexually transmitted diseases, or STDs).
2. **Pathogen Transmission by Direct Contact with Broken Skin.** This type of transmission can also include parasite entry through breaks in the skin. The reason for the skin break does not matter; it could be accidental, a surgical intrusion, a dog or mosquito bite, skin eruptions from a prior infection, a hangnail, or self-inflicted (like intravenous drug use). Most parasitic metazoans, like hookworms, gain entry to the body through breaks in the skin of the feet.
3. **Pathogen Transmission by Direct Contact with Intact Skin.** This method of transmission includes contact with someone who is infected with fleas, scabies, lice, ticks, fungi, poison oak, poison ivy, and poison sumac.
4. **Pathogen Transmission by Ingestion.** This includes the consumption of undercooked meats, food that has not been properly refrigerated or stored, and contaminated water.
5. **Pathogen Transmission by Inhalation of Airborne Pathogens via Droplets.** This mode of transmission includes infectious agents that are inhaled and absorbed through the mucous membranes of the lungs. Although no direct contact is made with infected mucous membranes, contamination occurs when the host comes into contact with airborne droplets of fluid arising from the respiratory tract and salivary glands of the reservoir host, primarily through coughing, sneezing, massaging, or talking within a 3-foot distance. Most respiratory diseases are spread by this method.

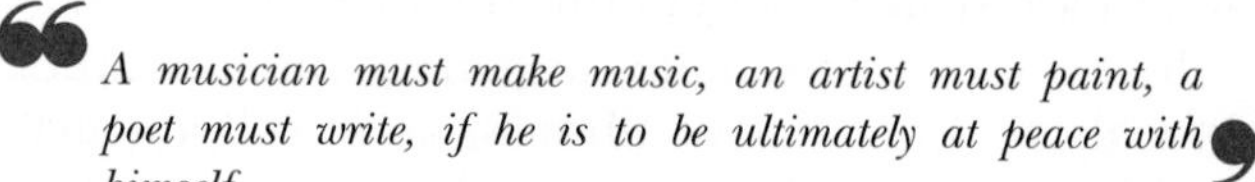

> *A musician must make music, an artist must paint, a poet must write, if he is to be ultimately at peace with himself.*
>
> —Abraham Maslow

Controlling Transmission

The best thing a massage therapist can do to control transmission of pathogenic organisms is to practice good hygiene and sanitation. Handwashing, using only clean linens and equipment, and noting breaks in your skin as well as the client's skin are commonsense measures. Many practices are routinely performed, while others are performed only when stricter standards are needed, such as gloves and disinfecting, to reduce the likelihood of contamination. Here are seven distinct ways in which you, as a massage therapist, can control the spread of pathogenic microorganisms.

1. Wash your hands often.
2. Disinfect equipment and supplies when needed, such as when in contact with an infected person or any body fluid leakage.
3. Use only clean linens.
4. Begin each day with a clean uniform or set of clothing.
5. Use a closed lubricant container with a dispensing mechanism.
6. Wear intact vinyl gloves, a bandage, or finger cot

when you have an open lesion or fungal or scabies infection on your hand.

7. Do not massage while you are ill or infected.

These safeguards will be explained in detail later in the chapter. Discuss these methods for controlling the transmission of infectious disease with other massage therapists. You may decide to incorporate other methods of sanitation in your practice. Remember that all the rules for sanitation are to protect the spread of infectious agents in any direction: from therapist to client, from client to therapist, and from one part of the client's body to another.

Universal Precautions

In December 1991, the Occupational Safety and Health Administration (OSHA) supported and helped to pass federal legislation that requires all healthcare workers who may be exposed to body fluids and/or wastes to adopt and prescribe to a plan to prevent the exposure to and spreading of blood- and fluid-borne pathogenic microorganisms. Body fluids that can carry harmful microorganisms are semen, vaginal secretions, blood, saliva, breast milk, urine, feces, and cerebrospinal, synovial, pleural, peritoneal, and pericardial fluids. From this legislation, the Centers for Disease Control and Prevention (CDC) established **universal precautions** to reduce the transmission of communicable disease. These precautions protect the client *and* the therapist.

Universal precautions include mandatory handwashing, vinyl gloves, protective eyewear, nose/face masks, protective clothing, laundering linens and uniforms, cleaning or disinfecting equipment, and observing proper methods for disposing of used medical supplies and biological material. Universal precautions are required when performing *invasive medical procedures* or when handling body fluids. Invasive medical procedures involve puncturing or penetrating body tissues or entering a body cavity.

How involved do massage therapists have to become with these medical precautions? The answer to this question varies according to your practice. Although massage therapists are not involved with surgical procedures, we do occasionally enter a body cavity such as the mouth for TMJ massage (where legal). Obviously, a therapist who works in a medical clinic or hospital has a greater exposure risk than the therapist who specializes in relaxation massage. In a clinical setting, the therapist may be required to perform rehabilitative therapy on patients who have pins, wires, stitches, staples, or open wounds near the treatment area. Each medical center will subscribe to strict standards in handling both clients and body fluids.

Contact with body fluids seldom occurs in a nonclinical massage therapy practice, but incidents do occur. A small blemish may break, lesions or minute scabs on recently shaved legs may drain, a client may cough or sneeze mucus, or a nauseated client may vomit. These and similar situations must be handled according to **aseptic protocol,** which involves the use of methods to eliminate the presence of pathogenic microorganisms and is outlined later in the chapter.

The use of intact gloves ensures client and therapist protection from transmission of disease. Massage therapists working with people who are HIV positive must be particularly careful not to infect their clients with something that could prove fatal in their weakened state. For more information on massage, gloves, and the HIV virus, read Chapter 21, Adaptive Massage and Client Management Issues.

If you must wear gloves during a massage, make sure they fit your hands well. Glove use may reduce your palpatory abilities. Performing massage with gloved hands also creates more friction, especially in thick body hair, and this may be uncomfortable for the client. Powder may be used as a lubricant in these cases. Most massage lubricants are oil based and break down latex glove material in seconds. *Do not mix latex gloves with oil-based lubricants. At the time of this writing, vinyl gloves are best when using lubricants.*

Inform the client directly about the use of gloves for safety and protection (e.g., open cuts). You may refuse to perform the massage if the client objects because some clients may be offended that you are donning gloves before the massage. Conversely, the client may refuse the massage if he suspects you have an open

When Should the Massage Therapist Use Gloves?

1. When handling any form of blood or other body fluid or secretions.
2. When working with a patient who has herpes lesions.
3. Anytime the therapist has a break in the skin or an infectious skin disease of one or both hands. If the injury or infection is only on the end of the finger, a finger cot may be worn.
4. For reasons of simple hygiene, such as internal TMJ massage.
5. Whenever the client requests that the therapist wear gloves.
6. Whenever the therapist does not feel comfortable without them.
7. If several of these conditions are present, then the therapist may decide that the risk factor is high enough to warrant double gloving or rescheduling the massage until the conditions change.

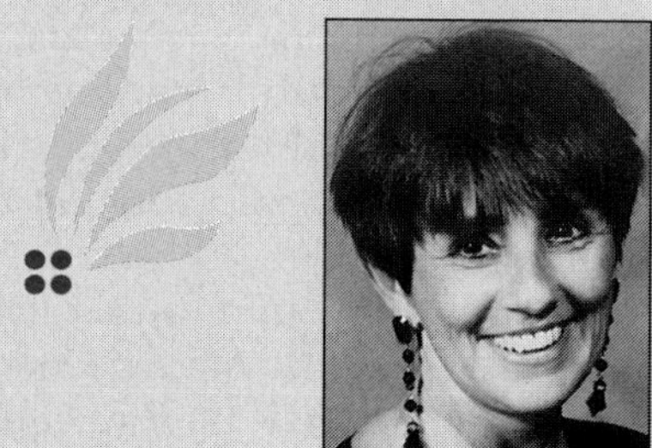

Tiffany Field

"The best pioneers are the ones actually out there doing massage. They get devotees just from having put their hands on them. That's what keeps the field alive and moving."

Tiffany Field has always been a woman on the move. As the daughter of an insurance executive and teacher, she lived in 12 different places when she was growing up, but now she's found her home and her life's calling—on the beach in Hollywood, Florida.

She's no massage therapist and she hasn't developed any particular massage modality; nevertheless, her work has dramatically affected the credibility of the profession. Tiffany Field is a professor of pediatrics, psychology, and psychiatry, and the director of the University of Miami School of Medicine's Touch Research Institute (TRI). TRI was established in 1992 and is the only center in the world devoted solely to the study of touch and its applications in science and medicine.

According to a recent article in *Massage Therapy Journal* by Mirka Knaster, Field has "a doctorate in developmental psychology, 20 years of research experience, a stack of publishing credits [300 plus], awards and research grants, editorial activity for 50 professional journals, and membership in more than a dozen professional organizations."

TRI evolved after her team's research findings supported touch as a factor that increased birthweight in premature infants. Preemies who put on weight with massage leave the hospital earlier. With 470,000 premature births in the United States each year, that could add up to $7.05 billion in annual savings.

The potential for cost cutting and Field's research landed the grant money to explore touch therapy further. Now her group is studying the effects of massage on all ages, from cocaine-exposed newborns to arthritic geriatric patients. There's a lot of hard work going on at TRI. Collecting data and presenting the findings may be an analytical person's dream job, but for many, statistical computations can be a little intimidating. Interestingly enough, one of the latest TRI research titles is "Massage Therapy Reduces Anxiety and Enhances EEG Pattern of Alertness and Math Computations."

Some of the work being examined at TRI is particularly groundbreaking. Still considered by many a contraindication for massage, an ongoing breast cancer study shows an increase in natural killer cells (cells that kill cancer cells) after massage. In a society that values scientific proof, such findings could eventually make massage therapy a component of mainstream medicine.

Field has a hectic schedule that involves lots of travel for fund-raising, overseeing projects, and writing grant proposals. To unwind, she swims daily, practices yoga, ballet, and tai chi when she has spare time, and of course she gets a massage whenever she can.

For the past decade Field has probably been one of the most instrumental individuals in helping gain respect for massage therapy, but she doesn't see it that way.

Her advice to beginning massage therapists is to "join a group practice to learn the ropes of operating a business."

wound or an infection (e.g., a cold or the flu). Before gloving up, wash and dry your hands using a thorough procedure. Glove up discreetly and quietly. If a glove is torn or damaged during a procedure, it must be removed, the hands rewashed, and a new glove replaced immediately.

Once the decision has been made to use gloves, care must be taken when removing and disposing of them to restrict possible contamination from the glove surface. One safe method of glove removal is to peel the first glove from the cuff to fingers so that it is inside out (Fig. 16–1A). Then, place the removed glove into the palm of the other hand (Fig. 16–1B) so that when you peel off the second glove, the first will be contained inside (Fig. 16–1C). Dispose of the removed gloves in a closed container. Even though you

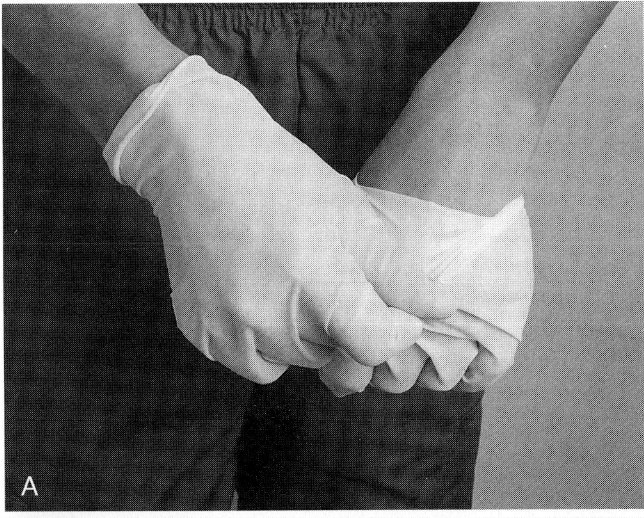

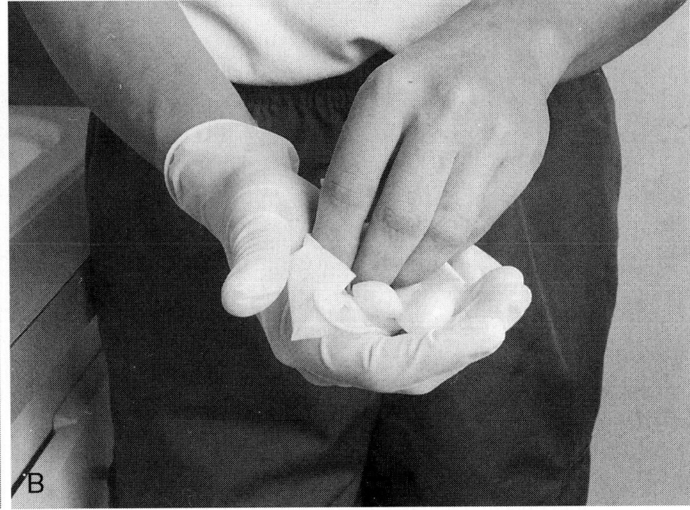

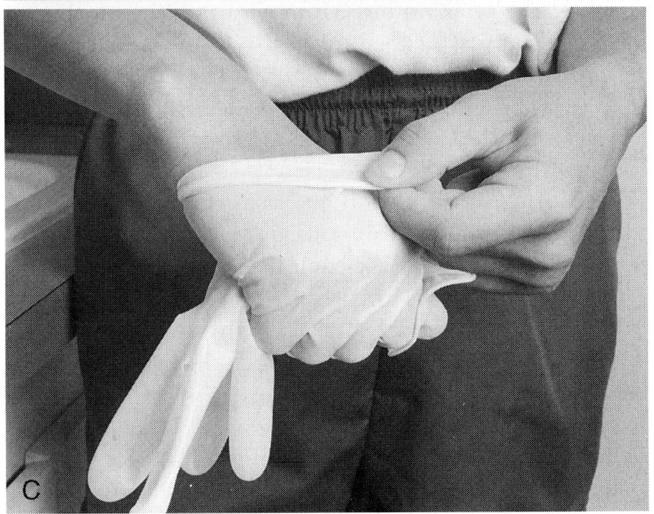

Figure 16•1 A,B,C Proper removal of vinyl gloves.

have been careful in removing and discarding the used gloves, wash your hands immediately.

SANITARY PROCEDURES FOR THE MASSAGE THERAPIST

One of the best gifts we can give to our clients is to follow the basic rules of sanitation. **Sanitation** involves the application of measures to promote a healthful, disease-free environment. For massage therapists to provide a sanitary environment, sanitary techniques, also known as medical asepsis, must be followed. **Medical asepsis** is the combination of water, friction, and soap or other disinfecting agents to eliminate pathogenic microorganisms. This can be accomplished chemically and/or mechanically. When you disinfect your massage table, you are using medical asepsis.

Sanitation. Because the protection of the client is a primary concern, sanitary procedures must be adopted and followed. This includes laundering the massage linens after each use, following a handwashing procedure, and cleaning and disinfecting massage equipment and supplies used for the client.

With handwashing or other aseptic techniques, pathogenic microorganisms are easily removed or destroyed from the forearms, hands, and nails. Other aseptic handwashing techniques include the use of special hand-cleaning solutions that are designed to be used without water. These high-alcohol content gels are designed for field use in sporting events and onsite chair massage appointments where handwashing may not be convenient or even possible. Be sure to follow the directions listed on the container. Because it is more difficult to remove microorganisms from small cracks and crevices found in ornate jewelry, wearing rings, bracelets, or wristwatches while performing massage therapy is not advisable. Long nails or cracked nail polish also provides hiding places for microorganisms and is not in keeping with sanitary standards. Long nails and jewelry can also potentially injure the client or break the protective barrier of gloves.

The garments you wear as you perform the massage, including your lab coat, must be laundered after being worn each workday. Wash your uniforms in hot water and detergent and dry them with hot air. If you suspect any uniform exposure to communicable disease, add ¼ cup of chlorine bleach to the detergent and washwater while laundering. Dry using hot air. Do not wear your massage uniform for other purposes. Short sleeves are more sanitary than long sleeves because they do not touch the client's skin.

Don't confuse "disinfection" with "sterilization." **Disinfection** is the removal of pathogenic microorganisms or their toxins from surfaces by a chemical or mechanical agent. This frequently does not remove many spores (the reproductive unit of the microorganism). Disinfection includes the use of antiseptics, which remove pathogenic organisms from the tissues of the skin's surface and mucosa without damaging or destroying the tissues, and retards pathogenic growth. **Sterilization** destroys microorganisms using heat, water, chemicals, or gases. In the practice of massage therapy, disinfection of hands, linens, and equipment is the aseptic procedure required by law in most states, and you can lose your license if you do not uphold these standards for clients.

In some circumstances, state law or employers require the massage therapist to be immunized against diseases such as hepatitis B, rubella, rubeola, poliomyelitis, diphtheria, and tuberculosis. Some employers of massage therapists, such as hospitals, may highly recommend vaccination, but they are not mandatory; however, if you choose to waive the immunization, then it is accepted practice that all nonimmunized employees be sent home for the duration of any outbreak. This will vary with the organism in question. Sanitation standards should be practiced at home. For example, always guard against the spread of pathogens by washing your hands when necessary and by keeping cuts and abrasions covered, even when you are not performing massage. The following rules for sanitation will guide you in using aseptic protocol to ensure the highest quality of healthcare possible.

Nine Rules for Sanitation (Aseptic Protocol)—The Louisiana Model

1. Exterminate all insects, termites, and rodents on the premises and maintain a pest-free facility.
2. Using an approved handwashing procedure, wash and dry your hands thoroughly before and after performing massage therapy. Some institutions have their own recommended handwashing procedure for healthcare professionals. One example is provided later in this chapter.
3. Vinyl gloves are to be worn anytime you, as the therapist, have a cut or open wound on your hands, when handling linens, or cleaning massage equipment that contains body fluids. A finger cot may be used over a bandage to keep the edges smooth or instead of a glove if the area of broken skin is contained to one finger.
4. Clean your massage table, face rest, arm shelf, and other table accessories at the start of each business day. However, if your massage table becomes soiled with blood or tissue fluids from seeping wounds, the table must be disinfected with a solution of chlorine bleach and water in a ten-to-one solution (ten parts water to one part chlorine bleach) before the next use.
5. Use only clean linens for each massage session, and launder all massage linens—sheets, towels, bolster covers, and face rest covers—after each session. If there is any blood or tissue fluid seepage due to any superficial wounds, remove the linens with gloved hands. According to the CDC, wash soiled linens separately in hot water, using laundry detergent and ¼ cup of chlorine bleach. Dry linens using hot air. Once soiled linens have been removed from the massage table, clean the table with a solution of chlorine bleach and water in a ten-to-one solution. Finally, wash your hands.
6. Wear a clean uniform each day. Avoid contact between used linens and your uniform. If your uniform becomes contaminated with body fluids or secretions, wash clothing separately in hot water, detergent, and ¼ cup of chlorine bleach. Dry using hot air.
7. To prevent lubricant contamination, use only closed dispenser-type containers. Jar containers run the risk of cross-contamination because the therapist must remove the lubricant from the jar, place it on the client's skin, and reach back into the jar for additional lubricant after touching the client. **Cross-contamination** (the passing of microorganisms from one person to another) can occur if the lubricant becomes contaminated. If a jar container is used, use a clean spatula or tongue depressor and remove enough lubricant for single-client use, placing it on a disposable palette or in a sanitary dish that can be sterilized.
8. Do not perform massage therapy while you are ill or have coldlike symptoms, such as sneezing, coughing, fever, or a runny nose. In these cases, it is preferred to cancel your clients or arrange for an associate to substitute, rather than to wear a surgical mask to prevent the spread of airborne pathogenic microorganisms. Protect your clients from infection!
9. Avoid massaging clients who are contagious.

HANDWASHING

The number one source of microorganism cross-contamination is by contact with human hands. It seems

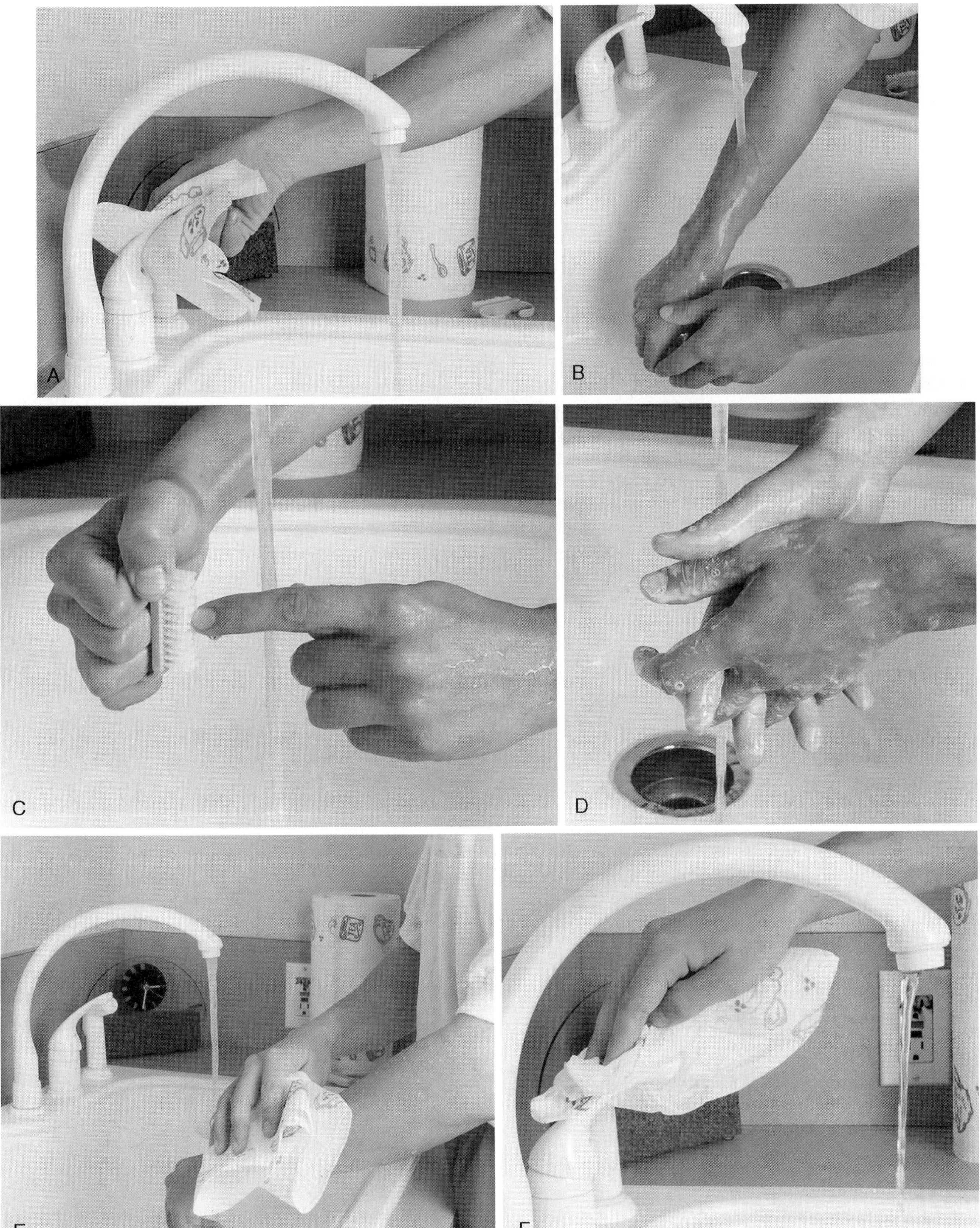

Figure 16•2 *A,* Step one: turning on the water. *B,* Step two: wetting hands, forearms, and elbows. *C,* Cleaning underneath fingernails. *D,* Step three: soaping the hands. *E,* Step four: drying the hands. *F,* Turning off the water.

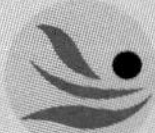

Handwashing Procedure

1. Approach the sink. Use paper towels to touch the valves (Fig. 16–2*A*), then turn them on. Adjust the hot and cold water valves until the water is a comfortable temperature and the water is not splashing in the sink. Throw away the paper towels.
2. Wet your hands, forearms, and elbows. Keep your hands lower than your elbows, or water, soil, and germs will run up your arms and onto your garments (Fig. 16–2*B*). Using a nail brush or orange stick, clean underneath the nails (Fig. 16–2*C*). A single-use nail brush or orange stick is preferred. Nails must be cleaned before hands.
3. Using soap, generate a lather in your hands, and rub the soap up the forearms using a firm, circular motion. Massage your soapy hands and forearms for 30 seconds. If you have performed an internal TMJ routine, have broken skin, or come into contact with body fluids, *increase the handwashing time to 2 minutes.*

   The friction created by rubbing your hands together is essential to emulsify the oils on the skin and to lift the bacteria and dirt from the skin's surface. These unwanted impurities become suspended in the lather, which will be rinsed away.

   When washing, include the areas between your fingers (Fig. 16–2*D*).

   Liquid antibacterial soap in a pump dispenser is preferred over bar soap because the soap does not become contaminated by direct contact and is therefore more sanitary. If you are using bar soap, rinse the bar before and after use.

   Liquid dishwashing soap can be used as an alternative to liquid hand soap.
4. Rinse the hands and forearms thoroughly, using tap water until all lather is removed. Allow the water to run from the fingers to the elbows. This rinsing technique ensures that the hands will be the most sanitary area. Do not skimp on this step. Leaving soap residue on the skin may result in chapped or dry skin.
5. Using paper towels, dry your hands and forearms well (Fig. 16–2*E*). Using the same paper towels, turn off the water valves (Fig. 16–2*F*). Continue to use the same paper towels to open door handles until you reach the room in which you will perform massage. Discard the paper towels.

reasonable that the best measure to prevent the spread of infection would be handwashing. Massage therapists must wash their hands before and after each massage—using gloves for massage therapy does not preclude handwashing (Fig. 16–2). The following handwashing procedure is recommended for healthcare professionals to ensure that appropriate steps have been taken to protect them and their clients.

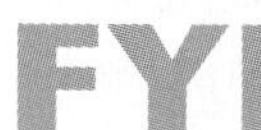

FOR YOUR INFORMATION

In 1843, Semmelweis, a Hungarian physician, reintroduced handwashing between patients to prevent the spread of disease.

HEALTH AND HYGIENE FOR THE MASSAGE THERAPIST

Hygiene can be defined as the collective principles of health preservation. Proper health and hygiene habits are important for massage therapists because we come into physical contact with our clients. In states requiring licensure of massage therapists, good grooming and hygiene are required by law. This is because proper hygiene habits not only preserve health but also help to protect the public from the transmission of microorganisms. The following list of tips has been compiled to aid you in practicing a health and hygiene regimen.

As you observe these hygiene tips, develop and maintain a respect for the diversity of different cultures found throughout the globe. What may be offensive to some are commonplace to others, and what is hygienic to some may be offensive to others. Each therapist must apply these tips to her own situation with her own common sense and knowledge of local customs.

Nine Professional Hygiene Tips

1. Bathe or shower daily. Use an antiperspirant or deodorant if necessary.
2. If you perspire heavily while performing a massage, wear sweatbands at the wrists and forehead to ensure that perspiration does not drip onto the client's skin.
3. Avoid perfumes, colognes, or scented lotions. Respect the client's allergies and sensitivities.

4. Brush your teeth at least twice a day, and floss to keep gums healthy. Regular brushing removes plaque and reduces the growth of bacteria. Because massage requires close contact with clients, you may elect to use a mouthwash or avoid food that can cause an offensive odor.
5. Wash your hair frequently. Choose a hairstyle that keeps hair out of your way during a massage; secure hair so that it does not touch the client. Because of its porosity, hair is a source of harmful microorganisms.
6. Keep nails clean, short, and neatly trimmed. Long nails can injure the client as well as hide bacteria.
7. Shave often or keep facial hair neat, trimmed, and well groomed.
8. Wash your hands thoroughly after using the toilet and before and after each massage session.
9. Do not chew gum or tobacco or smoke while in the company of a client.

These hygiene tips will enable us to be more effective healthcare providers. As such, we are making the statement that we care about health—the health of ourselves and our clients.

We usually use the word "health" in relation to our physical being, but health can supersede the physical realm. Health can be defined as the freedom from limitation. Freedom from limitation includes the freedom from the restrictions we place on ourselves, mind, body, and spirit. Richard Bach, author of *Jonathan Livingston Seagull,* wrote, "Argue for your limitations and they're yours." Nurture your mind, body, and spirit with "healthy," nonrestrictive thoughts and kind deeds. You and your clients will reap the benefits of these choices.

The simple fact is that we cannot give away what we do not have. The best gift we can give to our clients is by giving to ourselves first. "Charity begins at home" means that self-care is not "selfish" but self-nurturing in a way that allows us to pass along our gifts to others. The following health tips can be used to achieve good health in our own lives so we can become better gift givers. Additional information on activities to increase strength, flexibility, and stamina, as well as hand-developing exercises can be found in Chapter 17, The Science of Table and Body Mechanics.

Health Tips to Keep Fit for Massage and Model a Healthy Lifestyle

1. Exercise at least three times a week for 30 minutes. This helps you keep fit for massage therapy as well as burns calories and reduces stress.
2. Drink six to eight glasses of water a day for proper tissue hydration.
3. Eat foods that are low in fat and high in fiber, and maintain a balanced diet for your energy needs.
4. Limit your intake of salt, sugar, caffeine, and alcohol.
5. Avoid all forms of tobacco use. The smell of tobacco is often offensive to nonsmoking clients. While many smoking therapists are unaware of their tobacco odor, it can be detected on their clothes, hair, and linens.
6. Schedule "stress breaks" of at least 15 minutes to relax, especially on crowded days. Breathe slowly and deeply while allowing your body and mind to rest in a comfortable position. Morning meditation or "quiet time" is a good way to start the day and helps us avoid getting up on the "rat race" side of the bed.
7. Remember to schedule regular massage therapy for yourself.
8. Honor your emotions by expressing them appropriately. Keep a journal, see a counselor, or join a support group.
9. Stimulate yourself intellectually on a regular basis. Go to art galleries, museums, and concerts. Read a book, write poetry, see a foreign film. Talk about religion and politics with someone who has differing philosophies.
10. Laugh. Surround yourself with positive, happy people. Go to a comedy club. Tell stories with old friends. Watch a Monty Python or Marx brothers movie. It is best not to take yourself too seriously.

SAFETY PROCEDURES FOR THE MASSAGE THERAPIST

Safety procedures provide an environment that is hazard- and barrier-free. Safety has two aspects for the massage therapist; safety of the physical space or massage facility and of the procedure itself. A safe facility is accessible to all patrons, even those who are elderly or physically challenged. For the massage therapist to provide a safe procedure, knowledge of endangerment sites, human physiology and pathophysiology, first aid, and cardiopulmonary resuscitation (CPR) must be included in his training. Skill training and knowledge of the human body helps ensure that the massage therapist is safe and competent.

The following safety rules will assist you in providing a safe, germ-free and barrier-free environment for the practice of massage therapy. Once these safety rules have been followed, you and your client may proceed with the massage therapy with confidence. Check with state and local officials to be certain that you are within the standards set forth by these legal systems.

Rules for Facility Safety—The Louisiana Model

1. Comply with all state and municipal building fire and safety codes.

2. Establish and maintain current liability insurance coverage. The original or copy of this policy must be kept on the premises at all times and be available for inspection.
3. Maintain an operative fire extinguisher and heat or smoke detectors on the premises. Fire extinguishers must be located at eye level and in clear view (ratings specified by the city ordinance).
4. Have a fire escape route posted in the office, and clearly mark all building exits.
5. Provide safe and unobstructed human passage in the public areas. Safe passage includes level flooring. Uneven floor designs make wheelchair maneuvering difficult and dangerous. This safety feature is important for clients who have conditions that affect neuromuscular coordination or for those who are recovering from recent surgeries. Omit area rugs because they can be a slipping or tripping hazard.
6. Choose only nonslip flooring, especially in bathrooms and wet areas.
7. Provide an operative toilet and lavatory with hot and cold running water in a private restroom setting. Each restroom shall be equipped with toilet tissue, soap dispenser with soap or other hand-cleaning material, sanitary towels or other hand-drying device such as a wall-mounted electric hand drier, and waste receptacle. Massage establishments located in buildings housing multiple businesses under one roof such as a shopping mall or in hotels may substitute a centralized restroom. Facilities and fixtures shall be kept clean, well lit, and adequately ventilated to remove offensive odors.
8. Maintain clean shower facilities, as well as other equipment used to enhance the massage or for client use, such as a whirlpool bath, sauna, steam cabinet, or steam room.
9. Remove all trash from the premises daily.
10. Bathrooms should be accessible to the physically challenged and should include a wheelchair-height lavatory with lever-style faucets. Grab bars should be located near the toilet for clients who need assistance transferring to the toilet seat.
11. Lever-style door handles are required for physically challenged people. ***Note:*** Lever-style is the preferred handle for massage therapists as well. Round door handles are difficult to turn with oily hands.
12. Have a designated handicap-accessible parking space. There should be slopes, not steps, between the parking space and the building. The space should be marked with the international symbol of accessibility.
13. A ramp or lift should be available so that wheelchairs have access to the building. Exterior ramps should be designed so that they drain easily and do not hold water.
14. Public telephones should have an adjustable volume control.
15. Maintain a list of all emergency phone numbers by the telephone: the local fire station, police department, sheriff's department, local hospital or ambulance, and taxis.
16. The street address should be outside the building in clear view. This will make it easier for emergency assistance to locate your business.
17. Maintain all equipment used to perform massage services in safe condition. This includes checking and tightening your massage table hinges, knobs, and locks on your massage table and other equipment before each business day.

Rules for Client and Procedural Safety—The Louisiana Model

1. Obtain and maintain training or certification for first aid and CPR.
2. Keep a first-aid kit on the premises in a location known by all personnel.
3. After each massage, wipe the client's feet to remove the massage lubricant with a paper towel to decrease the likelihood of the client falling. You may wish to spray isopropyl alcohol on the client's feet and wipe it off with a paper towel to more effectively remove the lubricant.
4. Be able to identify endangerment sites and contraindications of massage therapy. Use this information in your massage therapy practice. For more information, read Chapter 19, Massage Physiology.
5. Do not perform massage therapy under the influence of alcohol or other recreational drugs.

SUMMARY

As healthcare professionals, we seek to improve the health and well-being of our clients through massage therapy and to ensure that there are no accidental injuries and no transmission of disease in our offices from client to client or from therapist to client. Protecting the client has many facets, some of which are understanding basic pathophysiology, practicing proper health and hygiene, and meeting safety standards for the massage facility.

Pathophysiology includes knowing the six causative agents of disease: bacteria, fungi, metazoa, protozoa, rickettsia, and viruses. There are also five types of disease: infectious, deficiency, metabolic, genetic, and cancerous. Infectious diseases are directly related to the causative agents, which can be transmitted through several different modes. Disease can be prevented by interrupting these modes of transmission. Transmission interruption is accomplished by following the basic rules of health, hygiene, safety, and sanitation, including handwashing, and using vinyl gloves, and the aseptic technique. Additional responsibilities are to provide equal access to your business and to prevent accidental injury to your clients by compliance with local building safety codes. The goal of health, hygiene, sanitation, and safety standards is to protect the client and the therapist by causing no harm.

SELF-TEST

Multiple Choice • Write the letter of the best answer in the space provided.

_______ 1. Some examples of infectious agents are
A. erythrocytes, leukocytes, thrombocytes, and bacteria
B. systolic, diastolic, parasitic, and vernacular
C. viruses, bacteria, leukocytes, and parasites
D. bacteria, fungi, protozoa, and viruses

_______ 2. Infections by fungal agents include
A. hookworms
B. ringworms
C. thrush
D. B and C

_______ 3. Which infectious agent can only replicate themselves within the cell nucleus of a living plant or animal host?
A. bacteria
B. fungi
C. viruses
D. parasites

_______ 4. Transmission of pathogens can occur by
A. inhalation of airborne pathogens via droplets
B. direct contact of mucous membranes
C. direct contact with broken skin
D. all of the above

_______ 5. What two primary functions do universal precautions serve?
A. protect the client and the therapist
B. protect the client and client's family
C. protect the therapist and the profession
D. protect the therapist and the U.S. government

_______ 6. Universal precautions may include which of the following?
A. mandatory handwashing
B. the use of vinyl gloves
C. laundering of linens and uniforms
D. all of the above

_______ 7. The number one source of microorganism cross-contamination is by
A. using unclean massage linens
B. contact with human hands
C. sitting on toilet seats
D. women sharing cosmetics

_______ 8. The most important hygiene habit to help protect the public from the transmission of microorganisms is
A. dental hygiene
B. clean garments
C. short hair
D. handwashing

_______ 9. Nail care includes keeping nails clean and
A. short and neatly trimmed
B. long and polished
C. short and ingrown
D. long and neatly trimmed

_______ 10. What is the combination of water, friction, soap, or other disinfecting agents to eliminate the presence of microorganisms called?
A. sterilization
B. inoculation
C. vaccination
D. medical asepsis

_______ 11. Handwashing or other _______ _______ destroy pathogenic microorganisms from the forearms, hands, and nails.
A. aseptic techniques
B. safety codes
C. unobstructed passages
D. health tips

_______ 12. Safety has two aspects for the massage therapist: safety of the massage facility and
A. safety of the procedure
B. safety of the office equipment
C. unobstructed passage
D. safety of the practitioner

_______ 13. For the massage therapist to provide a safe procedure, she must be trained in human physiology and pathophysiology, first aid, CPR, and
A. knowledge of endangerment sites
B. a current driver's license
C. aseptic techniques
D. sports massage

_______ 14. Which of the following is *not* recommended for the massage therapist to wear because it is more difficult to remove microorganisms from these items?
A. ornate rings
B. bracelets
C. wristwatches
D. all of the above

_______ 15. What is a process of removal of pathogenic microorganisms by a chemical or mechanical agent?

A. sterilization
B. safety codes
C. disinfection
D. hygiene

_______ 16. Which one of the following is *not* important in providing a safe, germ-free, and barrier-free environment for the practice of massage therapy?

A. safe and unobstructed passage
B. a hydraulic massage table
C. maintain a fire extinguisher
D. lever-style door handles

_______ 17. If there is any blood or tissue fluid seepage due to any superficial wounds, remove the linens with gloved hands and wash in

A. hot water, detergent, and chlorine bleach
B. hot water and detergent
C. hot water and chlorine bleach
D. hot water

_______ 18. The client may refuse the massage for sanitation reasons if

A. you have an open wound
B. you have an infection
C. you have a mole on your hand
D. A and B

_______ 19. To properly clean underneath the nails, use a(n) _______.

A. nail file
B. nail brush
C. orange stick
D. B and C

_______ 20. Massage your soapy hands and forearms

A. for 10 seconds
B. for 30 seconds
C. for 60 seconds
D. for 1 minute

References

Applegate, Edith J. *The Anatomy and Physiology Learning System: Textbook.* Philadelphia: W. B. Saunders, 1995.

Damjanov, Ivan. *Pathophysiology for the Health-Related Professions.* Philadelphia: W. B. Saunders, 1996.

Gould, Barbara E. *Pathophysiology for the Health-Related Professionals.* Philadelphia: W. B. Saunders, 1997.

Larson, E., T. Mayur and B.A. Laughon. Influence of two hand washing frequencies on reduction in colonizing flora with three products used by health care personnel. *American Journal of Infection Control,* issue 17, 1989.

Louisiana State Department of Social Services, *Uniform Federal Accessibility Standards Accessibility Checklist*—United States Architectural and Transportation Barriers Compliance Board, 1995.

Ogg, Suzie. Lafayette General Hospital, Lafayette, Louisiana, 1997, personal communication.

Torres, Lillian S. *Basic Medical Techniques and Patient Care for Radiologic Technologies.* Philadelphia: J. B. Lippincott Company, 1993.

Tortora, Gerald J. *Introduction to the Human Body: The Essentials of Anatomy and Physiology,* 3rd ed. New York: HarperCollins Publishers, 1994.

Hands are the heart's landscape.
—Pope John Paul II

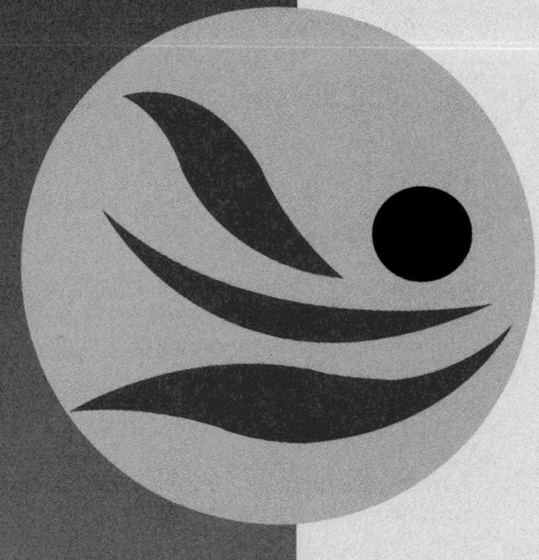

17 The Science of Table and Body Mechanics

Student Objectives

After completing this chapter, the student should be able to:

- Demonstrate hand exercises to develop strength, flexibility, and coordination
- Describe the basic elements of physical fitness
- Explain the rules for proper body mechanics and put these rules into practice
- Identify the two basic foot stances used in the practice of massage therapy
- Discuss ways to reduce the risk of repetitive motion injuries
- Use appropriate bolstering devices and position the client in the prone, supine, side-lying, and seated positions
- Properly drape the client with sheets and towels
- Maintain appropriate draping while the client rolls over
- Assist the client off the massage table while maintaining the appropriate drape

INTRODUCTION

In this chapter we will examine two important aspects of massage therapy that should be considered prior to and during the massage to your client. One set of preparations involves the use of **table mechanics** (e.g., draping, positioning the client, and the height of the massage table). The second set of preparations involves body mechanics (e.g., hand strength, preparation of the mind and body, breathing, body mechanics, and foot stances). Assisting the client on and off the table will also be addressed.

In order to ensure a successful long-term career in massage, maintaining good physical condition and using good body mechanics are important. Steps should be taken to prepare and maintain your physical stamina (massage is an active career choice). Take care to minimize the stress created on your body by reducing anatomical and physiological barriers. Anatomical and physiological barriers usually arise in muscles and joints and interfere with the massage through pain and loss of strength. Anatomical and physiological barriers can be circumvented by developing strength, flexibility, and coordination and by using proper body mechanics and practicing table mechanics.

HAND STRENGTH, FLEXIBILITY, AND COORDINATION

Massage therapists manipulate tissue using the entire body, but their hands must articulate the tissue through compression, lifting, twisting, rubbing, and squeezing. The strength, coordination, and flexibility of the hands will play an important role in how the massage is executed. Hand strength and flexibility may also reduce or prevent injuries that are a result of overuse. To illustrate this concept, let's examine one common injury in tennis. One way to rehabilitate tennis elbow is to strengthen the forearm flexors and extensors so they can better stand the stress of the racquet hitting the ball. Likewise, you can reduce the likelihood of injuries as a massage therapist by participating in activities that add strength, flexibility, and coordination to your hands. Ideally, the muscles acting on the hands are strong and the joints flexible. The hand and wrist are designed for articulation and dexterity, not weight bearing, so it is important that you perform exercises to strengthen these muscles and practice moderation when applying strokes. For example, you should not rest the weight of your body on a hyperextended wrist for long periods because you risk the possibility of damage. The following exercises are designed to assist the therapist in preparing her hands for the sensitive work involved in massage therapy.

Warm-up. Begin by rubbing your palms and fingers together, creating friction and warmth, then vigorously rub the backs of your hands and arms. Shake your hands and fingers at the wrists, then drop your hands to your sides and roll your shoulders forward for ten repetitions. Reverse the direction and rotate your shoulders backward. Do this movement sequence ten times. This quick warm-up is effective for preparing the hands right before a massage or before other hand-developing exercises. Remember to breathe as you move.

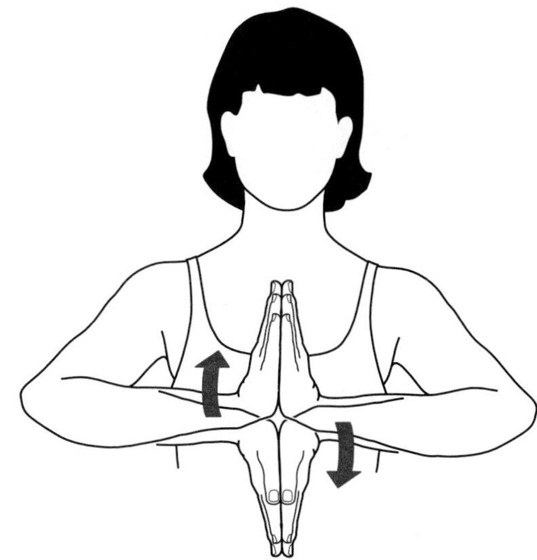

Figure 17•1 Hand swishing.

Hand Swishing. Press your palms and fingers together at chest level, with fingertips pointing up to your chin. Quickly rotate your fingers forward until they are pointing downward toward the toes, and then reverse back to the starting position (Fig. 17–1). This motion should be playful, quick, and vigorous. Note: The elbows and shoulders remain fixed while the wrists rotate together.

Digit Stretch. Press your fingertips together as you keep your wrists apart about 6 to 8 inches (Fig. 17–2).

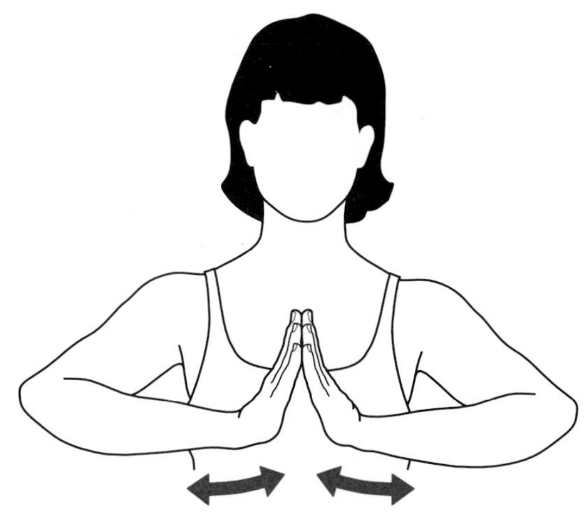

Figure 17•2 Digit stretch.

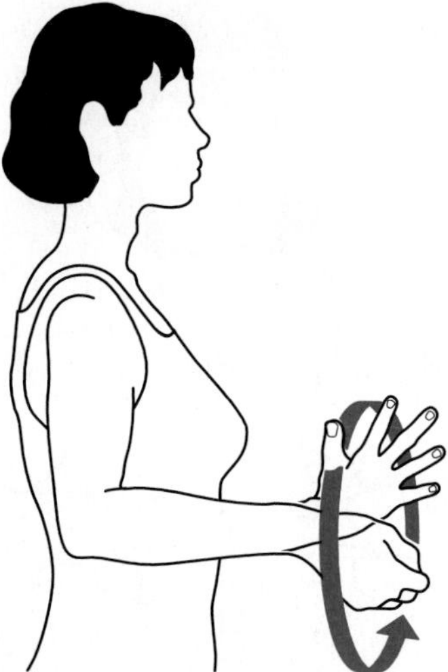

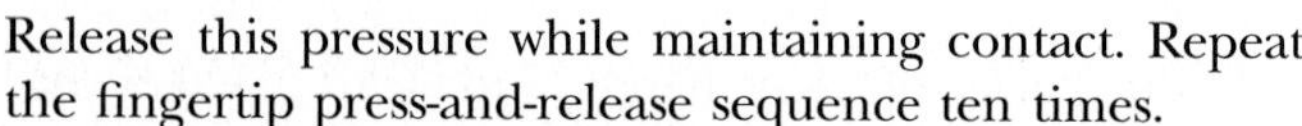

Figure 17•3 Wrist circles.

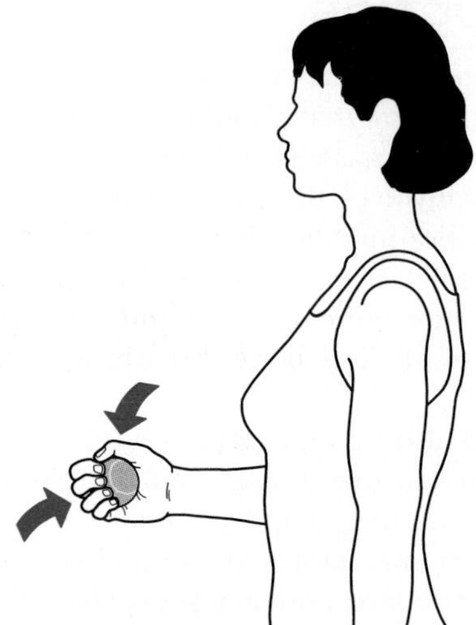

Figure 17•5 Ball press.

Release this pressure while maintaining contact. Repeat the fingertip press-and-release sequence ten times.

Wrist Circles. Begin with your arms at your sides. Flex the elbows while lifting your hands in front of you to chest level. With your fingers extended, circle both wrists in one direction for ten revolutions, and then reverse the direction for ten revolutions. Repeat the wrist circles in both directions, but this time, close your hands into a fist (Fig. 17–3). Do ten revolutions in both directions.

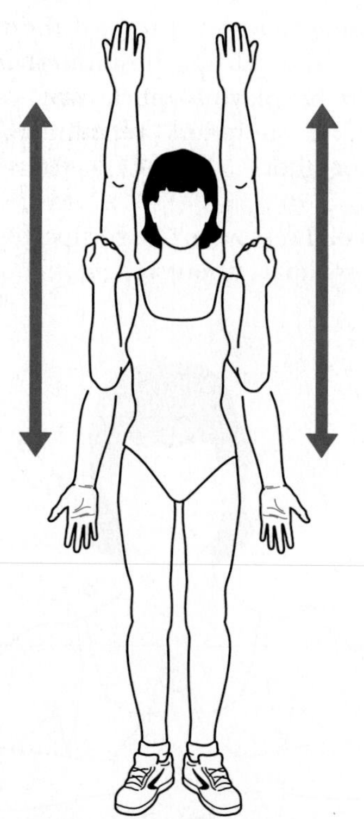

Figure 17•4 Grab and stretch.

Grab and Stretch. Start with your open palms at your sides. Pull your hands up to chest height, closing the palms into fists. Without stopping, continue the upward thrust of your hands over your head, stretching your fingertips out and inhaling simultaneously. Reverse the direction, bringing your arms back down. Close your hands as you pass your chest, and reopen them as they reach your sides, exhaling forcefully (Fig. 17–4). Keep your pace slow and your movements graceful. Repeat the sequence five times. Stop immediately if you become light-headed.

Ball Press. Place a tennis ball or a racquet ball in the palm of your hand, and wrap your fingers around it. Squeeze the ball as hard as you can for 10 seconds (Fig. 17–5). Repeat ten times. Switch hands, and repeat the sequence.

PREPARING THE MIND AND THE BODY

Bonnie Prudden, in her book *Pain Erasure: The Bonnie Prudden Way* (1980), classifies occupations into five categories, according to the degree of physical activity required to perform the job. These categories are sitting occupations, standing occupations, walking occupations, active occupations, and strenuous occupations. She lists massage therapy in the strenuous category because of the expenditure of physical energy and the use of torque (twisting and turning motions that occur in the torso). She adds, "Strenuous occupations all too often result in back pain." Taking steps to prepare our bodies and our minds will help us to avoid back pain because we will be stronger and not fatigue easily. Taking time to prepare ourselves will also help us become better therapists, as we will have more to offer our clients.

The term **physical fitness** is defined by the President's Council on Physical Fitness and Sports as the "ability to carry out daily tasks efficiently with enough energy left over to enjoy leisure time pursuits and to meet unforeseen emergencies." Being physically fit has many aspects. For discussion purposes, we can subdivide the elements of fitness into three components. The first consideration is balance and flexibility, the second is strength and stamina, and the third is grounding and centering.

Balance and Flexibility

The first elements are **balance** and **flexibility.** Balance and flexibility refer to the ability of the muscles, joints, and nerves to maintain static and dynamic stability while having the capacity to adapt to change. When your posture is balanced and flexible, you can shift your weight, move out from a foot stance to apply an effleurage stroke, and return with ease and grace. This is one reason why the bow stance is the most frequently used foot stance. The bow stance allows you to shift your weight and move out from your center of gravity (out of balance), to follow the excursion of the stroke, and then return to balance. Flexibility is needed to increase your range of movement.

Regarding movement, the concept of parts-to-whole is never ignored. Movement is initiated from the core outward and from the bottom up. The use of diaphragmatic breathing as you move will assist you in staying relaxed, paced, and focused. The lungs are located in the core of our bodies, and proper breathing can help fuel the muscles, relax the therapist, and pace the movement. Try to combine volitional (voluntary) breathing and massage therapy. As you massage, the strokes that require the therapist to reach may be accompanied by an exhalation, and the return strokes may be accompanied by an inhalation. Exercises that encourage balance and flexibility are certain types of yoga and martial art disciplines, such as tai chi and aikido.

Strength and Stamina

After developing balance and flexibility, the next elements of fitness are **strength** and **stamina,** consisting of the physical strength needed to apply the strokes and the stamina for performing the massage for extended periods. As a massage therapist, you may also be asked to assist your client on and off the table or to lift and move a client who is elderly or physically challenged. If you have not built adequate strength and stamina through exercise and proper diet, not only will you fatigue faster, you also may not have the strength to assist clients with special needs. Lack of strength and stamina may also set the stage for injury. In the chapter Health, Hygiene, Sanitation, and Safety Standards for the Massage Therapist, we discuss health tips to assist you in keeping fit. Additional complex carbohydrates added to a balanced diet are the best fuel food for keeping your energy level high. The best activities to add muscle strength to your body are floor exercises, such as sit-ups and push-ups, and weight training.

Grounding and Centering

The last components of fitness are **grounding** and **centering.** Embedded in the art of massage are these two concepts, which often refer to the mental, emotional, and the physical state of the therapist. The connection between the body and the mind is fundamental, and they are difficult, if not impossible, to separate. Being grounded and centered prepares the therapist's mind and body for massage. The best way to illustrate this intimate association between mind and body is to consider what happens to the body when you are under mental or emotional stress. The body responds by mirroring that state of mind; headaches and insomnia are not uncommon. Conversely, when people are ill or in chronic pain, it affects them mentally and emotionally. Many common tasks become difficult, and we often show our emotions too easily or not at all.

When you are grounded, you may feel the presence of God or your higher power and the presence of your client. You become part of a larger whole and recognize that you are just a vessel for positive change. The therapist imagines that all his tension is draining from his body, and he connects to the ubiquitous energy and power that brings life and peace. Using the "vessel" as a psychological reference point, the stress, tension, and excess energy that are released during a massage are not absorbed by the therapist.

Being centered means that you are in a body stance that is stable, yet responsive. Again, the martial art aikido is useful for guiding the massage therapist into useful application of movement principles. When teaching the concept of "centeredness" to students of aikido, masters often tell the students to place their weight underside and to allow themselves to feel light on top. Then the master can further shrink the focus to a space about the size of quarter 2 inches below the navel. This ancient "center of gravity" is called the **hara** or the **tan tien.** This is a topographical *and* meditative point of reference, known for thousands of years in many cultures as the center of physical and spiritual balance. A simple way to experience the power of this dynamic center is to allow your breath to move into and out of the tan tien. Upon exhalation, the therapist should contract the muscles of the pelvic floor in order to lower the center of gravity and splint the lower back muscles to help maintain a straight back. While practicing movement from both the bow stance and the horse stance, let movement be initiated from this center of balance. Being both grounded and centered will make a difference in how you deliver the massage; it will help you stay focused on what is at hand, and by clearing your mind and experiencing the moment, your body mechanics will be enhanced. The practice of yoga and the martial arts will enhance your ability to be grounded and centered for the practice of massage therapy.

When designing your fitness program, use a variety of exercises and activities. One type of exercise is not more important than another; they often complement each other. For example, strengthening the major muscle groups of the body will help build balance and contribute to stamina. It is significant to note that most members of our Western society focus on strength and stamina as the primary goal of their fitness program, seeing balance and flexibility as something that will come with time. The Eastern fitness philosophy focuses on building balance and flexibility first, and stamina comes with the discipline of maintaining a fitness routine. This philosophy views strength as not only muscle strength but also leverage. All fitness activities will help you explore the body's landscapes and build the body's natural energy, or bioenergy. Of course, anyone with serious health problems should consult a personal physician before initiating any exercise program, but generally if a person is healthy enough to do massage, then she is healthy enough to exercise.

MINI•LAB

Choose a partner. Have her stand with her feet 24 inches apart. Ask your partner to concentrate on her head. After a moment, give her a gentle push. Question her about how her body responds to the sudden change. Next, ask your partner to concentrate on an area between the fourth and fifth lumbar vertebrae on the front of the spine or about an inch or two below your navel. After allowing time for concentration, give another gentle push. Have your partner report on the difference she felt during each push. Which area of concentration felt more stable? Switch roles and allow your partner to gently push you. Compare experiences, noting similarities or differences. The area that felt more stable is the area from which you initiate your massage movements.

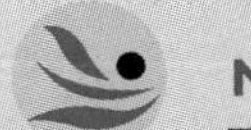

MINI•LAB

Generating Bioenergy: Begin by rubbing your hands together vigorously for 1 minute. Separate them about 5 inches, and be receptive to a light sensation between your hands. It may feel like the attraction or resistance of two magnets. Experiment by moving your hands very slightly, closer together and then farther apart. Let your right hand move in a small circle while your left hand is still. Reverse. Imagine a ball of energy between your hands. Move your hands back and forth, and imagine the ball becoming malleable. Breathe in and out slowly as your hands move. Imagine the ball growing as you separate your hands and compressing as you move your hands together (Fig. 17–6). Finally, separate your hands as far as possible, and turn the palms outward, allowing the ball of energy to dissipate.

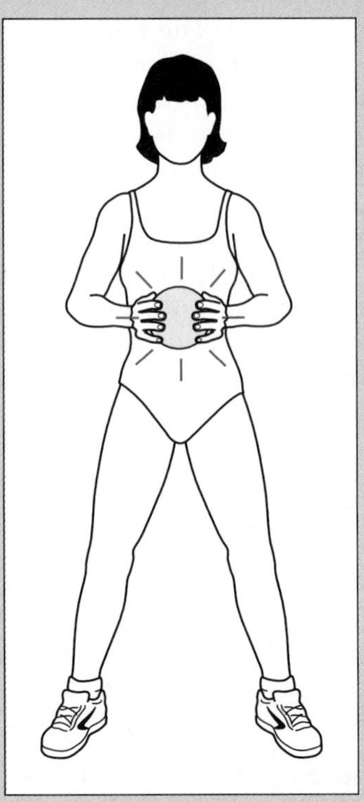

Figure 17•6 Bioenergy exercise.

FOOT STANCES FOR THE MASSAGE THERAPIST

Our physical world exists in three known dimensions: height (top to bottom), depth (front to back), and width (side to side). Massage movements are applied to the body using all three dimensions. We must be able to work up the leg, across the back, and under the scapula, just to name a few possibilities. We do not just massage with our hands; the whole body plays a role in how the massage is delivered. The placement of the feet is important to which massage stroke may be applied next. The lower extremities have two and a half times more available strength than the upper extremities, so it makes sense to use the body's natural strength to deliver effective massage with minimal strain on your joints. It is important to create a strong foundation with your feet because foot placement has a profound effect on body mechanics and keeping the body aligned.

The elements of a massage routine and the *kata* in martial arts are very similar in nature. To help us better understand these systems of movement, let's look at the ancient practices of kendo and aikido. Students of these martial arts are required to follow four basic principles: *eyes first* (for focus and attention), *footwork next* (foot position for weight transference), *courage third* (assessing timing, space, your opponent, and how you are going to initiate your movements), and *strength fourth* (body moves into action, or weight effort). It is important to note that strength and weight effort come last in the list. If we apply these principles to massage therapy, focus, foot stance, and assessment come before the massage strokes.

The massage therapist typically uses one of two basic foot stances when applying massage strokes: the *bow stance* and the *horse stance.* These two foot stances play an important role in length and direction of the massage stroke. If your feet are close together, you will not be able to traverse long distances; however, if your foot stance is wide (but not so wide that your body is unbalanced), you can move up the body while pressing and manipulating tissue, creating positive tissue response. Your foot stance can determine how far you can reach!

Both the bow stance and the horse stance provide a stable and balanced body posture. The foot stance used most frequently will depend on the style of massage you perform and the type of strokes you use most often. To prevent wear and tear on your knees, change you foot stance frequently. Besides the bow stance and the horse stance, other foot stances may be used, but these two provide the therapist with the widest range of massage strokes in all three dimensions.

The Bow Stance. Also known as the archer stance, the bow stance is frequently used when applying effleurage, or any gliding stroke where length may be important. The feet are placed on the floor in a 30- to 50-degree angle, one pointing straight and one pointing off toward the side. When your feet are positioned properly, they will look like the letter L, with the majority of the weight on the back leg while standing still. Another variation of the bow stance is with the weight distributed evenly on both feet; the foot pointing toward the side is turned slightly inward to provide greater comfort for the therapist (Fig. 17–7). In both variations, one foot is always pointing in the direction of movement. The distance between the two feet may vary from several inches to several feet. To move from

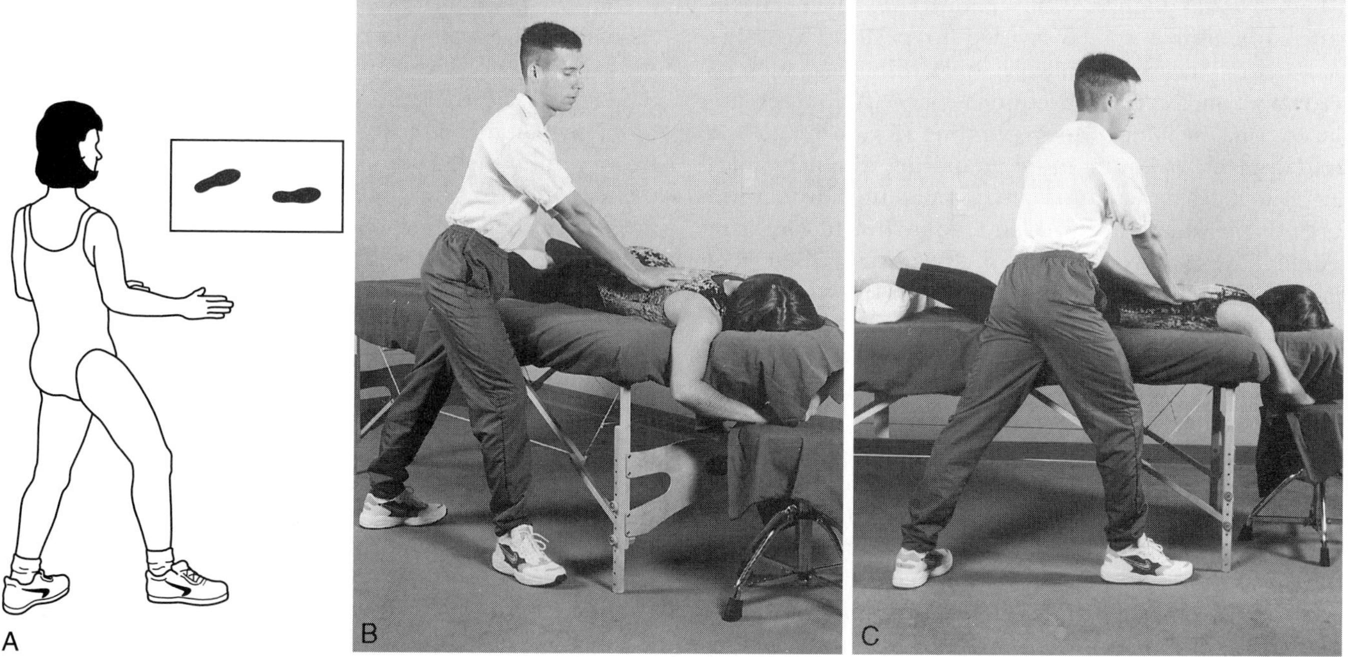

Figure 17•7 *A–C,* The bow stance.

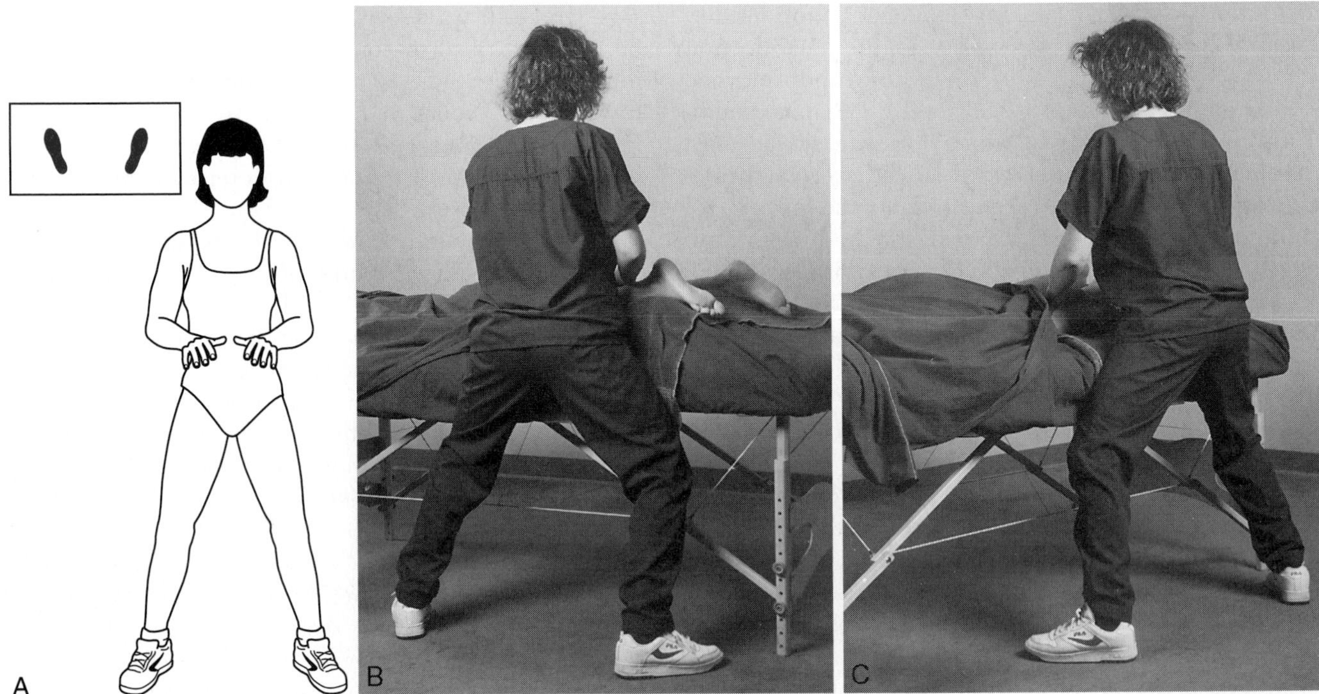

Figure 17•8 *A–C,* The horse stance.

reaching forward to moving back to your original position, simply shift your weight and flex the knees, while maintaining a *straight back.* If additional distance is needed to complete a stroke, step forward with your right and left legs, keeping your feet in the bow stance. With the bow stance, you will lean with your body weight and return to your original position, without losing contact with your client.

The Horse Stance. Also known as the warrior stance, the horse stance is used to perform massage strokes that traverse relatively short distances, such as petrissage and certain friction strokes. Both feet are placed on the floor, toes pointing forward (in the sagittal plane) a little more than hip distance apart (Fig. 17–8). The actual distance between both feet will depend on your hip size and your height. Shorter people have a lower center of gravity and their feet tend to be closer together. Taller people, who have a higher center of gravity, will place their feet farther apart. You may find that females, who often have wider hips, will place their feet farther apart.

If you are having difficulty maintaining balance, readjust your foot distance until maintaining the horse stance feels effortless. Once the proper foot distance is located, soften your knees by allowing them to flex slightly. Keep your hips pointed forward and your back straight. Your shoulders should be relaxed while your hands and arms perform the work. Pressure is added to the stroke by leaning forward. Shift your weight from one foot to the other as your hands move across the skin and muscles. This stance works particularly well for a two-handed alternating petrissage. If a lifting or lowering action is required to apply a massage stroke, raise or lower your body by bending your knees and *keeping your back straight.*

BODY MECHANICS FOR THE PRACTITIONER OF MASSAGE THERAPY

As mentioned in the introduction, certain barriers may reduce the effectiveness of the massage and even cause damage to the therapist's body. Anatomical and physiological barriers are self-limiting problems that arise from within the therapist, usually manifesting as pain or weakness in the joints or muscles. These barriers are generally due to incorrect working posture and techniques. Physiological barriers may take their toll from the duration of a single long workday or may develop slowly over the course of a career. Poor working posture and hand technique can increase stress on the joints, creating repetitive motion injuries. The solution to both of these problems is proper body mechanics.

Body mechanics is defined as the proper use of postural techniques to deliver massage therapy with the utmost efficiency and with minimum trauma to the practitioner. Also known as biomechanics, proper body mechanics will influence the execution of the massage, decrease fatigue and discomfort for the massage therapist during and after the massage session, and help

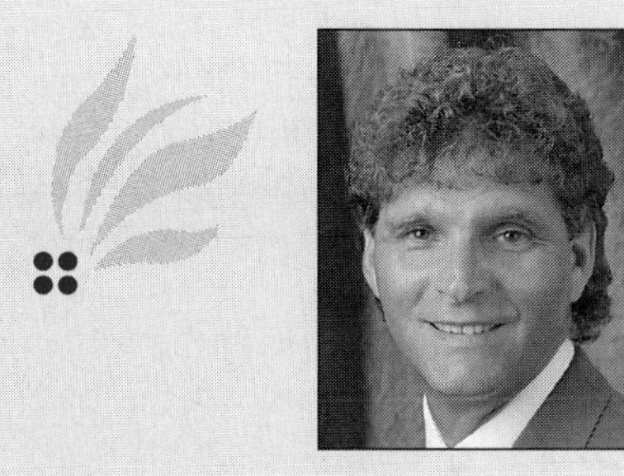

Paul St. John

Born: July 27, 1945

"Where all the growth is in this profession and in life is the line of most resistance. Oftentimes we resist so much of what life wants to teach us and why we're here."

The St. John Method of Neuromuscular Therapy is a comprehensive program of soft-tissue manipulation techniques that balance the central nervous system with the structure and form of the musculoskeletal system. On a more basic level it is the study of how form impacts function. The St. John Method can free the body to move, stand, and simply "be" the way it was created to be from a structural as well as a biochemical model.

Unlike some therapies that relax individuals and relieve minor pain, deep neuromuscular work zeroes in on the problem as well as the effect. According to St. John, the five principles of neuromuscular therapy are biomechanics, postural distortion, trigger points, nerve entrapment/nerve compression, and ischemia, all of which upset homeostasis.

Much of the charisma and commitment of Paul St. John, the man behind the method, was captured by Robert Calvert in an interview for *Massage Magazine.* St. John was 3 years old when his father, an illegal alien, was deported. He was a street kid and an average student who discovered later he had a learning disability. Playing high school football, he suffered his first injury, a broken back. Out of boredom one day he took an Army recruiter's aptitude test and did exceptionally well, but he wasn't quite ready to join. Instead he studied radiology, mainly because radiation therapy had helped his mother's cancer. While practicing radiology, he became disillusioned with medicine and voiced his concerns, which led to his being drafted in the middle of the Vietnam War. When his plane was shot down—his second bout with painful injuries—two Chinese doctors accomplished in minutes what the hospital had not been able to do in weeks.

Finally he was able to return home. His mother, like most, wanted him to get out right away and get a job. So he hitchhiked to Florida where he worked as a garbage man until his third accident. He began to have debilitating pain and, after spending a small fortune on doctors' visits, there was no improvement. That's when a chiropractic friend introduced St. John to the work of Dr. Raymond Nimmo, who developed a technique called receptor tonus. St. John learned as much as he could and soon began helping friends cope with pain. Not wanting to delay his career, he opted to attend massage therapy school. Now he is a teacher and practitioner who explains he never wants to lose touch with clients. It is as if his own encounters with pain, as well as his encounters with those in pain, fuel his desire to do even more. He is the perpetual student.

Today he is changing the quality of lives with his methods, giving hope to people who have not found relief through conventional means. "Why People Don't Heal" is the title of a particular St. John seminar that explores the relationship between form and function. "Medicine has unconsciously become totally function oriented," explains St. John. "It ignores form. But if you have someone with a collapsed diaphragmatic posture, peristaltic action and nutrient absorption is affected. The stomach collapses and loses tone. The medical community might suggest a laxative. You've got to treat the cause and not the effect. America spent over $4 billion for analgesics, medicines to suppress symptoms, this past year [1997]."

St. John shares the results of one of his latest cases: "A young woman, who was about to have a surgery to correct her scoliosis, spent some time at my clinic. Doctors were going to put a rod in her back. We corrected her curvature 27 percent and we have the x-rays to prove it."

He goes on to share other relationships between structure and disease. "Parkinson's patients almost all have a distortion in their cranium. In many stroke victims there is a forward head posture of 6 to 8 inches. This traps

continued on page 374

Continued

Paul St. John

the arteries. Patients with cardiac problems usually have a slumping shoulder posture. An abdominal posture affects the diaphragm, the aorta, the vena cava, and esophagus. That's why so many of these people develop hiatal hernias.

"Neuromuscular therapy is the best value for the money," says St. John. "If your carburetor needs fixing, you get it fixed, right? But we let our bodies stay broken down."

After treatment, St. John's clients ask, "Why hasn't my doctor done this? It makes so much sense!" Still, there are the skeptical. A man with a bad knee, who'd practically been dragged to the clinic, told St. John, "I know what's wrong with my knee. I'm 72 years old." So St. John pointed to the patient's good knee and said, "Oh yeah, so how old is that knee?

"He had a belief," explains St. John, "a belief in permanence creating a state of mind called inertia. So I created doubt by asking him about his good knee. Doubt is energy in itself. Once I created doubt in the permanence of his condition, it opened the door for me to point out that his right shoulder and pelvis were inferior, the knee was twisted and compressed, the left shoulder and pelvis were elevated."

St. John has many success stories, but because of his commitment to his work, little time. He has patients waiting. The interview is over with these words of advice for the beginning therapist, "Take personal responsibility. Specialize in a certain area if you really want to make a living. Techniques that work and work best conform to the laws of the universe. One-third medicine is intellectual, two-thirds is art."

In the Calvert article, St. John offers direction for anyone seeking success. "People who accomplish great things are ordinary people who have great dreams. It's not that they are more gifted and God has smiled upon them. People who become great have great work ethics and they put a lot of sweat equity into it. They aren't lucky people, you know, they work hard and they're committed."

prevent repetitive motion injuries for the therapist. Body mechanics include basic foot stances, posture, weight distribution, and joint stabilization when delivering pressure.

Proper body mechanics are a direct result of balanced static and dynamic posture during the massage. Although most massage movements are dynamic, static posture is often used to begin and end the massage while the hands are rested on the client's skin or on top of the drape. Proper posture takes into consideration structural alignment and physical principles of work (such as leverage) so as to minimize effort and reduce the likelihood of strain or injury. It is using the right tool in the best way to do the right job. While it is possible to drive a screw into a board with a hammer, substituting a nail for the screw or a screwdriver for the hammer will accomplish the job more efficiently. Proper body mechanics allow the therapist to take advantage of the natural design of the body's network of joints, tendons, ligaments, muscles, and other structures to accomplish small engineering feats.

Proper body mechanics also respect the laws of gravity. Gravity is the attraction of an object toward the center of a planetary sphere (Earth). When you are balanced in your gravitational field, less energy is expended during the massage. The center of gravity is the point at which the body is balanced, generally between the fourth and fifth lumbar vertebrae on the front of the spine, or an inch or two below your navel. Move your center of gravity slightly. Feel the body respond to keep balance. Move the center of gravity farther in space. Feel gravity pull you into a pattern of locomotion such as falling, walking, leaping, or running. Centering then, in the *physical* sense, is a state of balance in relation to all other living things. This principle can be expanded to an emotional/spiritual awareness or energetic experience of ourselves in relation to all our surroundings. This sensation of "peaceful energy" is experienced in the same place as our center of gravity. Using all these principles enables the therapist to *center* herself on all levels in preparation for a massage.

Balance and the distribution of weight vary according to the type of massage being performed. Lifting moves such as petrissage are more effective when the therapist's center of gravity is concentrated over his own feet, not over the client's body. This balanced stance allows for full freedom of movement. Deep-tissue work and downward strokes such as effleurage are more effective and demand less energy if the therapist shifts his center of gravity over the client. This facilitates downward pressure by making use of the therapist's own body weight, rather than exerting more pressure by using the arm muscles.

Author's Note

Often, while I am teaching massage, I will see a student in perfect balance. It is a beautiful thing—calm, simple, and direct. Balance through the bones produces minimal feedback in the nervous system—a curious state of low sensation because it is low stress.

Rules for Good Body Mechanics

1. If you are working on a table that is not yours or if someone else has borrowed your table, check the table height to make sure it is appropriate for you. A proper table height allows you to use your weight rather than your strength to develop pressure. Position the table accessories (e.g., head rest, arm shelf, and bolsters) to fit the client's body proportions, in order to give you optimum access to the various body parts with a minimum of strain. Other table height considerations are the size of the client (larger clients usually require a lower massage table), the type of massage you will perform (deeper massage usually requires a lower table), and the area of concentration (backwork typically requires a lower table and face- and footwork are more comfortable for the therapist on a higher table).
2. Always wear sensible supportive shoes with low or no heels and good arch supports. In addition, your clothing should be comfortable and professional. Cotton clothes are best because they absorb the body's perspiration, which helps keep the therapist cool.
3. Always warm up before giving a massage, especially on cold mornings and before strenuous routines such as active assisted stretching or body mobilization techniques. Warm muscles are less susceptible to injury. Stretching can be done as part of the warm-up, but make sure that some other form of warm-up has been used to increase the heart rate before stretching.
4. If you have to lift or move an object, keep the heaviest part close to your body. Use your legs, not your back, when lifting. Reduce friction by sliding a blanket under the object to be relocated.
5. Know your own limits. Do not try to lift a body part that is too heavy. Ask for assistance.
6. During the massage, use deep, full abdominal breathing. This will aid you in self-relaxation and will help you keep a steady pace with your massage strokes.
7. Find your *own* rhythm and then move *with* it. For example, petrissage can be done more efficiently in the horse stance with a side-to-side rocking motion. The rocking motion itself can be learned from an instructor, but the rate or rhythm is an internal component that originates within the therapist and is determined by the client.
8. Keep your movements smooth and flowing. What is jerky and rough for you is jerky and rough for your client as well.
9. Keep your feet planted firmly on the ground while standing, and let your feet reflect what your hands are doing. For example, use the horse stance for local work on a small area of tissue and the bow stance for gliding strokes.
10. Keep your knees soft and slightly bent to absorb shock better. Never lock the knees straight.
11. Keep your upper arm perpendicular to your upper body and your forearm parallel to the ground whenever possible. When your arms are far away from your body, they tend to fatigue faster. Avoid reaching across the table because this can strain your back. Your shoulders and upper back should be relaxed to help you keep your wrist and fingers in proper alignment. Avoid raising your shoulders to your ears.
12. Keep the wrists as straight as possible. At times it will be necessary to flex and extend the wrist, but remember that the greater the pressure, the straighter the wrist should be. Hyperextending the wrist while applying pressure can produce overuse injuries such as tendinitis and carpal tunnel syndrome.
13. Do not let the digits become hyperextended while applying direct pressure. Use braced finger techniques to avoid joint hyperextension (Fig. 17–9).
14. Instead of contracting your arm muscles to produce downward force, lean forward, using your body weight to create the pressure needed.
15. Keep your back straight by tilting your pelvis forward, which flattens out the low back and reduces an exaggerated anterior lumbar curve. Use the "penny-pinching" technique (see the Mini-Lab for specific instructions).
16. Keep your body in correct alignment by maintaining your head over your neck and shoulders. Keep your forward head posture to a minimum. When working on a muscle or group of muscles, keep

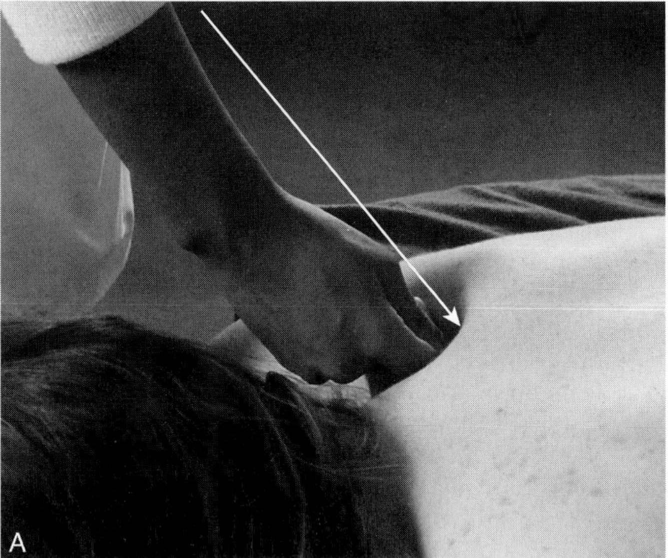

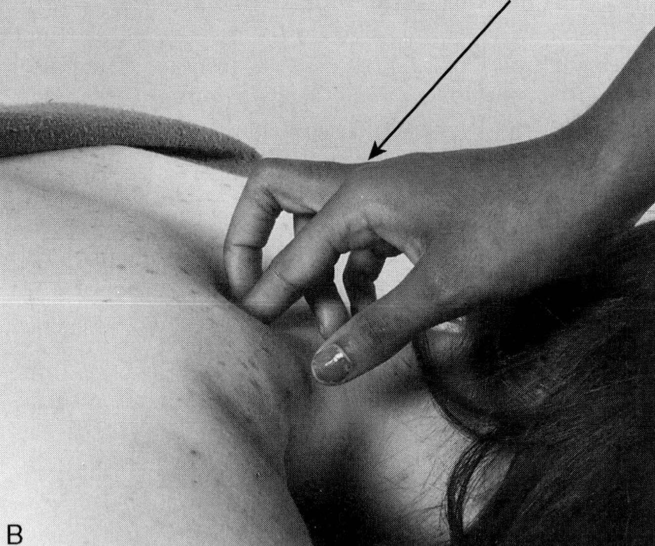

Figure 17•9 *A* and *B*, Braced finger technique.

your eyes forward, your neck straight, and your head erect. If you spend a great amount of time looking down, your neck may become stiff. If you must observe your work, lower yourself to the level of your hands (on your knees). Look up, out the window, or at the corners of the ceiling occasionally to stretch the anterior neck musculature. Another way to reduce the strain on your neck is to turn your head away from the direction of the massage stroke. Experiment with different head and neck positions for different massage strokes to discover which positions are more comfortable for you.

17. Take stretch breaks while walking from one side of the table to the other. Use this time to shake out your arms, stretch your neck, and relax. Clients usually do not see these breaks because they are either face down, have their eyes closed, or are asleep.
18. Between massage sessions spend a few minutes doing exercises to strengthen and stretch the muscles of the hands. The exercises at the beginning of the chapter can be used for this purpose.
19. Most massage routines are designed to protect the therapist from overuse injuries by varying the strokes and by changing foot and hand positions. Changing from effleurage to petrissage to tapotement to friction uses different muscle groups, thus reducing fatigue and repetitive motion injuries. As the therapist you must also listen to your own body. If the right forearm is fatiguing, use the left arm more; if compressive movements are irritating wrist and knuckle joints, change to a lifting move such as petrissage.
20. Avoid staying on your feet the entire day. Sit on a stool while performing foot or facial routines. Use the table for support when you need it; sit, lean, and brace yourself on the massage table. Allow enough time between massages for a sufficient break. If your body is going to make it to retirement, you have to be prepared to take care of yourself today.
21. Be aware of facial expression. Keep your jaw unlocked and your forehead relaxed.
22. Practice what you preach. Get regular bodywork yourself to keep your biomechanics working at optimum.

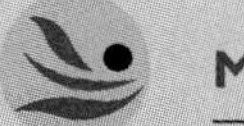

MINI•LAB

Stand in front of a full-length mirror. Place one foot 18 inches in front of the other and place your hands on your hips. Lunge forward, shifting your weight from the back leg to the front leg. As you move forward and backward, keep your shoulders and hips level. Look in the mirror to check your progress. Maintaining a good posture while you are in motion promotes a good working posture while performing massage therapy.

Body Mechanics Quick Check

Here's a list of questions to help you determine if correct body mechanics are used during the massage. Answer yes or no.

1. Is your massage table the correct height for you?
2. Are you warming up before your first massage of the day and stretching between massage sessions?

REPETITIVE MOTION INJURIES AMONG MASSAGE THERAPISTS

The number one reason why massage therapists decide to leave the industry is not professional burn-out or missed employment opportunities—it is injuries due to repetitive motions of the wrist and fingers. Our bodies were designed to be in motion. We begin to have problems when we start moving poorly. Even with understanding and use of proper body mechanics, body tissues will react negatively when the same motion is repeated excessively.

Repetitive motion injuries are caused by the repeated flexing and extending of a joint against resistance, which may result from activity or manual manipulation of tools or other equipment. The two most common types of repetitive motion injuries are carpal tunnel syndrome and ulnar neuropathy. The good news is that injuries can be prevented through understanding of cause and effect. Since this type of injury can shorten your career, let's examine repetitive motion injuries in detail.

Repetitive strain injuries (RSI), also known as repetitive motion injuries, encompass a broad spectrum of injuries that are related to inefficient biomechanics including general posture, sporting movements, and work habits. The constant single motion, combined with compressive forces, causes injury in the soft tissues. The symptoms and damage are progressive, unless the inefficient biomechanics or repetitive strain is altered. The general symptoms of RSI are related to the inflammation response: pain, redness, heat, and swelling. Initial symptoms are usually limited to the soft tissues. The progression of injury goes from muscle soreness to increased tonus to the formation of multiple trigger points, and in some cases to nerve entrapment. Chronic injuries may result in subluxation or trauma to the joints, including bursitis, arthritis, and even stress fractures of involved bones.

In sports, tennis elbow is a good example of a repetitive strain injury. The repeated rotation of the wrist while supporting the weight of the extended tennis racket causes a tendinitis irritation of the forearm extender muscles. Massage, ice, and a compression bandage can provide temporary relief. To properly assess the problem, seek the advice of a physician, physical therapist, or athletic trainer. Often the solution is to reduce the inflammation, to increase muscle strength through weight training, and to use a racquet of lighter weight.

For our clients, poor work habits are probably the leading cause of these types of injuries, and they are 100 percent preventable. All it takes is a little education. First, the client has to be made aware of the potential damage being done to his body, the warning signs and symptoms and the consequences. The client can then implement a new work habit. This again involves education of proper body mechanics, such as lifting and keyboarding. The only way to break a bad habit is to replace it with a good one. The worst thing about repetitive motion injuries is that they take time to occur. By the time they are symptomatic, we are already in the "habit" of doing an activity a certain way.

An example of an on-the-job repetitive motion injury is the secretary who holds the phone to his ear with his shoulder, which frees his hands to do other things. Years of this behavior, especially if he favors one shoulder, may lead to headaches, muscular tension, and eventually cervical disk herniation. In this case, an earphone with wraparound microphone or even a simple speaker phone may provide the relief he needs and still allow him to function efficiently.

But the great equalizer is *pain.* It eventually will get everyone's attention. Some examples of RSI in relation to the practice of massage therapy follow.

1. Inflammation in the wrist due to poor biomechanics, especially wrist hyperextension
2. Inflammation in the knuckle joints of the thumb and fingers, from digital hyperextension and the repetition of cross-fiber friction over a period of time
3. Numbness in the tips of the digits due to excessive trigger point work
4. Compression damage and nerve entrapment from incorrect technique during trigger point work with the olecranon process of the ulna (tip of the elbow)

The best ways for you to reduce the likelihood of RSI is to use a variety of strokes, to rest your hands by spacing your clients, to stretch between sessions, to adjust the height of the massage table, to avoid sustained pressure or delayed compression, to keep your body physically fit, and to use proper body mechanics.

3. Are you using proper lifting techniques?
4. Are you shifting your weight as you move, working with your whole body?
5. Are your knees slightly bent?
6. Are your feet firmly planted on the ground?
7. Is your upper arm perpendicular to your upper body?
8. Is your forearm parallel to the ground?
9. Are your wrists straight?
10. Are your thumb and fingers supported while applying direct pressure?
11. Is your back straight and your lower pelvis tilted forward?
12. Is your head centered over your neck and shoulder?
13. Are you using a variety of strokes in your massage?
14. Is a stool nearby to be used during facial and foot massages?
15. Is your face relaxed and your jaw unlocked during the massage?

If you answered no to one or more of these questions, you may be at risk for stress, strain, and injury due to poor body mechanics.

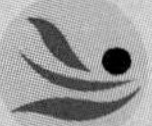

MINI•LAB

To experience a forward-tilted pelvis, try the "penny pinching" technique. While standing, imagine that you have a penny between your buttocks. To keep the penny from falling to the ground, contract your gluteal muscles and "pinch" the penny. This simple exercise straightens your back muscles, pulls in your abdominal muscles and tilts your pelvis forward.

Author's Note

A full-length mirror in your massage room can help you observe and adjust your body mechanics.

CLIENT POSITIONING

Once you have interviewed your client, and directed her to the massage table, you must determine how to position her while she receives the massage. First, in which position do you want the client to lie—the prone, the supine, side-lying, or the seated position? The next consideration is how you want the client's joints (e.g., neck, back, knees, and ankles) positioned during the massage. The last consideration is to determine if the client has any physical needs or limitations, such as a knee condition, that would require an adjustment to her position on the table or additional bolstering. But no matter which positions you and the client decide, it is a good idea to ask your client, "How can you become even more comfortable?" This process allows you to fine-tune the client's position and address her comfort needs.

The **prone position,** or lying belly-side down, is used when massaging the posterior side of the body. In the **supine position,** or lying backside down, you can massage the anterior side of the body. The **side-lying position** allows easy access to the neck and shoulders, arms, hands, medial and lateral thighs, and limited access to the back, anterior and posterior legs, and feet. Limited access is defined as access to a body area in a position that may be awkward for the therapist. Since the back, parts of the legs, and feet are approached from a vertical position, the therapist adjusts his body position for the best leverage, including squatting or kneeling down on the floor, while leaning or pushing to work these areas. The side-lying position is essential when the client is in the second or third trimester of pregnancy or if the client is elderly; has a colostomy, recent surgery, or vertebral fusion; or has any other situation in which use of the prone or supine position is limited or contraindicated.

The **seated position,** also known as the chair position, describes a massage given while the client is sitting in an ordinary chair or a chair that has been specially designed for client comfort and accessibility to major tension areas of the body. When an ordinary chair is used, the client leans forward and rests her head on a cushion placed on the top of the chair back or nearby table. The seated position may be preferable in one of the following situations.

1. The client prefers a chair massage or if the environment is more conducive to using a chair. This can be for a variety of reasons. A chair massage is often used when massaging a client at his office.
2. A massage table is not available.
3. There is not adequate physical space to set up a massage table and to use proper body mechanics during the massage.
4. The client has a condition (e.g., handicap, pain, mobility problem, or recent surgery) that makes it difficult to get on or off a massage table.
5. The client is in a wheelchair. Note: It may not be feasible for the client to transfer to a massage table or chair. Work with him in the wheelchair. Simply roll the chair up to the side of the massage table so that his legs are underneath. Lock the wheels in position, lean the client forward on a cushion, and proceed with the massage.
6. There is not enough time for a regular massage session. A regular massage session can last from 30 to 90 minutes.
7. The client has reservations about removing clothing for the massage.

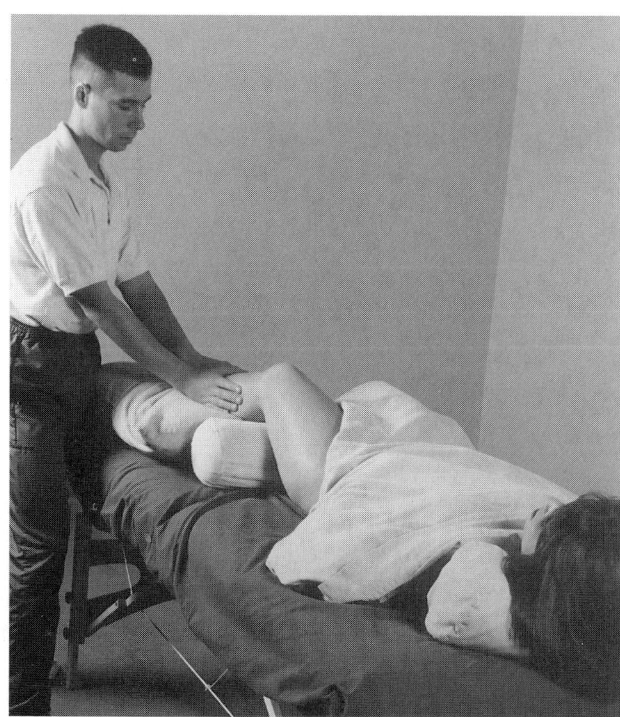

Figure 17•10 Client prone using an ankle bolster and demonstrating correct body posture for the therapist.

If you have determined that the seated position will best serve your client, refer to the information in Chapter 25, Seated Massage, for specific details on how to position your client for comfort and accessibility.

To provide greater client comfort and proper body mechanics in the prone, supine, or side-lying position, use cylinder-shaped bolstering devices. These cushions support the client's individual joints, which in turn more fully relaxes the muscles (Fig. 17–10). The three most commonly bolstered areas are the neck, ankles, and knees. In the absence of bolsters, as in you being away from your office while giving a massage, a rolled up towel, blanket, or pillow may be used.

Position the seam running lengthwise on the bolster away from the client's body. This will prevent any uncomfortable sensations or compression marks left on the client's skin. Always drape the bolster or pillow with a protective covering, such as a towel or specially designed bolster cover. These covers must be washed after each client use. The bolster may also be placed between the bottom sheet and the table surface. Remove the bolster before your client gets up off the massage table to dress. Clean your bolster at the start of each business day with a mild detergent (like dish soap). If the bolster or bolster sheet comes into contact with any body fluids, disinfect the surface with a solution of water and chlorine bleach in a ten-to-one solution.

Prone Position. The most frequently supported areas when the client is in the prone position are anterior ankles and the head/neck complex. If possible, use a face rest or specially designed prone pillow. This will allow your client to keep her neck straight while lying face down. If a face rest is not available, one or two standard-size pillows may be used, placing them either horizontally or diagonally under the head and shoulders. Large-chested women may need additional pillow support under the breasts or on the sternum.

A vinyl-covered 6- or 8-inch bolster under the anterior ankles allows the hips and legs to relax fully during the massage. Try both sizes to see which one works the best for each client. If the client complains of his low back feeling strained by lying prone, a pillow or soft cushion placed under the abdomen or pelvis reduces the anterior curve (lordosis), which may reduce the strained feeling. Clients who have mild to severe kyphosis may benefit from an additional pillow under

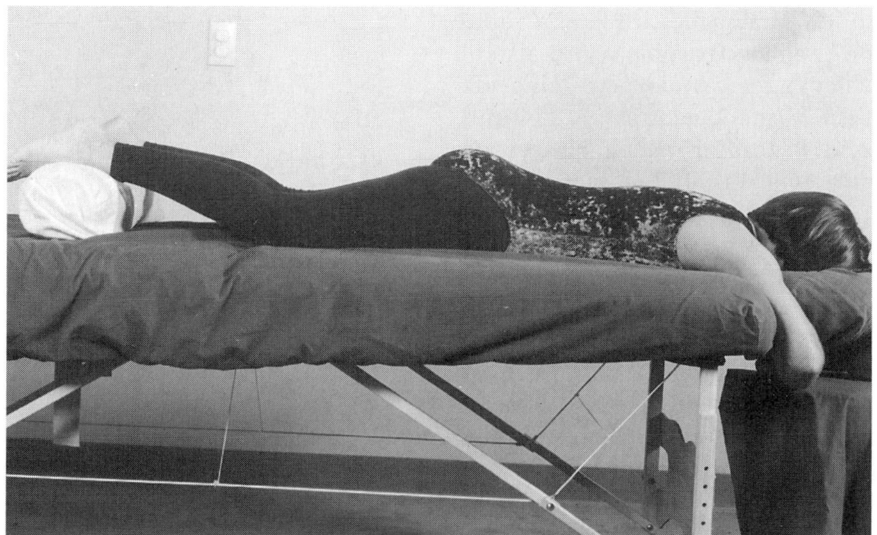

Figure 17•11 Ideal prone position using bolsters, arm shelf, and face rest.

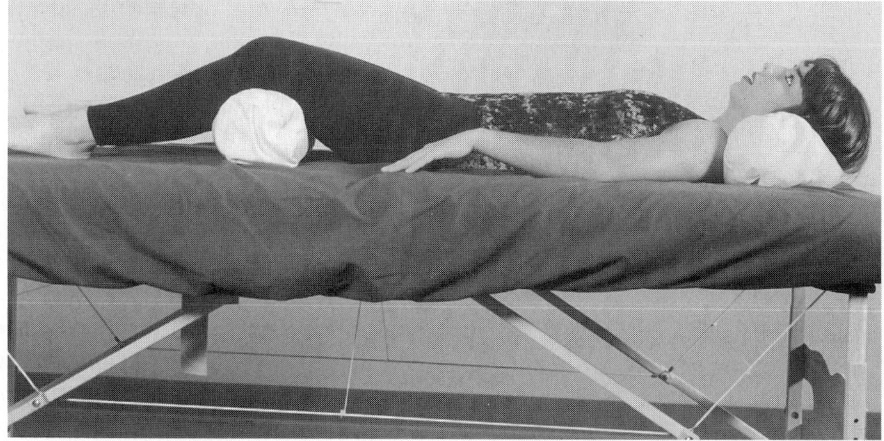

Figure 17•12 Ideal supine position using bolsters.

the clavicles while their faces are resting in the face rest cushion or on a standard-size pillow. For added shoulder and arm relaxation, an arm shelf or stool placed under the face rest can be used for a forearm rest (Fig. 17–11).

Supine Position. When the client is in the supine position, also known as the dorsal recumbent position, the most frequently supported areas are the posterior cervical region and the posterior knees. Use of a knee bolster helps to relax the low back. A soft cloth-covered cervical pillow is best; place it at the lower cervical region, not the occipital region (Fig. 17–12). A rolled-up bath-size towel can be used as a cervical pillow; fold both long sides toward the middle, leaving a 1-inch space down the middle before rolling the towel (Fig. 17–13).

While you are massaging the feet in the supine position, place a large pillow under the feet to elevate them to provide easier access to the feet and facilitate proper body mechanics for you. This added foot support also assists dependent drainage in cases of lymphedema. You may sit on the massage table or on a stool while massaging the client's feet. Avoid permitting the client to raise her own feet simultaneously because this may strain her low back. Instead, ask her to place one foot on the pillow at a time or lift her feet for her onto the pillow.

Side-Lying Position. Also known as the lateral position or lateral recumbent position, the side-lying position is preferred for pregnancy, for some elderly people, in cases of recent surgeries, and for various other conditions. The client may lie in either a right lateral or left lateral position. To facilitate the client's getting into a lateral or side-lying position from a prone or supine position, anchor the sheet on one side with your leg, and hold the sheet with your hand by reaching across the table. Instruct the client to roll to the side and to face either toward you or away from you. The direction usually is the side on which the client feels most comfortable, but you may dictate the direction. Use three or four pillows to allow the client to lie comfortably on her side. Place the first pillow underneath her head. The next pillow should be placed under the upper arm (the side of the body not against the table), supporting her arm and shoulder complex. The last is positioned under the upper knee and ankle complex; this pillow helps relax the hip and low back. If the hip, knee, and ankle are not all in the same horizontal plane, add another pillow until the proper

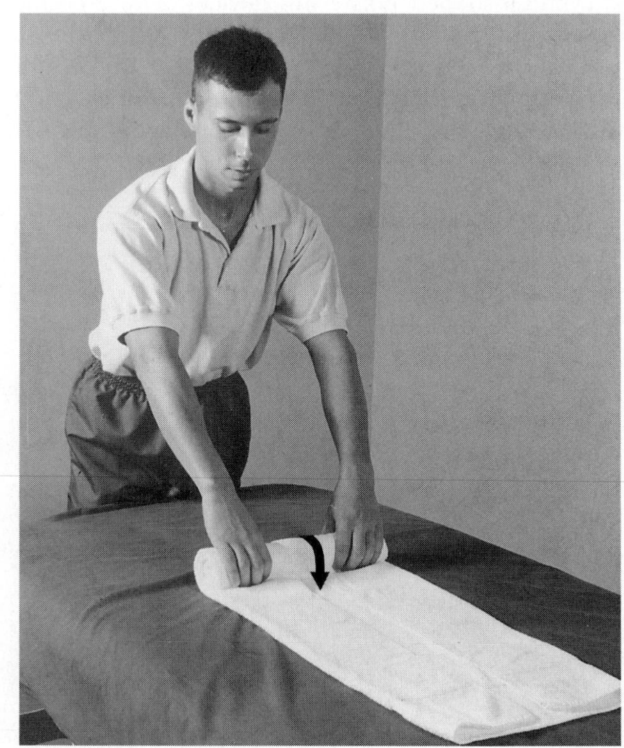

Figure 17•13 Rolling up a bath-size towel for a cervical pillow.

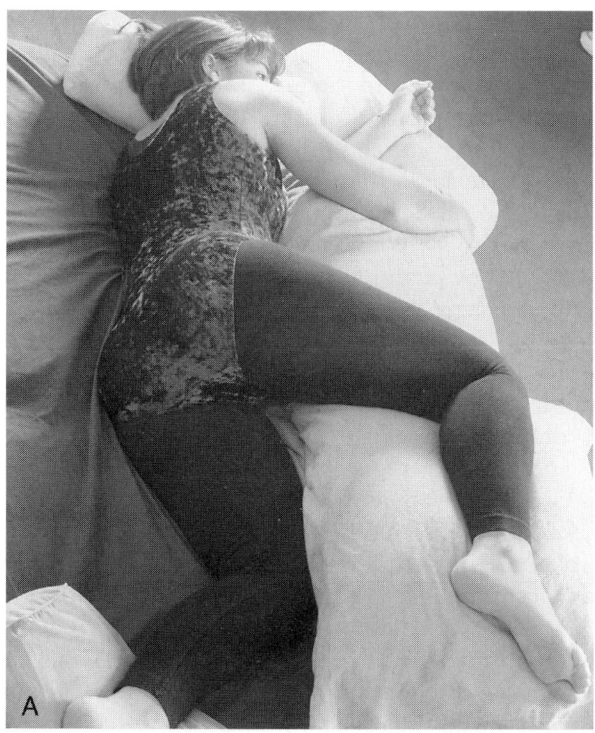

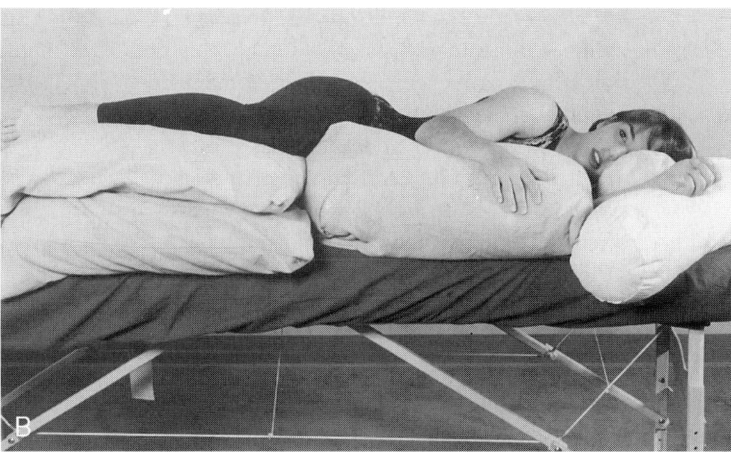

Figure 17•14 *A* and *B*, Side-lying position with pillows.

height is achieved. Two additional smaller pillows may be added under the wrist of the lower arm and under the lower ankle (side of the body touching the table). Before the side-lying massage is complete, the client will lie on both her left and right sides. See Figure 17–14 in this section, which demonstrates proper pillow postioning for the side-lying position.

Before your client changes positions, or before she gets up from the massage table after the session, remove all pillows and bolsters to reduce physical barriers that may impede her movement.

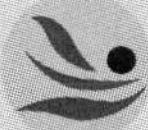

MINI•LAB

Acquire approximately six pillows of various sizes, a massage table, and a partner. Ask your partner to lie on the massage table in the supine position, and use the pillows to create a variety of comfortable positions. Once all possibilities are explored, remove the pillows from the massage table and ask your partner to turn over and lie on his side. Reuse the pillows to position your partner's arms, legs, and so on. Repeat the activity in the prone position. This discovery method will help you discover new and creative ways to work with pillows as bolstering devices.

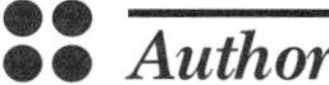

Author's Note

How do you begin the massage? Prone? Supine? How do you decide? What are the pros and cons of each method? Some therapists prefer to start their clients prone and end the massage with their clients supine or vice versa, while other therapists let the client decide. Here are some things to think about as you decide:

1. **Beginning Prone, Ending Supine.** Most clients complain of back-related pain. Beginning prone allows you to massage this crucial area first. Ending supine allows your client's sinuses to drain, otherwise she may leave your establishment with a stuffy head from being prone. Beginning prone also allows all genital regions of the body to be underneath the client's body and allows time for trust between the client and therapist to develop. Even with the best face rest, the client's neck may become stiff while lying prone. Beginning prone and ending supine allows the neck to be worked in the last half of the session to reduce or eliminate any neck stiffness that may have occurred from lying prone. Many therapists wrap their client up in the bottom sheet like a human cocoon. Ending supine allows this without disturbing the client by asking him to roll over supine.
2. **Beginning Supine, Ending Prone.** Clients often enjoy conversing with their therapists

but also enjoy silence during the massage. When you begin the massage supine, this position allows conversation and eye contact between the client and the therapist. When the client rolls onto her abdomen, this often signals a time of quiet rest. Ending prone also allows the back to be worked last, which is often the primary area of complaint.

After these considerations, weigh the pros and cons, and decide which position sequence you or your client prefers. You may even decide to finish the massage with the client in the side-lying position to allow her to rest before getting up off the table. The side-lying position also allows the client's back to be stretched; especially if you ask her to pull both knees to her chest into a fetal position.

DRAPING YOUR CLIENT FOR THE MASSAGE SESSION

The purpose of using a **drape** during massage therapy is to provide a professional atmosphere that supports the client's need for emotional privacy (modesty) and comfort, but also provide access to individual body parts. Covering up the body with cloth allows the client to be undressed while receiving the massage.

The primary comfort consideration is warmth. Clients may have difficulty relaxing if they are chilled, which may occur as the massage progresses because the parasympathetic nervous system is activated, causing a drop in basal body temperature. Always ask the client if he is comfortably warm at least twice during the session: once before you start the massage and halfway through. Even though you may have established communication during the consultation, an inquiry made about the client's comfort level will indicate to the client that he is special, as well as encouraging open communication. If he indicates that he is chilled, additional draping may be added by placing a blanket across the top sheet. If he becomes too warm, more body surface area can be exposed, provided the following areas remain draped at all times: the genital region on both men and women, the gluteal cleft, and in some areas of the United States, the breast area on females.

In addressing draping with regard to privacy or modesty of either the therapist or client, there are basically three rules that apply. The first rule is the state or local laws regarding draping—this is your minimum draping standard and you cannot drape with less than the law requires without endangering your license. The second rule is to honor the client's individual request for draping. As long as it does not conflict with your state laws, you may add extra draping or remove superfluous draping. For example, European and American customs contrast greatly concerning the female breast. European clients may object to an upper drape, while many American clients would refuse the massage without it. If your female client requests a lower drape only and there is *no conflict* with your state laws, then you may work her with the bottom drape only. The third rule is that the massage therapist has to be comfortable with the level of draping as well. For example, a client who lives in a state with no massage therapy legislation may be perfectly comfortable receiving a massage with no top drape. However, the therapist may be uncomfortable with this situation. The therapist may elect to use a more complete drape or refuse to perform the massage. For more information regarding draping and ethics, see Chapter 2, Professional Standards and Boundaries.

Expose only the body areas being massaged. For example, if you are massaging the back, both legs should be draped. If you are working on the posterior aspect of the left leg, the back *and* the right leg should be draped. By exposing only the areas that are being massaged, clients stay warmer, and physical and psychological boundaries are created, which gives a feeling of personal privacy. One reason why heavier sheet material such as flannel is preferred is because of the client's ability to feel heavier sheet material more easily, which is important while her eyes are closed.

The two main types of drapes are sheets and towels. Become proficient at utilizing *both* types of drapes because there may be times when you find yourself in a situation requiring the use of the one you do not normally use. Be patient with yourself while learning draping techniques; it takes time and practice and is considered an art in itself. A challenge for most new massage therapists is turning the client over while keeping the draping securely in place. It is in turning the client that most accidental exposures occur.

You have to do your work as if everything depends on you, then leave the rest to God.

—Mother Teresa

Towel Draping. Towels are often used as draping materials because they are thicker, heavier, more opaque than sheets, smaller, and easier to maneuver, but towel draping is more difficult to master. Typically, one towel is used for draping male clients, and two towels are used to drape female clients, but do provide more drape if a client requests it. An added benefit is that towel draping provides easy access to the abdomen. A flat or fitted sheet is used as a table cover below the client during towel draping.

Instruct the client to undress and lie face down (prone) on the table, draping himself crossways with the two towels, one across the back and one across the

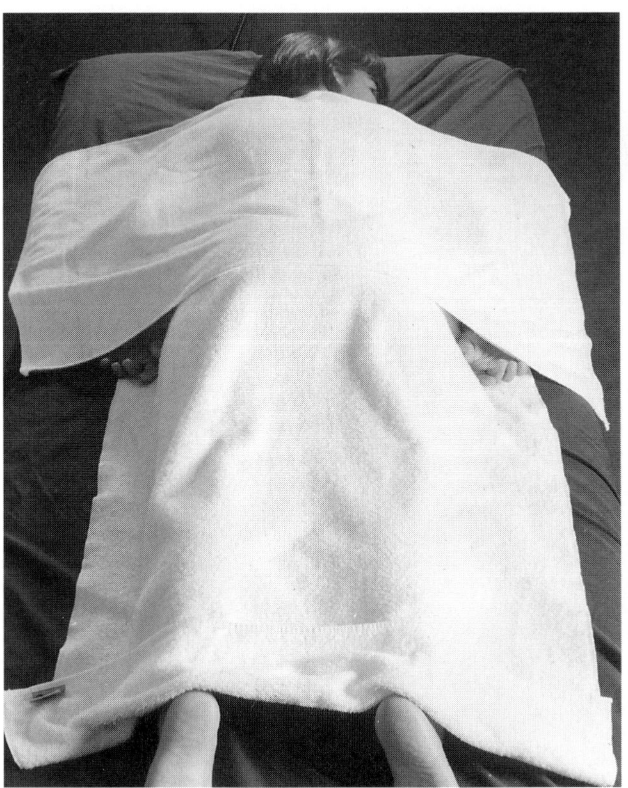

Figure 17•15 The towel T formation.

buttocks. The two towels are then parallel to each other, but perpendicular to the client's body, like an equals sign (=). After the therapist reenters the room, the bottom towel only is rotated 90 degrees, so that it is parallel to the body and creates a T where it meets the top towel (Fig. 17–15). The towels will be returned to the equals sign formation before the client is turned from the prone to the supine position.

When using towel draping, fold the towel back to reveal the area to be massaged (Figs. 17–16 and 17–17). In most circumstances, the towel will stay where it is folded, but it may be tucked underneath the body to provide a more secure draping. When instructing the client to lie down on the table and drape himself, give simple, clear directions. Use the illustrations provided to help you master draping with a towel.

Please note that towel draping is recommended for a pregnant client *only* when a pregnancy massage table is available and the towels are large bath-size towels. Towels should not be used for side-lying postures because they do not provide enough coverage.

Turning Your Client Over with Towels. Use the anchoring method. First, remove all bolstering materials before turning the client over (the towels should still be in the T formation). Rotate the lower towel back to the equals sign position using the following steps. Grasp the bottom corner of the towel with your lower hand and the top corner of the towel (opposite side of the table) with your upper hand. Keeping the center of the towel squarely over the genitalia, rotate the towel 90 degrees in a counterclockwise direction. The towels are now back in the equals sign position (Fig. 17–18*A*).

With the client in the prone position, instruct him to move down on the table so that his face is out of the face rest and he is onto the table proper, slowly guiding the towel down with him for proper coverage. His arms should be either above his head or by his sides under the top towel. The two towels should overlap each other at the abdomen by about 2 to 4 inches.

Once the towels are parallel, grasp the top corner of the top towel with your upper hand and the lower corner of the bottom towel with your lower hand. Anchor the overlapping corners at the middle of the table by leaning on them, thus securing them to the table. Instruct the client to turn to face you and continue turning (Fig. 17–18*B*) until all the way over onto his back (Fig. 17–18*C*). Return the towels to the T formation before proceeding with the massage (Fig. 17–18*D* and *E*).

To turn a client from supine to prone, use the above technique to rotate the bottom towel back into the equals sign formation. Instruct the client to turn to face *away* from you and continue all the way over until he is on his abdomen. The client may move up and make use of the face rest. Rotate the bottom towel back to the T position.

Sheet Draping. Sheets provide more coverage than towels. If you intend to use sheets as your draping material, choose an opaque fabric and color that does not reveal the client's body underneath. Two sheets are required for each client: one on the top and one on the bottom. Clients and therapists often prefer using sheets because they are already familiar with this arrangement; it is how beds are made. Twin-size sheets are preferred, but a double-size flat sheet folded in half works fine as a bottom sheet. The bottom sheet can be either flat or fitted, but the top sheet must be flat. Drape the top sheet neatly on the bottom sheet, folding the top edge down to reveal the bottom sheet, which gives the massage table an inviting appearance (Fig. 17–19). As you undrape specific areas of the body for massage, tuck the ends of the fabric underneath the client's body. Untuck the sheet, and redrape when moving to a different area for massage.

Sheet draping can be used to access all posterior body areas and most anterior body areas, the exception being the abdomen on female clients in the supine position. Two different methods can be employed to work the abdominal region on a female. First, the lower edge of the sheet can be pulled up to knee level, which creates a surplus of material around the

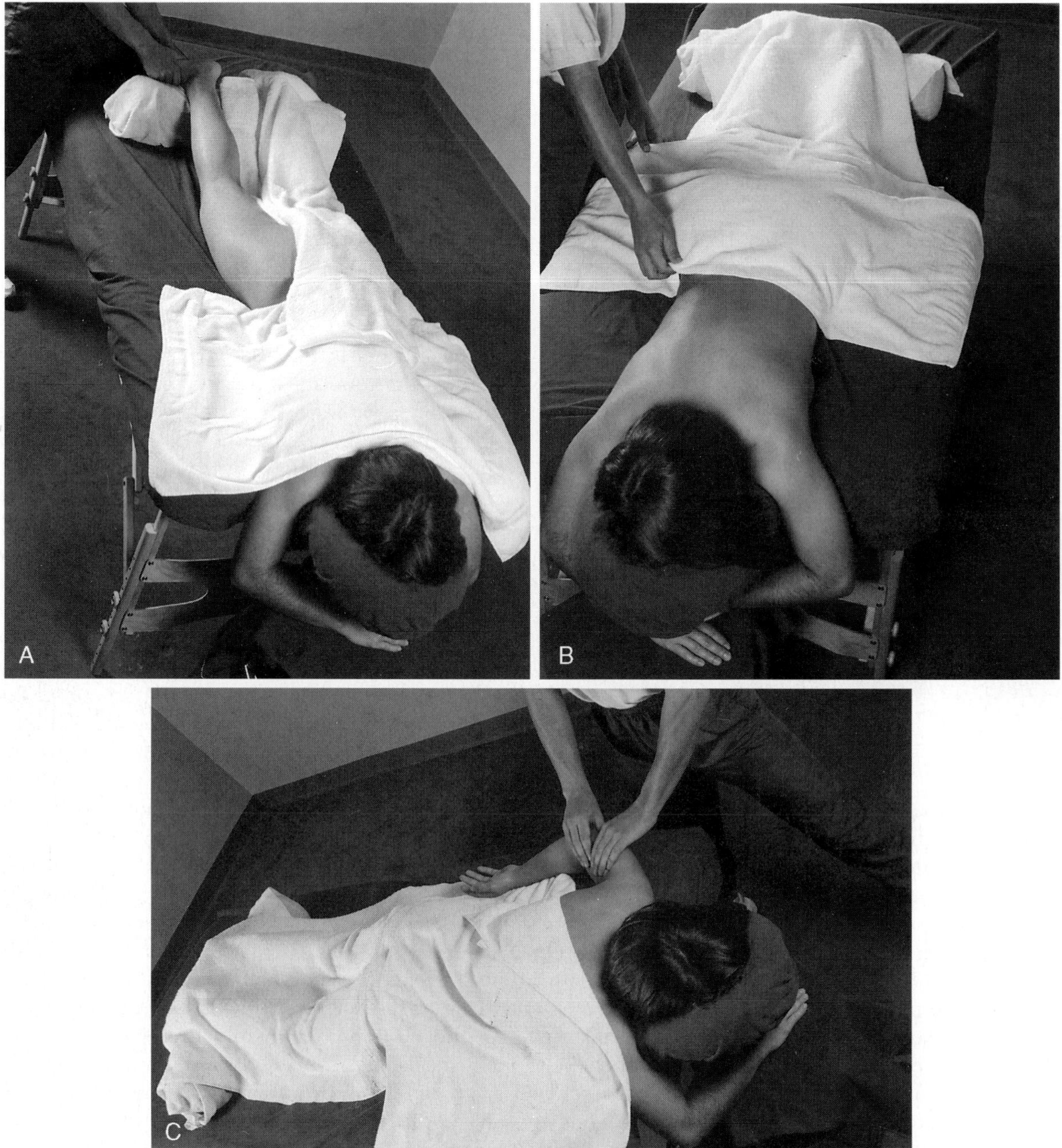

Figure 17•16 *A–C,* Towel access to posterior leg/buttock, arm, and back.

midsection. The sheet is then arranged in a C-shaped "window" to expose the abdominal area while keeping the pubic and pectoral regions covered. The second method requires the use of a towel or pillowcase. The towel is placed on top of the sheet, across the breasts, and perpendicular to the body. The top center edge of the towel is held at the superior border of the sternum with one hand. The other hand pulls the sheet out from under the towel without dislodging the towel from its position. Once the sheet is clear of the towel, the sheet is folded back to expose the abdomen, with the towel acting as a "bikini top." In both methods, care must be taken to keep the female breasts covered while the abdomen is being exposed. Figures 17–20 and 17–21 will assist you in using sheets as a drape during your massage session.

Turning Your Client Over with Sheets. Holding the sheet on the side of the table while the client turns over is called the anchoring method. It is the best method for turning the client over because it provides the best mobility and coverage. Before turning the client over, remove all bolstering materials. With the client in the prone position, instruct her to move

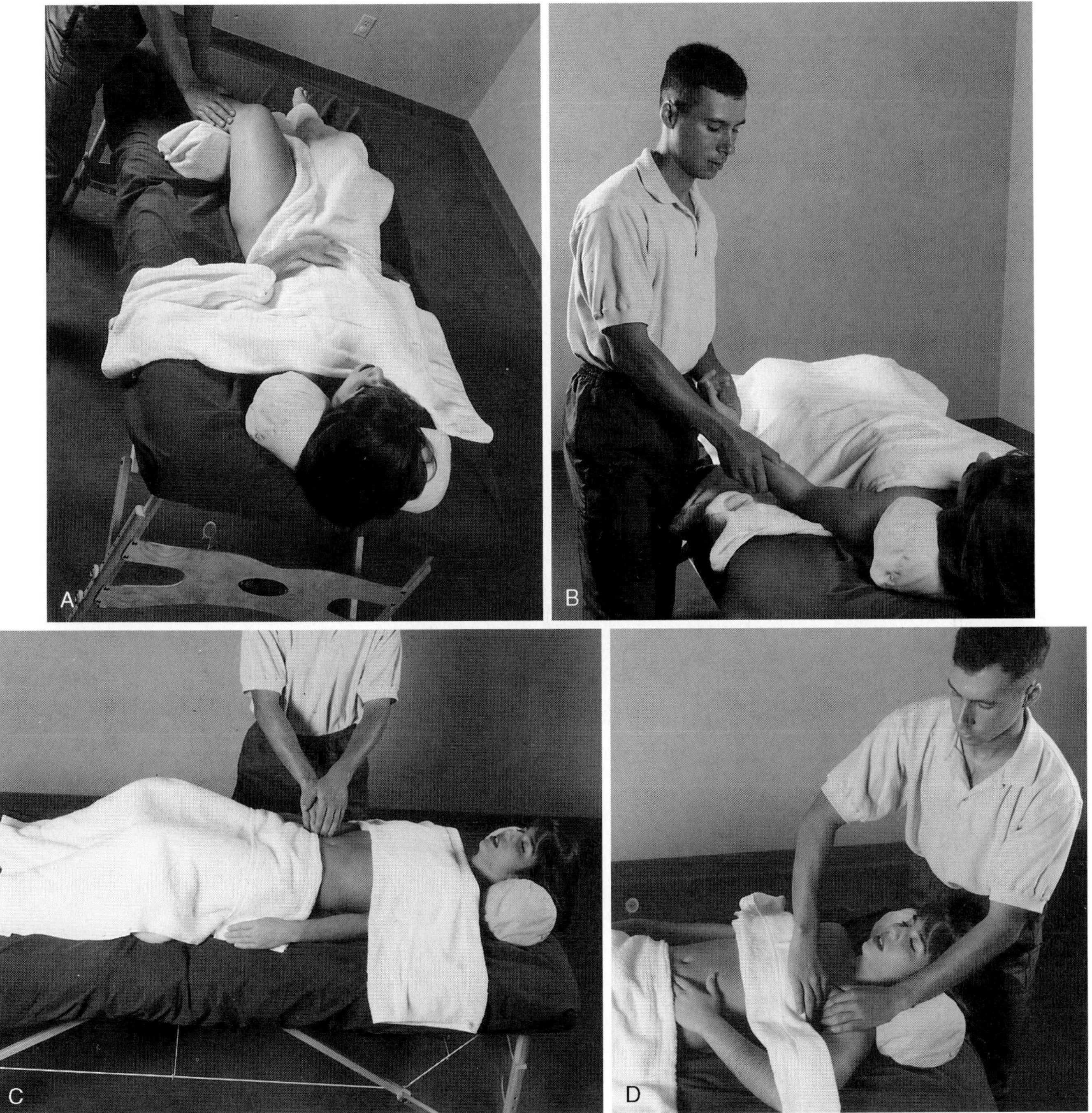

Figure 17•17 *A–D,* Towel access to anterior leg, arm, abdomen, and chest.

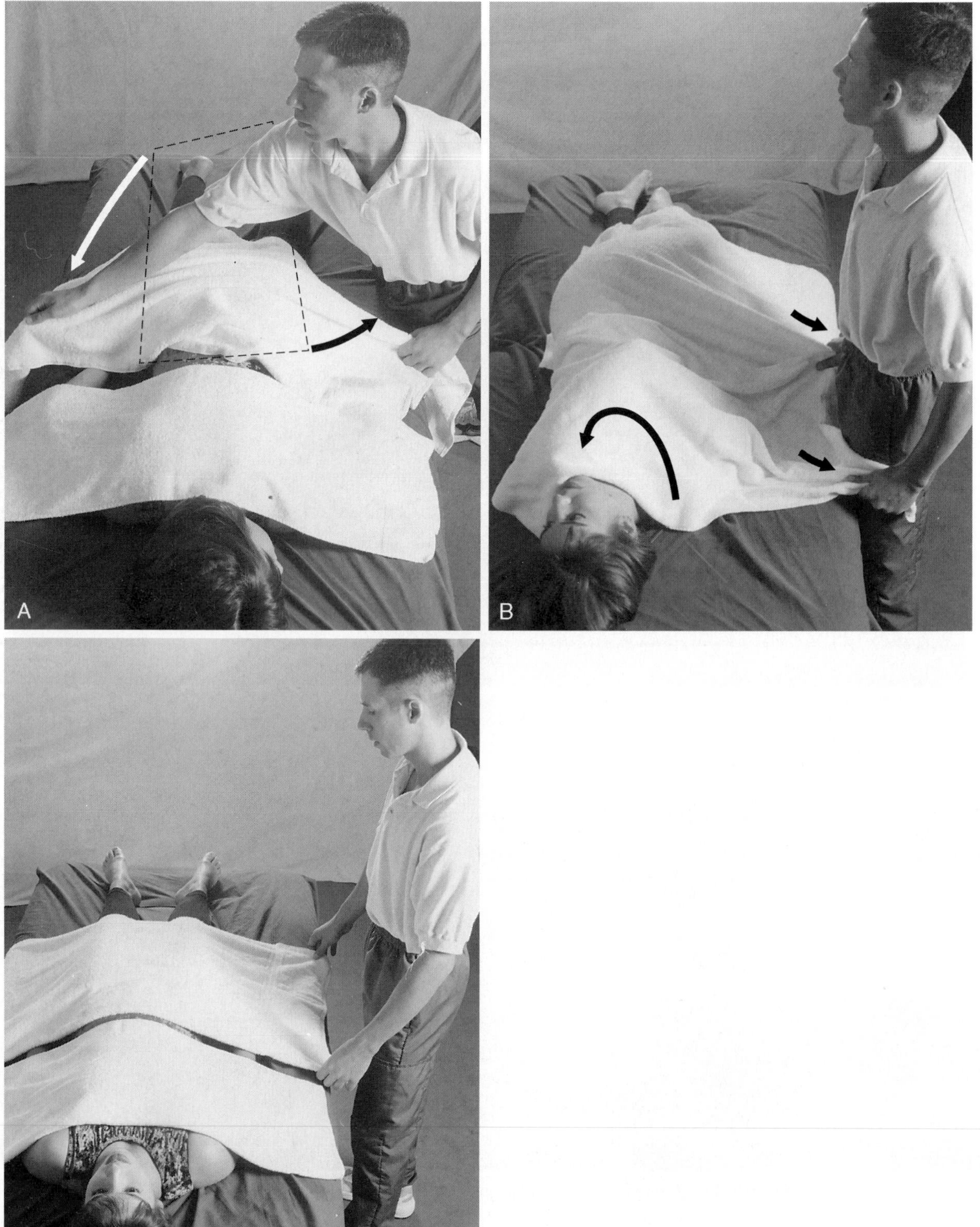

Figure 17•18 *A–E,* Series of illustrations showing turning motion in five steps using towels.

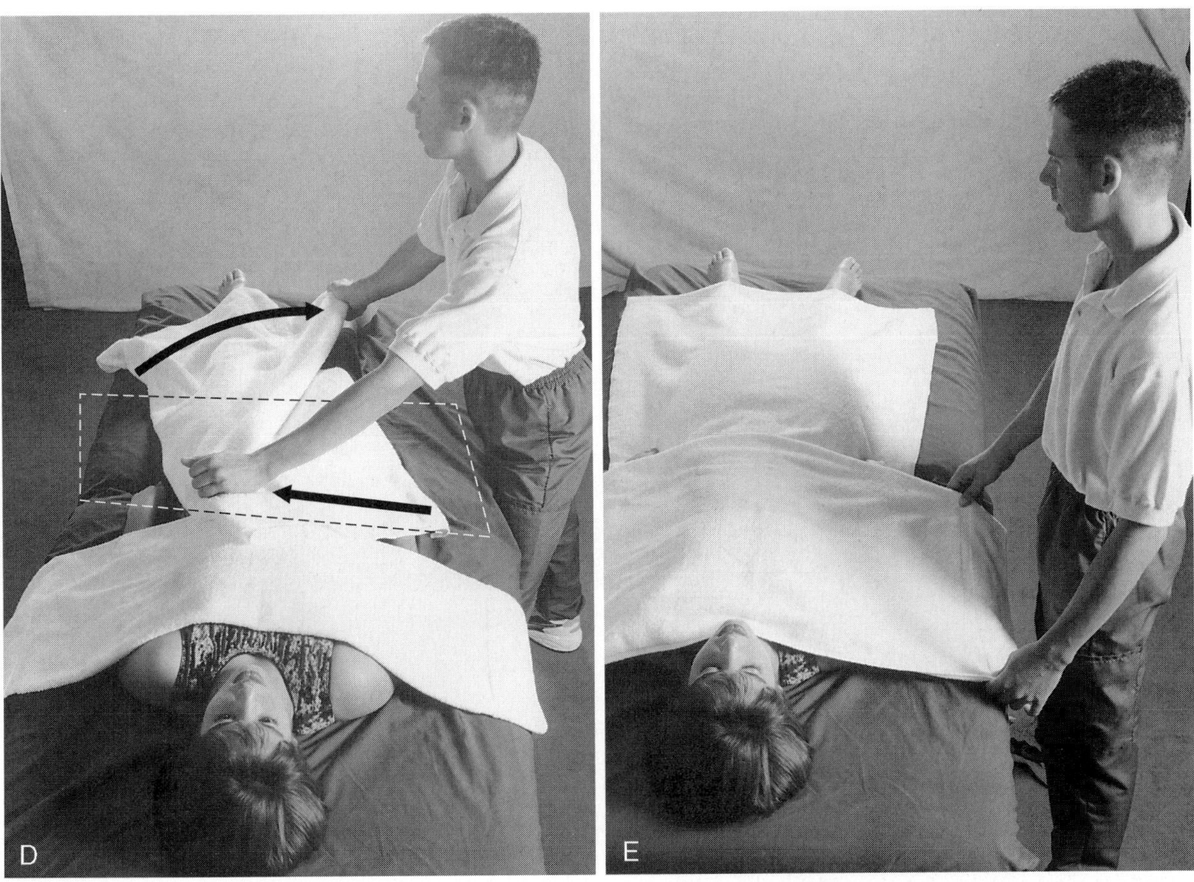

Figure 17•18 *Continued*

down on the table so that her face is out of the face rest and on the table proper. Her arms should be either above her head or by her sides under the sheets. Grasp the sheet along the opposite edge of the table, while anchoring the edge of the top sheet with your thighs on the side of the table closest to you. The therapist's hands are holding the sheet at the level of the client's shoulder and knee. Instruct the client to turn and face you and to continue turning until she is all the way onto her back (180 degrees). Sometimes it helps to pull a little extra top sheet material toward the therapist before beginning to turn the client.

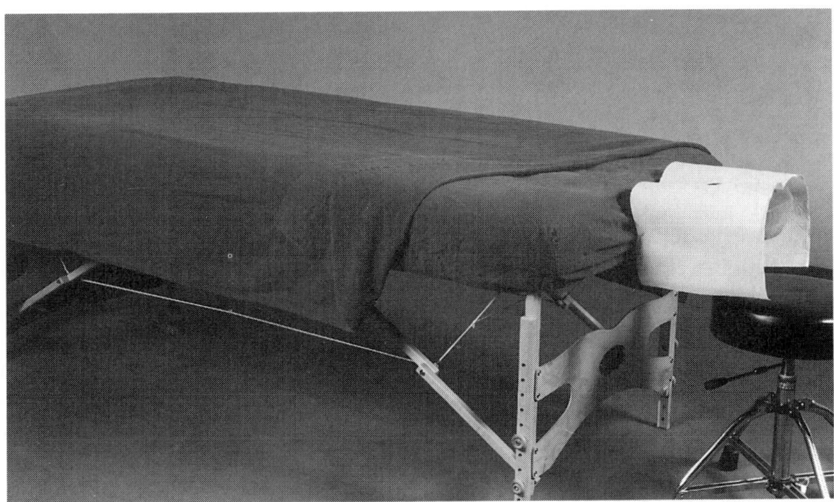

Figure 17•19 Sheet arrangement on the table without a client.

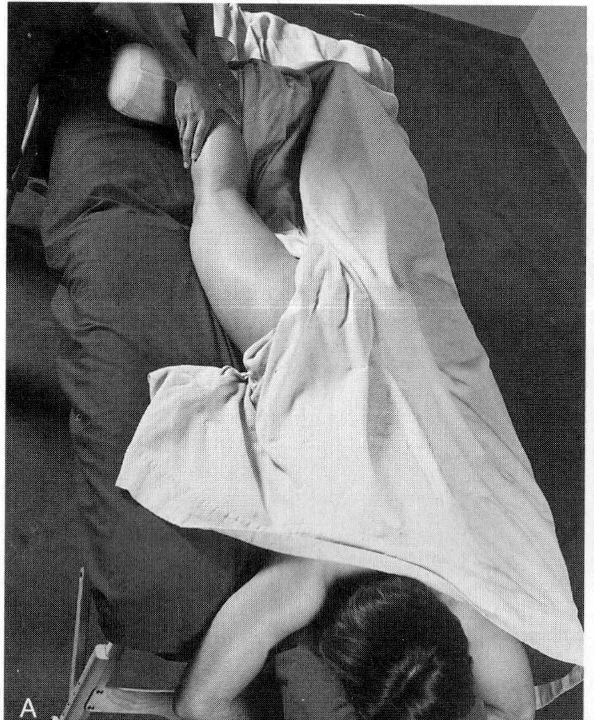

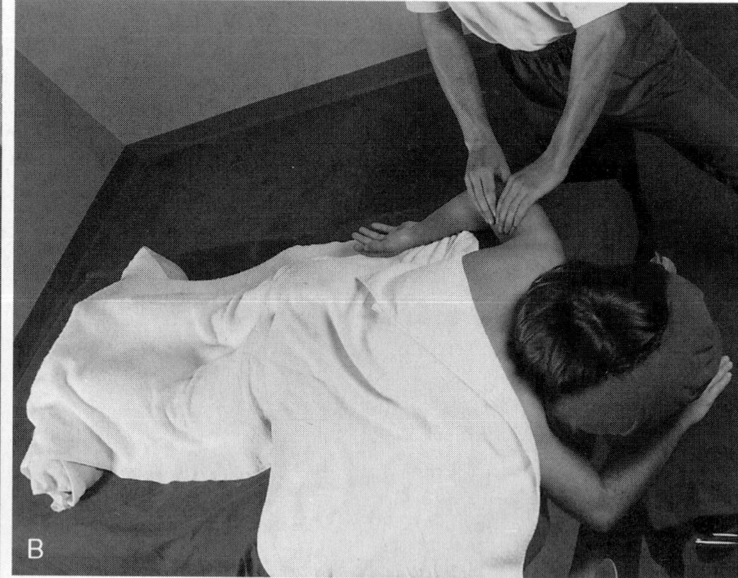

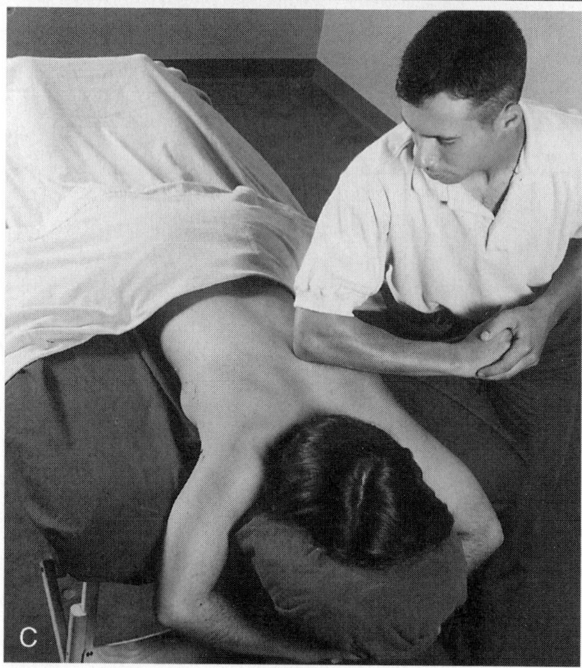

Figure 17•20 *A–C,* Sheet access to posterior leg/buttock, arm, and back.

To turn a client from supine to prone, repeat the procedure. Hold the sheet along the opposite edge of the table, while anchoring the edge of the top sheet on the side of the table closest to you (Fig. 17–22*A*). Instruct the client to turn toward you (Fig. 17–22*B*) and to continue all the way over until he is on his abdomen (Fig. 17–22*C*). Ask him to center himself on the table and to move up and to make use of the face rest. Be certain to communicate your instructions simply and clearly because the client may be groggy from the effects of the massage and may not easily comprehend your instructions.

It is important to note that the sheet not only constitutes the therapist's professional boundary, but represents the client's modesty boundary as well. It is inappropriate to lift, fluff, or move the sheet in such a way as to make the fabric leave the client's body. The sudden feeling of "air space" may violate the client's feelings of warmth, security, and privacy, thus detracting from the massage experience. Avoid lifting the sheet off the client's body for the turning over process. When the anchor method of turning is used, the client can feel the drape in contact with his body at all times and feel secure about his privacy.

Side-Lying Draping Technique Using Sheets. Side-lying draping is often used when a client is pregnant, elderly, or has had recent surgeries. The draping for the side-lying massage works best with sheets, because coverage must be provided on two or more sides of the body at once. Use the following steps to master side-lying draping.

1. Begin in the supine position. After massaging the anterior body surfaces, use the anchoring method for turning the client, only this time ask her to turn 90 degrees either toward you or away from you (a quarter turn).
2. Position the client on the side that is most comfortable to her; for pregnant women in the last trimester, spend most of the massage time on the right side because it prevents the weight of the baby from compressing the abdominal aorta.
3. Place a comfortable roll or bed pillow under the head, keeping the head and neck in a neutral position with the rest of the spine.
4. Use a large thick bed pillow placed underneath the sheet next to the client's chest for an arm support. The arm against the table either hugs the pillow or is tucked under the client's head pillow, according to her comfort.
5. The leg lying against the table is relatively straight and the upper leg is flexed at the knee, and the hip is at a 90- to 35-degree angle. Position a second thick bed pillow underneath the sheet to support the flexed upper leg at the ankle and knee, which should be at the same height to avoid hip rotation. Some clients with long legs may require two pillows to accomplish this.
6. Proceed with the massage as usual, exposing one area at a time.
7. When the back, neck, and shoulders are uncovered, use a towel folded in half lengthwise, and drape it over the client's side to anchor the drape. Keep in mind that this extra weight may be necessary to stabilize the drape because the side-lying posture is the least stable. The client's body moves more as pressure is applied.
8. For the bottom leg, drape as you would the anterior or the posterior leg.
9. For the top leg, undrape and tuck the sheet back around under the leg. This should ensure complete privacy as you massage.
10. Remove the pillows from the client. Turn the client over, and replace the pillows.

ASSISTING A CLIENT OFF THE MASSAGE TABLE

From time to time, a client may need assistance sitting up and getting off the massage table once the massage is complete. There are a variety of methods to accomplish this, while keeping the client comfortably draped and protecting the therapist's back. Prior to this procedure, follow these basic steps: wash your hands; collect the bolsters, lubricant, and other supplies used during the massage; and explain the procedure to the client. The client is supine, and you approach him from the side of the table closest to his clothes and personal belongings. If the client is male and doesn't have a top drape, use a paper towel in each of your hands to prevent grip slippage during the lift.

1. Stand with the lateral edge of your body against the massage table at the client's waist level.
2. Facing the client's head, place your closest arm under the client's closest arm and grasp his shoulder, securing the edge of the top drape with your fingers. Ask the client to reach under your arm and grasp your closest shoulder (Fig. 17–23*A*).
3. Continuing to secure the edge of the top drape with your fingers, slide your other arm under the client's back until you are supporting the opposite shoulder. Grasp the edge of the top drape while supporting the shoulder with your arm (Fig. 17–23*B*).
4. With the client assisting, raise him to a seated position. Use your legs, not your back, to lift.
5. Pull the sheet or towel loosely about his neck and shoulders. Leave your upper arm under the client's back and shoulders (Fig. 17–23*C*).
6. Reach over the client's knees, and cup your palm around and over his opposite knee (Fig. 17–23*D*).
7. While supporting the client's back with your upper arm, pull his knees toward you in a swivel so that his lower legs dangle off the table edge (Fig. 17–23*E*).
8. Maintaining your upper arm around his shoulders, use your other arm to support the client into a standing position (Fig. 17–23*F*). Never let go of the top edge of the drape until your client has it securely in his hand and drapes himself appropriately until you leave the massage room.

Author's Note

A small portion of the population (about 10 percent) finds it difficult to stand up after lying down for an extended period. This is due to insufficient cerebral circulation and a sudden drop in blood pressure that often occurs when moving into an upright position. Symptoms of this condition may include dizziness, im-

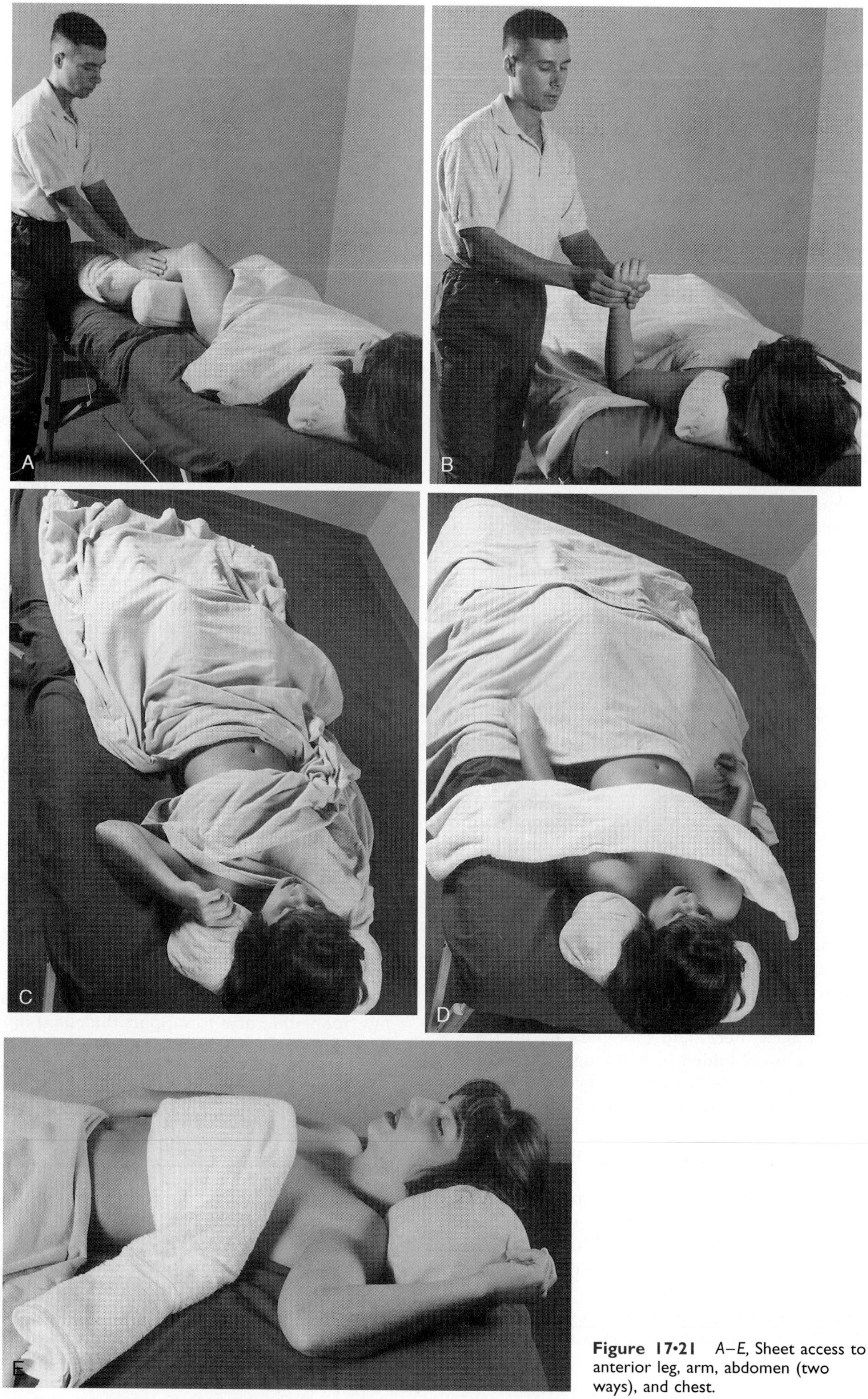

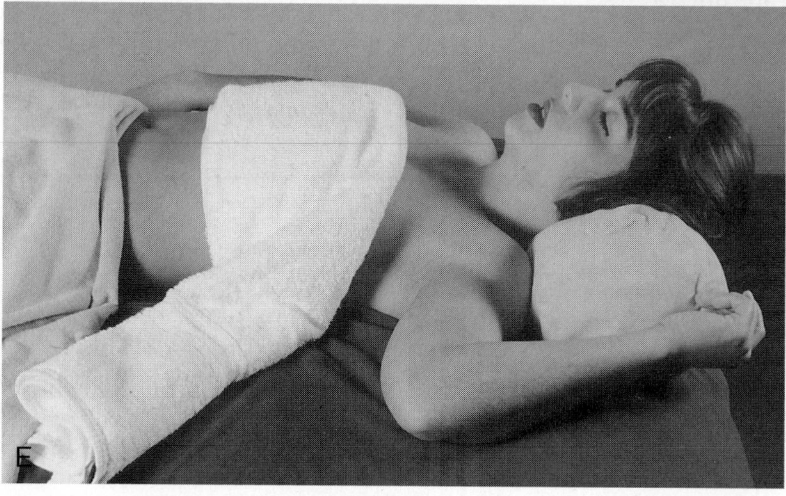

Figure 17•21 *A–E,* Sheet access to anterior leg, arm, abdomen (two ways), and chest.

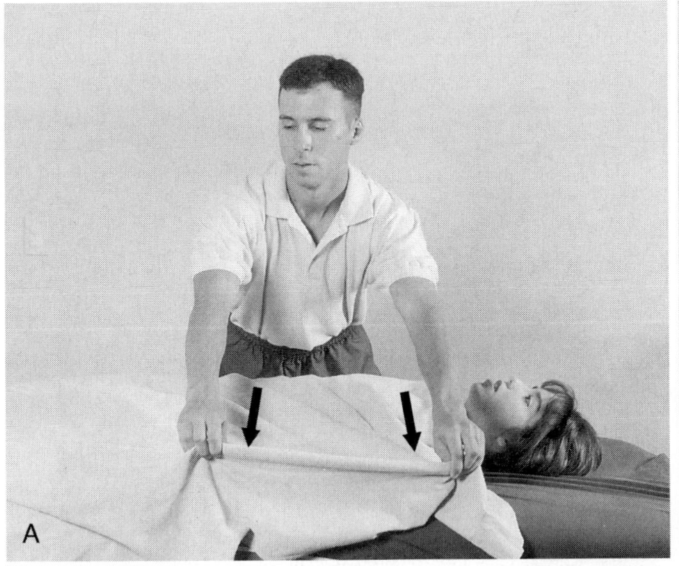

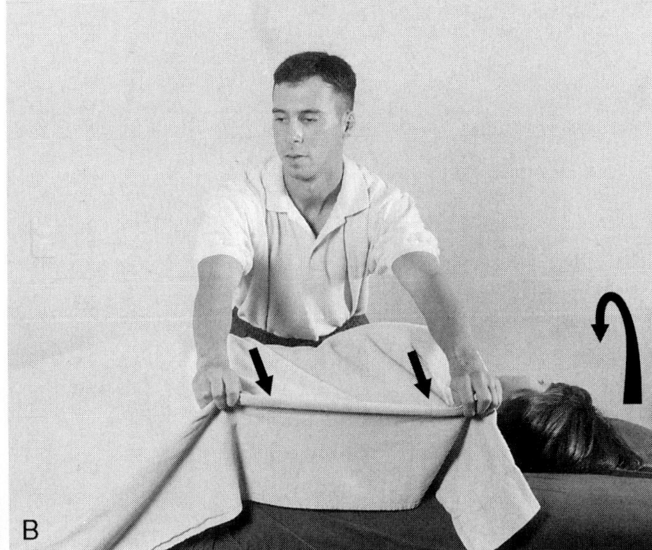

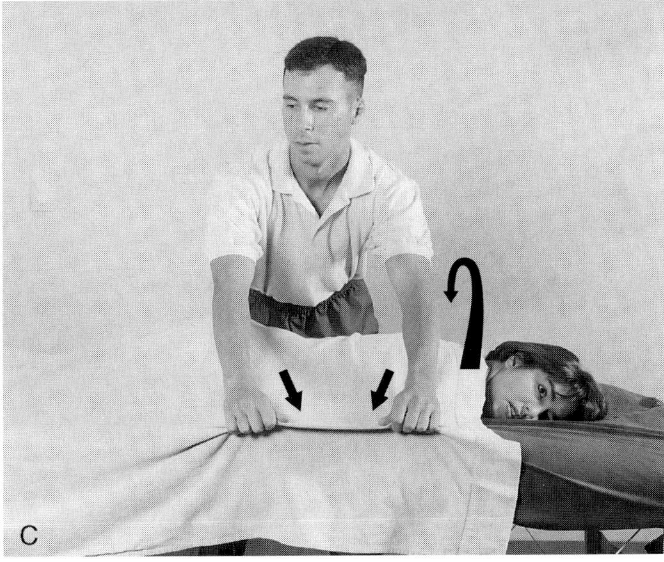

Figure 17•22 A–C, Series of illustrations showing turning motion in three steps using sheets.

paired vision, and buzzing in the ears. In more severe cases, fainting may occur.

With this in mind, it is helpful to do one of the following after the massage: remind your client to sit up for a few moments before standing or assist her into a standing position, pausing for a few moments to make sure she is oriented in the upright position.

Draping Tips for Sheet and Towel Draping

- Use verbal instructions *and* hand gestures such as tapping the table to direct the client which way to turn.
- Avoid situations that allow the client to feel air under the drape.
- If you accidentally expose the client, look away and redrape the exposed area. It is generally better to acknowledge your error with a simple "excuse me."
- If you use towels, pivot the bottom towel around the genitals so it lies perpendicular to the body before securing the towel and turning the client.

SUMMARY

As a precursor to giving the massage, we have explored two subjects that must be taken into consideration regarding both the client and the therapist. The first of these is the study of table mechanics, which comprises positioning, bolstering, and drap-

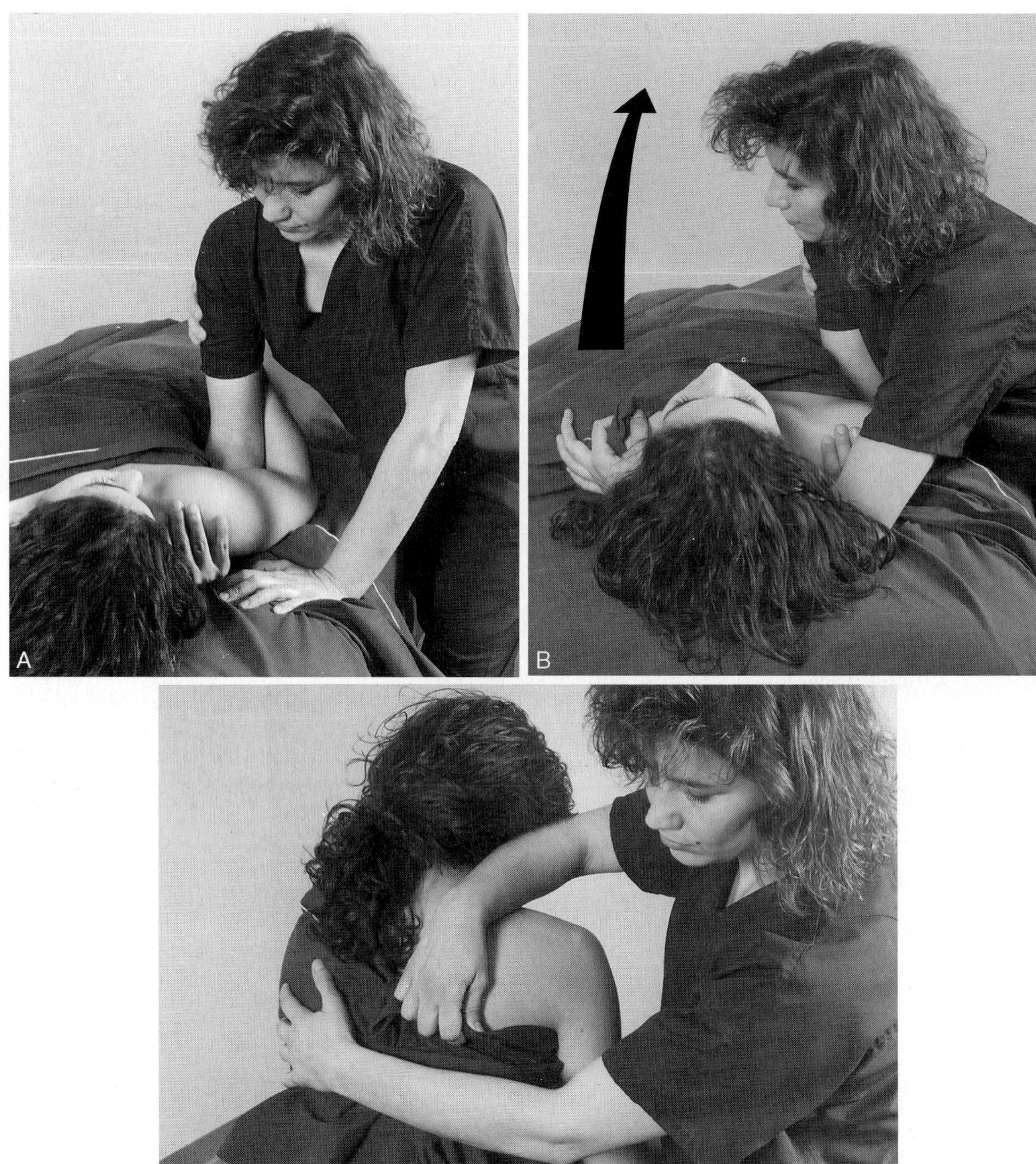

Figure 17•23 A–E, Therapist assisting client off the table.

ing the client. The second topic is body mechanics, which refers to the proper use of postural techniques to deliver massage therapy with the utmost efficiency and with minimum trauma to the practitioner. Table mechanics ensure that every step has been taken to provide a physically secure and emotionally comfortable space for the client. Positioning the client with table mechanics means being able to address all muscles in the prone, supine, and side-lying postures. Body mechanics reduce the physical toll taken on the therapist's body both on a daily basis and cumulatively over a long career. Specifically, body mechanics include hand strength, foot stances, hand position, preparation of the mind and body, flexibility, coordination, physical fitness, stamina, strength, balance, grounding, and centering. Each of these elements is essential to the success of the massage.

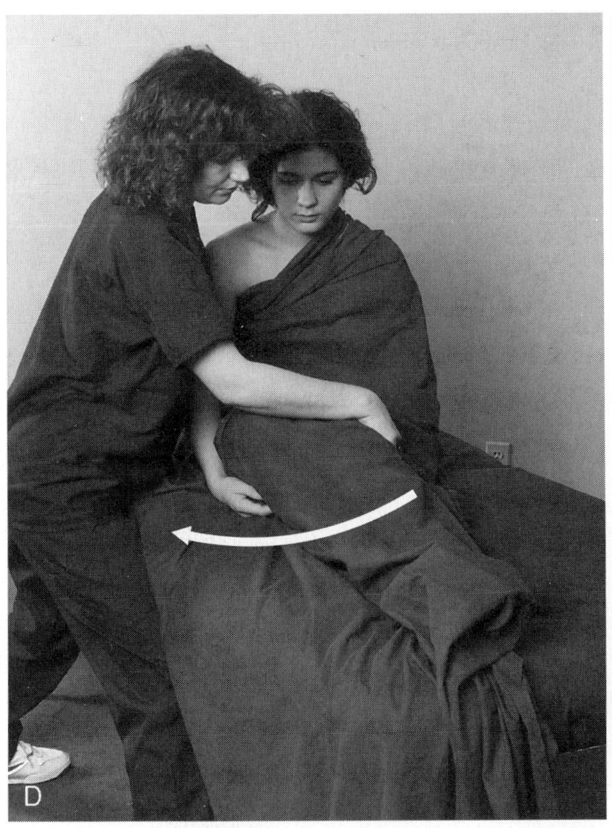

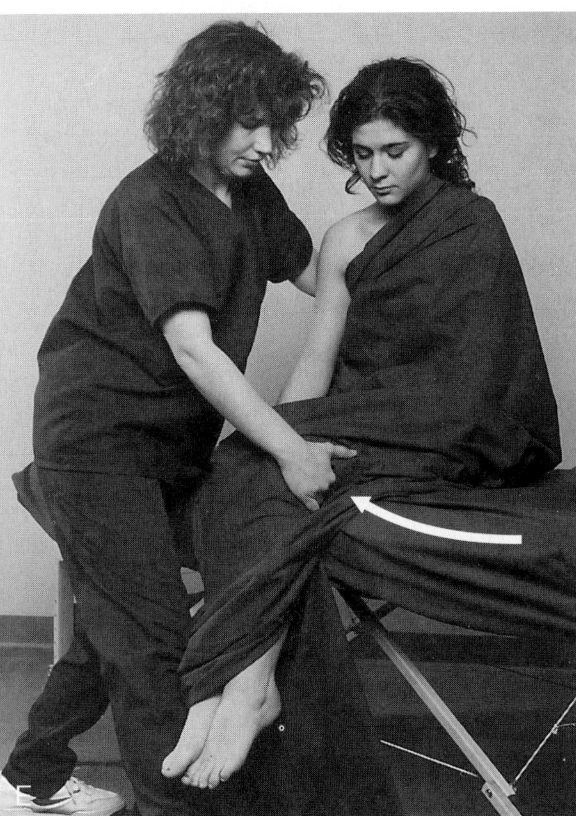

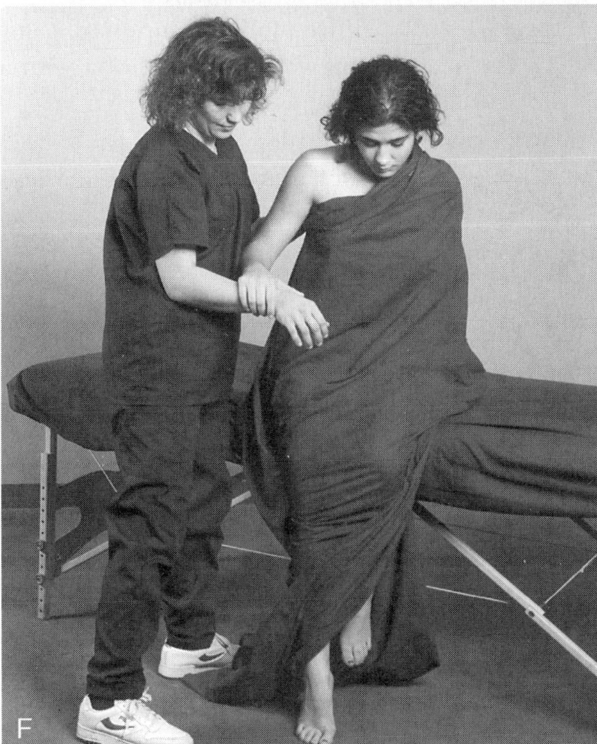

Figure 17•23 *Continued*

SELF-TEST

Multiple Choice • Write the letter of the best answer in the space provided.

_______ 1. Using bolsters, draping, positioning the client, and adjusting the height of the massage table are all elements of

A. body mechanics
B. table mechanics
C. massage mechanics
D. auto mechanics

_______ 2. The ability to carry out daily tasks efficiently with enough energy left over to enjoy leisure time pursuits and to meet unforeseen emergencies is the definition for

A. exercise
B. massage stamina
C. fitness
D. strength

_______ 3. According to Bonnie Prudden, massage therapists can the classified in which occupational category?

A. sitting occupations
B. standing occupations
C. active occupations
D. strenuous occupations

_______ 4. The ability of the muscles, joints, and nerves to maintain static and dynamic stability, while having the capacity to adapt to change is called

A. strength and stamina
B. balance and flexibility
C. grounding and centering
D. exercise and fitness

_______ 5. The "center of gravity," which is also a topographical and meditative point of reference located 2 inches below and behind the navel, is called the

A. chi point
B. tao center
C. massage region
D. hara or the tan tien

_______ 6. Another word for body mechanics is

A. table mechanics
B. biomechanics
C. joint mechanics
D. strength training

_______ 7. Poor working posture and hand technique can increase stress on the joints, creating

A. repetitive motion injuries
B. lordosis
C. fibromyalgia
D. the need for vitamins

_______ 8. The proper use of postural techniques to deliver massage therapy with the utmost efficiency and minimum trauma to the practitioner is called

A. body mechanics
B. table mechanics
C. massage mechanics
D. auto mechanics

_______ 9. The two most basic foot stances when applying massage are the

A. L stance and the bow stance
B. tai chi stance and the yoga stance
C. bow stance and the archer stance
D. bow stance and the horse stance

_______ 10. Which stance is used most frequently when applying effleurage or any gliding stroke where length may be important?

A. bow stance
B. horse stance
C. tai chi stance
D. yoga stance

_______ 11. Repetitive motion injuries are caused by

A. repeated flexing and extending of a joint against resistance
B. normal daily activities
C. manual manipulation of tools or other equipment
D. A and C

_______ 12. The two positional considerations during the massage are

A. position of the table; position of the client
B. position of the knee bolster; position of the neck bolster
C. position of the light source; position of the table
D. position the client should lie; position of the client's joints

_______ 13. Which of the following is *not* a consideration for a chair massage?

A. a massage table is not available
B. not adequate physical space to set up a massage table and use proper body mechanics during the massage

C. client has a muscle spasm in the trapezius
D. client is in a wheelchair

_______ 14. When the client is in the supine position, the most frequently supported areas are the
A. the anterior neck and the abdomen
B. the anterior ankles and the head/neck complex
C. the posterior cervical region and the posterior knees
D. the posterior cervical region only

_______ 15. The preferred position for pregnant women, the elderly, recent surgery clients, and a variety of other conditions is
A. prone position
B. supine position
C. side-lying position
D. seated position

_______ 16. What element of massage provides a professional atmosphere that supports the client's need for modesty and comfort, in a way that provides access to individual body parts?
A. pressure
B. body mechanics
C. face rest table accessory
D. draping

_______ 17. During the massage, expose only
A. the client's arms and legs
B. the area being massaged
C. the client's back, neck, and shoulder
D. the client's face

_______ 18. The best method for turning the client over because it provides the best mobility and coverage is the
A. anchoring method
B. hold and turn method
C. draping method
D. Saunders method

References

Barry, William. "Massage Body Mechanics." *Massage Magazine,* 60, March/April 1996.

Beck, Mark F. *Theory and Practice of Therapeutic Massage,* 2nd ed. Albany, NY: Milady Publishing Company, 1994.

Fritz, Sandy. *Fundamentals of Therapeutic Massage.* St. Louis: Mosby–Year Book, Inc., 1995.

Prudden, Bonnie. *Pain Erasure.* New York: M. Evans & Co., 1980.

Torres, Lillian S. *Basic Medical Techniques and Patient Care for Radiologic Technologies.* Philadelphia: J. B. Lippincott Company, 1993.

I do not understand. I pause; I examine.

—Montaigne

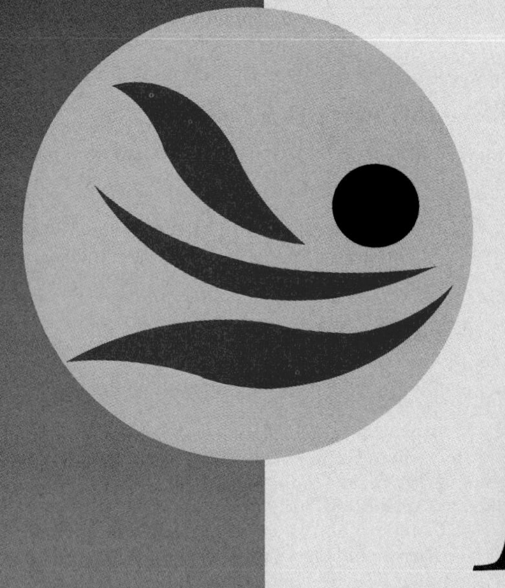

18 Classifying Swedish Massage Movements

Student Objectives

After completing this chapter, the student should be able to:

- Describe and implement the basic elements used in applying Swedish massage strokes: depth, pressure, excursion, speed, duration, flow, and sequence
- Describe and perform the five basic Swedish massage strokes and their variations: effleurage, petrissage, friction, tapotement or percussion, and vibration
- Identify and perform the ancillary techniques presented in this chapter, such as touch, nerve strokes, compression, trigger point work, stretching, and Swedish gymnastics

INTRODUCTION

Massage has been around for millennia, probably since early man hit his head on the roof of the cave and instinctively began to rub it to make it feel better. Massage in Asian countries developed according to Eastern philosophy, spirituality, theories of energy movement, and clinical practice. Massage in Western society was originally based on early religious and medical ideas, and has evolved under the influence of modern medicine, biology, and the sports models. For the purposes of this book, we will concentrate primarily on Western styles of massage.

Massage can be defined as organized, intentional touch. Its purpose is dependent upon the intent of the therapist and the goals of the client. Massage may be used for a variety of reasons: to bring a client to a deeper level of relaxation, to rehabilitate, or to prevent an injury or illness.

The era of modern massage began to develop in the early 19th century, when a wide variety of practitioners were advocating massage and developing their own systems. The most important of these writers was Pehr Henrik Ling (1776–1839), a Swedish physiologist and gymnastics instructor. Because of his nationality, Ling's system became commonly known as Swedish massage, and he became known as both the father of Swedish massage *and* the father of physical therapy.

The most widely known, prescribed, and utilized system of massage therapy in the United States is the Swedish system. There are five basic massage strokes or movements used to administer a Swedish massage: effleurage, petrissage, friction, tapotement, and vibration. Dutch physician Johann Mezger promoted Swedish massage using a medical model and is given credit for introducing and popularizing the use of French terminology into the profession. (For more information, see Chapter 1, A Historical Perspective of Massage.)

In addition to the five fundamental Swedish strokes and their variations, numerous ancillary, or supplementary, movements have emerged over the past few decades. These have been included for discussion in this chapter. Swedish and Western massage styles now include basic touch, nerve strokes, compression and trigger point work, stretching, and Swedish gymnastics. Note: Swedish gymnastics is part of the Ling system, but discussion of it has been included in the ancillary section because of its relationship to stretching.

Understanding the effects of these movements on the body is an essential prerequisite for the *scientific application* of massage. *Masterful application* requires the addition of one basic ingredient—practice, practice, and more practice. Recall any distinguished musical composer or performer; a musician practices scales before advancing to symphonies.

A master of massage, like a martial arts master, no longer has to think about the moves; she has totally integrated the science and the art, the physical, emotional, intellectual, and the spiritual aspects of her art into her own body. The massage therapist uses her whole being when practicing her craft. This includes using all of her sensory facilities, spatial awareness, and client "receptivity" for meticulous execution of massage strokes. Your skills of massage will evolve and mature as you evolve and mature as a therapist.

> *There is only so much you can learn about skydiving from standing on the ground.*
>
> —Joyce Maynard

ELEMENTS IN APPLICATION OF STROKES

During your study of massage therapy, you quickly discover that applying massage movements is much more than placing your hands on the body and manipulating skin, muscle, and fascia. Skillful application of massage strokes is a blend of the hand movements themselves and your body mechanics, as well as pressure and depth, excursion, rhythm and continuity, speed, duration, and sequence. These elements affect not only the body's response to massage therapy but also the intensity of the response.

As you begin your study of massage, your initial struggle is just to remember the names and order of the strokes. As you practice, your strokes will integrate these qualities (i.e., intention, depth, pressure, excursion, speed, rhythm, continuity, duration, sequence), which will vary within a session and from client to client, depending on the intent of the massage or the client's goals. Let's examine these concepts to deepen your understanding and then use them as you evaluate your own progress and digest the critiques of others.

Intention

Webster's dictionary defines intention as a "clearly formulated plan of action." All the other elements in the application of massage are dependent upon the intention of the massage therapist. This intention is generally based upon the needs the client has stated. As the therapist begins to palpate the tissue and administer the massage, the objective findings of the therapist are taken into account in altering the application. A general intention may be to give the client a stress-reduction and relaxation massage. As the massage proceeds, it may become apparent that the client may need some deeper work to release trigger points in his trapezius; the therapist's intent and approach are thereby altered.

Depth and Pressure

Depth is the spatial distance into the body's tissue that is achieved through pressure application. The therapist can control the amount of pressure exerted on the tissues, but the client often controls how much depth is achieved due to the amount of conscious or unconscious muscular relaxation. A tense, contracted muscle will prevent the therapist from going deep into the tissues. A relaxed muscle will yield and allow depth into the tissues. Hence, the depth achieved is a combination of the calculated depth and the muscle receptivity or resistance.

Pressure is the application of force (or thrust) exerted by the massage therapist on the client's body. Usually the therapist utilizes her own hands, elbows, or forearm to apply pressure; however, handheld tools can be used as well. Most massage tools are made of wood, rubber, glass, or stone. If a tool is used to apply pressure, it must be disinfected between sessions. For this reason, wood and rubber are less sanitary because they are porous and can pick up germs easily and cannot withstand repeated exposure to disinfecting chemicals.

The sensation of pressure can be stimulated by compressing the client's body surface. Initially, the pressure should be relatively light, gradually adding more pressure until the desired effect is achieved. The amount of applied pressure is ultimately determined by the intention of the massage. Pressure to affect lymph flow is very different than pressure to deactivate a trigger point.

Avoid applying pressure past the client's personal pain threshold. Pressure is often appropriate if the muscle responds by relaxing and does not contract. After tissue release has occurred, or the desired results have been accomplished, the pressure should be gradually released. Often an experienced therapist can sense tissue resistance better than the client. Ethically the therapist is bound to integrate her own palpatory findings with the client's input.

The amount of pressure that the therapist uses will also depend upon the following elements:

- The condition of the tissue prior to the application of a massage stroke
- The massage stroke the therapist is using
- The area on the body where the pressure is being applied
- The purpose or intent of the massage stroke
- The response of the client (i.e., reaching the client's pain threshold) during the application of pressure

If too much pressure is used, the client will react by tensing or muscle splinting, decreasing the stroke's effectiveness (i.e., very little depth will be achieved). An excessive amount of pressure may cause damage to superficial tissues before ever reaching the muscle tissue. Massage therapists typically develop good peripheral vision and are able to see a client tense up or raise a body part, even though their focus may not be on that area. As pressure is being applied, it is often helpful to watch the client's facial distortions or a change in breathing pattern. Distorted facial features or an alteration in the client's breathing (e.g., shallow breathing, holding the breath) often indicates pressure that is too great. Also, too much pressure will irritate the tissue and may cause soreness and bruising. Yet sufficient pressure must be used to create positive tissue changes as evidenced by hyperemia, softening of tight bands, and the deactivation of trigger points.

Pressure should be applied only to the desired level of contact in order to achieve the therapeutic intention of a given massage. This pressure equation must take into consideration the receptivity of the geographical area being worked. It is not desirable to use heavy pressure on delicate or thin-tissued areas such as the face, dorsum of the hand, and anterior throat. Thick muscular areas such as the back, legs, or hips are capable of withstanding far greater pressure. With appropriate training and good common sense, you will be able to make pressure judgments.

In exerting pressure on the tissues, it is important to remember to use your body weight and not to push. Apply pressure by leaning into the client's body. Leaning pressure is easier to deliver and not as taxing on your body. Keep your pressure consistent as your hands move over the skin, releasing pressure while maintaining contact when needed. The use of even pressure and anticipated motion will help you build trust with your client. It is easier for relaxation to take place when the client feels safe. If each long movement feels like a roller-coaster ride, the client will always be braced for the next unpredictable push.

Excursion

Excursion is the distance traversed on the client's body or the length of a massage stroke. Once the therapist has applied the desired pressure of a stroke, the next consideration is how far across the skin the movement should go. The therapist decides if the massage movement will cover the length of the muscle, the area of tissue restriction, or a topographical region, such as the lateral edge of the tibia or the vertebral border of the scapula.

Excursion has a relationship with body stance and foot placement. Longer strokes are best achieved with wider foot stances or by traveling with the stroke. For example, if the excursion of an effleurage is going the full length of the back, the therapist's feet must be placed several feet apart from each other or he will have to take a few steps to achieve the continuous movement up or down the full length of back. Foot placement is vital to ensure a smooth continuum of the excursion without a change in pressure or a break in flow.

Speed

Speed is also a consideration when contemplating rhythm and continuity. **Speed** refers to the rate of motion (how fast or slow a massage movement is being executed). The therapist determines the speed based on the purpose of the massage (e.g., pre-event sports massage is delivered with more speed than a relaxing massage). Some general rules apply.

- If the massage moves are too fast, the client will not be able to track the movement across his skin.
- Massage strokes delivered too quickly may alarm the client and cause a tensing reaction. Fast massage movements may also fatigue the client.
- If the rate of hand speed is too fast, the therapist cannot palpate and assess the soft tissues of the body.
- Massage moves that are too slow may prevent the therapist from distinguishing ischemic tissue.

In general, fast movements stimulate and slow movements sedate and relax.

Rhythm and Continuity

An ordered repetition of strong and weak elements in the delivery of the massage strokes is **rhythm.** Rhythm is affected by excursion, speed, and pressure. The basic rhythm of a massage should fit your client's needs. The most favorable rhythm for a massage depends on the intent of the massage; a slower, more fluid technique is more relaxing. The concept of **continuity** in massage refers to the uninterrupted succession or flow of strokes and to the unbroken transition from one stroke to the next. It is more difficult for the client to relax when the massage lacks a smooth rhythm and continuity. During the massage, the therapist should keep his hands relaxed and flexible, which allows them to be lifted, without losing contact, around the bony regions and contours of the body. Rhythm and continuity come not only from what the hands are doing, but also from what the rest of the therapist's body is doing (e.g., foot placement, distance between the client and the therapist) and the height of the table. Both rhythm and continuity are learned skills and will come with experience.

Duration

The length of time you spend on an area, or **duration,** may be difficult to determine. There are physiological components that affect duration, such as achieving a release in tight tissues. We must also consider how much time the client has allotted for the massage and the client's goals. If your client requests that you focus on her low back, spend most of the session massaging her low back. Once again, intention comes into play. Most massage sessions last from 30 to 60 minutes, but shorter and longer sessions are used in certain settings. For example, orthopedic massage in a clinical setting may be 15 minutes long, and multimodality massage (e.g., combining Swedish massage with reflexology and/or shiatsu) can last for 90 minutes.

Some massage therapists use a system by which a certain number of massage strokes are used on a particular area and are repeated a certain number of times. For example, a therapist performs six effleurage strokes, ten petrissage strokes, then returns to three effleurage strokes on the client's hamstrings. Other massage therapists initially assess the condition of the tissue and work until the tissue responds. This method assumes that the therapist has the skill and experience needed to make this type of decision. An area can easily be overworked if the therapist cannot detect muscle guarding (muscle contracting to protect itself from an unwanted intrusion) or track the client's response. Using a combination of these two methods is recommended.

Sequence

A **sequence** is a succession of strokes. In a Swedish massage, the sequence is physiologically designed to increase circulation of blood and lymph by applying strokes to proximal areas first and proceeding to the more distal areas; the strokes also progress from superficial to deep. The various strokes are not random but are specifically sequenced in order to prevent repetitive motion injury to the therapist and to create physiological effects within the client's body. Have a sequence in mind as a basic plan, but continually listen to the client to make appropriate decisions.

The Routine

The union of these elements, along with how the therapist's body is positioned in space, results in a routine, which can be further broken down into its various massage movements, depending upon the style of the massage. The delivery of these strokes may be adjusted through the use of pressure, depth, excursion, rhythm, continuity, duration, and speed. For a discussion of the massage routine, please see Chapter 22, Putting It All Together.

CLASSIFICATION OF SWEDISH MASSAGE MOVEMENTS

There are probably as many different massage styles as there are massage therapists; each therapist has her own "flavor" and style. Western massage is typically composed of a set of fundamental and traditional Swedish massage strokes and a set of ancillary movements. The following five Swedish massage strokes have been categorized into groups according to their application. These groups are effleurage, petrissage, friction, tapotement, and vibration. The classifications of each stroke are thoroughly described and illustrated. Also included are details exploring technique and stroke variations. At times, it may seem as if the description of these moves is like describing a kitten; you have a better chance of understanding them through sight and touch. Hence, learning these strokes will take more than a book. Rely on your experienced and caring instructor(s) to demonstrate properly each move, to model technique as you go, and to guide your practice (Fig. 18–1).

Effleurage

The first and most frequently used Swedish stroke is effleurage (*ef*-flur-ahzh). The term comes from the French word *effleurer,* which means "to flow or glide" or "skim the surface." The **effleurage** stroke is an application of purposeful, gliding movements that follow the contour of the client's body. These strokes are, in effect, a "pushing" of the tissue both downward and away from the therapist. This stroke may be applied to the client's body with the hands, fingers, forearm, or elbow; the pressure may be either superficial (gentle) or deep. Deep effleurage is also known as "ironing." Effleurage movements are unbroken repetitions of gliding strokes across the skin and are well suited for extended parts of the body, such as the back, arms, and legs.

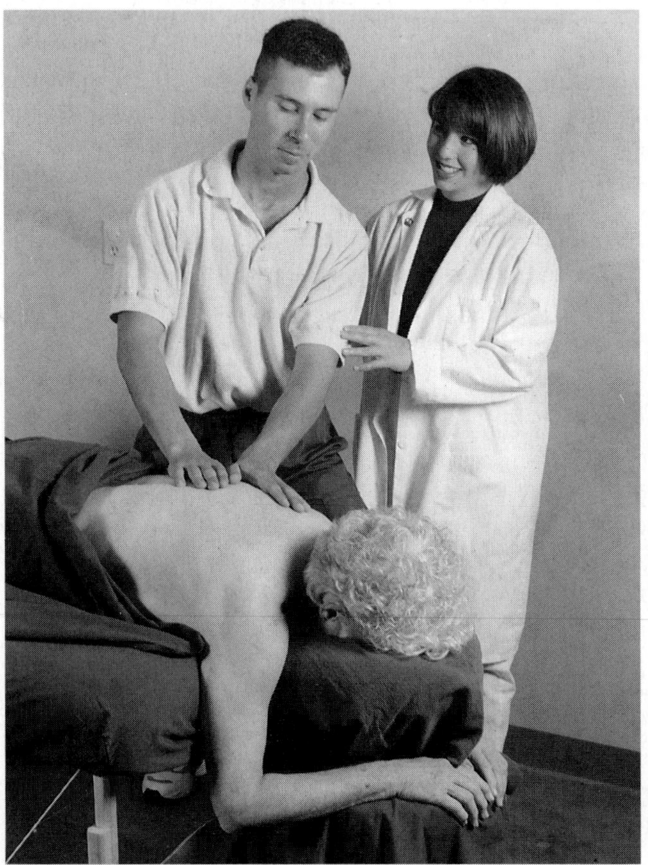

Figure 18•1 A student practices giving a professional massage with an instructor nearby.

Effleurage Techniques

Effleurage is delivered using a "lean and drag" technique. Place your hands on the client's body, and *lean* with your body weight, pushing down and away from you. In the application of Swedish massage, pressure strokes must be applied toward the heart or **centripetally.** When working the extremities, it is necessary to work the area most proximal to the trunk first, proceeding distally, stroking in the direction of the heart. For example, the thigh is massaged from the knee to the hip first and then the calf from the ankle to the knee. If a stroke has several phases or progressions up the leg or arm, apply more pressure when gliding from distal to proximal. When applying effleurage on the back, centripetal application does not apply because the heart is centrally located.

Once the excursion is complete, *drag* your hands back to their original position; use no added pressure, just the weight of your hands. Remember to maintain contact during each repetition. More pressure may be applied simply by changing your body position to put more (or less) of your own body weight into the stroke or by lowering (or raising) your massage table. Additionally, a deeper effleurage is more effectively delivered by going more slowly.

When performing the effleurage stroke, keep the angle of the wrist between 100 and 180 degrees. Hyperextension of the wrist may eventually lead to repetitive motion injuries (damage to the nerves and joint capsule) such as carpal tunnel syndrome. The therapist's hands, arms, shoulders, back, and legs should all be aligned along path of movement in order to reduce injuries and increase the ease of stroke application (Fig. 18–2).

The wrists must be flexible, the hands relaxed, and the movement even. If the palmar surface of the hands is used, mold them to the contours of the client's body. As you lean and extend your hands, keep your hands and fingers relatively still; the returning hands may travel a little faster. Gradually increase the pressure with each repetition. Effleurage is often repeated six times on an area, or until the desired effect is achieved (e.g., hyperemia, release of taut bands of tissue, etc.). Remember to apply pressure in only one direction or you will cause friction.

Massage increases venous and lymphatic circulation;

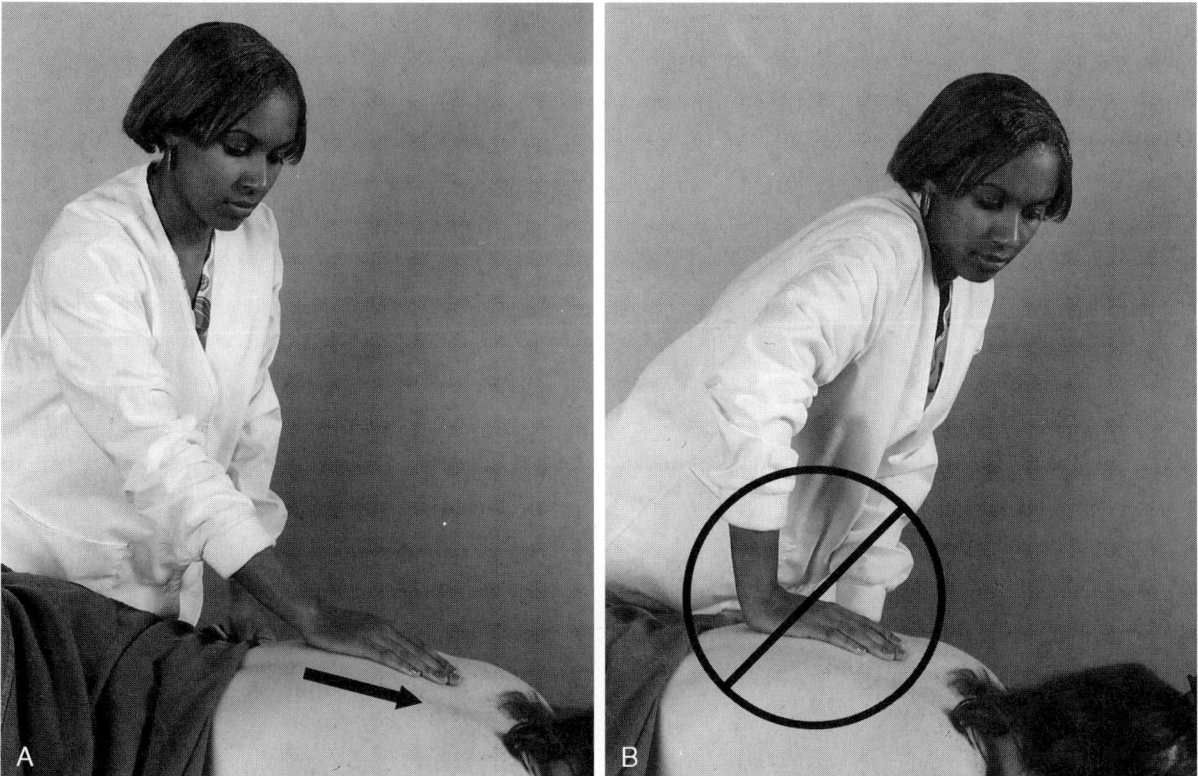
Figure 18•2 *A,* Correct wrist angle. *B,* Incorrect wrist angle.

many veins and lymphatic vessels are located close to the surface of the skin. Effleurage movements are applied with the force of pressure centripetally because this path follows the direction of venous blood flow. Valves in the veins maintain the direction of blood flow toward the heart and prevent backflow. Massaging away from the heart can damage the valves and contribute to varicosities.

Variation: Circle Effleurage

Circle effleurage can be performed around the ball-and-socket joints of the shoulder (glenohumeral joint), hip (iliofemoral joint), and on the abdomen. As one hand circles a region, the other hand moves behind the first hand in a half circle or a crescent shape (Fig. 18–3). Continue these circular repetitions for 6 to 12

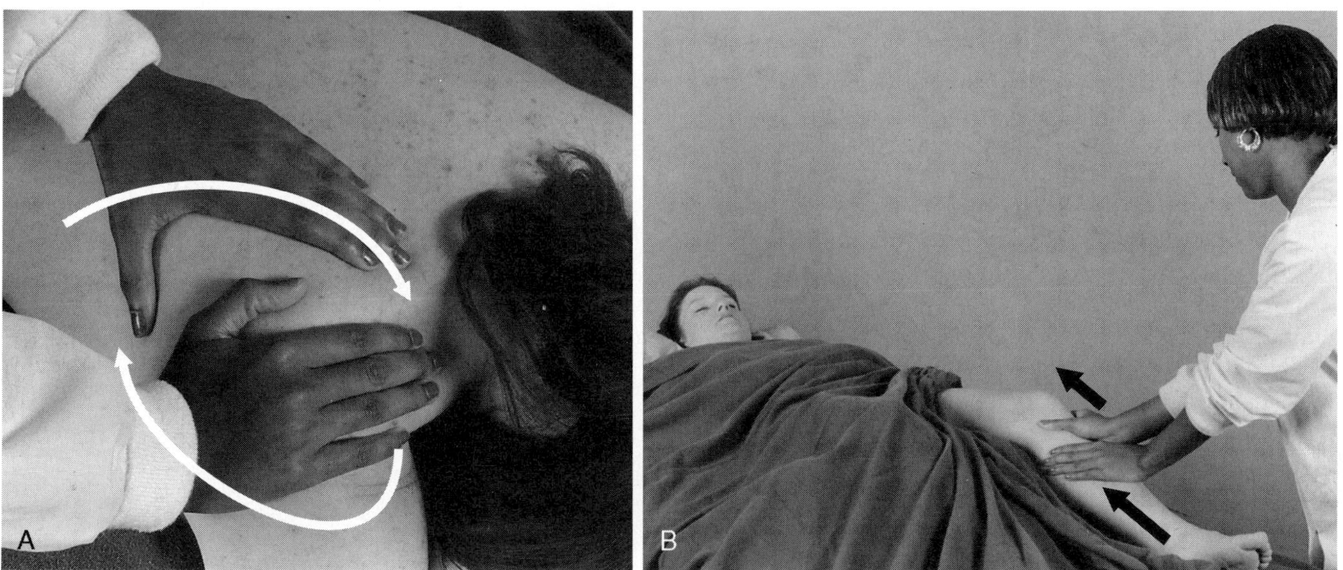
Figure 18•3 *A, B,* Circle effleurage on the shoulder and gliding effleurage on knee joint.

times, or until the desired effect is achieved. Because of the full- and half-circle sequence, this variation is also known as "sun-moon."

Effleurage is the stroke of choice to begin and end a massage therapy session because it is so proficient at moving blood and lymph. Effleurage can be used to prepare tissue for deeper massage and to flush out the tissue after using other strokes. It can be used on virtually every type of body surface, making it the preferred "transition" stroke to use between other strokes. It is also an excellent stroke for assessing tissues, which enables the therapist to discover anomalies when exploring the underlying tissues.

Benefits of Effleurage

- Repeated effleurage warms the tissue and makes it more extensible.
- It relaxes the client and prepares the area for deeper strokes.
- Effleurage soothes an area after deep work.
- It soothes places too painful for deep work.
- It aids in moving wastes out of a congested area (also known as flushing).
- Effleurage creates length in a muscle, if applied with fiber direction, while broadening and stretching the muscle and fascia and provides passive stretching to superficial muscle groups.
- It dilates capillaries and increases circulation.
- It increases lymphatic circulation if applied with light pressure.
- Effleurage spreads lubricant.
- It soothes tired, achy muscles.
- Effleurage aids in the relief of insomnia.

Petrissage

The term "petrissage" (*peh*-tre-sahzh) comes from the French word *petrir* meaning "to mash or to knead." In a Swedish massage routine, petrissage typically follows effleurage strokes. The application of **petrissage** consists of a cycle of rhythmic lifting of the muscle tissues away from the bone or underlying structures with the hollow of the palm(s), followed by firmly kneading or squeezing the muscle with a gentle pull toward the therapist, ending with a release of the tissue. This kneading or milking of the muscle may be accomplished with one hand or by alternately using both hands. It helps to imagine that the palm of your hand is a suction cup and that you are "slurping" up the tissue. The focus is on *lifting* the tissue rather than *pinching* it. Some petrissage variations, such as ocean waves, combine lifting and squeezing followed by a downward compression. Petrissage is the stroke of choice to "milk" the tissue of metabolic wastes and to draw new blood and oxygen into the tissues. It is important to repeat the effleurage stroke following petrissage in order to flush the stirred-up waste from the area and back into the circulatory system. The petrissage stroke can also be followed with friction, then with effleurage strokes.

Petrissage Technique

Grasp a fold of skin with the hands in a C formation. Lift up the skin and the underlying muscle tissue with the palm of one hand and compress. This movement should raise the muscle from its usual position, away from the bone. Next, lighten the grip enough to allow the muscle tissue to be released while still remaining in contact with the skin. As you relax the grasp, repeat the first move with the opposite hand (Fig. 18–4). Repeat the lifting, compressing, and releasing using both hands intermittently. Do not lose contact with the skin while you are switching hands.

In general, pressure should be applied in a rhythmic circular pattern to achieve alternate compression and relaxation of the muscle. On large muscular areas, such as the back, use as much of the hands as possible. Enough pressure must be used to engage the muscle, but not so much that you cause pain. On smaller

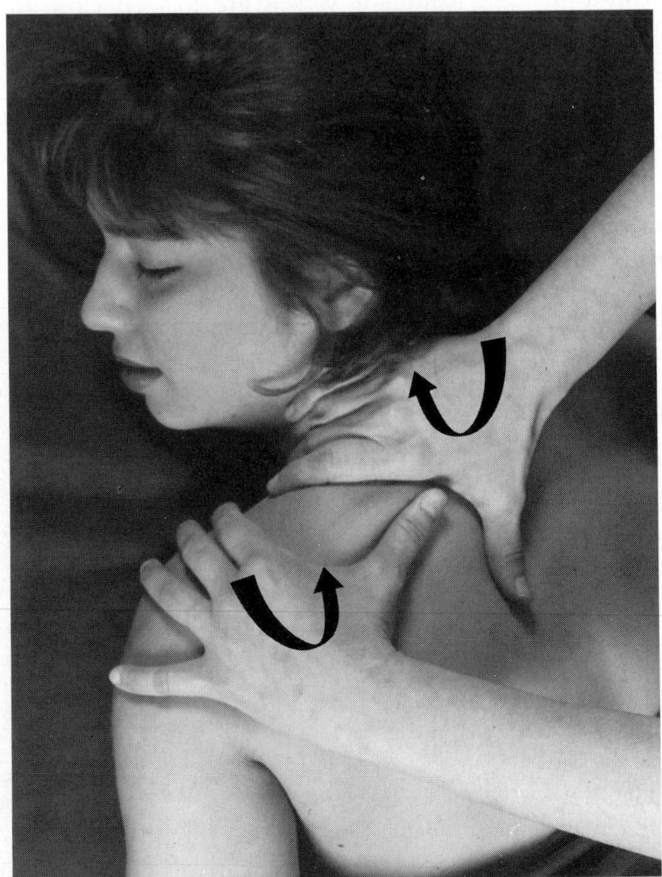

Figure 18•4 Kneading petrissage.

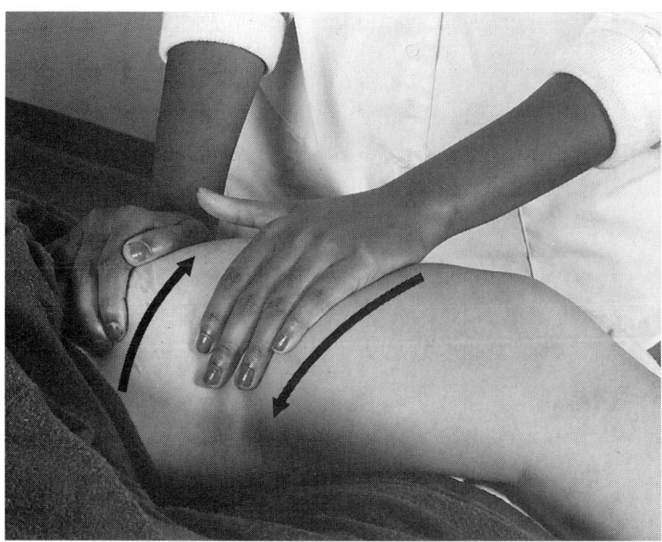

Figure 18•5 Ocean waves.

areas, such as the top of the trapezius or the anterior forearm, use only the pads of the fingers and thumb.

Variation: Ocean Waves

Ocean waves petrissage involves rolling the tissues against the bone before they are squeezed and lifted away from their usual position. Apply this variation in a back and forth movement while the hands oppose each other. Because the hands are moving across the body, covering both the top and sides of an area, press down toward the bone. This variation is typically applied across the muscle belly to broaden the tissue (Fig. 18–5).

Author's Note

If your client has a lot of body hair, a circular petrissage may matte and pull the hair. As an alternative, use the back and forth pattern (as in ocean waves) instead of a circular pattern or perform the petrissage movement on top of the sheet. Some massage therapists have had limited success using talc to overcome this problem of pulling body hair. A lotion and oil combination may also address the problem.

Variation: Fulling Petrissage

Fulling petrissage is effective for broadening muscles and their related tissues. Because of this, fulling petrissage is often referred to as broadening. Broadening strokes mimic the movement of a muscle when it contracts. Grasp the tissue with both hands, lift it up away from the bone, and spread it out laterally (Fig. 18–6).

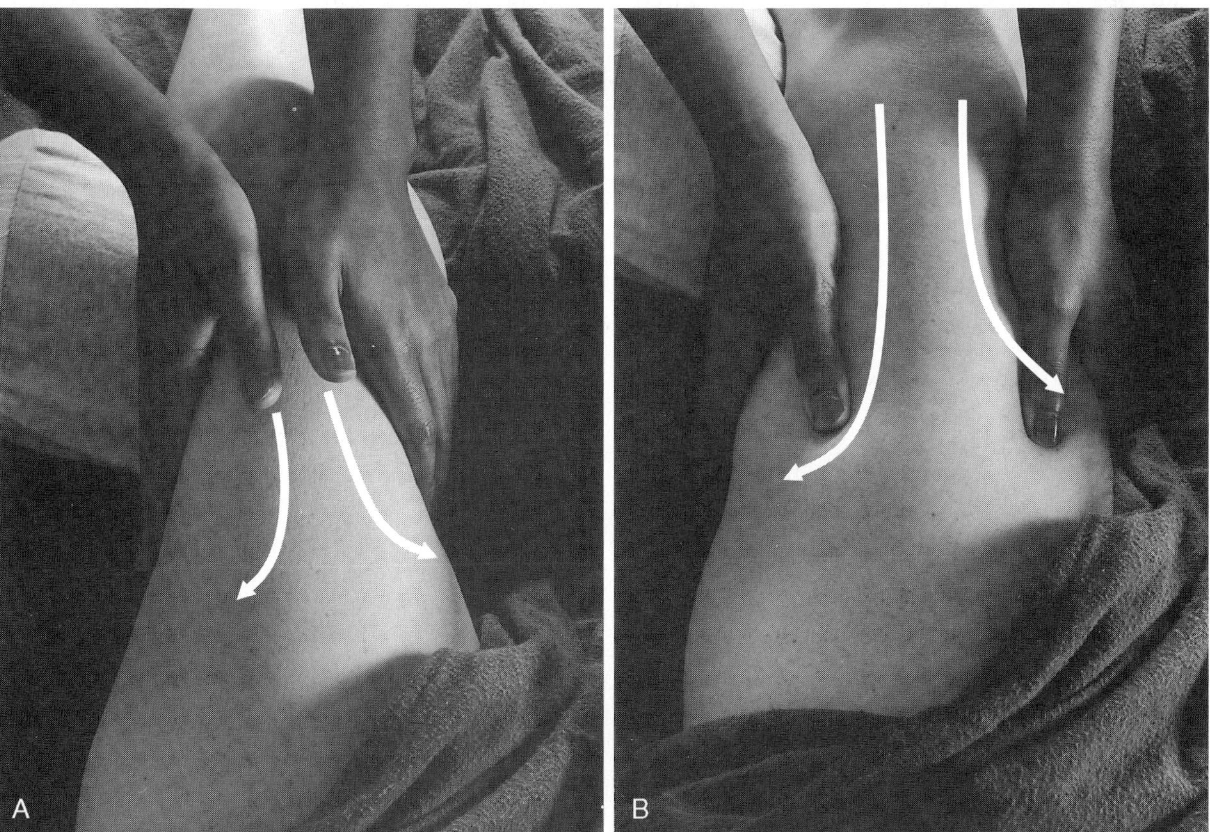

Figure 18•6 *A* and *B*, Fulling.

Repeat the fulling movements until the tissues feel warm and elastic.

Variation: Skin Rolling

Skin rolling involves manipulation of the connective tissues located on the body's surface. Tissues are lifted and compressed to release myofascial restrictions. Skin rolling is a technique essential to Bindegewebsmassage (connective tissue massage) and to myofascial release. Because no downward force is used, skin rolling is one of the few massage techniques that may be applied over bony areas. It may be initially uncomfortable for the client as the therapist loosens the adhesions between the superficial layers of skin and the deeper myofascial components. Therefore, move gently and respect the client's pain threshold because these areas are vascular and sensitive and overworking an area may leave the client bruised and sore.

Do not apply lubricant to the skin. Grasp and lift the skin between the fingers and thumbs, compressing the tissue. Roll the skin as though you were rolling a pencil, using your fingers to scoop up the skin as you move across the skin (Fig. 18–7). Continue the rolling technique until the designated area has been treated. Because the superficial fascia lies in several directions, lift and roll the skin in several directions over one body area. If the skin is not lifting, do not force the tissue into this position. It is recommended that you address the area two or three times in a session, allowing time between each application. Hot packs may be used to prepare the skin and fascia.

Benefits of Petrissage

- Petrissage increases blood flow.
- It works out toxins.
- It reduces local swelling.
- It relieves general fatigue.
- Petrissage improves cellular nutrition.
- It mechanically relaxes the muscle.
- It lifts muscle belly away from the underlying bone, stretching and broadening the muscle.
- Petrissage psychologically creates a sense of space in the muscle.
- It has a deeper circulatory effect than effleurage and addresses tension *under* the surface.
- It reduces muscle soreness and stiffness.
- Petrissage invigorates or stimulates the nervous system.
- It softens superficial fascia and can loosen adhesions.
- Petrissage skin rolling produces analgesia by stimulating the release of pain-relieving chemicals, such as endorphins.

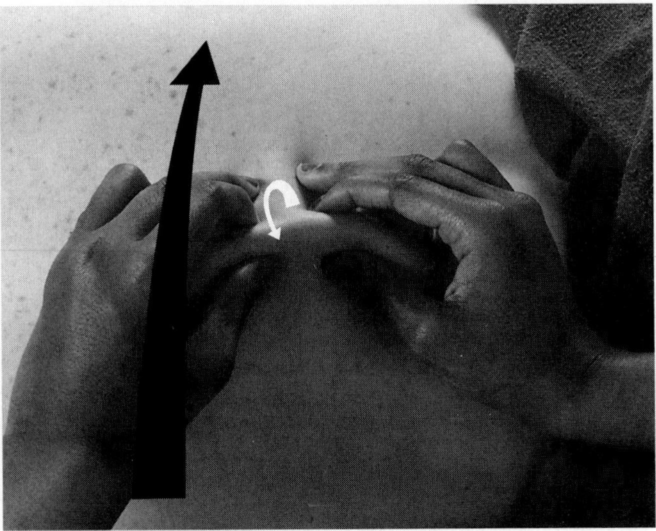

Figure 18•7 Skin rolling.

Friction

The term "friction" comes from the Latin word, *frictio,* meaning "to rub." Friction typically follows petrissage in a sequential order of Swedish massage strokes. **Friction** massage is a brisk, often heat-producing compressive stroke that may be delivered either superficially to the skin or to deeper tissue layers of muscle, depending upon the intention of the therapist. Friction strokes are typically done using little or no massage lubricant. In superficial or general friction, heat is produced by the drag of the hands contacting the skin's surface. In deeper friction strokes, the therapist's hands do not slide over the skin; they take the skin with them, applying pressure to the muscle tissue underneath. Heat is generated when the therapist rubs one layer of muscle fiber against another.

Deep frictioning techniques such as cross-fiber friction and circular friction appear to soften hyperplasia, break down adhered scar tissue, and rearrange muscle and collagen fibers in a more biofunctional pattern. This is accomplished by *stressing* the scar formation at the injury site, using mild, controlled pressure in a specific direction. Stress, in this instance, is defined as a physical factor that requires a physical response. Deep frictioning increases circulation to areas that normally have little or no blood supply, such as ligaments and tendons.

The six types of friction are straight (or general) friction, rolling, chucking (linear), wringing, cross-fiber, and circular. The friction variations may be applied in either a circular motion or linearly with a reciprocating movement. Friction may be applied with one or two hands, or specific work may be done with the thumb, forefinger, elbow, or forearm. General friction requires the sparse use of a lubricant; greater amounts are used in proportion to the amount of body hair. The desired rate of speed for the stroke is also a factor in determining quantity of lubricant. Faster friction strokes may require more lubricants, and deeper variations of friction require little or no lubricant. Unwanted lubricant can be removed with a towel.

Variation: Straight or Longitudinal Friction

Also known as a heat rub, straight friction is superficial and is performed using very little pressure. The heat generated is significant, but affects superficial layers only. Place both your hands palm down on the client's back (or other body part). The fingers of the hands should be together firmly. Move the hands simultaneously in opposite directions, one toward you and one away. As you reach the maximum length of excursion, reverse the direction (Fig. 18–8). The hands should pass each other in midstroke and continue to alternate like pistons. Begin to pick up speed and to build friction heat. The muscles of the shoulder and upper arm are used to propel the hands, thus reducing the stress on the therapist's hands. General friction may be applied using the ulnar or palmar surface of one or both hands.

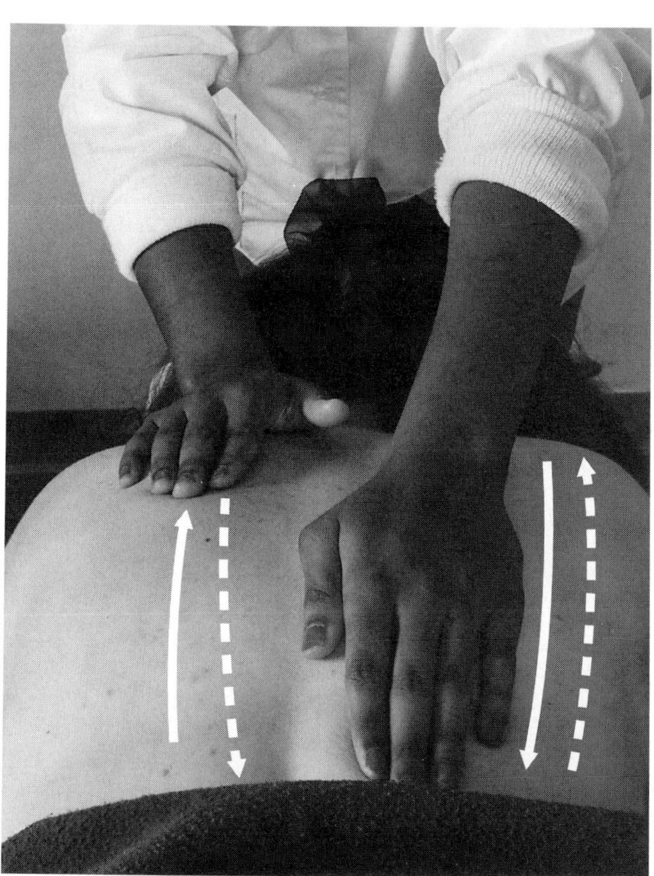

Figure 18•8 General friction.

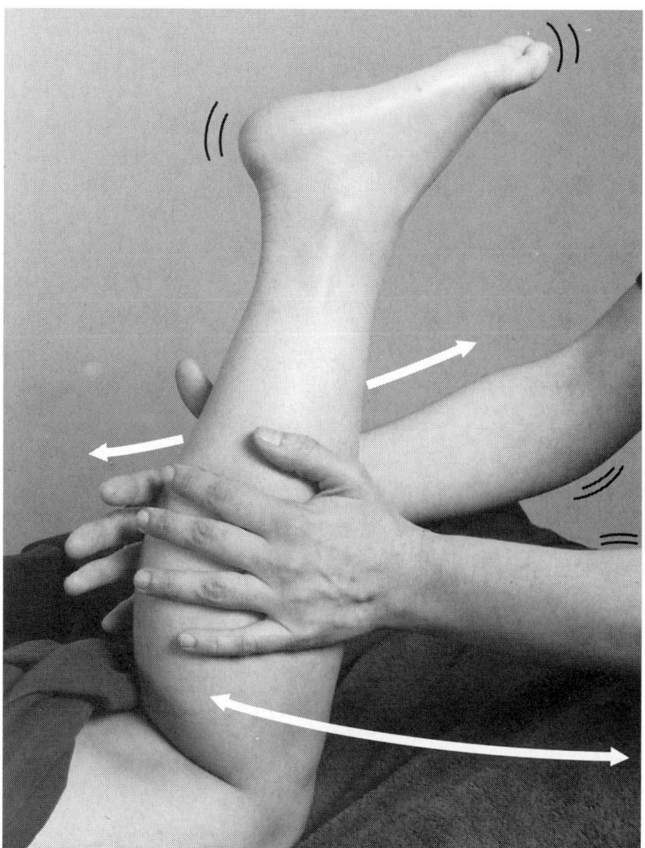

Figure 18•9 Rolling friction.

Variation: Rolling Friction

Compress the tissue firmly with the open palms and extended fingers of both hands. Roll the skin, muscle, and surrounding tissues around the bone, moving both hands in opposite directions. As you roll the tissue around an extremity, use a back and forth movement (Fig. 18–9). As you compress and roll the tissue, slowly move your hands from distal to proximal. The client may assist by holding the limb still.

Variation: Chucking Friction

Also known as linear friction, chucking requires the therapist to rub his thumb or fingers back and forth, moving the superficial tissue over the underlying structure. Chucking is usually performed one-handed, while the other hand is supporting the limb that is being massaged. This movement is usually on the belly of a muscle or between bony areas (e.g., metacarpals, metatarsals, forearms, and lower legs) (Fig. 18–10).

Variation: Wringing Friction

While compressing the tissue on all sides with the palmar surfaces of the hands and fingers, move the hands in opposing directions. Slide the hands down toward the trunk of the body during the massage

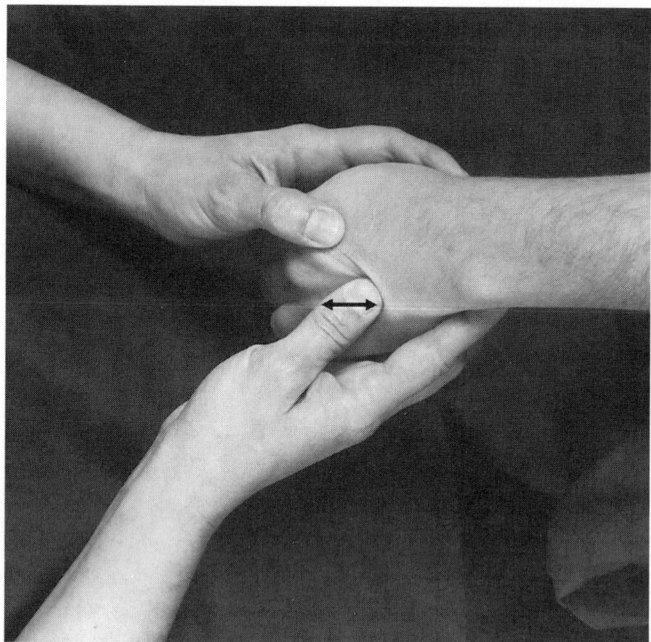

Figure 18•10 Frictional chucking.

movement (distal to proximal). Wringing friction is performed vigorously, like wringing water out of a cloth (Fig. 18–11). This movement is best suited for arms, legs, and fingers. To wring the fingers and other small body areas, modify your technique; compress the tissue using only the fingers rather than your entire hand.

Variation: Cross-Fiber Friction

Also known as deep transverse friction and digital friction, cross-fiber friction is a very precise and penetrating form of friction popularized by Dr. James Cyriax of London, England. Success of this method depends upon the therapist's ability to identify contracted or injured tissue by palpation and then to apply the technique. Cross-fiber techniques are extremely beneficial when following compression or trigger point work.

One or more fingers are placed on the skin at the exact site of a *lesion* (a pathologic change or abnormality in body tissue). Applying firm, consistent pressure in one or both directions, move the fingers in a back and forth motion across the affected structure. The direction of movement should be across and perpendicular to the direction of the muscle fibers (Fig. 18–12). The fingers and skin must move as one unit, or a blister may form and you will not affect the tissue you want to reach. Apply moderate to heavy pressure, according to the client's tolerance, for several minutes. This is somewhat uncomfortable at first, but the dis-

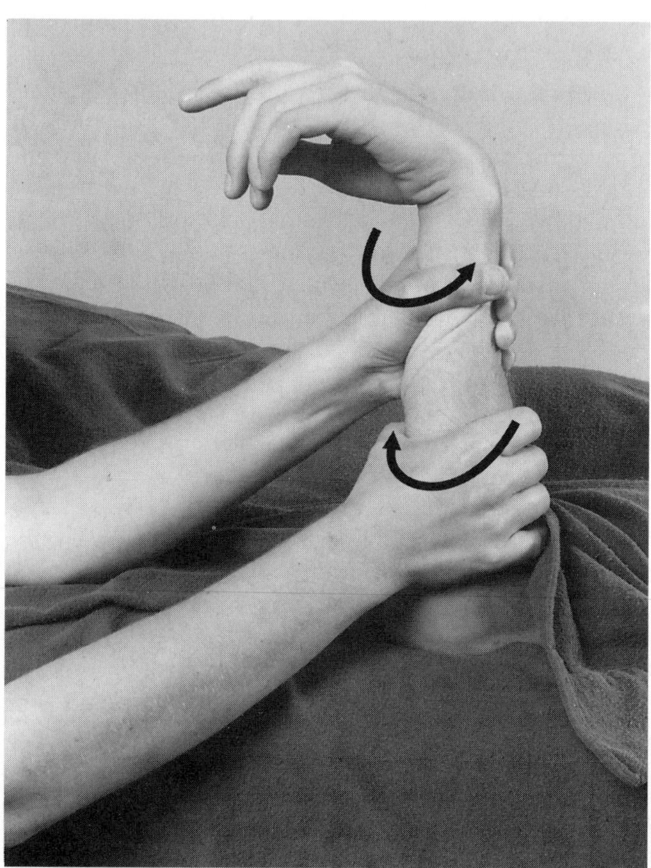

Figure 18•11 Wringing friction.

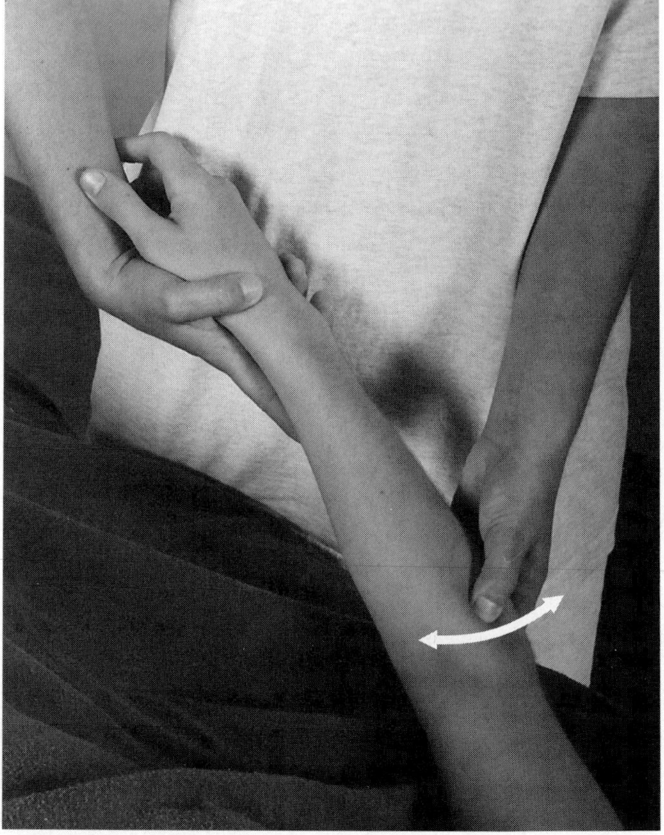

Figure 18•12 Cross-fiber friction.

comfort diminishes as the treatment progresses. The release of endorphins and enkephalins may be responsible for the anesthetic response. This massage movement is a rehabilitative or corrective stroke, and is remarkably effective in treating most muscular, tendinous, or ligamentous injuries and when adhesions and fibrosis are involved. Cross-fiber is often combined with ice for an additional vasodilation and anesthetic effect. Refer to the hydrotherapy chapter for specific ice application methods.

Variation: Circular Friction

Circular friction is applied in the same manner as cross-fiber friction, but instead of the back-and-forth motion of the thumb or finger, the digits are moving in a circular direction (Fig. 18–13). As in cross-fiber friction, the skin tissue is moved over the deeper structures. This movement is particularly useful around joints and in bony areas.

Benefits of Friction

- Friction generates heat.
- It dilates capillaries and increases circulation (hyperemia).
- It loosens stiffness in joints by relaxing muscles.
- It improves the glandular action of the skin.
- Friction reorganizes collagen and facilities its proper parallel pattern.
- It mimics muscle broadening and stretching that occurs in normal muscle movement.
- It reduces trigger and tender point activity.
- Friction breaks down and coaxes apart adhered tissue, freeing restricted areas.

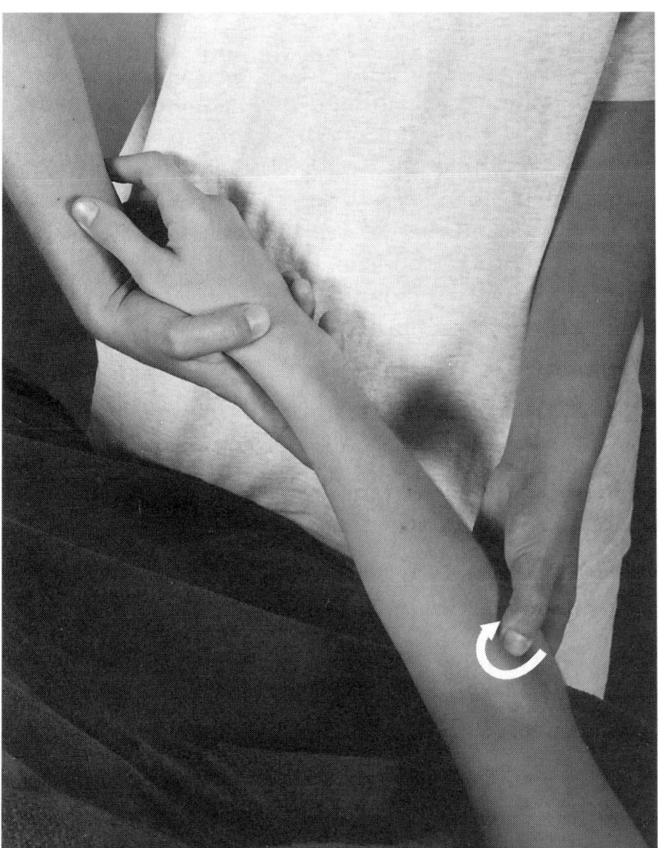

Figure 18•13 Circular friction.

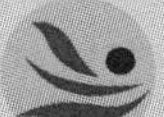

MINI•LAB

To illustrate how cross-fiber friction can have an effect on scar tissue repatterning, do the following activitiy. Place 50 toothpicks in a haphazard formation under a thick towel. Lay your hand, palm down, on the towel and begin moving your hand in a back and forth motion. Continue doing this for several minutes and notice what happens to the toothpick arrangement. Do they remain haphazard or do they line up straight? How does this relate to applying cross-fiber friction on restricted fascia or a scar?

Write your conclusion and share it with your class.

Percussion or Tapotement

The word "percussion" comes from *percussio* which means "a striking." The synonym **tapotement** (tap-ot-mon) is a French derivation of an Old French term *taper* that means "a light blow," which in turn was derived from the Anglo-Saxon *taeppa,* meaning to "tap," in the sense of draining fluid from a cavity. At first, this may seem like a strange etiology, but interestingly enough, the mechanical impact of the tapotement techniques is still used by respiratory therapists and nurses to loosen phlegm congestion in the lungs. **Percussion** involves repetitive staccato striking movements of the hands, simultaneously or alternately, with loose wrists and fingers, for the purpose of stimulating the underlying tissues.

The technique variations are tapping, cupping, beating, slapping, and hacking. The style of the percussion depends on the location where it is employed and the desired effect. Muscular areas such as legs and hips may absorb more force in the delivery, and thin-tissued or delicate areas such as the face require a lighter tap. Proper percussive techniques should be learned under the supervision of a qualified instructor because percussion delivered with too much force can bruise a client. Avoid the application of tapotement after exercise because this stroke can activate muscle spindles and stimulate cramping. Avoid applying percussion over the kidneys because they are not adequately protected by soft tissue. Percussion may be applied directly to the skin or through the drape.

General Technique for Tapotement

Tapotement consists of a series of successive strikes delivered to the skin with either one or two hands. The stroke may be delivered with the ulnar surface of the palm, the tips of the fingers, the open palm, the cupped palm, or the back or ulnar surface of a loosely closed fist.

When applying tapotement, begin with a soft and slow hand strike, gradually building to a more forceful and quick stroke, finally diminishing in speed and depth to end the series of blows. The stroke is delivered rhythmically with your hand or fingers, allowing your hands to spring back after contact. To avoid bruising, keep your wrists loose and your fingers relaxed while making skin contact.

Variation 1: Tapping Tapotement

Using your fingertips, strike the body's surface, using one or both hands. This variation of tapotement is appropriate for use on the head, face, feet, chest, arms, legs, and back. Tapping may also be referred to as *punctuation* (Fig. 18–14).

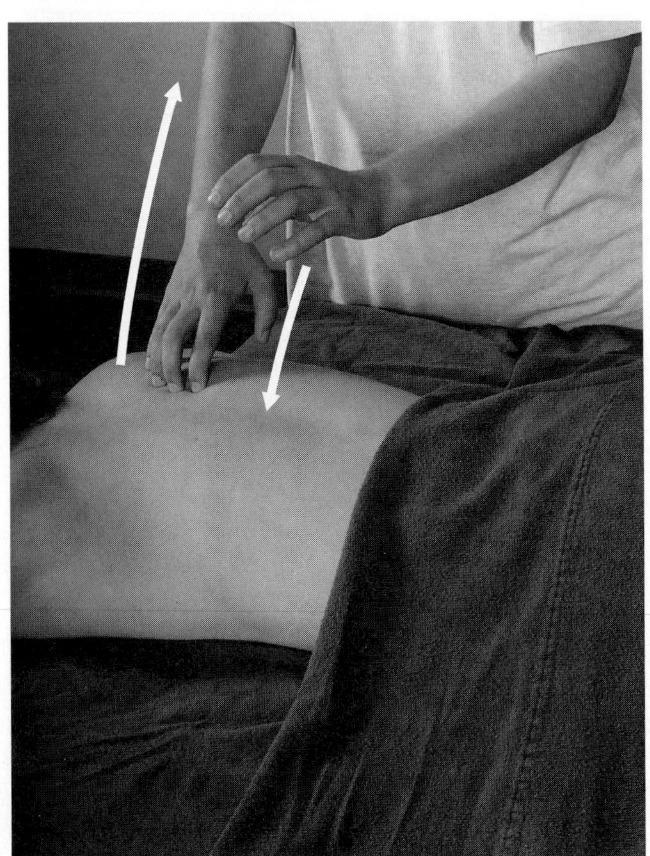

Figure 18•14 Tapping tapotement.

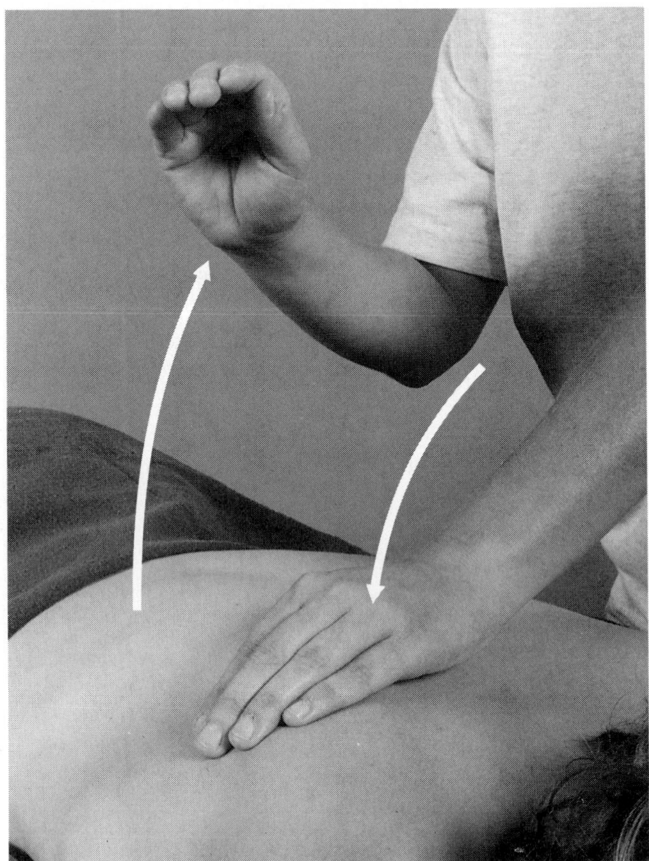

Figure 18•15 Cupping tapotement.

Variation 2: Tapping Tapotement

This variation is performed one-handed, with an alternate deep and light tap; the light tap is generated by landing the fingertips on the skin that is bouncing back from the deep tap. The deep tap is comparable to a full note and the light tap is comparable to a half note. The sound produced by the soft and hard tap reverberates like the sound or feel of a beating heart (lubb, dubb, lubb, dubb).

Variation 3: Tapping Tapotement

Each fingertip of the hand strikes the skin lightly at a different time. This variation is called *raindrops* and is commonly used on the face or scalp.

Variation: Cupping Tapotement

Curve the palmar surface of the hand into a cup, as if holding water. Strike the client's skin with the edges of a cupped surface, making a muffled horse-hoof sound (Fig. 18–15). A vacuum is created when lifting the palm of the hand from the surface of the skin, hence, the hollow sound of suction. Cupping is often used on large areas such as the back or legs. This is the stroke of choice for loosening mucus and phlegm in the thoracic region. You may want to warn the client about the loud noise that often accompanies cupping tapotement. Additionally, it is a very vigorous stroke and may induce coughing. Therapists using this type of stroke therapeutically should interrupt the technique to allow for coughing and have plenty of tissues on hand for the client. Often it helps to orient the client with the head lower than the chest by using pillow bolsters under the abdomen and chest to induce positional drainage. Make sure you end this section with several soothing strokes. This type of tapotement may not be considered a pleasant experience, so make sure that you thoroughly explain the procedure and obtain an informed consent.

Variation: Loose Fist Beating Tapotement

Also known as *pounding,* loose fist beating tapotement is performed with loose fists, contacting the skin alternately. These blows are delivered rhythmically using moderate pressure (Fig. 18–16). Loose fist beating is used on large, muscular areas such as the posterior legs and the hips.

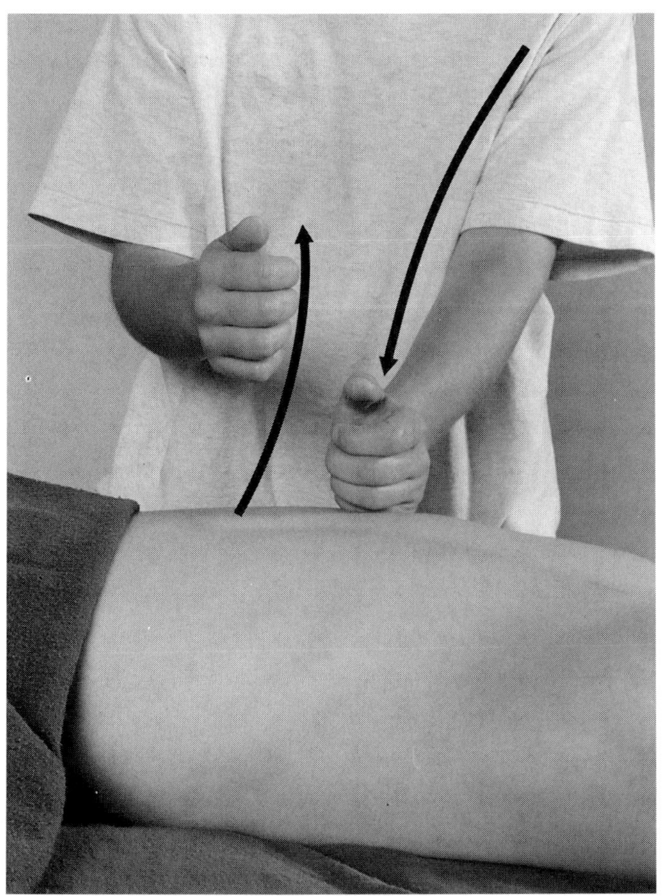

Figure 18•16 Loose fist beating.

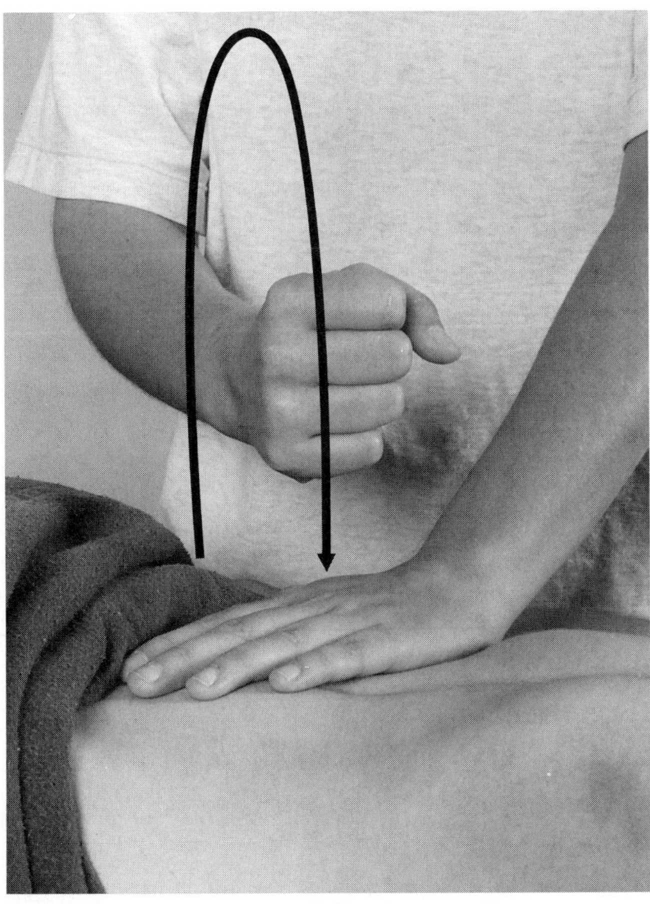

Figure 18•17 Diffused tapotement.

Variation: Diffused Tapotement

Lay the palmar surface of one hand on the client's skin. Using a relaxed fist, strike the dorsal surface of your open hand to diffuse the force (Fig. 18–17). Diffused tapotement is commonly used over the abdominal region.

Variation: Slapping Tapotement

Slapping is performed with the palmar surface of the hands and fingers, striking the skin with alternate strokes (Fig. 18–18). A loud smacking sound will be heard if done correctly. Use slapping on large areas such as the lower back, hips, and gluteals or on thick, hard surfaces such as the soles of the feet. A light upward slapping may be done on the sides of the face. This variation stimulates the sebaceous glands in the skin to secrete oil or sebum, which lubricates and softens the skin. While it is often an invigorating stroke, slapping tapotement is not recommended for use on clients who are known to be survivors of abuse as it may trigger painful past episodes of abuse.

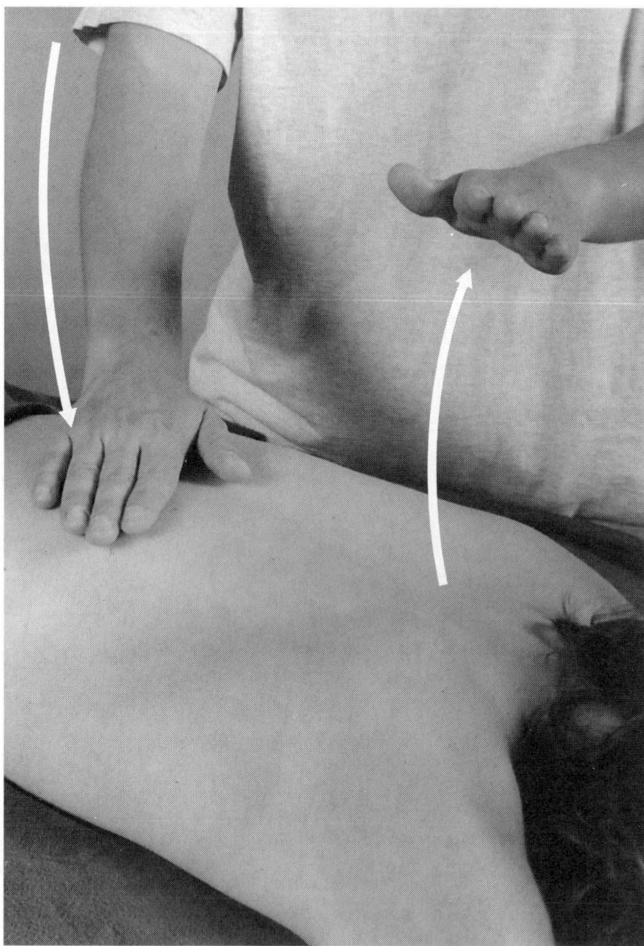

Figure 18•18 Slapping tapotement.

Variation: Hacking Tapotement

Using the ulnar edge of the hands, alternately strike the surface of the client's skin. The hands should be held loosely with the finger slightly spread. Upon contact, the momentum of the stroke will cause each finger to contact the one below it, creating a pulsating effect. This will produce a slight vibratory action coupled with the percussive action of hacking.

Hacking may be applied down the muscle fibers or across the muscle fibers. Hacking *along* muscle fibers, with the fingers parallel, will produce relaxation in the muscle (Fig. 18–19). Hacking applied *across* large muscles, with the fingers perpendicular (across the grain), will stimulate muscle spindle activity (Fig. 18–20). Minute contractions of the muscle will be the result.

The therapist may use the perpendicular striking technique to energize a muscle in preparation for a sporting event or may repeat the stroke in order to lead the muscle into a state of fatigue or exhaustion. This stimulatory action is one of the therapeutic principles behind electric muscle stimulation or galvanic stimulation.

Benefits of Tapotement

- It stimulates nerve endings initially, becoming more sedative if continued.
- It aids in decongesting the lungs by loosening and mobilizing phlegm in the respiratory tract.
- Tapotement tones atrophied muscles if applied briefly.
- It increases local blood flow (histamines and acetylcholine vasodilators are released).
- It accesses deeper structures such as hip rotators.
- It creates an "ultrasound" effect manually.
- It relieves pain, perhaps due to the gate theory.
- Tapotement can desensitize a hypersensitive area because of the release of corticosteroids from nerve axons after about 15 minutes of tapotement stimulation.

Author's Note

Ultrasound is acoustic mechanical vibration of high frequency that produces thermal and nonthermal effects. Therapeutic ultrasound is unique because it falls

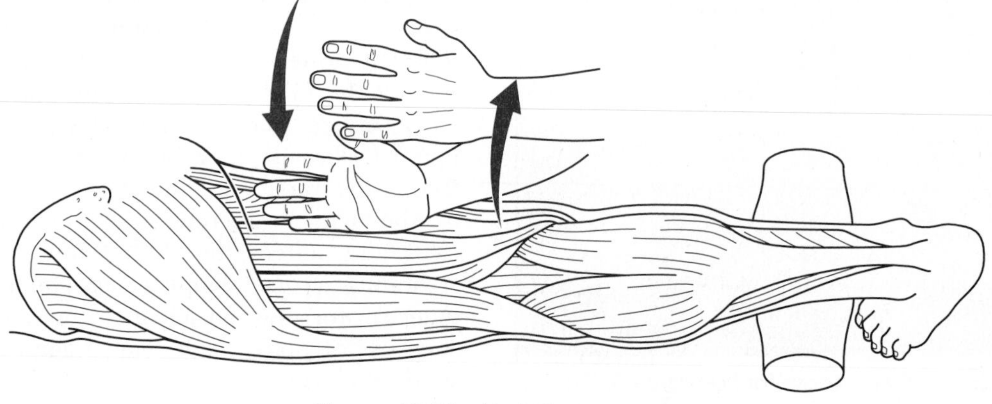

Figure 18•19 Hacking percussion.

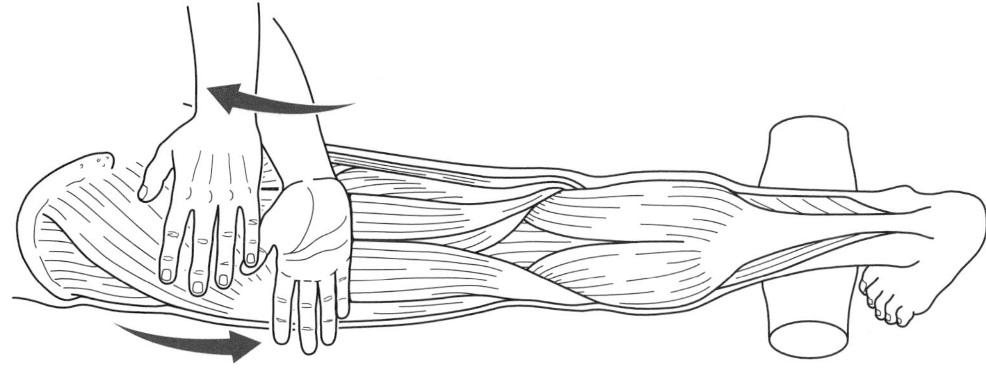

Figure 18•20 Perpendicular hacking.

within the acoustic spectrum and not the electromagnetic spectrum. Sonic (sound) energy can be transmitted into the body during tapotement delivery. Therapeutic ultrasound is known for its thermal effects, but its acoustic pressure changes are the most important. Doctors of physical medicine and physical therapists often refer to therapeutic ultrasound as "micromassage." It is also interesting that lower frequencies of sound penetrate farther into the tissue.

Vibration

The term vibration comes from Latin for "a shaker." **Vibration** is rapid shaking, trembling, or oscillating movements that are applied with full hands, fingertips, or a mechanical device for the purpose of inducing relaxation. Vibration differs from tapotement in that the hands do not break contact with the client's skin in vibration (except for the rocking techniques). Additionally, vibration is bidirectional whereas tapotement has a unidirectional impact. The therapist's hand may remain in one location or glide around an area, such as the stomach, while applying the trembling movement. Performing vibration correctly requires coordination and practice. During vibration, you will be able to observe the tissue moving near the area of contact. There are three basic categories of vibration: fine, coarse, and rocking.

Variation: Fine Vibration

Place the fingertips on the skin and begin a trembling movement by rapidly contracting and relaxing the arm, keeping the fingers and wrist stiff. Fingers should be moving up and down (like a piston), or side to side, while maintaining contact with the skin (Fig. 18–21). This type of vibration is especially useful over the abdomen to increase peristalsis.

Another way to apply fine vibration is to compress and lift the tissue. Once this is done, begin trembling the hand that is in direct contact with the tissue. The stroke feels as if you are slurping up the tissue in your hands.

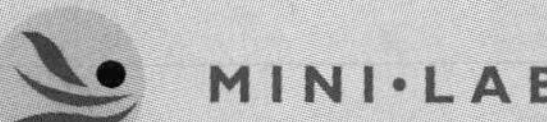

MINI•LAB

To demonstrate the ability to relax the body during vibration, do the following. With a partner, decide who will be the giver and who will be the receiver. Stand about 18 to 24 inches apart. The giver will grasp the receiver's wrist and pull, using moderate force. Note the response of the receiver's body. Let go and again grasp the receiver's wrist. Pull, using moderate force, only this time rock or shake the arm as you do so. Note the response of the receiver's body. Ask the receiver to share his experience with both techniques. Do the exercise again, reversing roles. Is it more difficult to tense up and resist the forward movement while your body is being rocked? Could the rocking movement also be providing a distracting element, interfering with the body's tendency to stiffen?

Variation: Coarse Vibration

Coarse vibration, or *jostling,* is applied by grasping a limb and shaking it rhythmically with a small degree of traction (Fig. 18–22). This vibration type is typically applied to the ball-and-socket joints of the shoulder and hip. Coarse vibration can loosen up muscles that surround a joint.

Variation: Rocking Vibration

The gentle rocking in a mother's womb or in a parent's arms is probably the first motion your body experiences. Even as adults we find comfort in this sensation.

Rocking vibration requires a "pitch and catch" mo-

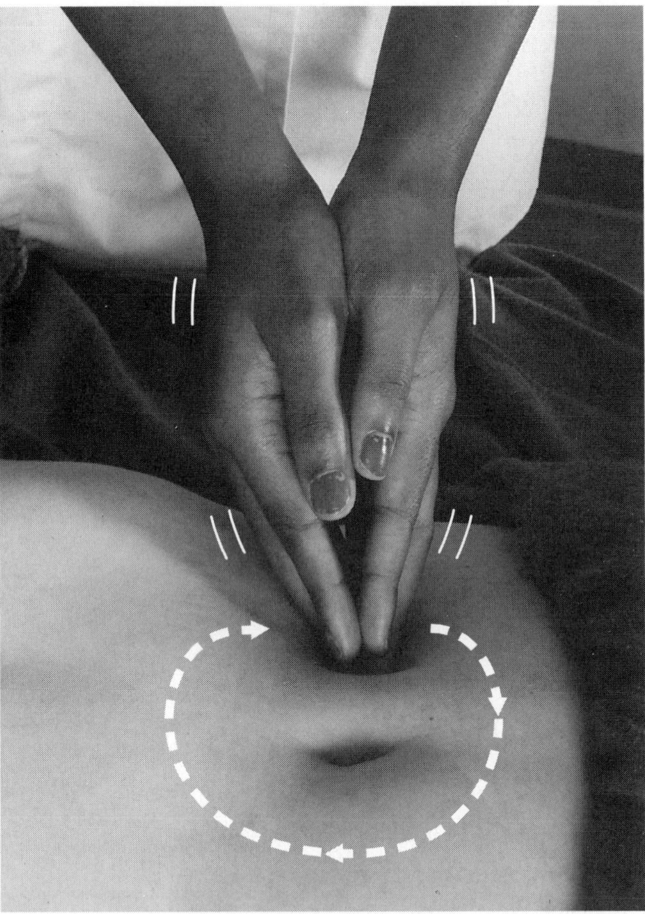

Figure 18•21 Fine vibration.

tion. Push, or "pitch," the body with both hands, retrieving, or "catching," it as the body swings back toward you (Fig. 18–23). Pitch and catch the body until it begins to move easily or fluidly. You can also pitch and catch the body using one hand on each side of the body. One of the best places of contact is the lateral aspects of the ilium to rock the hips. A wonderful bodily sensation for the client, rocking is often physically taxing to the therapist, who should closely monitor her own personal exertion for setting the duration of the stroke. Not unlike pushing someone on a swing, the timing of this stroke is everything.

Author's Note

When rocking a client, you will notice that each body has its own type of movement pattern depending upon the size of the body, the tissue density, and the health of the joints. Some bodies tend to have a quicker "rattle," whereas others have a slow, full rock. You must support the client's own movement pattern, whether it is a rattle or a rock. Avoid imposing an unnatural rhythm on the body.

Variation: Vibratory Mechanical Devices

Place a towel between the client's skin and the mechanical unit for a more comfortable delivery of electrical vibration. The cord must be long enough to reach the area of treatment from an electrical outlet. Also make sure the cord does not touch the client. If the cord is long enough, drape it over your shoulder while holding the appliance. Never leave the appliance on the floor or the cord stretched out for someone to trip over. Check the cord often for wear, and replace it immediately if it is frayed.

The three types of vibration provided by electronic devices are orbital, oscillating, and percussion/vibration. The orbital unit uses a circular, or orbital, mo-

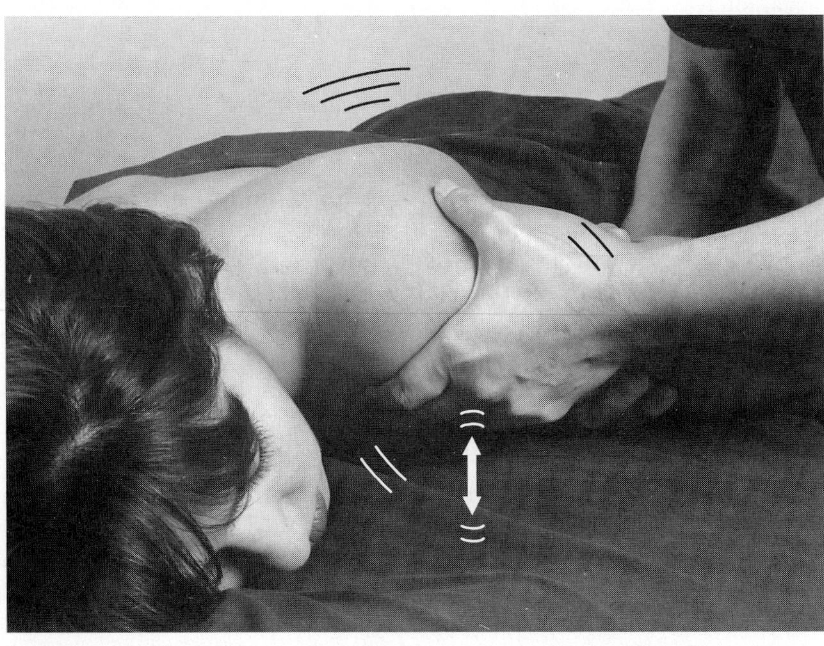

Figure 18•22 Coarse vibration.

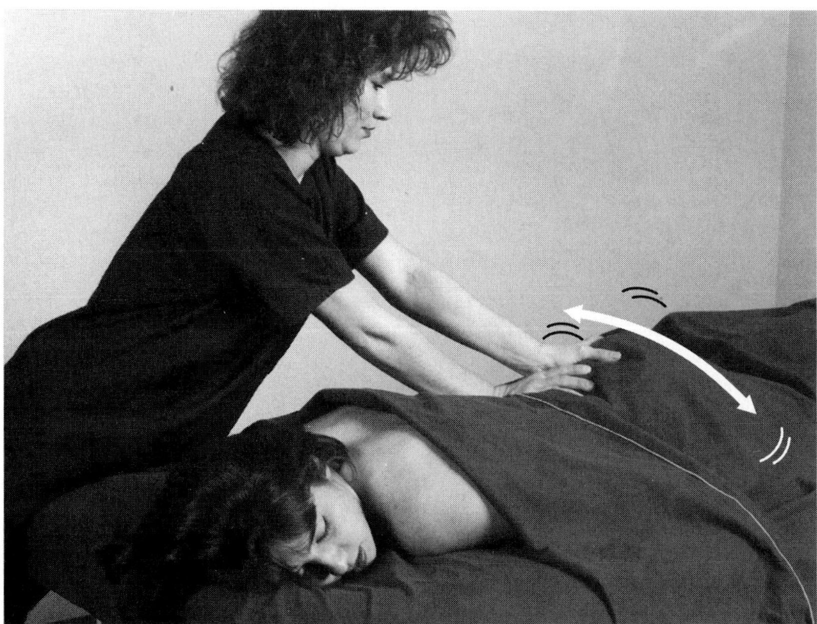

Figure 18•23 Rocking.

tion. As the contact pad moves over the skin, it produces a shaking action to vibrate the tissues. The popular Jeanie Rub electric massager (Morfan, Inc., 3002 N. Home St., Mishawaka, IN 46545) uses an oscillating vibratory action like a sander, but this type of massager does not penetrate very far into the tissue. The brand name Thumper (Wellness America, 1241 Denison St., #40, Markham, Ontario, L3R4B4, Canada) is the most popular percussion/compression electric appliance. Not only does it go up and down (as opposed to a side to side or circular direction), producing the percussion action, but the unit is heavy, adding valuable pressure to the motion. The combination of pressure and percussion/vibration is felt deep into the tissues.

The use of handheld vibrators or electric vibrators that strap to the back of your hand should be kept to a minimum. New research indicates that prolonged use of these appliances has a harmful effect of the nervous system of the therapist. Vibration applied on one area for more than 15 minutes will create an unpleasant numbing sensation. After a 20-minute vibratory session, a rash may appear, indicating tissue irritation. Often, massage therapists who use handheld electric vibrators suffer nerve damage of the hand. In one case, the nerve damage was so severe that opening a jar lid was difficult and painful.

Benefits of Vibration

- It enhances general relaxation.
- It increases circulation.
- Vibration stimulates muscle spindles, thus creating minute muscle contractions.
- It relieves pain, perhaps due to the gate theory.
- It relieves upper respiratory tract congestion, including sinus congestion.
- Abdominal vibration stimulates peristalsis of the large intestine.
- Abdominal vibration diminishes gas in the lower gastrointestinal tract.
- It stimulates synovial fluid production in joints when applied with traction.
- It accesses deeper structures such as hip rotators.
- Vibration relaxes myofascial tissue.
- It desensitizes trigger points.

ANCILLARY MOVEMENTS

The word **ancillary** refers to something that is auxiliary or supplementary to a standard. In the case of massage therapy, the Western standard is the five strokes of Swedish massage. But just as every therapist develops her own style and modification of the fundamental Swedish moves, modified techniques have evolved into effective and popular ancillary strokes, some of which have been developed into whole new systems of massage therapy in themselves. The ancillary movements discussed here have been grouped into the following classifications: touch, nerve strokes, compression, trigger point work, stretching, and Swedish gymnastics.

Often the hands will solve a mystery that the intellect has struggled with in vain.

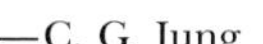

—C. G. Jung

Touch

Touch is the medium of massage and a powerful therapeutic tool. For purposes of distinction between touch and massage movements, **touch** is defined as laying the hands on the skin without movement. The more sensitive we can become, the more powerful our touch can become.

Touching the client on the head, feet, or back is one of the best ways to begin and end a massage session (Fig. 18–24). Often, a moment of quiet accompanies your initial contact with your client, giving him the opportunity to become accustomed to you without distracting conversation.

Benefits of Touch

- Touch increases the hemoglobin count of red blood cells.
- It decreases blood pressure (temporarily).
- It reduces anxiety.
- Touch can activate growth hormone.

Nerve Stroke

Nerve stroking, or feather stroking, is a finishing stroke in massage therapy and is typically the last move to be applied (excluding basic touch). The **nerve stroke** is a light fingertip tracing over the surface of the skin to signal psychologically the end of the massage session to the client. This ancillary stroke is often classified as light effleurage.

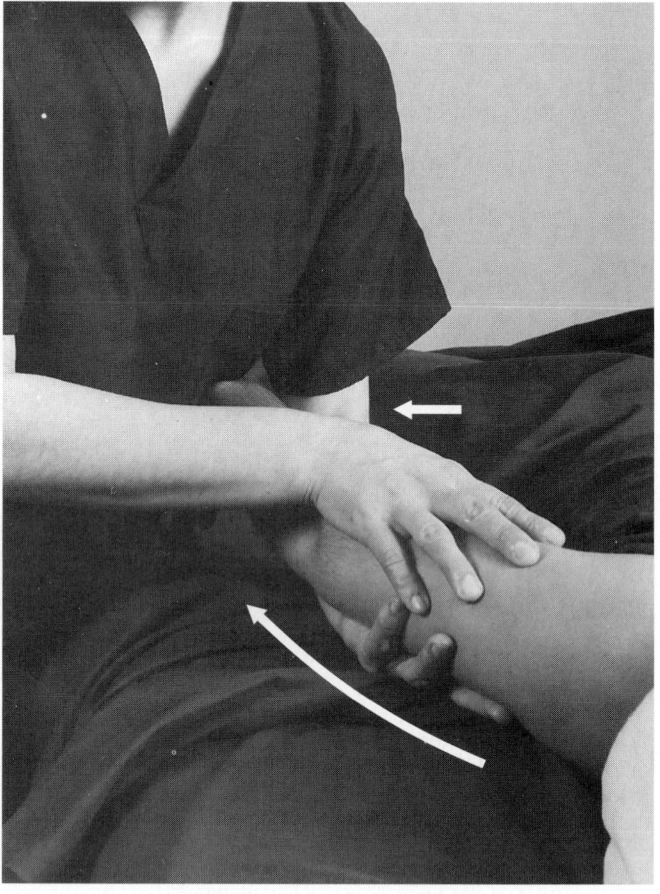

Figure 18•25 Nerve stroke.

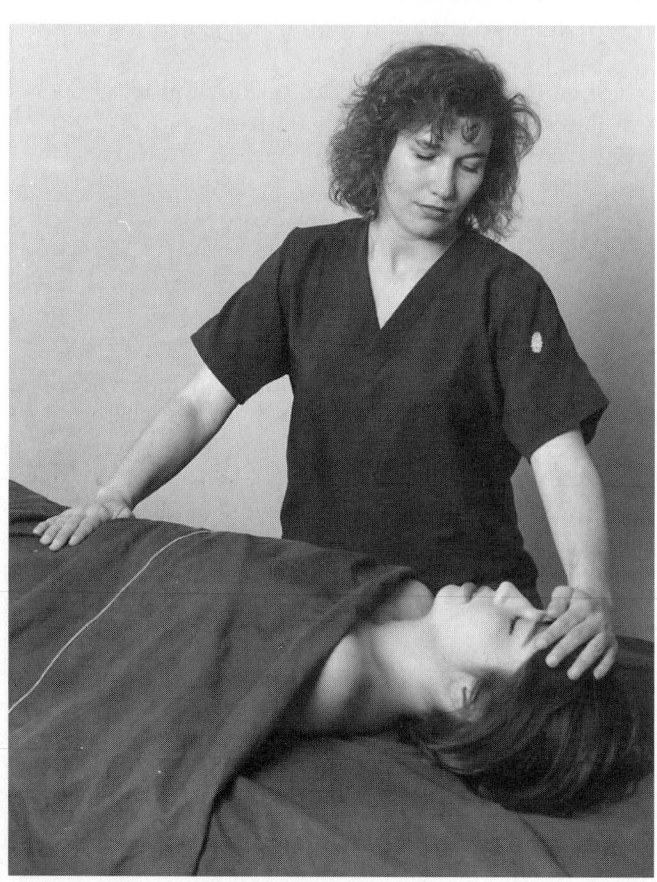

Figure 18•24 Touching.

Avoid pressure that is too light because it may be perceived as ticklish or produce goosebumps. The stroke may be applied to bare skin, to clothed clients (sports or seated massage), and through drapes. The back, arms, and legs are areas where nerve strokes are most often applied. Many therapists consider nerve stroking as the icing on the cake. Of course, each client is different; not all will find this sensation pleasant. Ask the client for his opinion; your last touch should be pleasant for him.

Technique 1

Using just the weight of your hands or fingers, use a gliding stroke down the body (Fig. 18–25).

Technique 2

This technique is frequently used in applying chair massage or over a draped client in the prone position. Extend the index and middle fingers of both hands in a V formation. Place the tips of these two fingers on either side of the spine. Using a quick, downward, whipping motion, forcefully brush the fingertips from the shoulders down the back to the buttocks. Repeat this stroke several times.

Benefits of Nerve Stroking

- It soothes the nervous system when done slowly.
- It stimulates the nervous system when done quickly.

Compression

Compression massage is a rhythmic mechanical pumping on a muscle belly over bone to create a sustained increase in circulation and muscle relaxation. In the 1950s, compression massage became an independent classification of massage movements. Many pre-event sports massage techniques use compression as the main technique because it is nonspecific, light, and warming. Compression massage can be done over a clothed client, if the client is ticklish, or when lubricant is inconvenient or contraindicated (see Technique). Application of progressively stronger compression on a trigger point often eliminates the trigger point's tenderness and hyperirritability. Application of pressure typically blanches the compressed tissues, and they become hyperemic on release of the pressure. There are three variations: palmar compression, fist compression, and forearm compression.

Technique

For proper application of compression, the muscle belly must be pressed perpendicularly into the underlying bone. Press your palm or fist into the muscle and release. Compression massage uses a *rhythmic pumping* action. Because the direction of the stroke is perpendicular to the tissues (not linear or parallel), lubricant is not necessary. Some therapists may elect to use a lubricant in order to combine this move with other strokes that require a lubricating medium.

Compression is generally applied with the palm, fist, or forearm. To apply palmar compression, use the palmar surface of your hands and press into the muscle belly using about 7 to 10 pounds of pressure (Fig. 18–26). Keep your fingers loose. Fist compression requires use of the proximal digit surface of a closed fist to apply the pressure. To deliver forearm compression, apply pressure to the belly of the muscle with the ulnar surface of the forearm.

Avoid applying intermittent compression directly on a muscle spasm—this will only serve to increase the spasm. Instead, apply even compression and maintain constant pressure for 8 to 12 seconds. Please consult the section on trigger point work for more information on sustained pressure.

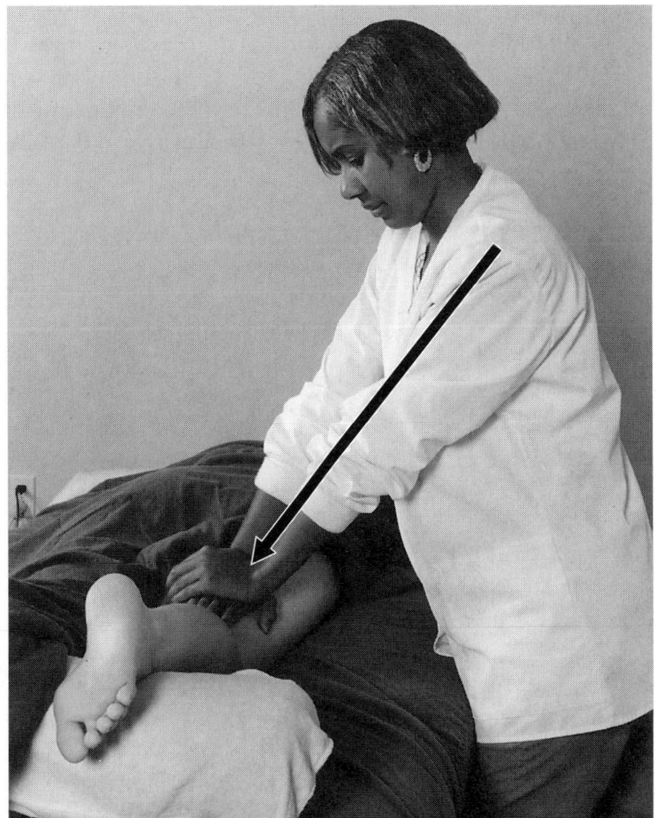

Figure 18•26 Compression.

Benefits of Compression

- It serves as a capillary flush (hyperemia).
- It increases local cellular nutrition.
- Compression softens superficial fascia through increased circulation.
- It spreads and broadens muscle.
- Sustained compression reduces muscle spasm.
- It interrupts the pain-spasm-pain cycle.
- Compression stimulates the release of histamines and acetylcholine (vasodilators) to produce a sustained increase in local circulation.

Trigger Point Work

Trigger points are hypersensitive (taking little stimulation to contract) areas in muscles, fascia, tendons, and ligaments that refer pain to distal regions of the body. Muscles become tense when strong stimuli affect the nervous system. Trigger points can also be described as the point of strongest motor return from the central nervous system back to the spinal cord and can be the result of repetitive or stressful motion, trauma, or poor posture. Dietary, environmental, and emotional stress can also create these localized areas. Many physiologists dispute exactly what trigger points are and what causes them; as a result, there is no single universal explanation. If an area is locally sensitive but stimulation of the site causes no referred sensations, it is not considered a trigger point but a **tender point.**

The **referred pain,** or autonomic, phenomenon, can be subjectively experienced as a variety of sensations (e.g., pain, tingling, numbness, itching, aching, heat,

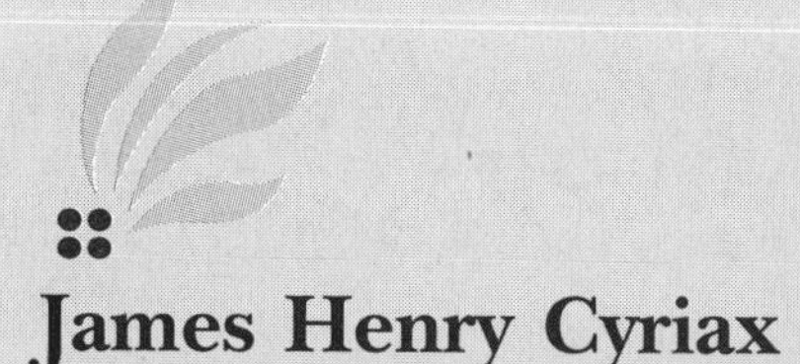

James Henry Cyriax

Born: 1904; died: June 17, 1985.
Physician. Father of orthopedic medicine.

"He could often be seen walking backwards along Lambeth Palace Road round to the bus stop on Westminster Bridge 'so as to keep an eye on the oncoming buses.' "

James Cyriax was born in London, England, the son of Edgar and Annyuta (Kellgren) Cyriax, both of whom studied medicine. Of note is the fact that his mother's family utilized exercise and manipulation in the treatment of musculoskeletal disorders, something that was not in common practice at the time, and which became very influential in James's medical career.

Young James was educated at University College School (Gonville) and Caius College (Cambridge) before finally graduating from St Thomas's Hospital Medical School (London). Soon after passing his qualifying medical exams, Cyriax became affiliated with St. Thomas's Hospital in the department of orthopedic surgery. He is generally given credit for coining the term "orthopedic medicine" and was probably one of Great Britain's most noted orthopedic practitioners. In 1938, Cyriax transformed the massage department at St. Thomas's into the first department of orthopedic medicine. His new department did much to help transform the art of manipulation into a science that was practiced by trained medical doctors and physical therapists.

Especially important in Cyriax's contributions was his system of soft tissue diagnosis. According to his *Textbook of Orthopedic Medicine* (1982 edition), Cyriax had a four-step process for determining problems of soft tissues: 1. active motion (to assess the patient's range of motion, strength, and willingness to move the affected area); 2. passive motion (to assess the degree of motion available and the direction of limitation, the use of palpable sensation at the end of passive motion [which Cyriax called "end-feel"], and the determination of resistance felt by the practitioner during the end-feel testing); 3. resisted contractions (to determine the reaction of the muscle, tendon, and bony attachments to contraction); and 4. palpation (to confirm involvement of the structures suggested by the preceding three steps in the diagnostic procedure (Hayes et al., 1994).

In efforts to determine the exact location of a soft tissue lesion, Cyriax's work is extremely important (although not without numerous critics) in that it helps therapists identify the tissues causing the pain and, consequently, select the best methods of treatment to diminish the pain. In general, Cyriax advocated the use of manipulation, deep friction massage (without the use of creams or oils), and the injection of selected drugs in the treatment of soft tissue lesions. Even though Cyriax's ideas were (and remain) controversial, he provided the first systematic diagnostic approach to determine the cause of a patient's soft tissue disorder.

It is important to note that Cyriax was a firm believer in deep-tissue massage (deep transverse friction), either alone or in conjunction with passive or active movements, for the treatment of muscular, ligamentous, and tendinous lesions. In his *Textbook of Orthopedic Medicine* (1982 edition), he wrote, "Deep transverse friction restores mobility to muscle in the same way a manipulation frees a joint. Indeed, the action of deep transverse friction may be summed up as affording a mobilization that passive stretching or active exercises cannot achieve."

According to Cyriax's obituary in the *British Medical Journal* (July 1, 1985), he was apparently persona non grata within the British medical establishment because of his nontraditional views and consequently never

Continued

elected a fellow of the British Royal College of Physicians. His work continues to be scrutinized, as an examination of the various journals within the physical medicine profession will attest. He was an individual who brought out the extremes in individuals, with both his supporters and critics being very adamant about their views. Regardless, Cyriax was instrumental in advancing the concepts of manipulation and massage in the medical profession, and made incalculable contributions to those professions.

A key indicator of the importance of James H. Cyriax's contributions is the fact that his *Textbook of Orthopedic Medicine* is presently in its ninth edition.

and cold). When working a trigger point reveals a pattern of referred pain, that area of referral should be massaged as well. The referral zone of one trigger point can be responsible for activation of satellite trigger points within that zone. A **satellite trigger point** is a tender area that lies within the referred pain zone of the primary trigger point.

Trigger point work is sustained digital pressure applied to trigger points to relieve pain and discomfort. In the book *Myofascial Pain and Dysfunction, The Trigger Point Manual,* Travell and Simons (1983) referred to trigger point work as *ischemic compression.* Trigger point work may be used between other strokes during the massage session when localized pain is found and is indicated for chronic pain arising from the trigger point–referred pain phenomenon, the degree of which is directly related to the activity of the trigger point. In general, the farther the referred pain sensation travels, the more "active" the trigger point is and the more it needs to be addressed. Other deep-tissue techniques, such as myofascial release, may be indicated for chronic pain arising from fascial adhesions, lesions, and general ischemia.

Trigger point work is contraindicated for clients who are on large doses of blood thinners because it may induce bruising due to the weakened response of their clotting abilities.

The premassage interview will help you gather information about where to look for trigger points. The client may report persistent localized pain—areas in the body where pain comes and goes. Although a client may not be able to determine whether a specific pain is local or referred, she may often report having injured her rotator cuff muscles and unexplained pain down the arm. As the levels of localized excitation build, the client eventually becomes overwhelmed with perceiving painful sensations accurately. As her nervous system continues to be bombarded with hypertonicity and pain, it eventually reaches a state in which these sensations spill over into distal references (the referred pain phenomenon).

Palpation is the key for locating trigger points. Healthy tissue should feel firm but yielding and neither hard nor flabby; it is typically smooth, warm, and does not elicit sensations of pain when therapeutic levels of pressure are applied to it. The unhealthy tissues that surround or contain trigger points might be described as ropy, stringy, knotted, tight, thickened, waxy, or mushy. Trigger points may show up as taut bands of fibrous tissue, and you may be able to feel a firm nodule in the muscle. Occasionally, the trigger point can be located by an audible or palpable click or crunch in the soft tissues. A trigger point map may be used to assist you in locating these general areas on the body (Fig. 18–27). Then, using the client's reports of pain, you can locate the trigger point. A very common trigger point area is the tendon attachment of the levator scapulae muscle at the scapula.

Other indications that a trigger point has been found are the local twitch response and the jump sign. The **local twitch response** is an involuntary firing or twitching in a muscle (a reflex motor output), in response to the sensory stimulation (pressure) on the trigger point. The **jump sign** is a spontaneous reaction of pain or discomfort that may cause a client to wince, jump, or verbalize upon application of pressure. More information concerning trigger points can be found in Chapter 26.

Technique

It is important to warm up the tissue first before treating trigger points. Areas where trigger points are located are often ischemic and need manual assistance to increase blood flow and tissue temperature. Warm-up strokes (e.g., effleurage, petrissage, friction) also provide the therapist an opportunity to begin making contact that is comforting and relaxing for the client, sensing pressure tolerances, tissue textures, and patterns.

Once the tissue has been warmed up, use one of the following for pressure application: the tip of the

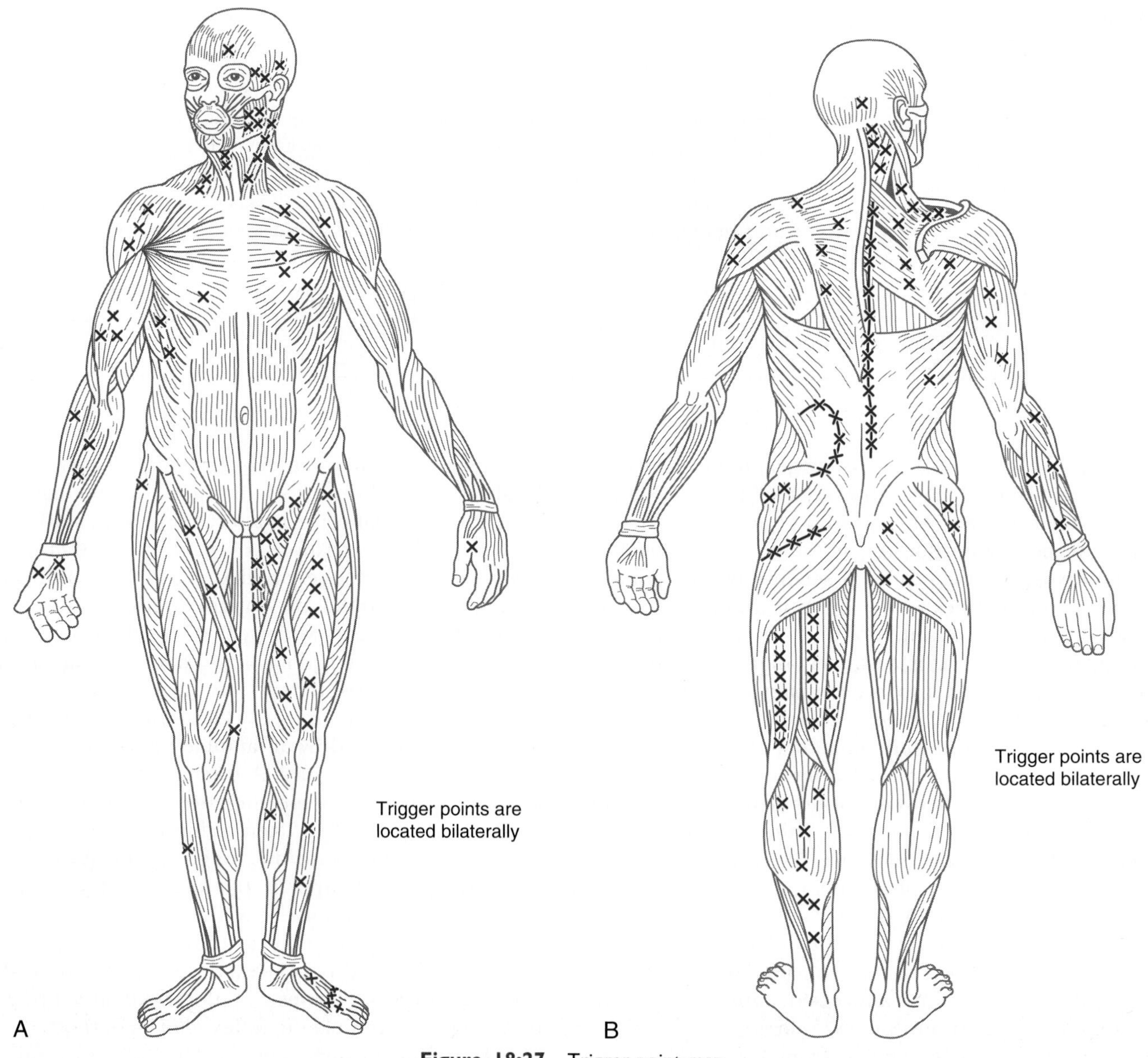

Figure 18•27 Trigger point map.

thumb, a braced finger, palm or heel of the hand, a fist, a knuckle, the forearm, an elbow (see note on body mechanics below), a knee, or a foot. A handheld tool may also be used, but is discouraged since the therapist may risk overtreatment by the inability to detect local tissue changes by palpation.

The therapist applies pressure to the client's tolerance while being aware of the client voluntarily tensing in response to the pressure. The therapist may encourage deeper breathing or may offer a visualization that suggests softening, a sense of ease, melting, or releasing. Using open-ended contact statements like "How is this for you?" or "What is happening for you now?" can offer your client opportunities to express his experience of the work. Hold the pressure for 8 to 12 seconds. Repeat the application of pressure two or three more times, if necessary.

Increase the amount of pressure the second and third time, according to the client's tolerance. Ask your client to calibrate the pain. Create a scale of discomfort using 1 to indicate no pain and 5 to indicate excruciating pain. Try to stay between 3 and 4.

The client may feel a decrease in sensitivity and pain as the treatment progresses and the therapist may notice reduced spasticity as the muscle releases. Once spasm has been eliminated, the target muscle should be stretched in order to reset the muscle spindles. This will decrease the likelihood that the trigger point will return immediately or soon after the session is complete.

Once an area has been treated, it is usually a good idea to do some general relaxation work such as Swedish massage for at least 3 to 5 minutes before reapplying the trigger point work. This allows the nervous system to "quiet down" from high levels of excitation.

One to four treatments per area per session is recommended. It is important for a therapist to continually monitor the balance between general work and specific trigger point work.

Like all other injury treatment modalities, do not use trigger point therapy during the acute stage of the injury; wait 24 to 48 hours, depending upon the severity of the injury.

When applying pressure to trigger points, you should consider two basic rules of body mechanics: Do not let the digits become hyperextended while applying pressure, and instead of contracting your arm muscles to produce downward force, lean forward using your body weight to create the pressure needed.

It is important to inform our clients that they may be sore for up to 48 hours after trigger point work. Applying ice, increasing water intake, and stretching may be recommended to decrease this time. If the client experiences little or no residual soreness, you may be inclined to increase your pressure in the subsequent session. Generally, if the client is sore for more than 48 hours, the client was worked too deeply or too long. The issue of overtreating is an important one to discuss in conjunction with lengthy periods of soreness. Many therapists prefer to space trigger point sessions at least 48 hours apart to give the client time to recover from any soreness.

Application Strategy: Locating TPs

Bonnie Prudden, the developer of myotherapy, uses a compass method of locating trigger points. Place your finger or thumb into the general location of the trigger point. Without moving the thumb over the skin, move the thumb up and down, then side to side (or north, south, east, and west). When the hypersensitive area is located, maintain the pressure for 8 to 12 seconds (Fig. 18–28). Follow the application of direct pressure with compression massage or effleurage. Repeat if necessary.

Benefits of Trigger Point Work

- It stimulates the release of histamines and acetylcholine (vasodilators).
- It stimulates local blood flow.
- It broadens muscle tissue by means of direct pressure.
- It interrupts the pain-spasm-pain cycle.

Stretching

Stretching is such a vast and complex field of study, a small section of one chapter will not do this subject justice. Physical therapists spend more than a year studying stretching as compared with a week or less studying massage. The purpose of this section is to give the beginning massage therapist a basic understanding of the importance and the mechanisms of stretching, as well as to foster a desire for further learning. Additionally, massage therapists should check their state's definition of scope of practice for the inclusion or exclusion of stretching modalities.

Also known as *myotasis,* **stretching** involves elongat-

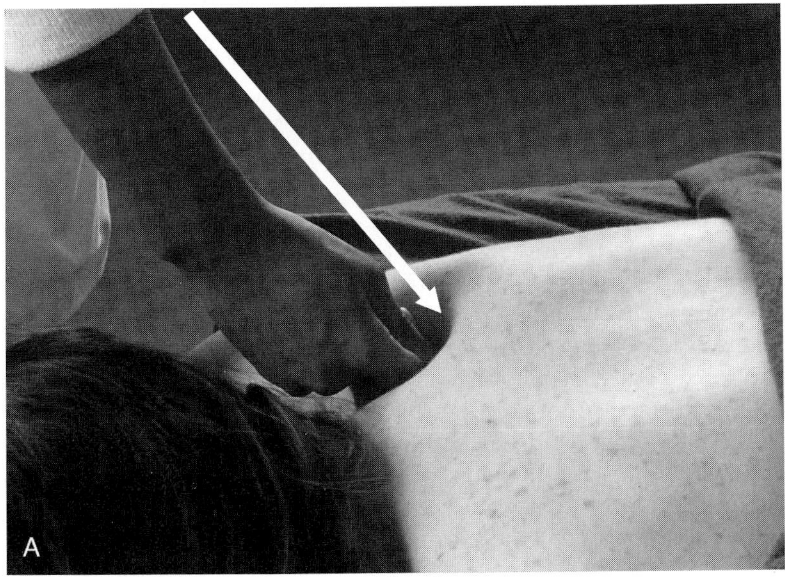

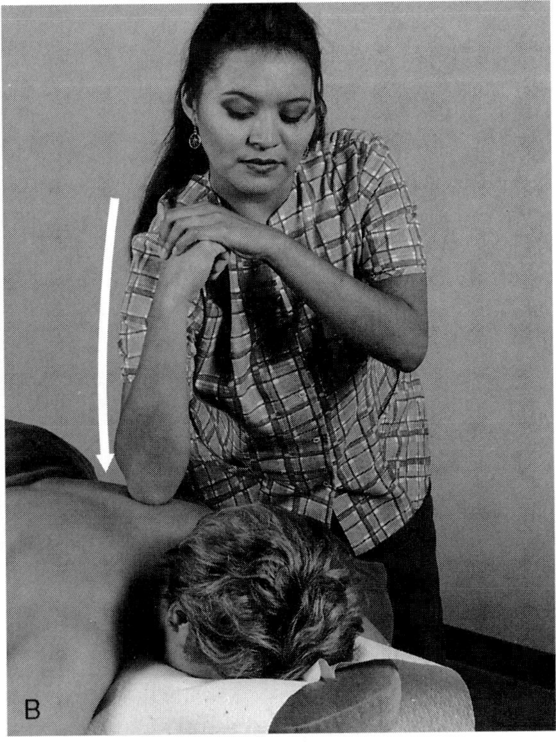

Figure 18•28 Sustained pressure.

ing or extending the muscle tissue to its full length. How far a muscle can be stretched depends upon numerous factors including the client's flexibility, the health of the involved joint, fascial restrictions, and the autonomic nervous system response of muscle guarding. *Flexibility* is the ability of muscles and other soft tissues to lengthen and shorten through the range of motion for which they are intended. While factors such as genetic limitations in joint mobility may limit one's ability to stretch, we can use massage therapy and stretching to decrease the amount of tension in the muscle, decrease the fascial restrictions, and reduce autonomic nervous system guarding, thereby increasing flexibility.

Therapeutic stretching is performed by changing the joint position in order to lengthen the specified muscle. This positional change removes the slack from the affected muscle and allows a sufficient amount of leverage to bring the muscle into a stretch. There are different variations of stretching. It can be done passively by the therapist with no assistance from the client; it can be done actively by the client with no assistance from the therapist. Stretching that is a combined effort between the therapist and client is known as **active-assisted stretching.**

Many massage movements, such as deep effleurage or ironing, stretch muscle tissue. Often those techniques can be combined with a simple range of motion. For example, to stretch the hamstring muscles by ironing, ask the client, lying prone, to flex the knee. With a closed fist, the therapist applies pressure above the popliteal space and glides with deep pressure up the posterior thigh to the ischial tuberosity as the client extends the knee. This engages the muscle in active gymnastics and is sometimes referred to as "pin and stretch." The excursion should be timed so that the entire hamstring has been traversed by the time the knee arrives at full extension.

In order to achieve optimum effectiveness with stretching, you must be able to tell where the pulling action is happening. Most stretching advocates recommend that once a comfortable maximum stretch is achieved you allow the muscle to maintain this position for a specified time, which length varies with the type of stretch being done. Static stretches may take 30 seconds of holding at maximum stretch, whereas active-assisted stretches may only hold for 1½ to 2 seconds. A number of repetitions of the stretch are recommended depending again on the type of stretch being used. It is helpful for the client to relax and breathe deeply while the muscle is being stretched.

Avoid overextending a muscle and creating pain. It is important that the muscle be warm and full of blood before attempting to stretch, which can be accomplished through light activity or massage. The principle is simple. Like clay, warm tissues are pliable and will stretch without tearing. Cold tissues tend to be rigid and less malleable, making them more susceptible to injury. If a person stretches every day, it's like taking out a little insurance. Although stretching does not guarantee that he will not get stiff and sore, it decreases the likelihood.

Stretching routines are not range of motion exercises. A range of motion exercise involves moving a joint through its entire movement capability. A stretch involves a single muscle (and its synergist) being drawn out to its fullest length.

Stretch Reflexes

Stretch reflexes initiate muscle contractions and are of primary importance in maintaining posture and protecting muscles from overstretching. Stretching that is too far or too fast can tear muscles, tendons, and supportive structures. This is especially true when the stretch is too quick or extreme. There are two types of reflexes associated with stretching and corresponding sensory nerves that initiate each reflex. Both of these two reflexes are safeguards that are activated by extremes. There are agonist/antagonist reflexes that govern most normal-range activities of muscle. Safe stretching techniques should engage neither reflex response.

One of the neurological reflexes governing stretching is the **myotatic stretch reflex,** activated when a muscle is pulled and the muscle contracts. Receptors located within the muscle belly, *muscle spindles,* detect the stretching motion and speed of this motion. A sensory impulse is sent to the spinal cord, where the sensation triggers a motor response back to the muscle, telling it to contract. The force of the muscle contraction is somewhat related to the force and speed of the stretch that triggers it. This reaction is designed to protect the joint from further movement in that direction and the muscle from overstretching by causing the muscle to contract. Muscle spindles do not "fire" unless there is a sudden or extreme stretch in the muscle.

The second stretch reflex is called the **inverse stretch reflex,** or the **autogenic inhibition.** The inverse stretch reflex is mediated by the *Golgi tendon organs,* mechanoreceptors that measure a change in distance or degree of tensile force between the fibers of the muscle/tendon junction. When Golgi tendon organs are stimulated by slow, low-force stretches, they inhibit regular muscle contraction, which relaxes the entire muscle, allowing maximum stretching. The goal is to optimize the best tension length relationship between the agonist and antagonist musculotendinous unit.

Ballistic, Static, and Proprioceptive Neuromuscular Facilitation Stretching

There are several types of stretching techniques: ballistic, static, and proprioceptive neuromuscular facilita-

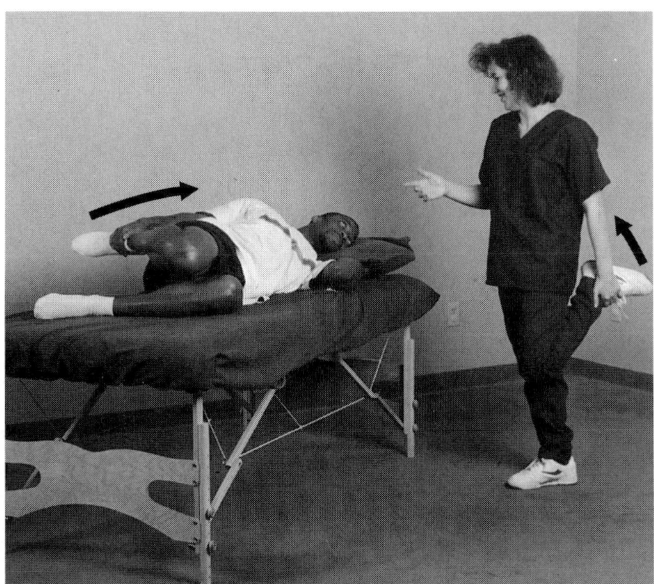

Figure 18•29 Active stretching.

tion. These stretches can be assisted or unassisted. **Ballistic stretching** is achieved by high-velocity, forceful repetition of a bouncing or bobbing motion, each successive bounce increasing the extension of the muscle. An example of a ballistic stretch is a bouncing split. Ballistic stretching has lost popularity in past years because of the high potential of damage to the tissue. *A succession of ballistic movements can cause irritation or even tear the muscle, fascia, tendons, and ligaments. Damage can also occur in the joint capsule itself.* Since the stretch reflex is triggered by muscle spindles that measure both degree and rate of elongation, the quick changes in muscle length associated with ballistic stretching are more likely to trigger the reflex and cause damage to the tissue.

Static stretching, or slow, held stretches, which have been used for centuries in disciplines such as yoga, consists of bringing a muscle to full extension and then maintaining the pressure necessary to keep the muscle in extension from 1 to 30 seconds, depending on the stretching ideology involved. Static stretching is safer than ballistic stretching because there is less likelihood of muscle and connective tissue tearing when the muscle is moving into a lengthened position *slowly.* In other words, static stretching is achieved not *only* by increased muscle length but *also* by the *speed* of the lengthening.

Proprioceptive neuromuscular facilitation (PNF), or contract-relax technique, is based on the neurological phenomenon of *reciprocal inhibition.* PNF involves stretching a muscle through active participation of the client and a 6-second sustained isometric contraction by the attending therapist. Then the muscle is further stretched and its action is resisted. The procedure of stretching and isometric contraction cycles is repeated for 1 minute. In this way, the agonist relaxes the antagonist.

Active and Passive Stretching

Active stretches, or therapist-instructed stretches, involve the therapist describing or demonstrating the stretch while the client *actively* follows along (Fig. 18–29). When the client reaches his natural limit, he has hit the *physiological barrier,* which can be caused by structures such as fascia, the muscle fibers themselves, and scar tissue. This barrier prevents the muscle from stretching as a result of limited function within a muscle or surrounding muscles. Active stretching has two variations: active assisted and active resisted or isometric.

Active-assisted stretches are stretches in which the client contracts the agonist to stretch the antagonist while outside forces assist in the lengthening action. The contraction of the agonist takes advantage of the reciprocal inhibition phenomenon to achieve a greater stretch. The outside force can be a therapist applying leverage pressure to the area being stretched (Fig. 18–30). The outside force can be the other muscles of the client himself, such as using the hands to grasp a piece of rope looped over the foot in order to help stretch the leg.

Active-assisted movement combines active stretching with external assistance. The client is instructed by the therapist on a particular stretch while the therapist assists the client for a maximum stretch. Once maximum stretch has been achieved, the position is held for 1½ to 2 seconds. It is important to limit the maxi-

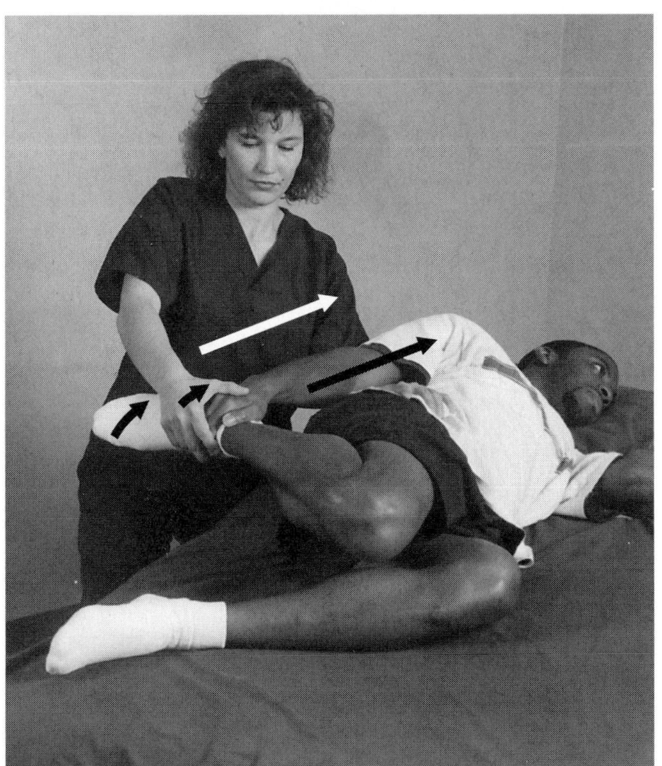

Figure 18•30 Active-assisted stretching.

mum stretch to only 2 seconds in order to honor the myotatic stretch reflex. Several repetitions should be administered in a cycle of stretch, release, stretch, release, stretch, release. Active-assisted stretch expert Aaron Mattes (1995) recommends between 8 and 10 repetitions. Upon release, the stretched muscle should be brought to the opposite extreme of range of motion to pump blood to the muscle.

Active-resisted, or **isometric, stretches** involve the therapist applying gentle resistance while the client is actively engaging in the stretch (Fig. 18–31). Even though isometric stretches do not constitute a muscle stretch, they do enhance flexibility by encouraging local blood flow and stimulating the tissue, which results in a relaxation of the muscle after contraction. When performing active-resisted stretches on yourself or a client, repeat the resistance three to six times.

Passive stretching involves slow, steady movement using gentle force to lengthen tissue. During passive stretching, the client remains relaxed (or passive) and makes no contribution while the therapist applies the stretch (Fig. 18–32). When the therapist and client cooperatively reach the limits of the muscle stretch, she has hit the *anatomical barrier*—the joint structure (soft tissue or bone) that is preventing the joint from mobilizing any further. A muscle passively stretched will extend to a greater length than one actively stretched. A passive stretch is achieved by exerting an outside force on the joint in order to stretch the muscle, for example, an athlete who uses her hand to pull her heel back to touch her gluteals without contracting the hamstrings, flexing the knee passively so that quadriceps group is stretched.

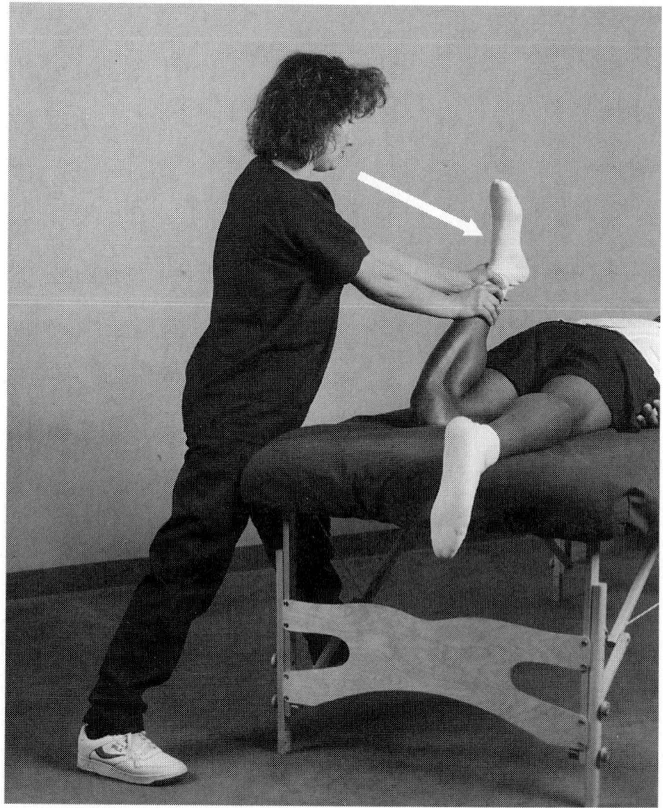

Figure 18•32 Passive stretching.

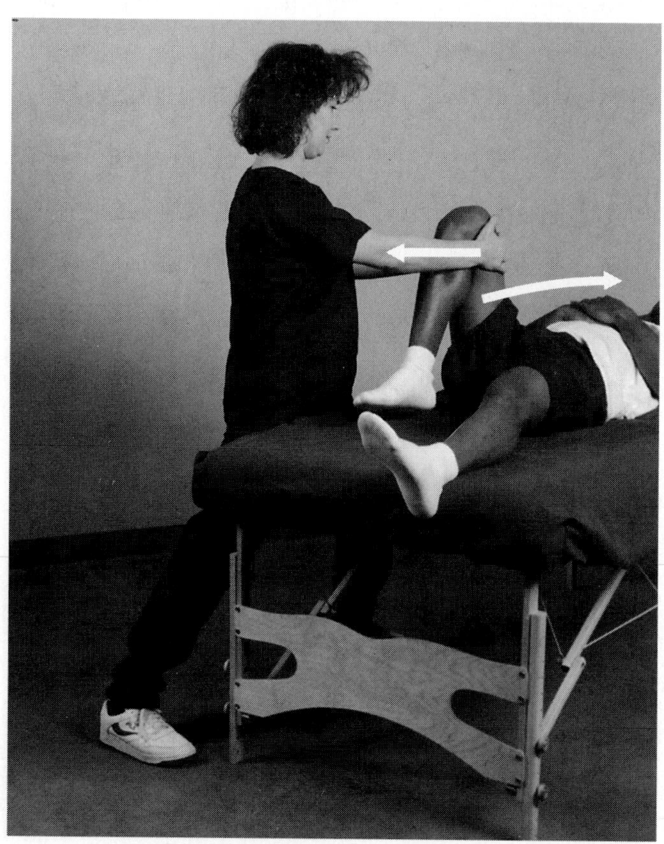

Figure 18•31 Active-resisted stretching.

MINI•LAB

Place your hand, palm down, on your anterior thigh. Keeping your hand flat, raise up your index finger and notice how high it can go. Now raise your index finger again. But this time, use your other hand to lift your finger to its fullest extent. Notice how much farther your index finger can go with active assistance.

Author's Note

Use caution when applying an active-assisted or a passive stretch. Stretching and joint mobilizations are physically demanding upon the therapist, particularly when the client is large. Use proper body mechanics when applying stretching or joint mobilizations. When the client tells you that the muscle is at maximum comfortable stretch, stop the movement. Honor the

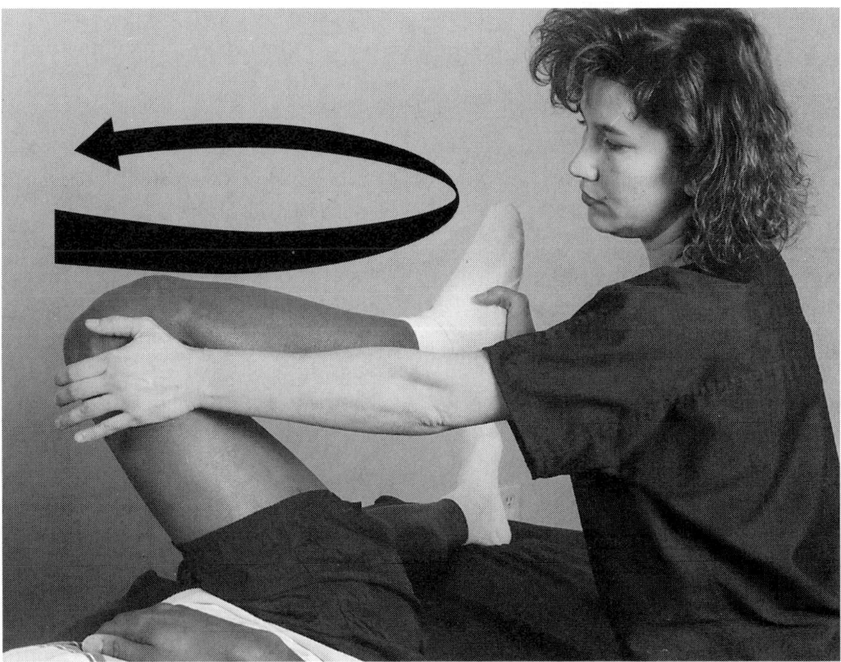

Figure 18•33 Swedish gymnastics of the hip joint with the knee and hip flexed.

myotatic reflex, and remember that overstretching or stretching improperly may cause injury.

Benefits of Stretching

- Stretching promotes relaxation and relieves soreness in the muscle.
- It aids in rehabilitation and recovery.
- It prepares muscles for activity and returns them to resting length after activity.
- Stretching mechanically elongates fascia and muscle tissue, increasing flexibility and making tissues more elastic.
- It resets the muscular tone around a joint, increasing joint mobility.
- It squeezes the blood vessels, activating circulation through movement.

Swedish Gymnastics

Ling's system of Swedish massage included the practice of **Swedish gymnastics**—active, passive, and resistive movements of the body's various joints and muscles. Most often Swedish gymnastics include the artful and fluid presentation of *passive* range of motion. Swedish gymnastics are also known as Swedish movements, remedial gymnastics, table stretches, joint mobilizations, and range of motion exercises.

For more effective range of motion, the movements are applied after the body has been warmed with added blood flow via massage. Be familiar with the joint and its movement before it is mobilized. The sweeping motions should be gentle and not induce pain (Fig. 18–33). The objective is to take a joint through its full range of motion through mild traction. Take the joint through three range-of-motion, repetitions and do not overtreat. See Chapter 7 for a discussion of major joints.

Benefits of Swedish Gymnastics

- They assist the therapist in assessing tissues.
- They decrease pain in a joint.
- They elongate soft tissue.
- Swedish gymnastics enhance joint nutrition and promote synovial fluid production in mobilized joints.
- They help to increase and maintain range of motion in a joint.
- They promote relaxation.

SUMMARY

Massage may be used to relax the body or to rehabilitate an injury. Swedish massage is the grandparent of most Western forms of massage therapy. It utilizes five main strokes—effleurage, petrissage, friction, tapotement, and vibration—and several ancillary strokes to influence positively a client's health and well-being. Execution of these strokes can be measured by several qualities, including intention, depth, pressure, excursion, speed, rhythm, continuity, duration, and sequence.

MASSAGE THERAPIST'S SELF-ASSESSMENT GUIDE

- Are the movements smooth and easy for you to do? Are the movements jarred, rough, or abrupt?
- Are your transitions smooth?
- Is your own body as fluid, easy, and open as the movement qualities you want to give to the client?
- Do you pause enough? Do you leave time for the client to respond?
- Do you know how far a stroke needs to go? Are your excursions long enough or are they too long?
- Is there an awareness of the tissues and not just a repetition of learned movements?
- Is there depth without force, invasion, or intrusion?
- Do you know when to stop so as not to overwork part of the body?
- Do you use your body well (positioning, stance, leverage, and wrist angle)? Are your body mechanics complementing your massage movements?
- Are you working within an appropriate amount of time?
- Is the session feeling whole and integrated?
- Are you beginning to glimpse the possibilities of the work?
- Does your client feel honored and invited?
- Are you enjoying yourself and the work?

Ancillary strokes may be incorporated into the therapist's repertoire. These ancillary movements include touch, nerve strokes, compression, trigger point work, stretching, and Swedish gymnastics. These movements are the tools with which we build massage routines.

SELF-TEST

Multiple Choice • Write the letter of the best answer in the space provided.

_______ 1. Which of the following are used when applying massage strokes?
A. intention, pressure, and excursion
B. rhythm and continuity
C. speed, duration, and sequence
D. all of the above

_______ 2. The distance traversed on the client's body or the length of a massage stroke is called
A. pressure
B. depth
C. speed
D. excursion

_______ 3. The spatial distance into the body's tissue that is achieved through pressure application is
A. fascial massage
B. depth
C. speed
D. excursion

_______ 4. An ordered repetition of strong and weak elements in the delivery of the massage strokes is
A. pacing
B. percussion
C. rhythm
D. sequence

_______ 5. Which of the following refers to the rate of motion or how fast or slow a massage movement is being executed?
A. speed
B. depth
C. pressure
D. excursion

_______ 6. The application of force (or thrust) exerted by the massage therapist on the client's body is called
A. speed
B. depth
C. pressure
D. excursion

_______ 7. When applying pressure, it is important to
A. not exceed the client's personal pain threshold
B. cause muscle relaxation, not muscle contraction
C. take into consideration the area on the body where the pressure is being applied
D. all of the above

_______ 8. As pressure is being applied, it is often helpful to watch the client's face for distortions or for changes in his breathing pattern. Distorted facial features or an alteration in the client's breathing often indicates
A. a need for a tissue
B. pressure that is too great
C. a need to void
D. pressure that is too light or ticklish

_______ 9. The best way to learn massage strokes is from
A. a videotape
B. a book
C. an experienced and caring instructor
D. a book on cassette tape

_______ 10. An excellent stroke for assessing tissues is
A. effleurage
B. petrissage
C. friction
D. tapotement/percussion

_______ 11. A brisk, often heat-producing compression stroke that may be delivered either superficially to the skin or to deeper tissue layers of muscle, depending upon the intention of the therapist, is referred to as
A. effleurage
B. petrissage
C. friction
D. tapotement/percussion

_______ 12. Which of the following consists of a cycle of rhythmic lifting of the muscle tissues away from the bone or underlying structures with the hollow of the palms, followed by firmly kneading or squeezing the muscle with a gentle pull toward the therapist, ending with a release of the tissue?
A. effleurage
B. petrissage
C. friction
D. tapotement/percussion

_______ 13. A rapid shaking, trembling, or oscillating movement applied with full hands, fingertips, or a mechanical device for the purpose of inducing relaxation is
A. effleurage
B. petrissage
C. vibration
D. percussion/tapotement

_______ 14. Application of purposeful, gliding movements that follow the contour of the client's body is

A. effleurage
B. petrissage
C. friction
D. tapotement/percussion

_______ 15. Which of the following is *not* a benefit of effleurage?

A. directly lifts the muscle belly away from the underlying bone
B. relaxes the client and prepares the area for deeper strokes
C. creates length in a muscle
D. soothes tired, achy muscles and aids in the relief of insomnia

_______ 16. Variations of petrissage are

A. circular, cross-fiber, and digital
B. hacking, tapping, and diffused
C. ocean waves, fulling, and skin rolling
D. oscillating, compressive, and vibratory

_______ 17. Variations of friction include

A. circular, cross-fiber, and straight
B. hacking, tapping, and diffused
C. rolling, chucking (linear), and wringing
D. A and C

_______ 18. Which of the following is a benefit of friction?

A. dilates capillaries, increases circulation, and reduces swelling
B. loosens stiffness in joints by relaxing muscles
C. breaks down and coaxes apart adhered tissue, freeing restricted areas
D. all of the above

_______ 19. Variations of percussion/tapotement are

A. circular, cross-fiber, and straight
B. hacking, tapping, and cupping diffused
C. rolling, chucking, and wringing
D. fine, coarse, and rocking

_______ 20. When applying percussion/tapotement

A. avoid after exercise because it can activate muscle spindles
B. avoid applying percussion over the kidney area because it is not adequately protected by soft tissue
C. use as much force as you can generate
D. A and B

_______ 21. The three basic categories of vibration are

A. circular, cross-fiber, and straight
B. hacking, tapping, and cupping diffused
C. rolling, chucking, and wringing
D. fine, coarse, and rocking

_______ 22. When using electrical units to provide vibratory massage

A. make sure the cord does not touch the client
B. never leave the appliance on the floor or the cord stretched out for people to trip over
C. avoid applying vibration on one area for more than 15 minutes
D. all of the above

_______ 23. Which of the following is *not* a benefit of vibration?

A. creates length in a muscle
B. stimulates the muscle spindles, thus creating minute muscle contractions
C. relieves upper respiratory tract congestion, including sinus congestion
D. stimulates peristalsis of the large intestine with abdominal vibration

_______ 24. The word *ancillary* refers to

A. a position near or beside a reference point
B. something that is auxiliary or supplementary to a standard
C. a circular movement used in friction
D. a tool used when applying pressure

_______ 25. Which of the following is a term used to describe the laying of hands on the skin without movement?

A. compression
B. stilling
C. touch
D. massage

_______ 26. Also referred to as light effleurage, which of the following ancillary stroke is a very light fingertip tracing over the surface of the skin and is often a finishing move in massage therapy?

A. pennate massage
B. feather friction
C. nerve stroke
D. finale feathering

_______ 27. A rhythmic pumping on a muscle belly to create a sustained increase in circulation and muscle relaxation is called

A. trigger point work
B. compression
C. frictional pumping
D. ballistic stretching

_______ 28. Sustained digital pressure on specific areas in the muscle (trigger points) to relieve pain and discomfort is known as

A. trigger point work
B. compression
C. frictional pumping
D. ballistic stretching

_______ 29. Localized, sensitive ischemic tissue that is hypersensitive to touch but does not cause referred sensations is called

A. trigger point
B. satellite point
C. tender point
D. tsubo

_______ 30. Involuntary firing or twitching in a muscle in response to the sensory stimulation (pressure) on the trigger point is

A. local twitch response
B. jump sign
C. peripheral firing
D. ischemic twitch response

_______ 31. A spontaneous reaction of pain or discomfort that may cause a client to wince, jump, or verbalize upon application of pressure is the

A. local twitch response
B. jump sign
C. peripheral firing
D. ischemic twitch response

_______ 32. Also known as myotasis, which of the following involves elongating or extending the muscle tissue to its full length?

A. Swedish gymnastics
B. remedial elongation
C. stretching
D. flexibility

_______ 33. Stretching can be done _____ by the therapist with no assistance from the client or _____ by the client with no assistance from the therapist.

A. passively; actively
B. actively; passively
C. ballistically; statically
D. statically; ballistically

_______ 34. Stretching that is a combined effort between the therapist and client is known as

A. active-passive
B. passive-active
C. active-assisted
D. static-active

_______ 35. Stretches that are high-velocity, forceful repetitions of bouncing or bobbing motions which may cause tissue damage are called

A. active-bobbing
B. ballistic
C. static
D. barrage

_______ 36. Slow, held stretches, consisting of bringing a muscle to full extension and then maintaining the pressure necessary to keep the muscle in extension from 1 to 30 seconds, depending on the stretching ideology involved, is

A. active-bobbing stretching
B. ballistic stretching
C. static stretching
D. PNF stretching

_______ 37. Stretching that involves the therapist's applying gentle resistance while the client is actively engaging in the stretch is

A. active-assisted
B. ballistic
C. resisted or isometric
D. static

_______ 38. This reflex is activated when a muscle is pulled and there is a resultant contraction of the muscle.

A. inverse stretch reflex
B. myotatic stretch reflex
C. autogenic inhibition
D. A and C

_______ 39. Mediated by the Golgi tendon organs, this stretch reflex is stimulated by slow, low-force stretches, inhibiting regular muscle contraction, which allows for maximum stretching.

A. inverse stretch reflex
B. myotatic stretch reflex
C. autogenic inhibition
D. A and C

_______ 40. A system of active, passive, and resisted movements of the body's various joints and muscles, most often just the artful and fluid presentation of passive range of motion is called

A. active stretching
B. table gymnastics
C. Swedish gymnastics
D. passive stretching

References

Anderson, Bob. *Stretching.* Bolinas, CA: Shelter Publications, 1980.

Beck, Mark F. *Theory and Practice of Therapeutic Massage,* 2nd ed. Albany, NY: Milady Publishing Company, 1994.

Drez, David. *Therapeutic Modalities for Sports Injuries.* St. Louis: Times Mirror/Mosby College Publishing, St. Louis, Missouri 1989.

Fritz, Sandy. *Fundamentals of Therapeutic Massage.* St. Louis: Mosby–Year Book, Inc., 1995.

Hayes, K. W., et al. "An Examination of Cyriax's Passive Motion Tests with Patients Having Osteoarthritis of the Knee." *Physical Therapy,* Vol. 74, No. 8, pp. 697–708, 1994.

Juhan, Deane. *Job's Body, A Handbook for Bodyworkers.* Barrington, NY: Station Hill Press, 1987.

Kendall, Florence, and Elizabeth McCreary. *Muscles: Testing and Function.* Baltimore: Williams & Wilkins, 1983.

Krieger, Dolores. "Therapeutic Touch: The Imprimatur of Nursing." *American Journal of Nursing,* Vol. 99, May 1975.

Mattes, Aaron. *Active Isolated Stretching.* Self-published by Aaron Mattes, 1995.

Mennell, J.B. *Physical Treatment,* 5th ed. Philadelphia: Blakiston Publisher, 1945.

Moore, Keith L. *Clinically Oriented Anatomy,* 2nd ed. Baltimore: Williams & Wilkins, 1985.

Prudden, Bonnie. *Pain Erasure.* New York: M. Evans & Co., 1980.

Reed, Brian, and Jean M. Held. "Effects of Sequential Connective Tissue Massage on Autonomic Nervous System of Middle-Aged and Elderly Adults." *Physical Therapy,* Vol. 68, No. 8, August 1988.

St. John, Paul. *St. John Neuromuscular Therapy Seminars Manual I.* Largo, FL. 1995.

Taber's Cyclopedic Medical Dictionary, 13th ed. Philadelphia: F. A. Davis Company, 1977.

Tappan, Frances M. *Healing Massage Technique, Holistic, Classical and Emerging Methods.* Norwalk, CT: Appleton & Lange, 1988.

Travell, Janet G., and David G. Simons. *Myofascial Pain and Dysfunction, The Trigger Point Manual.* Baltimore: Williams & Wilkins, 1983.

Voss, Dorothy E., Marjorie K. Ionta, and Beverly J. Myers. *Proprioceptive Neuromuscular Facilitation.* Philadelphia: Harper & Row, 1985.

Williams, Ruth E. *The Road to Radiant Health.* College Place, WA: Color Press, 1977.

Massage has the power to repair the complicated machine known as the human body.

—*M. Rawlins, author of* A Textbook of Massage: For Nurses and Beginners (1930)

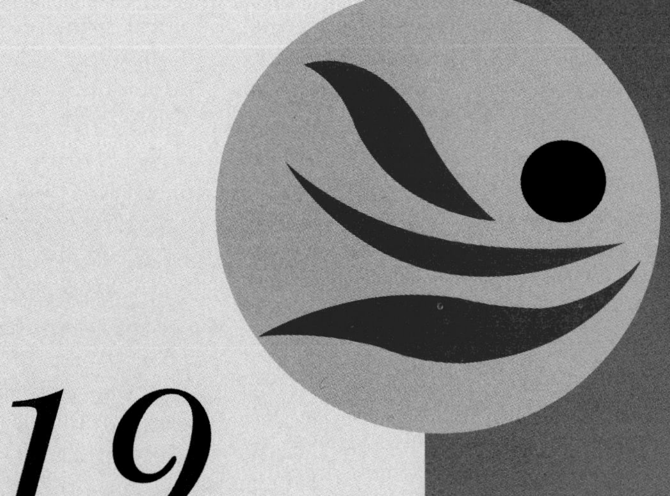

19 Massage Physiology—Benefits, Indications, Contraindications, and Endangerment Sites

Student Objectives

After completing this chapter, the student should be able to:

- Compare mechanical and reflexive responses of massage
- Discuss the benefits of massage in various body systems
- Using the gate theory, discuss how massage relieves pain
- Identify at least 15 indications for massage therapy
- Identify at least 15 contraindications of massage therapy
- Recognize and avoid vascular, nervous, osseous, and other miscellaneous endangerment sites

INTRODUCTION

To understand better how massage therapy benefits the client, we first need to understand how the body physiologically experiences the massage. Through years of scientific observation, experimentation, and speculation, the medical community has defined and refined what massage can and cannot accomplish. This chapter will introduce you to the effects of massage.

While many people are aware of the positive effects of massage on sore muscles, few are familiar with other conditions that massage can benefit, such as temporomandibular joint dysfunction, carpal tunnel syndrome, and fibromyalgia. These and other indications for massage are outlined in this chapter.

Although massage is beneficial for many body ailments, there are a few conditions for which massage is *contraindicated.* If massage therapy is to be administered safely, the prudent professional will know how to screen clients to rule out these conditions.

There are also various anatomical landmarks for which caution is recommended or massage should be avoided. These topographical regions are known as *endangerment sites,* regions in the body where nerves, blood vessels, and other fragile structures lie near the surface of the skin. Locations and descriptions of the major endangerment sites are included in this chapter.

MECHANICAL AND REFLEXIVE RESPONSES TO MASSAGE

Massage movements cause two types of responses in the body. One is the **mechanical response** (direct response brought on by force or pressure) and the other is the **reflexive response** (reaction to a stimulus that is governed by the nervous system). A massage response can be primarily mechanical or reflexive in nature, but both responses are closely related and often occur simultaneously. Reflex responses to massage frequently occur due to mechanical stimulation of nerve receptors.

A mechanical response occurs as a result of pressure and range of motion. Tissue is pulled, lifted, rubbed, compressed, and manipulated to produce mechanical effects. Examples of mechanical responses are increasing blood circulation, reducing swelling, and breaking up of scar tissue.

To create a reflex response in the body, nerves must respond to a stimulus, such as decreased arousal of the sympathetic nervous system (general relaxation), or triggering of nerve receptors (e.g., muscle spindles). Reflex responses include increasing the diameter of blood vessels, reducing blood pressure, and general relaxation.

BENEFITS OF MASSAGE

The massage stroke and the response it creates within the body have the capability to affect physiology in the circulatory, skeletal (connective), integumentary, respiratory, reproductive, muscular, excretory, nervous, endocrine, and digestive systems. While some claims made about the benefits of massage therapy are due to scientific experiments, most are from empirical clinical observations and speculation based on known physiological principles. By examining the beneficial aspects of massage on each body system, we can understand the scientific application of massage therapy.

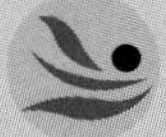

MINI•LAB

Imagine that you have two uninflated balloons—one is small and the other is twice the size of your first. Place a cup of water in each balloon. Which balloon has the lesser amount of pressure? The smaller or the larger? The larger one has the lesser pressure. This illustrates how massage can lower blood pressure through reflex action and increasing the parasympathetic response. By increasing the diameter of the vessel, the pressure inside the vessel decreases (Fig. 19–1).

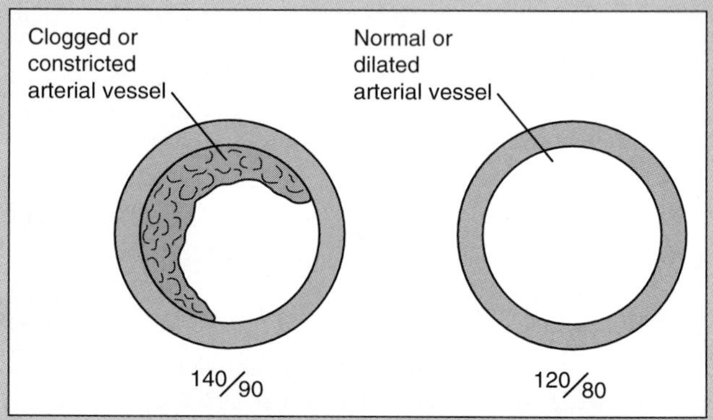

Figure 19•1 Blood pressure and blood vessel diameter.

Cardiovascular (Heart, Vessels, and Blood)

1. Deep stroking improves circulation by mechanically assisting venous blood flow back to the heart. When deep stroking (effleurage) is applied, compressive forces propel blood through the veins; the effect is similar to squeezing a toothpaste tube. In the area that has been compressed, the veins are emptied, and there is less resistance in the empty veins than there is in the nearby veins that were not com-

pressed by massage. The empty veins become the path of least resistance and therefore are more receptive to blood flow. Backflow of blood from the heart is prevented by the valves in the veins. The hands of the massage therapist basically act like a "second heart," which increases circulation only in the area being worked (Mennel, 1945).

The body responds to light and deep effleurage reflexively by dilating the blood vessels, which increases blood circulation and lowers blood pressure. (It has been documented that circulation increases during massage up to three times more than circulation at rest). Massage also stimulates tissue release of histamines and acetylcholine.

The release of these chemicals causes dilation of the blood vessels and **hyperemia,** which is the observable reddened skin that results from increased blood flow. *In areas where arteries are superficial (e.g., the front of the throat), deep massage is generally contraindicated.*

2. Because blood circulation is enhanced (venous blood flow directly and arterial blood flow indirectly), the delivery and removal of products in the blood (i.e., nutrients, oxygen, and metabolic wastes) are improved. Improved circulation affects **capillary beds** (collections of capillaries). Not all capillary beds are active (i.e., transporting blood) at the same time. Because some may become dormant for a time, particularly in fat storage areas, dormant capillary beds as well as active ones, are affected by massage (Pemberton, 1939).
3. Blood pressure is temporarily decreased by dilation of the capillaries, affecting the permeability of capillary walls. This increase in permeability is due to the stimulation of vasomotor nerves and to the release of local vasodilator substances. These effects last approximately 40 minutes after the massage session (Barr and Taslitz, 1970).
4. Massage temporarily increases systolic stroke volume. As the heart rate slows due to decreased activation of the sympathetic nervous system, there is more time for the cardiac ventricles to fill with blood. The result is more blood volume being pushed through the heart with each ventricular contraction, thereby increasing stroke volume (De Domenico and Wood, 1997).
5. Also known as the "relaxation response," massage decreases heart rate through decreased stimulation of the sympathetic nervous system,
6. The number of functional red blood cells and their oxygen carrying capacity are increased by the application of massage. This effect is achieved by
    - Promoting the spleen's discharge of red blood cells
    - Stimulating visceral circulation; excess blood is recovered from engorged internal organs and recruited back into circulation
    - Stimulating stagnant capillary beds; by reawakening these dormant beds, the red blood cells are returned to general circulation, which increases the count

    These data suggest that massage may be good for individuals with anemia (Mitchell, 1904; Pemberton, 1939).
7. The presence of white blood cells in the capillaries increases following massage. Apparently the body perceives the massage itself as a microtrauma and recruits additional white blood cells into the bloodstream. The increase in white blood cell count and the local availability of white blood cells enable the body to more effectively protect itself against disease (Pemberton, 1939).
8. Gentle but firm massage strokes also increase the number of thrombocytes (platelets) in the blood (Lucia and Richard, 1933).
9. Massage reduces ischemia. **Ischemia,** a decrease in blood supply to an organ or tissue, is believed to be the major cause of muscular pain (Fig. 19–2). Ischemia is also related to trigger point phenomena and their associated pain referral patterns. It has been documented that digital compression techniques not only bring about a reduction of ischemia but also create a temporary period of hyper-

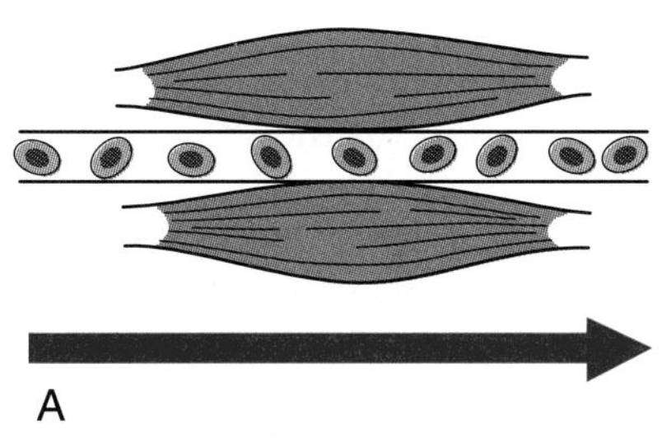

A

Capillaries running between two relaxed muscle fibers; round forms are red blood cells.

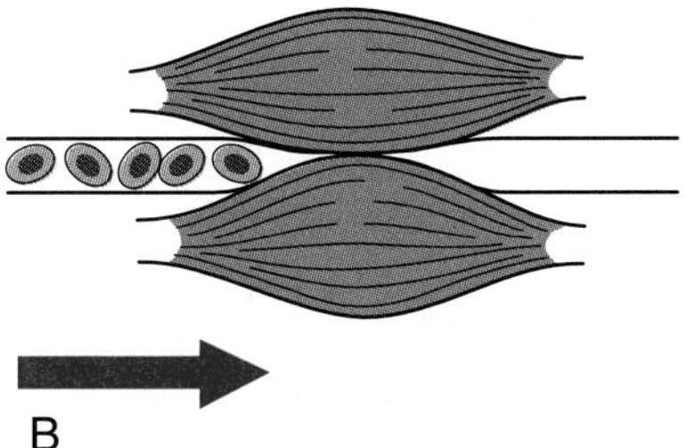

B

Capillary is compressed —squeezed— by the shortened thickened fibers of contracted muscle.

Figure 19•2 "Please don't squeeze the capillaries."

emia and a reduction in local and referred muscular pain (Travell and Simons, 1983; Fassbender, 1975).

Lymphvascular (Lymph and Vessels)

1. Massage reduces lymphedema (swelling) by mechanically stimulating circulation to the lymphatic system, which helps remove waste from the system more effectively than either passive range of motion or electrical muscle stimulation. Lymph is a viscous fluid that moves slowly within its system of vessels. Lymphatic circulation depends upon mechanical forces, such as pressure exerted on the walls of the lymphatic vessels (e.g., muscular contraction and respiration) (Bell, 1964; Cuthbertson, 1933).
2. The presence of natural killer cells and their activity increased with massage to individuals infected with the HIV virus, suggesting that massage may strengthen the immune system (Field et al., 1992).

Integument or Skin

1. Massage stimulates sebaceous glands of the skin, causing an increase in sebum production. This added sebum improves the skin's condition, texture, and tone. Clinical observations have determined that massage also improves the appearance (i.e., color and texture) of the skin (Krusen, 1941) (Fig. 19–3).
2. Through increased circulation, massage strokes increase insensible perspiration by stimulating the sudoriferous glands located in the skin. **Insensible perspiration** is the constant evaporative cooling that occurs as microscopic beads of perspiration evaporate from the skin's surface (Krusen, 1941).
3. Creating increased circulation and heat, massage stimulates vasomotor activity in the skin. As superficial blood vessels dilate, the skin appears hyperemic (reddish pink) and feels warm to the touch. This increased skin circulation brings added nutrients to these tissues (Cuthbertson, 1933).
4. Massage applied to scar tissue helps to reduce the formation of superficial keloids in the skin and excessive scar formations in the soft tissues beneath the site of massage application (Bodian, 1969).

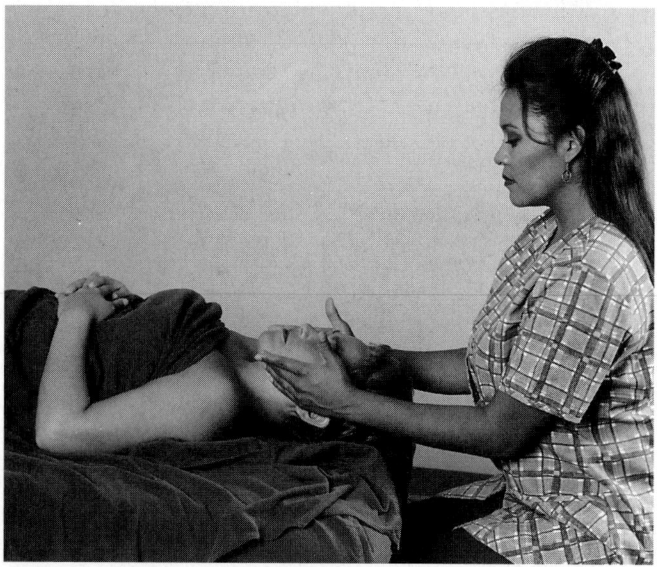

Figure 19·3 Close-up of a facial massage.

Nervous and Endocrine Systems

1. Massage activates sensory receptors and can stimulate or soothe the nervous system. Results depend on the massage stroke you choose and on the pressure applied. Slow, light, and rhythmic movements are soothing to the nerves because such movements produce a low level of excitement to the nervous system. Vigorous movements applied in short duration stimulate the nervous system due to their high level of excitation. The stimulatory massage movements are deep petrissage, friction, vibration, and tapotement. Sedative massage movements are light effleurage, light petrissage, light friction, and light vibration (Goldberg et al, 1994).
2. Massage decreases pain by the release of endorphins (endogenous morphine), enkephalins, and other pain-reducing neurochemicals. General relaxation brought on by massage therapy has a diminishing effect on pain (De Domenico and Wood, 1997; Meek, 1993).
3. Massage inhibits pain by interfering with nociceptive (pain) information, which enters the spinal cord through stimulation of cutaneous thermo- and mechanoreceptors (e.g., Pacini's corpuscles and Meissner's corpuscles). Only a certain amount of sensory information can be received by the nervous system at any given time. Sensations produced by a massage have the potential to suppress painful stimuli. Activation of cutaneous mechanoreceptors also can occur through mechanical vibration and transcutaneous electrical nerve stimulation (TENS). For more information, see the informational block in this section on the gate theory (Wall and Melzack, 1965).
4. Massage relieves pain caused from hypersensitive trigger points or referred pain, presumably by increasing circulation to the tissue (reactive hyperemia), thereby reducing ischemia-related pain (Travell and Simons, 1983).
5. Massage mechanically stretches and broadens tissue. These changes are detected by mechanoreceptors (e.g., Golgi tendon organs) and reflexively alter the contraction signal. Massage retrains the

tissue *from* a contracted state *to* an elongated state. This principle is one of the theories of *neuromuscular re-education.*

6. Muscle spindle activity is increased during abrupt massage strokes, such as tapotement and some forms of vibration. These strokes create minute muscle contractions to help tone weak muscles, which are particularly beneficial in cases of prolonged bed rest and flaccidity (De Domenico and Wood, 1997).
7. Research shows that massaged individuals who received a 15-minute massage twice a week had an increase in delta wave activity and a decreased beta wave activity (EEG determined). These individuals performed better on math tests and completed problems with increased accuracy (50 percent fewer errors) and speed (approximately half the time) (Field et al., 1998).
8. Massage stimulates the parasympathetic nervous system, thus promoting relaxation, decreasing insomnia and improved sleeping patterns (Mennell, 1945; Field et al., 1993).
9. Through numerous studies conducted by the Touch Research Institute, massage has been proven to reduce norepinephrine and cortisol (stress hormones) levels by activation of the relaxation response (Field et al., 1998).
10. Massage recipients show an increase in dopamine and serotonin levels. This suggests a decrease in stress levels and depression (Field et al., 1998).

Muscular System

1. Massage relieves muscular restrictions, tightness, stiffness, and spasms. These effects are achieved by direct pressure on the spasm by manipulating the tissue that sends messages of "length" to the central nervous system and by the increase in circulation. Results are more flexible, supple, and resilient muscle tissues (Bell, 1964).

   Because massage promotes muscular relaxation, massage has also been shown to increase muscle length and flexibility. A finger-to-floor test was given to 25 individuals to assess the flexibility of the back and posterior leg muscles. The group members who had received massage instead of passive rest had an increase in flexibility (Nordschow and Bierman, 1962).
2. Massage enhances blood circulation thus increasing the amount of oxygen and nutrients available to the muscles. Increased oxygen and nutrients reduce muscle fatigue and postexercise soreness. As a result of circulation, massage improves muscular nutrition (Smith et al., 1994; Despard, 1932).
3. Massage promotes rapid disposal of waste products and replenishment of nutritive materials through increased circulation, further reducing muscle fatigue and soreness. A fatigued muscle recuperates 20 percent after 5 minutes of rest and 100 percent after 5 minutes of massage (Cuthbertson, 1933; Evans, 1980).
4. Massage interrupts the pain cycle by relieving muscular spasms, increasing circulation, and promoting rapid disposal of waste products.
5. Massage helps to maintain muscles in the best possible state of nutrition, flexibility, and vitality, thus hastening muscle recovery and enabling them to function at maximum. Muscle tissue examined microscopically after injury proves that a massaged limb is more normal looking, contains no fibrosis around the blood vessels, and appears larger (less atrophy) than nonmassaged muscles (Mennell, 1945).

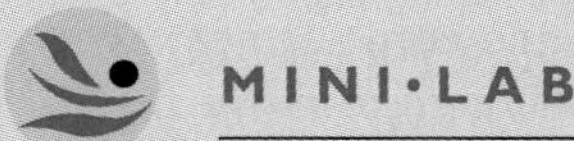

Sit in a chair with your feet flat on the floor. Moving only your head and neck, look over your left shoulder, and notice how far you can comfortably move. Do the same, looking to the right. Take your right hand, and grab the top of your right shoulder. As you apply pressure, slowly move the shoulder up and down ten times. Maintain the pressure, and roll your shoulder back ten times, then forward ten times. Do this same movement with the left shoulder. Squeeze the back of your neck. Without releasing the pressure, turn your head (as if saying no), nod your head (as if saying yes), and circle your nose clockwise and counterclockwise ten times each. After the "squeeze and move" activity, look over your right and left shoulders again. Notice how much farther you can go. This increase is due to self-administered massage.

Connective Tissue (Bone and Soft Tissues)

1. Especially when performed locally on stable fractures, massage increases the retention of nutrients such as nitrogen, sulfur, and phosphorus in bones. When a bone is fractured, the body forms a network of new blood vessels at the break site. Although the precise mechanism is not understood, local massage seems to provide an increase in circulation around the fracture, leading to increased deposition of callus to the bone (Mock, 1945).
2. Theoretically, massage flattens out adipose globules located under the skin and makes the skin seem smoother. Cellulite, a type of adipose tissue, appears as groups of small dimples or depressions

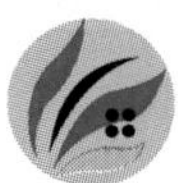

THE GATE THEORY

In 1965, Wall and Melzack postulated the gate theory of pain relief, which explains why massage, ice, and heat are effective in the treatment of pain. The gate theory refers to the exclusion of certain nerve impulses, when multiple impulses are competing for the same synaptic "gate" or entry into the central nervous system. To understand this, we will examine the two types of nerve fibers.

The sensory transmitters for pressure, temperature, and sharp acute pain lie close together in large concentrations near the body's surface. Their nerve pathways are composed of long, fast type A nerve fibers, which are important for protecting the body from external harm. Strong stimuli to these surface transmitters create a quick sensory input to the cord segment, where a reflex-motor impulse is generated to move the affected body part out of harm's way. Touching a needle or a hot pan elicits this type of immediate reflex response.

The sensory transmitters for deep aching pain, such as myofascial pain, originate in the deeper tissues. These nerve pathways are composed of short, slow type C nerve fibers, which tend to transmit pain that has been present for some time and requires no immediate protective action (i.e., headache or muscular pain). These nerves transmit stimuli that are of lesser importance and lesser consequence to the body. The purpose of type C nerve pathways is to make the conscious mind aware that a problem exists, which can be used to prevent overuse or dependence on an injured body part.

Suppose that an Olympic gymnast is having her performance compromised by pain in her right Achilles tendon. This pain originates from the deeper, slower type C nerve network. When a pressure stimulus such as massage is applied to the calf, the new sensory input travels along the faster, longer type A nerve network and bridges the synaptic gap ahead of the type C sensory input. The synaptic gate is closed, thus excluding the pain information from entry to the spinal cord. The body experiences the pressure of the massage stroke as interruption of pain (Fig. 19–4).

Massage therapists can use the gate mechanism a number of ways: (1) in the application of cold; (2) in the application of heat; (3) in the application of pressure; (4) in the application of vibration; (5) in the application of percussion; and (6) in the application of superficial rubbing or light stimulation of cutaneous tissue. Any of these applications has the potential to interfere or interrupt pain signals.

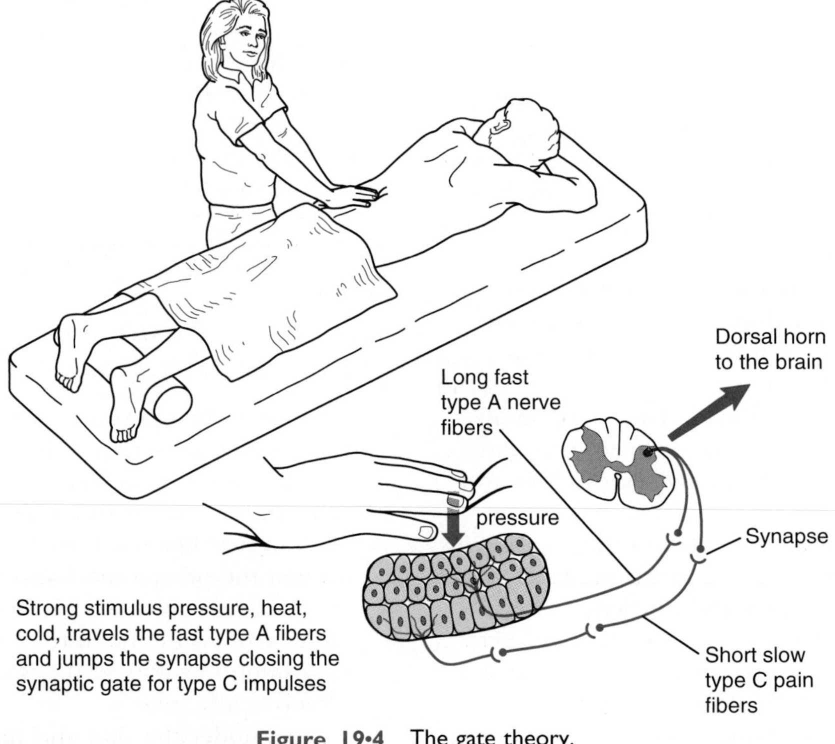

Figure 19•4 The gate theory.

under the skin, caused by an uneven separation of fat globules below the skin's surface, which is displaced by manual manipulation. Massage does not reduce the amount of cellulite below the skin; instead it temporarily alters the shape and appearance of cellulite.

3. Massage can make the body more mobile by reducing hyperplasia (thickening) of connective tissue and freeing fascial restrictions. Because posture and fascial tension are so closely related, releasing and minimizing fascial restrictions can improve posture. If you imagine the human skeleton, a tensile force upon one region will cause that region to shift. By releasing fascial restrictions, many posture distortions disappear (De Domenico and Wood, 1997).
4. Deep massage displaces adhesions and rearranges scar tissue. Deep friction can create an appropriate scar that is strong yet does not interfere with the muscle's ability to broaden as it contracts. Massage therefore helps to restore normal, pain-free motion of the affected joint if restrictions are due to adhesions (Bodian, 1969; Cyriax, 1984; Hammer, 1993).

Author's Note

The pain-cycle is initiated when painful stimuli result in reflex muscle contraction and localized muscle splinting or guarding. The localized muscle guarding restricts movement and decreases local circulation, which restricts the amount of oxygen available to the tissues and the removal of metabolic wastes. The subsequent swelling creates more pain. From this point, muscle splinting is intensified and the cycle repeats itself. A more generalized secondary pain results that outlasts or exceeds the original discomfort. Massage interrupts the pain cycle on all levels (Fig. 19–5).

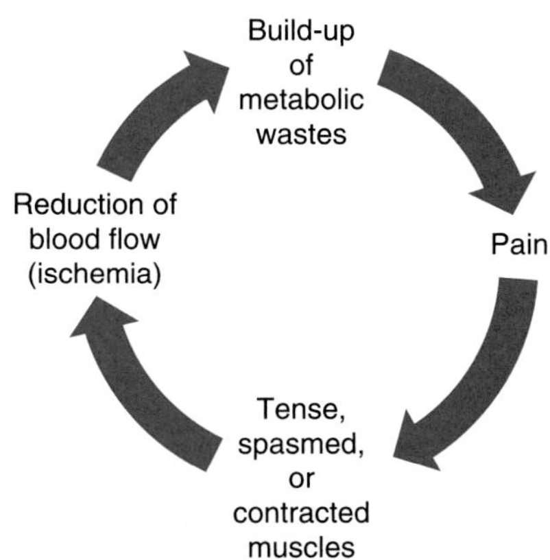

Figure 19•5 Massage interrupts the pain cycle.

Respiration

1. Massage slows down the rate of respiration via reduced stimulation of the sympathetic nervous system.
2. The mechanical loosening and discharge of phlegm in the respiratory tract increases with rhythmic alternating pressures. Tapotement (cupping) and vibration on the rib cage are often used to enhance this effect. Phlegm loosening and discharge is further enhanced when combined with postural drainage (promoting fluid drainage of the respiratory tract through certain body positions) and when the client is encouraged to cough (Cyriax, 1984).
3. By freeing tight respiratory muscles and fascia, massage can be used to increase vital capacity and pulmonary function (Field et al., 1998).

Digestion and Elimination

1. Massage promotes excitation of peristaltic activity in the large intestine, helping to relieve colic and intestinal gas (De Domenico and Wood, 1997).
2. Provided that the direction of massage follows the normal intestinal flow (clockwise), massage can promote evacuation of the colon, thus relieving constipation (Mennell, 1945).
3. Massage also promotes activation of the parasympathetic nervous system, which stimulates digestion.

Urinary and Excretory

1. Massage, especially abdominal massage, increases urine output by activating dormant capillary beds and recovering lymphatic fluids for filtration (Cuthbertson, 1933).
2. Massage promotes the excretion of nitrogen, inorganic phosphorus, and sodium chloride. The levels of these metabolic wastes are elevated in urine after massage (Cuthbertson, 1933).
3. Massage promotes autonomic nervous system functioning, promoting general homeostasis and increasing urine output.

Psychological Effects

1. Massage therapy reduces stress and anxiety through relaxation of body and mind.
2. Individuals diagnosed with attention deficit hyperactivity disorder (ADHD) who receive massage were observed to be less fidgety and hyperactive, and spent more time completing an assigned task (Field et al., 1998).
3. Massage enhances well-being and body awareness through relaxation and cutaneous stimulation, and improved body image (Field et al., 1993).

4. Because of the close relationship, massage helps to satisfy the needs for intimacy, caring, and nurturing touch.
5. Elderly individuals who gave massages reported enhanced self-esteem and an improved lifestyle (e.g., more social interaction) (Field et al., 1998).
6. Massage can assist the ease of emotional expression through relaxation.
7. Massage given to victims of rape and spousal abuse was reported to produce a reduction in touch aversion (Field et al., 1998).
8. Massage increases mental alertness by relaxing the body and by removing unwanted stress.
9. Clinically depressed adolescents reported decreased feelings of depression and anxiety after 5 weeks of massage, twice a week (Field et al., 1993).
10. Many clients experience a sense of renewed energy after massage by taking a break from the stresses of the day.

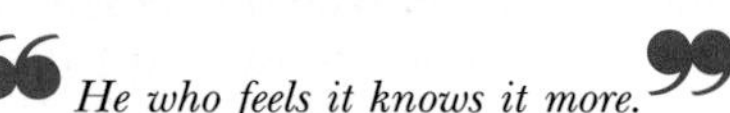

—Bob Marley

INDICATIONS FOR MASSAGE

Below is a list of conditions for which massage is indicated.

1. Most headaches (muscular, cluster, eye strain, sinus, etc.) can be relieved by reducing tension.
2. Insomnia is alleviated by inducing relaxation.
3. Stress and anxiety are reduced by decreased activation of the sympathetic nervous system and promotion of the relaxation response.
4. Fatigue and muscular soreness are relieved by flushing out the tissue and by drawing in oxygenated blood.
5. Mental fatigue is reduced by inducing relaxation and increasing circulation. More nutrients (e.g., oxygen, glucose) are available to the brain when circulation is improved.
6. Pain associated with musculoskeletal conditions, fibromyalgia, and myofascial syndrome is reduced.
7. Poor circulation and some types of anemia are aided by virtue of the circulation benefits of massage.
8. Skin problems such as mild dryness can be alleviated due to the increase of sebum production and blood circulation.
9. Stiffness due to fascial restrictions, muscle tension, and muscle soreness is reduced.
10. Digestive and elimination problems, including colic, can be relieved through massage.
11. Swelling due to lymphedema can be reduced with massage if it is not a result of inflammation or disease. Edema due to traumatic inflammation may be aided with techniques such as manual lymphatic drainage massage.
12. The muscular component of temporomandibular joint (TMJ) dysfunction can be eased.
13. Respiratory drainage is encouraged through cupping tapotement and vibration.
14. Massage can speed the healing of overuse injuries, sprains, and strains.
15. Postural deviations can be alleviated if their sources are myofascial pain, discomfort, connective tissue restriction, and/or limitation.
16. Conditions of nerve entrapment that occur when soft tissues constrict the nerve, such as carpal tunnel syndrome, thoracic outlet syndrome, and sciatica, are relieved by release of the myofascial component.

Once you know the benefits and indications of massage, an understanding of contraindications and endangerment sites becomes simple. For instance, by increasing lymph circulation, massage affects the tissue and fluids of the body. Since massage increases the circulation of blood, thrombosis (the tendency for the blood to form clots) must be a contraindication.

CONTRAINDICATIONS FOR MASSAGE THERAPY

This section will consider pathologies and symptoms that may contraindicate massage. The professional therapist must exercise caution in some situations and under certain conditions. During the intake process prior to massage therapy, the therapist conducts a consultation with the client to establish goals, to note precautions, and to determine any preexisting conditions that might affect the treatment. It is the duty and obligation of the therapist to rule out the presence of any conditions in which massage may have detrimental effects.

Conditions in which massage is inappropriate, is not indicated, and may be harmful are known as **absolute contraindications.** If contraindications exist, massage therapy is not advised; however, there are very few absolute contraindications. The "no massage" rule generally refers to massage that is not applied to the affected area.

Most contraindications are referred to as **partial** or **relative contraindications.** These are conditions or situations that merit caution and adaptive measures to ensure that the massage is safe and that the client is comfortable. An example of a partial contraindication is poison ivy or an abrasion; you must avoid the lesions. Examples of other partial contraindications are cancer and rheumatoid arthritis. Massage can be administered, but the therapist should ask clients (and perhaps their physician) about their conditions to determine the appropriateness of massage. Massage,

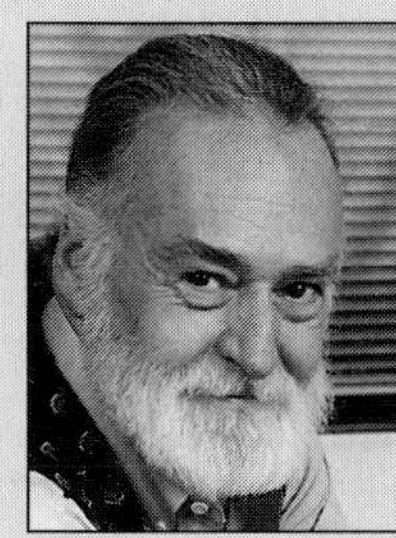

John F. Barnes

Born: February 3, 1939

"The master therapist is real, calm, nonjudgmental, intelligent, sensitive, strong yet flexible, supportive, compassionate, empathic, and joyful."

One of the major differences between myofascial release and many other forms of bodywork is that—at its best—it allows the therapist to bring more to the table. It is systematic, physiologically grounded, and intuitive without apology. Its founder, John Barnes, is a physical therapist and teacher who values a wide range of modalities like the work of Ida Rolf, Milton Trager, John Upledger, and Paul St. John.

Barnes's father died when he was 3, and he was raised by his mother. He remembers enjoying being alone in the forest and learning to be so quiet that the wildlife would venture out. He studied karate and, as a result, learned about the role of ki. As a junior in high school he knew he wanted to be a physical therapist.

With warm eyes, a burly build, and a full beard, he looks like a guy who should live in a log cabin and love nature. He does. He's been called an "old soul" and doesn't scoff at the label. He doesn't believe in assembly-line quick fixes. How could he? He knows how insidious pain can be.

As a teen, Barnes was weightlifting and couldn't get out of a dead squat, so he turned a backflip and landed on his tailbone with an extra 300 pounds to boot. It wasn't long afterward that his back locked up just as he was about to kiss a girl he was crazy about. Nevertheless, he didn't pay much attention to his condition. He had youth on his side and charged on, until a skiing accident left him in worse condition than many of the patients he treated. Surgery made a big difference, but the pain left an indelible scar.

In an article about Barnes written by Robert Calvert, owner of *Massage Magazine,* Barnes is quoted: "I don't really mean this should happen, but in a way, every physician or therapist should be severely injured, and not just hurt for a week or two or a month, but a couple years. It's a whole different story when you are a prisoner in your own body. I felt broken and I was broken. It was a horrible, horrible experience."

Yet another injury led him to explore the advantage of alternative therapies that hadn't been offered in his traditional physical therapist training. He began to blend experience with principles from different disciplines and discovered how fascia and energy flow are connected. Basically, myofascial release is based on understanding the role of fascia, a web of interconnected tissue that travels the body without interruption. It surrounds individual cells, organs, systems, and then wraps it all up in one huge package, head to toe. This network also serves as the communication medium from cell to cell and organ to organ. Trauma, posture, or inflammation can change the consistency of the web, solidifying and shortening fibers and blocking the flow of messages that are necessary for homeostasis. This web, pulled too tightly in one place, can leave other areas restricted, creating pressure on nerves, muscles, organs, and bones.

As a physical therapist, Barnes's style had always been focused, slow, and rhythmic. Sometimes his touch was light. Sometimes the tissue beneath his hands granted him deeper access. He didn't know he was practicing "myofascial release" per se until he attended a physicians' course on connective tissue. Afterwards he began to see—and treat—the interrelationship of the whole body (including the mind or spirit) rather than the isolated sore neck, bum knee, or other body part. This shift in thinking enhanced the results of his work, but stirred up emotions that demanded his attention. As his work evolved, so did Barnes. (The goal of myofascial release is not necessarily to incite emotional response, but considering the pervasive nature of myofascial system and the complex nature of humans, many forms of bodywork are considered—and may eventually be proven—therapeutic for emotional as well as physical trauma.)

continued on page 438

Continued

John F. Barnes

Barnes started teaching others his form of bodywork in the mid-1970s. His task begins by reawakening the therapist's ability to "feel" what's happening with the body. Then he teaches the techniques to evaluate and release restricted areas in a systematic way. In his opinion, a comprehensive program should also include exercise and flexibility programs, movement awareness facilitation techniques, instruction in body mechanics, mobilization and muscle energy techniques, nutritional advice, biofeedback, and psychological counseling.

Even with such a systematic and comprehensive approach, Barnes is realistic about results. Therapists do not "fix" clients or patients. We can offer tools for change not only in the form of bodywork but "mindwork" as well. When it gets right down to the nitty-gritty, we can't help our clients unless they're ready to help themselves. That's a humbling thought, yet being proficient as well as humble is a good starting point.

Barnes's advice for beginning massage therapists is to continue learning advanced methods after graduating from the typical 500-hour program. Just reading about a bodywork concept or simply being introduced to a modality isn't sufficient to practice it successfully and in some cases may lead to learning bad habits or faulty techniques. Barnes suggests learning as many forms of bodywork as possible in order to adapt to the wide range of client needs.

which is generally helpful in reducing anxiety and stress, can usually be administered to areas of the body that are not affected. Many situations and conditions that require adaptive positions or techniques are addressed in Chapter 21, Adaptive Massage and Client Management Issues.

Always exercise good judgment and use common sense when identifying these situations. You may decide, after determining contraindication, to refer your client to his personal physician for further evaluation and treatment recommendations. As a rule, the therapist should be conservative. If there is any doubt about a specific condition or injury, ask the client to obtain written medical clearance from his personal physician.

During the massage, monitor the client's response continuously. If the client reports that his pain has increased either during or after the massage session, modify or discontinue the massage treatments until further evaluation.

The following is a list of conditions that may contraindicate massage therapy (note that may of these conditions are relative contraindications).

1. **Fever,** or pyrexia, is a contraindication for massage therapy because of the risk of spreading infection as a result of increased circulation. During fever, the body temperature rises as a result of foreign bacteria or viruses. Massage gives these foreign agents an extra "push" through the body, and fever may rise (this principle works also when you exercise while feverish). Fever may also be a symptom for other conditions, especially infectious ones.
2. **Vascular conditions.** Do not massage a client who has a vascular disease without the approval of his physician because there is a tendency toward bruising, clots, thrombus formation, or rupturing of blood vessels. Vascular conditions include varicosities, embolus, phlebitis, thrombosis, aneurysm, atherosclerosis, hypertension, and Raynaud's phenomenon. When a client has distended varicosities, or damaged veins, do not massage distal or directly on the area; however, you may work proximally to the area. Do not massage a client if he has a history of embolus or thrombus because the increased circulation may move it to the heart. Avoid the medial thigh and the anterior neck because these areas are the ones most likely for clots to form. It is also best to avoid the use of mechanical vibrators and tapotement on the posterior and medial surfaces of the legs of clients with vascular disorders. Do not administer massage if the client has phlebitis, thrombosis, arteriosclerosis, or an aneurysm because the vascular system lacks integrity. A client with Raynaud's phenomenon may experience peripheral numbing, paresthesia (decreasing sensation), and the inability to give feedback regarding pressure and discomfort. Clients with hypertension (high blood pressure) should receive a massage that is soothing and sedating. Hypertension is defined as blood pressure that is consist-

ently above 140/90 mmHg (although this figure may be adjusted for the patient's age). Clients with high blood pressure, even if they are on medication, should have medical clearance prior to massage due to their susceptibility to form blood clots. Some clients may be taking aspirin or prescription anticoagulants such as blood thinners for heart or stroke therapy. Realize that these clients are more susceptible to bruising and deep-tissue modalities should be avoided. Purpura, or spontaneous bruising, may be a sign of edema, severe vitamin deficiency, or may be a side effect of certain medications. Strong localized pressure is a contraindication because it can leave a substantial bruise. You may elect to use full palmar pressure instead of digital pressure.

3. **Severe heart condition.** The increased circulation typical of massage treatments can overburden a failing heart and can increase the risks of thrombus and embolus. Get medical clearance before beginning massage treatments.
4. **Skin abnormalities and conditions (infectious, viral, fungal, or bacterial). Rashes, poison ivy, poison oak, sumac, impetigo, athlete's foot, ringworm, scabies, blisters, abnormal lumps, warts, herpes simplex, herpes zoster, large or loose moles, lymphogranuloma venereum, and skin ulcerations** should not be massaged. These conditions may be worsened, may spread by massage, and can be contagious. Remember, massage lubricant provides an excellent medium for the spreading of transmittable skin problems. Pruritus or severe itching is contraindicated if the onset of the massage aggravates the condition. Massage is avoided on areas that contain eczema only because it is typically hypersensitive, not because it is contagious.
5. Do not massage over areas where foreign objects such as glass, pencil lead, or metal are embedded in the tissues. Massage can cause further damage to these tissues by virtue of pressure and movement. Where the protective barrier of the skin is broken, there is risk of infection to the client and body fluid contamination to both client and therapist. Refer the client to a clinic or physician for removal of the foreign body.
6. Avoid areas of redness or warmth. This suggests an acute inflammation and alteration in the health of the skin or deeper tissues.

Author's Note

Acute refers to those conditions that last for a short time (usually a few days to a few weeks), and **chronic** refers to conditions that have a long duration (in some cases, a lifetime).

7. Abrasions, cuts, hematomas, and contusions should be avoided because massage could further damage the healing tissue, expose the client to infection, and expose the therapist to bodily fluids.
8. **Cancer** is a massage contraindication. Because many cancers spread lymphatically and massage increases circulation of lymph, you must obtain medical clearance. Massage may also aid in the metastasis of the cancer. However, many physicians do prescribe massage for patients who have cancerous conditions because it relaxes and nourishes the body and supports the immune system. Consult with the client and her physician and make a collective decision. Massage is often used as palliative care (therapy that eases or reduces pain or other symptoms).
9. **Recent injury.** Wait at least 72 hours before massaging minor injuries due to the possibility of internal vascular bleeding. Ice may be applied to the injured area in cases of recent trauma once medical clearance is received.
10. **Recent surgery.** After surgery, obtain medical clearance before massage therapy begins. Massage can be helpful in reducing scar formation, but these techniques require advanced and specialized training.
11. **Infectious diseases** (e.g., cold, flu, scarlet fever, measles, tuberculosis, and mumps) are contraindicated. Infectious diseases are caused by a biological agent, such as a virus or a bacterium, and can be highly contagious. Refer to the sanitation chapter for a discussion of transmission routes of diseases.
12. **Multiple sclerosis.** Many clients with multiple sclerosis experience alterations in sensation and are unusually sensitive to touch. Because of nerve damage, do not apply external heat. The client may require a shorter massage because an hour massage may cause the client to feel overstimulated. After massage therapy the client may feel awkward or clumsy from relaxation.
13. **Diabetes** is a contraindication, requiring medical referral, because clients with diabetes are prone to atherosclerosis, high blood pressure, and edema, and because they typically lose sensation in extremities in advanced stages. Any loss of sensory nerve function must be taken into consideration. Stroke pressure, especially tapotement and vibration, must be carefully monitored and administered carefully; however, massage can be beneficial by stimulating circulation in the extremities. If the client is receiving insulin therapy by injection, avoid massage on recent injection sites.
14. **Local and general acute inflammatory process.** These conditions include Crohn's disease, systemic lupus erythematosus, and cystitis. Obtain medical clearance and avoid local areas of inflam-

mation. Clients with rheumatoid arthritis can receive a massage only when the disease is in remission from the elevated level of systemic inflammation; avoid the affected joints because they can be reinflamed. In areas of gouty arthritis, massage may be administered excluding the affected area.

15. **Fractures.** Because massage therapy is usually applied with pressure and motion, clients with healing fractures should avoid massage in the affected area. Ideally, the broken bone ends will heal correctly if left undisturbed. Medical clearance will protect the therapist and ensure that he does not interfere with proper bone healing or cause rebreaking.
16. **Preeclampsia,** or toxemia, which is a bacterial toxin in the blood and albumin in the urine, is a complication in pregnancy. The pathological condition is characterized by edema of the lower extremities, vomiting, diarrhea, and high blood pressure. Because of the complexity of this condition, massage is not indicated unless okayed by the attending physician. Eclampsia occurs in 2 percent of pregnancies. The cause is not known.
17. Clients with **umbilical hernias** or **abdominal diastasis** should not receive deep abdominal massage because the integrity of the tissues is compromised. A hernia is the protrusion of an organ through the surrounding tissues, and a diastasis is the separation of two tissues that are normally joined. These conditions require corrective surgery, and massage should not be applied until clearance is granted by the client's primary physician.
18. **Severe pain.** This contraindication is usually at the judgment of the therapist. Be a cautious and conservative therapist.
19. **Psychological issues.** Unless you are a massage therapist *and* a licensed counselor or mental health technician, all psychological issues should be referred to a licensed professional. Touching may aggravate some conditions and is contraindicated for other psychiatric diagnoses (manic depressive psychosis, schizophrenic psychosis, paranoid conditions). However, massage does have a significant role in the treatment of dissociative disorders, post-traumatic stress disorders, and some abuse disorders.
20. **Hepatitis.** Massage is generally contraindicated because the increased circulation only stresses an already debilitated liver and should be performed only with the approval of the treating physician. If medical clearance is obtained, universal precautions must be taken. Therapists should also develop an awareness about touching their own faces, especially the mouth and nose areas, because the infection in people may not be diagnosed.

I have spent many childhood summers with my grandparents. I feel very close to them, so this story strikes close to home.

I received a call from my grandmother early one afternoon. She asked me if I would make an emergency house call. PawPaw had gone for his afternoon walk and somehow managed to "throw his back out." She was frightened because she had never seen him in so much pain. I could hear him talking to MawMaw in the background and knew from the sound of his voice that the situation was more than I was comfortable handling. I urged my grandmother to take him to the doctor immediately.

Later that evening, I got a call from my aunt. The family was all at the hospital with PawPaw. He had an abdominal aneurysm that had ruptured. The blood pooling in the peritoneal cavity was causing massive referred back pain. After talking to the doctors, I learned that a massage in this situation could have been fatal. ••

21. Do not work on anyone who *will not* disclose his medical history.
22. Do not work with anyone **under the influence of prescription** or **over-the-counter drugs that reduce pain, alcohol,** or **any other substance** that would *inhibit or distort the client's response or ability to give feedback regarding discomfort or pain.*

ENDANGERMENT SITES

Endangerment sites are areas that contain certain anatomical structures that are prone to injury. Direct or sustained pressure should not be used while applying massage therapy on or near these areas. Endangerment sites include such structures as nerves, blood vessels, organs, and small, prominent bony projections. Compression of nerves may cause loss of motor control and may create pain or numbness. Pressure upon vascular endangerment sites may cause bruising or damage to vessels in the affected area, a reduction in blood flow, and may possibly affect blood pressure. Compression of certain sharp or fragile bony areas may cause pain, bruising of surface tissues, and in some cases fracture of the bony projection. Pressure to organs may cause nausea, sharp pain, or temporary or permanent dysfunction.

The following specific locations of each different type of endangerment site can be located on the endangerment site map (Fig. 19–6). All endangerment sites are bilaterally symmetrical with the exception of those located on the midline of the body.

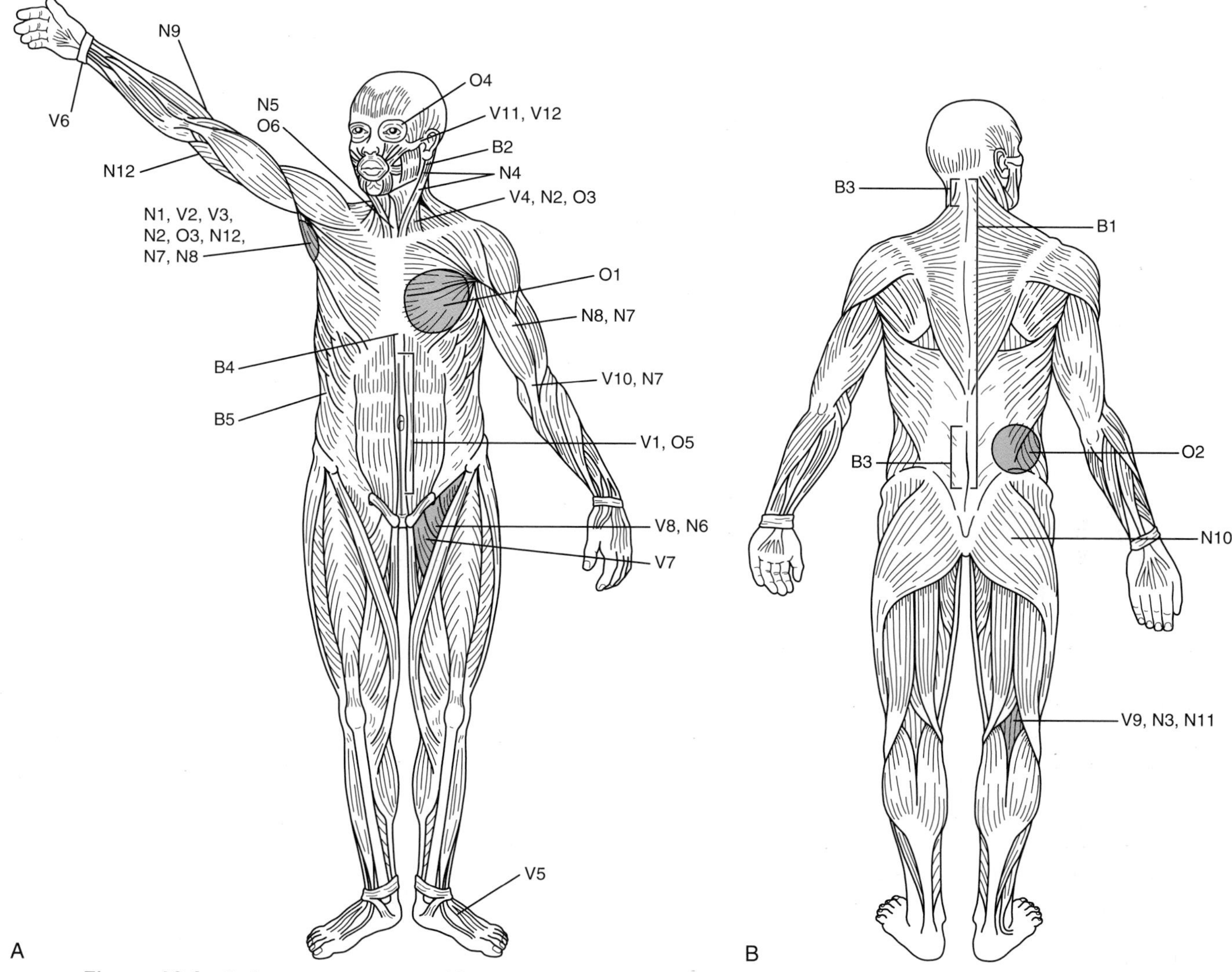

Figure 19•6 Endangerment site map. Massage therapists should exercise extreme caution when working these areas.

Vascular Endangerment Sites

The following list of vascular endangerment sites does not differentiate between arteries and veins with the exception of the great saphenous vein and the jugular vein. Arteries and veins of the same name lie in proximity to each other, and caution of one generally reflects caution of the other. Many of these vascular endangerment sites are common pulse point locations.

V1. Abdominal and descending aorta (abdominal region)
V2. Axillary artery (axilla)
V3. Brachial artery (axilla)
V4. Carotid and external carotid arteries (anterior neck)
V5. Dorsalis pedis (top of the foot)
V6. Ulnar artery (ulnar side of wrist)
V7. Femoral artery (femoral triangle)
V8. Great saphenous vein (femoral triangle)
V9. Popliteal artery (popliteal fossa or posterior knee)
V10. Radial artery (cubital area or anterior elbow)
V11. Temporal artery (anterior ear)
V12. Transverse facial artery (anterior ear)

Author's Note

When massaging an area where there is a known or suspected superficial artery, apply light pressure and feel for a pulse. If a pulse is felt, avoid the specific pulse location.

When applying a deep stripping pressure over a superficial vein, *always* move from distal to proximal, or you may promote varicosities. Varicose veins, or damaged veins, lack a sufficient interior valve system. Pressure in the wrong direction promotes improper blood flow.

Author's Note

There are several neuromuscular techniques in which massage is performed in certain endangerment site areas (e.g., the anterior throat). These techniques take into account the inherent danger for each site and use specialized techniques to avoid injury. It is not advisable to work an endangerment site area without special training in these advanced techniques.

Nerves and Nerve Plexus Endangerment Sites

These noted structures are to be avoided.

N1. Axillary nerve (posterior axilla)
N2. Brachial plexus (neck, posterior triangle, and axilla)
N3. Common peroneal nerve (lateral popliteal fossa)
N4. Lesser and greater auricular nerves (lateral throat)
N5. Vagus nerve (throat, deep abdomen, and sternal notch)
N6. Femoral nerve (femoral triangle)
N7. Median nerve (axilla, anterior elbow, and medial brachium)
N8. Musculocutaneous nerve (axilla and medial brachium)
N9. Radial nerve (lateral epicondyle of the humerus)
N10. Sciatic nerve (medial gluteal region and posterior thigh)
N11. Tibial nerve (popliteal fossa)
N12. Ulnar nerve (axilla and medial epicondyle of the humerus)

Osseous Endangerment Sites

Pressure that is swift or sudden and high-velocity thrusts are contraindicated and are outside of the massage therapist's scope of practice. Deep pressure to certain bony areas is also contraindicated.

B1. Spinous process of the vertebrae (medial spine)
B2. Styloid process of the temporal bone (anterior to insertion of the sternocleidomastoid and posterior to the angle of the mandible)
B3. Lateral border of the transverse process of the cervical and lumbar vertebrae
B4. Xiphoid process of the sternum
B5. Floating ribs, especially the lateral surface

Organ and Miscellaneous Endangerment Sites

The following areas are also to be avoided.

O1. Breast area (repeated pressure can break down breast tissue and is illegal in many states)
O2. Kidney region (avoid heavy tapotement; kidneys are retroperitoneal)
O3. Lymph nodes (anterior or posterior neck, axilla, and inguinal areas; avoid when enlarged)
O4. Orbital region (avoid direct pressure to the eyeball)
O5. Linea alba (connective tissue band running down the abdominal wall): it can herniate; exercise extra caution during pregnancy
O6. Trachea

SUMMARY

Massage has a powerful impact on the health and functioning of the body and has beneficial effects on virtually every body system. Yet it is not the preeminent answer for all problems and ills. The massage therapist who has studied and learned the indications and contraindications inspires confidence in his clients by demonstrating a strong grasp of anatomy and physiology. This includes the science of how massage provides pain relief through such mechanisms as the gate theory. There is no greater gift that can be given a client than the attention and caution to contraindicated conditions and to vascular, nervous, osseous, and other miscellaneous endangerment sites. In this way the therapist also demonstrates an appreciation for his own abilities, an awareness of his own limitations, and an unflagging reputation for acting in the best interest of his clients.

Author's Note

When in doubt, don't.

SELF-TEST

Multiple Choice • Write the letter of the best answer in the space provided.

_______ 1. Which one of the following responses results from pressure during a massage (tissue being pulled, lifted, rubbed, compressed, and manipulated)?

A. metabolic
B. mechanical
C. reflexive
D. psychological

_______ 2. Which one of the following responses is an indirect or involuntary reaction to a stimulus governed by the nervous system?

A. metabolic
B. mechanical
C. reflexive
D. psychological

_______ 3. What is the term used to describe an observable reddening of the skin resulting from increased blood flow?

A. hyperemia
B. ischemia
C. hypoxia
D. anemia

_______ 4. Blood pressure is temporarily decreased by dilation of the _______ and by affecting the permeability of capillary walls.

A. alveoli
B. nephron
C. blood capillaries
D. myofibril

_______ 5. The number of functional red blood cells, as well as their oxygen-carrying capacity, is increased by the application of massage by

A. promoting the discharge of red blood cells by the spleen
B. stimulating stagnant capillary beds
C. increasing lymphatic circulation
D. A and B

_______ 6. A decrease in blood supply to an organ or tissue is referred to as

A. hyperemia
B. ischemia
C. hypoxia
D. anemia

_______ 7. Through stimulation of the circulation by massage

A. heat is generated, and the skin feels warm to the touch
B. the skin appears hyperemic
C. added nutrients are available to tissues
D. all occur as benefits of massage

_______ 8. Slow, light, and rhythmic movements are soothing to the nerves because they produce a low level of excitement to the nervous system, whereas vigorous movements

A. cause nerves to go numb
B. stimulate the nervous system
C. decrease synaptic transmission
D. excite nociceptors only

_______ 9. Through stimulation of cutaneous thermo- and mechanoreceptors, massage inhibits pain by interfering with nociceptive information entering the spinal cord. This phenomenon is called the

A. gate theory
B. dorsal horn phenomenon
C. pain reduction theory
D. inhibitory phenomenon

_______ 10. Certain massage strokes create minute muscle contractions by

A. increasing circulation
B. increasing muscle spindle activity
C. increasing lymph flow
D. decreasing respiration rate

_______ 11. Massage can temporarily alter the shape and appearance of _______ by flattening out adipose globules located under the skin, making them seem smoother.

A. cellulite
B. warts
C. freckles
D. moles

_______ 12. Deep friction can create an appropriate scar that is strong, yet does not interfere with the

A. circulation in the extremities
B. calcium deposits on bones
C. broadening of muscles in contraction
D. nerve supply to the affected area

_______ 13. Which one of the following is *not* a benefit of massage?

A. helps relieve colic and intestinal gas
B. promotes evacuation of the colon
C. increases urine output
D. all are massage benefits

_______ 14. Which one of the following is *not* an indication for massage therapy?
A. stress, anxiety, and insomnia
B. phlebitis, thrombus, and varicosity
C. muscular soreness and fatigue
D. myofascial pain

_______ 15. Conditions or situations that merit caution and adaptive measures to ensure the massage is safe and that the client is comfortable are called
A. partial or relative contraindications
B. endangerment sites
C. absolute contraindications
D. indications

_______ 16. Which of the following groups of conditions are not contraindications for massage therapy?
A. arteriosclerosis, aneurysm, Raynaud's phenomenon, hypertension, multiple sclerosis, diabetes, and fever
B. rashes, poison ivy, poison oak, sumac, impetigo, athlete's foot, ringworm, scabies, blisters, abnormal lumps, warts, herpes simplex, herpes zoster, large or loose moles, lymphogranuloma venereum, and skin ulcerations
C. areas where foreign objects are embedded in the tissues, abrasions, cuts, hematomas, and contusions
D. all of the above are contraindications for massage therapy

_______ 17. Areas of the body that contain certain anatomical structures prone to injury, such as nerves, blood vessels, organs, and small, prominent bony projections, are referred to as
A. partial or relative contraindications
B. endangerment sites
C. absolute contraindications
D. indications

_______ 18. Which one of the following is *not* an endangerment site?
A. femoral triangle
B. brachial plexus
C. origin of the adductor magnus
D. styloid process of temporal bone

References

Barr, J. S., and N. Taslitz. "Influence of Back Massage on Autonomic Functions." *Physical Therapy,* Vol. 50, 1970.

Bodian, M. "Use of Massage Following Lid Surgery." *Eye, Ear, Nose, and Throat Monthly,* 1969.

Bell, A. J. "Massage and the Physiotherapist." *Physiotherapy.* JCSP, 1964.

Cuthbertson, D. P. "Effects of Massage on Metabolism: A Survey." *Glasgow Medical Journal,* 1933.

Cyriax, James. *Textbook of Orthopedic Medicine,* vol. 2, 11th ed. "Treatment by Manipulation, Massage, and Injection." London: Bailliere-Tindall, 1984.

De Domenico, Giovani, and Elizabeth Wood. *Beard's Massage.* Philadelphia: W. B. Saunders Company, 1997.

Despard, L. L. *Textbook of Massage and Remedial Gymnastics,* 3rd ed. New York: Oxford University Press, 1932.

Evans, P. "The Healing Process at a Cellular Level: A Review." *Physiotherapy.* JCSP, Vol. 66, 1980.

Fassbender, H. G. *Pathology of Rheumatic Diseases.* New York: Springer-Verlag, 1975.

Field, Tiffany, Connie Morrow, Chad Valdeon et al. "Massage Reduces Anxiety in Child and Adolescent Psychiatric Patients." *American Academy of Child and Adolescent Psychiatry,* Vol. 31, 1992.

Field, Tiffany, Connie Morrow, Chad Valdeon et al. Touch Research Institute Studies. 1998.

Fraser, J., and Janet Ross Kerr. "Psychophysiological Effects of Back Massage on Elderly Institutionalized Patients." *Journal of Advanced Nursing,* Vol. 18, 1993.

Fritz, Sandy. *Fundamentals of Therapeutic Massage.* St. Louis: Mosby–Year Book, Inc., 1995.

Goldberg, J., D. Seaborne, and S. Sullivan. "The Effects of Therapeutic Massage on H-reflex Amplitude in Persons with a Spinal Cord Injury." *Physical Therapy,* Vol. 74, No. 8, 1994.

Hammer, W. I. "The Use of Transverse Friction Massage in the Management of Chronic Bursitis of the Shoulder and Hip." *Journal of Manipulative Physiological Medicine,* Vol. 69, 1993.

Helbing-Sheafe, Hannelore. "Guidelines for the Therapeutic Massage Practice." *Digest of Chiropractic Economics,* Vol. 7, January/February, 1988.

Juhan, Deane. *Job's Body, A Handbook for Bodyworkers.* Barrington, NY: Station Hill Press, 1987.

Kresge, Carol A. "Massage and Sports." In *Sports Medicine, Fitness, Training, Injuries.* Baltimore, Urban and Schwarzenberg, 1987.

Krieger, Dolores. "Therapeutic Touch: The Imprimatur of Nursing." *American Journal of Nursing,* Vol. 5, May 1975.

Krusen, F. H. *Physical Medicine.* Philadelphia: W. B. Saunders, 1941.

Lucia, S. P., and J. F. Richard. "Effects of Massage on Blood Platelet Production." *Proceedings of the Society for Experimental Biology and Medicine,* 1933.

Meek S. "Effects of Slow Stroke Back Massage on Relaxation in Hospice Clients." *IMAGE: Journal of Nursing Scholarship,* Vol. 25, 1993.

Mennell, J. B. *Physical Treatment,* 5th ed. Philadelphia: Blakiston, 1945.

Mitchell, J. K. *Massage and Exercise in System of Physiological Therapeutics.* Philadelphia: Blakiston, 1904.

Mock H. E. "Massage in Surgical Cases." *American Medical Association Handbook of Physical Medicine.* Chicago: Council of Physical Medicine, 1945.

Moore, Keith L. *Clinically Oriented Anatomy,* 2nd ed. Baltimore: Williams & Wilkins, 1985.

Nordschow, M., and W. Bierman. "Influence of Manual Massage on Muscle Relaxation: Effects on Trunk Flexion." *Physical Therapy,* Vol. 42, 1962.

Pemberton, R. "Physiology of Massage." In *American Medical Association Handbook of Physical Therapy,* 3rd ed. Chicago: Council of Physical Therapy, 1939.

Prudden, Bonnie. *Pain Erasure.* New York: M. Evans & Co., 1980.

Reed, Brian, and Jean M. Held. "Effects of Sequential Connective

Tissue Massage on Autonomic Nervous System of Middle-Aged and Elderly Adults." *Physical Therapy,* Vol. 68, No. 4, August 1988.

St. John, Paul. *St. John Neuromuscular Therapy Seminars, Manual I.* Largo, FL 1995.

Scull, C. Wesler. "Massage—Physiological Basis." *Archives of Physical Medicine,* March 1945.

Smith. L., et al. "The Effects of Athletic Massage on Delayed Onset Muscle Soreness, Creatine Kinase, and Neutrophil Count: A Preliminary Report." *JOSPT,* 1994.

Taber's Cyclopedic Medical Dictionary, 13th ed. Philadelphia: F. A. Davis. 1977.

Tappan, Frances M. *Healing Massage Technique, Holistic, Classical and Emerging Methods.* Norwalk, CT: Appleton & Lange, 1988.

Tortora, Gerald J. *Introduction to the Human Body: The Essentials of Anatomy and Physiology,* 3rd ed. New York: HarperCollins Publishers, 1994.

Travell, Janet G., and David Simons. *Myofasical Pain and Dysfunction, The Trigger Point Manual.* Baltimore: Williams & Wilkins, 1983.

Voss, Dorothy E., Marjorie K. Ionta, and Beverly J. Myers. *Proprioceptive Neuromuscular Facilitation.* Philadelphia: Harper & Row, 1985.

Wakim, Khalil G. *Manipulation, Traction and Massage.* New York: Robert E. Krieger, 1976.

Wall, P. D., and R. Melzack. "Pain Mechanisms: A New Theory." *Science,* Vol. 150, 1965.

Williams, Ruth E. *The Road to Radiant Health.* College Place, WA: Color Press, 1977.

The body tells the story. It is, in fact, a living autobiography.
—Elaine Mayland

Susie Ogg Cormier

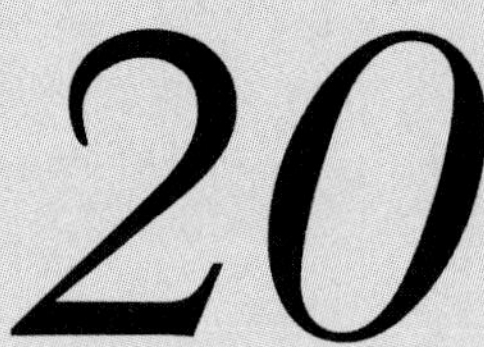

20

Professional Communication, Assessment, and Documentation

Student Objectives

After completing this chapter, the student should be able to:

- Explain and demonstrate basic verbal communication skills used in structured interviews
- Identify categories of health information; define subjective and objective data for each
- State how data collection enhances the client-practitioner relationship and massage therapy
- Using selected joints, record a baseline postural analysis and ROM assessment of a fellow student
- Using data, formulate massage therapy goals
- Write subjective and objective information via the SOAP format
- Using the SOAP format, document the sequence and techniques in a massage session
- Describe and document changes resulting from the therapeutic massage
- Through analyzing plan responses, client homework and lifestyle changes
- Evaluate a client's response to massage, alter the therapy plan, and document changes
- Learn the criteria that must be met for massage to be considered "medically necessary"
- Use status and narrative reporting to communicate with other health professionals

INTRODUCTION

Professional communication is an interaction between the massage therapist and the client (or agents of the client) for the collection, recording, and transmission of data for therapeutic purposes. Professional communication includes assessing the client's health, needs, priorities, and anticipated response to massage therapy. Good communication means informing the client about benefits and potential side effects of massage, informing clients of their rights, and obtaining consent for therapy. The client may also be informed about the therapist's massage specialties and the policies and procedures involved in service.

Professional communication is a critical skill that enhances feelings of connection and trust between the client and therapist, which forms the basis of a positive, committed, and cooperative working relationship. An effective therapist listens carefully to the client to identify her needs, desires, and expectations. Using his unique talents, the therapist then customizes the massage based on assessment. This chapter will examine professional standards for communication, assessment, and documentation.

COMMUNICATION SKILLS

Communication skills are used in listening, speaking, writing, and assessing nonverbal messages. The verbal and assessing skills are used throughout the professional therapeutic process: greeting the client; explaining and informing the client of services and procedures; collecting and reviewing the health history and intake form; gaining informed consent; goal planning; and room orientation. We use written skills to prepare forms for client use, to document client information, and to document progress and response to therapy.

Communication skills are both a science and an art. The science of communication involves systematically obtaining information and imparting it to others. We use written forms, direct questioning, observing body language, and listening for helpful information to communicate. The art of communication is twofold. First, like any other art it can be achieved through natural ability and practice. Second, we must have the desire to communicate. Our clients often speak through a filter of emotions that delivers the message in a way that has meaning for *them.*

Successful communication leaves the client feeling that she has been listened to. The massage therapist can hear what the client is saying, interpret the message, give feedback or helpful directions, and perform the massage session based on the information that was subjectively and objectively received. Patience, guidance, and skillful communication techniques can help establish a positive and authentic professional relationship.

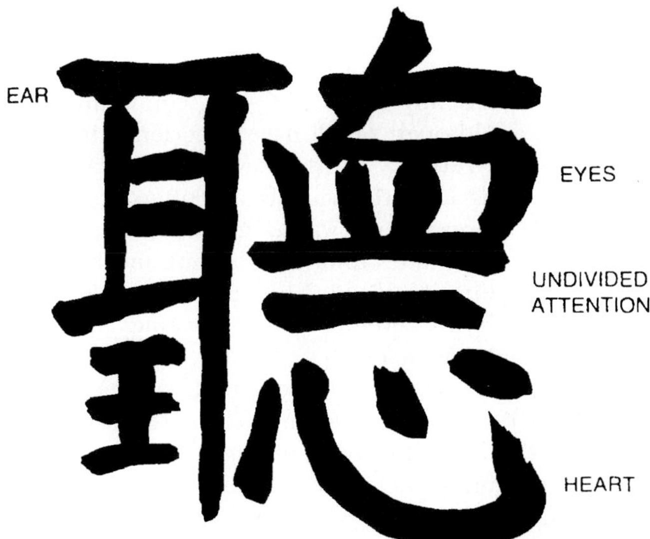

Figure 20•1 Calligraphy depicting communication. (From Adler RB, Towne N: Looking Out/Looking In, 7th ed. New York: Holt, Rinehart and Winston, 1993. Calligraphy by Angie Aw.)

When exchanging information with your clients, you will use three types of communication techniques: verbal, nonverbal, and written (Fig. 20–1).

VERBAL COMMUNICATION

Verbal communication—speaking—involves sending and receiving information by both parties. For clarity choose words to convey your intent clearly, concisely, and tactfully.

An effective speaker also considers the background or education of the receiver and uses words that are understood by the receiver. Using anatomical names and medical terminology may be inappropriate for clients who do not have the background or training in these areas.

Verbal communication is a cooperative effort. The effective speaker pauses and asks for periodic feedback to verify that the message she intends is the message being received. In this way, alterations, or corrections can be made. Pausing allows the listener to comment or to let the speaker know how the message is perceived. This feedback alerts an effective speaker that she needs to adjust the message to suit the listener.

The speaker's main objective is being heard and understood. It is the speaker's responsibility to be clear in intent, to frame the intent with words in an effective manner, and to deliver the message with supportive body language. After the listener has received the message, it is the speaker's responsibility, using listening skills and reflective responses, to determine that the message sent is actually the message received.

Verbal Communication: Effective Listening

Massage therapy involves one-to-one communication and contact. Although we all have experience in relating to people, very few of us know how to relate professionally. Massage professionals are often characterized by their respectful, warm, genuine, open, and understanding attitudes toward the client and have developed "listening hands and hearts." With a little insight, skill can be developed in cultivating "listening ears and minds" as well.

Although skill in speaking is helpful, the most critical skill for developing an optimal client relationship is listening. Through effective listening we can customize therapy to achieve the client's goals and expectations for the session. Most of us falsely assume that we are listening when we hear. Hearing actually requires little or no effort on our part; usually volume ensures adequate reception, but hearing does not mean that we comprehend verbal information. Effective listening means understanding the language used, the emotional state of sender and receiver, and focusing attention on receiving the message.

As a therapist it is your responsibility to focus and to facilitate the client's communication. You need information that is clear and accurate upon which to base decisions regarding therapy. The massage therapist uses listening skills to receive the information, checks to make sure he understands the information as the client intended, and interprets the information to customize the therapy session.

To ensure accuracy in collecting information, the client needs to feel that the therapist is actively interested in listening. You need to consider that your body language and attitude are also being observed. Authenticity and presence are conveyed nonverbally by maintaining eye contact and by occasional nodding or using appropriate facial expressions that coincide with the tone of the message. Verbal phrases or sounds, such as "really," "uh-huh," "hummmm," show interest and encourage the speaker to continue.

The client perceives the therapist's openness and senses a safe environment for disclosure of sensitive or private information. Listening in a nonjudgmental and empathic manner helps the speaker to reveal honest thoughts and feelings; this is known as **self-disclosure.** Self-disclosure is usually guarded unless the therapist has established a measure of trust. Being nonjudgmental requires that the therapist withhold personal evaluation of the speaker and the message being conveyed. Suspending judgment respects the client's right to have his own life experiences. Genuine acceptance is evidenced by receiving the message as is without rebuttal, argument, or additions.

Being empathic requires that the therapist put herself in the client's shoes, seeking to understand information from the client's point of view. Listening with empathy requires the therapist to consider the client's words, feelings, and intent. The sender will feel a deeper sense of safety if the message is acknowledged. Assisting the client to be present in the moment and to experience a safe environment allows the client to attend to her own needs within the session.

Verbal Communication: Checking Listening Effectiveness

A reflective response verifies that the listener has understood the feelings and content of the speaker's message and mirrors this understanding back to the client. The client can then correct or modify the listener's perceptions. Unless time is taken to reflect and receive feedback, the therapist may make incorrect assumptions that lead to inappropriate planning and goal setting, ultimately resulting in client dissatisfaction. Common reflective techniques are paraphrasing, clarifying, summarizing, exploring, and redirecting.

Paraphrasing involves stating in your words what you believe the client has said. You may use phrases such as "What I hear you saying is . . . ," "In other words . . . ," "So basically how you feel is . . . ," and so on. The client may acknowledge that you heard him correctly, or he may send the message again with additional information.

Clarifying involves asking the client for additional information because you are not sure if you understood the intended message. Because they are symbols, words have a wide interpretation from person to person. The client can report symptoms with words that are vague, and the therapist needs additional clarification. The meaning of a word such as "pain" varies significantly from one person to another. Is the pain mild, moderate, or severe? Does it occur every day, all day, only with certain movements or activities? Words like "a lot," "all the time," and "always" require clarification and feedback to ensure that the therapist understands the client's experience.

Summarizing involves briefly stating the general feeling and content of the client's message. Recapping can be used when the therapist has an idea about what the client is trying to say. The therapist needs feedback from the client to affirm that the summary is accurate.

Exploring and *redirecting* are types of clarification. The therapist assists communication by providing an intake form. The therapist's verbal review of the intake form can clarify or uncover facts that would be helpful in determining treatment plans and goals, contraindications, and needed referrals. Using a written form also serves as a reminder to the therapist to redirect the conversation to the areas that need further investigation.

Usually open-ended questions allow the client to reflect and to clarify his own thoughts and feelings, thus producing more accurate subjective information. Closed questions are more direct and can keep the client's responses focused on the agenda. The therapist must use care not to suggest answers or responses, but must focus on asking questions that will benefit the therapy session.

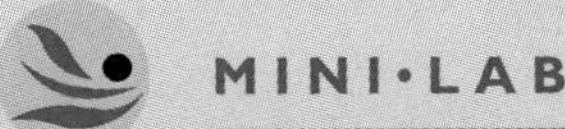

MINI•LAB

Dividing them into groups of two, choose one of the 12 roadblocks in the left-hand column, and consult books on communication in your local library or bookstore. Design a skit in which the therapist/interviewer uses the roadblocks to interfere with communication while interviewing the student client. Following the skit, the class will guess which roadblock was demonstrated. End the exercise by giving helpful hints to avoid the group's particular roadblock.

Verbal Communication: Barriers to Effective Listening

Barriers to good communication can come from the therapist or the client. An effective therapist wants to listen to the client and is interested in receiving accurate information regarding the client's health and concerns. If a therapist lacks a skill in professional communication, he may not establish a basic connection with the client. Planning and adequate preparation for the interview will help avoid scanty or faulty information collection, which can result in poor communication and difficulty meeting the client's expectations. If the therapist believes that her perceptions will give her all the client information she needs, communication is nonproductive. Collection of information without clarification usually contributes to guessing and assumption. The therapist may ask yes/no questions, finish sentences, and in other ways block effective communication with the client.

Sometimes therapists are unable to set their own personal or professional issues aside and cannot be present and available to their clients. A therapist can also rely on biased generalizations based on personal assumptions, which may result in his determining a plan to achieve the goals he assumes are best for the client. For example, a client with chronic cervical pain requests a stress-reduction session because of job-related events. A therapist not tuned into the client's message may spend too much time in the cervical area at the expense of a deeply relaxing session.

A client barrier to effective communication may arise when the client is excessively stressed, depressed from chronic pain, or in acute pain. An intensely emotional client will need a therapist who remains calm and centered and who listens through the screen of emotions. Patience, guidance, and skillful communication can often smooth the situation and begin positive interactions. Awareness of potential problems can help us modify our behavior.

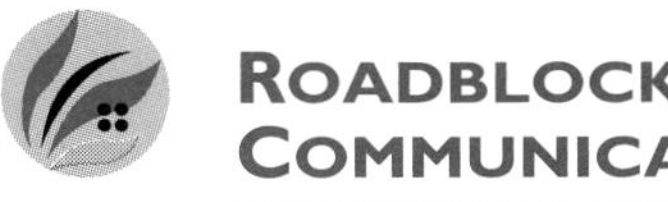

ROADBLOCKS TO COMMUNICATION

- Ordering, directing, and commanding
- Warning, admonishing, and threatening
- Exhorting, moralizing, and preaching
- Advising, and giving solutions or suggestions
- Lecturing, teaching, and giving logical arguments
- Judging, criticizing, disagreeing, and blaming
- Praising and agreeing
- Name calling, ridiculing, and shaming
- Interpreting, analyzing, and diagnosing
- Reassuring, sympathizing, and consoling
- Probing, questioning, and interrogating in excess
- Withdrawing, distracting, humoring, and diverting

Verbal Communication: A Sample Interaction

During verbal communication the client may say, "My migraine headaches have returned. I'm really stressed out. We lost my mother last week after a 6-month bout with cancer." The therapist might reply: "I'm really sorry to hear about the loss of your mother. I know that must be very painful and stressful for you. Am I correct in understanding that the migraines are your biggest physical discomfort at this time?"

The client may say: "I've got a failed lumbar fusion and am in constant pain. My friend Gary told me that I needed to get some deep-tissue work from you, but he said it would hurt. I'm really desperate for relief but don't think I can take any more pain right now. But old Gary has a lot of faith in you. He talks about you all the time."

Since the client is now focusing on a lengthy story about Gary, the therapist might interrupt and redirect: "Well, I sure appreciate the fact that Gary referred you to me. And I understood you to say that you're experiencing a lot of pain as a result of a failed surgery and that you don't want to hurt more. Is that so?" (Silence.) "We don't have to start with deep-tissue techniques, we can begin with a milder treatment and see if it brings you relief. Would you like to do that?"

Notice how each scenario brings the conversation back to therapy.

NONVERBAL COMMUNICATION

Nonverbal communication involves message transmission by means other than the spoken word. Nonverbal messages are sent by the person's body, often without the speaker's awareness. For this reason nonverbal communication is also known as body language. We communicate with others in five ways: (1) words; (2) tones; (3) gestures; (4) posture; and (5) facial expressions. Effective speakers and listeners consider and use nonverbal communication to enhance and reinforce their overall communication.

Nonverbal messages are also an important part of communication. Just as tone conveys information about the emotional state of the speaker, so does body language. The listener may be distracted if you are speaking in a way that says she is important while you are glancing at the clock and ruffling through papers as if you are in a hurry. Being aware to match gestures, expressions, and muscular movements to the message also helps the message to be understood clearly. Generally the strongest message, the message the listener will receive and remember, is the unspoken one because it is perceived to be the most honest.

Nonverbal communication accompanies the speaker's words and even occurs when conversation has ceased. Because four out of five methods of communicating are nonverbal, body language often gives the therapist more complete information than the spoken word. Nonverbal cues indicate how the client is feeling and her internal state. Body language includes

1. Facial expressions such as grimaces, frowns, puckers, rapid blinking, and eye contact.
2. Gestures such as making fists, clawing or gripping the table, fidgeting, and nodding.
3. Sudden movements such as the toes coming up off the table, buttocks tightening, change in breathing, lifting of the head, and looking down.
4. Sounds such as sighs, grunts, groans, hummm, and uh-huh.
6. Posture in relation to others (when one is seated higher than another, or one is standing and one is sitting; usually the higher person is more important or more power is implied).

So how does nonverbal communication help? Often the client may not tell you that a certain massage move or pressure is too intense or uncomfortable. Body language will communicate his unspoken discomfort. Sometimes the client may be unaware of conflicting emotions associated with certain stressful events. Look for congruency between what the client says and what his body language tells you.

For example, (1) a client, while frowning, tells you a story and declares how glad he is about the event; (2) a client answers your question verbally by saying no, while enthusiastically nodding her head affirmatively; (3) a client who was in a horrible accident tells the whole story while smiling or laughing. All these examples, while extreme, demonstrate that their verbal communication is incongruent with their body language. The perceptive massage therapist notes the nonverbal discrepancy and includes this information in her assessment of the client if clarification is not appropriate. If the client winces but then denies that the pressure or touch is uncomfortable, the therapist should immediately seek clarification or change her touch, whichever seems most appropriate.

Report your observations. Telling the client what you observe often improves the communication process because what you are observing can be affirmed or denied. For example, if you notice that your client is holding the muscles in his face tightly, you might say, "I notice that you're wrinkling your forehead. Are you feeling tense today?" He may say, "Why, yes, it has been a hectic day to this point." Always use personal inquiry over assumed meaning.

Remember that, whether consciously or unconsciously, the client is also reading your body language. The information you project with your body language may affect therapeutic relationships. For example, you may promote the benefits of regular massage therapy in stress reduction, while obviously stressed out and in need of a session yourself. The prudent therapist is aware of his own body language and uses this information to note discrepancies between his own emotional and intellectual realities. If you consciously project an open, caring, professional image by nonverbal body language, you then strengthen the weight carried by your words. When actions match words, the result is an increased feeling of authenticity, comfort, and security for the client.

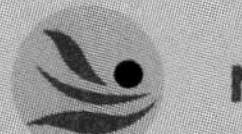

MINI·LAB

Visit your local library or a bookstore. Using resources describing body language, make a list of nonverbal cues and describe some of the possible meanings. The class may play "guess the meaning" as each one acts out a cue from the list for the class.

WRITTEN COMMUNICATION

Written communication for professional purposes includes gathering and recording subjective information, our objective findings, and any other information that is necessary to assist treatment. Since written information is recorded on paper, or **documented,** the therapist can reread it to aid recall and review. This may be one reason that the written word is the communication of choice in the professional world. Much discussion centers around the use of records in litigation; even written contracts and other legal documents are hotly debated and subject to interpretation by those who read them. The chief purpose of documentation is to assist in rendering better professional services.

Written forms of communication include the client intake form, consent to therapy, written reports, prescriptions from medical and chiropractic physicians, your own treatment notes, any other recorded information related to therapy, and correspondence with attorneys or insurance companies. These written communications will ultimately verify the information your client has shared and justify the treatment she has received. Accurate records provide supportive documentation that treatment was within acceptable and safe boundaries and protect you from malpractice claims, which occur rarely. More importantly, the record gives you a full accounting of the client's healing process in response to massage therapy. The key is to document, continue to document, and do it as specifically as possible.

There is no single adopted standard of assessment and documentation for massage therapists. The American Massage Therapy Association, the National Certification Board for Therapeutic Massage and Bodywork, and the National Association for Nurse Massage Therapists are proposing guidelines through codes of ethics and professional practice standards, which includes systematic and ongoing documentation.

There has been much debate on the rationale for requiring written assessment and systematic documentation. Recording the client's health history and obtaining consent ranges from none to verbal to written at the therapist's option. In the past the client was a passive recipient, but today clients are choosing a variety of massage therapies for specific health benefits; they are choosing to be educated partners in their healing processes. Progress awareness and informed choices in the modalities and management of her specific concerns, create a treatment team of the therapist and the client. The client's record reflects the documentation of progress toward her goals.

Massage is moving into a wider practice environment: from home and private office to sports events, to public retail spaces (in grocery stores, airports, etc.), to business places, to physical therapy and chiropractic clinics, and to other health settings such as hospitals. It is our emerging professionalism that drives the need to collect and document systematically the ongoing client care commitment that we have. Through our written record, we confirm our educated assessment, choice of massage, and the evaluation of the client's progress toward health. Written versus verbal communication is an important step in defining ourselves as professional practitioners. Through effective written records, we can help increase respect for our professional findings and therapy in improving client health status. As the effectiveness of our work becomes increasingly recognized, other healthcare practitioners are adding massage therapists to the therapeutic team. Insurance coverage for our services is increasing, and because we assess the tissues directly, our physical findings may be sought in legal proceedings; therefore, we need to document our findings for attorneys, health practitioners, and insurance representatives.

Many states are mandating systematic collection and ongoing documentation through their state boards of massage therapy. Licensed practitioners are increasingly required by law to comply, and client records may be used in peer review, licensing determinations, and other legal proceedings. Formal clinical groups often require random selection and review of client records on file for completeness and accuracy. Random sampling demonstrates that the therapists are maintaining professional standards concerning all clients. Licensing increases our accountability to the public and carries the potential for litigation from negligence, injury, breach of confidentiality, or other offenses.

Another reason to document treatment sessions is that our memory is limited. Initially, when you have only a few clients, you may remember your clients and many particulars regarding their sessions; however, when you are seeing 15 to 30 clients per week, you will have more trouble remembering the needs and particular details of each client. Relying on memory is poor record keeping. Written notes serve to jog your memory and to remind you of particular details you want to review before the next session; the more detailed and specific your treatment notes are, the more accurate your assessment and planning.

Author's Note

I like to look at documentation as a type of insurance coverage. I can purchase minimal insurance by recording general impressions, or, with a little time and effort, I can have a million-dollar policy by recording specific details. When you need insurance the coverage is never too much! Recording specific details ensures the highest quality of recall and therapeutic continuity.

THE MASSAGE CONSULTATION

We establish a positive, trusting, and therapeutic relationship with a potential client through the massage consultation. Time spent in establishing this working relationship often results in client satisfaction and continued patronage. Success in building a client relationship is possible through thoughtful preparation and planning for the interview. Knowledge of listening skills previously discussed will greatly enhance verbal interaction.

Regardless of setting, the therapist's goal is to achieve the greatest warmth, safety, and comfort possible for the client. To encourage concentration and relaxation, give attention to the physical environment by providing privacy from distractions such as the phone, radio, TV, and other people. Attend to the physical comfort of the room by adjusting such details as lighting, temperature, and seating. Provide for physiological comfort and decreased apprehension of a first-time client by using an easily manipulated pen and clipboard. You may also choose to attend to esthetic details of the assessment process such as paper quality, attractive layout of printed material, a fine writing pen, music, and choice of aromatherapy to make the experience more enjoyable for the client, or you may conduct the interview verbally and record the information yourself. You alone will decide what your environment will be like. Ask yourself if your environment reflects you in a unique and memorable way. A therapist who is empathetic and genuinely concerned for the client can do a lot to "warm" even the most clinical (such as a hospital) or busy (such as a salon) environment.

The reasons for the client's visit can also modify the massage consultation phase. A client coming to receive massage for a recent injury or painful symptom may need a more lengthy symptom discussion and a focused evaluation of posture, gait, or ROM. The generally healthy client with no specific complaints, by comparison does not require a lengthy assessment. Additional time may be needed to record information for clients involved in legal, insurance, or physician-referred massage, which needs a clear initial understanding of therapy goals prescribed, evaluation, and follow-up. To help allay therapist stress, anticipate variables and be as flexible as possible.

Following the initial consultation, prepare for future sessions by briefly reviewing your client records and health history. These activities assure the client of your attention to her care; they also provide for client safety as you review any health concerns and lack of progress that may necessitate modification of the original plan. As a mark of professionalism and to ensure continuity of care, physicians and other healthcare providers are always careful to review the client's record prior to greeting the client. Likewise, prepare for future sessions with a brief review of your client's records and health history. Project your professionalism through attention to detail and through systematic and continuous collection and documentation of information (Fig. 20–2).

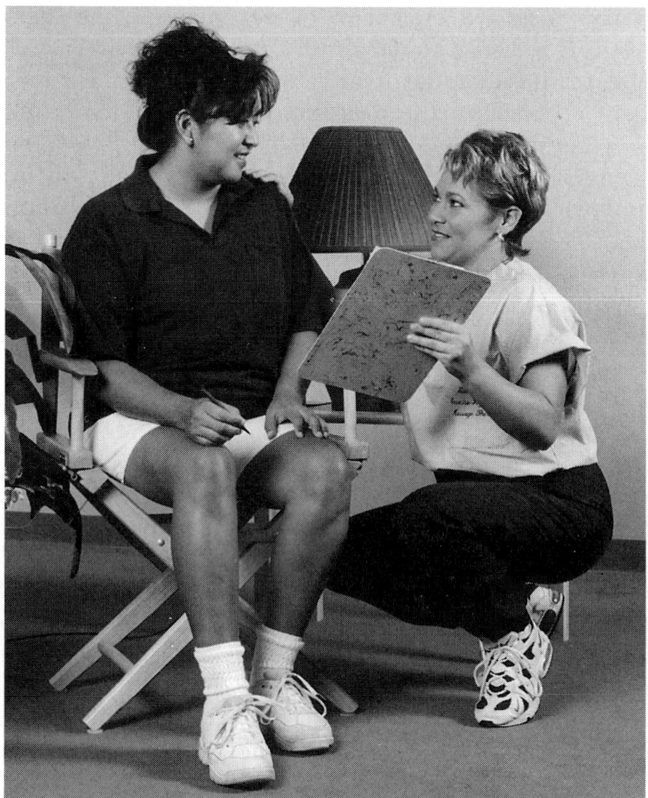

Figure 20•2 Prepare for future sessions with a brief reivew of your client's records and health.

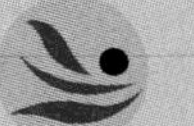

MINI•LAB

Visit a massage therapist's office. What is the initial impression you have approaching the door? List words to describe how you feel. Is the mood serene, businesslike, busy, chaotic, impersonal, cluttered? What do you hear or smell?

Author's Note

Many clients will ask you how many massages you have done today and if you are tired, or after noting the physical nature of our work, will ask if the hands become tired. I believe what they are really asking is: Do you have enough energy for me? I assure them that I have stamina and endurance built up from frequently doing massage and that when my hands do feel tired, I massage them back to happiness. At this point they seem to be less fearful and greatly relieved.

SUBJECTIVE ASSESSMENT VIA THE INITIAL INTAKE OR HEALTH HISTORY

Systematic record keeping begins with collecting information from the client, pertinent others, and healthcare personnel. These data are collected by questionnaire, interview, and records when deemed necessary by the therapist (be sure to send a signed consent for release of records with the request). For continued collection and updating of the initial baseline of information, complete a treatment record or client visit report after each successive visit.

All client information is usually organized in **SOAP format:** Subjective assessment information; Objective assessment information; Application of massage or therapy and response; and Plan. This information includes assessment of client status, therapy or massage application, evaluation, goal setting, and planning. There is some variation in each category, but all records contain a baseline of information that is standard care for each of your clients. *Systematic recording* of a baseline gives you criteria by which to measure positive changes resulting from therapy and needed modifications to overall goals. You may also choose to use special assessment forms for your client to measure progress, the initial goal being to achieve a holistic picture of the client's health. This picture is the basis for planning and goal setting.

In general, a client will not want to spend more than 10 minutes filling out your health questionnaire. You may need an additional 10 to 15 minutes to review and clarify the information you have requested. Carefully select questions to collect a baseline of information that will benefit you most in addressing the concerns of the client. There is no one perfect form that meets the needs for all kinds of massage sessions and therapists, so choose one that you think will collect the data you need and then tailor it to match your needs. The main purpose of using a form is to ensure that nothing will be forgotten or overlooked.

Suggested considerations for intake forms (Fig. 20–3):

1. Readability. Is the type large enough?
2. Organization. Is it organized logically?
3. Convenient. Can the client check off or circle quickly those that apply?
4. Necessary. Is the information requested relevant and important for the therapist to know?
5. Flexible. Is there adequate space to write personal information that is important for this client?

Keeping the form to no more than one page helps to decrease the client's stress. You may wish to send the health history, policy and procedure form, and consent to the client before the scheduled appointment. You may advise the client to come 20 to 30 minutes early or tell him that the first session will be extended 20 to 30 minutes to allow for adequate time. Some therapists opt to do a verbal intake interview and to record the client's responses in interview style, with only the consent and policy and procedures to be signed. These strategies may relax the client since he will not worry if the paperwork and interview will take away from the massage time he is expecting. If your evaluation is lengthy, be sure that the client is informed concerning the potential benefits of this process and that he agrees to pay for the evaluation as part of the first session, if this is your policy.

Designing the Initial Intake or Health History Form

General biographical information is a standard part of all information forms. This includes the client's name and address, home and work phones, date of birth/age, date at which the baseline is being reported, and referring person. Other facts to include are occupation, marital status, sex, height and weight, number of children, the person's social security number, person who is responsible for the fees, and person to contact in an emergency.

Determine what information you need for the type of massage therapy you practice and include questions on your initial intake form that reflect your data needs. Information collected directly from the client is subjective in nature (i.e., from his viewpoint). The first thing you want to know is what the client's chief concern is today. This information will reflect her perception of her current health status and what she needs to receive from today's massage session. Be clear about what motivated today's visit. If you do not hear the reason, find it, and then work on the problem area. If you do not understand the client's goals, you will not meet her expectations for the session and probably not get another chance.

Sample Questions for Chief Concerns/Priorities

1. What is your major concern today? Other areas of pain or concern?
2. What type of massage would you prefer? (Relaxation? Deep-tissue? Other?)
3. What results do you want from your massage sessions? What would you like to achieve with our work?
4. Is there any area where you would like extra time spent, any area where you seem to hold a lot of tension?

Include assessment questions that ask how the client is using her muscles daily. Investigate her frequent activities at work and home such as sitting, standing,

INITIAL INTAKE FORM FOR MASSAGE THERAPY

Name ______________________ SS# __________ Birth Date _________ Date __________
Address ______________________ Ph.wk. __________ Ph.hm. __________
______________________ Referred by ______________________

What is your major concern today? ______________ Other areas of concern ______________

How would you describe your discomfort? ______________________

Intensity: ___Mild ___Moderate ___Severe ___Other: ______________________

Duration: ___Constant ___Intermittent ___ With certain motions ______________________

How long does the discomfort last when it occurs? ___min. ___hrs. ___days ______________

When did you first notice pain or discomfort? ______________________

What activities are difficult or painful to do? ______________________

What activities are helpful to do? ______________________

Are you currently under the care of a health practitioner for any reason? ___ no ___ yes __________

Has there been a medical diagnosis? ___ no ___ yes ______________________

What are your most frequent activities involved in work and home? ___sitting ___standing ___lifting
___other exercise and frequency: ______________________

Healthy Diet? ___ Always ___Frequently ___Sometimes ___Infrequently ___Rarely

Adequate Sleep? ___Every Night ___ Most Nights ___ Difficulty Sleeping ___ Use Sleep Aid

Sleep Position? ___ Back ___Side ___Stomach ___Still ___ Restless, many positions

Habits? ___Coffee/Tea ___ Sugar/Sodas, etc. ___Tobacco ___Alcohol

In which part(s) of your body do you feel stress most often? Check all that apply. ___ Head ___ Neck
___Shoulders ___Back ___Digestive ___Extremities ___Other: ______________________

Is a portion of your day set aside for relaxation? ___yes ___ no What kind? ______________
____

Previous injuries, including broken bones, NOT requiring surgery: ______________________
____

Previous surgeries with approximate dates: ______________________
____

Please review this list and circle any illness and/or medical conditions which apply.

diabetes	contact lenses	ruptured/bulging disc
arthritis	heart condition	elevated cholesterol
seizures	skin disorder	high blood pressure
cancer	varicose veins	infectious conditions
stroke	phlebitis	autoimmune disorder
contacts	scoliosis	previous MVA/trauma
headache	loss of balance	fatigue/depression
pins/needles	bruxing/grinding	painful joints

Other: ____

Medications: ___Vitamins ___Herbs ___ Aspirin/Anti-inflammatories ___Muscle Relaxants
___Pain Reducers ___ Anti-anxiety/Depressants ___Sleeping Pills

Figure 20•3 A sample initial intake. (Permission is hereby granted to reproduce this form in its entirety, including the copyright notice, for commercial or instructional use but not for resale.)

chasing small children, or carrying heavy books. Assess general soft-tissue health by asking how much and what kinds of regular exercise or sports activity she participates in. Habits such as diet, adequate sleep, or use of tobacco and alcohol also affect tissue health. Questions about these issues help the client begin to make connections between how she feels and her lifestyle choices. You will gain information concerning muscle health, potential areas of muscle stress, and expected tissue response and recovery time after your massage. You may even modify your original plan based on this information.

Sample Questions Related to Soft-Tissue Conditions

1. Do you follow a regular exercise program? What kind?
2. Do you use alcohol, coffee, or tea? Is your use heavy, moderate, or light?
3. What are your frequent activities? Occupation?
4. What are your sleep habits. (every night, most nights, difficulty)? What is your sleep position? Is your mattress comfortable?
5. What is your diet like?
6. Do you use orthotics such as heel lifts, sole lifts, arch supports, inner soles?
7. How many glasses of water do you drink daily?

If stress reduction is your focus, you may need to add questions related to the amount of overall stress that the client is experiencing and how long she has been under prolonged stress. Chronic stress can result in the development of various autoimmune conditions as the person becomes exhausted. Use information about stress to anticipate body findings as well as to stimulate discussion and solicit the client's partnership in committing to lifestyle improvements.

Sample Questions Related to Stress

1. In which part(s) of your body do you feel stress most often (check all that apply: head, neck, shoulder, back, digestive, extremities, other)?
2. Is a portion of each day set aside for relaxation? What kind?
3. Have you ever had a massage? What is your previous experience with professional massage?
4. Do you have a music or aroma preference?
5. For stress reduction I use prayer, meditation, guided imagery, exercise, energetic therapies, or _____.

A **symptom** may be anything the client notices as unusual and uncomfortable. If symptom reduction is your massage focus, you will need questions to collect information that describes symptoms completely. You can fill in any missing information through the interview process.

Sample Questions for Symptom Analysis

1. List and describe the symptom (include description of the character or quality). What is the pain like?
2. How severe or uncomfortable is the symptom for you?
3. What is the location of the symptom? How much of the body is affected?
4. What is the onset? When did your problem begin? When did you first notice the symptom? What brought it on? What makes it worse? How long does it last? Is the symptom getting progressively worse? Is it constant or intermittent (comes and goes)? Is there a pattern?
5. Describe one episode—number of times per hour, day, week, month.
6. What activities help or make the symptom worse? What activities are altered or have to be avoided or decreased (shopping, housekeeping, self-care, child care, work, sleep)?

When a symptom affects a person's ability to maintain the usual daily activities, massage therapy can be added to the care the healthcare provider has recommended. You may need thorough investigation and frequent follow-up to document that massage has made measurable change toward restoring the client's level of functioning. You may also wish to have the client complete **self-report forms** to evaluate his progress periodically (Fig. 20–4). The self-report form describes the client's perception of his symptoms; he answers questions or indicates on a body map the area of discomfort. This form contains simple pictures of a body (front and back) for the client to mark or circle areas in which there is discomfort. Use self-reports periodically to note progress and symptom resolution at the beginning of any session.

Questions Related to Mobility and Ability to Perform Various Activities

1. What have you done to get relief? What home remedies have you used to get relief?
2. What body positions are most comfortable? Do you use over-the-counter medications? Which ones? In general, what makes your pain better?
3. Have you been or are you under a physician's care for this symptom? Has there been a diagnosis? Do you have a physician's prescription for therapy?
4. What does this problem mean to you? This last question allows the client to relate the feelings and emotions surrounding the problem; these feelings are important to the person as a whole but are often neglected by focusing on the part of the person that is seen as the problem.

Since the client does not always know what information is important to the therapist, your information

SELF-REPORT FORM

Optional Self Report Form

Athlete's Name (Print) ______________________ Event: ______________________

I understand that sports massage is designed to be a complementary health aid. I agree to immediately inform my therapist of any discomfort or unusual sensation so pressure or strokes may be adjusted to my level of discomfort. I have read this form and freely give my permission to be massaged.

______________________ ______________________ __________

Signature of Therapist | Signature of Athlete | Date

*Circle the area of most concern:

Label #1

*Circle the area you would also like to include, time permitting:

Label #2

Brief Medical History:

List Injuries or Surgeries with Dates:

____

____

____

ATHLETE'S EVALUATION OF THE MASSAGE

Duration of the massage (circle one) 8-10 min., 15-20 min., 30+ min.

Do you feel the massage you received was a positive experience? ______________________

The massage helped (mark one or more): Relieve Cramping _____ Relax _____

Revitalize _____ Decrease soreness _____ Other ______________________

Have you ever had a massage (pre) (post) event before? yes _____ no _____

Was the sign in, waiting, or therapist connection helpful and realistic?

Comments: ______________________

Additional comments or areas of evaluation not measured by this form. ______________________

____

____

My Therapist was: ______________________

Figure 20•4 A sample self-report form. (Permission is hereby granted to reproduce this form in its entirety, including the copyright notice, for commercial or instructional use but not for resale.)

may often be incomplete. You may want to list several symptoms and conditions that can assist the person to remember and report. Important symptoms such as headaches, fatigue/depression, pins and needles in the extremities, painful joints, loss of balance, stiffness, loss of strength, edema, constipation, diarrhea, and heartburn are helpful to know.

Massage therapists need to be sure that massage will be appropriate and beneficial (or indicated) for the person, considering her overall health status. You must therefore assess if the client has any contraindications for massage (a contraindication is any condition for which massage would not be appropriate or beneficial). Serious contraindications include susceptibility to easy bruising or hemorrhage, forming clots, or having conditions in which a clot could be easily dislodged. If, because of medication use, the client cannot judge the therapist's pressure, massage is not appropriate. Having a condition in which there is decreased sensation to the therapist's touch can constitute a contraindication to massage of areas such as the feet or legs. Usually the therapist asks the client to list previous injuries, surgeries, illnesses, medical conditions, and medications to help determine other contraindications for massage. You may use a specific list for the client to check.

The practitioner can ask the person to explain in detail about any unfamiliar conditions or medications. Acquiring and referring to a pathology text with massage applications can be useful. The therapist may wish to secure a release from the primary healthcare provider if the client is currently receiving medications and periodic checkups. If you are using aromatherapy or other skin products, ask the client about any allergies.

Sample Questions to Discover Possible Contraindications

1. Are you currently under the care of a health professional? If so, for what condition(s)?
2. What is your provider's name/phone? Do I have permission to contact your provider?
3. List any other types of therapy or medical care you are receiving (a list such as the following for quick scanning will be helpful).
   - pregnancy
   - contact lenses
   - diabetes
   - arthritis
   - ruptured/bulging disk
   - previous MVA/trauma
   - autoimmune disorder
   - varicose veins
   - seizures
   - TMJ disorder
   - heart condition
   - cancer
   - stroke
   - kidney disorder
   - elevated cholesterol
   - high blood pressure
   - phlebitis
   - infectious conditions
   - skin disorder
   - scoliosis
   - other ____

Another option is to request the client to list conditions and surgeries with approximate dates.

1. List your previous injuries, including broken bones, *not* requiring surgery. Include dates.
2. List your previous surgeries with dates. Did you have any residual effects?
3. List any previous illnesses and medical conditions with dates. Are you having residual effects?
4. List current medications such as Aspirin/Anti-inflammatories—Sleeping Pills—Painkillers—Anti-anxiety/Stress-Reducing Medications—Muscle Relaxants—Blood Thinners.
5. Allergies to medications, nuts, oils, or scents.
6. Other information: mental or emotional status, psychological, social, or spiritual health may be pertinent to your therapy but is hard to assess by questionnaire because of the emotional component that may be involved. Since certain areas are sensitive, they may best be used by the advanced practitioner.

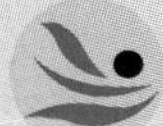

MINI•LAB

Using the preceding questions and suggestions, design a one-page form that you could use in your type of massage practice. To help customize your session, begin by selecting a particular type of therapy, such as stress reduction, and select questions from each category that would yield helpful information. Select font style and size. Decide how the client will complete the form (fill in the blank, check boxes, circling, etc.). Create a layout for your intake form. Practice using your form for the next several clients you massage, and ask them for feedback regarding the ease and readability of the form.

Interview

After the client has completed the initial intake forms, review the information on it. Usually the client's chief motivation for the visit will be his most pressing concern. Often verbal communication is reflected in the client's gesturing. When people describe pain, they

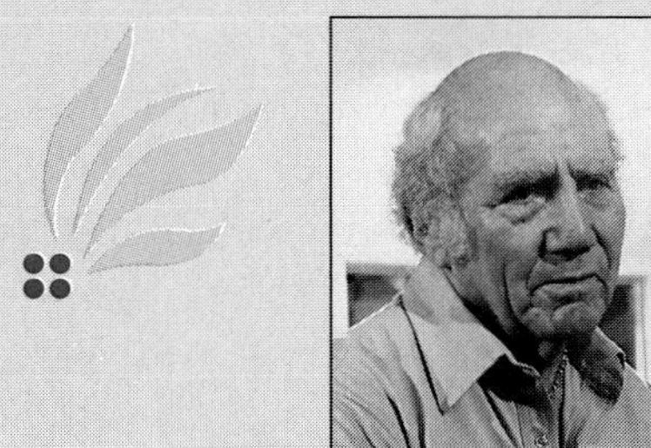

(Photo courtesy of the Trager Institute, Mill Valley, CA.)

Milton Trager

April 20, 1908 to January 20, 1997

"Not until we experience it is it more that just words. After we experience it, there is no need for words."

It is the roaring '20s in sunny Miami. But for a high school dropout who lied about his age to get the $.65-an-hour post office job, it's all work. He barely has time to breathe—until today. Today the posted health tip instructs him to do so and to sign his name indicating that he has done so.

Milton Trager slowly inhaled, then exhaled. He had no idea that he possessed a talent that would develop—without outside influence—into a revolutionary method of bodywork. That one deep breath put Trager in touch with his body for the very first time. "It was the beginning of me," he recalls. Soon he started working out at the beach, doing acrobatics, developing his muscles, and listening to the waves as he swayed to their ebb and flow. Fascinated by the movements of boxers in the ring, he took up the sport. One day he offered to "turn the table" and massage his trainer. His trainer was stunned at his ability. From there he went home to massage his father, who had severe sciatic pain. Four treatments and the pain was gone, never to return.

At 19, Trager helped a child walk who hadn't walked in 4 years. The proverbial 90-pound weakling had grown into a strong, agile young man whose acrobatic antics along his mail route captured the attention of the Hollywood studios. However, his unique mode of hands-on therapy went virtually unnoticed.

He enlisted with the navy medical corps. After his release, he decided it was time to get the credentials that would make doctors take notice of his work. But the only medical school that would accept a 42-year-old was in Guadalajara. So he headed south with his wife and embarked on the arduous task of earning a medical degree in a completely Spanish-speaking environment.

Establishing a medical practice was difficult for someone with his background, but the Tragers finally settled in Honolulu. Sadly, the medical community remained deaf and blind to his work, but Trager didn't need their blessing to know what he was doing was right. His method of holding, listening to, rocking, and freeing the body continued to evolve.

By chance, a well-known psychologist experienced Trager's methods and convinced him to demonstrate at Esalen, a workshop and meeting place for developing human potential. Jack Liskin, Trager's biographer, writes: "And so it was that an aging and unusual doctor with an unusual talent, unattached to any movement, New Age or conventional, came face-to-face with the California counterculture." (From Liskin J: Moving Medicine: The Life and Work of Milton Trager, M.D. Barrytown, NY, Station Hill Press, 1996.)

The Trager Approach uses nonintrusive movements to lull the body into a better, more mobile, lighter state of being by releasing deep-seated physical and mental patterns.

Essential to Trager work is a state that's been termed "hook-up," which means that the practitioner becomes so totally focused that she achieves a hypersensitivity to body cues. It's as though the practitioner's mind/body communicates, without using words. And what is being said to the receiver is, though you may have hidden them from your consciousness, you hold the keys to unlock patterns that are holding you physically and mentally hostage. I'm just here to give your body the cues to gently remind you of your own potential—nothing more.

A Trager session doesn't end with tablework. Mentastics reinforces the results. Mentastics is Trager's term for "mental gymnastics," the gentle, mindful movement exercises that help the body recall positive physical or mental changes that occurred on the table and reinforce these changes.

Continued

Though Trager never cared for explaining his work, those who experienced, practiced, and witnessed its results have filled in the gaps.

"The practitioner uses the vast sensory capacities of the skin and deeper tissue to transmit messages. Using wavelike, moving rhythms that are at the core of all forms and matter of life, it communicates its messages thousands of times during a session to break habitual patterns," writes Liskin in *Moving Medicine, The Life and Work of Milton Trager, M.D.*

Trager never cared to be referred to as a genius, guru, or healer, claiming instead to have a talent. But his talent touched lives and changed minds about what was possible.

For instance, Betty Fuller, a frequent seminar leader at Esalen, was prepared to live the rest of her days in chronic pain. When Trager reached out to examine her, she practically shrieked: "No one touches my neck." But he persisted in his gentle but unyielding manner. Soon she was pain-free and became Trager's first instructor. In Trager she saw the same deep reverence for the mind's ability to heal the body that she'd experienced as a student of Moshe Feldenkrais. It was to Fuller that Trager turned to protect his name and his work, and in April of 1980 the Trager Institute was founded (From Massage Magazine, Issue 67, May/June 1997.) Today practitioners all around the world are using the Trager Approach and Mentastics Movement Education to ease headaches, back pain, and the debilitating effects of Parkinson's, cerebral palsy, polio, and multiple sclerosis.

tend to touch and rub it, unaware that they are doing so. Watch your client as he describes pain to determine the exact location. Be sure to verify your perception by asking him if it is the right shoulder that hurts, for example, if that is where he touched. Since your form systematically collects information concerning symptoms, read each question and response; explore and reflect when additional input is needed. Determine if there are any contraindications for local or general massage or if a referral to his health practitioner for clearance is needed. He may also be referred to another massage therapist with skills suitable for a particular type of therapy that you do not practice, such as energy therapy, manual lymphatic drainage, or reflexology.

The *right of refusal* by the therapist is based upon the information gleaned through the health history and interview process, during which the therapist may discover a particular condition for which massage is contraindicated. These conditions are stated as contraindications based on the alteration in biophysical status caused by a disease process. Since contraindications are varied and many, the practitioner, when in doubt, may consult a text of massage pathophysiology, an experienced mentor, peer, or other healthcare practitioner. When such a contraindication is suspected, the therapist has a right, responsibility, and even an obligation to refuse to treat the client or the local area involved until the client obtains a written or verbal okay to proceed from a qualified health practitioner. At that point the therapist has the additional responsibility of adjusting the technique or of referring the client for a technique that is appropriate and safe for the client. This is also an excellent time to document. If no contraindications exist, proceed to the informed consent.

Determine the client's goals and expectations for the massage session in light of her subjective reporting. What is the desired outcome? What must happen for her to be satisfied? Are her expectations reasonable? You may have to educate and negotiate with some conditions. Advise her of the modalities of massage that you practice that you think would obtain the outcomes she desires. Discuss the benefits and possible risks of the procedure you are advising.

For example, if the client has moderate discomfort in the right shoulder, would she like a targeted massage that would focus on the back, shoulder, arms, and neck? Inform her that this approach could take up to an hour on the upper body alone, could result in some discomfort, could give only minimal relaxation, and could carry the potential for bruising (because the client has been on anti-inflammatories). Another result could possibly be some exercise-like soreness following the massage. The potential benefits would be decreased pain and discomfort and increased range of motion. The client might opt for less pain reduction work and prefer a full-body Swedish massage, with extra attention to the shoulder area. Perhaps she has had a very stressful week that has contributed to her sense of pain in the shoulder. The client may not want to give up the full-body relaxation for targeted work that you think would benefit her in fewer sessions.

Your goal is to adopt the client's choice of therapy based on her priorities in this mutually cooperative way. The client is responsible to make a decision based on the education and information you provide regarding your services. In fact, remember, it is her legal right to do so. "The client also has the right to refuse, modify, or terminate a procedure at any time. When this occurs the therapist will comply, regardless of prior consent." (NCTMB ethics statement) Review your policies and procedures, and answer any questions the client may have. The consent is then signed.

Informed Consent and Plan of Care

An informed consent contains the information from which the client can make an educated/knowledgeable decision for her own protection. Most consent forms stress the voluntary nature of the process and state the client's right to alter or terminate the therapy (Fig. 20–5).

An informed consent also advises the client of potential benefits and possible undesirable effects of the particular massage modality that you will use. According to the definition of informed consent, unless both benefits and risks are listed, the consent is not a valid, legally sound document. Additionally, through the consent process, the client receives information on how massage and bodywork can influence her symptoms.

Many client information forms have a place for the client's signature, which verifies voluntary consent for massage therapy. Often policy and procedural issues are also included. Although this approach may save time, it can result in both policy and procedure information being abbreviated and incomplete. Collection of the signature testifies that the client has read and agreed to the terms included. If the client signs without reading, it is the therapist's responsibility to read or review the contents with the client.

It is our professional/ethical responsibility to collaborate with the client in designing the plan of care to suit her needs and desires. If we feel we know a particular technique that would benefit her, we are bound to tell the client about potential benefits and undesirable side effects or discomfort that may result. This information is called possible treatment reactions or responses. You are obliged to honor the client's wishes regardless of your disagreement with her choices. Failure to honor these boundaries may form the basis for civil, criminal, or professional disciplinary proceedings. Danger of infringements may be encountered when the client and therapist do not agree on the focus of the session.

Assure the client that you do not diagnose medical conditions and that your services are not a substitute for medical treatment. As a therapist, using your training and expertise you actually advise and cooperate in the formation of a plan of care with the client. Be careful to keep the client's specific desired results and goals clearly in mind. It is often difficult for the practitioner to know, given the variable of client response, how often and how many massages may be needed to achieve the client's desired results/goals. In general, the initial period consists of frequent sessions, tapering off as symptoms subside. For example, an eight-session treatment plan could begin with every other day (three) the first week, two the next week, then one a week for 3 weeks. Periodic evaluation as a basis for renewing the therapeutic contract is standard in the health profession. With experience, you will be able to make more accurate recommendations regarding treatment plans or protocols. A **treatment protocol** describes the steps used to form the therapy plan.

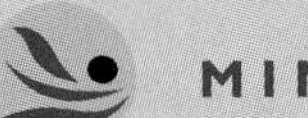

MINI•LAB

Find an article from a professional massage journal related to a particular symptom that a client has experienced. Record the protocol suggested. If you find more than one, contrast and compare the options. If you cannot find an article, read about a pathology or symptom that your client has experienced, and devise a treatment protocol based on your knowledge of the benefits of massage and bodywork. Review this plan with an instructor or experienced massage therapist.

CONSENT FOR THERAPY

- The unclothed body will be properly draped at all times for your warmth, sense of security, and as a mark of massage professionalism.
- Focused attention and manual therapy will be given as agreed upon by therapist and client for the predetermined goals of stress reduction, relief of muscular discomfort, and or health promotion. My therapist has discussed the potential benefits and possible side effects of this therapy. I have been given an opportunity to ask questions.
- I as client agree to provide complete and accurate health information and notice of health changes at successive appointments as appropriate.
- I understand that massage therapy is designed to be an ancillary health aid and is not suitable for primary medical treatment.
- Written referral is requested from your primary care provider if
  1) you are currently receiving care or
  2) you have a specific medical condition or symptoms for which you take medication or receive periodic evaluation or treatment.
- I will immediately inform my therapist of any unusual sensation or discomfort, so that the application of pressure or strokes may be adjusted to my level of comfort.
- I understand that this professional massage is therapeutic in nature and is performed by a trained, state-licensed therapist. During the initial interview, the therapist has informed me of her credentials.
- I understand that the massage is not sexually oriented in any way and that any illicit or suggestive remarks or behavior on my part will result in immediate termination of the session.
- I understand that by signing this form, I give my consent to receive the treatment discussed in this and all future sessions and agree that my presence at subsequent sessions shall be construed to be validation of this written consent.
- I have read this form and hereby freely give my permission to be massaged.

Date:____________ Name:____

Cancellation notice as far in advance as possible is appreciated.

You may also choose to add your own individual items to suit your needs, such as:

- I verify that I am not involved in any active or pending legal process related to my physical symptoms.

Figure 20•5 A sample consent for therapy form. (Permission is hereby granted to reproduce this form in its entirety, including the copyright notice, for commercial or instructional use but not for resale.)

A Sample Therapy Protocol for Tension Headache

1. If the client is under a healthcare provider's care, consult the client's provider to request clearance for therapy. You may need to explain proposed therapy, rationale, and the results desired. The client may need to sign a release for records, indicating his permission for the therapist to discuss his health history with the healthcare provider. The client may also contact his own provider to secure the release for therapy. Written or verbal receipt is documented, along with the name, date, and time you receive the information.
2. Goals: Ideally you hope to see a decrease in the frequency and severity of the client's symptoms. You also hope to see education in self-care such as ice packs, stretching, and posture to prevent recurrence, so that the client takes responsibility for maintenance of therapeutic progress.
3. Assessment for tension headache may include general stress level, posture, cervical range of motion (ROM), palpation of potential contributing muscles, severity on a ten-point scale, and statement of frequency.
4. Plan of Care: two hours a week for 2 weeks, tapering to once a week for the first month. The plan evaluation is to demonstrate 25 to 50 percent progress to your goal. Make adjustments in the plan as needed. Evaluate possible sources of reinjury or barriers to progress.
5. Technique: Initially 20 minutes of craniosacral release or mobilization, followed by cervical ROM to establish baseline; Swedish massage to warm the tissues for 10 minutes; neuromuscular massage of targeted muscles for 15 minutes; 10 minutes of calming techniques such as proprioceptive neuromuscular facilitation, vibration, or Swedish massage to finish; and evaluation of the therapy session using cervical ROM.

Your standard informed consent form will be for your most frequently used modality such as Swedish massage, with benefits, possible undesirable effects, and recommended duration and interval to realize maximum benefit. Some therapists give the client an information sheet on care after massage to avoid undesirable effects such as soreness. A suggested list can be found in the chapter, Putting It All Together.

If there is another modality that would be beneficial for a specific client concern, you may want to have information sheets for each massage type to attach to your basic consent. Your treatment protocol takes the following form: healthcare provider clearance; desired outcome/goals; treatment modalities; duration of sessions; frequency of sessions; number of sessions; evaluation; and maintenance. The educational process and final decision regarding protocol are made at the time of the interview when mutual goals are established or following the initial therapy session and evaluation of client response to therapy. Obviously more than 5 minutes would be required to establish a treatment- or goal-oriented series of massages.

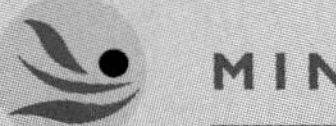

MINI•LAB

Role-play an initial consultation using the intake form or health history, consent, and policy and procedures form with another student. Note how long it takes. The student may select a personal or assumed chief concern. The student acting as therapist responds to the process using the skills discussed. Exchange roles. When both have had an opportunity to be therapist and client, have them exchange and evaluate the records with each other, using the following evaluation criteria.

Evaluation Criteria

1. Does the client feel as if an accurate picture of her status is reflected in the data collected?
2. Did the therapist clarify vague reports of symptoms with terms denoting quality or quantity?
3. Did questions or concerns arise that were not addressed by the form or the interview process?
4. Did the chosen therapy reflect consideration of the client's preference and expectations?
5. Were both the benefits and risks clearly explained?
6. Were the policies and procedures briefly but clearly explained? If written and reviewed with a signature, did the therapist verify that they were understood?
7. What was the client's response to the process? How long did the process take?

THE TREATMENT RECORD

The primary purpose of the **treatment record** is to provide a journal of treatment sessions that contains the client's information and responses to therapy in SOAP format for each session. It may also include diagrams of the body for visual summary of findings, as well as written notes (Fig. 20–6). In light of planned goals, the client's response to therapy and progress are available for quick review and evaluation. You may make adjustments during the review and during the update at the beginning of each session. Written documentation always supports the professional therapist should records be requested for legal or medical reasons. If a referring physician requests information, the written record becomes ready reference for completing progress reports. The treatment record contains the client's name, date of birth, social security

TREATMENT RECORD FOR MASSAGE THERAPY

Name:____________________ DOB________ SS#__________ PH __________

Healthcare Provider__________________ DX/Codes________________________

Notes: ____

Date Seen: - - Time: AM PM Length

Therapist:________________________

S

O

A

P

Date Seen: - - Time: AM PM Length

Therapist: ________________________

S

O

A

P

Date Seen: - - Time: AM PM Length

Therapist: ________________________

S

O

A

P

Date Seen: - - Time: AM PM Length

Therapist:________________________

S

O

A

P

S=Update & Description of Symptoms & Goals

O=Visual & Palpable Observations Findings & Tests

A=Massage Application: Modalities & Response

P=Plan & Comments, Education & Activities

Mark the areas where you are feeling discomfort on the figures below.

R L

L

R

L R

Figure 20•6 A sample treatment form. (Permission is hereby granted to reproduce this form in its entirety, including the copyright notice, for commercial or instructional use but not for resale.)

number, diagnosis, and referring healthcare provider (if applicable), and the name of your clinic in the heading. Many therapists find schematic views of the body helpful on one side of the page. Several sessions are noted on one page; include the date of the session, time of day, length of session, and name of the therapist. As a prompt, the letters SOAP are arranged vertically on the left, opposite which information applicable to each category in this sequence is written. The format is not important, but you should have a system for recording your information.

SOAP information is stated concisely and may be abbreviated. Many medical dictionaries abound for discovering standard accepted abbreviations. A list of the most frequently used abbreviations are located in the Appendix. If you originate your own list, be sure to provide a legend when your records leave your office for any reason. If at all possible, collect several sessions on one page to save space and paper.

Author's Note

All client records must be kept indefinitely.

Documenting Subjective Information on the Treatment Record

Through the initial interview and review of the client's health history, the therapist and client agree on the goal for the session, which will be listed besides the "S" on the client's treatment record. A session's goals needs to be realistic within the confines of the time allowed for the session. Short- and long-term goals can be determined following the first session, after the therapist's palpatory assessment and evaluation of the client's response to therapy. Both the client's self-report and the therapist's palpatory findings compose the initial evaluation from which the therapeutic plan and goals are formulated.

The documentation of information can vary from general and nonspecific to detailed and precise. Obviously the more qualitative and quantitative information recorded, the better the written data serve the therapist's recall of what occurred with the client.

For future sessions you will want to update the record by collecting the client's subjective assessment of his current status and of how much progress was made toward his goal. Documentation may also include how long relief was experienced, which areas are feeling better, which still need attention, and if the client experienced any adverse effects such as soreness or bruising. You will want to note what the character of discomfort is today.

If the client has had a personal crisis or is experiencing a headache, his current needs may supersede his previous therapy plan, and you may agree upon a different therapeutic approach for that session.

For example, an "S" note that reads "painful right shoulder" tells you the symptom "pain" and the location "right shoulder." What you do not yet know is how severe the pain was for the client before therapy, if the pain involved moving the right arm, how long the client was in pain, what the cause of the pain might have been, and what pattern of pain was experienced (constant or intermittent). An inexperienced therapist may not collect enough information to paint a detailed picture. Post-therapy assessment (before the client leaves) can demonstrate the effects of therapy to the client and can measure the client's initial response to that therapy. When the client returns for the next session and states he still has pain in the right shoulder, if the original recording was too general, you will not be able to suggest or document the impact of the initial therapy. Without an accurate descriptive baseline, documentation that shows change will be impossible.

Contrast the above with an "S" note that reads severe pain, constant for 2 weeks in the right shoulder, horizontal abduction of right arm causes increase in pain. A postsession note that pain was reduced to moderate and that horizontal abduction was accomplished without increase in pain is specific, useful information. Prior to the next session, the client reports his right shoulder is still painful, but upon palpation the client reports the pain is only moderate. Many times a client who is feeling better does not remember how much discomfort he was feeling and may attribute improvement to other supportive measures he is using. At worst, he may not be able to note that any improvement has been made. Refer to the collection of information related to a symptom in the initial intake form.

Objective Assessment

The therapist gathers objective information **empirically** (measurable and verifiable by use of the senses) through visual and palpatory assessment of the client. During the interview and health history, you may uncover reports of pain or discomfort that the client identifies as priorities for the session. The client's report may prompt the therapist to suggest an evaluation of gait or posture before the massage, to enhance the therapeutic goals of the client, who may wish to focus only extra attention to these painful areas during a general session. At your option, you may assess painful areas before the actual massage to provide a logical basis for therapy and to create short- and long-term goals.

A competent massage therapist keeps in mind that, although she may recognize signs and symptoms of a particular condition such as bursitis, stating that the client does in fact have bursitis constitutes malpractice. Since bursitis is the name of a medical condition/ disease process, only a certified healthcare provider can diagnose it. What is permissible for the massage therapist is to note the specific signs and symptoms that she observes and to assess without labeling a condition. You might view the problem as suspicious or abnormal, and you would encourage the client to seek further assistance from a qualified healthcare provider. For example, the client may be referred to a physician who will use her knowledge and skill to evaluate the history of the disease process, to assess the signs and symptoms, to collect laboratory data, and to order special tests before she determines that it is in fact bursitis. When the client refers to a condition using a medical diagnosis given to her by her healthcare provider, the therapist may also refer to the condition in those terms.

To understand the difference between objective and subjective findings, let's look at the following example. If a client comes into a massage therapist's studio and enters his height and weight on the intake form, this is subjective information. If the therapist uses a tape measure and a scale to determine the client's height and weight, it is objective information. Since most objective measurements require precision, record the information at the time of collection.

Visual Assessment

Visual assessment begins when you greet the client. You will be able to observe the client's prevailing mood, obvious deviations in posture, muscle guarding, ease, depth, and rate of breathing, and of course, gait. These assessments may alert you to various areas that need special attention during the massage. By noting the prevailing mood, you have an opportunity to check for accuracy of perceived feelings through asking for verification of your perceptions. Visual observation may also alert you to educational or lifestyle enhancements that may be beneficial to the client. During the massage, you may observe the condition of the skin, hair, and nails, or you may note a suspicious mole on the client's back that needs the attention of a healthcare provider. Although massage therapist do not diagnose, their education in physiology and pathophysiology assists them in recognizing a potential deviation that should receive proper care.

Author's Note

I usually acknowledge bruises (which I avoid) during the massage to the client. The client may not notice a bruise's presence until after receiving massage, at which time you may receive the credit!

Palpatory Assessment

Palpatory assessment is assessment through touching with purpose and intent. Palpatory assessment is an essential skill. Assessing the tissues includes locating the muscles from origin to insertion and feeling the difference between different types of tissues (muscles, tendons, ligaments). The general condition of the same types of tissues can be determined through palpation. For example, are the muscles flexible, tight, or lacking in tone? What is the difference between well-exercised healthy muscle tissue and hypertonic tissue? Alterations in the consistency or texture of the same tissue, such as an area of restriction or contraction, can also be determined through touching. Your fingers are your eyes. Are the tissues above the muscles, such as the adipose and skin layers, free and pliable, or are they solid, boggy, dense, and stuck to the muscles?

Temperature is also significant. Decreased circulation or interference with neurological health are two frequent causes of cool fingers and toes. Exercise frequency and metabolism may also play a role in alterations in temperature. Temperature is commonly increased with fever/infection, inflammation, and irritation. Alterations in body temperature may warn the therapist of possible restrictions within the tissues, of contraindications for certain styles of massage, and of the need for the avoidance of local massage. The therapist uses whatever words best describe what he is feeling to record palpatory findings. Consult a medical dictionary to aid in describing what is palpated.

What is the client's response to areas of altered tonus or to other unusual tissue findings? Usually the client responds to pressure differently in an area of altered tonus or spasm. Take note of various tissue responses that the client reports, such as burning, stabbing, or sensations that refer to other parts of the body. The therapist may investigate or assess what the extent and character of the alteration are in order to see if they can be "normalized" within the comfort level desired by the client. Often the client assumes that it has to hurt to be released. He may need to be

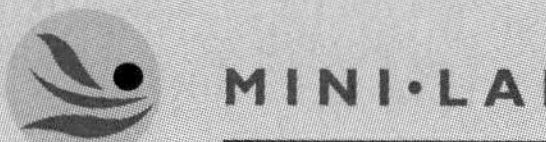

Using a medical dictionary (Dorland's, Miller-Keane) or a reference book such as Travell and Simons' *Myofascial Pain and Dysfunction,* find and define words that could be used to describe a knot or ropiness, tonus or tension, thickening or swelling, tenderness or discomfort, and numbness. Use these appropriately in the objective portion of your treatment record.

educated that if the muscle is under stress and hurting it may not release if painful pressure is used. This explanation can help you in getting good client feedback to control the maximum pressure level response to a "good hurt" or mild discomfort. *Always adjust assessment pressure to the client's desired level.*

Objective Tests and Measures

Through use of assessment tests and measures, we can evaluate the tissues involved in movement and their impact on the body structure. Basic assessment tests and measures include postural analysis, range of motion, and gait. While strength and other tests of muscle, tendon, and ligament integrity are within our scope of practice, usually these skills are learned through advanced training in areas such as sports massage, neuromuscular massage, and myofascial release.

Often we record these findings on a specialized report form, such as a postural analysis sheet or body map of some kind. The client's treatment record may also be used if it contains anatomical figures. We may ask the client's permission to record observations via voice-activated recorder and later transcribe them to text to be included with the record. Some therapists find Polaroid photographs of the client helpful in assessing posture.

Range of Motion

The **range of motion (ROM)** is a measure of possible joint movement from the least to the greatest by a particular joint. Range of motion is a powerful tool when used to assist you in determining which muscles, tendons and ligaments to target during the massage. You can also use ROM to provide instant feedback to the client and to help you monitor changes in status due to massage. Range of motion also provides a baseline for measuring restoration of function for insurance and other payers. Education of the client into the value of ROM assessment may result in her opting to include it as a helpful service.

You will find ROM to be very useful within the session to assess a single joint that may be problematic for the client. For example, if the client complains of neck pain, you may simply ask him to demonstrate the movement in which pain is experienced and to stop when he feels tension. Observe as the client demonstrates this single range of motion. You can then work on the muscles involved, moving the neck in that particular range (i.e., the scalenes and semispinalis capitis for lateral flexion). Then ask the client to repeat the movement. You thereby can show him how massage therapy directly and immediately improved his problem. Of course, supportive measures such as posture and factors responsible for the spasm need to be considered as well.

Active ROM measures the client's movement using his voluntary muscles. Passive ROM measures movement while the client assists by relaxing or disengaging voluntary muscle control. The therapist moves the joint slowly and gently until slight resistance is felt or until the full range is accomplished.

To assess the range of motion of a joint, first consider how to get the most objective results. A fearful client will not move a tender point easily. To provide an atmosphere of safety and trust, you must establish a protocol for assessing the ROM of any joint. In general, active movement is preferred to passive for assessment, especially for muscles, tendons, and tendon sheaths. Passive ROM and stretching are preferred during the massage session and for testing ligaments, joint capsules, and some tendon injuries. Therapist discretion and appropriateness are the overriding criteria for choosing to use active ROM or passive ROM.

1. **Explain Why.** Explain to the client that examining the movement of a particular joint will give you information about hypertonic and spastic muscles and about tendon or ligament involvement.
2. **Therapist Demonstration.** Demonstrate the exact movement desired and how to isolate the precise movement. Assist the client in performing the movement correctly; he will have less apprehension knowing exactly what is expected.
3. **Move the Unaffected Side First.** First, ask him to repeat the demonstration on the uninjured or less injured side of a bilateral joint. This will give you a baseline for his "normal" range.
4. **Move the Affected Joint.** Ask him to move the affected joint. Stress that you do not want him to move the joint if there is discomfort. Educate him so that you gather sufficient information to guide therapy by moving the joint into tension, but with no pain. If he encounters any pain, note this in your record.

A chart of joint movements and their range of motion in degrees can be found in the skeletal system chapter. Many texts of kinesiology and muscle testing have baseline degrees of joint mobility, and some books state which muscles are involved in each range of motion. There will be slight variations from author to author. Being too exact is not the focus that will help guide therapy for the beginning practitioner; rather, being consistent in the guidelines you choose is crucial. Unless the student is trained in the use of a **goniometer** in which actual degrees are measured, it is recommended that the beginning practitioner note only variations from normal, both in increased mobility and in decreased mobility; you can use a bilateral joint to establish a normal baseline. You may note ROM using symbols: plus (+) and minus (−), arrows up for increased (↑), arrows down for decreased (↓), and checkmarks (✔) for normal. Some therapists expand the scale by adding minuses to indicate moderate or severe decrease in a joint's range of motion. The therapist may use letters or abbreviations to indicate mild, moderate, or severe increase or decrease in a normal range, with normal denoted as WNL (within normal limits; a standard medical abbreviation). Again, attach a legend when originating a system of notation.

The most common error massage therapists make in charting is to state that "massage increased range of motion." There is no note of what joint has improved or of what particular movement was enhanced. Often there is no assessment and only a general feeling that the client is more flexible because the muscles are relaxed and therefore must have greater range of motion. The objective soft-tissue findings should be congruent with what actually happens in the body. ROM is an objective test. ***Unless it is measured, it cannot be stated.***

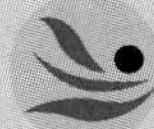

MINI•LAB

Using the joint movement reference chart in the skeletal system chapter, assess a joint in all its ranges using the preceding protocol. Note the findings using a three-point scale for hypo-, hyper-, and normal mobility. Remember to move the joint to tension with no discomfort. If discomfort is present, indicate this with your documentation. Example: Active—Cervical—Left Lateral Flexion—WNL—with slight discomfort. If you are going to assess many motions in a particular joint, use a chart format with the joint assessed, and whether movement was active or passive; list motions individually, and give headings for left and right when applicable. Also you can add a column for comments, noting discomfort or weakness.

Posture Assessment

Posture is the position of the body in space, such as sitting, standing, lying supine, and lying prone. We usually consider standing as the baseline measure of balance and alignment because this posture is maintained through the strength and tone of the muscles against gravity. Movement of the body off the physiological planes or misalignment of the structure is frequently found to be a source for continued or chronic pain. The body is designed so that muscles and other contractile tissues effectively maintain its alignment to oppose gravity. Alteration in posture, such as a spasm, produces alteration in body function and movement; the body cannot efficiently dissipate momentum. Modalities that work to restore postural support and alignment from the uneven pull of various muscle groups, tendons, ligaments, fascial distortions, and skin involvement may be needed to address underlying problems.

Train your eyes to evaluate the physiological structure by taking baseline measures in several planes of the body to find deviations. A plumbline and other aids may be used, but a good baseline measurement may be made without these items if you use your observational skill (Fig. 20–7). Observe major postural signs of imbalance, such as a pelvic bowl, which "spills" the abdominal contents, knees locked back or overly bent, shoulders rolled forward and in, forward head posture (Fig. 20–8), faulty base of support from collapsed arches or feet rotating out or in, high or low ear position on one side, and uneven facial features. Many things that are long-standing with a person are often taken as "normal" or uncorrectable deviations; the client's discomfort serves as a "mystery." Chronic pain or traumatic injury may also result in difficult symptom patterns, which are maintained by postural imbalance; if not detected, the imbalance may block therapy goals.

After observing the obvious distortions in body planes (see Fig. 4–8), chart these deviations on the

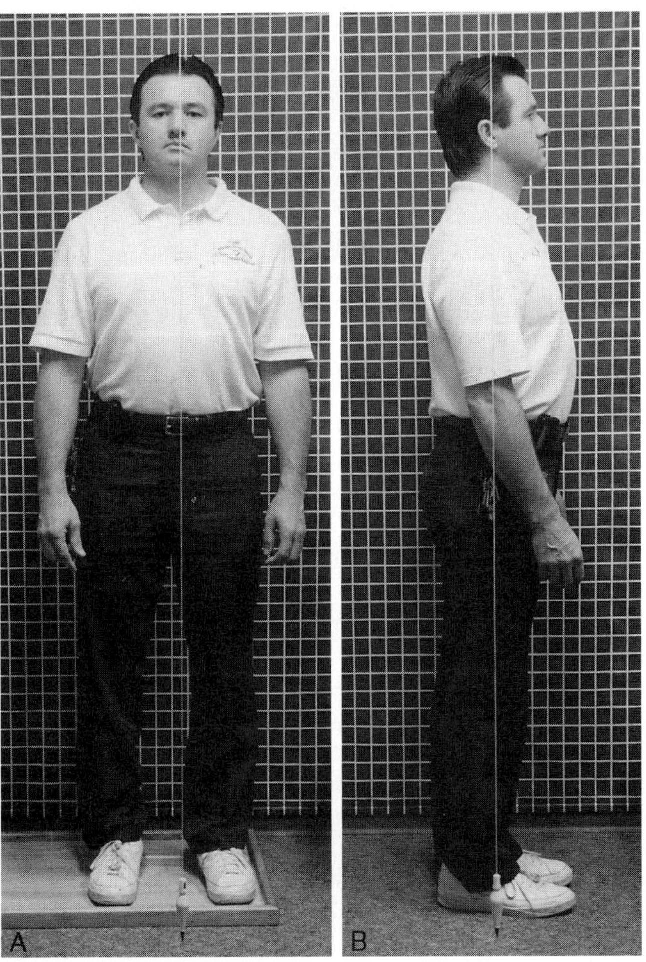

Figure 20•7 Postural analysis.

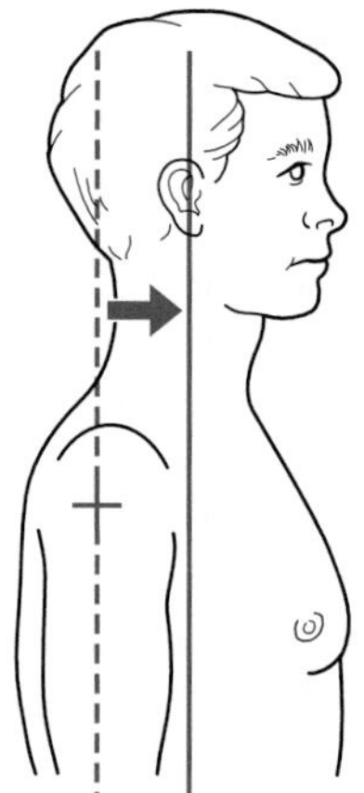

Figure 20•8 Forward head posture.

paper figure. During the massage, note where you found muscle tension to be greatest. With practice, you will become more skillful in focusing your efforts on problem areas and gain additional therapy techniques through continuing education, which uses postural analysis as a guide to focus massage. Educating your clients in realigning posture will greatly enhance soft-tissue resolution and will prevent reinjury.

Another avenue to explore is the science of ergonomics. Ergonomics is the scientific study of individual anatomy and physiology as it relates to performing work. Ergonomically designed products support the alignment and balance of the body while we use them in daily activities. Information about these products will help clients to decrease reinjury from repetitive tasks or activities. A basic understanding of the principles of kinesiology will also be beneficial. Remember to focus on the maintenance of healthy body mechanics and prevention of injury in the client's everyday life.

Gait Assessment

Gait simply refers to a person's walking pattern. A normal gait pattern is smooth, coordinated, and rhythmic. A person's posture can be described as erect, with eyes looking forward, the arms extended to her sides and swinging forward in opposition to the leg. The toes point forward with the feet positioned slightly apart (Fig. 20–10).

Common abnormalities in gait, which are learned movement patterns, result from muscle weakness, postural imbalance, pain, and connective tissue restriction. Abnormalities in gait are found throughout the postural chain and result in a multitude of soft-tissue compensations. Further study in the components of gait will help you as a therapist to locate and resolve soft-tissue alterations.

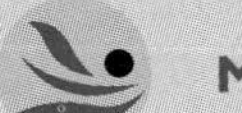

MINI•LAB

Work in pairs and have one student stand barefoot and at ease, facing forward. Assets symmetry by placing your index finger on the following landmarks and drawing an imaginary line bilaterally. With your eyes at the level of your imaginary line, determine if the bilateral points are level. Assess the following nine horizontal landmarks (Fig. 20–9):

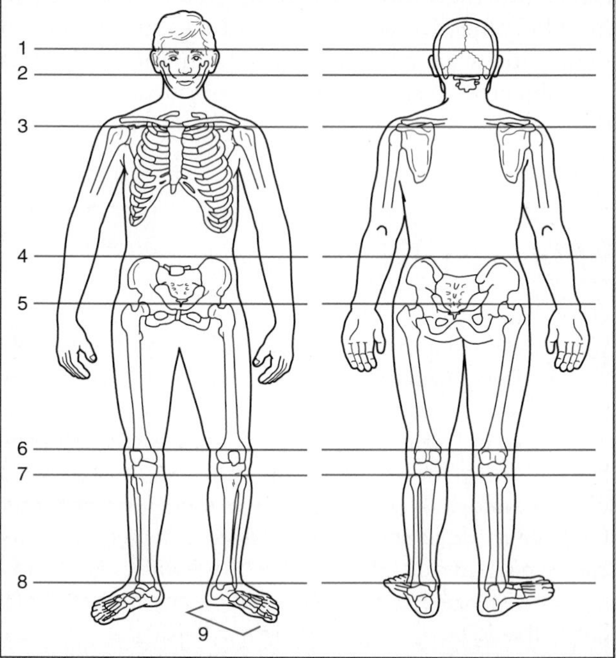

Figure 20•9 Horizontal landmarks.

1. The ears
2. The ramus of the mandible
3. The top of the acromioclavicular joints
4. The top of the iliac crests below the flank
5. The top of the greater trochanter of the femur (ask the student to extend the leg laterally and abduct the femur to aid in finding this point)
6. The top of the patellas
7. The top of the fibular heads
8. The tip of the medial malleolus of the tibia
9. The foot arches (examine and describe them)

After all horizontal landmarks are assessed for bilateral symmetry and charted, massage your partner. Note the areas of alteration in tone, sensitivity, and spasm, and draw these on the paper figures. Was there a difference right to left? Reverse roles. Compare your drawings with others in the class who found similar alterations in horizontal bilateral symmetry.

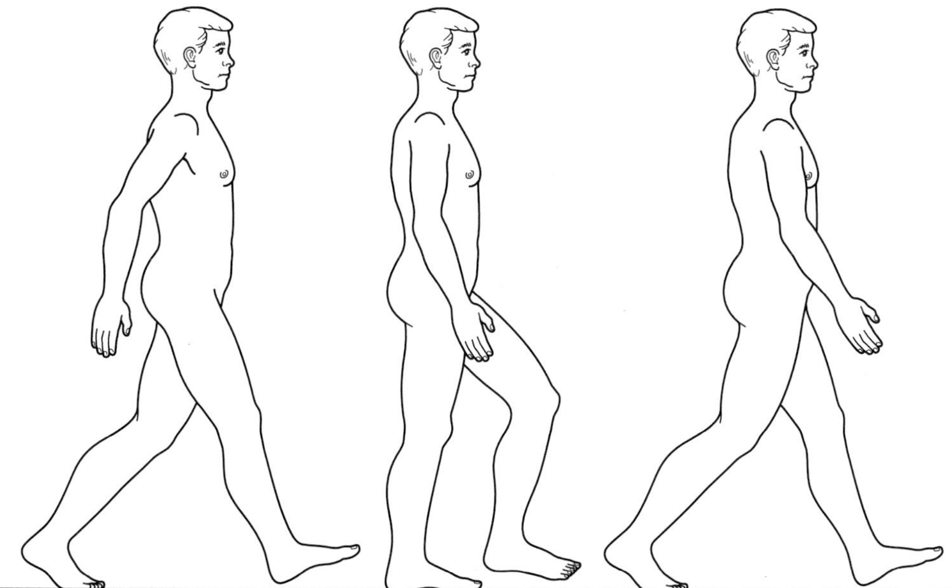

Figure 20•10 Straight-on gait sequence.

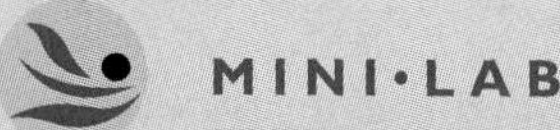

MINI•LAB

Work in pairs and have the student client, using a normal pace, walk "normally" about 20 feet away from the student therapist, turn around, and walk back. Have the student client repeat the walk slowly, then briskly. As the therapist, describe (1) the movement and placement of the feet, (2) the movement and placement of the hands, (3) movement of the hips, and (4) movement of the knees.

Documenting Objective Data on the Treatment Record

Begin by recording, in abbreviated summary style, any visual assessments you made. Note, for example, if the client appears to be holding back a flood of tears, obviously tense or stressed. The "O" note could read "tearful, appears tense." Record alterations in posture, such as "the neck almost touching the shoulder with a subjective report of cervical pain." Document changes in ROM or gait. The "O" note could read "moderate R lateral flexion," or "MOD, R, LAT FLEX," or "MOD, R lateral flexion." Report the results of any tests performed prior to the massage that are used to guide therapy (and refer to the sheet dated and enclosed with the record).

Include a detailed report of any abnormal palpatory tissue findings. State the location and describe the symptom. The "O" note may state "moderate hypertonus, R scalenes" or "MOD, HT, R, Scalenes," or "MOD. hypertonus R, scalenes." Using a ten scale or three scale as described in symptom analysis, note any degree of discomfort the client experienced. The "O" note would reflect "severe pain, 8, moderate, hypertonus, R scalenes" or "S, P, MOD, HT, R, Scalenes," or "P, 8, MOD, HT, R, Scalenes." Describe any referral or sensation patterns that accompany the symptoms; state the area to which pain is referred. The "O" note might read "severe pain, 8, moderate hypertonus, R scalenes, trigger point to R shoulder," or "S, P, MOD, HT, R, Scalenes, TP to R, SH." List muscles individually when there are several involved. If there is significant tissue involvement, you may refer to a group of muscles with the same action, such as forearm flexors or leg adductors. If the symptoms are not found bilaterally, be sure to specify "left" or "right." Capture the highlights.

A good massage therapist, like a good detective, is always looking for signs or clues. Learn to think beyond the problem; develop "thinking fingers" along with an "inquiring mind."

Application or Assessment

The "A" of SOAP may be used for recording "Application," that is, to record the techniques used during therapy, if not previously described. The "O" may be used for "Assessment" in which case the "O" note would be used to record the reassessment of the client following massage or the client's response to treatment. Healthcare practitioners who use the "Assessment" approach are traditionally assessing, applying a treatment, and then reassessing. Massage therapists assess, apply therapy, and reassess or evaluate, in a continuous and interconnected process throughout the massage session. As the massage therapist touches the client, she observes tissue alterations and responds to them using massage. Discussion of the alteration and the changes from application of massage are both objective assessments. Since there is no mandated standard, the choice is up to the individual practitioner.

Massage therapists who practice a variety of massage and touch modalities benefit from recording which therapies were chosen for the particular client. If the client returns for her next session stating that whatever the therapist did last time worked well and she would like more, a note reflecting what was applied may be very helpful. Healthcare providers may prescribe a massage modality for their patients. Healthcare payors require the recording of the modalities or types of massage therapy used, according to CPT code designations, in order to process the patient's claims. The "A" portion of the SOAP note is a convenient place to document these needed notes.

Prescriptive Directions

When a healthcare provider wishes to include massage as part of her patient's healing process for a particular medical diagnosis, she may write a prescription indicating that she considers the therapy necessary to healing. Insurance companies and other payors accept this prescription as indication of legitimate need for services and will often reimburse the client for cash out of pocket if massage is a covered expense.

The **prescription**—which literally means "take thou this"—is a written order by a licensed healthcare provider that must specify massage therapy as opposed to physical or occupational therapy. "Massage therapy" indicates that the provider is a massage therapist. Using the simplest form, the physician may prescribe evaluation and treatment at the discretion of the therapist, or she may prescribe a specific modality such as soft-tissue mobilization or massage. She may also state how the massage is to be "taken or administered." Massage is "taken" in increments known as sessions, with a specific time frame such as 60 minutes ("strength"). The prescription may also specify frequency, such as once a week, and duration such as 6 weeks ("dosage").

At the end of the prescriptive period, the client returns to the referring healthcare provider for follow-up and evaluation. The provider may request a progress note or status report to aid in the evaluation process. To be prudent, request additional information or precautions to assist in meeting the referring healthcare provider's expectations for her client and the client's particular disease process. Often the provider has expectations but does not know enough about the particulars of massage therapy to be exact. Remember, there is even great variation among practitioners who use similar modalities.

Modalities

A **modality** is a general term used to denote any technique, procedure, or product that produces a positive response for the client. As we discussed in informed consent, each type of massage has specific benefits and sometimes risks that need to be considered in relation to the client's goals and current health status. Products, as a modality, include such things as aromatherapy, hydrotherapy, various oils, creams, and lotions, use of magnets, mechanical vibrators, and music. A procedure or protocol uses a combination of techniques or products in a specific order.

When using modalities on a client, we expect that they will result in positive change and improve function. Careful documentation of our direct (one-on-one) interaction with the client and the chosen modality will aid in reimbursement through insurance and other payors. These systems use modality codes (CPT codes) listed by the American Medical Association that are thought to be effective.

CPT stands for current procedural terminology, and the codes are published in book form yearly by physicians through the American Medical Association. These codes define which modalities are reimbursable in the nonacute, outpatient, or professional office setting. A general brief description (and for some, the duration of application) may also be specified. The modalities listed are broad categories under which many techniques apply. For example, "myofascial release" and "soft-tissue mobilization" applies to any procedure that focuses on the elongation, manipulation, and treatment of the connective tissue. There is also a category for unspecified modalities. You need to document that the chosen modality was effective in increasing function and health; be sure that the modalities you list are within the parameters of your massage therapy scope of practice (which varies from state to state). Generally, other modalities can be added to enhance or modify the treatment, but not without the healthcare provider's direct consent.

Insurance companies and other reimbursement systems operate strictly on the basis of modalities via the CPT code designation. Modalities used must fall within the parameters of the code in both application and duration. Tie your progress notes directly to the modalities chosen. If the client is regaining function (i.e., able to do more of his daily living activities), the therapy is regarded as **necessary** and appropriate **care.** Therapy that eases or reduces pain or other symptoms toward increased function is called **palliative care;** this is not reimbursable as a medically necessary service in most instances.

Documenting Application Information on the Treatment Record

To capture the session, create a word picture or summary of the session flow. What was the position of the client during the massage? If you work only supine and prone, which side was massaged first? Which side does the client prefer first? Did you do a targeted neuromuscular massage with the client left lateral, supine, then right lateral? Did you start at the head or feet? Did you use specific positioning devices? Was there any specific client response that should be noted, such as a client who does not tolerate prone positioning? For example, an "A" note may state "start prone, moderate sinus activation relieved in supine position," or "start PRON, MOD sinus activation relieved in SUP POS."

What techniques did you use in the client's therapy session? By documenting the techniques applied, you can better communicate with healthcare providers and payors. What techniques were helpful for this client and which were not? If you note the techniques you used, you can eliminate what was not helpful. Documentation may also give you valuable information concerning therapy for all clients with similar symptoms or diagnoses. For example, an "A" note may read "soft tissue mobilization myofascial release, vibration; responds well to vibration," or "STM/MFR, VIB responds well to VIB."

Do you apply specific protocols that are recorded? You can simplify your recording by referring to a protocol that may be retrieved if records are requested for any reason. A flow sheet of techniques that are listed vertically and checked off is another convenient way to note session flow and sequence when working with a specific protocol. If the protocol is performed in its entirety, the note would state "CST I" for the craniosacral technique.

Protect yourself by documenting a client's local contraindications for generalized massage. Noting what areas of the body were avoided and for what reasons decrease the therapist's legal liability.

Include documentation of client preferences for adjunctive modalities in the "A" section of the treatment record. The choice of music, aroma, hydrotherapy, support devices, and even special linens such as flannel sheets fall in this category. Did you try an eye pillow on a client who finds it difficult to focus or relax during the session? Was it effective in achieving this goal? Clients may express enjoyment of a particular selection of music. Noting this and offering it again to the client is a way of enhancing the customer service component of your business. Use of progressive relaxation sequences, guided imagery, and focused breathing, if not part of your routine for each client, should be recorded.

Plan

The plan section of the SOAP format is where the assessment ("S" and "O"), application, and response to massage are used to note short- and long-term therapy goals. This section is also used to note if progress toward long-term goals is proceeding. The term outcome is also used to describe the client's response to therapy and progress toward short- or long-term goals.

You may also note education and lifestyle modifications that you have suggested in the therapeutic plan section. These suggestions support and enhance therapy outcomes, which will need to be followed up and evaluated in subsequent sessions. The plan section is also useful to document reminders of things you wanted to get to but did not (perceptions shared by the client late in the session and needing investigation in a future session; evaluation or observations following the initial session that will modify the planned timeline).

Short-Term and Long-Term Goals

You will find setting goals with the client to be challenging, but a competent therapist has a sense of what his particular skills can accomplish in a given time frame with a client who has a unique array of soft-tissue involvements, activities, and supportive environments.

The projected pace of therapy, barring client reinjury, will influence therapy progress. The therapist will continue, modify, or change the modality for future sessions, depending on how the tissues respond to chosen modalities. The amount of resolution may suggest additions to the plan, such as hydrotherapy before massage, education in prevention of reinjury, or lifestyle modification in the sleeping posture, or referral to an appropriate healthcare provider, for example.

Typical short-term goals involve decreasing discomfort in a specific area or of a particular symptom, such as headache, by the end of the session. A long-term goal would be to eliminate discomfort in a specific area or to decrease the frequency or intensity of a symptom such as headaches. Short-term goals are increments of progress toward a larger goal. Descriptive words such as "decrease" and "increase" suggest an expectation that positive change will occur. Depending on the involvement and extent of deviation from normal, short-term goals generally focus on a client's immediate problem; long-term goals focus on restoration of normal or enhanced function. Because spasm, hypertonus, and discomfort are decreased, the person is able to improve in his level of functioning. In fact, his rate of tissue recovery may be enhanced by avoidance of reinjury and by self-care activities, resulting in strength, endurance, and performance enhancement.

Continually evaluate therapy goals using client feedback. The therapeutic plan is modified to reflect assessment of reinjury, to uncover educational needs, and to gain involvement of the client between sessions in lifestyle modification. Many times initial goals are unrealistic and unachievable due to the extent of injury and the client's inability to avoid reinjury from daily activities such as child care or work. If the client is not invested in the healing process, she may be unwilling to support the therapy with positive lifestyle change. This usually results in periods of remission and exacerbation with little overall change. Consistent data keeping will help you document the factors affecting outcomes for each client.

Client Education

Client education holds great potential for empowering the client to manage her own preventive or wellness practices. Areas of education include ergonomics, musculoskeletal self-care activities, exercises, and postural adjustments.

It is vital for the client to understand all the factors that can play a part in her healing process. Insight is explored in areas that need support since the last session. What is the client doing after and between sessions? Typically a client will be so happy to have a few hours of relief that she will overdo following a session, or she will not be aware that the tissues have been worked and need care following massage. Increased water, light activity and/or rest, and use of ice may be appropriate.

It is important to assess the receptiveness of the client to making lifestyle changes. A client who is interested in what she can do to support her healing process may invest the necessary time, energy, and expense. Remember that injury or long-term chronic stress narrows a client's perceptions and is usually accompanied by a degree of anxiety and depression. Care must be taken not to overwhelm the person, no matter how helpful you feel the change would be.

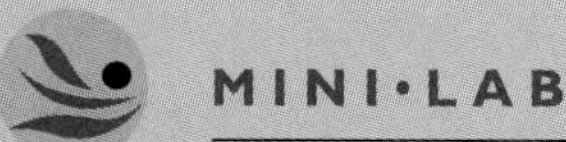

MINI•LAB

Create a notecard-size educational list of ways to protect and preserve the client's massage for take-home use.

Suggest an activity for home use that would be most beneficial to the client and her goals within her current schedule and budget limitations. Try to suggest a change that would fit easily into the day and that would tie into an activity that is done daily; you might suggest gentle stretching of the neck under the shower. Frequent checks may uncover the need for additional clarification, demonstration, or alteration to increase cooperation and success. Once the activity is regularly used, additional ones may be added to enhance the client's goals. Document all client recommendations in the Plan section of your SOAP notes, or note recommendations in your client progress report.

Realize that the client may not yet be in a place to self-motivate or to take responsibility for herself. What may be workable for her is to evaluate activities that are not supportive of the healing process and to modify those. She may be open to modifying sleeping posture, to using cold, or to getting a phone head set. Again, by exploring options, the client may be able to identify what she is willing and able to do.

Ergonomics education (how to support the body's balance and alignment throughout daily activities) frequently prevents reinjury and greatly supports symptom resolution. Posture education and kinesiology are basic to client improvement. Standing erect, sitting, sleeping postures, and movement are all areas that can support the client in regaining and maintaining soft-tissue health. Books to educate yourself and your clients are found in local bookstores and libraries.

Education in self-care activities (e.g., meditation, stress reduction, breathing exercise, yoga, tai chi) supports the healing processes by moving the person into the rest mode or by parasympathetic stimulation. To introduce these methods, acquire informed consent to incorporate and demonstrate these methods; discuss with the client the possible benefits of the demonstrated method. If you observe that the person's stress level is impeding the healing process and you do not feel qualified to offer these other modalities, cultivate a referral base of practitioners to assist you.

Education in flexibility and muscle elongation activities is very helpful to the motivated client. Take care not to encroach on the professional boundaries of other practitioners involved in the client's care. If a physical therapist is assigning and working with exercise, it would be inappropriate for you to add more or different activities. Likewise, avoid commenting negatively on the assignments from another practitioner. If the physician has given the client exercise, do not add or change the regimen. What is appropriate is to network directly with the client's physical therapist or healthcare provider to discuss any concerns you have regarding the client's exercise and tissue findings.

Author's Note

Many times, clients do assigned exercises incorrectly. They crank out the required number of repetitions without feeling that they are exceeding their limitations.

They may fail to make progress because they are constantly reinjuring tissues or are trying to develop strength and endurance in an injured muscle. Help your clients to be connected with their bodies; teach them to listen for the cues that would indicate time to rest and time to proceed. Remind your clients of the importance of the long-term health of the tissue.

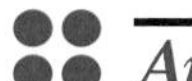

Author's Note

Complete the treatment record immediately following the client's session. Information is easily and quickly forgotten as you refocus your attention on the next client or on the concerns of the day. Book enough time between appointments to take care of paperwork, to change linens, and to center yourself for the next client.

Documenting the Plan in the Treatment Record

To record the outcome of a session is to evaluate the effectiveness of the therapeutic plan in accomplishing short-term (session) goals and long-term (prescriptive period or projected timeline) goals. A "P" note may read "40% decrease in hypertonus of muscles listed in 0," or "40% DEC in HT of MS (listed in 0)" or "MS cont ↓ HT, 40%"

A statement such as "hypertonus of symptomatic musculature was decreased 70 percent" is much more descriptive than "client was pleased" or, in the client's words, "my neck feels looser." Client statements are always appropriate and are best recorded verbatim if memorable, but these direct quotes are not always reflective of tissue change.

Specific evidence may also be provided to support positive outcomes. For example, common responses following a Swedish massage are due to the relaxing parasympathetic effects of massage and bodywork and may include deeper breathing, slower breathing, the "big sigh" at the end of the massage, stomach rumbles and noise, snoring, snoozing, sleeping, and chilling down as the circulation is returned to the "core."

At the end of the session, you may be overwhelmed by the amount of time and paperwork necessary for adequate documentation of the first session. Typically, you will make some decisions regarding whether you will comply entirely with all the documentation suggestions. Minimum paperwork will consist of a health history or intake form, a consent, and a treatment record. However, observational test forms, policy and procedures, and therapy protocols are recommended for professional practice. Additional paperwork will be needed if you plan to assist the client with insurance or other forms of reimbursement. As a private practitioner, you may not be subject to internal review and record audit. If your state has a massage practice law, the massage board may exercise the right to request a sample of the forms you routinely use as evidence that you are complying with the law. Quality assurance is routinely verified by large organizations, such as hospitals by pulling an estimated number of records completed that month and by verifying that all information was collected.

NETWORKING THROUGH CLIENT REPORTS

You may use client reports to communicate your initial evaluation and summarize progress. Legally, you must obtain the client's verbal consent or have him sign a release of records when information regarding treatment is transferred to another person. This information may be released only to the specified provider who is directly involved in the client's care or to legal authorities.

Write the **initial evaluation** from your SOAP notes of the first session. You may wish to include the plan of care suggested by the physician's diagnosis, which you and the client have agreed upon. Also include a statement acknowledging that he will be referred back to the healthcare provider for evaluation at the close of the prescriptive period.

A progress report summarizes the client's progress to date. One type is called a **narrative report** because it can be lengthy, stretching through many sessions and prescriptive periods. Usually the initial baseline session and the latest session are chosen as the measures to show improvement. The application of massage therapy and the client's responses are discussed in detail; to resolve symptoms, to continue progress, or to maintain progress currently achieved, you may present justification for continuing therapy, if appropriate.

Sample Narrative Report

Letterhead

Date

Person Requesting Narrative Report
Address

Dear Healthcare Professional,
Re: Client's Name

Mrs. Ouch was first seen Month, Day, Year as a referral from Dr. Feelgood, with a diagnosis of tension headache. The initial prescription included massage to neck and shoulders for 60 minutes, twice a week for 8 weeks.

The client is being referred back to Dr. Feelgood for follow-up evaluation. Mrs. Ouch describes the onset of headaches following a front-end MVA on Month, Day, Year, in which she remembers gripping the wheel and being thrown forward and backward. She states she was wearing a seatbelt. She does not remember hitting any structure in the car. Mrs. Ouch initially presented with the following complaints:

- constant, severe neck pain
- shoulder pain, moderately severe on the right, and on the left
- inability to look over her shoulders, difficulty driving
- inability to lift her arms above her shoulders, difficulty dressing, and grooming
- generalized neck and shoulder tension
- daily headaches that increase in intensity in the posterior region of the head and that interfere with work, sleep, and daily activities

Evaluation of Mrs. Ouch revealed postural distortions that traditionally exacerbate cervical discomfort, notably

- a 1½- to 2-inch forward head posture
- internally rotated shoulders
- high right shoulder
- high left iliac crest

ROM is significantly decreased bilaterally in lateral flexion and rotation R>L. Palpatory findings revealed acutely tender and severely hypertonic muscles in the following areas:

- posterior cervicals; anterior cervicals; scalenes; anterior and posterior rotator cuff; erector spinae; trapezium; triceps; and coracobrachialis

There is significant involvement of the fascial system and superior soft tissues that contributes to boggy, congested tissue, and to extreme tension in the cranial fascia.

Initial treatment consisted of a myofascial approach to begin restoring elasticity and circulation to the superior tissues. Swedish massage was used to warm and prepare the tissues for neuromuscular therapy. Progression in therapy depth was based on positive tissue response and client comfort. Additionally, myofascial therapy for the cranial fascia and craniosacral work to calm the nervous system was found effective in achieving therapy progress.

Presently Mrs. Ouch reports the following:

- intermittent, mild to moderate neck pain
- shoulder pain, mild on the right
- full cervical lateral rotation, increased lateral flexion with no pain
- ability to lift arms carefully above her shoulders as needed
- decreased neck and shoulder tension
- occasional headaches; which are decreased by half following the first week

Current palpatory findings reveal mild to moderate hypertonic muscles in the following areas: scalenes; erector spinae; trapezium; subscapularis; anterior serratus; and pectoralis minor. Mrs. Ouch has residual postural distortions contributing to cervical discomfort; there is a forward head posture of 1 inch.

Based on Mrs. Ouch's positive response to therapy, I feel continued therapy would contribute to resolution of her residual symptomology. My therapy plan would focus on continued release and depth progression, adding gentle proprioceptive neuromuscular facilitation activities for long-term maintenance of progress to date. Eight sessions tapering in frequency based on Mrs. Ouch's resolution to date may bring her to at least 75 percent of her preinjury state. A maintenance plan of massage once a month for 6 months is also recommended.

Thank you for referring Mrs. Ouch. If you have further questions or comments, please feel free to contact me at your earliest convenience.

A **status report** describes how the client is doing at a point in time or over a short duration of time, such as a prescriptive period. It is brief and concise, using the last SOAP note with an estimate of progress to date or since the last progress report, and may include other measures of client progress, such as compliance with exercise or lifestyle changes. Stating the client is noncompliant with recommendations may result in loss of payment and termination of therapy.

A paragraph for each component of the SOAP note is introduced, along with a general greeting stating how the client relationship was established. This example is a physician referral by prescription: "Mr. Client was first seen on (date). He was referred for massage therapy, 1 hour twice a week, for 1 month, by Dr. Complimentary Care, with a diagnosis of iliolumbar ligament strain."

In the "S" paragraph, describe his symptoms and related information as you recorded them on the date he was first seen. Use the "O" paragraph to describe your findings. The "A" paragraph describes the therapy modalities you used and their results. In the "P" paragraph, describe your estimate of the client's progress toward a preinjury state or resolution, factors that assist (or hinder) therapy, and your recommendation of what therapy would be required to maintain the progress achieved.

To be courteous, a closing statement offering availability to review what you have written or to answer questions is appropriate.

Since the report is being "sent," use a classic letter format. Things that can increase the ease and speed of reading are lists with bullets for multiple items of the same type and check-off style forms. A letter that is well organized and easy to read increases the likelihood that the receiver will review the report. By using standard forms, you will save time in report writing. Figures 20–11 and 20–12 are examples of reports using a check-off, fill-in-the-blank report style.

Report writing can increase your professional growth through networking with other healthcare professionals, who also become more educated regarding the potential benefits and value of including us in their therapeutic team.

Date: ____________________

To: ____________________

Client's Name: ____________________

Diagnosis: ____________________

Prescription of Medical Necessity: ____________________

INITIAL EVALUATION AND THERAPY BY: ____________________

Client Reports:

Stress due to: ____________________

Pain location: ____________________ Description: ____________________

Other symptom(s) location: ____________________ Description: ____________________

Decreased ROM. Joint(s): ____________________ Movement(s): ____________________

Therapist's Findings:

Posture and Gait (visual): ____________________

Palpatory R/T Diagnosis: ____________________

Application of Massage:

Therapeutic Massage Techniques: ____________________

_____ Stretching for Flexibility _____ Visualization & Imagery _____ Other:

_____ Use of Ice Packs _____ Use of Hot Packs

Continued on next page

Figure 20•11 Examples of reports using a check-off, fill-in-the-blank report style. (Permission is hereby granted to reproduce this form in its entirety, including the copyright notice, for commercial or instructional use but not for resale.)

Page 2

INITIAL EVALUATION AND THERAPY FOR: ______________________________

Client Response:

_____Decrease in Stress/Parasympathetic Effect:

____

_____Decrease in Pain & Other Symptoms:

____

_____Increase in ROM with Decreased Discomfort:

____

_____Posture

____

Therapeutic Plan & Goals:

_____Re-establish posture (balance between musculoskeketal and nervous system)

_____Normalize the musculoskeletal tissues by extinguishing triggerpoints, spasms, hypertonicities, etc.; thereby increasing flexibility, ROM and functional activity

_____Prevention of re-injury via self-care education

_____Stress reduction, awareness and education

Suggested Therapeutic Plan:

____

____

____

____

____

____

For questions or comments please feel free to contact the Therapist:

In the Journey Toward Health,

Figure 20•11 *Continued*

CERVICAL ROUTINE/PROTOCOL

Date ____________

Client Name: ______________________ Diagnosis: ______________________

Notes: ____

____

Postural Assessment Standing

____

____

____

____

____

ROM Assessment:

	Active R L	Discomfort R L	Passive R L	Discomfort R L
Lateral Flexion				
Rotation				
Flexion				
Extension				

Swedish Massage: ____________________

Craniosacral CV-4
Stillpoint, other: ____________________

Myofascial Release: Area: ____________________

Neuromuscular Massage:

- Anterior Cervical
- Anterior Rotator Cuff
- Posterior Cervical
- Posterior
- Rotator Cuff
- Trapezius
- Levator Scapulae
- Other:

Proprioceptive Neuromuscular Facilitation
Passive/Area: ____________________

Swedish Massage: ____________________

Active ROM Assessment by the Client--Note Change: ____________________

Figure 20•12 Sample treatment protocol using check-off list. (Permission is hereby granted to reproduce this form in its entirety, including the copyright notice, for commercial or instructional use but not for resale.)

Author's Note

These items comprise a typical client record.

I. Suggested Paperwork: The consent and policy and procedure are often combined on one form. When all three are combined on one form, quality, as well as quantity, needs to be considered.
   - Client Intake Form or Health History
   - Consent
   - Policy and Procedures
   - Treatment or Session Record

II. Optional Paperwork: These are written forms with a signature and date that resemble a contractual agreement. Current practice is verbal explanation and agreement with documentation in the treatment record.
   - Information Sheet and Consent for each modality you practice
   - Therapy Protocol

III. Paperwork completed when requested by insurance, legal agency or referring healthcare provider or at the therapist's option
   - Release of records signed by the client before releasing any records or summaries of records
   - Initial Evaluation: may include proposed treatment plan or other requested information
   - Progress or Status Report: a summary of progress from the date of the last report to the present. If the prescriptive period is 8 weeks, write a progress report after session 8. If the prescription for massage was renewed, the next progress report would be written after session number 16 and would cover the progress from session 8 to session 16
   - Narrative or Summary Report: a survey or summary traditionally in letterstyle spanning the first to the last client visit

SUMMARY

Good communication skills are useful to introduce and ease the client through the massage therapy environment. Verbal interview skills are used to review, complete, and verify the therapist's understanding of the client's wants, needs, and expectations. By assessing and understanding the client's current health status and chief concerns, you can determine the appropriate massage therapy to enhance his health and wellness. Through this process you create a cooperative working relationship with your client.

Document health history, review policies and procedures, obtain informed consent, and list therapy modalities to systematically provide a journal of therapy. Written communication also helps us preserve information as a reference for networking with other healthcare professionals through report writing.

The cooperative nature of the process is evidenced by the formation, evaluation, and modification of therapy goals. Participation by the client in self-care such as posture, ergonomics, and therapeutic activities is encouraged. A commitment to maintaining appointments and to evaluating progress is a natural outcome of open communication and cooperation in therapy. Success in using professional communication will result in a comfortable and therapeutic experience that the client will want to repeat and recommend.

SELF-TEST

Multiple Choice • Write the letter of the best answer in the space provided.

_______ 1. Professional communication is an interaction between the massage therapist and the client (or agents of the client) for the collection, recording, and transmission of data. Which of the following is not a purpose of professional communication?

A. forming a client receipt and statement
B. giving the client information about the massage such as benefits and potential side effects
C. informing clients of their rights as well as obtaining consent for therapy
D. anticipating the client's response to massage therapy

_______ 2. In SOAP charting, SOAP stands for

A. subjective information, objective findings, assessment, and practice
B. subjective objectivity, objective subjectivity, assessment, and procedure
C. subjective information, objective findings, application, and plan
D. subjective information, objective findings, analysis, and procedural application

_______ 3. The purpose of collecting subjective data through written intake and interview is to

A. determine client needs and goals
B. determine if massage is safe for the client
C. determine client expectations
D. all of the above

_______ 4. Clients reporting on their problem, beliefs, attitudes, and biases is known as

A. client-biased information
B. objective information
C. subjective information
D. propaganda

_______ 5. Updating the client's "S" note before the start of the following session is necessary for

A. determining the effect of the previous session
B. determining if the massage plan needs adjustment
C. determining if the client was satisfied
D. A and B

_______ 6. Empirical information gathered by the therapist is called

A. client-biased information
B. objective information
C. subjective information
D. propaganda

_______ 7. Information assessed and documented by visual observation includes all of the following *except*

A. gait
B. mental and emotional status
C. muscle spasm
D. skin integrity

_______ 8. Information assessed and documented primarily by palpatory observation includes all of the following except

A. location of the muscles involved
B. identification of the soft-tissue problem
C. postural symmetry
D. response to pressure

_______ 9. The rationale for testing the uninjured/unsymptomatic joint first includes all of the following except

A. increased trust in the therapist
B. decreasing fear of the unknown
C. increased muscle guarding
D. providing a baseline for comparison

_______ 10. The primary thing to keep in mind when planning therapy goals is

A. remaining flexible
B. using published milestones
C. remaining constant and focused
D. avoiding biased client feedback

_______ 11. CPT codes (current procedural terminology) published yearly by physicians through the American Medical Association define which modalities are reimbursable in the nonacute, outpatient, or professional office setting. An example of a modality approved for reimbursement is

A. craniosacral massage C. sports massage
B. myofascial release D. pregnancy massage

_______ 12. Prescription for massage therapy includes
A. frequency of sessions
B. total number of sessions
C. length of individual session
D. date of session

_______ 13. Considerations for designing home therapy support (homework) for clients with demonstration and return demonstration by the client includes all of the following except
A. simple, use of only those beneficial and necessary
B. fit the client's time, energy, and means
C. challenge the client
D. provide immediate noticeable results

_______ 14. To verify that the listener has understood the feelings and content of the speaker's message, a reflective response may be made. A type of reflective response is
A. paraphrasing C. sympathizing
B. interpreting D. advising

_______ 15. The therapist may refuse to massage in part or in total a client based upon
A. the physical appearance or behavior of the client
B. information gleaned through the health history and interview process
C. inappropriate language or behavior of a sexual nature
D. all of the above

_______ 16. The most important aspect of the plan section is
A. establishing a timeline for therapy
B. follow-up and evaluation of therapy
C. management of goals to produce desired outcomes
D. reminders and session notes

_______ 17. The SOAP format is also used in report writing. A report that covers the period from prescription through the first session, is known as
A. initial evaluation C. progress report
B. status report D. narrative report

References

American Massage Therapy Association: Code of Ethics, Evanston, IL, 1994.

Bolton, Robert. *People Skills.* New York: Simon & Schuster, Inc., 1979.

Burley-Allen, Madelyn. *Listening: The Forgotten Skill.* New York: John Wiley & Sons, Inc., 1995.

Davis, Neil M. *Medical Abbreviations: 7000 Conveniences at the Expense of Communications and Safety,* 5th ed. Huntington Valley, PA: Neil M. Davis Associates, 1990.

Dolan, David W. *Objective Structural Findings in Massage Therapy: Key to Insurance Reimbursement & Specially Physician Referrals.* Jacksonville, FL: Advanced Therapeutics America, 1995.

Ignatavicius, Donna D. and Marilyn Varner Bayne. *Medical-Surgical Nursing: A Nursing Process Approach.* Philadelphia: W. B. Saunders, 1991.

Lowe, Whitney W. *Functional Assessment in Massage Therapy.* Corvallis, OR: Pacific Orthopedic Massage, 1995.

McKay, Matthew, Martha Davis, and Patrick Fanning. *Messages: The Communication Skills Book.* Oakland, CA: New Harbinger Publications., 1987.

National Association for Nurse Massage Therapists: Standards of Practice. February 16, 1992.

National Certification Board of Massage Therapy: Code of Ethics. McLean, VA, 1995.

Sohen-Moe, Cherie. "Taking Care of Business: The Ultimate Client Interview." *Massage Therapy Journal.* Fall 1996. pp. 133–136.

Thompson, Diana L. *Hands Heal: Documentation for Massage Therapy.* Seattle: Diana L. Thompson, 1993.

Torres, Lillian S. *Basic Medical Techniques and Patient Care for Radiologic Technologies.* Philadelphia: J. B. Lippincott Company, 1993.

It is only with the heart that one can see rightly. What is essential is invisible to the eye.
—*Antoine de Saint-Exupéry*

21 Adaptive Massage and Client Management Issues

Student Objectives

After completing this chapter, the student should be able to:

- Learn modifications for the client's position on the massage table when someone requires variation from the norm
- Adjust massage techniques to suit the client's various health conditions
- Adapt massage therapy for pregnant clients
- Accommodate clients who have visual, auditory, or speech impairments
- Adjust massage to accommodate someone physically challenged or in a wheelchair
- Discuss emotional releases, and describe ways they can be appropriately handled

INTRODUCTION

The standard massage routine is designed to suit the needs of the average client, who probably represents the majority of your clientele. However, you will encounter individuals who have unique situations that include physical, emotional, and health-related challenges, and you must accommodate these and modify and adapt massage therapy to fit their special needs. These needs may range from postsurgery and scar treatment to amputations or terminal illnesses.

The most important way in which you can assist individuals who need adaptive massage is to view them as people first and their special need only as a secondary consideration. Many clients who have special needs may be touch-deprived, and massage can go a long way to provide safe touch and to provide psychosocial as well as physiological needs. Adopting this attitude will set the stage for a therapeutic relationship that will be fulfilling to both of you.

When adapting your massage for these special populations, keep in mind that the massage strokes themselves may not change. The alterations come in how you modify your pressure, speed, the duration, and frequency of the massage; how you position your client on the massage table; and other safety precautions you must take.

Conditions that demand accommodation may include clients with large breasts or breast implants; large clients; clients during menstruation or pregnancy; age-related special needs in pediatric or geriatric clients; the chronically or terminally ill; communicable diseases; diabetes, spinal abnormalities, and osteoporosis; postsurgery and scar tissue; amputations; clients who are visually, hearing, speech, or locomotion impaired such as paraplegia, quadriplegia, hemiplegia; and those recovering from substance abuse, sexual abuse, and emotional difficulties. Each of these areas will be covered in detail, with specific recommendations on tailoring the massage for the client's needs.

It is always a good idea to consult the client's managing physician before proceeding with the massage. If you know ahead of time what kind of condition your client has, educate yourself on his condition and be prepared when he arrives; spend a few minutes looking up his condition in a pathophysiology book or a medical dictionary.

The best way to obtain information about the special need is to ask the client directly during the premassage interview. Each situation will be different and you must be willing to be open-minded, patient, tolerant, and flexible. Each client will teach you, if are willing to observe and to listen. Although each client will have different needs in the delivery of the massage, the therapist's boundaries should always be consistent. Refer to Chapter 2, Professional Standards and Boundaries, for an in-depth discussion of personal and professional boundaries and confidentiality issues for the massage therapist.

The following list will give you a few guidelines and procedures to help you make necessary accommodations.

LARGE BREASTS OR BREAST IMPLANTS

When massaging a woman with large breasts or breast implants, there are several options available to make the client more comfortable while lying prone. You may give the client a rolled-up towel or cylindrical pillow to be placed under, above, or between the breasts, whichever is most comfortable. Many clients prefer a supportive device both above *and* below the breasts. Several commercial devices provide longitudinal support for the sternum; this may provide comfort without compromising the cervical spine. Several massage table manufacturers now carry tables fitted with breast recesses that allow the client to lie prone more comfortably (Fig. 21–1). When not in use, two small, round cushions fill the breast recess spaces.

In the supine position, it is sometimes difficult to access muscles in the chest area of full-figured women. If massage is needed in the pectoral region, the serratus anterior, or in the walls of the axilla, you may ask the client to cup the breast tissue in her hand and retract it medially. This technique allows a safe boundary to be established between client and therapist.

MASSAGING THE LARGE CLIENT

When massaging the client who is large (i.e., obese or the somatotype known as an endomorph) or who has generous amounts of fragile subcutaneous tissue, two areas require special consideration. The first consider-

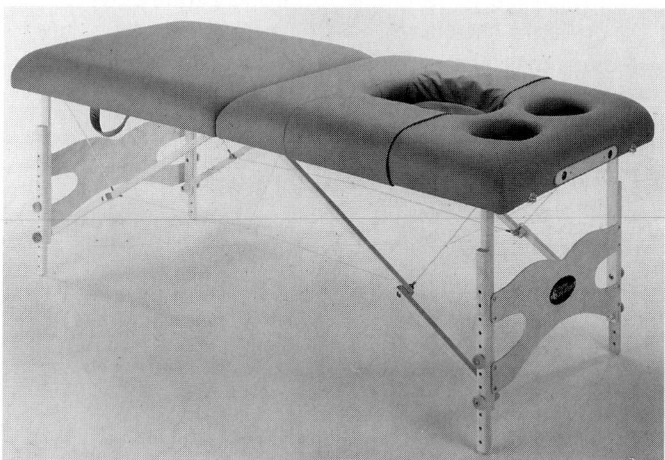

Figure 21•1 Massage table with breast recesses and pregnancy option.

ation is psychological and requires approaching the client with an attitude that is compassionate, caring, and nonjudgmental because large clients typically have a history of verbal abuse from society in general and other healthcare providers in particular. Never badger a client about his weight or blame excessive size or weight on lack of morality or self-control. No one has a body that is perfect in all aspects. Make the accommodations necessary for his comfort, and proceed with the session.

The second consideration is physiological in which pressure must be applied carefully to areas that contain high quantities of adipose tissue to reduce tissue damage. Adipose tissue is extremely vascular, with each pound of tissue containing approximately 1 mile of capillaries, the most fragile of vessels, making adipose tissue extremely susceptible to bruising. Avoid deep stroking of adipose tissue because it can damage and break these vessels. He may have large amounts of soft subcutaneous adipose tissue and yet still have rock-hard back and shoulder muscles that have become overdeveloped to support the extra weight. The back, neck, shoulders, hips, and sometimes legs of many larger clients may require extra massage work.

Palpation must be used to discern the difference between muscle and adipose tissue. If muscle fiber cannot be felt with gentle pressure, avoid working deeply into the tissue. You can ask the client to contract a specific muscle or muscle group. If the tissue does not respond with an increase in tone, it is probably adipose tissue, and deep work should be avoided. Sometimes it is possible to gently retract adipose tissue in order to access muscle tissue underneath. Clients who have had recent weight loss may have areas that tend to hang in folds until the skin tightens. These areas should never be worked deeply or pinched; folds can be moved to the side while working on adjacent muscle and may be flattened out against the area to be worked so that the therapist can work through it.

Inquire about the client's activity level. Just because someone is large does not necessarily mean that he is sedentary. Many large clients are very active and will prefer deep work. For those who are inactive, watch for signs of edema.

Another area of consideration when working with larger clients is the therapist's body mechanics and efficiency. It may help to either lower the table height prior to the client's visit or have a small platform to stand on to gain height and leverage. Most table manufacturers offer electric lift or hydraulic tables that can be raised or lowered to a comfortable height.

To assist your client's need for emotional security, use a sheet or an extra-large towel as a top drape to provide adequate coverage. A client who is obese or excessively large may feel awkward or unsafe getting on and off the massage table. Have a foot stool available, and be willing to offer assistance. If you have an electric or hydraulic lift massage table, set it in the lowest position while the client is getting on and off. If the client does not feel comfortable on your massage table, he may need to receive his massage on the floor. Provide a comfortable floor mat for such an instance.

MASSAGE AND MENSTRUATION

When a female client is menstruating, she often feels physically and emotionally uncomfortable. Since she will be wearing some kind of feminine protection (e.g., pads or tampons), it is not uncommon for undergarments to be left on. Keep feminine protection items on display in your restroom in case your female clients require them. Should any breakthrough bleeding occur while she is on the massage table, wash contaminated linens separately in hot water with detergent and a quarter cup of chlorine bleach after the massage. Dry them using hot air. Your massage tables and related equipment should then be wiped down with a solution of one part chlorine bleach to ten parts water.

Many clients cancel previously made appointments during this time of month. If they do keep their appointment, forgo deep abdominal work, particularly if they are having cramps. A fomentation (hot moist) pack placed on the abdomen when the client is supine or placed on the low back while the client is prone can help soothe the achy feeling associated with menses. Some extra time spent massaging her low back may offer some pain relief.

Author's Note

The following information can be found throughout this manual:

- Transdermal medicated patches—Integumentary system chapter
- Central venous catheter—Circulatory system chapter
- Massage for upper and lower respiratory congestion—Respiratory system chapter
- Colostomy, ileostomy, urostomy—Digestive system chapter

MASSAGE AND THE PREGNANT CLIENT

During the premassage interview, inquire about the female client's current as well as past pregnancies, breasts soreness, and nausea. If there is a history of spontaneous abortion (miscarriage), avoid massage in the first trimester because everything, including massage, is suspected should she miscarry. If she is cur-

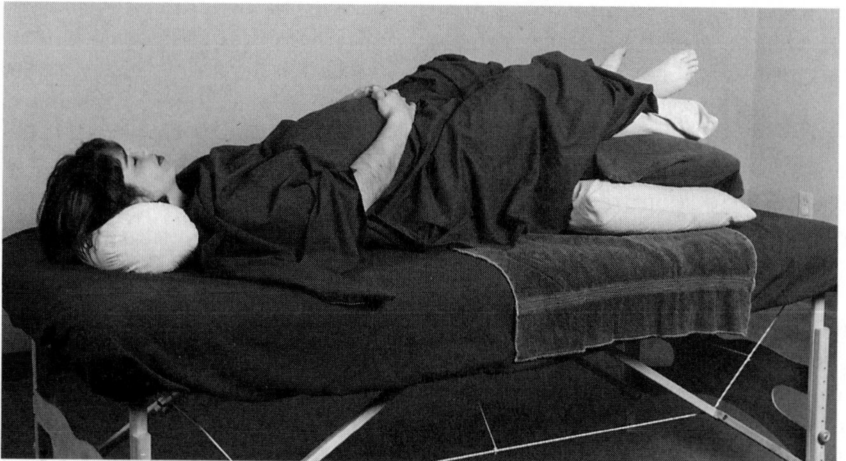

Figure 21•2 Pregnant client showing knee and foot elevation.

rently experiencing eclampsia (toxemia), massage is not indicated unless ordered by her physician. If your pregnant client reports that she is healthy with no past complications, proceed with the massage. In the first trimester, the client's position on the table is not a concern unless she is uncomfortable lying in a specific position. Avoid deep abdominal massage during the entire pregnancy and for 3 months following childbirth. If the client has breast soreness, make modifications to her position while prone (refer to previous section on Large Breasts or Breast Implants). If the pregnant client is experiencing nausea, reduce or omit rocking from your routine.

Expectant mothers in their second and third trimesters should receive a massage in the supine and side-lying positions. Other positioning methods allow the pregnant client to lie prone—discuss these with your client and make a joint decision. Typically, the supine and side-lying positions are the most comfortable. Due to the pressure exerted on the abdominal blood vessels by the growing fetus, massage the pregnant mother in the supine position on an angle for only 15 to 20 minutes. Ask her on which side she feels more comfortable lying and allow her to spend most of the time during the session in that particular position (most pregnant clients report that the left side is more comfortable).

Due to the presence of the hormone relaxin (which affects *all* connective tissue), avoid overstretching muscles and overmobilizing joints and ligaments because it can create permanent laxity. Pregnant women tend to urinate frequently because of the fetus pressing on the urinary bladder. Suggest to your pregnant client that she visit the restroom before getting on the massage table and perhaps about midway through the session. Most pregnant women are also sensitive to stuffy rooms and high temperatures; avoid heating blankets and hot packs. She may be more comfortable if you keep a fan blowing in a corner of the room during the massage. If the pregnant woman has swollen ankles, elevate her knees and feet using a bolster and pillows while she is supine; the feet are positioned higher than the knees. (Fig. 21–2).

THE PEDIATRIC CLIENT

Children, or **pediatric** clients, are defined as young people between 3 and 18 years of age. They are often accompanied by anxious parents because most pediatric massage addresses specific tissue problems due to injury or illness, resulting in pain to the client. During the premassage interview, explain the procedure to both the parents and the child, but informed consent must be obtained from the parents or legal guardians. In some states, a parent must also supervise while the massage is in progress (Fig. 21–3). If the child is between the ages of 16 and 18, parental permission is not necessary; however, it is sometimes prudent to keep the parent in the room while massaging a child of the opposite sex. This is especially true, for example, when working in a sensitive area such as a pulled adductor injury in a young athlete.

In younger children, the massage session may last only 30 to 45 minutes due to the child's smaller stature, short attention span, short neural reflex, and increased metabolism. Use the extra time to establish a rapport with the client.

Use special caution when working with adolescent boys. The reflexive sexual erection response is often very sensitive; peripheral stimulation (i.e., massage) on the thighs and belly can trigger this reflex. It is helpful to keep the top drape bunched up in the groin area to disguise any physical response to the massage. If you are comfortable with approaching the subject, you can educate the child and parent, while making appropriate acknowledgment of normal body physiology.

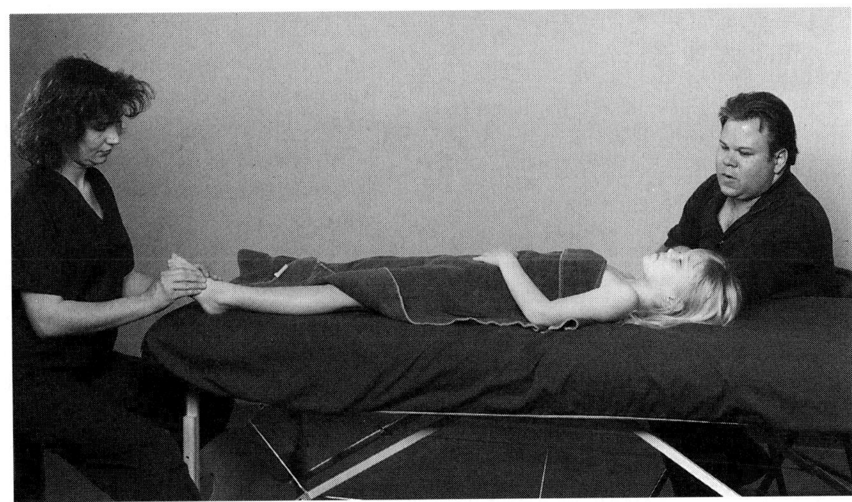

Figure 21•3 Child receiving a massage.

THE GERIATRIC CLIENT

Geriatric refers to elderly clients who are 70 years of age and older. Geriatric clients represent the fastest growing population groups in the country. Many massage therapists offer discounts to elderly clients because most are living on fixed incomes.

During the premassage interview, assess the geriatric client's condition and provide adaptations to ensure her comfort and safety. Establish rapport by acclimating her to her surroundings to help her feel safe and secure. Use a soft, clear voice, and face the client when speaking. When explaining procedures, tell her what parts of the body you will be massaging using simple, nonanatomical terms. Be sure your client understands what is being said, and allow time for asking questions. Guard against chilling by using blankets over the client's body and, if appropriate, an external heat source such as a portable heating unit.

Many elderly clients live or feel alone because their spouses have passed away or because family members are busy raising their own families. It may be important that you provide an opportunity for elderly clients to talk and share their thoughts with you. Depression may also affect the elderly client. Be attentive and sensitive to the client's emotional needs.

The health and physical condition of the elderly decline with age, but this varies from person to person. As we age, certain changes occur to all the body systems.

1. Nerve and reflex reaction time is shorter, and there may be a loss or increased sensitivity to pain. More time is typically needed to perform tasks (note adjustments during the premassage interview).
2. There is typically a loss in hearing and vision (especially nearsightedness) that must be taken into consideration.
3. A decrease in strength and muscle tone is often noted.
4. The bones are not as strong and flexible. Joints begin to wear down and osteoarthritis is common. A mild kyphosis may be noted (dowager's hump).
5. The skin appears pale and wrinkled and becomes thinner, looser, and more frail. Age spots (purple macules and senile purpura) may appear on the skin due to blood leaking from damaged and weak capillaries. Liver spots (senile lentigo) may be seen on the skin of older people, especially those who have been exposed to excessive sun.
6. In the case of inactivity, circulation may not be efficient. Atherosclerosis is fairly common among elderly people.
7. There may be an increase in incontinence resulting from loss of muscle tone in the urinary and gastrointestinal tracts.

When massaging an elderly person, deep work should be avoided unless order by her physician. Because elderly people may tire easily, massage for shorter periods. Because of decreased reaction time, to possible insensitivity to pain, and to thinning of the blood vessels and skin, it is easy to damage the skin or cause bruising. Avoid extreme neck mobilizations, because of loss of bone integrity.

Many elderly people experience a sudden drop in blood pressure (hypotension) when they move from a recumbent position to an upright position. The massage therapist should assist the geriatric client into a sitting posture on the table (for more information, see Chapter 17, The Science of Table and Body Mechanics), allowing time for the client to adjust to the change in position. You may choose to spend this time massaging her neck and shoulder region while she is seated on the massage table. Help her to her feet, if needed; otherwise, she may become dizzy while transferring off the table, lose her balance, and fall.

THE CHRONICALLY OR TERMINALLY ILL PERSON

A **chronic illness** is a condition of the body for which there is no known cure such as multiple sclerosis, chronic fatigue syndrome, fibromyalgia, Parkinson's disease, lupus, and rheumatoid arthritis. When a client has a chronic illness, massage therapy can reduce his suffering and increase his personal comfort. Clients who are critically ill may experience good days and bad days. For the critically ill, not getting any worse is an improvement. Obtain medical clearance, and administer the massage more gently, more frequently, and for shorter periods. Constantly monitoring these clients is required because massage therapy can be tiring for them.

A **terminal illness** is a type of chronic illness in the sense that there is no cure, and the client is expected to die. Examples of terminal illness are AIDS, leukemia, and other cancers. As with the chronically ill, massage therapy can reduce their suffering and increase their comfort level. Follow the same basic guidelines used in massaging the chronically ill client. For instance, massage gently, with more frequency, and for shorter periods.

It is helpful to address your own feelings about death and dying if you work with a terminally ill person. You may attend workshops that are part of a local hospice program and read books on the subject. Several authors who have written wonderful books on the subject are Elisabeth Kubler-Ross, Stephen Levine, and Bernie Siegel. These may be helpful in working with the chronically ill because they are facing grief issues as well.

Before you decide to work with a client who is terminally ill, make a personal commitment to stay with him until death because abandonment is very difficult to face at this time. Know that you will probably become attached to the client, cry when death comes, mourn, and grieve. And grow.

CLIENTS WITH HIV AND AIDS

The human immunodeficiency virus (HIV), which is transmitted through the exchange of certain body fluids, is partially responsible for the acquired immune deficiency syndrome (AIDS). People who have the virus are said to be HIV-positive; people who have AIDS have three or more opportunistic viruses, and/or a T cell count below 100. In order to become infected by the HIV virus, three elements must occur simultaneously:

1. The virus must be in a *proper environment* to survive. The virus may be found in blood, semen, vaginal secretions, and mother's milk. It has also been found in tears, sweat, and saliva.
2. The HIV virus must be in *sufficient quantity* when entering the body. The only body fluids that contain high concentrations of the virus are blood, semen, vaginal secretions, and mother's milk. Tears, sweat, and saliva do not appear to contain enough of the virus to cause infection, as there are no known reported cases of transmission by these body fluids. It has been speculated that it would take 6 to 10 gallons of saliva to have enough concentration for the virus to be transmitted.
3. The virus must have a *port of entry*. It can enter the human body of a noninfected person through unprotected intercourse or blood-to-blood contact with an infected person. The HIV virus cannot be transmitted by simple contact with an infected person. Intact skin is adequate protection from the virus.

Author's Note

There have been no known reported cases of a massage therapist contracting the HIV virus from a client while performing massage.

The massage for an HIV-infected client is not that different from any other client. Inquire about the areas that need to be avoided, including the most recent site of bloodwork. If the HIV-infected client has Kaposi's sarcoma, deep massage is contraindicated because it can cause internal bleeding. Even light massage may be contraindicated around lesions, which can be extremely painful even if superficial.

When massaging a client who has AIDS, the therapist may take into consideration the client's general vitality, any secondary conditions, and limit any Swedish gymnastics and other range of motion exercises if the client is bedridden because this can affect bone integrity. If you are giving the massage in the hospital, check with the doctor or nurse about additional information needed to serve the client most effectively. Work carefully around tubes, catheters, needles, monitors, and other medical equipment. Under these circumstances, rarely is a 1-hour Swedish massage needed to bring comfort to an HIV-infected client.

If there is any spillage of body fluids while the client is on the massage table, wash the contaminated linens separately in hot water with detergent and a quarter cup of chlorine bleach. Dry linens with hot air. Disposable linens may be used, depending on your preference. After your client leaves, the massage table and equipment can be wiped down with a solution of one part chlorine bleach to ten parts water. If you accidentally come into contact with body fluids, immediately wash the area of contact with a disinfectant. Since it is not always possible to tell if linens have come in contact with body fluids, some therapists tend to treat all sheets as "hot" or a possible exposure hazard. Refer to

The Great Glove Debate (Related to HIV)

Standard universal precautions used by the medical profession are too extreme for the massage therapy profession. It is unnecessary to wear gloves, face mask, and goggles while giving a massage. It's a bit like wearing a life preserver in the bathtub—you are overprotecting yourself. The only precaution used (and debated) by massage therapists is medical gloves.

There are several schools of thought surrounding the use of gloves. One group of massage therapists bases glove use upon risk, and adopts the following selective, rather than universal, precautions. Gloves should be used only if the therapist has small cuts, splinter punctures, broken blisters, or other skin breaks from the wrist down; if the client has fresh sutures, open lesions, or other breaks in the skin, wear gloves.

Some massage therapists will even wear two sets of gloves when they have a bad cut. They claim that the first glove acts as surrogate skin, since their own skin is damaged, and the second glove functions as the protective barrier.

Another group of therapists advocates no glove use at all. They say that the best preparations for massage are the standard hygiene precautions that involve handwashing before and after the massage with an antibacterial soap or Betadine solution. Damaged tissue, such as open wounds, should not be massaged under any circumstances. In this regard it does not matter whether the client is infected with the HIV virus—you are going to avoid these areas anyway.

Each therapist must make this decision for herself. It is best to examine the issue from all sides, to discuss it with colleagues, and even with those who are infected with HIV virus, before deciding how to handle this sensitive issue.

Chapter 16, Health, Hygiene, Sanitation, and Safety Standards, for more information.

If you believe you have been exposed to HIV, contact your local HIV/AIDS foundation for testing, information, and free counseling.

Sanitation and cleanliness are important for the client *and* the massage therapist. Because the immune system of the HIV-infected client is not fully functional, he is more susceptible to contacting infections through simple exposure. If and when secondary complications occur, assess it as a separate and individual condition.

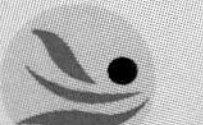

Discussion

AIDS and HIV are socially and emotionally charged issues today. Discuss with your classmates how you feel about these subjects. Begin by stating what you think the problem is, then how it affects you as a massage therapist and what precautions you will take.

Should massage therapists be routinely tested for HIV virus? Examine the legal, ethical, and medical ramifications. Perhaps it might be based on personal and professional risk factors. What if you, as a massage therapist, discover that you are HIV-positive? Should it restrict you from performing or receiving a massage? There are no right or wrong answers—only points of view.

MASSAGE AND THE DIABETIC CLIENT

Diabetes refers to a disorder of carbohydrate metabolism characterized by an elevated blood glucose (sugar) level. Long-term complications such as peripheral vascular disease and neuropathy may develop as the disease progresses. Massage can be beneficial to clients with both peripheral vascular disease (poor circulation in hands and feet) and neuropathy (decrease or change in sensation in the hands and feet).

Massage therapists must be very careful with these clients to ensure that any loss of sensory nerve function is taken into consideration. It is the massage therapist's duty to inform diabetic clients of any bruises or breaks in the skin, especially since they may not be able to see or feel all parts of their bodies. Encourage them to check their feet daily for redness, hot areas, ingrown toenails, and breaks in the skin, any of which should be reported to their physician immediately.

Other complications the diabetic client may experience are atherosclerosis, high blood pressure, blindness, and thrombosis. If your client is taking insulin, massage should not be done on or around the site where their insulin shot was given. The increased circulation will speed up insulin absorption, possibly causing a low blood sugar reaction. Vigorous massage, especially tapotement and vibration, must be carefully administered because it can damage already compromised blood vessels.

POSTOPERATIVE CLIENTS AND SCAR TISSUE

Following surgical procedures, massage can be used to promote healing and relaxation or to reduce scar tissue and adhesion. However, it is generally wise to

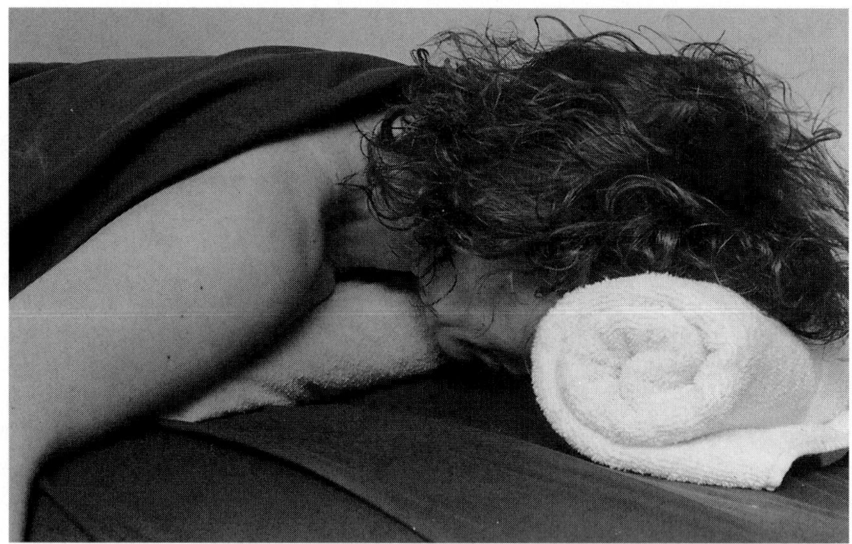

Figure 21•4 Client with kyphosis.

avoid massage therapy in the affected area until the client receives medical clearance from his attending physician.

When massage does begin, make sure to consider the reason the surgery took place as well as the physician's and patient's opinion of how successful it was. Use lighter pressure when massaging clients using anticoagulants because they tend to bruise easier. Get a verbal update on medication at every massage following surgery.

Avoid massaging scar tissue, within a 2-inch diameter, for 6 to 8 weeks and then only if all stitches and staples have been removed. Avoid any areas that are bright red, moist, or oozing or scar tissue that is not completely healed and is scabbed over. When massaging scar tissue, use a lubricant that contains any of the following: natural oils, cocoa butter, vitamin E, aloe vera, and arnica. Work the scar using friction techniques both with the fiber and across the fiber. Deeper scars from tears or muscle sutures can be accessed using deep cross-fiber friction. Stay within the client's pain tolerance.

Regardless of the type of surgery involved, the cross-fiber techniques can significantly reduce keloid scarring and break up the uneven lumps or knots that are sometimes associated with stitches. Layers of adhered tissue can be separated by using myofascial release techniques.

POSITIONING THE CLIENT WITH SPINAL ABNORMALITIES: KYPHOSIS, LORDOSIS, AND SCOLIOSIS

When massaging a client who has spinal abnormalities, positioning or table mechanics will provide a way in

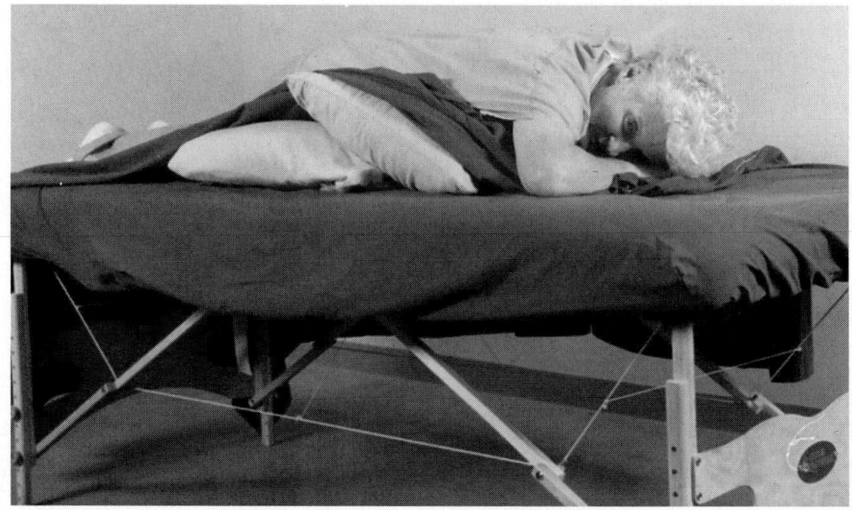

Figure 21•5 Client with lordosis.

which the client can relax in a recumbent position. Massage is effective in relaxing the affected and neighboring muscles.

Clients who have a spinal condition called *kyphosis,* or humpback condition, may be uncomfortable lying in the prone position. Place a supportive device under the clavicles and offer a standard-size pillow or a face rest for his head when your client is in the prone position (Fig. 21–4). In this way, your client can further relax and enjoy the massage.

Lordosis, or swayback, is common in clients who are overweight or who have flaccid abdominal muscles. A pillow under the anterior superior iliac spine (ASIS) while the client is in the prone position may relieve low back discomfort (Fig. 21–5). Additionally, a bolster under the ankles and using pillows to correct externally rotated femurs may help to release the hips. A bolster behind the knees while the client is lying supine may also relieve pain associated with lordosis.

Scoliosis is a spinal distortion that occurs mostly in females (60 to 80 percent). Because the abnormal curve is in the thoracic region, the ribs and hips will have distorted positions. There are different degrees of spinal distortion, so offer your client with scoliosis several pillows and suggest that she position them until she feels supported and comfortable (Fig. 21–6).

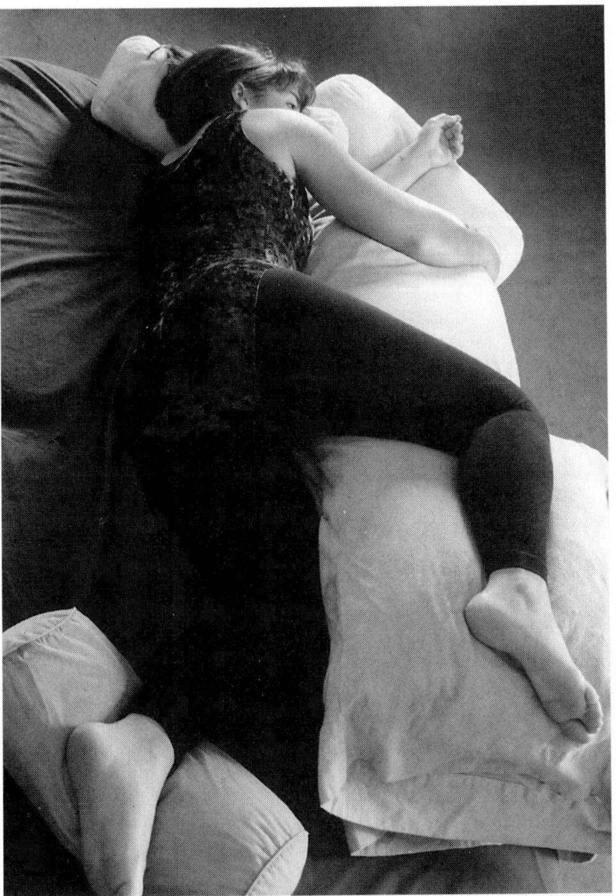

Figure 21•6 Client with scoliosis.

More information on spinal abnormalities can be found in Chapter 6. If any of these atypical spinal positions are present in your client, or if comfort cannot be found using supportive devices, you may elect to forgo massaging in the prone position.

CLIENTS WITH PARAPLEGIA, QUADRIPLEGIA, HEMIPLEGIA, AND OSTEOPOROSIS

Loss of muscle function (motor paralysis) or loss of sensation (sensory paralysis) can be due to a variety of causes such as trauma and disease. The massage pressure for clients with paraplegia (paralysis of the lower extremities and trunk), quadriplegia (paralysis of the arms and legs), hemiplegia (unilateral paralysis), and osteoporosis (thinning of bone) must be light due to the increased porosity of bone tissue. Limit all range of motion exercises, especially on the neck, spinal column, and hip joint. Assist the client on and off the table. Most clients with these conditions will be in a wheelchair (for further information, refer to the section in this chapter, Clients in Wheelchairs).

MASSAGE AND THE PERSON WITH AMPUTATIONS

If your client has an amputation, inquire about the actual surgical procedure during the premassage interview. Most clients will know this invaluable information. For instance, if a midhumeral amputation has a smooth stump with no protruding bone, it helps to know if the triceps or biceps was used to wrap the stump end. This information will help you find trigger points. Before you massage the stump, obtain permission from the client. If the client concedes, ask if the stump is sensitive or numb. Avoid areas of broken skin; use light tapotement or electrical vibration to desensitize the area. Many practitioners of energy work, such as polarity and Reiki, treat the energy field of the missing limb as if it were still present.

Approximately 70 percent of all people with amputations experience phantom limb pain (feeling pain and other sensations in all or part of an amputated limb). The onset of pain is generally within the first week but may occur several months or years after the amputation. One possible explanation of this phenomenon is that neuromas (a tumor found in nervous tissue) form on the terminal severed nerve ends of the amputated limb. Another theory states that abnormal sensory input along the afferent nerve in the amputated area enters the higher centers of the brain, resulting in pain. Another postulation is that the nerves in the central nervous system still send out signals to the length of the missing limb. Clearly phantom limb pain is complex and does involve both the peripheral and the central nervous systems. However, the calming effects of massage generally have a positive outcome on phantom limb pain regardless of the suspected pathology.

THE VISUALLY IMPAIRED CLIENT

Massage helps visually impaired people because of their need for tactile stimulation; touch is one of the most important ways they define their world. During the initial consultation, allow extra time to give and receive information. The best source of information when adapting your massage for a client who is visually impaired is the client himself. Ask your client to explain his impairment and what assistance, if any, is needed. Do not feel offended if he declines your offer for help; this is true for any client who is physically challenged.

Keep your facilities as barrier-free as possible; the floor in your office, hallway, bathroom, and massage room should be free from clutter.

Announce your presence, and speak in a normal tone of voice. Begin by addressing the client by name, then state your name. When transferring a visually impaired client from one area to another, stand just in front or to the left. He may choose to touch your right elbow and follow you. Be a gentle guide and give useful, meaningful directions. It may be helpful to describe the surroundings, using the face of a clock as a reference. Rather than saying, "There is a table in front of you," say, "There is a table at two o'clock." Go into detail about what you are going to do and what you would like him to do. Never begin a massage on a client who is visually impaired until he knows that you are in the room, and maintain contact throughout the massage as much as possible.

If your client has a service dog, do not feed, pet, or interact with the dog without permission from the client. This kind of interaction distracts the dog, making his important task more difficult.

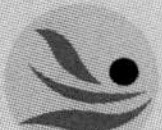

MINI•LAB

Sensory Deprivation Gather a blindfold (scarf or king-size pillowcase) and a dollar bill. Locate a partner. You will be the "explorer" first. Take the dollar bill and stick it in your pocket. Your partner will be the "attendant." Ask your partner to blindfold you.

The attendant will guide the blindfolded explorer, on foot and in silence, to a nearby store to make a refreshment purchase. After you walk back blindfolded, remove the blindfold and reverse roles. You are now the attendant and your partner is the explorer. Return to your starting point by a different route.

Share your experiences with each other. This activity is designed to experience what it is like to be without sight. You may notice a heightened sense of awareness in your other senses, such as hearing and skin sensations.

If a store is not a convenient destination, allow the students to walk a few blocks from the school and back. This activity can be done with ear plugs as well as blindfolds.

UNDERSTANDING THE CLIENT WHO HAS SPEECH DIFFICULTIES

If your client has difficulty articulating speech, or enunciating words, ask him to repeat anything that is unclear or that you do not understand. It is helpful to repeat what you heard to the client and give him an opportunity to give you clarification or further instructions.

During the premassage interview, inquire about any accommodations that can be made in his behalf. Be direct and inquire about the speech difficulty. It may be due to a physical abnormality such as cleft palate, aphasia (abnormal neurologic condition causing difficult speech and verbal comprehension) resulting from a stroke or head injury, a regional dialect or accent, dementia due to drug usage or illness, or inadequate pronunciation due to deafness (see the following section on the hearing impaired client). If a client speaks a foreign language that you do not understand, ask him if it is possible for him to bring a support person to act as an interpreter.

All feelings, both positive and unpleasant, come out of the same faucet. To turn down the faucet on pain is to slow the flow of pleasant feelings as well.

—Gay and Kathlyn Hendricks

THE HEARING IMPAIRED CLIENT

It is important to remember that hearing impaired clients communicate perfectly well; they just receive and interpret sounds differently from those of us whose hearing is intact. Be aware that even a small hearing impairment can hamper a person's ability to understand what you say. It also helps to know whether she can lip read.

Clients with long-term loss may rely heavily on lip reading. The following ideas will help the therapist to better communicate with a client who lip reads. When initiating conversation with a hearing impaired client, get her attention before you begin to speak. Eye contact is considered a sign of attention. It is perfectly acceptable to tap a person lightly on the shoulder or arm, or to wave a hand in the person's direction to attract her attention. This will be especially important

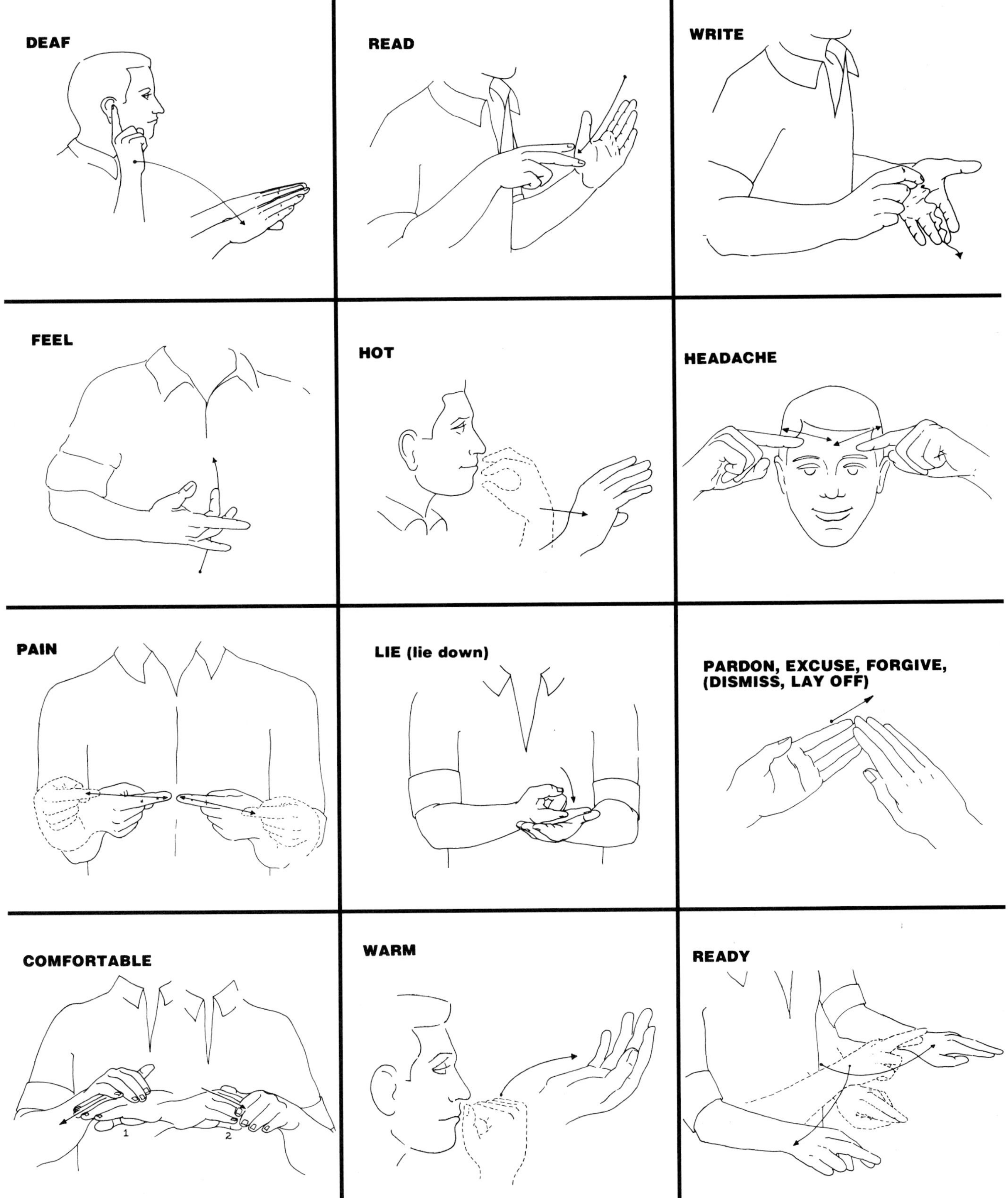

Figure 21•7 Manual skills communication. (From a Basic Course in Manual Communication, revised edition, Silver Spring MD, National Association of the Deaf, 1973.)

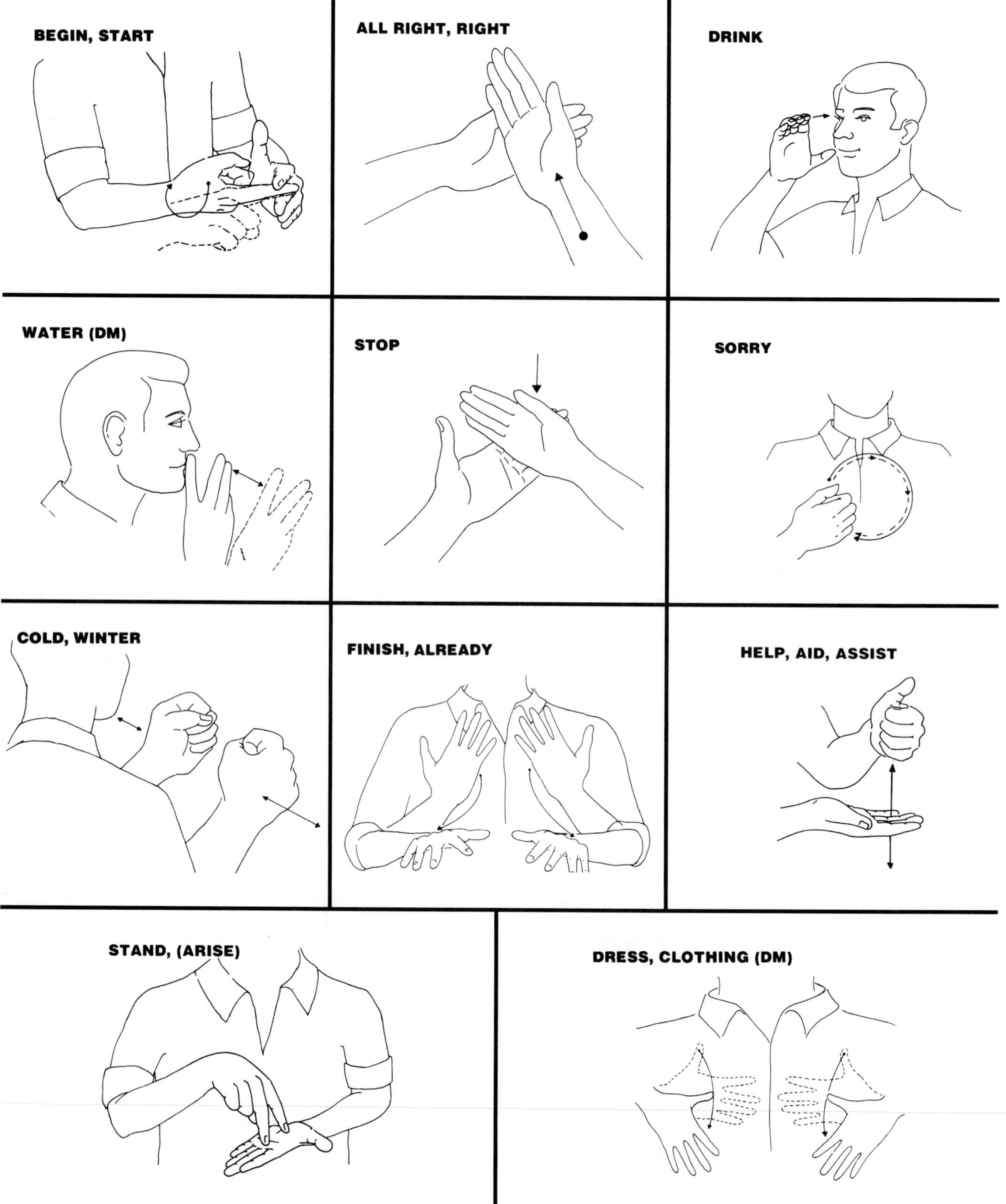

Figure 21•7 *Continued*

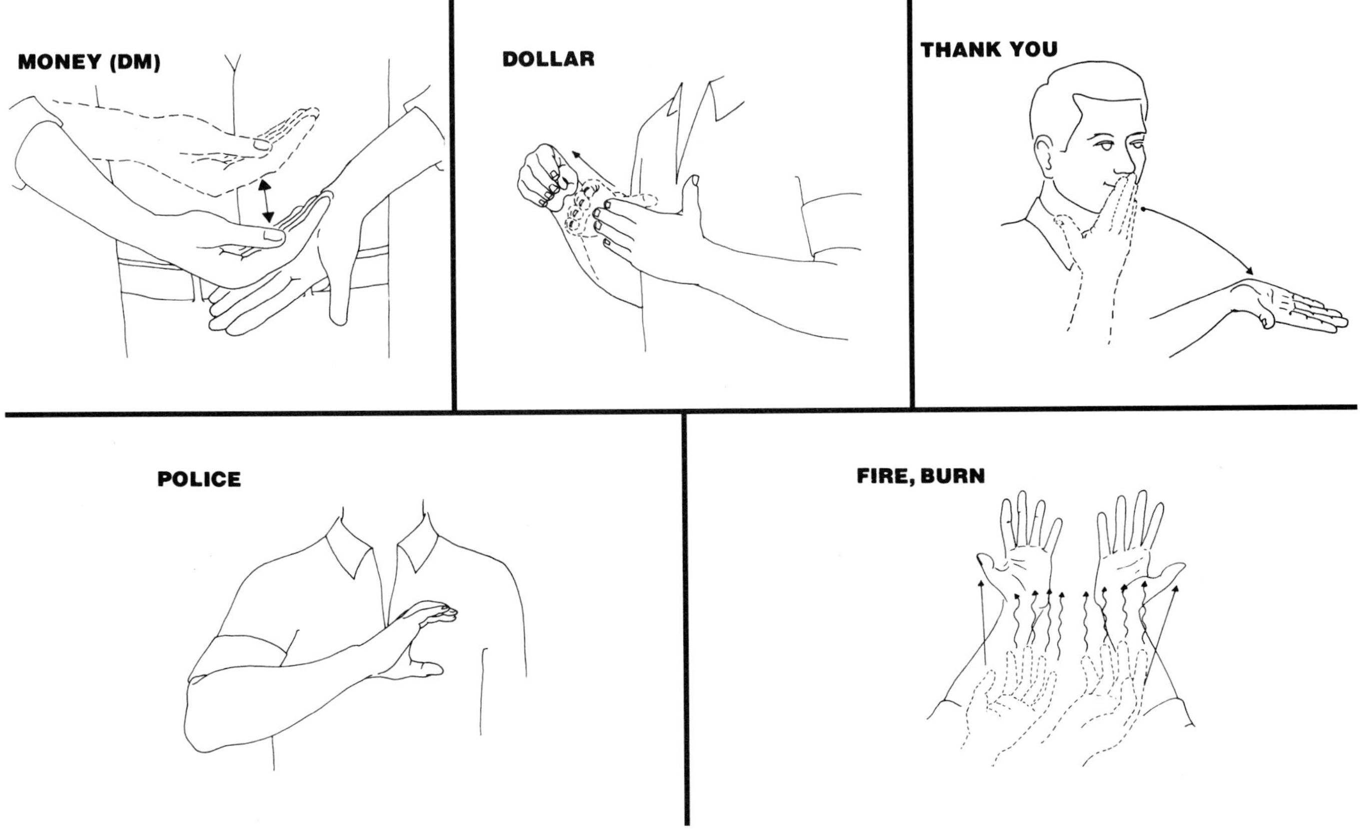

Figure 21•7 *Continued*

when the client is lying face down in the face cradle and cannot see the therapist. Face the client and maintain eye contact through the conversation. Enunciate clearly and normally, but do not exaggerate your lip movements. Use facial expressions and body language to clarify your message. Don't be embarrassed to be expressive. If she has a sign language interpreter, do not direct your conversation to the interpreter; make eye contact and talk directly with the person with the hearing impairment. Stand close and do not let any object obstruct the person's view of you. Do not eat, smoke, chew gum, or hold your hands in front of your mouth while you talk. Stand in a well-lighted place. Avoid standing with your back to a light source such as a lamp or window because this throws your face into a shadow and makes it difficult for lip movements to be clearly seen.

Allow more time during the premassage interview (refer to Chapter 22, Putting It All Together, for methods of communication that require gestures). Rephrase any sentence that the deaf client does not understand; do not just repeat the same words over and over in the same sequence. Allow time for her to respond. If you have a regular client who is hearing impaired, it may be a good investment to attend a class on sign language to be used during the interview process (Fig. 21–7).

Many people try to compensate for their hearing loss through the use of hearing aids. Do not assume that a hearing aid corrects hearing loss; it may just improve it slightly. If your client is wearing a hearing aid while she is on the massage table, avoid moving your hands close to her ears. Proximity to the hearing aid will generate feedback, producing an uncomfortable squeak in her ear. Some clients are embarrassed to use a hearing aid and may remove it before or during the session.

Remember that those clients who lost their hearing early in life may often have speech difficulties as well. When the cause of the speech difficulty is hearing loss, the client may pronounce words incorrectly. Many people make the mistake of assuming that someone with a speech problem is mentally retarded. It helps to remember that the client is *only deaf, not stupid.* Talking very slowly or using exaggerated lip movements only serves to frustrate the client. Give her the dignity you would afford any intelligent adult in normal conversation.

Many medical establishments use a flash card system for communicating with both hearing and speech impaired clients. The system consists of a single card listing a set of simple questions. The answer area of the card has a "yes" and "no" block. The client responds by pointing to the appropriate answer. This principle can be used to create a pain tolerance level flash card for massage clients.

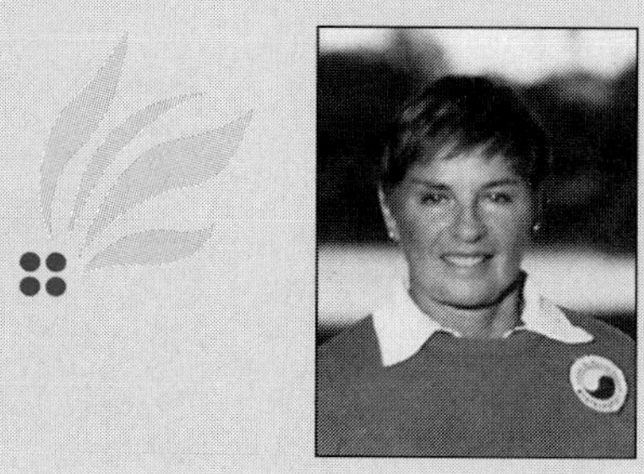

Bonnie Prudden

Born: January 29, 1914

"Seeing ahead is fun. But pushing is very hard work."

The next time your hands grasp a taut trapezius, remember this: There is a woman, who, if she would have had her way, would have changed our physiological history. At the tender age of 2, your client would have already begun an exercise and strengthening program, supervised by Mom. The body on the table would be flexible, coordinated, and toned—and so would your own.

She is Bonnie Prudden, known in massage circles for her groundbreaking work in myotherapy, but her vision was to change the course of physical education and to develop stronger bodies from the very beginning, rather than provide pain relief for bodies unable to cope with the physical and emotional stress of everyday life.

Why should an individual—and a woman at that—be so passionate about jumping jacks and push-ups long before fitness became a fad? As a survivor of the Depression, alcoholic and abusive parents, an orphanage, and a stint in Marymount Convent (which she said was like trying "to lock a wild horse in a closet"), Bonnie Prudden found the outlet she so desperately needed in physical training. She was angry, and that anger fed her boundless, but undisciplined, energy. Prudden says she has physical educators to thank for teaching her the lessons of truth and honor. By contrast, Prudden laughs that her longtime assistant recalls learning nothing more from her physical education classes than the rules for 21 games.

Her fight for better bodies began in the early 1940s. Prudden was part of a team that tested the physical fitness level of children all over the world. Conclusions were frightening. American children were some of the weakest and were getting weaker.

"We are de-evolving physically," she explains. "Children ride the bus to school, sit down for class, ride the bus home, then sit in front of the TV or play video games until it's time to go to bed. We are a dying nation," Prudden claims, "dying from the inside out."

Ironically, Prudden was unable to recruit physical educators to join her crusade for better health and fitness. However, armed with passion and statistics, she did convince President Eisenhower to start the President's Council on Fitness. (Remember those tests you took in junior high to earn your patch from the president and how you yearned to be the fastest one up and down the rope, the longest distance jumper, the strongest to throw the softball?)

To some, implementation of such a program would have been considered a milestone. To Bonnie Prudden it was a compromise. She knew children could—and should—be stronger. She responded by publishing book after book on the subject and even introduced the first infant exercises in *Sports Illustrated* as early as the 1960s.

But it was completely by accident that she "hit upon" myotherapy. Through a combination of seeking relief from her own pain after a skiing accident and familiarity with the work of Dr. Hans Kraus, Dr. Janet Travell, and Dr. Desmond Tivy, myotherapy was born. Travell says it was sheer serendipity. Though it happened over years, here are some of the highlights: One morning Prudden woke up for a mountain climb with a neck so stiff it threatened to change her plans. While examining her neck, Dr. Kraus, an associate eager to get on with the climb, grabbed a spot and and Prudden said, "I thought my eyeballs might pop out of my head, it hurt so bad." But when he let go, her neck was straight.

During work with Dr. Tivy, Prudden's job was to circle the patient's painful area for the doctor to inject—a method pioneered by Janet Travell—then show the client how to exercise the area to prevent further problems. During one of these sessions, Prudden "marked the spot" and

Continued

voila! the pressure itself took care of the pain *without* injection. These events, coupled with her knowledge of anatomy and physiology, led to the study and development of myotherapy.

At the most basic level, myotherapy (*myo* meaning "muscle," *therapy* meaning "service to") involves the application of noninvasive pressure to painful muscular areas or specific prescribed points that may cause pain in another location (referred pain or satellite pain). Pressure is applied to these areas—using the finger, elbow, or a special tool—long enough to cut off or limit the oxygen supply to the area and/or fatigue the muscle, thus effecting change.

These painful areas or trigger points are consistently located irritable spots in a muscle that contribute to pain. This recurring pattern allowed Travell and then Prudden to map these points. (For a more scientific definition of trigger points, Prudden quotes Janet Travell, M.D., coauthor of *Myofascial Pain and Dysfunction.* Travell laid much of the groundwork for myotherapy. Therapists and students interested in trigger point therapies can benefit from the excellent illustrations and body mapping found in this text, as well as the medically oriented approach to, and definitions of, myofascial pain disorders.)

Prudden's textbooks on this subject, unlike Travell's, are written in laymen's terms. Basically, any number of things can cause trigger points. It could have happened the summer you were 8 and the hay bale came crashing down on your head or just the other day when you lifted the desk to move it a couple of inches away from the wall. It may have even happened during your trip from your mother's womb into your new world. Regardless of the injury or insult to the muscle, trigger points may lie dormant until an emotionally or physically stressful event becomes the proverbial straw that breaks the camel's back. The muscle spasms, and the autonomic nervous system reacts and compensates by sending more spasm to the affected area to prevent further threat. This spasm-pain-spasm cycle shortens the muscle. Myotherapy returns the muscle to its lengthened, relaxed state.

But myotherapy doesn't stop there. Injured and insulted muscles were probably weak or shortened muscles to begin with. That's why exercise, which includes stretching, is as integral to the success of myotherapy as the application of pressure to prescribed trigger points.

Massage therapists across the country are beginning to combine different styles of massage, including myotherapy, to address the special needs of clients. For instance, some massage therapists use traditional Swedish massage strokes to warm up the tissue and locate trigger points during the first half of the massage session. Later in the session, they return to these painful areas to apply deeper work, such as myotherapy, concluding with effleurage to flush out toxins that may have been released during the deeper work.

Prudden's advice for massage therapists? What else—Exercise and stretch religiously. "You can't help people if you're not in good condition yourself," she warns. She also acknowledges the emotional toll of full-time massage therapy work and recommends a creative outlet such as dance, drawing, or sculpting, which she has incorporated into her school curriculum. She adds that it's important for students to get out and teach the community what they've learned about taking care of the body and managing pain.

Today the 84-year-old Prudden takes exercise as seriously as ever, though

continued on page 496

Continued

Bonnie Prudden

she has reluctantly heeded her body's message to slow down, which means she doesn't expect a body with two hip replacements to scale any major mountains. (According to a recent article in *Massage,* "No woman has yet surpassed Prudden's place in climbing history.") She personally teaches and inspires students at the Bonnie Prudden School for Physical Fitness and Myotherapy in Tucson, Arizona. To learn more about myotherapy, check out Prudden's books on the subject: *Myotherapy, Bonnie Prudden's Complete Guide to Pain-Free Living* and *Pain Erasure.*

CLIENTS IN WHEELCHAIRS

The first consideration when working with a client in a wheelchair is how he will enter your massage establishment. Most municipalities require businesses to be barrier-free, but if yours is not, schedule a home visit and perform the massage off-site.

When you speak to a client who is in a wheelchair, sit down in a chair or a stool, or kneel down on the floor to be able to speak to him at his eye level. Inquire about his particular limitations. Avoid making assumptions—just because your client is in a wheelchair does not necessarily mean that he is paralyzed. He may be inactive, unable to walk long distances, depressed, or have a short-term injury such as a broken foot.

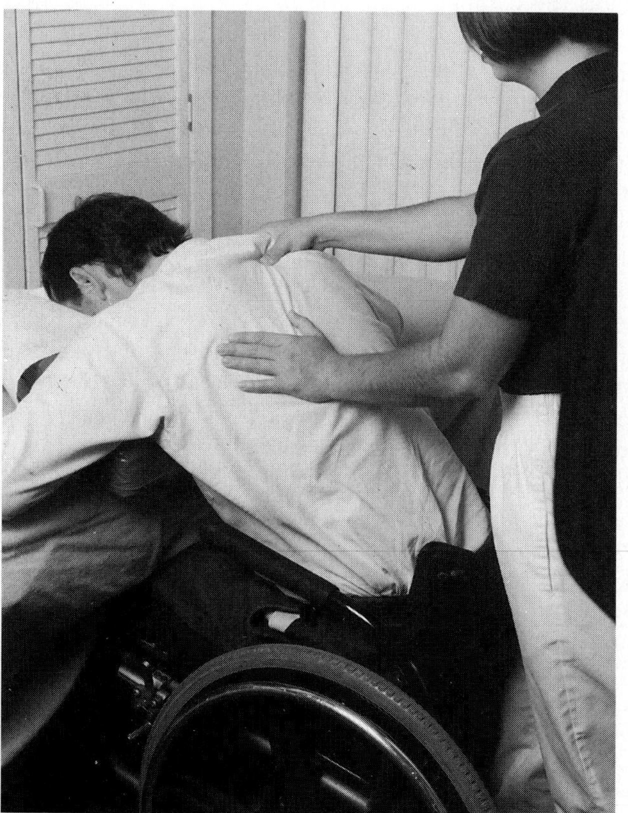

Figure 21•8 Client in a wheelchair receiving a massage.

During the massage, it is important to remember that being paralyzed does not mean that the client cannot detect pressure and vibration. Ask him directly for valuable feedback regarding pressure, body warmth, and how he feels positioned on the table. You may be required to massage the client while he is in the chair (Fig. 21–8). Modify your massage techniques and body mechanics as needed. Trigger points may be located in the shoulders and chest area from moving about in the chair. Range of motion exercises can be administered to active joints safely.

Never push a wheelchair without permission from the person in the chair. When moving the client from the chair to the table, he can give you the best instructions on how to proceed. Usually the person in the wheelchair has learned how to "transfer" or move himself in and out of the chair.

MASSAGE AND CLIENTS WITH SUBSTANCE ABUSE AND DRUG ADDICTION ISSUES

Addictive or compulsive disorders develop when the individual starts using a mood-altering chemical as a temporary chemical "escape" from unpleasant emotions. Some of these uncomfortable feelings are pain, inadequacy, sadness, loneliness, anger, and fear. The behavior continues to escalate until the consequences of the addiction exceed the pain of the original experience, trapping the person with the disorder in a cycle of pain and escape. Examples of chemical dependency disorders range from nicotine and caffeine addiction to alcohol and narcotic abuse.

Massage therapy may be part of the recovery process for clients with addictions because it is effective for relieving stress and flushing out the lymphatic system during chemical withdrawals. Deep work should be avoided because it releases toxins into the system and this may tax an already burdened detoxification period. During episodes of **recidivism** (relapse into the previous condition such as substance abuse), massage can be used for its psychological as well as physiological benefits.

While massage can assist the recovering addict through relaxation and increased body awareness, education and support are probably the best tools for overcoming this disorder. Most massage therapists are not licensed to provide counseling services, but can offer these special clients acceptance and moral support as a part of their recovery.

WHAT IF A CLIENT HAS BEEN SEXUALLY ABUSED?

It is likely that you will meet clients who are survivors of sexual abuse. Abuse crosses all population barriers, with both perpetrators and survivors being male and female, straight and gay, old and young, poor and wealthy. The majority of these incidents tend to be perpetrated by family members, extended family members, friends of family members, or friends of the survivor (e.g., date rape). Many survivors require special consideration during massage therapy, and in some cases, massage may even be contraindicated. This is generally up to the client, but she may need an extended period to build rapport with the therapist before any massage work actually begins. She may be unable to accommodate any touch and benefit more with some form of energy work. In any case, treatment can best be provided by a massage therapist who has an understanding of the dynamics of abuse as well as of the steps to take to make massage therapy emotionally and physically safe.

One of the reasons that sexual abuse is so traumatic is because sex is such a powerful experience. It has the potential of being the ultimate expression of intimacy or one of the worst bodily assaults possible. Many survivors become people of extremes, often developing other addictions, such as to food. These survivors may overeat to a point of obesity, cocooning themselves from others emotionally and physically by hiding inside excess body weight. Other survivors may relate to their body as the source of self-esteem and become compulsive about exercise and diet. To anesthetize the pain of the abuse, many will develop alcohol, nicotine, caffeine, and narcotic dependencies. Frequently it is depression or chemical addictions that get most survivors of sexual abuse involved in counseling. As the survivor begins to peel back different layers of various issues, she discovers incidences of abuse underneath, or she may have always been aware of the abuse.

The "extreme" behaviors may also involve sexual inappropriateness. Many survivors may fear or encourage sexual interactions; they may have difficulty understanding appropriate sexual boundaries. For a victim of sexual abuse, part of the healing process is to be in contact with positive role models. As massage therapists, we must be aware of our own issues surrounding sexuality and possess good boundaries so we can role model this behavior. If you are not clear about your own boundary issues, or if you experience feelings of sexual attraction toward a particular client, refer her to another therapist.

If a client confides in you that he has an abusive history, take extra precautions to ensure a nurturing, safe, and healing environment. Some suggestions are to close window blinds, turn off the telephone, and reduce noises that may trigger a startled response. *Ask the client if he knows what his triggers are.* Common triggers are perfume, certain body positions, touch in a particular area, lightning, the color red, and certain kinds of music. Allow the client to set the boundaries from one massage to the next and reassure him that he has control of the session. Examples of boundaries are draping issues, areas to be worked on, speed and depth of massage, and length of time an area is to be worked. Ask for a contact person who knows of the client's abuse history. She can be contacted if the client needs care beyond the scope of the massage. This person may be a counselor or a support group member. Often massage itself may act as a trigger mechanism for old abuse issues.

Occasionally a client's physical body may "remember" a past traumatic event while receiving a massage. These repressed memories come to the conscious mind by a mechanism called **state-dependent memory,** which is triggered by duplicating the original position of a client, location or amount of pressure, body movements, emotions, and nervous system activation at the time the experience occurred. When your body assumes a particular position or a certain set of circumstances, your body recalls the past experience, for example when climbing on a bicycle for the first time in 20 years.

Some survivors of abuse cope with the original trauma by "leaving the body," to not feel, or to believe that the abuse was happening to someone else. This coping mechanism is called **dissociation.** Clients may relive abuse memories during a massage and repeat the dissociation. Signs of dissociation are the client becoming unresponsive, a distant look in the eyes, shaking, disorientation, loss of clarity between the present and the past, and a shift in breathing pattern.

It is not our job to change the coping mechanism by reminding the client to remain aware of her body. Neither is it our job to remove a coping skill or to use guilt for the coping skill. It takes time to learn to cope differently, and we must honor the ways in which the client has learned to survive. We must also honor her need for emotional release. Do not massage when it has just retriggered the client because further dissociative touch can be traumatizing.

Emotional Release

Occasionally, survivors of abuse will release physical or emotional tension during a massage session. These releases can manifest themselves as a deep sigh, a stream of tears, laughter, shaking, uncontrollable muscle twitching, or in rare cases, a thrashing temper tantrum. These emotional expressions may be an indication of pain, sadness, anger, or even rage. The causes of these releases may be suppressed emotions that are "locked" in the muscles and released through massage therapy. Muscle twitching may be a physical manifestation of "body memories" that are trauma induced during the time of the abuse and may occur at any time, not just during a massage. Some clients let down their defenses (or walls) and release emotions during massage because of the high level of intimacy and safety they experience with their therapists.

If the client is in counseling, her emotions are typically closer to the surface, and she is more likely to experience emotional releases. The most common form of emotional release is tears or crying. Chances are that the tears are not about physical pain. Here are some tips on handling your client's tears. If the client is aware that she is likely to experience a release during the session, it is better to orient her by explaining the following process in advance.

1. Approach the emotional expression with the attitude of total acceptance. Do not interfere with questions.
2. Discontinue the massage and make touch contact in an area that is neutral to the abuse (shoulders, arms, feet; this should be determined before the massage begins). Most clients prefer to stop the massage because their bodies have another job now—crying. Avoid leaving the massage room unless instructed to do so by the client. Leaving the room may be interpreted as abandonment. Help provide a safe place for your client to experience and release these emotions without explanation or judgment.
3. Don't be quick to offer facial tissues. Drying someone's tears or offering the tissue too fast can be taken as disapproval of crying and of the feelings beneath it.
4. When appropriate, remind your client that the tears, shaking, or fear is all right, that she is in a safe place. Ask the client if she would like to take a short break, would like for you to offer a comfort measure, would like her hair stroked, or would like to end the massage session.
5. No matter which option she chooses, be calm and accepting of the response, and never encourage or repress the response.
6. Get in touch with your own feelings about others expressing emotions. You must be willing to witness another person's pain without interrupting him. While we may either feel empathic or uncomfortable with the client's tears, we need to give him time and the place to experience the emotion without interruption.
7. We are not counselors, but we can support the client emotionally. You can be supportive with comments such as, "It's all right to cry; in fact it's good to cry," or "Tears are part of the natural cleansing process of the body."
8. In most instances, it is best to continue the massage. This allows the body to integrate the information. Clients may ask that the massage continue, but to a less emotionally charged area, such as the hands or feet.

After the Storm: Responding to Your Client's Emotional Release

1. If the client asks for an explanation of what happened, mirror back to her what you observed. Do not offer your personal interpretation or analysis, but you might mention your understanding of state-dependent memory.
2. Dissociation typically leaves the client in an emotional void. Many clients will be self-conscious. They may want to leave before they are ready to go back to the "real world." Provide a safe, private space for them to do some integrating of the experience, whether with yourself, by themselves, or on the phone with their counselor. Avoid asking the client to leave while she is in a raw, open, wounded, or disassociated state.
3. When appropriate, refer the client to a qualified mental health counselor.

If you are truly uncomfortable with the client's emotional release, be honest with yourself. Support her through the experience as best as you can while she is on the table. Later, share your feelings of apprehension with a counselor, fellow therapist, or a peer support group. Process your feelings and see if you can get past your apprehension.

If you choose not to work with survivors of sexual abuse, discuss your limitations with your client during a consultation. It is inappropriate to discuss how uncomfortable you are while she is on the massage table or immediately after the emotional release when she may feel vulnerable. Simply communicate only that you cannot provide the care the client needs. Make sure that *you* take ownership of the limitation or boundary, then refer the client to a massage therapist who is trained and comfortable in dealing with these issues.

Working with survivors of sexual abuse requires special skills and much empathy. If you are planning on working specifically with survivors, familiarize yourself with these issues through reading (obtain copies of *The Courage to Heal* and *Allies in Healing* by Ellen Bass and Laura Davis), seminars, or taking an introductory class at a university. Another resource is a support group called *Survivors of Incest Anonymous.* Although there are many support programs available, there is no substitute for a qualified psychotherapist who specializes in sexual trauma. Find out who the good ones are in your area and do referral work with them.

As is true with all of your clients, always remember that confidentiality is a sacred trust. Everyone has painful psychological issues at some point in their lives. Protect the anonymity of your clients. It is their right alone to divulge personal information.

SUMMARY

Massage is a very adaptable medium of therapy; the diversity of routines are so great and so rich that there are endless variations. By applying specific combinations of these variations, we can reach out to assist those individuals with special needs who fall outside the average treatment session, including physical, emotional, and health challenges. These can be met by using adaptive massage techniques and basic client management to ensure client safety and to eliminate restrictive barriers.

Client respect is the primary focus of adaptive massage. Whether you understand the client's condition, respect for him is essential before a therapeutic relationship can be established. The patients themselves are almost always the most valuable source of information. Once respect and communication have been firmly established, adaptive massage techniques can be used to heal and enrich the lives of your special clients. Working in this type of practice requires commitment, patience, discipline, and flexibility. It can also be one of the most gratifying areas of the profession.

SELF-TEST

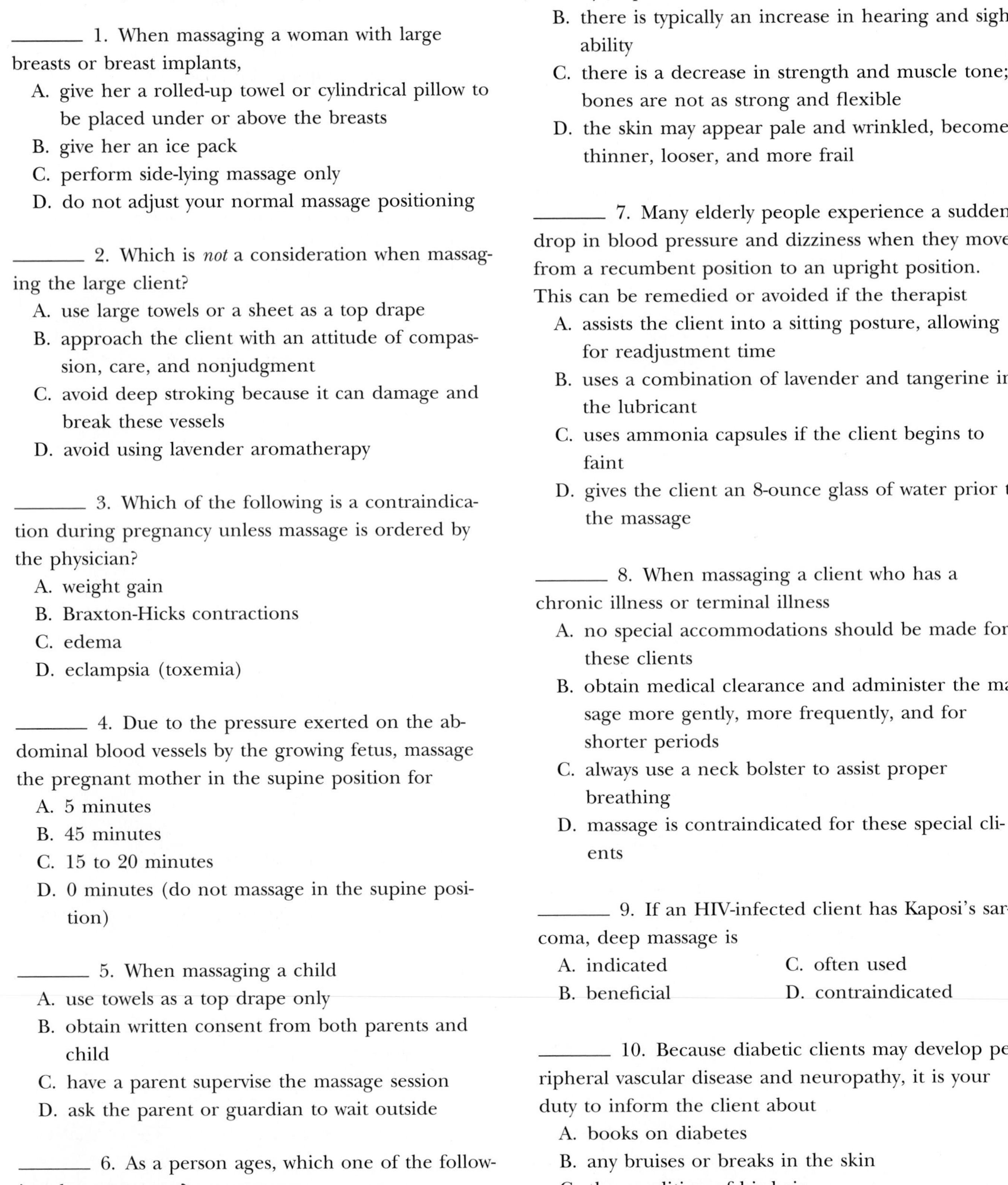

Multiple Choice • Write the letter of the best answer in the space provided.

_______ 1. When massaging a woman with large breasts or breast implants,
- A. give her a rolled-up towel or cylindrical pillow to be placed under or above the breasts
- B. give her an ice pack
- C. perform side-lying massage only
- D. do not adjust your normal massage positioning

_______ 2. Which is *not* a consideration when massaging the large client?
- A. use large towels or a sheet as a top drape
- B. approach the client with an attitude of compassion, care, and nonjudgment
- C. avoid deep stroking because it can damage and break these vessels
- D. avoid using lavender aromatherapy

_______ 3. Which of the following is a contraindication during pregnancy unless massage is ordered by the physician?
- A. weight gain
- B. Braxton-Hicks contractions
- C. edema
- D. eclampsia (toxemia)

_______ 4. Due to the pressure exerted on the abdominal blood vessels by the growing fetus, massage the pregnant mother in the supine position for
- A. 5 minutes
- B. 45 minutes
- C. 15 to 20 minutes
- D. 0 minutes (do not massage in the supine position)

_______ 5. When massaging a child
- A. use towels as a top drape only
- B. obtain written consent from both parents and child
- C. have a parent supervise the massage session
- D. ask the parent or guardian to wait outside

_______ 6. As a person ages, which one of the following does *not* occur?
- A. nerve and reflex reaction time is less than normal and there may be a loss or increased sensitivity to pain
- B. there is typically an increase in hearing and sight ability
- C. there is a decrease in strength and muscle tone; bones are not as strong and flexible
- D. the skin may appear pale and wrinkled, become thinner, looser, and more frail

_______ 7. Many elderly people experience a sudden drop in blood pressure and dizziness when they move from a recumbent position to an upright position. This can be remedied or avoided if the therapist
- A. assists the client into a sitting posture, allowing for readjustment time
- B. uses a combination of lavender and tangerine in the lubricant
- C. uses ammonia capsules if the client begins to faint
- D. gives the client an 8-ounce glass of water prior to the massage

_______ 8. When massaging a client who has a chronic illness or terminal illness
- A. no special accommodations should be made for these clients
- B. obtain medical clearance and administer the massage more gently, more frequently, and for shorter periods
- C. always use a neck bolster to assist proper breathing
- D. massage is contraindicated for these special clients

_______ 9. If an HIV-infected client has Kaposi's sarcoma, deep massage is
- A. indicated
- B. beneficial
- C. often used
- D. contraindicated

_______ 10. Because diabetic clients may develop peripheral vascular disease and neuropathy, it is your duty to inform the client about
- A. books on diabetes
- B. any bruises or breaks in the skin
- C. the condition of his hair
- D. your experience with diabetes

_______ 11. After a surgical procedure, avoid massaging scar tissue for

A. 24 hours
B. 72 hours
C. 6 to 8 weeks
D. 1 to 2 weeks

_______ 12. Which massage stroke can significantly reduce keloid scarring and break up uneven lumps, once the scar is properly healed?

A. cross-fiber friction
B. nerve stroke
C. vibration
D. tapotement

_______ 13. A client with lordosis may experience a reduction in low back discomfort if a pillow is placed

A. under the abdomen in the prone position
B. under the clavicles in the prone position
C. under the feet in either the prone or supine position
D. under the head in the prone position

_______ 14. Clients with scoliosis should be offered pillows to be placed

A. under the abdomen in the prone position
B. under their clavicles in the prone position
C. under the feet in either the prone or supine position
D. wherever they feel supported and comfortable

_______ 15. Prior to massaging a client with an amputation

A. obtain all surgical records
B. obtain permission from the client
C. take a course in polarity or Reiki
D. wash hands with Betadine solution

_______ 16. When working with clients who are visually impaired, which one of the following is *not* an appropriate adaptive measure?

A. announce your presence in a loud, clear voice
B. orient them to their surroundings
C. tell them what you are going to do and what you would like them to do
D. begin the massage after they know that you are in the room, and maintain contact throughout the massage as much as possible

_______ 17. If your hearing impaired client is wearing a hearing aid, avoid

A. deep pressure on the pectoralis major muscle
B. loud music and bright overhead lights
C. moving your hands close to his ears
D. the use of hot and cold packs

_______ 18. When your client is in a wheelchair, which one of the following is a suitable accommodation?

A. sit down in a chair or a stool, or kneel down on the floor so you can speak to him at eye level
B. inquire about his particular limitations
C. be prepared to massage him in the chair, if needed
D. all the above

_______ 19. Massage therapy can be used as part of the recovery process for clients with addictions because of its effectiveness in relieving stress during chemical withdrawals, but deep work should be avoided because it

A. stimulates endorphin production
B. releases toxins into the system which may tax an already burdened detoxification period
C. may cause episodes of recidivism
D. may cause numbness and tingling down the extremities

_______ 20. Occasionally a client's physical body may "remember" a past traumatic event while receiving a massage. These repressed memories come to the conscious mind by a mechanism called

A. state-dependent memory
B. precognition
C. dissociation
D. telepathy

_______ 21. One way the survivors of abuse cope with the original trauma is to "leave the body" or to believe that the abuse was happening to someone else. This coping mechanism is called

A. state-dependent memory
B. precognition
C. dissociation
D. telepathy

_______ 22. Which one of the following is *not* appropriate when confronted with a client's emotional expression of tears?

A. leave the room immediately and check back in 5 minutes

B. approach the emotional expression with the attitude of total acceptance
C. discontinue the massage and just lay your hands on her shoulders or back
D. remind your client that the tears are all right and that she is in a safe place

_______ 23. Even though most massage therapists are not counselors, you can

A. advise clients on personal matters
B. share with clients your interpretation of their expressed emotions
C. use the DSM-IV to offer clients a psychiatric diagnosis
D. support clients emotionally

References

Barstow, Cedar. *Tending Body and Spirit: Massage and Counseling with Elders.* Self-published book. 1985.

Bass, Ellen, and Laura Davis. *The Courage to Heal.* Philadelphia: Harper & Row, 1988.

Fritz, Sandy. *Fundamentals of Therapeutic Massage.* St. Louis: Mosby–Year Book, Inc., 1995.

Gould, Barbara E. *Pathophysiology for the Health-Related Professions.* Philadelphia: W. B. Saunders, 1997.

Ignatavicius, Donna D., and Marilyn Varner Bayne. *Medical-Surgical Nursing: A Nursing Process Approach.* Philadelphia: W. B. Saunders, 1991.

McKay, Matthew, Martha Davis, and Patrick Fanning. *Messages: The Communication Skills Book.* Oakland, CA: New Harbinger Publications, 1987.

Rounseville, Cheryl. "Phantom Limb Pain: The Ghost That Haunts the Amputee." *Orthopedic Nursing,* March/April, 1992.

Tortora, Gerald J. *Introduction to the Human Body: The Essentials of Anatomy and Physiology,* 3rd ed. New York: HarperCollins Publishers, 1994.

Fish will be the last to discover water.

—Albert Einstein

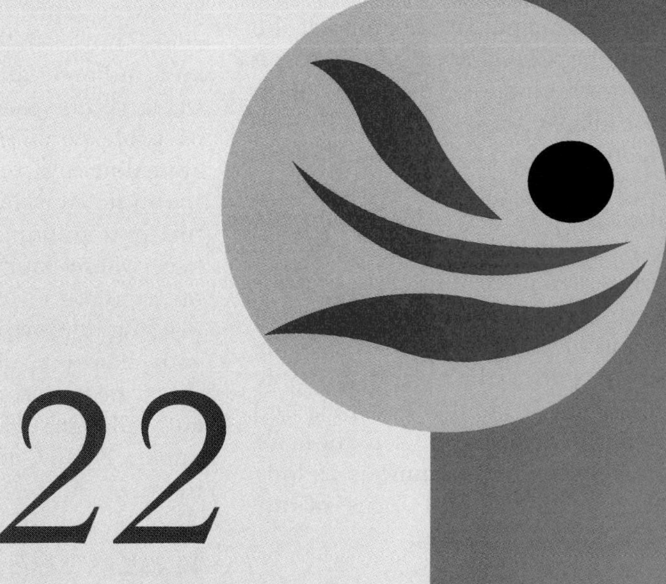

22 Putting It All Together

Student Objectives

After completing this chapter, the student should be able to:

- Prepare a workspace before the client arrives
- Demonstrate how to greet a client and prepare him for the massage
- Get ready for the massage session with movement and breath work
- Role play, addressing the client's care and comfort needs and show how communication and feedback will be handled during the massage
- Give a massage using the elements discussed in this textbook
- Design or locate follow-up information, to be dispensed to the client after the massage

INTRODUCTION

This chapter is designed to put all you have learned into practice by simulating a representative massage session. Realizing that there is no such thing as a "typical" session, we will concentrate on common elements that do exist. The union of these elements, as discussed throughout this textbook, is a routine.

In this chapter we will dissect our massage routine into its various segments and will also discuss the therapist's duties during each segment. The sections of the massage are (1) Before the Client Arrives, (2) When the Client Arrives: Room Orientation and Preparation for Massage, (3) Before the Massage Session, (4) During the Massage Session, and (5) After the Massage Session.

Massage is not a fixed process. A routine is simply a road map to help you learn your way around. As we discuss a massage routine, keep in mind that there is room, and even a need, for creativity. You can invent massage strokes. For instance, you can massage the palm of the hand and the sole of the foot at the same time! You could try massaging around the scapula and up the neck simultaneously for a unique sensation for your client. Your session will indeed be unique as long as you keep the client as the central focus of the massage.

BEFORE THE CLIENT ARRIVES

If possible, try to arrive at least 30 to 60 minutes before your first appointment. Check your answering machine or answering service, and take care of any calls. You may want to call each person the day before the scheduled massage to verify the appointment. This will reduce any confusion and minimize "no shows." Look over your schedule, and review any client intake forms. If you are expecting a first-time client, have the blank intake form and any literature ready.

Clean all the massage equipment. Prepare the table and the ambiance in the massage room before the client arrives. If you have prepared your massage room the day before, inspect the room for any unexpected items (e.g., dead insects that may have appeared while you were away). When your client enters the massage room, music should be playing, lighting should be soft and indirect, and the room should be inviting and warm (both visually and thermostatically). It is a mark of professionalism to have the massage area visually appealing and ready to go (bolsters, linens, lubricant). If you do not allow enough time between massages for this preparation, have a place (e.g., waiting room, office) where your client can wait while you prepare the massage room.

Using a mirror, critique your own appearance. Is your hair out of your face? Are your nails trimmed short, neat, and clean? Are your pockets empty of keys and change? Have you removed your jewelry and watch? Finally, add a friendly smile, and you are ready to go.

> Katie and I go back years. She is my friend, my colleague, and was the matron of honor in my wedding. One day she told me a story about the importance of providing adequate lighting during a massage.
>
> Stressed and ready for some pampering, a client came in for a massage. Katie wanted to create a relaxing ambiance, so she included the warm glow of candlelight and soothing background music. As she finished what was possibly one of the finest Swedish sessions she had ever given, she turned on a lamp so her client could dress. As she turned around to tell her client "thank you" and "goodbye," she was aghast to discover that her client's back had a skin rash!
>
> The moral of the story is look before you leap. Ambience is wonderful, but have enough lighting to survey for skin conditions before and during the massage.

WHEN THE CLIENT ARRIVES: ROOM ORIENTATION AND PREPARATION FOR MASSAGE

This section is concerned with the time frame beginning with the client's actual arrival until she begins to undress for the massage. Greet your client by name at the door whenever possible. Introduce yourself (if this is your first time as her therapist) and escort her to the area where all the paperwork and interviewing will take place (refer to Chapter 20, Professional Communication, Assessment, and Documentation for this procedure). If there are any special considerations that must be addressed, discuss how the massage will be adapted to suit the client's special needs (see Chapter 21, Adaptive Massage and Client Management Issues for more discussion). The client may be overwhelmed by all the information that is needed to prepare for a safe and well-tailored massage session. It may be helpful to ask the client to show up 15 minutes early for her first appointment, or you may want to mail out in advance all the forms that you require (e.g., initial intake, consent, and brochure of your practice or policy and procedures). This packet may be titled "What to Expect" or "What a Massage Is Like." The purpose of this procedure is to decrease the client's stress and anxiety and save you time.

One approach is to direct your client to your music selection, tell him what is currently playing, and ask him to make a selection if he prefers a different kind of music. Next, direct him to your massage lubricant selection and ask him to make a choice. Point out the most popular lubricant to make the selection process easier. Take into consideration any skin sensitivities and allergies. The use of aromatherapy can help the client to unwind. These topics are addressed in Chapter 3, Tools of the Trade and the Massage Environment.

Even though draping is discussed in the premassage interview, there are often many emotions associated with disrobing and with touch that will distort the client's perspective, making directions and instructions difficult to hear. Simple directions and concise instructions will best assist the client in the transition from the mental focus of the initial consultation to the physical and emotional focus of a massage session. Be sure to allow the client time to settle into the space provided for him before giving directions on location of the massage linens (if they are on a shelf and not on the table), before positioning on the table, and before indicating when and how you will return to begin the massage. Remembering that questions may be indirect; allow time for the client to process information and ask questions. It may be necessary to show the client how to close the door to the massage or dressing area or how to draw a privacy curtain. This will only take a few moments and will lessen the chance of confusion. Every precaution should be taken to ensure the client's comfort, physical and emotional safety, and privacy. (Further discussion may be found in Chapter 2, Professional Standards and Boundaries.)

Before you exit the room, address any comfort needs your client may have. Offer the client a glass of water and suggest a trip to the restroom. Show her where to place her clothes and personal items, and explain to her any special procedures you use to handle these items. Tell the client how to lie on the table (either to get underneath the top sheet or to drape towels over her body). Tell her that you are going to leave the room so she may disrobe in privacy and that, when you reenter the room, you will knock before you open the door. This will alleviate any apprehension she may have about your unannounced return.

Client empathy is one of the reasons it is so important that you, as the therapist, receive massages from other therapists. By getting back in touch with what it is like to be a client, you will be a more attentive and sensitive therapist.

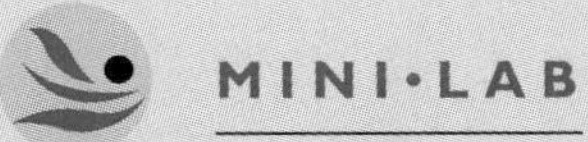

MINI•LAB

When feasible, get a massage from a therapist you do not know. For many therapists, this activity may only be possible when traveling out of town. During the massage intake, do not reveal to the therapist that you are a massage therapist or student of massage therapy. In this way, you will get the full experience of what it is like to be a client. Along with helping you learn what to do and what *not* to do, this activity will also reinforce the things you are doing that work well for the client. Role reversal can be an eye-opening experience.

Care of the Client's Belongings

Clients often wear a watch, jewelry, and bring a purse, wallet, or other valuables to the massage establishment. Since most jewelry and watches are removed before the massage begins, care must be taken to safeguard these items. Large articles, such as purses, should not leave the client's sight. For smaller items, use a large envelope or small container (e.g., basket or bowl) to accommodate the client's belongings (Fig. 22–1). A portable container allows these items to remain with the client if he must move from one room to another. A locker or locked box may also be used to store these items safely during the massage.

If the therapist removes jewelry or wristwatches for the client, it is in the therapist's responsibility to make sure the client leaves with these items. The therapist may simply indicate where the items have been placed before leaving the room for the client to dress. In the

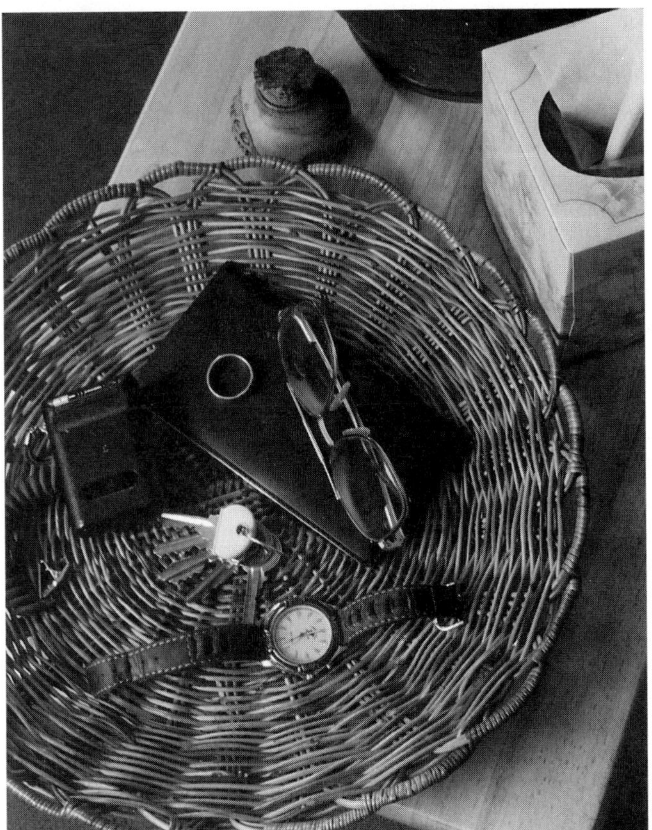

Figure 22•1 A basket or bowl for personal items.

case of a client who is physically unable to put the jewelry back on herself, the therapist should offer to assist. You may use a towel to remove the bulk of the massage lubricant from your hands before attempting to fasten watches, bracelets, and necklaces.

Often, a client may be disoriented after a massage and may accidentally forget these items while in your massage establishment. Forgetfulness is less likely to occur if the client was given an envelope in which to place her personal belongings, but a friendly reminder is always best. If you do discover personal articles in a room after a massage, place them inside an envelope and seal it. Write the date, the item, and the owner of the item. If you do not know who owns the item, call the clients who were there that day and ask them if they left anything in your studio. It is generally best to let them tell you what they are missing and give a complete description before returning the item.

Author's Note

If you remove a client's eyeglasses while she is on the massage table or if a client gives you her eyeglasses before the massage, hand them back to the client *before* she gets off the massage table and *before* you leave the massage room to allow her time to redress. If you neglect this important procedure, you may be liable if the your client trips or falls in your massage room and incurs injuries because she was unable to see clearly.

BEFORE THE MASSAGE SESSION

While the client undresses and gets onto the table, wash your hands and forearms. If you need a quick review, refer to Chapter 16, Health, Hygiene, Sanitation, and Safety Standards. Because your hands may become cool from the handwashing, warm them using direct heat or friction before the massage begins; this will warm the massage lubricant too.

You have spent much time and energy learning a craft and preparing your massage room; spend a little time preparing your mind, body, and spirit. Grounding and centering yourself before the massage is an integral part of your therapy session. If you feel distracted and not present with your client, you will not be able to give the best massage possible. Learning how to clear your thoughts, how to prepare your body, and how to ground and center yourself will help you be a more skilled and sensitive therapist.

Breathing and body movements are some techniques you can use to prepare yourself before the massage begins. No matter what style of massage you practice, you will expend energy. Before you enter the massage room, move and stretch your body while practicing deep breathing. If all you have is a few seconds, simply squat down to stretch your low back (do this only if your knees can do this comfortably), and stand up to shake out your entire body (Fig. 22–2). If you have a minute, you might want to try the following 60-Second Energy Snack. There are no calories ingested, and it's loaded with energy.

There are numerous ways to prepare yourself before the massage session. Choose what works best for your body. Breathing is discussed in the respiratory chapter, and body movements are addressed in Chapter 17, The Science of Table and Body Mechanics. As you utilize deep breathing and movement techniques, clear your mind. This does not mean forgetting everything you know about the client or his condition, but allow a new calm to exist in your thinking—a space for new pieces of the puzzle to emerge. Massage is a client-focused service and, as such, the session should center on the client's needs.

Some massage therapists choose to incorporate elements of their own spirituality into the massage. If this choice works for you, this is a good time to engage in a spiritual prayer. Some therapists choose to turn their skills and the direction of the massage over to the care of God (or a higher power). A simple prayer, verbal or silent, of gratitude for the opportunity to work with this client will help create the atmosphere for healing to occur (most massage therapists prefer to pray in silence). If you decide to pray in the massage room while touching the client, it is ethical to ask permission before praying over the client. Some clients will be fine with prayer; others will consider it too personal an issue and may be uncomfortable.

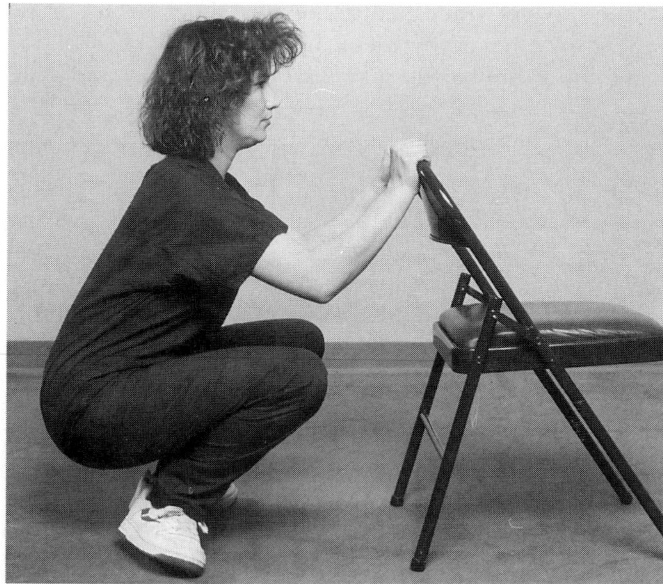

Figure 22•2 Massage therapist stretching before entering the massage room.

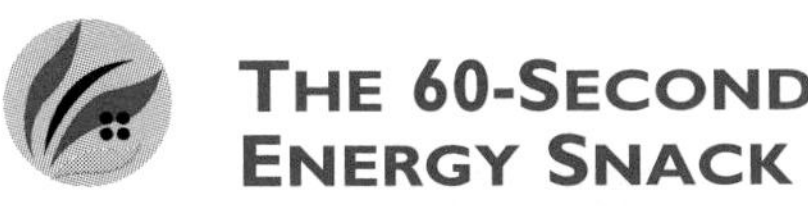

The 60-Second Energy Snack

1. Slap the palms of your outstretched hands together, and rub them rapidly for 5 seconds (out of earshot of clients, please).
2. Hold your warmed palms over your cheeks and eyes for 5 seconds.
3. Make your hands into claws and apply vigorous tapping tapotement to the scalp for 5 seconds.
4. Apply loose-fist tapotement up and down each arm for 10 seconds.
5. Gently grasp the hyoid bone, and mobilize it from side to side to stimulate the thyroid gland.
6. With your right hand, cup your palm around the back of your neck and squeeze firmly about 10 times.
7. Repeat #6 with the left hand while nodding the head at the same time.
8. Repeat #6 with the left hand while shaking the head at the same time.
9. With the right hand reach across the midline of your body and grasp the top of your left trapezius and squeeze firmly about 10 times.
10. Repeat #9 to the right trapezius with the left hand.
11. Do three sets of shoulder rolls forward and three backward.
12. Pincer-grip the thumb web of each hand and hold for 3 seconds (omit this step if you are pregnant).
13. Shake the hands out.
14. Stomp the feet several times.

You are now energized and ready to go!

*No one is useless in this world who lightens the burdens of another.*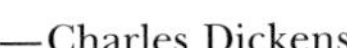

—Charles Dickens

DURING THE MASSAGE SESSION

This section of the chapter addresses the time frame that begins when the massage therapist reenters the room and ends when the massage therapist leaves the room after the massage is complete.

Before you begin the massage, address the client's care and comfort needs one more time. Ask your client if the room temperature is comfortable. It is difficult to relax while you feel chilled. Place bolsters or pillows underneath the areas of the body that require additional support (e.g., neck, knees, ankles). Remind the client about the importance of being relaxed and offering feedback during the massage. If he is uncomfortable in any way, he may not become or stay engaged with the massage.

Begin by making physical contact with the client, perhaps with quiet and still touch. Once you and the client are ready, proceed with a massage routine. There are dozens of methods for massaging the body, each effective in its own way, that are best learned in the classroom under a skilled and caring instructor.

Sometimes as you massage, you may notice the client's body becoming tense. You may silently respond to tension by changing your pressure or rhythm. If the client remains tense, ask for feedback. Reiterate how important communication is during the massage. You may discover that the client is feeling tickled or is in pain and therefore is splinting, or contracting, his muscles. Or perhaps he may have to use the restroom. Address his needs, and then continue with the massage. Be patient and caring; enhance your client's ability to relax.

Avoid becoming too talkative because this may distract from the client's overall relaxation. One guideline is to talk only when answering the client's questions and when addressing the client's comfort needs. Otherwise, stay silent and follow the client's lead. If one of your clients falls asleep during the massage, you may need to stop doing deep work and begin more relaxing massage moves. A client who is asleep will be unable to offer helpful feedback on pain and discomfort.

Designing and tailoring the session to the client's individual needs are the hallmarks of a proficient massage therapist. Every body responds differently to massage. The more you learn and practice, the greater the number of massage styles you can offer your clients. Know all your options and honor your limits. As your experience increases, you can incorporate new moves into your routine. Like any art, mastery is a lifelong process.

The following are a few general guidelines to be considered as you are applying massage. Blank lines have been added so that you can add other guidelines.

1. Work from general to specific, then back to general.
2. Be thorough and complete. Always connect body parts to themselves and to one another.
3. Stroke lightly over joints and endangerment sites.
4. Work deeply enough to contact and release tension but not so deep that you cause tension and pain! "Above all, do no harm."
5. Stay present with the person; be focused, and respect the client.
6. Use good body mechanics and table mechanics.
7. ______________________________
8. ______________________________

9. ______________________________

10. ______________________________

Communicating and Giving Directions During the Massage

Communicating and giving directions during the massage is a little different from normal conversation because eye contact is infrequent. When a client is lying prone, the head is to one side or in a face cradle; when a client is supine, either the eyes are closed, or a client must strain her neck muscles to obtain eye contact. Establish a method of communication in the premassage interview, and reinforce your instructions during the session when needed. The most important feedback a massage therapist needs is how the client is receiving the massage. More specifically, the therapist must know if there is any pain or discomfort caused by the massage. The following is an abbreviated system of communication developed by massage therapist Ralph Stephens. This system is also featured in Chapter 25, Seated Massage; it is particularly helpful in establishing and maintaining communication and in building rapport with your client during the session.

When It Hurts or If the Pressure Is Too Hard. Tell the client, "Be sure to tell me whenever I find a tender area. Will you do that for me?" or "If at any time I am working too hard, be sure and tell me right away. Will you do that?" Quantitative measuring scales you can use are:

1. Ask the client to simply raise a hand if pain is felt.
2. Use the 1 to 5 scale: 1 represents "no pain" and 5 represents "excruciating pain." You will know, by the number vocalized or the number of fingers raised, how she is responding to the pressure. A 1 to 5 scale is necessary to allow easy one-handed response.
3. Establish a "thumbs up–thumbs down–okay" gesture system. Thumbs up means that more pressure is needed (Fig. 22–3). Thumbs down means that less pressure is requested. An "okay" symbol (index finger touching thumb with other fingers extended) means the pressure is perfect.

When It Gets Better. Tell the client: "When I find these tender places, I will stop and maintain the pressure. This sustained pressure will cause the nervous system to respond by relaxing the tender area. It may feel to you like I am letting up on the pressure, or it's beginning to feel better. Will you let me know when it gets better?"

If It Refers. Tell the client: "When I am examining or maintaining pressure on an area of tissue, you may experience some sensation somewhere else. It could be a pain, tingling, numbness, aching, or some other sensation somewhere besides right where I am massaging. These may be trigger points that need to be massaged as well. Will you tell me if you feel anything other than pressure where I am working?"

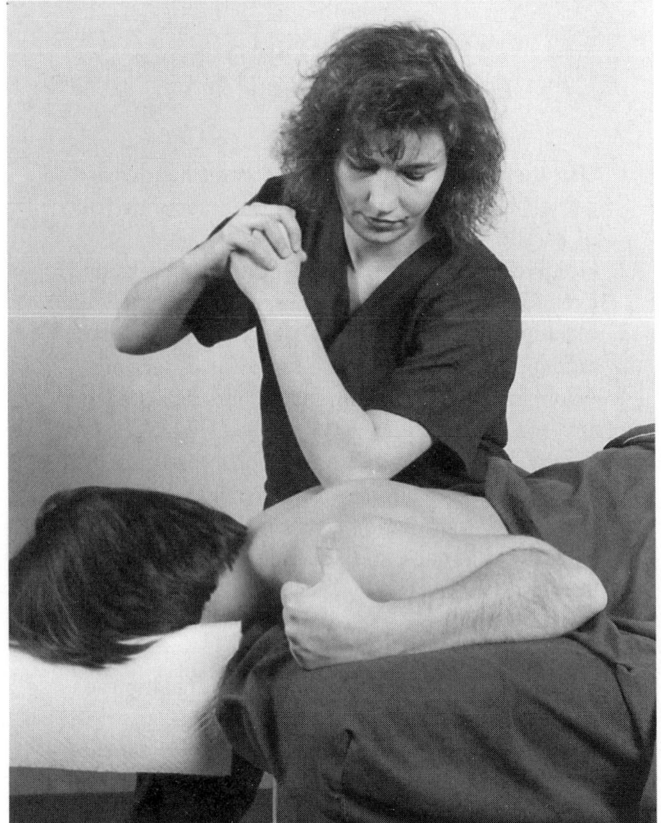

Figure 22•3 Client giving a "thumbs-up" during a massage.

Regardless of which system of feedback you use for assessing pain and pressure, use your peripheral vision, and look for physical signs of discomfort. Some clients do not voluntarily report feedback for pain. They may be accustomed to denying pain and discomfort, or they may have a different sensation and perception assigned to pain. However, the body rarely lies. Body gestures may indicate that you are working too hard; the client begins to pull away from you or contracts muscles to limit your access into the tissues. Other signs are general squirming, eyebrows rising up, holding the breath, white knuckles, and raising the head up off the table.

Another helpful tool to use when giving directions is to use tactile cues and gestures. For example, as you ask the client to scoot over to the edge of the table, gently touch her shoulder or tap the tabletop on the side you want her to move toward. This method can be used when you need the client to move up or down the table, as well as when to turn the head to one side or another. Think of it as the massage therapist's version of the neonatal "rooting reflex," a touch that causes an infant to turn toward light stimuli in order to nurse a nipple. When asking a client to turn over, if eye contact is possible, supinate or pronate your hand to indicate the direction she should roll. When giving directions in which a client should place her arms or other body part a certain way, demonstrate it first. If you need the client to raise her head, feet, or knees to accommodate a bolster, supply a gentle lifting motion with your hand. Your client may be so relaxed that verbal directions are processed slowly. These kinetic cues will help the client understand what you need her to do, so that you can provide the best massage possible.

Avoid hurrying the client off the massage table. In fact, invite her to rest a few minutes. Because the client has been in one position for an extended period, it is often helpful to ask her to roll over on her side and bend her knees to her chest. Place a soft pillow under her head, and ask her to lie in this position for a few minutes before she gets up to dress. If she is afraid of falling asleep and losing track of time, tell her that you will be back in 5 minutes to remind her to get up. This short rest period allows the client some quiet time devoid of stimuli to integrate the physical and emotional aspects of the massage, as well as transition time to move from internal focus to external focus before rescheduling, leaving, and driving. Before you leave the room, remove the bolsters and wipe off any excess lubricant from the soles of your client's feet.

You may find it necessary to instruct the client on how to get up off the table. Once lying on her side, suggest that the client allow her lower legs to fall off the edge of the table. She can then use the arm that is not lying against the massage table to push her upper body up into a seated position. Avoid letting the client sit straight up from a supine position because she may strain her back or neck. Remind the client that the best way for getting up off the massage table is also the best way to get out of bed in the morning! If your client requires assistance getting off the table, refer to Chapter 17, The Science of Table and Body Mechanics, for a discussion of an efficient method.

As you leave the massage room, let the client know if she is to wait in the room for you to return or if she needs to exit the room to find you in another area.

AFTER THE MASSAGE SESSION

This last section concerns the therapist's activities from the time he exits the massage room following the massage until the client leaves the premises. While your client is dressing, wash your hands and write any case notes, if possible. Make sure the lighting in the post-massage area is not too bright or too noisy because this type of environment is not very relaxing. Provide a transitional space. Take a few deep breaths, and prepare to greet the client with a smile.

Have ready any parting information that you wish to give the client. Information sheets can be anything from tips on how to use ice, self-massage, relaxation techniques, and theories about muscle soreness to how to preserve and prolong the effects of the massage. Without the educational element of massage therapy, the massage session may be no more than an expensive aspirin or bandage. Avoid just putting out fires; show clients how to prevent them. Clients really appreciate this added service of information on items such as how to alter sleeping positions to reduce muscle strain or how to sit in a chair more comfortably. Be familiar with your scope of practice to make sure "client education" is legal for a massage therapist in your state.

Collect fees, if you have not already done so, and ask the client if he would like to reschedule. Offering the client another glass of water is a nice touch. After the client has gone, ready your room for your next client, take a few deep breaths, and stretch out your muscles.

Some clients may want to stay and talk after the massage. If the conversation is related to the massage and the client's health and progress, the therapist should make some time to address the client's concerns. If, on the other hand, the conversation is just a friendly chat, the therapist may have other priorities. Often the massage therapist may need to tend to phone messages, wash linens, ready the massage room

10 Daily Steps for Preserving and Prolonging the Effects of Your Massage

- Drink 2 quarts of fresh water daily (for soft-tissue irrigation)
- Maintain a neutral sleeping posture by using pillows to bolster the extremities in order to keep the spine straight
- Practice movement therapies or stretches
- Apply ice packs on painful areas (10 to 15 minutes each)
- Practice postural awareness during the day
- Decrease the intake of caffeine and sugar as much as possible (these neurostimulants can increase pain perception and dehydrate the body)
- Breathe slowly, extending the exhale
- Develop a positive attitude
- Simplify/prioritize and take stress breaks
- Love yourself

©1993 Karen Zurlinden Photography

Deane Juhan

Born: April 18, 1945

"The principle is elegantly simple. We learn to love by being loved, we learn gentleness by being gentled, we learn to be graceful by experiencing the feeling of grace."

Deane Juhan is a bodyworker, one of the first Trager-trained instructors, an anatomy teacher/lecturer for the Trager Institute, and author of *Job's Body, a Handbook for Bodyworkers.* As the title suggests, the book offers an answer to the age-old question of "why" regarding the Old Testament book of Job, but that's just for starters. *Job's Body* explores "the various ways through which intuitive and informed touch can positively affect a wide variety of symptoms and help to change people's lives for the better."

The book was 9 years in the making, which is surprising considering the manner in which Juhan's words cascade mellifluously during casual conversation. (Indeed, he's the one of those rare individuals who could pronounce and use the word mellifluously without missing a beat.)

Born to a woman who "had poor taste in men" and a soldier who didn't hang around to become a father, Juhan was adopted. He grew up as an only child in Glenwood Springs, Colorado, which, as he puts it, "its only claim to fame is that it's 40 miles from Aspen." His father worked for the state and Juhan recalls when he got that "big" raise from $400 a month to $425 a month. Nonetheless, his parents were wise about using resources, and were determined that their only child's education receive top priority.

Juhan describes himself as an underachiever in high school. The University of Colorado introduced him to a whole new way of living and he admits to being caught up in the novelty of this hip, liberal atmosphere until his junior year of college when "his rudder finally bit the water," he says. It was then he became interested in the aspects of art, science, and civilization.

He "encountered" Esalen, a workshop and meeting place for developing human potential in Big Sur, California, while working on his dissertation in literature. In fact, he sneaked in and eventually began doing massage. He was so good at it, he just sort of hung around. His first experience in anatomy was developing slides and lectures for Structural Integration for Rolfing lectures. But when he witnessed Milton Trager he was hooked and abandoned all other methods to learn the Trager Approach.

"It was love at first sight," says Juhan. "I was attracted to his quality of being. It was his rich avuncular benevolence without all the preliminary folderol that made me want to learn to do what he did, so I threw myself into it and gave it my all."

But it didn't come easy for this hard-pushing 6-footer. His strength had always been—well—his strength. Nonetheless, he broke down and cried when he saw his first Trager demonstration. Then, as he clumsily applied himself to unlearning everything he ever thought he knew about bodywork, Trager reduced his ego to ashes, hollering at him during training, slapping his hand away and taking over, always admonishing him to work lighter . . . softer . . . and to quit trying so hard to get the job done.

Juhan points out that Trager's use of inducing a transcendental meditation state during a session, which has been termed "hook-up," is one of the things that sets Trager apart and makes the work so effective. It is during this hook-up that messages are communicated that have nothing to do with verbal and nonverbal interaction as we know it, and it's this exchange that's key to long-term change.

For the bodywork session, the goal is to connect with the client's sensory information, process what the practitioner helps the client discover or rediscover, then help the client "wake up" to the possibility for long-term change through movement. The practitioner lays down new patterns by repeating a movement message again and again. The feeling finally becomes etched on the client's awareness, creating an experience of length, relaxation, and pain-free movement.

Continued

Before this can be achieved, however, the bodyworker needs to understand how the body works and what this "preverbal" language is all about. Juhan also argues for bodywork to "redress some of the underdevelopment and dysfunction we find associated with various pathological conditions." But most important, he wants to change the way we think about our bodies.

In short, Juhan asserts, we've stopped "listening to the only reliable source of self-regulation and preservation we have available. It's the direct result of century-long programming that has debased our subjective awareness." When we're in pain or simply feeling bad, rather than confront what's at the root of our problem we seek help outside the wisdom of our own bodies. We go running to the doctor, the shrink, the psychic, the minister, and the self-help section of the nearest bookstore. And of course, there's nothing wrong with any of these things, but Juhan reminds us that the only thing we truly know about the world is the way our body is responding to it. And no one can know how we're responding to stimuli the way we can. In short, we are to a very great degree, responsible for our own well-being.

Juhan writes in *Job's Body:* "For Job this was revelation—the perception that God was in his very flesh, in the throbbing of his heart, in the singing of his nerves, in the coiling of his muscles, to be touched and felt more intimately than an embrace."

As a beginning massage therapist, you're probably not seeking a revelation so much as direction. You can probably guess that Juhan's advice is to look within. Choose the modality that will, according to Juhan, "flower in your psyche or experience. Look for what turns you on, look for what you love, not what the market says is hot."

for the next client, or have a bite to eat and recharge her own batteries. Usually, simply walking the client to the door, perhaps even stepping outside with him, saying thank you and goodbye, and walking back in the office is enough (Fig. 22–4). You may have to say something such as, "I really enjoy talking with you, but I have a few things to take care of." Setting a boundary is necessary to take care of yourself and to serve

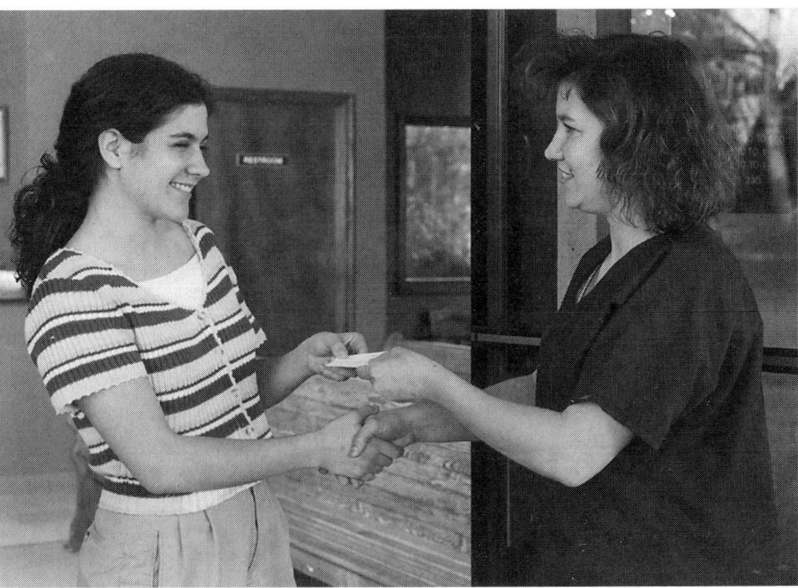

Figure 22•4 Telling a client goodbye.

MINI•LAB

The following exercise is designed to increase your level of sensitivity as a massage therapist and to strengthen your proprioception. Select a partner, and decide which of you will be the giver and which will be the receiver. Sit facing each other, and raise your hands to shoulder level. Gently flex your fingers; allow your fingertips to touch your partner's fingertips. Both the giver and the receiver then close their eyes (Fig. 22–5).

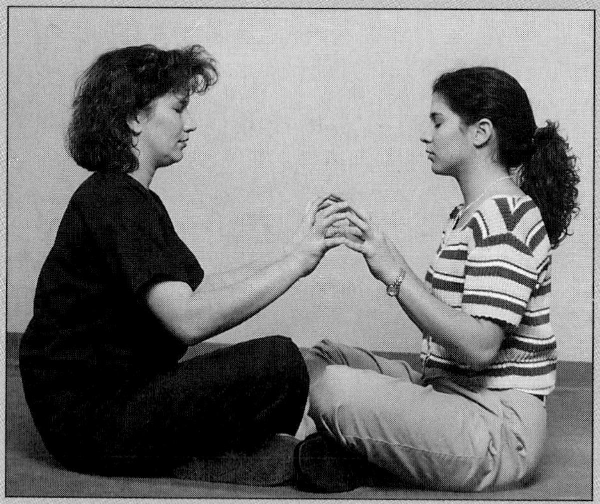

Figure 22•5 Demonstration of the position needed for push hands.

The designated giver slowly begins to move his hands in space, allowing the receiver to follow his hands while remaining connected by fingertips. This may feel awkward at first, but as the receiver expands his awareness, it begins to feel as if the two are dancing. After a minute of practice, the giver says, "switch," and the roles are reversed.

After the exercise, ask yourself the following questions. How confident were you as the giver? How did you feel as the receiver? When you were the giver, did your receiver relax and follow you, or did he tense up? There is sometimes a tendency to follow by anticipating the moves instead of experiencing the moves. The more sensitive the receiver becomes, the easier it will be to follow the giver. How can this type of sensitivity apply to massage therapy?

the other clients you have scheduled for the rest of the day.

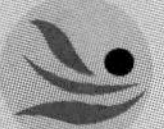

MINI•LAB

Once you have learned a basic massage routine, perform a massage blindfolded. The recipient on the table may have to assist with the draping and turning aspects of the massage because these may be too difficult for you without your sense of sight. This activity will help you get out of your head and intellect and into your hands and feeling skills.

SUMMARY

This chapter dissects the massage routine into basic components and defines responsibilities for each time frame. Before the client arrives, the massage therapist should take care of equipment cleaning, room preparation, paperwork, and personal appearance. When the client arrives, the therapist should introduce herself, gather initial intake information or get an update, explain the procedures, and answer questions. Before the massage, the therapist should wash her hands using appropriate hygiene techniques, and prepare herself emotionally, mentally, and physically. During the massage, the therapist continually addresses the client's needs by initiating contact, responding to muscular tension, and following the client's lead. The most important part of the massage process is establishing and maintaining a comfortable level of rapport with the client. After the massage, the therapist should again wash her hands, prepare the outside environment as a transition for the client, prepare any handouts for the client to take home, collect fees, and offer to schedule another appointment. Following these protocols enables the therapist to provide optimum care for the client.

Throughout the process, the massage therapist should cultivate and maintain an attitude of respect and courtesy toward her client.

SELF-TEST

Multiple Choice • Write the letter of the best answer in the space provided.

_______ 1. When you arrive at your massage therapy office, to which of the following should you attend?
A. check your answering machine, taking care of any calls
B. look over your schedule and review any client intake forms from your files
C. clean all the massage equipment and prepare the massage room
D. all are important elements

_______ 2. When you greet your client at the door, you should
A. introduce yourself if this is your first time as her therapist
B. compliment her and her hair and attire
C. greet her using her name
D. A and C

_______ 3. Telling the client that you are going to leave the room so she may disrobe in private, and that you will knock before you reenter the room, helps to
A. conduct an intake
B. signal the time to get on the massage table and drape herself
C. alleviate any apprehension she may have about your unannounced reentering the room
D. signal the beginning of the massage

_______ 4. Which of the following is *not* recommended as a way to safeguard your client's jewelry and valuables during the massage?
A. ask her to lock all valuables in her car or allow large personal items such as purses to stay in the massage room
B. place all client belongings in your pocket for safekeeping
C. provide a basket or bowl to accommodate the client's belongings
D. provide a locker or locked box to store items safely during the massage

_______ 5. Before beginning the massage, the therapist may choose to ground and center himself by using which of the following techniques?
A. breathing and body movements
B. burning incense
C. spraying a fabric softener in the room
D. all of the above

_______ 6. Sometimes as you massage, you may notice the client's body repeatedly becoming tense; you may
A. stop the massage
B. ask directly for feedback and reiterate how important communication is during the massage, changing the application if needed
C. perform light effleurage and nerve stroke for the rest of the massage
D. ignore the client's tension

_______ 7. In general, during the massage session
A. talk only when answering the client's questions and when addressing the client's comfort needs
B. ask the client to stay silent during the massage because conversation can distract the therapist
C. engage in as much conversation as possible, as long as the client discusses his problems
D. ask the client to stay silent during the massage because conversation limits his enjoyment of the music

_______ 8. When applying massage therapy, it is often best to
A. work the area of complaint only
B. work from general to specific, then back to general
C. avoid the area of complaint
D. work from general to specific, then end the massage

_______ 9. When addressing pressure with the client during the massage, it is helpful to
A. ask the client to simply raise a hand if pain is felt
B. use the 1 to 5 point scale: 1 represents no pain and 5 represents excruciating pain
C. ask the client to stand as much discomfort as possible—more pain, more gain
D. A and B

_______ 10. Which of the following sensations are *not* associated with the trigger point referred sensation phenomenon?

A. aching or pain
B. tingling or numbness
C. intense itching
D. burning or electrical shock sensation

_______ 11. To aid in your client's comprehension of directions during the massage, it is often best to

A. use tactile cues and gestures
B. talk louder
C. use telepathy
D. use questions written on note cards

_______ 12. As your client is leaving, it is a good idea to

A. get feedback about the massage session
B. ask her if she'd prefer to rebook now or call for her next appointment
C. send her home with self-help handout sheets
D. all of the above

UNIT FOUR

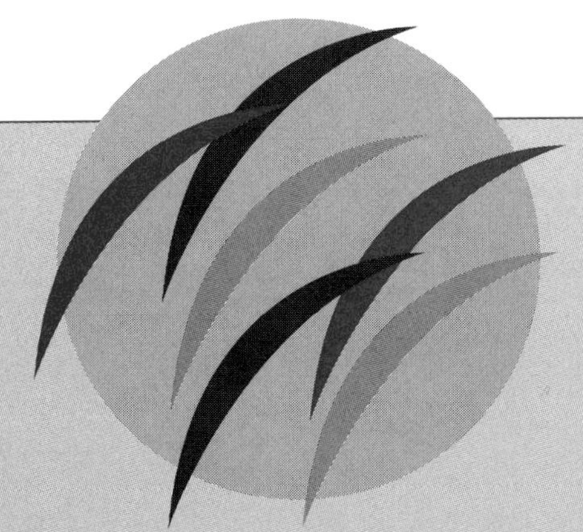

A User's Guide to Alternative and Adjunctive Therapies

Nothing on earth is so weak and yielding as water, but for breaking down the firm and strong it has no equal.

—Lao Tzu

23 Hydrotherapy, Cryotherapy, and Thermotherapy

Student Objectives

After completing this chapter, the student should be able to:

- Define hydrotherapy, cryotherapy, and thermotherapy
- Describe the three physical states of water
- Explain sanitation and safety procedures for hydrotherapy, cryotherapy, and thermotherapy equipment
- Name the benefits and contraindications for hydrotherapy
- Demonstrate or explain a salt glow, a Swedish shampoo, and a sitz bath
- Name the benefits and contraindications for cryotherapy
- Discuss the hunting response
- List the four sensations felt by the client during an ice treatment
- Demonstrate or explain a cold immersion bath, an ice pack, ice massage, cryokinetics, cold mitten friction, and the contrast method
- Name the benefits and contraindications for thermotherapy
- Demonstrate or explain a warm immersion bath, a whirlpool bath, paraffin bath, hot pack, steam bath, sauna bath, and the use of liniments
- Contrast and compare the physiological differences between ice and heat

INTRODUCTION

From the time of written history, water has been used to maintain health, manage pain, and treat physical and emotional ailments. The Babylonians, Romans, Greeks, Chinese, Japanese, and Egyptians utilized and advocated the healing effects of water in the form of various baths. Temperatures of the baths were adjusted to suit the needs of each bather. In Sparta, laws were passed that made frequent bathing mandatory. Water, in its various forms, continues to be employed to enhance the health and well-being of individuals and can be used to add therapeutic value to massage therapy. Hydrotherapy is a natural way for massage therapists to add diversity to their practice.

Water can be used in its liquid form, frozen, or heated to a vapor (Table 23–1). What physical energy can be added or removed to change water to all three states? That's right—heat! Adding heat to ice will excite the molecules and cause them to move farther apart, changing a block of ice into a puddle of water, and a puddle of water into a cloud of water vapor. Removing heat from water will turn vapor and water into ice. The word "hydrotherapy" finds its roots in the Greek word "hydro" meaning water. "Hydro" as a prefix is defined as "fluid" or "liquid." Let's consider each physical state briefly (Fig. 23–1).

- **Solid.** A substance that does not flow.
- **Liquid.** Water or a watery substance that flows freely.
- **Gas or Vapor.** A substance whose molecules flow freely and quickly fills all dimensions of its container.

To help students comprehend the scope of hydrotherapy, this chapter is divided into three other sections: hydrotherapy, cryotherapy, and thermotherapy. Hydrotherapy is the external therapeutic use of water and complementary agents, such as soap and salt, at temperatures close to normal body temperature. Cryotherapy refers to the application of cold, such as ice, icy water, frozen gel, or chemical cold packs. Thermotherapy includes the application of heat in its various forms, such as whirlpools, moist heat packs, and steam baths as well as paraffin baths, saunas, and steam baths. The effects of each modality are different, depending on the temperature and duration of treatment. A comparison chart is included for you to explore further the uses of ice and heat. Presenting classic hydrotherapy studies in smaller sections will help the student to understand how to use these powerful therapies more effectively.

Table 23–1
Temperature Ranges

Fahrenheit	Description	Celsius
212°	boiling point of water	100°
110°–120°	painfully hot	43°–49°
104°–110°	very hot	40°–43°
100°–104°	hot	38°–40°
92°–100°	warm	33°–38°
80°–92°	tepid	27°–33°
70°–80°	cool	21°–27°
55°–70°	cold	13°–21°
32°	freezing point of water	0°

It may be helpful to review the list of specific indications and contraindications of these modalities. As therapy applications are presented, you will find some descriptions are instructional and some are simply informative. If the modality method is lengthy or complicated, a step-by-step guide will assist you in the proper usage of each method.

Because extreme hot and cold can harm your client, the massage therapist must always be aware of the temperature of the water. Water temperatures below 32°F or above 124°F can cause tissue damage (Table 23–2). It is helpful to test the water temperature using your fingertips but for a more accurate reading, use a thermometer (thermometers can be purchased at a pool or spa supply store). Bear in mind when using hot water from a faucet that most water heaters are set at about 140°F.

Many healthcare and allied healthcare practitioners,

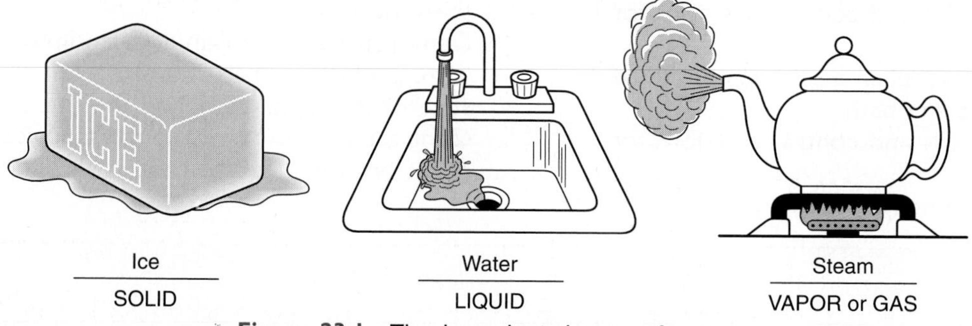

Figure 23•1 The three physical states of water.

Table 23–2
Temperature Conversion Table

Fahrenheit to Celsius	Celsius to Fahrenheit
Subtract 32, then multiply by 5⁄9 (°F − 32) × 5⁄9 Example: (212°F − 32) × 5⁄9 = 100°C	Multiply by 9⁄5, then add 32 (°C × 9⁄5) + 32 Example: (0°C × 9⁄5) + 32 = 32°F

from emergency room technicians to physical medicine experts, are frequent users of hydrotherapy, cryotherapy, and thermotherapy. All agree that these treatments are beneficial to the body. As with other forms of therapy, there are certain cautions and parameters to observe. Know your treatment. For example, use care when applying heat or ice to clients who have generous amounts of subcutaneous tissue. Adipose tissue is a good insulator and may hinder the transfer of thermal energy to the tissues that require treatment. However, do not extend the treatment time. It may be necessary to reduce the duration of hot or cold treatment to prevent tissue damage to the skin.

SANITATION AND SAFETY PROCEDURES FOR HYDROTHERAPY, CRYOTHERAPY, AND THERMOTHERAPY EQUIPMENT

Maintain your hydrotherapy equipment in good working order, and clean each item at the beginning of each workday with mild soap and water. Surfaces that come in direct contact with the client, as well as all reservoirs that collect perspiration or exfoliated skin cells, must be cleaned after each treatment. If body fluids (blood, genital secretions, mother's milk) come into contact with therapy equipment, a solution of water and chlorine bleach (ten parts water to one part chlorine bleach) can be used to disinfect the equipment.

Maintain hot tubs, spas, steam cabinets, and whirlpools in compliance with public and multiple-use standards. If water collects on the wet room or bathroom floor, wipe it up immediately to prevent accidents. If hydrotherapy equipment is kept in the massage room, make sure it is not in a high-traffic region of the room. If a client accidentally touches a hot hydrocollator unit, it will probably burn his skin. It may be more

CHECKLIST FOR PREPARATION OF HYDROTHERAPY AREA AND GENERAL GUIDELINES FOR APPLICATION

- ☐ Plan ahead and assemble all necessary articles.
- ☐ Cover furniture, rugs, and other objects that may be damaged during treatment.
- ☐ Check and monitor the temperature of the water.
- ☐ Ask the client not to eat one hour before the hydrotherapy treatment.
- ☐ Allow at least twenty minutes after the treatment for the body temperature to return to normal.
- ☐ Explain all hydrotherapy procedures, quietly announcing what is coming next and what effect is desired.
- ☐ Remain with the client or within close range (easy calling distance).
- ☐ Place a towel on equipment that will be in direct contact with the client, such as wet tables and steam cabinets.
- ☐ Use a timer to limit the duration of all hydrotherapy treatments. Do not overtreat.
- ☐ Clean steam cabinets, tubs, wet tables, and shower stalls after each use; clean all bath surfaces and flooring at the start of each business day.
- ☐ If water collects on the floor, wipe it up immediately. This will reduce tripping hazards.
- ☐ ____________________
- ☐ ____________________

Figure 23•2 Thermotherapy checklist. (Permission is hereby granted to reproduce this form in its entirety, including the copyright notice, for commercial or instructional use but not for resale.)

convenient to have hydrotherapy equipment in the treatment room, but safety must come before convenience.

Even though water is a powerful modality by itself or with massage therapy, it can easily damage massage tables, floors, and walls. Preventive measures can be taken such as not splashing water and covering furniture with a protective cloth. Use the checklist in Figure 23–2 to help you prepare your workspace for hydrotherapy application.

HYDROTHERAPY

Hydrotherapy is the external therapeutic use of water and complementary agents, such as soap and salt, at temperatures close to normal body temperature. Water is valued for its pressure effect and as a means of applying physical energy to the tissues. Even though hydrotherapeutics include the use of ice and heat, these methods will be addressed in the cryotherapy or thermotherapy sections. Only the hydrotherapy treatments that involve the use of water and other complementary agents, such as salt glows and Swedish shampoos, are included in this section.

When hydrotherapy is not used for the desired effects of cold or heat, this therapy becomes a tool for enhancing skin tone, producing mild, pleasant stimulation of the skin. Hydrotherapy also promotes relaxation and health. Soaps, scents, minerals, and healing agents are frequently added to the water to enhance therapeutic value. The indications and contraindications will assist you in applying these special baths safely and effectively in your practice of massage.

Benefits of Hydrotherapy

- It cleans and exfoliates the skin
- It improves skin tone
- It increases cutaneous circulation
- It stimulates nerve endings, creating an invigorated feeling
- It can also produce a calming, relaxing effect

Hydrotherapy Contraindications

- Topical infections and skin rashes
- Open or weeping wounds
- Freshly shaved skin (salt glow)

Hydrotherapy Applications

Hydrotherapy, or water therapy, can be applied using water, salt pastes, and herbs, shampoos, and the like. These treatments can be used exclusively or as part of the massage therapy session. Most clients will agree that hydrotherapy stimulates the skin and blood circulation while creating a relaxing effect. Most of the supplies needed for hydrotherapy are affordable and easy to assemble. For best results, use a large shower or a specially designed table with a drain. Another application method is to sit the client on a water-resistant stool in a room that has a floor drain. For variation, try administering salt glows, Swedish shampoos, and Turkish shampoos outdoors. Make sure it is a clear and warm day, and choose an area that is quiet and private.

Swedish Shampoo. Swedish shampoo, or **body shampoo,** involves brushing the body with a brush dipped in warm soapy water. A circular or linear motion is used on the skin to work the soap into a lather. After the body shampoo, pour a pail of water at 105°F over the client's skin. Follow this procedure with a lukewarm shower. A **Turkish shampoo** is the same thing as a Swedish shampoo, with one exception. After the 105°F pail pour, conclude with a 90°F pail pour (Fig. 23–3).

Sitz Bath. A sitting bath with the water covering the hips and coming up to the navel is called a **sitz bath** (Fig. 23–4). The bath chamber is usually designed so the legs can remain out of the water. The water temperature will range from 90°F to 102°F. The duration is 3 to 8 minutes for a tonic or stimulating treatment and 20 to 45 minutes for a sedative, calming effect. Healing agents such as salt or alum usually accompany the bathwater.

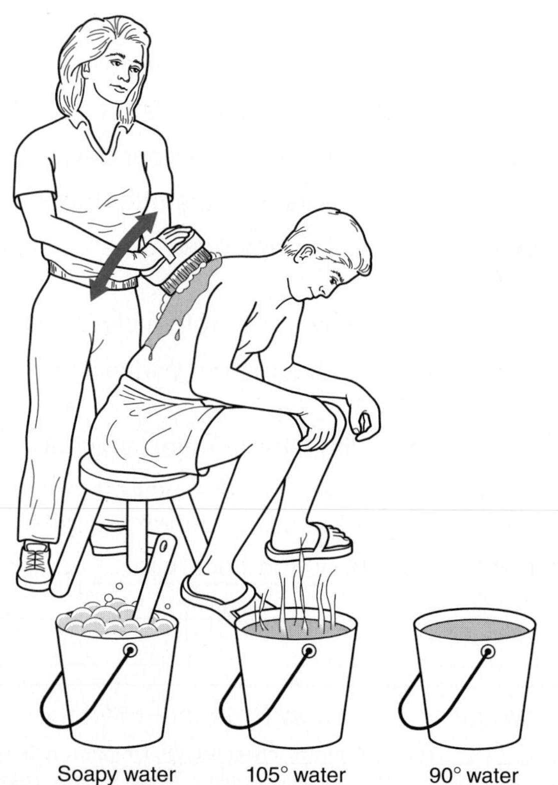

Figure 23•3 Swedish shampoo and Turkish shampoo.

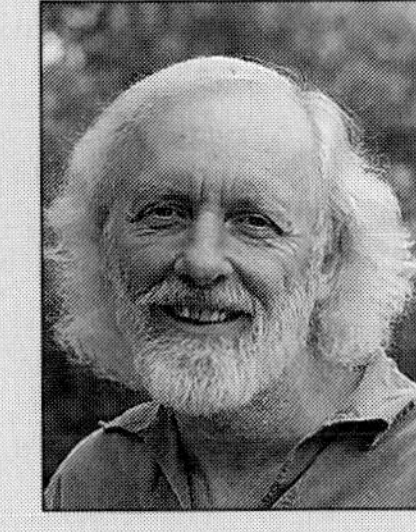

Harold Dull

Born: December 18, 1935

"The body is movement. Breath is life. And the base of our being is the support of others."

There seems to be no direct path to a career in facilitating health. So it's no surprise that a physics major who decided to become a beatnik poet is the man behind one of the latest forms of hands-on therapy. It's called Watsu, which is the combination of water and shiatsu. The wonderful name was coined by wordsmith and bodyworker Harold Dull. Developed 15 years ago, it is a hybrid of Zen shiatsu, flotation, joint mobilization, and stretching.

Harold Dull was born in Seattle, the oldest of four boys. His parents were in real estate. Bored by high school, he attended the University of Washington with the intention of studying physics . . . or prelaw . . . or philosophy. He wound up studying poetry instead, became a writer, and was part of the poetry renaissance.

"At age 40 I had never had a massage," Dull says, "but I decided to begin studying Zen shiatsu in San Francisco with Wataru Ohashi and Reuho Yamada." Dull finally traveled to Japan to complete studies with world-renowned master Shizuto Masunaga. When he returned home he began teaching others the ancient Japanese art and later hit on how to combine shiatsu with the hot spring therapy he'd enjoyed at Harbin Hot Springs Resort in California. In its earlier incarnation, Watsu was dubbed Wassage. Dull used a board set up in a hot tub. In time, however, he dived right in and began doing his unique form of bodywork in Harbin's hot springs.

In Watsu the water is the medium as well as the message. Its buoyancy helps practitioners and clients by supporting body weight, so small practitioners are able to handle large clients. The water also helps the therapist "see, feel, and listen" to what's going on with the client's body. As the body rises and falls with each breath, the water helps the practitioner identify areas that need work. The water, maintained at body temperature, also soothes the client, releasing tense muscles and taking the load off joint articulations, helping increase flexibility and range of motion.

Step into a conventional massage room and you may not feel the result of your massage until after the therapist begins, but immerse yourself in water and you immediately feel different—lighter. As you relax into your breathing pattern, supported by your therapist, you gradually let go as the tickle of the water filling your ears silences a chaotic world and lulls you into a heightened state of relaxation.

Here's how one writer describes her experience with Watsu: "The surprise, for me, was just how profound this was. It has become a cliché to say that a therapy works 'on many different levels,' but that is actually an excellent description of Watsu. Deeply rooted physical tensions and ailments are worked on more easily, while the experience of being safely held and moved through the water also touches profound emotional and spiritual levels." ("Watsu, Flowing Free in Water," by Diana Brueton for *Kindred Spirit Quarterly*.)

Dull notes that it is "the unconditional acceptance that is so powerful. So many injured people are treated as less than what they once were." In addition to its emotional impact, Watsu has reportedly helped headache pain. Muscle spasms disappear and chronic lower back pain and spine misalignment have been corrected.

Dull's vision is to make the therapeutic value of his work—and especially the added benefit of the sense of unconditional acceptance it brings—available to everyone. "From an equipment standpoint you need a 10-foot diameter pool with about 4 feet of water, which should be maintained at body temperature," he explains and adds that new ways will be discovered to heat water at a lower cost.

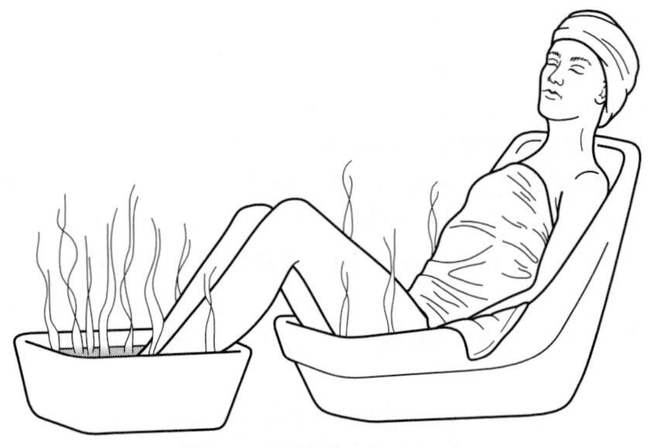

Figure 23•4 Sitz bath.

As an alternative, the feet may be placed in a tub of water that is warmer than the sitz bath. This provides a contrast that increases circulation.

Cover the client and tub with a dry sheet for the feeling of comfort and protection. A 30-second cold shower, plunge, or pour may be used at the end of the bath. A sitz bath is often indicated for relief of painful menstruation; however, it is contraindicated in cases of pelvic inflammation.

Salt Rubs, or Salt Glows. A **salt glow** is the rubbing application of wet salt on the skin (Fig. 23–5). Salt glows can be used to exfoliate the skin and are beneficial if the client is undergoing a fast or any type of self-cleansing regimen. This procedure should not be used on freshly shaved legs, cuts, abrasions, or skin rashes because the salt will burn. The massage stroke used to apply the wet salt mixture is brisk back-and-forth friction. Use a light application, and avoid salt glows on clients who have ruddy or thin skin because superficial blood vessels can be prone to injury with this type of treatment.

Salt Glow Procedure

1. Ask the client to lie on a large towel or use a specially designed table or stool for water treatments. If the client is more comfortable standing, allow her to do so.
2. Put about ½ cup of salt in an unbreakable quart-size dish. Use a mixture of kosher salt or Epsom salts, and ordinary table salt in a 1:1 ratio. If this mixture is unavailable, use whichever you have on hand; however, a coarser grade of salt is preferred.
3. Add just enough water to make the grains stick together, but not enough to dissolve the salt. It should be the consistency of slush.
4. After moistening the skin, take approximately 1 heaping tablespoon of the moistened salt in the hands, and distribute between your palms. Hold an extremity (arm or leg) in one hand, and use a brisk upward and downward movement with the other while the client holds the extremity stiff. Rinse the area off with warm water, and proceed with the salt application and rinsing until the entire body is complete.
5. Use a cool shower or a pail pour to cleanse the skin at the end of the treatment. The water should be at a pleasant temperature. Rub the skin vigorously during the rinsing, with the client assisting.
6. Use a vigorous friction motion with the towel to dry the client.

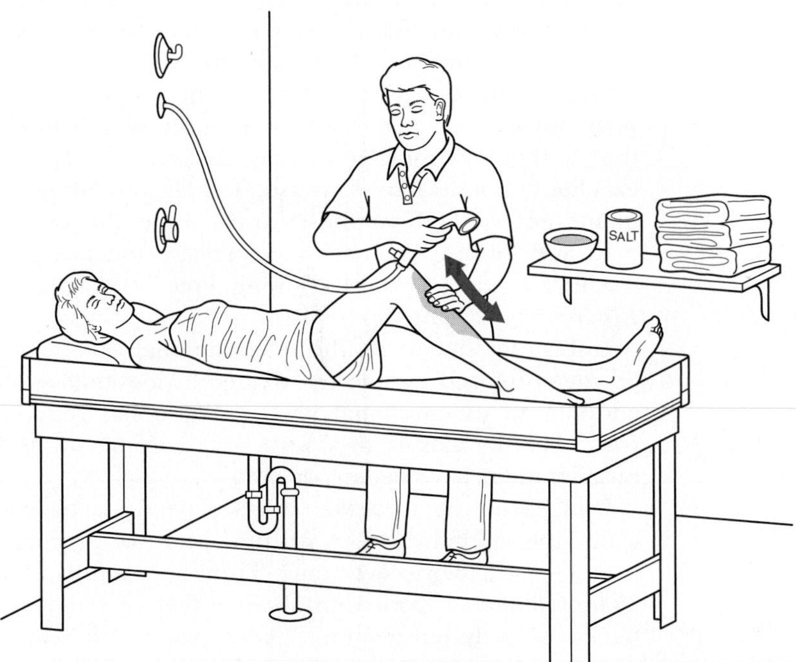

Figure 23•5 Salt glow.

CRYOTHERAPY

Cryotherapy is the external, therapeutic application of cold. Ice is the safest, simplest, and most effective method for reducing pain and swelling in injuries and has replaced the use of heat in many rehabilitation clinics. *Cryotherapy is not to be confused with ice as a first-aid treatment* (the traditional ICE or *i*ce, *c*ompression, *e*levation). Massage therapists can only use cryotherapy because treatment of initial injuries is beyond our scope of practice.

The beauty of ice therapy is that it lends itself to self-administration and is one of the best things we can teach clients to do for themselves at home. Ice is cheap, does not have to be manufactured, requires no special packaging, is safe, and is nonaddictive. But many people have an aversion to ice because they do not think it feels good.

Most of us are conditioned to use heat for pain; for example, we are taught to "warm up" before activity. A warm-up will raise the body's temperature and bring blood into the muscles about to be used. Because warming up the body before exercise reduces the risk of injury, it is easy to see why many individuals believe that warming up an injury with external heat will aid healing. But this is often one of the worst things you can do. Heat application following a soft-tissue injury will accelerate inflammation, increase swelling, and irritate injured tissues.

The application of ice has several very distinct physiological effects. During the first 9 to 16 minutes of cold application, the area undergoes a reduction of blood flow through reflex *vasoconstriction.* This reduction in the size of the blood vessels will cause the skin to appear blanched or pale; local edema is reduced, and hematoma formation is controlled.

If ice application continues, a sudden deep-tissue *vasodilation* occurs. This can last from 4 to 6 minutes. This increase in the diameter of the blood vessels is a thermoregulatory response to restore homeostasis and will raise local temperature. After a few minutes, vasoconstriction will resume and the cycle continues. One cycle of vasoconstriction and vasodilation takes about 15 to 30 minutes. This up-and-down cycle is the **hunting response** (Fig. 23–6).

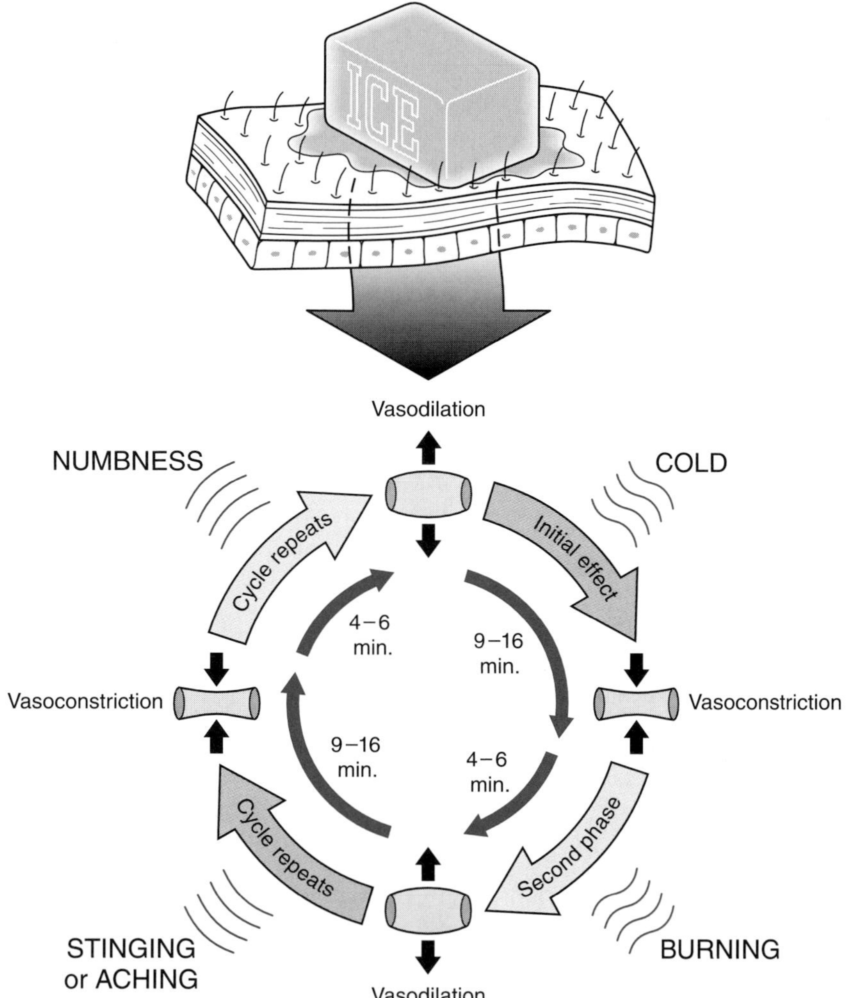

Figure 23•6 The hunting response.

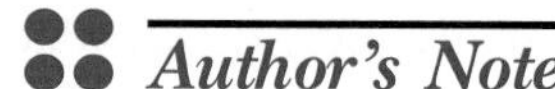

When in doubt, use ice.

The alternating action and reaction of the body to cold application brings blood into and out of the area, flushing out tissue debris and bringing in much needed oxygen. This cycling between vasoconstriction and vasodilation creates a "vascular pump" or "vascular gymnastics," which creates an increased deep local circulation, one of the most important effects of cryotherapy.

So what is the client feeling? During the ice treatment, four very distinct sensations will be experienced; (1) coldness or cooling, (2) burning, (3) stinging or aching, and (4) numbness. Allow ice to remain on the body until the fourth and final phase (this may take anywhere from 5 to 20 minutes). Remove the ice immediately after numbness to prevent tissue damage from excessive cold.

Some types of massage movements (e.g., friction, deep effleurage, petrissage, and tapotement) create the same vascular reactions as cold applications. Pressure during a massage may cause a brief period of ischemia or blanching of the skin. Upon the release of pressure, vasodilation occurs, producing hyperemia. This is why the skin appears pink or red. The following two sections discuss the benefits and effects of ice, as well as contraindications for its safe and responsible use.

Benefits of Cryotherapy

- It decreases cell metabolism, temporarily decreasing local oxygen supply (hypoxia)
- It interrupts pain-spasm-pain cycle, reducing muscle spasm
- It reduces swelling
- It decreases tissue damage
- It reduces blood clot formation
- It reduces muscle spindle activity, resulting in reduced muscular spasticity
- It reduces pain by creating an anesthetic effect through reduced nerve conduction velocity
- It stimulates vasodilation, which speeds nutrients to an area and encourages debris removal
- It draws heat out of an area, thus reducing inflammation

Cryotherapy Contraindications

Do not use on clients who have:

- Asthma (it can trigger wheezing in asthmatics)
- Raynaud's phenomenon, ischemia of the extremities of the body caused by cold exposure or emotional stimuli; most prominent in the fingers, toes, ears, and nose
- Cold or plastic allergies
- Open wounds
- Skin rashes
- Rheumatoid conditions
- Had CVAs (*c*erebro*v*ascular *a*ccidents or strokes)
- Sensory impairments, individuals who cannot report subjective reactions (e.g., infants or elderly people), or when the client has the inability to react appropriately to excessive temperature changes (e.g., infants, elderly people, people with diabetes, those who are mentally handicapped, clients who have multiple sclerosis)
- An aversion to cold

Author's Note

Caution must be used when applying ice. If local or general application is prolonged (more than 20 minutes), tissue damage may result in the form of frostbite and/or hypothermia. Both conditions are harmful to the client.

Cryotherapy Application

Cryotherapy or ice therapy applications include, but are not limited to, cold immersion, ice packs, ice massage, cold mitten friction, or cryokinetics. Become familiar with all the following popular methods of application. If the client is already chilled prior to the cryotherapy treatment, do not apply cryotherapy. It may be helpful to administer a hot foot bath to help the client feel more comfortable before proceeding with the cryotherapy.

Cold or Ice Immersion Baths. Cold immersion baths involve soaking an affected area in a container of icy water. This method is ideal for hands and feet. To apply cold immersion baths, immerse the affected area in a tub of tepid water, then add ice. Because this procedure is often uncomfortable, clients may elect to leave their fingers or toes out of the icy water, or they may choose to dip their hand repeatedly into the icy water until they are accustomed to the temperature. Once the immersed area is numb, instruct the client to draw pictures or trace the alphabet with his fingers or toes in the water. Keep the area immersed in cold water for 5 to 10 minutes, but no longer than 20 minutes.

Ice Packs. Ice packs are plastic or cloth bags filled with ice or icy water and placed on an affected area. The use of a noncommercial ice pack is preferred over commercial ice packs for several reasons. First, commercial ice packs, which are typically filled with chemi-

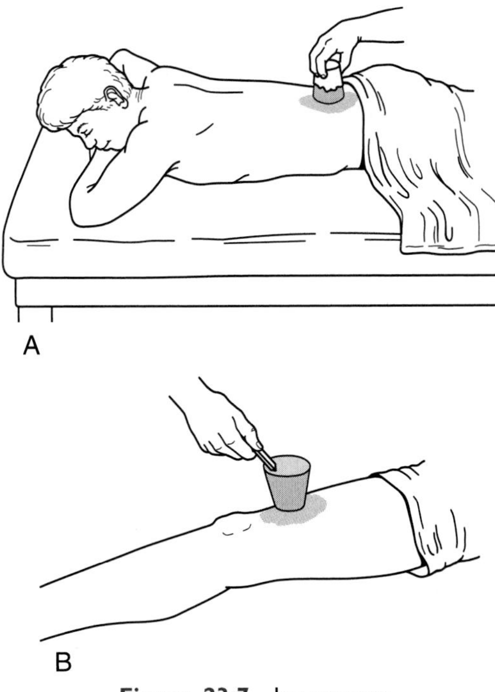

Figure 23•7 Ice massage.

The first time I used ice massage was quite memorable. I had prepared an ice cup the night before it was needed. I located a 20-ounce paper cup, filled it with water, leaving one inch at the top for expansion during freezing.

The following day my client arrived and took off his shirt for the ice massage treatment. After tearing off the top portion of the cup, I placed the ice cup on his exposed shoulder and began the massage. To take his mind off the cup of ice on his back, we engaged in some light conversation and he began to relax.

A few minutes later, I heard a "crack" and then a "whoosh." He began to scream and a look of horror swept across my face. My ice cup was not frozen solid! My cup runneth over! ••

cals, are prone to rupture and can damage clothing. Second, many commercial ice packs, being colder than homemade ones, can chill the skin too fast and cause tissue damage. No matter which is used, a thin cloth or paper towel must be placed between the ice pack and the client's skin. If the cloth is too thick, the effectiveness of the treatment is reduced. Apply ice packs for 20 minutes.

Two methods of ice application are crushed ice in a towel or slushy ice water in a zipped plastic bag. A solution of two-thirds water and one-third alcohol may be mixed in a zipped plastic bag and kept in the freezer. The alcohol will prevent the water from freezing solid, and this homemade ice pack will conform easily to the affected area. Be sure to double-layer the plastic bag to prevent water leakage.

Ice Massage. Ice massage combines the use of cryotherapy with circular friction. To begin, fill a 6- or 8-ounce styrofoam cup or paper cup two-thirds full with water, and place it in the freezer until the water has turned to solid ice. Tear the edges of the cup to expose the ice, leaving the bottom portion of the cup to protect your fingers (Fig. 23–7, top). Place the ice on the client's skin, and rub in small, circular motions. Continue the ice massage over the affected area for 5 to 10 minutes. A "Popsicle" can be made by placing a tongue depressor in the cup, so that after the water freezes, the ice cube has a handle (Fig. 23–7, bottom).

Cryokinetics. The application of cold followed by full range of motion of the affected area is called **cryokinetics.** When using cryokinetics for rehabilitation and reconditioning, our goal is full functional use of the affected area. When a client is in pain, it may be difficult to convince her that movement of the affected area will hasten recovery, but the longer a muscle or joint is immobile the harder it is to get it working again.

The solution is to combine ice with motion to facilitate full functional use of muscles and joints. The pain-reducing effects of ice allow the client to push through the discomfort barrier and to achieve range of motion faster and easier. The resulting movements encourage decongestion of the injured area and free restricted muscles.

Cryokinetics Procedure

Apply an ice pack, cold immersion bath, or ice massage to chill the affected area. Allow the ice to remain on the client's skin until numb. This usually occurs within 10 to 15 minutes, but the sensations felt by the client will ultimately determine the length of treatment.

Once the area is numb, the client exercises the body part (Fig. 23–8). Movement continues until the tissue

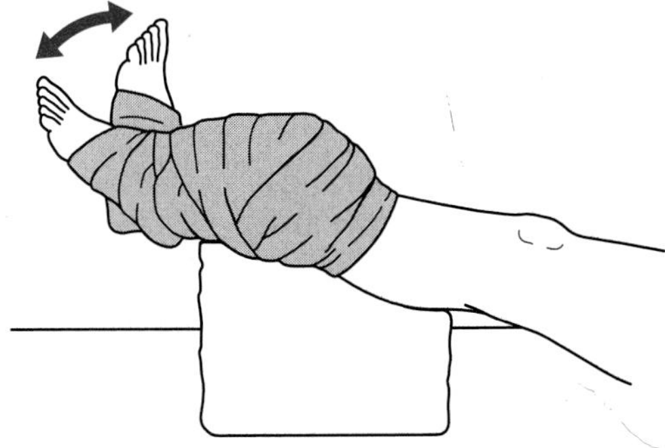

Figure 23•8 Ice applied to an injury while the client is doing active range of motion.

warms up and feeling is restored, which takes about 3 to 5 minutes, then reapply the ice until the client experiences numbness. The injured area can be iced and exercised from three to five times. Active range of motion or isometric (resistive) exercises are preferred over passive range of motion. Instruct the client to mirror back to you the demonstrated movements as you emphasize circular, diagonal, and spiral motions. Never use a motion that causes pain. Maintain communication so progress can be monitored.

Cold Mitten Friction. **Cold mitten friction** is an application of cold accompanied by friction movements generated at a force of 5 to 10 pounds of pressure. This treatment is also called a tonic treatment because it is thought to aid in the prevention of colds, low energy and endurance, poor resistance to infections, poor circulation, and anemia. Ice application through cold mitten friction causes blood vessels to contract and dilate (vascular gymnastics), promotes heat production, and reduces swelling. As you recall, these are all physiological effects of friction. Combining cryotherapy and friction will intensify the vascular benefits.

Cold Mitten Friction Procedure

Place your client on a table designed or modified for wet treatments. Have the following items near the treatment area before your client arrives: (1) two or more towels; (2) friction mitts (you may use a washcloth wrapped around the hand [tuck in the edge] or make mitts by simply sewing along the sides of a folded washcloth); and (3) a pail of ice water 50° to 60°F or less.

Dip the mitts into the icy water and squeeze out the excess water. Arrange the mitts on your hands. Begin at the legs and work up with vigorous to-and-fro friction movements (Fig. 23–9). Dip the mitts again and repeat the process. Quickly remove the mitts. Cover the area with a towel, and rub vigorously over the skin until it is thoroughly dry. Coarser mitts or a loofah sponge may be used for greater friction.

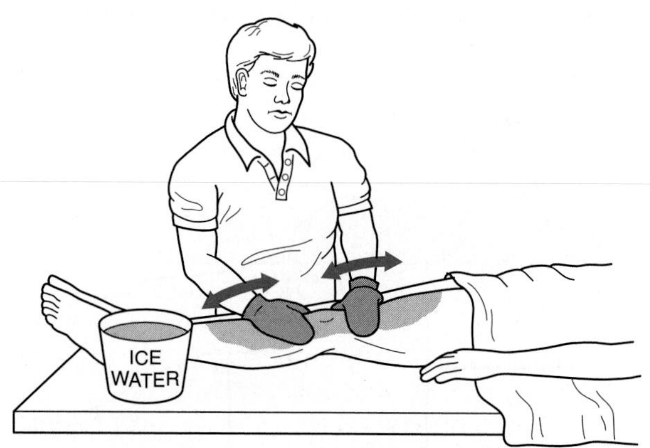

Figure 23•9 Cold mitten friction.

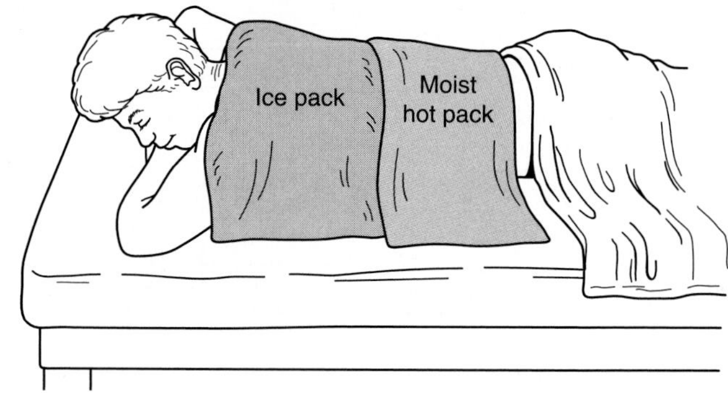

Figure 23•10 The contrast method.

Contrast Method

The most potent technique in the therapeutic use of cold is to combine its use with heat. The application of both ice and heat is known as the **contrast method** or the **contrast bath.** There are two variations: the **alternate contrast method** and **simultaneous contrast method.** The alternate contrast method is the most commonly used variation. It involves the application of ice on the client's skin for 10 to 15 minutes. The ice is then removed and heat is applied for about 10 minutes. Ice is reapplied for a final 10- to 15-minute period. Repeat the alternate contrast method two to three times. Alternating cold and heat applications intensifies the circulatory effect on the tissues.

An ice pack is placed on the area of complaint and a heat pack is placed at the same time next to the ice pack; this is the simultaneous contrast method (Fig. 23–10). For example, a painful rotator cuff injury could be treated with the client lying prone with a hot pack under his shoulder and an ice pack on the top of his back covering the shoulder. Not only do the heat impulses interfere with the cold impulses, but the sensation of heat comforts the client and induces relaxation. Cycles of vasoconstriction and vasodilation that ice and heat create will help remove metabolic waste.

THERMOTHERAPY

Thermotherapy is the external application of heat for therapeutic purposes. Heat is transferred into the body using one of three methods of delivery: conduction, convection, and radiation. *Conduction* involves the exchange of thermal energy while the body's surface is in direct contact with the thermal agent (e.g., hot packs). *Convection,* a more rapid process than conduction, involves the body's surface contacting heat energy through a fluid or gaseous medium (e.g., whirlpool bath or steam bath). *Radiation* is the transfer of heat energy in electromagnetic rays through a conducting medium (e.g., infrared lamps). Moist heat is transferred by conduction and convection, dry heat often is transferred by radiation. The best form of heat for inducing general relaxation is moist heat.

Physiological changes produced in the body by heat application are superficial, at best. This is because we are homeotherms (Gr. Homos—same, and therm—heat), which is another way of saying that we are warm-blooded creatures. Our bodies maintain a relatively constant internal temperature (98.6°F or 37°C). This temperature is achieved through a constant dynamic balance between heat loss and gain. Most of this maintenance is accomplished through the mechanisms of the skin (sudoriferous glands and blood capillaries).

When our bodies encounter heat, we respond in one of several ways to create heat loss. One of the following events will occur:

1. Stimulation of perspiration through sudoriferous or sweat glands. This pushes sweat onto the skin's surface, and evaporation cools off the human machine.
2. Cutaneous vasodilation. Blood vessels near the skin's surface begin to dilate, and excess heat is dissipated through the skin. During this process, the skin will appear flushed due to hyperemia.
3. Our behavior will be altered. Feeling hot makes most of us uncomfortable, so we tend to make appropriate environmental adjustments, such as turning down the thermostat on the air conditioner or wearing cooler clothing.

These body thermostat reactions respond to limit the depth of thermal penetration into the tissues. It is easy to see how the application of heat only affects the skin surface and superficial structures of the body. The skin's redness during heat application is the body's way of dissipating unwanted heat. Heat offers little or no circulatory benefits to deeper muscles because it is dissipated by the body in the superficial layers of skin and muscle. It also may create swelling and irritate tissues, so why use heat at all? There are a number of reasons.

Benefits of Thermotherapy

- Heat soothes, sedates, and comforts your clients, and it can relieve pain or discomfort, as long as inflammation is not present. When pain is masked by the heat, the muscles begin to relax.
- It alleviates pain. The brain also produces a "comfort" hormone (endorphin) during the application of heat.
- General heat (whirlpool, steam, and sauna) produces an artificial fever that increases white blood cell count, stimulating immune system response. The increased body temperature (between 102° and 104°F) inhibits the growth of many bacteria and viruses.
- Heat reduces muscle spasms by activating the relaxation response and by temporarily inhibiting the nerve activity in the muscles. Heat is indicated for general relaxation of tense, spasmed muscles.
- Heat awakens closed capillary beds in cutaneous tissues, increasing blood volume. As a result, these tissues are provided with increased oxygen and nutrition.
- The single most important clinical benefit of thermotherapy is its effect on the body's fascia. Following an application of a hot compress, a whirlpool bath, or a sauna, the superficial fascia distends, softens, and becomes more supple. The added thermal energy alters the state of the gelatinous/solid fascia, just as the heat created by handling modeling clay makes it more pliable. Massage manipulations are much more effective after the tissues have been prepared by heat; however, heat should not be used in many conditions and circumstances. The following list of contraindications will help you use heat safely.

Thermotherapy Contraindications

Most of the following conditions are contraindicationed for thermotherapy because of the effect heat has on the circulation of blood and swelling. Heat may irritate certain conditions. Taking into consideration the guidelines at the beginning of the chapter, do not apply heat in the following circumstances.

- Immediately after an injury because of the possibility of internal bleeding (hemorrhage)
- Over a fresh hematoma (bruise)
- Over a tumor
- Directly over the eyes or external genitalia
- Edematous conditions (swelling)
- Phlebitis
- Hypertension
- Diabetes
- Cardiac impairment
- CVA survivors (cerebrovascular accident)
- Fever
- Recent burns, including sunburn
- Malignancy
- Skin infections and open wounds
- Sensory impairments, individuals who cannot report subjective reactions (e.g., infants or elderly people), or when the client has the inability to react appropriately to excessive temperature changes (e.g., infants or elderly people, people with diabetes, mentally handicapped clients, clients who have multiple sclerosis)
- Pregnancy, with the exception of paraffin baths
- Clients who have an aversion to heat

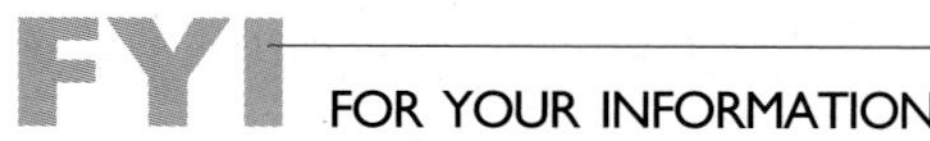

FOR YOUR INFORMATION

The unit used for measuring heat energy is the calorie.

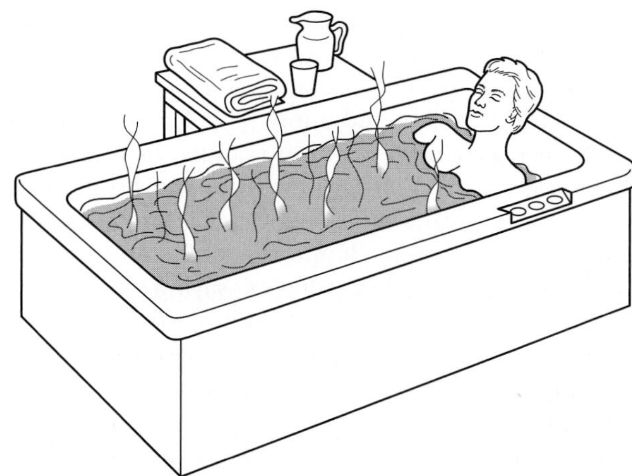

Figure 23•11 Whirlpool immersion.

Thermotherapy Applications

Thermotherapy or heat therapy application includes, but is not limited to, whirlpool or warm immersion baths, paraffin baths, hot packs, spinal packs, saunas, and steam baths. Most of these methods are simple and affordable, but others require commitments of space and capital expenditure. Regardless of which are better suited to your practice, familiarize yourself with all of these applications.

Warm Immersion Baths, Whirlpool Baths, Hydrotherapy Tubs, or Spas. By definition, **warm immersion baths** and **whirlpool baths** are tubs for soaking or for receiving jets of water against the skin, draining the water after each use. **Hydrotherapy tubs** or **spas** are similar to immersion baths and whirlpool baths, but the water is treated to remain clean and sanitary for multiuse.

All forms of immersion baths are used when an area is to be soaked in warm to hot water. The soaking time can range from 15 to 20 minutes, depending on the water temperature and client's comfort (Table 23–3). Hotter water temperatures require shorter treatment times. In healthy clients, immersion baths and whirlpool baths can be taken once or twice a week. Additives may be used, such as salt, to add to the therapeutic value. Epsom salts (named for the mineral springs in Epsom, England) or commercial bath salts, like Batherapy, turn the immersion bath into a mineral bath.

Whirlpool baths, or spa treatments, include full or partial body immersion with agitated water mixed with air (Fig. 23–11). Because of the heat and pressure effects on the tissues of the body, whirlpool baths are also known as *hydromassage treatments.* If using a whirlpool bath soon after an injury, adjust the jets to push water toward the sides of the tank and not on the affected area and use tepid to warm water. The addition of hot water and pressure may exacerbate an injury.

When warm water immersion is combined with light exercise, a Hubbard tank is used. Named after its inventor, Carl Hubbard, this tank is often used in rehabilitation clinics because the buoyancy of the water allows easier movement and produces a soothing sensation. This is more comfortable for individuals with weak or painful muscles or joints.

Table 23–3
Recommended Durations for Whirlpool Treatments at Various Water Temperatures

Fahrenheit	Time Interval	Celsius
100°	20 minutes	38°
102°	15 minutes	39°
104°	10 minutes	40°
106°	5 minutes	41°

Whirlpool Procedure

A shower must be taken prior to treatment because the spa is a soaking and not a cleansing chamber. Before placing a client in a whirlpool, take her pulse rate and check it every 5 minutes. If the pulse rate increases 20 beats or more per minute, or if the client feels weak or dizzy, stop the bath immediately and assist her out of the bath.

Assist your client into and out of the spa. While the client is soaking, offer her a cup of tepid water in a nonbreakable cup and a cool washcloth for her face. If she becomes too warm, but is not ready to leave the spa, she may lift her arms out of the circulating water, exposing a greater surface area of the skin to allow for evaporative cooling.

Author's Note

The best use I get out of a whirlpool bath is to use it *before* a massage session. A 20-minute soak in the circulating water slows clients down mentally so they are ready to receive a massage. Another way a soak before massage is helpful is the effect on the superficial fascia. Massage movements that may be slightly uncomfortable become pleasant when fascia is softened and pliable.

Paraffin Baths. Paraffin baths use a petroleum-based waxy mixture that is white and odorless. Paraffin wax treatments are used to apply heat energy to the tissues and are particularly useful with injuries to the more angular bony areas. Wax conforms well to hands, wrists, elbows, knees, ankles, and feet. These treatments soften the skin and are used for pain relief. Paraffin baths are used on clients who have painful, arthritic joints or bursitis. Recalling the contraindications for thermotherapy, do not apply to joints that are hot and swollen. Paraffin baths are often used by cosmetologists to soften the skin and remove body hair. When these dead skin cells and body hair are removed, they remain in the waxy mixture until it is discarded. Unless you discard the wax after each application, your procedure is not sanitary.

Paraffin Bath Procedure

The paraffin wax is kept in a thermostatically controlled vessel at 126° to 130°F. To reduce the ability of the wax to stick to the skin, add heavy mineral oil to the waxy mixture in a 5:1 solution (5 pounds of paraffin wax to 1 pint of mineral oil). The molten wax can be applied as a pack, painted on the affected part, or as a dip, the latter being most widely used.

Clean and dry the treatment area thoroughly before the wax dip. Lotion or alcohol can be applied to the treatment area to help remove hardened wax. The client dips the body part into and out of the wax bath quickly, allowing time for the wax to dry between dippings. The process is repeated 6 to 12 times or until a layer of wax is formed ½ inch thick or is opaque. Be careful; hot wax can burn.

Wrap the waxed area with a plastic sheet (plastic wrap) and then with a towel (the towel serves as insulation). Allow the treated area to rest for up to 30 minutes or until the client reports that he can no longer feel heat.

Allow the client to remove the wax covering from his hands and form the wax into a ball (squeezing the ball is good exercise for the hands and forearms). Replace or discard the paraffin bath unit.

Hot Packs. Other names for hot packs are hydrocollator packs, fomentation packs, hot compresses, and hot dressings. **Hot packs** are moist heat applications used for pain relief. Most hot packs used in clinical settings are inexpensive, simple to use, and sanitary. A hydrocollator pack's canvas pouches are filled with silicon granules, which holds the heat in the pack for about 30 minutes. The temperature range in the hydrocollator kettle is between 140° and 160°F. Hot packs are often used by massage therapists in preparing an area for massage because heat will soften the fascia and dilate the superficial blood vessels. One disadvantage for hot pack use is that the packs can burn the skin if left on too long or if insulating material is not placed between the pack and the client's skin. Hot packs also block the therapist's access to and observation of the treatment area.

Hot Pack Procedure

Prepare the hot pack by wrapping it in up to six layers of terry cloth to prevent burning (¼ to ⅜ inch of padding is recommended to prevent the pack from burning the client's skin). Place the wrapped pack on the client's skin, making sure that the temperature of the pack is comfortable. Never allow the client to lie on the hot pack, unless the pack is specially designed to be placed under the body. To modify the intensity of the heat, add or subtract cloth layers between the pack and the skin. Periodically check the skin under the pack to make sure it does not show signs of irritation or damage.

Allow the pack to remain on the treatment area for 20 minutes, during which you may proceed with the massage routine. If the client begins to perspire, place a cold compress on the forehead or back of the neck (Fig. 23–12). As the pack begins to cool, you can remove a layer or two of insulation to extend the exchange of heat to the skin.

A **spinal pack** is a long, narrow fomentation pack applied directly on the spine (Fig. 23–13). These packs are used primarily to soothe and relax clients during the massage session. Fold a towel lengthwise to achieve a 3- or 4-inch width and place the hot pack in the insulating towel. Place the pack along the entire length of the spine. Leave the pack on the spine until pack is cool (about 10 minutes).

Steam Baths, or Wet Sauna. Steam baths are hot vapor baths given in specially designed chambers where temperatures are maintained at 105° to 130°F at 100 percent humidity. A steam cabinet that allows the

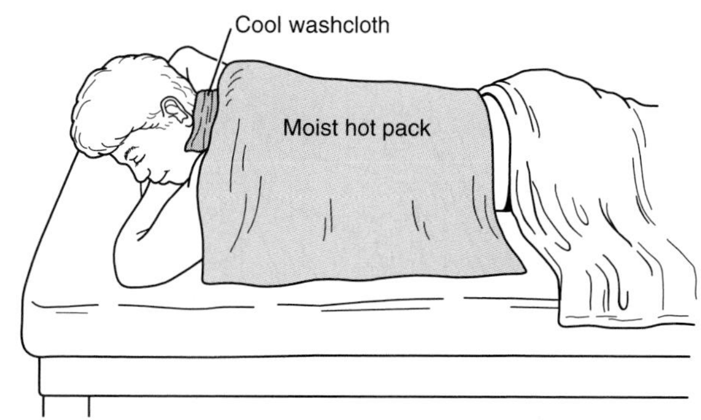

Figure 23•12 Client lying prone using a hot pack across the shoulders and a cool washcloth across the neck.

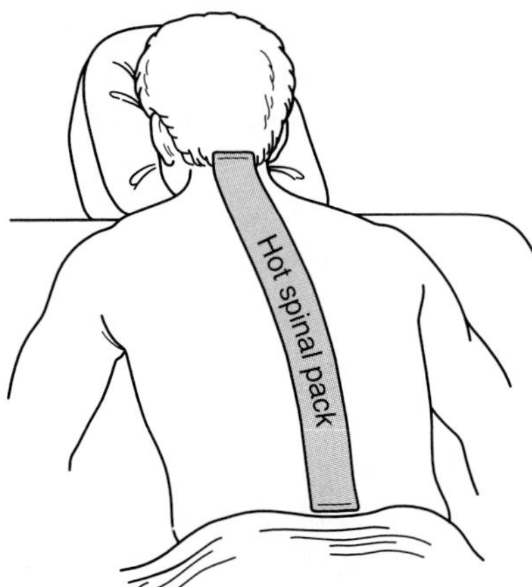

Figure 23•13 Spinal fomentation pack.

head to be exposed is called a **Russian bath** (Fig. 23–14). The average time in a steam bath is 15 to 20 minutes, but the client's comfort level can be used to determine treatment time. By increasing perspiration, steam baths are used to increase the removal of toxins from the body. The client typically feels relaxed and sedated following the treatment. Clients may take a steam bath once or twice a week.

Offer a shower to the client before he enters the steam cabinet or room. It is recommended that the client drink fresh water and use cool compresses over his forehead during the treatment. The steam bath is often followed by a plunge in cool water or a cool shower. Because hot vapor baths cause the pulse rate to rise, take the client's pulse rate before and during the bath. If the pulse rate rises 20 beats or more per minute, discontinue the session immediately. Place the client in a supine position for 10 minutes or until his pulse rate is normal.

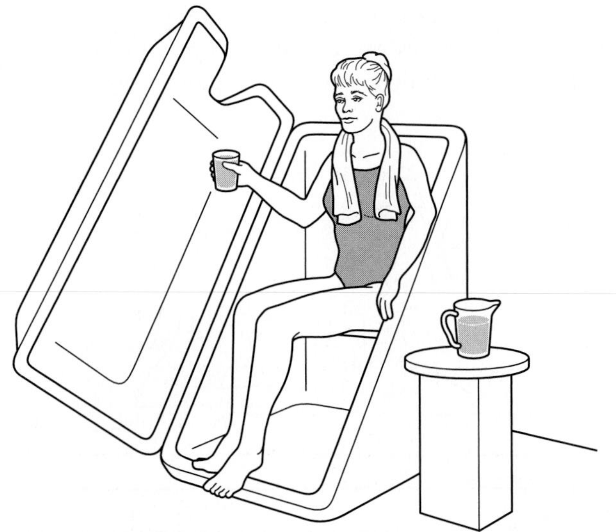
Figure 23•14 Steam cabinet, or Russian bath.

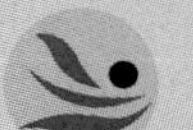
MINI•LAB

Choose one of the following hydrotherapy applications. Administer the treatment to a classmate and write a narrative report.

A. Salt glow
B. Swedish shampoo
C. Turkish shampoo

Choose one of the following cold applications. Administer the treatment to a classmate and write a narrative report.

A. Cold immersion bath
B. Ice pack
C. Ice immersion

Choose one of the following heat applications. Administer the treatment to a classmate and write a narrative report.

A. Hot pack
B. Russian bath
C. Warm immersion bath

Author's Note

Light-complexioned people, as a rule, cannot withstand intense moist heat; conversely, darker pigmented people are able to endure hotter temperatures.

Sauna Baths. A **sauna bath** is a hot-air bath with temperatures ranging from 160° to 180°F in 6 to 8 percent humidity. A special chamber must be built or purchased to withstand and hold these intense temperatures. The client can remain in the sauna for 20 to 30 minutes. As with any thermotherapy treatment, instruct the client not to eat 1 hour before a sauna and allow time for a cool shower and a cool-down period for the temperature of the body to return to normal. A dry sauna induces sweating and is indicated for general tension and insomnia, but it also increases metabolism, increases circulation, and aids in the removal of toxins. Because of the intense heat and minerals lost during the sweating response, limit the sauna bath treatments to once a week.

Liniments. Liniments are alcoholic, oily, or soapy agents used in massage to create the sensation of heat. All liniments are *rubefacient,* which means they redden the skin because of the counterirritation caused by the ingredients. As the skin is irritated, the vessels become dilated, and the supply of blood increases. Liniments can also produce an analgesic effect. Avoid using lini-

The Great Temperature Debate: Which Is Better, Heat or Ice?

So, how does the massage therapist choose between ice and heat? If a client complains of a stiff neck, do you reach for an ice pack or a hot pack? Before we can answer these questions, let's review the effects of ice and heat.

The best way to approach this dilemma is first to reexamine the body's response to each modality. The next step is to compare the effects of ice and heat to highlight any similarities or note any striking differences. The last step is to incorporate this information with actual massage situations. Use Table 23–4 to gather and record information. Space has been provided for your own additions and conclusions.

In comparing the effects of heat and ice, it is fair to say that both are highly therapeutic and have significant value in the field of massage therapy. Ice is usually preferred if inflammation is present or suspected, or if an area is swollen. Because postmassage soreness is common following a deep-tissue session, cryotherapy can be used to cool and calm down these areas.

Heat is the best choice to warm the client, in preparation for massage, and to generally relax the client before or during the massage.

Ice? Heat? The great temperature debate may come down to personal preference.

Table 23–4
Comparative Effects of Ice and Heat

Physiological Response	Initial Effect of Ice	Prolonged Effect of Ice	Initial Effect of Heat	Prolonged Effect of Heat
Heart rate	increases	decreases	decreases	increases
Vascular response	contraction	dilation	dilation	contraction
Depth of action	superficial	deep	superficial	superficial
Pain-spasm-pain cycle	interrupts		interrupts	
Muscle tissue volume	decreases		increases	
Fascial response	unchanged		softens	
Tissue damage	decreases			
Analgesic	no	no	yes	yes
Anesthetic	no	yes	no	no
Inflammatory response	decreases		increases	
Renal response	stimulates		inhibits	
Digestive response	stimulates		inhibits	
General response	excites	relaxes	relaxes	intense heat excites
________	________	________	________	________
________	________	________	________	________

ments or liniment-type lotions on a client's hands or near mucous membranes.

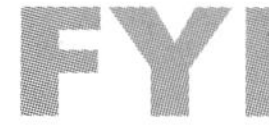

FOR YOUR INFORMATION

In 1785, Antoine Lavoisier proved that water is composed of two parts hydrogen and one part oxygen.

MINI•LAB

Arrange a meeting with a local physical therapist. Ask her how and why she uses ice, heat, and water in rehabilitation. Prepare a summary and present it to the class.

SUMMARY

Hydrotherapy is one of the oldest forms of therapeutic pain relief known to man. The large variety of therapies available encompasses water in all three of its physical states, solid (ice), liquid (water), and gas (vapor). These therapeutic modalities can be further classified on the basis of temperature, with hydrotherapy containing those methods closest to normal body temperature. Hydrotherapy applications include salt glows, sitz baths, Turkish shampoos, and Swedish shampoos. Cryotherapy is the external application of cold and is regarded as the most effective of these therapies. It includes ice packs, ice massage, cold immersion baths, cryokinetics, and cold mitten friction. The last category is the application of heat: thermotherapy. Thermotherapy encompasses both moist and dry therapies, including whirlpools, liniments, paraffin baths, hot packs, spinal packs, steam baths, Russian baths, and saunas.

Both cryotherapy and thermotherapy may be used alternately or simultaneously, to achieve a contrast effect. All of these therapies can stand by themselves or be used in combination; however, the greatest benefit to the client may be derived when they are used as adjuncts to massage.

SELF-TEST

Multiple Choice • Write the letter of the best answer in the space provided.

_______ 1. Hydrotherapy is defined as the therapeutic use of

A. massage in humid conditions
B. massage with water-based lubricants
C. water and complementary agents, such as soap and salt
D. water that is ingested during the massage

_______ 2. Cryotherapy refers to the application of

A. cold
B. electrical currents
C. heat
D. liniments

_______ 3. Thermotherapy includes the application of

A. cold
B. electrical currents
C. heat
D. petrissage

_______ 4. Temperatures beyond which temperature range can cause tissue damage?

A. 32° and 124°F
B. 45° and 110°F
C. 40° and 120°F
D. 50° and 98.6°F

_______ 5. Clean each item at the beginning of each workday with

A. lavender
B. an abrasive cleanser
C. an autoclave
D. mild soap and water

_______ 6. Surfaces that come in direct contact with the client as well as all reservoirs that collect perspiration or exfoliated skin cells must be cleaned

A. after each treatment
B. once a week
C. every 72 hours
D. once a month

_______ 7. Ask clients not to eat

A. after 8:00 P.M. the day before their scheduled appointment
B. 1 hour before the hydrotherapy treatment
C. the day of the hydrotherapy treatment
D. food intake is not a consideration

_______ 8. Which is *not* a benefit of hydrotherapy?

A. cleans and exfoliates the skin and improves skin tone
B. increases cutaneous circulation
C. decreases swelling and inflammation
D. produces a calming, relaxing effect

_______ 9. Which is *not* a contraindication of hydrotherapy?

A. tension headaches
B. open or weeping wounds
C. topical infections and skin rashes
D. freshly shaved skin

_______ 10. The application of wet salt on the skin used as an exfoliant is called a

A. salt glow
B. Swedish shampoo
C. brine massage
D. sitz bath

_______ 11. The principal massage stroke used to apply the wet salt mixture is

A. tapotement
B. friction
C. petrissage
D. vibration

_______ 12. Which hydrotherapy treatment involves brushing the body with a brush dipped in warm soapy water and a pail pour of water at 105°F?

A. salt glow
B. Swedish shampoo
C. brine massage
D. sitz bath

_______ 13. A sitz bath is a type of bath in which

A. the client's hands and feet are immersed
B. the client is is lying supine, water is at the level of the ischial tuberosity
C. the client's head is immersed
D. the client is sitting in water up to her navel

_______ 14. During the application of cold, cycles of vasoconstriction and vasodilation occur. This is known as the

A. up-and-down response
B. cyclic response
C. hunting response
D. cold response

_______ 15. The sensations experienced by most clients during cold application are felt in which order?

A. coldness, burning, stinging or aching, and numbness

B. burning, stinging or aching, coldness, and numbness
C. coldness, numbness, stinging or aching, and burning
D. numbness, coldness, burning, and stinging or aching

_______ 16. Which of the following is *not* a benefit of cryotherapy?
A. interrupts pain-spasm-pain cycle, reducing muscle spasm
B. exfoliates the skin
C. reduces swelling, tissue damage, and blood clot formation
D. reduces inflammatory response as ice draws heat out of an area

_______ 17. Which of the following is *not* a contraindication of cryotherapy?
A. Raynaud's disease
B. rheumatoid conditions
C. clients with sensory impairments or the inability to react to excessive temperature changes
D. local inflammation

_______ 18. Cold immersion baths involves soaking a/n
A. nonaffected area in a container of icy water
B. affected area in a container of icy water
C. nonaffected area in a container of tepid water
D. affected area in a container of tepid water

_______ 19. Ice massage combines the use of cryotherapy with
A. effleurage C. petrissage
B. deep breathing D. circular friction

_______ 20. The application of cold, followed by full range of motion of the affected area is called
A. cryokinetics C. dynamic freezing
B. cold mitten friction D. icicle

_______ 21. The application of cold accompanied by friction movements generated at a force of 5 to 10 pounds of pressure is called
A. cryokinetics C. contrast bath
B. cold mitten friction D. ice massage

_______ 22. The most potent technique in the therapeutic use of cold is to combine it with heat. This is called
A. cryokinetics C. contrast bath
B. cold mitten friction D. hot and cold friction

_______ 23. Thermotherapy is the external application of
A. water for therapeutic purposes
B. heat for therapeutic purposes
C. hot and cold water for therapeutic purposes
D. heat and aromatherapy for therapeutic purposes

_______ 24. The delivery method that involves the exchange of thermal energy while the body's surface is in direct contact with the thermal agent is
A. convection C. radiation
B. conduction D. diffusion

_______ 25. A rapid process of heat transfer in which the body's surface is in contact with a heated fluid medium is called
A. conduction C. radiation
B. convection D. osmosis

_______ 26. The transfer of heat energy in electromagnetic rays through a conducting medium, such as air, is called
A. convection C. radiation
B. conduction D. diffusion

_______ 27. Which of the following is *not* a benefit of thermotherapy?
A. soothes, sedates, and comforts
B. relieves pain
C. reduces inflammation
D. distends and relaxes superficial fascia

_______ 28. Which of the following is *not* a contraindication of thermotherapy?
A. muscle spasm C. cardiac impairment
B. phlebitis D. skin infections

_______ 29. Water that is agitated, mixed with air, and directed against an immersed, affected part, is called
A. a whirlpool bath
B. hot packs or fomentation packs
C. a paraffin bath
D. a steam bath

_______ 30. The type of heat application that uses a petroleum-based waxy mixture that is white and odorless, is a

A. whirlpool bath
B. hot pack or fomentation pack
C. paraffin bath
D. steam bath

_______ 31. A moist heat application used for pain relief is called a

A. whirlpool bath
B. hot pack or fomentation pack
C. paraffin bath
D. steam bath

_______ 32. Hot vapor baths given in specially designed chambers where the temperatures are maintained at 105° to 130°F at 100 percent humidity are

A. whirlpool baths
B. saunas
C. paraffin baths
D. steam baths

_______ 33. An alcoholic, oily, or soapy agent used in massage to create the sensation of heat is called a

A. poultice
B. liniment
C. painkiller
D. anti-inflammatory

References

Barnes, Lan. "Cryotherapy — Putting Injury on Ice". *Physician and Sportsmedicine.* Vol. 7, No. 6, June 1979, pp. 130–136.

Drez, David. *Therapeutic Modalities for Sports Injuries.* St. Louis: Times Mirror/Mosby College Publishing, 1986.

Klafs, Carl, and Daniel D. Arnheim: *Modern Principles of Athletic Training.* St Louis: CV Mosby, 1981.

Knight, Kenneth. *Cryotherapy: Theory, Technique and Physiology.* Chattanooga, Tennessee: Chattanooga Corporation, 1985.

Lawrence, D. Baloti. *Waterworks.* New York: Putnam Publishing Group, 1989.

Leibold, Gerhard. *Practical Hydrotherapy.* Wellingborough, England: Thorson Publishers Limited, 1980.

Mellion, Morris B. *Sportsmedicine Secrets.* Philadelphia: Hanley and Belfus, Inc., 1994.

Nikola, R. J. *Creatures of Water.* Salt Lake City: Europa Therapeutic, 1997.

Tepperman, Perry S., and Michael Devilin. "Therapeutic Heat and Cold; A Practitioner's Guide." *Postgraduate Medicine.* Vol. 73. No. 1. January 1983, pp. 69–76.

Thrash, Agatha, and Calvin Thrash. *Home Remedies: Hydrotherapy, Massage, Charcoal and Other Simple Treatments.* Seale, Alabama: Yuchi Pines Institute, 1981.

When the only tool you have is a hammer, every problem looks like a nail.

—Albert Einstein

Cathy Allen

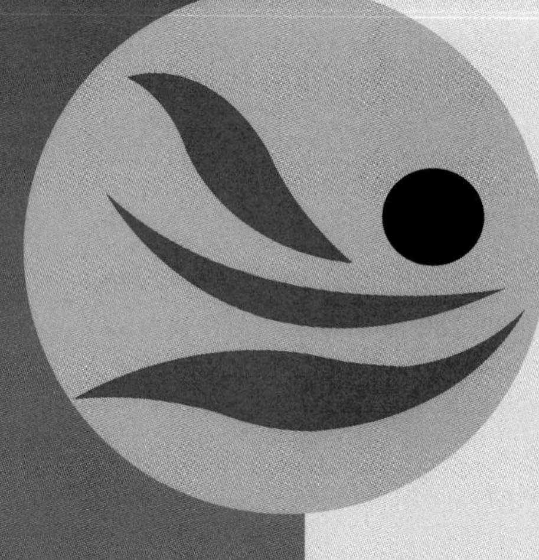

24 Foot Reflexology

Student Objectives

After completing this chapter, the student should be able to:

- Discuss the theories of how foot reflexology works
- Identify the ten zones and the horizontal landmarks on the foot
- Explain the importance of relaxation techniques prior to the foot reflexology session
- Locate all the reflex points on the feet and ankles
- Perform the basic techniques used in foot reflexology

INTRODUCTION

Historically, feet have been revered and considered sacred in most countries and most cultures. Jesus washed the feet of his disciples, and Asian students traditionally kissed the feet of their spiritual teacher. Native Americans believed the feet were sacred because they are our contact with the earth's energy; therefore, feet should be uncovered to receive her life force.

Sometimes feet were not so revered. In some oriental cultures, the feet of women were bound from birth to prevent growth; tiny feet were considered feminine. And yet we do not have to travel back in culture and time to experience the misuse of the feet. How many of us stuff our feet into ill-fitting shoes that look stylish but deform our toes and impair our circulation?

So why does it seem that we have such a strong fascination and reverence for our feet? According to ancient Eastern healing principles, the feet accumulate human energy and healing force. If we compare reflexology to shiatsu, acupuncture, and many other body therapies, we discover that this energy, or chi, exists as a specific and significant force in the body. In our polarized world, energy fields surround our bodies just as magnetic fields flow between the North and South poles. We are all enmeshed in this life force. Just as iron filings form a specific configuration when a magnet is held over them, many believe that energy travels through the body in a specific pattern.

In foot reflexology, these energy pathways are called **zones.** Foot reflexology is basically energy work brought down to the scale of the foot (although reflexology principles are applicable to the hands as well, the focus on this chapter will be on foot reflexology). In this section we will study the arrangement of reflex zones on the feet and learn the benefits and contraindications of reflexology as well as the specific techniques for improving the health of a reflex point.

HISTORY OF REFLEXOLOGY

Reflexology originated over 5,000 years ago, when pressure therapies were seen as preventive and therapeutic medicine. Indeed, the use of pressure points on the feet and hands may be older than acupuncture itself (Fig. 24–1). Reflexology is rooted in the same theory that energy pathways exist throughout the body; however, in reflexology the pathways begin in the feet; blockages lead to illness and disease.

One of the earliest pieces of evidence we have concerning the existence of reflexology dates back to 2,500 B.C. It is a pictograph from an Egyptian physician's tomb, depicting a physician performing both hand and foot reflexology to ease his patient's pain. Underneath the pictograph is carved the words "Do not hurt me." To this, the physician replies, "I will act only to help you."

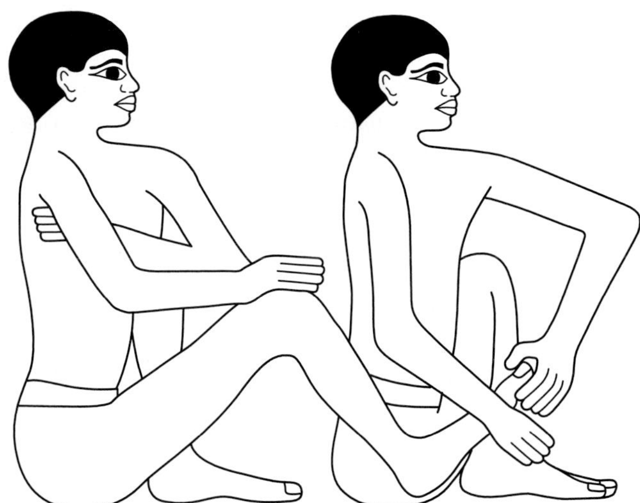

Figure 24•1 Hieroglyphics of reflexology.

At about this same time, other historical tracts show reflexology springing forth from the Far East. The path of reflexology's growth can be traced from India to China to Japan. Early statues from India of the Hindu god Vishnu depict Sanskrit symbols placed on his feet at the same location where modern reflexologists locate reflex points.

Over centuries, knowledge of this art form spread, and reflexology was used around the world to ease aches and pains. Modern reflexology developed out of zone therapy and the research and writings of Dr. William Fitzgerald in the early 1900s. It was popularized in North America by Eunice Ingham, a physiotherapist, who is affectionately referred to as "the mother of reflexology." She spent most of her life mapping the exact location of reflexes on the feet. She was an untiring disciple whose primary focus was to spread the word of this art form through teaching, writing, and demonstrating reflexology on as many people as possible.

Today in many parts of Europe and China, reflexology is an accepted form of medical treatment that offers health benefits for relief from conditions ranging from a simple headache to diabetes mellitus. In these countries, reflexologists are encouraged to design and prescribe viable treatment plans. The practitioner works in concert with other healthcare professionals to enhance the well-being of patients. In the United States, reflexologists can only legally provide clients with stress reduction through deep relaxation and improved circulation.

HOW REFLEXOLOGY WORKS

Foot reflexology is based on the theory that our entire body, including organs, glands, and body parts, have reflex points located on the feet. Through applied pressure, one can release blockages around the corresponding body part and rebalance the entire body. You can think of the feet as a scanner screen recording body function. Disease in the body will manifest itself on the feet. Stimulating a reflex point can balance the body when it has drifted from a state of health.

The reflexes in the feet are actually "reflections" of the body parts. Reflex locations and relationships to each other follow a logical anatomical pattern that closely resembles that of the body itself. Glancing at a reflexology chart, imagine that you are laying the feet alongside the body, with the toes next to the head.

Foot reflexologists believe there are ten zones or energy pathways in the body, which run vertically from the toes to the head. There are five zones beginning on each foot, with all ten zones meeting on the head. These zones pass through every part of the body; consequently, all organs, glands, and body parts will fall into one or more of the zones. If you were to draw a line starting at the big toe and continuing straight up to the head, everything within that line would be considered zone 1. For example, zone 2 is aligned with the second toe, zone 3 the third toe, and so on. By working the zones, you could affect the entire body.

Congestion or tension in any part of the zone will affect the entire zone. Sensitivity to pressure in a specific zone or reflex point signals that there is something manifesting in an organ or body part. Direct pressure will affect the entire zone; by directing life force along its natural pathways to untangle "energy knots" caused by physical or emotional stress, tension can be relieved.

There are channels of energy coursing through the body. When the body is in a state of health, this life force is free-flowing energy. Disease or pain is a block or imbalance in the life force. The life force does not differentiate between physical and emotional pain, which are simply expressions of blocked life force.

Another theory suggests that by pressing on the feet, toxins and impurities are released by increasing local circulation. The feet are the most distal region of the body. Venous circulation may not be adequate to push all the fluid back to the heart, and the lymphatic circulation may be sluggish. Consequently, a pooling of heavier toxins such as lactic and uric acid can develop around the nerves and blood vessels in the feet, blocking vital body functions. Reflexology can act to push these toxins back into the circulation of blood and lymph. At the same time, vital connections between the feet and the corresponding body parts are stimulated and energized.

There are over 7,200 nerves enervating each foot. Each organ and muscle is connected by a network of nerves to a tiny point on the foot, where the energy terminates. Many people think that when you apply pressure to reflex points on the feet, the nervous system carries messages to the corresponding body area, stimulating it electrochemically.

Thus far no one has been able to explain scientifically why or how reflexology works. However, for many years, many reflexologists have worked successfully to offer relief using this technique, and the results cannot be denied.

BENEFITS AND CONTRAINDICATIONS

Reflexology offers deep relaxation, and relaxation is the first step toward physiological and psychological normalization. Since stress is a frequent reality for most of our clients, reflexology can serve as a preventive program. If reflexology never accomplishes anything more than combating stress with relaxation, it serves humanity well. However, for those who practice reflexology, the benefits go far beyond relaxation.

One of the reasons reflexology is so favored over other forms of massage is that there is no undressing and no problems with towels and oils. This massage can be practiced virtually anywhere that is comfortable for both the practitioner and the client.

Reflexology is safe to use with most of your clients and there are very few contraindications. Unlike massage therapy, reflexology is safe for clients living with cancer, unless a tumor is located on the foot. However, cancer patients who are receiving chemotherapy or radiation therapy should be given shorter, more frequent treatments because their body systems are already taxed. Elderly clients or clients who are weak from a long illness should be treated with lighter pressure. Other structures and situations to avoid are pressing directly on varicose veins or corns; avoid working on the feet if the client has any contagious or infectious disease such as athlete's foot or any open wounds or sores on the foot. Clients with diabetes often have neuropathy (decrease or change in sensation in the hands and feet); lighter pressure should be used. Avoid inflamed joints, especially in clients with gouty arthritis.

BEFORE AND AFTER REFLEXOLOGY

One of the joys of reflexology is that it can be practiced anywhere. Your client may be seated or lying down prone or supine during the session with bare feet. Although reflexology can be performed through socks and stockings, the therapist's fingers, thumbs, or knuckles tend to slide off the reflex points, and the client's skin may become irritated from the cloth fibers. In addition, certain reflex points located between the toes are difficult to approach through socked feet. Bare feet are best because skin-to-skin contact between the therapist and the client provides a concrete connection. The important thing is that you and the client are both comfortable.

The therapist needs freedom of movement and a sense of grounding; the body should not be unnecessarily bent and contorted or the wrists at extreme angles. The client should not have to hold up his body weight, but be resting comfortably. Ideally, his feet should be resting on a clean towel, but paper towels will suffice.

Conduct an interview to rule out any contraindication and to establish the client's needs. For a discussion of this process, see Chapter 20. Show the client to the area where the reflexology session will take place, and discuss the procedure, answering all questions to the best of your ability. Wash your hands before and after each session.

To relax the muscles of the feet, begin the foot reflexology session with a foot bath; use cool water on a hot day or warm water on a cold day. Use an astringent or a few drops of your favorite essential oil (lavender is good for insomnia or sage for detoxification). A mist of green alcohol is refreshing to feet that have been cooped up in workboots all day. An alternative (if you own a microwave) is to heat up two damp hand towels, sprinkle them with the essential oil, then wrap the client's feet. Allow the client to sit back and relax.

After the session, stimulate the feet with a dry brush, and dust with a foot powder. Help your client put on his shoes and socks, if appropriate. Always be within arm's reach as the client is transferring to and from the table or chair where the session takes place. It is helpful to ask the client to drink plenty of fluid, namely clean water, for a day or two following the session.

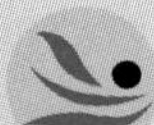

MINI•LAB

The following activity is designed to help you achieve self-relaxation and can be used to center yourself before a reflexology session.

Sit comfortably in a chair, feet flat on the floor, sensing the connection between your feet and the earth. Take a few deep breaths through your nostrils, imagining that you are drawing air up from the earth through your feet. As you exhale, allow the breath to exit through your mouth; imagine the exhaled air as it moves out of the top of your head and down your arms and out through the palms of your hands and your fingertips. In energetic bodywork, the exhaled breath is potential energy.

For the next few minutes, sit and continue to follow your breathing, anchoring your thoughts in the breath. Sense each inhalation and exhalation as it flows through your nostrils and mouth. When the mind wanders, gently anchor your thoughts with the breath. Your thoughts can be like a playful puppy who cannot be still. Over time, with this simple meditation practice, your mind will become more focused. It is like flexing new muscles. Imagine with each exhalation that the breath traveling down your arms becomes a warm, healing ball of energy in your palms, and the exhalation feeds that ball, sending the flames out through your fingertips.

Having taken the time to center yourself, you can now connect with your client. You may choose to rest the palms of your hands on the client's feet, knowing that you are grounded in the earth's energy and are allowing this energy to flow through your palms and into the client's feet. Imagine the energy continuing out through the top of her head, until both of you are part of a continuous circle of energy, with no beginning and no end.

Author's Note

Bringing yourself into the moment is vital for doing client-centered work. Our minds tend to wander, and unless we take time to become present, sensitive to our client's needs, we can perform an entire session that is technically proficient, yet does not touch on the intuitive skill required to listen to the body's subtle messages.

THE LUBRICATION SITUATION

As a rule, reflexologists do not use oils, creams, or lotions when giving a reflexology session. However, some reflexologists use a light lotion or cream. It is a matter of personal preference. You may use a lubricant to warm up the feet during foot relaxation, then wipe off any excess lubricant before you begin the point work. Warming up the foot with a lubricant also gives the hands a much needed break; many reflexologists complain that the joints in their hands ache from prolonged pressure. Foot powder or talc can be used as a substitute for cream.

By using oil or heavy lotion or cream, the foot becomes slippery and your fingers and thumbs may slide off reflex points. Because the bottom of the foot has a leathery quality, oil creates the sensation that the therapist's hands are trying to slide over rubber. The best choice is an oil-free cream that does not absorb so quickly that you have to reapply it often, yet that is not so greasy it never absorbs and you glide over the foot in the most superficial way. Read the label on lubricant bottles or contact manufacturers for product samples. Ask reflexologists in your area for their recommendations.

If you use any lubrication, wipe off any excess and apply ethyl alcohol before the client walks on the floor; this may prevent accidents from slips and slides. However, ethyl alcohol has a drying effect; avoid using ethyl alcohol or perfumed lubricants if your client has dry or cracked skin on her feet.

GENERAL GUIDELINES AND RELAXATION TECHNIQUES

Generally, a reflexology session begins with a relaxation technique such as deep breathing, guided imagery, or visualization. The reflexes will be more accessible if the client is relaxed and if the tissue feels pliable. As a rule, pressure does not have to be excruciatingly deep. Electrical intensity of the nerve impulse depends on the size of the nerve rather than the strength of the stimulus. If the foot is worked too deeply, the body will splint around the painful area, using muscular tension to protect from the invasion of the painful stimulus, which makes it more difficult to stimulate the reflex point. It is more effective to warm up the area well with noninvasive pressure and to increase pressure as the client can tolerate it, while staying attuned to deeper levels of softening and tissue release. By doing this the client's body will become relaxed and stay that way.

Relaxation techniques, also called "desserts," for relaxing the feet before, during, and after a reflexology session are shaking the feet from side to side, taking the foot through range of motion, sliding your knuckles down the bottom of the foot, or "wringing out the foot" (imagine the foot is a wet cloth and you are wringing out all the excess water). If you do whatever feels good to you while you are receiving a reflexology session, it will also feel good to the client. Clients enjoy their feet being kneaded and stroked. Do not be afraid to have fun and become inventive. You will discover that your hands and your client's feet work well together.

SELF-REFLEXOLOGY

Use a golf ball or tennis ball to massage your feet for those times when you are tired and your feet ache. Simply roll the bottom of your foot over a ball placed on the floor, pressing down on areas that feel good. Maintain a comfortable pressure for 15 seconds. Return to these areas for additional work as needed.

Author's Note

Many of the foot relaxation techniques are derived from watching children play with their own and others' feet.

REFLEXOLOGY TECHNIQUES

Reflexology is performed with the fingers, thumbs, or knuckles; however, if you were to browse through some of the earlier books on the subject, you would see examples of elastic bands and clothespins used to give sustained pressure to the points! Press to the point of dull sensitivity, not pain. Eye contact is a good measuring tool. Watch for signs of tension in the client's face, hand clenching, or body rigidity, then apply less pressure.

For pressure on the dorsum (top) of the foot, the fingers are generally used, as there is less padding on the fingertips, and thumb pressure is too strong. The thumbs are used on the plantar surface of the foot because the thick padding located there requires more intense pressure. On the thick skin of the heel, bend your index or middle finger over and use your knuckle. Avoid overtreating by working an area too long; working a reflex point for 15 to 30 seconds is fine, but use your own judgment. It is actually better to undertreat than to overtreat to prevent overstimulation of the body area. You may elect to go back and rework a reflex point.

The basic method is a walking technique, which requires that you inch the thumb along, bending and straightening at the interphalangeal joint. This is good for working the ten zones because there are so many reflexes along its path. Holding the foot firmly with one hand, slowly move the thumb and cover each area of the foot thoroughly; this ensures that all the reflexes on the foot are stimulated. To find the correct side of the thumb to use, rest your hand on your thigh and notice how the lateral (some texts call this the medial) edge of your thumb is the side in most direct contact with your leg. Begin to walk your thumb from your upper thigh toward your knee, bending and straightening at the most distal joint. As you move your thumb up in small increments, you should feel as if you are hitting reflex points. Try the same technique with your finger. The fingertips are used for hard to reach areas such as between the toes, where the thumbs are too big to be effective.

After you have mastered the thumb walk, you can try some specific techniques to work the reflexes. The first is direct pressure applied by your thumb, which can be increased by rotating, or flexing, the foot onto the point. The other is a hooking action in which you sink in with your thumb, then flex your knuckle like a bottle opener. Try it on your palm of your hand. If you break the hooking action into three parts, it looks like this: Locate the desired reflex, sink into the reflex with the thumb bent to apply pressure, then flip the knuckle over as if you are pushing the tissue aside and going deeper. This technique is used for hard to reach areas such as the pituitary reflex, which is deeply embedded in the great toe. If your hands tire, begin the relaxation strokes. After a few moments, return to the pointwork.

HOW THE FOOT IS MAPPED

There are ten zones in the body through which energy travels: five zones on each foot (Fig. 24–2). Imagine a line passing from the center between each toe directly down to the base of the heel, then continuing straight up to your head. Everything in this area in your body, including glands, organs, and body parts, is found in that particular zone located on your foot. If you follow zone 2 from the center of the second toe up through the body, you will pass through the kidneys and eventually the iris of the eyes. Zone 1 passes through the great toe, zone 2 passes through the second toe, and so on, until you reach the smallest toe, which is classified as zone 5. Each of these zones travels straight up through the body to meet on your head; therefore the head has all five zones from both feet. Any reflexology work done in that zone on the foot would affect anywhere along that part of the body.

Visually locate the four horizontal landmarks that are important aids in locating the foot reflexes. The first horizontal landmark is the neck/shoulder line located at the base of the toes, more specifically, at the space where the toes meet the ball of the feet. This is an important area to work for shoulder or neck pain. The next landmark is the diaphragm line, which is located where the ball of the foot meets the arch. In the diaphragm line, you will notice a change in skin texture and color. The edges of the foot rise up until they converge in the center. This line is shaped like the costal arches of the rib cage, which it represents. Just as you can slide your fingers up under the rib cage, you will get the same sensation when working the diaphragm reflex; you can easily slide your fingers

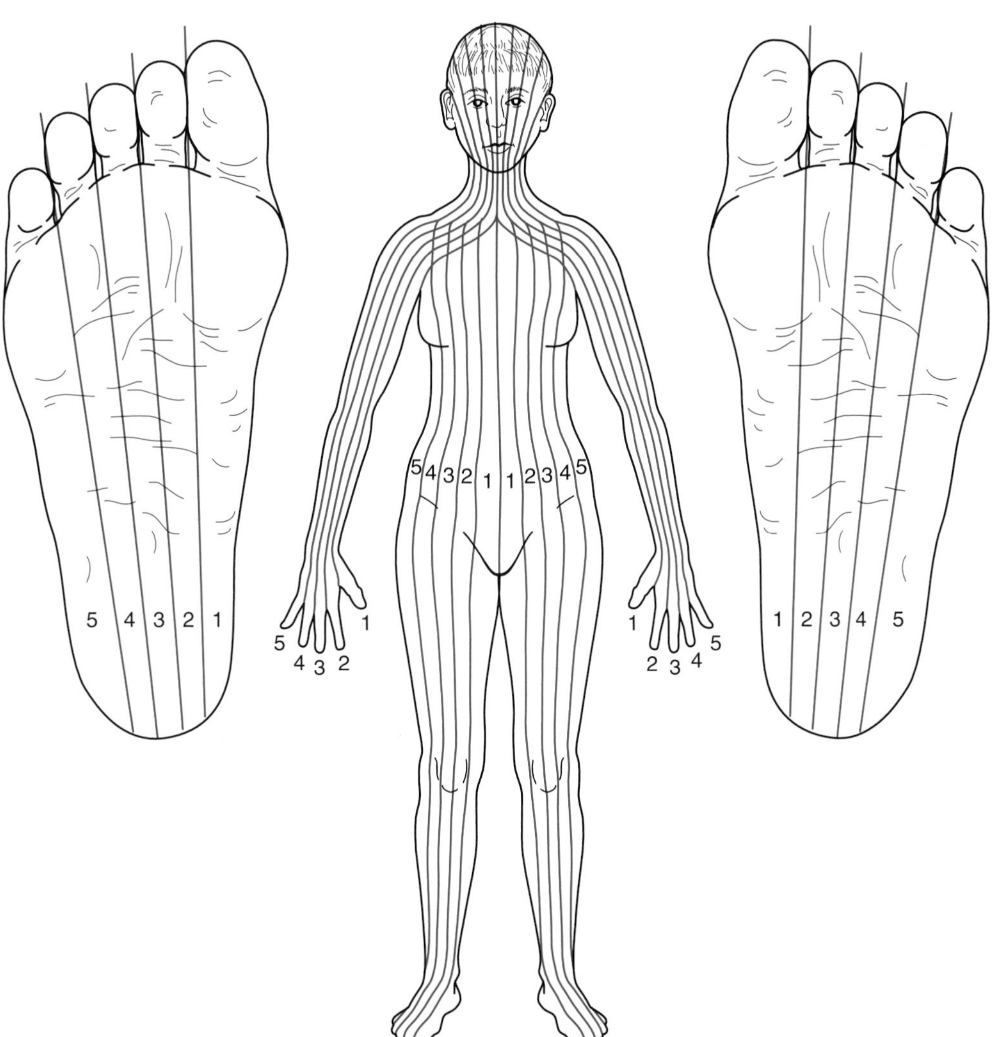

Figure 24•2 Horizontal demarcations.

up underneath the ball of the foot. The third landmark is the waistline. To locate this horizontal landmark, begin at the toes, and slide your middle finger down the lateral side of the foot until you hit a bump at about the middle of the foot. This bony protrusion is the proximal edge of the fifth metatarsal, as well as the waistline demarcation. The last landmark is the pelvic line, and it is located where the heel line joins the bottom of the foot.

LOCATING THE REFLEXES

Once you have an understanding of the zones and horizontal landmarks, locate the foot reflexes. When learning reflexology, you can divide the foot into six areas: the head, the chest, the abdominal, the pelvic, the reproductive, and the spinal areas. In review, the foot is laid out anatomically the same as the body (Fig. 24–3).

Head Area

With this in mind, logically the big toe is the head reflex. The brain, the pituitary gland, the mouth reflexes are all found on the big toe. The pituitary reflex is referred to as the "master reflex" because it plays such an important role in all hormonal activities of the body. An effective method of locating this reflex is to look for the center of the swirl on the big toe and sink into that point with your thumb. Often you will feel a small pea-shaped area here. This is an effective reflex to work if you need an added boost of energy to get you through your day or for any glandular problems, due to its importance in the endocrine system.

Squeeze the toe padding to stimulate the sinus reflexes. During early spring when the pollen count is so high, this is the reflex most often requested for additional pointwork.

Chest Area

The entire ball of the foot is the reflex area for the lungs and the heart. In our bodies, the heart is two-thirds on the left and one-third on the right, as it is on the foot. You will find the heart reflex primarily on the left foot, with a small section on the right. This area is important to work for asthma and other respiratory conditions. In the ball of the foot, between the first and second toe, is the bronchial reflex. Use a pincer technique and grasp the area between your thumb and index finger. Using the thumb-walking technique, work between the metatarsals as well as on the bones themselves. If a client is particularly congested, it is effective to jiggle the metatarsals, changing the relationship of the bones. Creating space in the interosseous membranes is like opening and creating space in the intercostal spaces.

If a client is suffering from shoulder pain, grasp the ball of the lateral side of the foot (the little toe side) between your thumb and index finger and give it a firm squeeze. Ask your client to unlock his jaw at the same time.

This diaphragmatic area is an important demarcation. Working it early in the session allows the client to breathe with ease, encouraging deeper states of relaxation and a more effective reflexology session.

Another important reflex in the chest area is the solar plexus, which experienced reflexologists refer to as the "key to relaxation." In the body, it is often referred to as the "abdominal brain" because it contains a large number of nerves. It is located under the ball of the foot between the second and third toes; occasionally it is found closer to the great toe and the second toe. Your client knows exactly when you land on the point and will reward you with a generous sigh of relief. Of all the reflexes, return to this reflex often because pressing it returns the client to a place of relaxation, especially after much deep pressure. It helps to have the client breathe deeply into the solar plexus area of the body while you hold the point on the feet (Fig. 24–4).

Abdominal Area

Slide your middle finger along the lateral side of the foot to the proximal edge of the fifth metatarsal (the demarcation for the waistline). Everything between this line and the diaphragm line is laid out as it is in your body. The spleen and stomach are located on the left side of the body, and the liver and gallbladder are on the right side. Work the spleen reflex on individuals who have anemia and who experience blood deficiencies, because the spleen plays such an important role in blood formation and storage (as does the liver). Having more than 500 functions, the liver is one of the most complex organs of the body. The liver reflex can be worked for everything from blood sugar to cholesterol to skin problems. Another important reflex to stimulate is the pancreas. It is located on the right foot just behind the stomach. Both the liver and the pancreas should be worked thoroughly on anyone with diabetes mellitus. Avoid overworking the reflexes of the abdominal area in the initial 4 weeks of treatments because the reflexology in this area may leave the client feeling overwhelmed and exhausted.

Pelvic Area

Continuing on down the foot toward the heel, just below the waistline demarcation, is the pelvic area, which houses all of the lower abdominal organs. On the right foot, note the ascending colon and part of the transverse colon; on the left foot are the descending colon and the other half of the transverse colon.

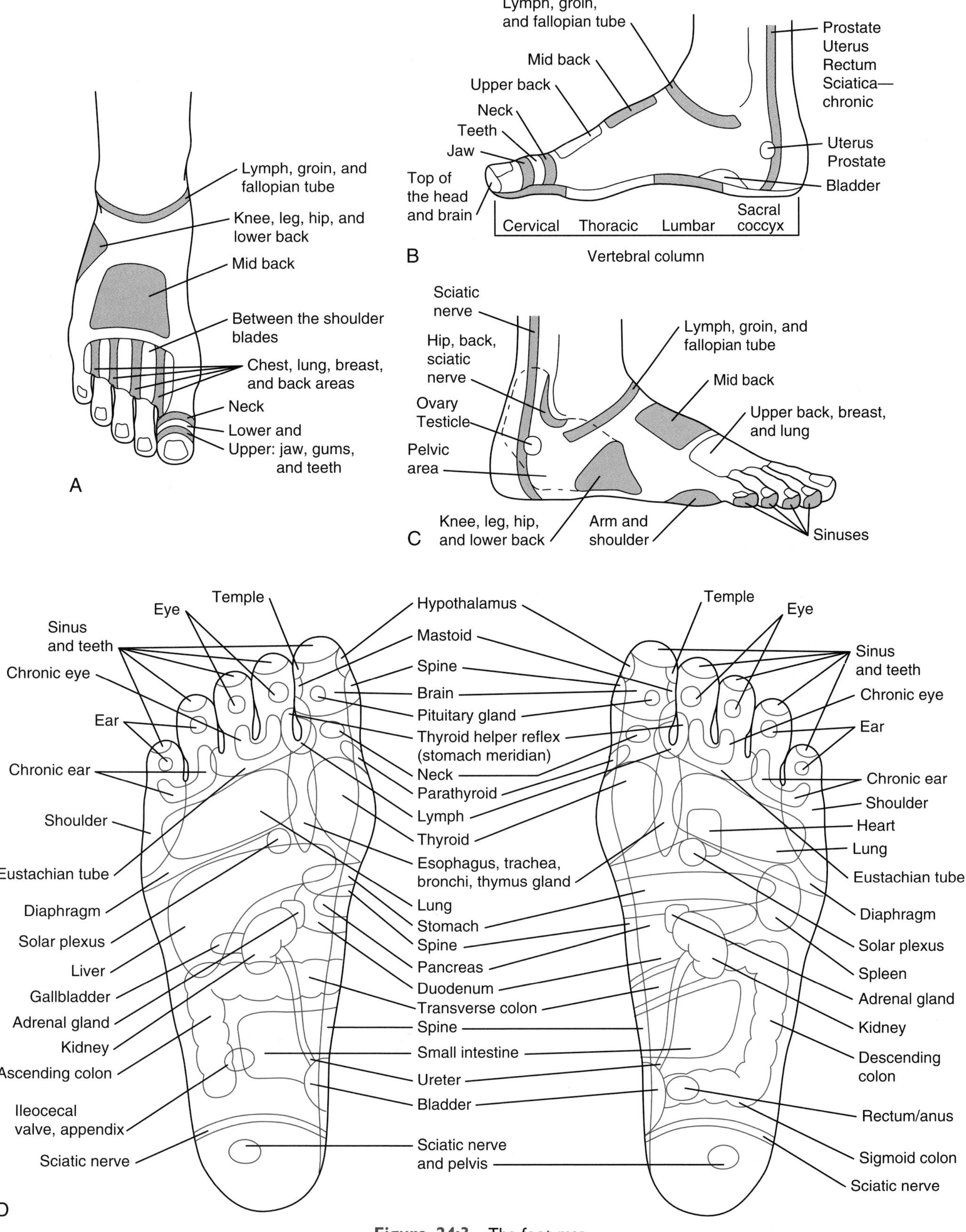

Figure 24•3 The foot map.

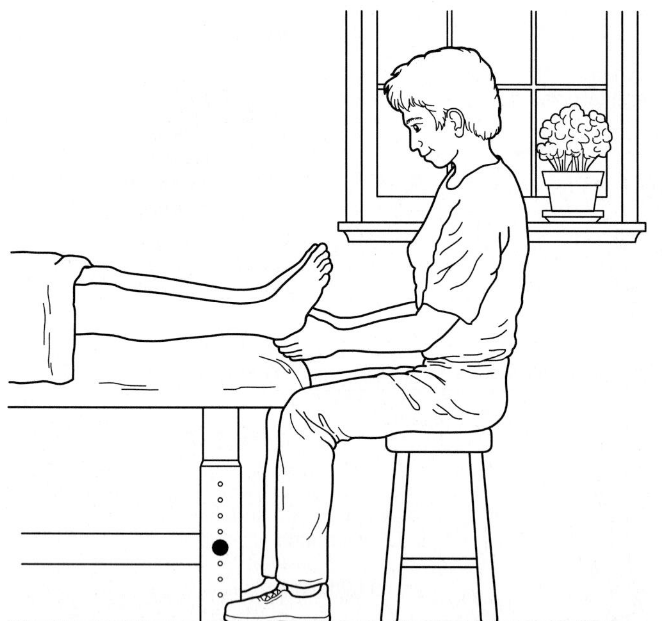

Figure 24•4 A therapist sitting in a chair holding the solar plexus points; she is relaxed, with her feet firmly planted on the ground.

The large intestine surrounds and is a continuation of the small intestine. The pelvic area is important to work on individuals experiencing intestinal inflammatory conditions such as back pain.

The organs of the urinary system are also located here in the pelvic area. You may notice a puffy area where the pelvic line meets the arch of the foot. This is the urinary bladder reflex. Sometimes redness and puffiness here suggest an imbalance in this reflex. If that is the case, warm up the area first with light massage strokes, then gently sink your thumb into the point. Work this area briefly, then continue with the rest of the foot, returning to work on it throughout the session. After you have come back to the urinary bladder several times, the initial tenderness decreases and the reflex point may look less swollen! You may use this approach of working and reworking on any blocked reflexes on the foot.

The kidneys are also located in the pelvic region of the body. The kidney reflex point is located along the waistline demarcation, between the second and third toes. Because of the kidney's role in filtering toxins from the blood and producing urine, this reflex can be worked for cystitis, blood pressure problems, and to encourage the body to rid itself of toxins.

Reproductive Area

One of the last areas worked in reflexology is the reproductive reflexes, the heel. More specifically, the medial heel is the location of the uterus/prostate reflexes, and the lateral heel is the location for the ovaries/testes reflexes. To locate the reflex for the uterus/prostate, measure from the high point of the medial malleolus to the base of the heel; in the middle of that diagonal line you will find the reflex. Use the same measuring procedure to find the ovaries/testes on the outside of the heel. Avoid using your thumb to stimulate these reflexes—they tend to be hypersensitive. They may be worked when women are suffering from emotional imbalances as well as premenstrual syndrome (PMS). Work these areas on men if they are experiencing prostate problems.

The next set of foot reflexes worked is the sciatic nerve. Working on this reflex can reduce sciatic pain. To locate it, imagine a stirrup running from the inside of the calf, medial to the Achilles tendon, to about 4 to 6 inches above the ankle bone. Because this is the actual path of the sciatic nerve, hypersensitivity may be experienced by the client, especially if she has low back or sciatic pain.

Spinal Area

The last set of reflexes, and one of the most important, is the spinal reflex located in the spinal area on the medial aspect of the foot. As you look at the arch of the foot, you will notice that it has four distinct curves, just like your vertebral column. If a client has a flat back, chances are he also has flat feet. Likewise, if he has a high arch, chances are he has an exaggerated lumbar curve.

There are 31 pairs of spinal nerves that feed virtually every part of the body. By working the spinal reflex you can affect the entire body; this reflex is therefore worked in every session. Walk your thumb along the spine reflex, pressing on and under the bones of the arch continuously from the base of the heel to the tips of the great toe. If you only have a few minutes to work on the feet, perform the thumb walk on the entire spinal reflex.

Two of the goals of reflexology are to assist health maintenance by preserving homeostasis within the entire system and by promoting deep relaxation. Just because someone is experiencing pain or discomfort in a specific area of the body does not always mean blockage will be found in exactly that same place on the foot. You may find tenderness anywhere in the body system of which the affected organ is part. Therefore, it is important to work the entire system thoroughly when tender reflexes are detected. For example, if a client complains of stomach discomfort, you may find tenderness in the liver reflex, which is part of the digestive system.

DOCUMENTING YOUR REFLEXOLOGY SESSION

Documentation is a useful tool for mapping your client's progress. Before the initial session, take a thor-

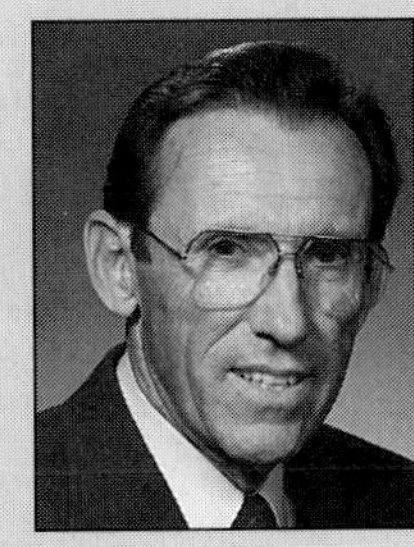

Dwight Byers

Born: February 10, 1929

"You may be walking on the solution to many of your health problems."

Dwight Byers claims he was one of the guinea pigs for his aunt's early work in reflexology. His aunt, Eunice Ingham, a physical therapist and member of the New York Medical Massage Therapist Association, worked during the early 1930s for a doctor who had a passing interest in the art of "zone therapy." Zone therapy was a predecessor of reflexology and was introduced in the early 1900s by Dr. William H. Fitzgerald, who successfully used different devices to place pressure on certain points on the hands to relieve pain.

Eunice Ingham took this work a step further and put her own mark on this ancient healing art, which was practiced as far back as 2,330 B.C. According to Byers, his aunt was strong-willed, extremely intuitive, and totally dedicated to easing suffering in her fellow man.

Along with a compassionate heart, Ingham had a keen mind. Her time-honored techniques are the result of experiment, research, and copious notes. She threw out what didn't work and perfected what did. For a more detailed review of her results, check out her books: *Stories the Feet Can Tell Through Reflexology* and *Stories the Feet Have Told Through Reflexology*.

It was Ingham's dedication to helping relieve suffering that proved inspirational to her young nephew, who was at first skeptical. His skepticism—as well as his hay fever and asthma—vanished after experiencing his aunt's healing touch firsthand.

"At first we kind of laughed at her," remembers Byers, as he shares the stories of traveling with his aunt as she conducted seminars on reflexology throughout the United States. "I helped her carry her bags and set up. But soon I became fascinated, and eventually my sister and I began helping her teach."

Byers's background as a medic in the army and later his experience in mortuary science helped hone some of his anatomy skills as he was practicing reflexology part-time. When his aunt died in 1974, Byers formed the International Institute of Reflexology to help preserve the original Ingham method. In 1983 he published his book, *Better Health With Foot Reflexology* for the same reason.

This book defines reflexology as "the science that deals with the principle that there are reflex areas in the feet and hands which correspond to all the glands, organs, and parts of the body. Reflexology is a unique method of using the thumb and fingers on the reflex areas to help relieve stress and tension, improve blood supply, promote the unblocking of nerve impulses, and help nature achieve homeostasis."

Basically, every aspect of your body can be "found" on the bottom of your feet and these locations correspond roughly with anatomy, thus the term "zone therapy." For instance, the gallbladder is located in your upper torso to your right. On the bottom of the right foot, its corresponding point is to the upper portion of the right foot. But it's not enough to know where particular organs are located. Reflexologists are also trained in physiology to understand how different body systems interface. For instance, while working with someone who might have gallstones, added emphasis is placed on the entire digestive system. Studying the correct pressure and type of motion to employ on the feet or hands is also vital.

"Reflexology sends a message to the organs to normalize, to decrease or increase hormonal levels," explains Byers. His results have been phenomenal. But even he admits that he doesn't have all the answers to why this method works.

In the forward of Byers's text, Dr. Ray C. Wunderlich Jr. offers some compelling theories to account for reflexology's success:

continued on page 546

Continued

Dwight Byers

Quite probably, it will eventually be shown that foot reflexology alters energy flow in the body. . . . There are 7,200 nerve endings in each foot. Perhaps this fact, more than any other, explains why we feel so much better when our feet are treated. Nerve endings in the feet have extensive interconnections through the spinal cord and brain with all areas of the body.

—From *Better Health With Foot Reflexology* by Dwight Byers, 1983.

Byers, whose favorite adage is "Experience is the father of all knowledge," claims that the best results are obtained by those who practice, practice, practice. You've got to work on thousands of feet. My advice for beginning massage therapists is to master your art. Don't be a jack-of-all-trades and master of none."

It's also essential that the therapist is really the type that wants to help people and not someone who thinks of money first. "You've got to give a lot," he says. This isn't idle lip service from Byers. He has done his share of throwing in an extra free visit and has helped out senior citizens with discounted sessions.

He is a man who understands people. He's down to earth and pragmatic. So are his seminars. The final is "hands-on" and it's his feet that are up for grabs after about a 200-hour program. His criterion for grading? "Would I pay to have this treatment done?"

Massage therapists who become certified in reflexology use it to enhance their business. Beginning the session with reflexology can induce relaxation and increase circulation, which benefits muscles, glands, and internal organs from the inside out.

ough medical history. This can provide a better understanding of the client's state of health. Moreover, the history can provide information as to what may be causing imbalances that you palpate on the feet.

For all ensuing sessions, carefully record any sensitivities experienced and/or reactions to the visit as well as changes in the client's health status. Documentation becomes a useful tool to reference as sessions continue. Typically, when consistent records are kept regarding the client's progress, certain patterns emerge, for example, a young female client who may experience hypersensitivity on her feet only when she is ovulating. During this time, almost without fail, the reflexes of the endocrine glands are more sensitive than usual, especially the ovarian reflex. Likewise, just before she begins to menstruate, her feet may become more swollen than usual and more sensitive to touch. This pattern becomes evident only through documentation.

REFLEXOLOGIST'S DON'T LIST

Reflexologists do not prescribe or adjust prescription medications. Medical conditions are referred to a licensed physician.

Reflexologists do not diagnose. No one can be 100 percent sure what is causing tenderness on the foot.

Reflexologists cannot treat specific conditions or illnesses. Always work both feet during a session, and let the body heal itself. Any attempt to diagnose or prescribe could land a well-meaning reflexologist in court!

WHAT TENDERNESS MAY MEAN

Overall, a reflexology treatment should be a pleasurable experience. Although hypersensitivity on the feet will no doubt occur, it can be caused for a variety of reasons. Generally speaking, if only pressure is felt, one can say the reflex is healthy. When the feeling of slight discomfort or pain is present, it may mean the reflex and/or corresponding body area is under stress. Often your client will leave the session feeling deeply relaxed and will report back next session how wonderful he felt after the work.

However, a client might experience a headache or an increase of elimination through the skin, bowels, or urination. She may even experience a flare-up of an illness that had never really healed. All of these symptoms can be classified as a healing crisis. It is the body's way of throwing off excess toxins or impurities.

More than likely, most of these symptoms will go away in a few days, but of course if the client has any questions or concerns, refer her to her physician.

Imbalances on the feet can be experienced in a number of ways. As you palpate a reflex, you may feel a lumpy or grainy deposit, known as "crunchies." It is believed these are crystal deposits of uric and lactic acid that accumulate and pool in the feet. They create congestion and blockage around vital nerve functions and interfere with blood circulation to the feet. It is believed that massage of these areas breaks them down to a substance that the body can reabsorb into the lymph system and release from the body.

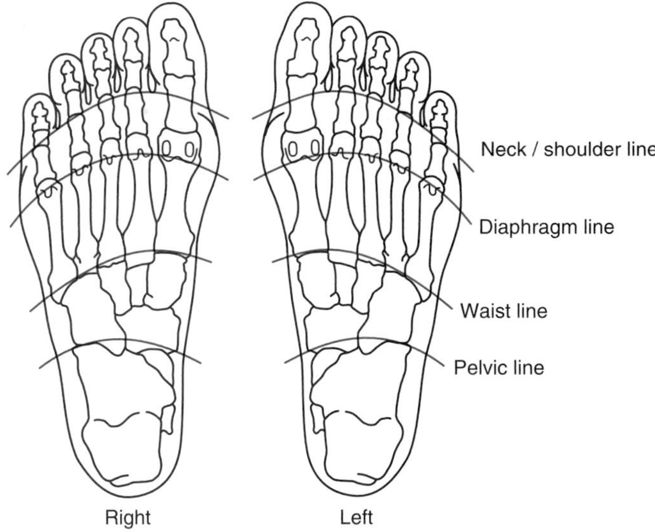

Figure 24•5 The ten zones.

SUMMARY

The manual manipulation of the feet has been practiced in one form or another for thousands of years. The importance of the feet has been well documented in different customs and cultures throughout the ages. Modern foot reflexology has its roots in the ancient theory and practice of shiatsu, acupuncture, and energy work. The routines we use today were popularized by Eunice Ingham, a physiotherapist of the 1900s. Reflexology postulates that there are specific points on the feet where a reflex mechanism exists for each organ or area on the entire body. There are five vertical zone patterns in each foot for a total of ten zones. The reflex for each zone corresponds to the body parts located above it. Problems in an organ are reflected to the reflex point and are manifested as sensitive "energy knots."

One way to locate the foot reflexes is by using a series of horizontal landmarks found on the foot (Fig. 24–5). By using firm but gentle pressure, the reflexologist assists the body to a state of health.

The massage therapist can use reflexology to balance the body system and facilitate homeostasis. Only the client can heal herself; the therapist can act as a catalyst by using reflexology techniques to unblock the river of energy that stagnates at tender reflexes.

Reflexology is safe and convenient to use. No draping is required, and there are few contraindications. Reflexology can be done in a regular chair, a recliner, or on a massage table. No lubricants are needed. Reflexology is a natural addition to the massage therapy practice (Fig. 24–6).

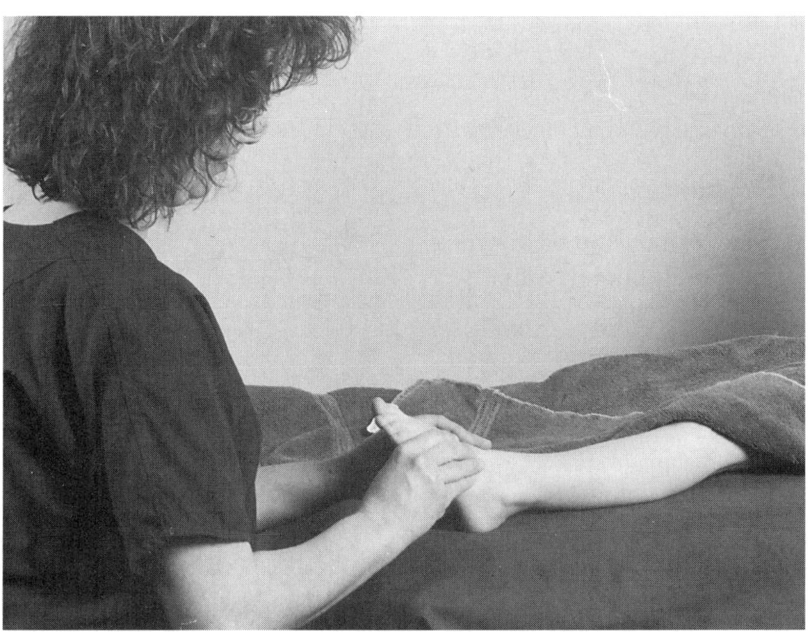
Figure 24•6 Therapist giving a foot reflexology session.

SELF-TEST

Multiple Choice • Write the letter of the best answer in the space provided.

_______ 1. In shiatsu and acupressure, energy pathways are called meridians and in foot reflexology, they are called

A. chi lines
B. zones
C. bipolar demarcations
D. Tao pathways

_______ 2. One of the earliest pieces of evidence we have concerning the existence of reflexology dates back to

A. 5,000 B.C.
B. 50 B.C.
C. 2,500 B.C.
D. 1877

_______ 3. The evidence was a pictograph found in a tomb in what country?

A. Greece
B. China
C. Manchuria
D. Egypt

_______ 4. Modern reflexology developed out of zone therapy and the research and writings of Dr.

A. William Fitzgerald
B. Petre Ling
C. Tiffany Field
D. James Cyriax

_______ 5. Foot reflexology is rooted in the theory that our entire body, including organs, glands, and body parts, has

A. trigger points in the muscles
B. reflex points located on the feet
C. tsubos along meridians
D. lactic acid buildup in myofascial structures of the body

_______ 6. The locations and relationship of the reflex points follow a logical anatomical pattern that closely resembles

A. ancient Oriental writings
B. the earth's bipolar gravitational field
C. the human body
D. the theory of evolution

_______ 7. Congestion or tension in any part of the zone will affect the

A. entire zone
B. the adjacent zone
C. all the zones in the foot
D. every other zone

_______ 8. Sensitivity in a specific part zone or reflex point signals that there is something going on

A. in the cosmos
B. in the organ or body part
C. in that body system
D. in the immune system

_______ 9. Direct pressure will affect the entire zone by directing life force along its natural pathways to

A. interfere with the pain-spasm-pain cycle
B. reduce insomnia by inducing sleep
C. untangle "energy knots" caused by physical or emotional stress
D. open up the subconscious mind

_______ 10. One of the reasons reflexology is so appealing to people over other forms of massage is

A. there is no undressing
B. it can be practiced almost anywhere
C. there are no towels or lubricants
D. all of the above

_______ 11. Which of the following is *not* a contraindication for reflexology?

A. clients living with cancer
B. varicose veins, corns, or calluses
C. any contagious or infectious disease like athlete's foot
D. any open wounds or sores on the foot

_______ 12. Ideally, reflexology is performed

A. through socks and stockings
B. through shoes with cloth soles
C. after Swedish massage
D. on bare feet

_______ 13. Which of the following is *not* done before reflexology?

A. conduct an interview to rule out any contraindication
B. establish the client's needs
C. answer all questions to the best of your ability and wash your hands
D. all are important before reflexology

_______ 14. After reflexology, it is often helpful to your client to put on his shoes and socks and to

A. be within arm's reach as he is transferring to and from the table or chair where the session takes place
B. have him schedule another appointment
C. give him a reflexology map
D. clean his shoes with a high-quality shoe cleaner

_______ 15. If the foot is worked too deeply, the body will

A. relax
B. heal faster
C. splint around the painful area, using muscular tension to protect from the invasion of the painful stimulus
D. eliminate toxins

_______ 16. Reflexology is performed with the

A. fingers
B. knuckles
C. thumbs
D. all the above

_______ 17. For pressure on the dorsum (top) of the foot, use the

A. fingers
B. knuckles
C. thumbs
D. all the above

_______ 18. When working on a reflex point, it is better to

A. use steady pressure
B. undertreat than to overtreat
C. use a wooden tool
D. use intermittent pressure

_______ 19. The basic technique used in reflexology is the

A. walking technique
B. point technique
C. running technique
D. Egyptian technique

_______ 20. The _______ are used for hard to reach areas such as between the toes, where the _______ are too big to be effective.

A. knuckles; fingertips
B. thumbs; fingertips
C. fingertips; thumbs
D. thumbs; wooden tools

_______ 21. The four horizontal landmarks, from toes to heel, are the

A. pelvic line, waistline, neck/shoulder line, and diaphragm line
B. waistline, pelvic line, diaphragm line, and neck/shoulder line
C. neck/shoulder line, pelvic line, diaphragm line, waistline
D. neck/shoulder line, diaphragm line, waistline, and pelvic line

_______ 22. When learning reflexology, you can divide the foot into six areas. These are the

A. head, chest, abdominal, pelvic, reproductive, and spinal areas
B. head, torso, diaphragm, bowel, back, and front areas
C. head, costal, diaphragm, bowel, back, and front areas
D. head, face, neck, torso, leg, and feet areas

_______ 23. After each session, the therapist should carefully record

A. the client's height and weight
B. any sensitivities experienced and/or reactions to the visit as well as changes in health status
C. any peculiar remarks made by the client that relate to the profession
D. the therapist's personal feelings about the client

_______ 24. There may be times during reflexology treatments when a client experiences a headache or an increase of elimination through the skin, bowels, or urinary system. She may even experience a flare-up of an illness that never really resolved. All of these symptoms can be classified as a/an

A. chronic illness
B. malignancy
C. infectious disease
D. healing crisis

References

American Reflexology Certification Board Study Guide, P.O. Box 620607, Littleton, CO 81062, 1993.

Berkson, Devaki. *The Foot Book.* New York: HarperCollins Publishers, 1977.

Byers, Dwight C. *Better Health With Foot Reflexology: The Original Ingham Method.* St. Petersburg, FL: Ingham Publishing, Inc., 1996.

Dougans, Inge *The Complete Illustrated Guide to Foot Reflexology.* Boston: Element Books, 1996.

Norman, Laura. *Feet First.* New York: Simon & Schuster Publishers, 1988.

Weil, Andrew. Self Healing Newsletter. Self Healing, 42 Pleasant St., Watertown, MA 02172. May, 1997.

We can be knowledgeable with another man's knowledge, but we cannot be wise with another man's wisdom.

—Michel De Montaigne

Ralph R. Stephens

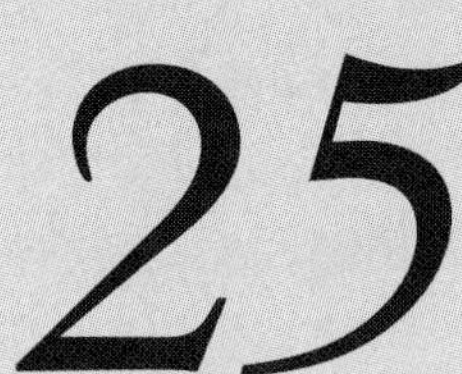

25

Seated Massage

Student Objectives

After completing this chapter, the student should be able to:

- List five considerations when purchasing a massage chair
- Describe five types of seated massage equipment
- State six reasons a massage therapist might choose to massage a client in the seated position
- Explain and demonstrate procedures of sanitation and hygiene
- Properly adjust the massage chair for the client
- Describe proper body mechanics and safety considerations for the massage therapist who uses a massage chair
- Use adaptive professional communication to effectively communicate with the client before and during the massage
- Perform a basic seated massage routine

INTRODUCTION

Massage, in a chair, with clothes on and no oil? To rub someone's shoulders as he is sitting in a chair is an instinctive thing to do. It makes sense to take advantage of this natural urge and to develop it into something therapeutic. In North America, seated massage, often referred to as chair massage, came to prominence through the efforts of David Palmer, whose vision was to make massage therapy safe, convenient, and affordable for anyone, anywhere, anytime. He introduced seated massage in the workplace in the early 1980s. Working at corporations such as Apple computers and Pacific Bell, he developed the idea for a chair to complement the massage. In 1986, he introduced the first special massage chair and coined the term "onsite massage." Palmer adapted the traditional Japanese system of massage, called amma, to create massage routines performed on the client in a special portable chair. Amma routines use acupressure techniques and percussion (tapotement).

Seated techniques have made massage more accessible to the mainstream public by making it as convenient and affordable as a haircut. Enterprising therapists have expanded this concept to shopping malls, beauty salons, day spas, airports, sporting events, locker rooms, even street corners. Sessions are typically short (from 5 to 15 minutes), although they can last as long as 30 minutes. The cost is usually $10 to $20, averaging about a dollar per minute (1997 statistics). Some individuals not familiar with massage find seated massage more acceptable than table massage. There is no need to disrobe, and oils or lotions are not used. People generally feel less vulnerable seated in a chair than lying on a table, and the time commitment is considerably less, especially when the therapist goes to the client's place of business, or onsite.

Seated massage may be done onsite or in the thera-

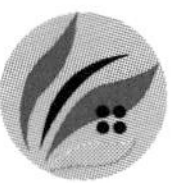

How To Select A Massage Chair

There are many different massage chairs on the market today. Just as with a massage table, different features appeal to different people (Fig. 25–1). The following are things to keep in mind when purchasing a massage chair:

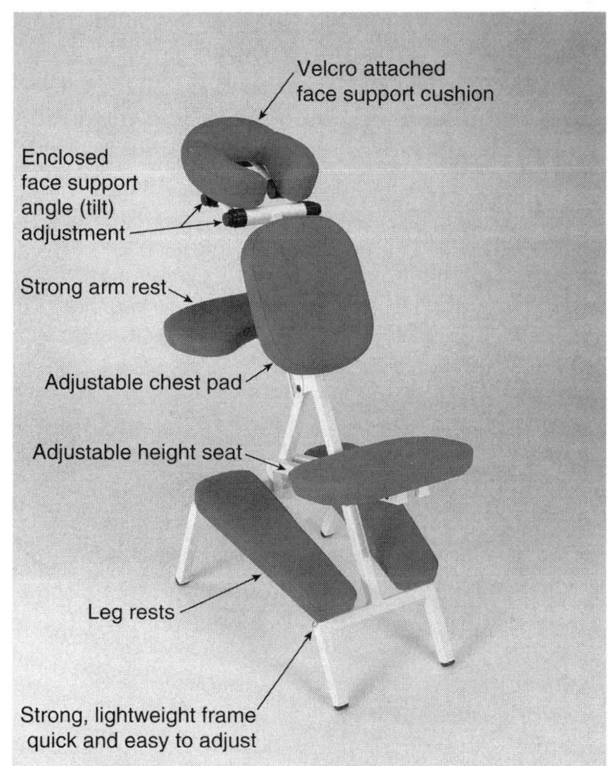

Figure 25•1 A massage chair highlighting the stress points and adjustable joints. (Courtesy of Golden Ratio Woodworks, Emigrant, MT.)

- The massage chair should be lightweight because you may be moving it from location to location.
- It should be quick and simple to set up and take down.
- It should have enough adjustments to fit a variety of body styles, but not so many adjustments that you spend a lot of time adjusting the chair. Avoid massage chairs requiring a series of smaller adjustments after making a major adjustment. Simple is better; simple and quick is best.
- It should be sturdy and strong. A creaky or wobbly chair makes the person sitting in it feel insecure and unsafe.
- Be sure the arm rest is strong enough to withstand deep compression and friction techniques performed on the client's arm.
- Face support adjustments on massage chairs should be completely enclosed. Exposed latches and locking mechanisms can pinch therapists' fingers and catch clients' hair. Exposed latches and locking mechanisms can also come loose if bumped by the client or therapist and are difficult to keep clean and sanitized.
- The chair manufacturer should offer a trial period during which the chair may be returned for a full refund if the therapist is not completely satisfied. The chair should come with a 5-year or more warranty.
- It is generally best to buy from a manufacturer that is well established. It usually provides better customer service. Recognized brands usually have better resale value should you decide to sell your chair.

pist's office. In seated onsite massage the therapist takes a massage chair to the recipient's location; in seated office massage the therapist is in a fixed location and recipients come to that site, such as an airport, salon, or private office. One therapist may work part-time in several different locations. Many therapists use seated massage to promote their table massage practice; others practice seated massage exclusively. The chair is as versatile as your imagination.

Seated massage is most often used for stress reduction and relaxation, as a "stress-buster break"; however, routines can be adapted to address specific complaints such as low back pain, headaches, neck-shoulder tension, and arm-wrist overuse injury. Combining Swedish massage techniques with amma techniques gives the therapist the option of doing clinical massage in the seated position in either an onsite or private office setting. Individuals are more likely to participate in a program of seated massage if it provides reduction of painful complaints and injuries. Employers are more likely to allow employees to participate if they believe it will prevent injuries, improve morale, and enhance productivity in the workplace.

In research published in 1996, Dr. Tiffany Field, at the Touch Research Institute in Miami, found that individuals who received a 15-minute seated massage twice a week showed increased cognitive ability, performed better on math tests, and completed problems with increased accuracy and speed. These individuals also experienced a significant decrease in tension compared with individuals who practiced traditional relaxation techniques while seated in a chair without receiving massage. Massage doesn't cost, it pays.

A massage chair takes up less room than a table, making it more adaptable to space limitations. This, coupled with the "through-clothes" technique, has brought the chair into therapy areas, athletic training rooms, and into many massage therapists' treatment rooms as an adjunct to their tables for specific work. It is well worth the massage therapist's investment of financial resources and time to acquire a massage chair and learn how to use it effectively.

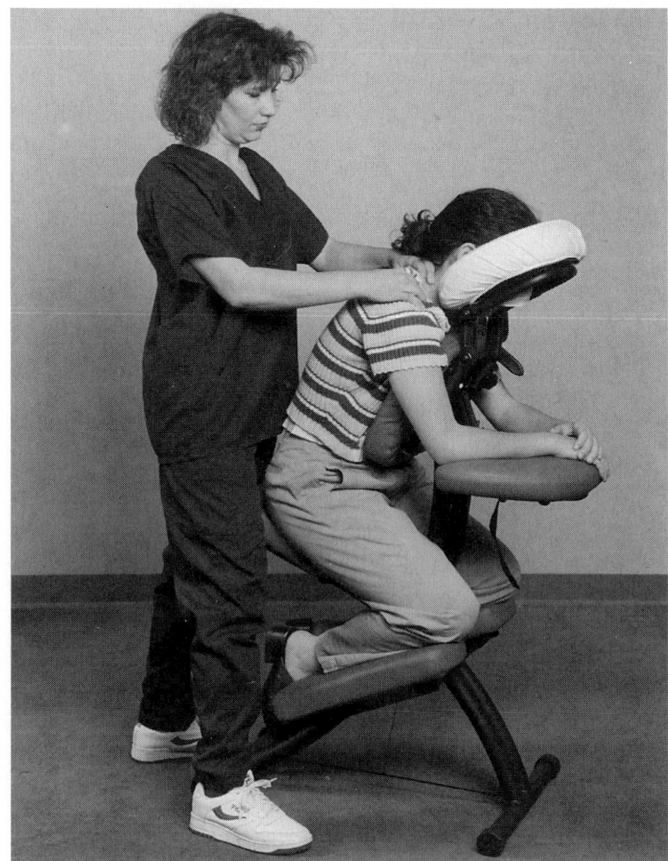

Figure 25•2 Full length of therapist (body mechanics) with client in chair.

TYPES OF SEATED MASSAGE EQUIPMENT

There are several types of seated massage equipment as well as ways to accommodate clients who want a massage in a seated position:

- The massage chair (Fig. 25–2)
- Desktop face support, which is typically the face support from a massage chair designed to be clamped to or balanced on the edge of a counter, table, or desk; some of these have chest pads that hang vertically over the edge of the desk
- A system of specially designed cushions that can hang over the back of an armless chair; these are often the same cushion system used for positioning and support on a massage table top
- A stack of pillows on a table or chair
- A stool or chair (this arrangement provides no support for the head, upper body, or arms)

MASSAGE THERAPISTS USE THE CHAIR FOR A VARIETY OF REASONS

- Massage therapists may use seated massage techniques as their primary modality and source of revenue.
- Massage therapists may use a massage chair as their secondary modality and supplemental source of revenue.
- Seated massage can be used as a promotional tool to introduce the public to massage therapy in a safe, nonthreatening way, thus promoting the therapist's practice in particular and the profession in general.
- Massage chairs are often used at sporting events. Other opportunities include fund-raisers and conventions.

- Onsite massage services may be used at offices and other workplaces for stress reduction, pain relief, and injury prevention.
- Seated massage is used by therapists in their offices for short treatments of the upper body.
- The massage chair is ideal for clients who have difficulty getting on and off a massage table.

SANITIZATION AND HYGIENE CONSIDERATIONS

The need for hygiene for the massage therapist and sanitization of the massage chair cannot be overemphasized. The public is very aware of the importance of cleanliness, and your clients will notice and appreciate that you keep your equipment sanitary and your work environment clean.

When doing table massage in an office setting, the massage therapist must wash his hands before and after each client. However, with the shorter treatment protocols, it is not economically feasible to take time between clients to wash the hands twice. When working onsite, washroom facilities may be very inaccessible. Seated massage therapy procedures must be self-contained, including hygiene.

Seated massage therapists can purchase antimicrobial disposable towelets from a medical or massage supply business. Use these disposable towels to sanitize your hands as well as the face support, arm rest, and chest pad of the chair between clients. Sanitize the leg rests if the client was wearing shorts or a skirt. These wipes are specially treated to destroy microscopic organisms that can cause diseases, such as staphylococci, streptococci, common cold and flu viruses, herpes virus, HIV, and tuberculosis. As a rule, if a disinfecting agent destroys tuberculosis bacteria, all other microbes will be destroyed as well. These cleansers help protect the therapist and the client by preventing the spread of contagious pathogens.

It is very important to keep your hands clean. The most common way to spread germs is from touching the eyes, ears, and nose. Keep your fingernails short and clean. Using an antimicrobial skin barrier further protects your hands. These come in creams or foams that when rubbed onto the skin dry to form a barrier. Protect yourself and your clients.

Use a cover on the face cradle to make your clients feel more comfortable, as well as to facilitate keeping the face support cushion clean. These covers help keep makeup off the vinyl. Face cradle covers feel more comfortable on the face than vinyl fabric. One type of cover is a "nurse bouffant cap," available through medical or massage supply businesses. Other types of covers are paper towels and specially designed paper covers, the latter available through massage supply sources.

SAFETY CONSIDERATIONS AND BODY MECHANICS FOR THE SEATED MASSAGE THERAPIST

To prevent repetitive motion injuries, it is essential to use proper body mechanics at all times. Before you set up your massage chair, select an area that allows you to move completely around the chair during the massage (Fig. 25–3). If you use a massage chair carrying case, place it out of the way. Provide a clear, unobstructed pathway for your clients to and from the chair.

Work in the lunge position, keeping the feet and body pointed in the direction of the force you are applying. Keep your back straight and your head erect. Your movement and pressure will be generated from the pelvis as you shift your weight from back leg to front leg. As you massage, the front knee is flexed and the arms stretched in front, elbows only slightly flexed (Fig. 25–4). For the majority of seated massage techniques, the wrists should not be extended more than 45 degrees.

When using the thumbs, maintain proper thumb alignment by "stacking the bones." This means that the bones of the thumb are in relatively straight alignment with the bones of the wrist and arm. If you look straight down your arm, the thumb will be pointing

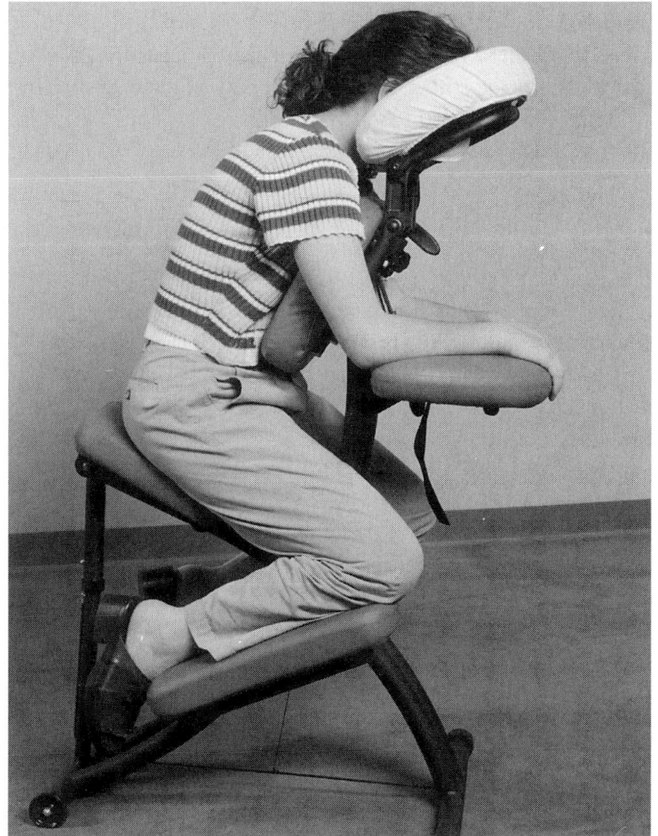

Figure 25•3 Client in a massage chair with proper chair adjustments.

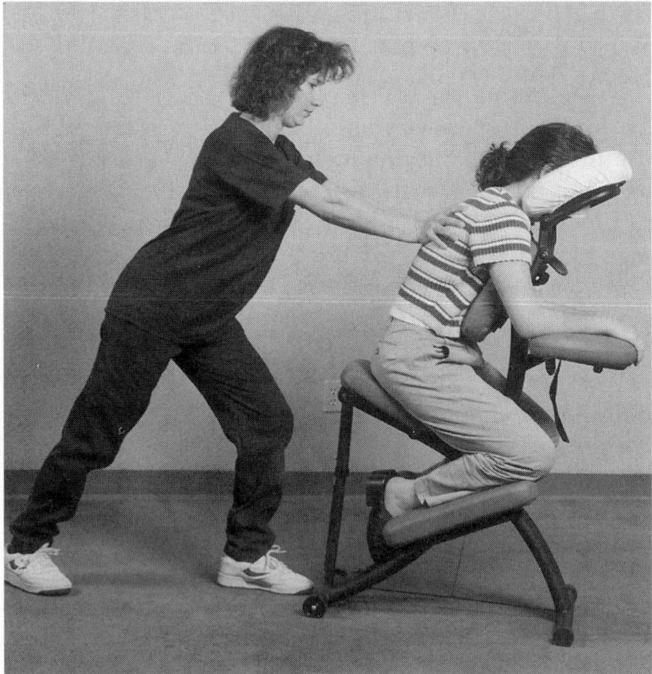

Figure 25•4 Proper body mechanics with a massage chair in an unobstructed area (paraspinal compression).

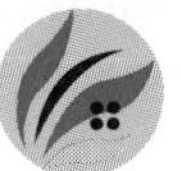

YOU KNOW WHEN THE CHAIR IS PROPERLY ADJUSTED TO THE CLIENT WHEN . . .

1. The client's back is straight and her chest is relatively flat against the chest pad
2. The face cradle is centered around the face and tilted to allow the therapist access to the posterior cervical muscles, without subjecting the client to excessive flexion
3. The arm rest is at a height that does not elevate the client's shoulders; the shoulders should be at a natural height, with the elbow lightly touching or just a few millimeters above the arm rest
4. After asking the client if there is anything you can change to make the chair more comfortable, she has no further suggestions or requests.

straight ahead. As you use your thumb, the fingers of the working hand may be open or loosely closed. You may also use your fingertips, palm of the hand, or elbow to apply massage techniques. This gives your thumbs a needed break and varies the quality of touch for the client. However, be sure to maintain proper body mechanics at all times. Spread your feet farther apart as you work closer to the floor. Avoid bending the back and neck.

BEFORE THE SEATED MASSAGE BEGINS

If this is your client's first time to sit in the massage chair, physically demonstrate how to do it properly. As you are sitting in the chair, orally explain what you are doing. For example, "I am sitting in the chair placing my knees and lower legs on these cushions, while my forearms rest on this shelf and my face is supported by this crescent-shaped pillow." You will be amazed how many positions your clients will assume without directions. Some sit on the chair backward whereas others climb onto it as if it were a motorcycle. Although this is entertaining, the client could upset the chair and be injured. Be specific with your directions and actions.

Most massage chairs have adjustments so they can properly support any body size or type. Before the seated massage session, adjust the chair to each client; do not expect the client to conform to the chair. The primary adjustments are the seat height, the chest pad height, the face support height and angle (tilt), and the arm rest height. A client will typically arch her back or slump if the chair is improperly adjusted to her body. Be sure the client's back is straight and that the arm rest is low enough so the client's shoulders are not raised. The proximal end of the forearm is just slightly off the arm rest. The most comfortable position of the face cradle, for most clients, is when the neck is slightly flexed forward. Once the chair is completely adjusted to the client, the therapist then asks, "If you could change anything what would it be?" If the therapist asks, "Is that all right?" most clients, who do not know how the chair should feel, will say yes. However, if given the option to make it better, they will point out any area of discomfort. This simple question takes a few seconds and has a significant impact on the session.

MASSAGE STROKES USED FOR SEATED MASSAGE

Seated massage routines use Oriental and Swedish massage strokes (without oil) as well as ancillary massage strokes. These strokes include compression, sustained pressure (acupressure), stretching methods, deep and superficial friction, petrissage, effleurage, nerve stroke, and tapotement. The strokes used will vary according to the training of the therapist.

Compression. Compression is effective on the muscles of the forearm and back. Apply firm pressure primarily from the heel of the hand or loosely clenched fists. During compression of the forearm, you face the client, and your relaxed fingers are pointed toward the client's elbow. Apply pressure straight in and straight out, while maintaining contact. Instruct the client to exhale as you apply pressure to the back and to inhale as you release. Avoid applying excessive pressure on the floating ribs and the lumbar region due to the kidneys as well as any previous injuries.

Sustained Pressure. Also known as ischemic compression or acupressure, sustained pressure is usually applied with a finger or thumb, elbow, or a handheld tool. Direct sustained pressure displaces fluids in the tissues being compressed, spreads muscle fibers, and relieves muscle spasms. It is primarily used to relieve trigger points and tender points found using palpatory strokes, such as deep friction and petrissage. In Oriental techniques, pressure is applied to points in a pattern to improve or balance energy flow in the meridians.

Deep Friction. Deep friction is applied with the thumb, finger, elbow, loosely clenched fist, palm, or heel of the hand. During friction, engage the skin through the client's clothes and move the skin over the underlying structures. Avoid sliding on the client's skin or clothes. "Deep" does not denote hard pressure, but the effect of shifting the skin over deeper structures.

Superficial Friction. A warming, stimulating stroke, superficial friction is applied with the palms of both hands, in a rapid back-and-forth movement on the superficial tissues. A variation is to use the ulnar sides of the hands in a "sawing" motion. This variation is effective for reducing muscular tension around the shoulder joint on either side of the spine and across the top of the upper trapezius.

Petrissage. Petrissage involves grasping, lifting, and kneading the tissues, or rolling the tissues between the thumb and fingers. This massage movement is used primarily in the neck and top of the shoulders.

Effleurage. Effleurage, or light stroking, is applied over the client's clothing for relaxation and sedation. Nerve strokes can also be used.

Tapotement. Toward the end of the seated massage, tapotement can be used on the back, head, arms, and hips. Hacking and beating are best for the torso, hips, and arms, while tapping with the fingertips is best on the scalp. Do not use tapotement over areas where trigger points were found and treated because it can cause them to re-form.

ADAPTIVE PROFESSIONAL COMMUNICATION

Spoken communication with the client is very important in seated massage. Because eye contact is impossible when the client is in the face cradle, a method of communication must be established in the initial interview before beginning the treatment. Following is a recommended way to establish communication.

- ***When It Hurts.*** Explain that you will be examining the tissues of the back, neck, and arms, looking for areas that are tight and contracted. When these areas are located, they will be tender. You should say something like, "Be sure to tell me whenever I find a tender area. Will you do that for me?" Not only does this give the client permission to tell you that something is tender, but she agrees to do so.
- ***When It Gets Better.*** Continue by saying, "When I find these tender places I will stop and maintain the pressure. This sustained pressure will cause the nervous system to respond by relaxing the tender area. It may feel to you like I am letting up on the pressure, or it's beginning to feel better. Will you let me know when it gets better?"
- ***If It Refers.*** Then add, "When I am examining or maintaining pressure on an area of tissue, you may experience some sensation somewhere else. It could be a pain, tingling, numbness, aching, or some other sensation somewhere besides right where I am massaging. These are trigger points. Will you tell me if you feel any sensation radiating anywhere other than where I am working?"
- ***If It's Too Hard.*** Say, "If at any time I am working too hard, be sure and tell me right away. Will you do that?" This is very important because it gives the client permission to tell you that you are working too hard. Often the client will not tell you this, because she thinks you are the professional and you must be doing it right. She may think it is supposed to hurt. Some clients will endure anything if they believe it may make them better. Another way to put this is, "Let me know if what I am doing feels good or if it hurts, especially if it hurts, because this work should not be painful."

During onsite massage, the massage area may be noisy, making it difficult to hear the client. In this case, ask the client to communicate by raising her hand if she is in pain. If more specific information is needed regarding pain, establish a pain-measuring system on a scale from 1 (no pain) through 5 (excruciating pain). You will know, by the number of fingers raised, how she is responding to the pressure (Fig. 25–5). This system may be used in quiet places, too.

Some people will not tell you that something hurts.

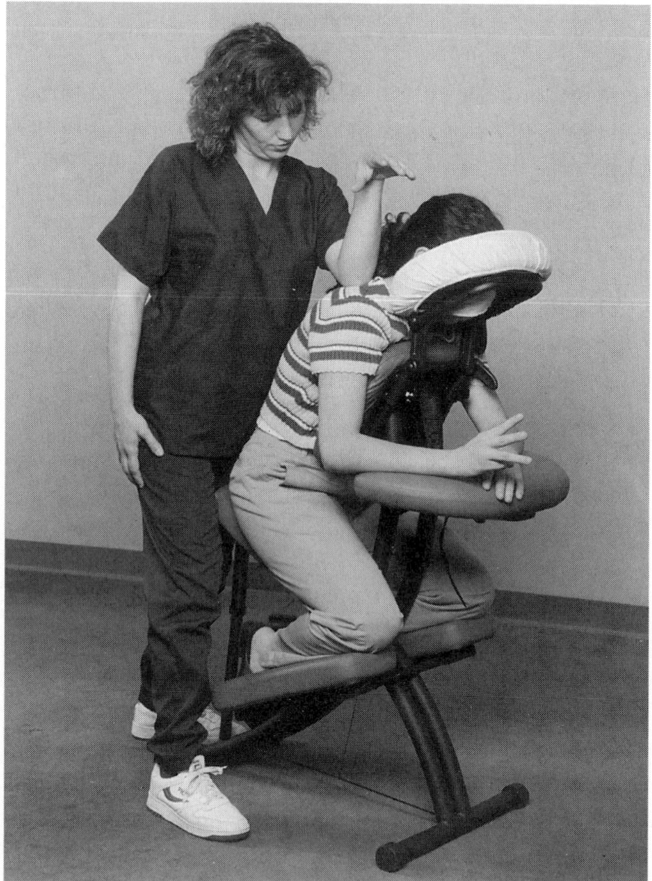

Figure 25•5 Client showing the three-finger hand signal for good pressure during elbow trigger point compression.

They are accustomed to denying pain or they may have a different sensation and perception assigned to pain. However, the body never lies. You can always tell that you are working too hard when the client begins to pull away from you or unconsciously contracts muscles to limit your access into the tissues. If he is tensing up, squirming, or pulling away, *you are using too much pressure.*

RECORD KEEPING

It is uncommon for seated massage therapists to keep full SOAP notes for each client; however, it is prudent to keep a record of each session and to note any unusual findings or observations. Even in seated massage, have your clients fill out a basic intake form, and obtain informed consent. The initial interview with your client may be brief, but the form should ask questions regarding medications, eye conditions that could be affected by the face cradle (contacts) and any medical conditions for which they are being treated. Establish your client's primary and secondary complaints.

Specific seated massage treatments require keeping more detailed notes. Treatment notes document progress and remind the therapist of what procedures were performed and which treatments were helpful. In legal situations, proper documentation is helpful for you and your clients. Also, unless you give each client a receipt, it may not be considered a legal transaction by taxation authorities. To save time, receipts may be prepared in advance with a place to fill in the client's name, the date, and the amount.

SAMPLE SEATED MASSAGE ROUTINE

The following basic routine is a suggested protocol that you will be able to accomplish in 15 minutes. Use it as a guide, but remain creative and intuitive. Accomplish as much as you can for each client within the time allowed. Concentrate the majority of the time on the area of her main complaint, which is usually the low back, neck, or shoulders. However, in the workplace, forearm, wrist, and hand complaints are quite common. Start with some general strokes to acquaint clients with your touch and to establish their sensitivity. Gradually become more specific, focusing primarily on the main complaint with some attention to any secondary complaints. You cannot resolve everything that has been wrong with a client for years in one treatment. Even recent injuries usually require multiple treatments. In a 15-minute session, if you can reduce the main complaint and accomplish some general relaxation, you have accomplished a great service for the client. Complete the seated massage treatment with general techniques. Work from general to specific, then back to general.

The Upper Back and Neck

Begin the treatment with compression strokes to the paraspinal muscles. Use the heels of the hands or loosely clenched fists. It is important to have the client breathe in rhythm with the compression. Ask your client to take a deep breath, and as he exhales, apply firm pressure to the tissues on either side of the spine (it is best if the therapist breathes along). Begin between the scapulas and move inferior a hand width at a time until the ilium bones are reached. Then move back superior a hand width at a time until the starting point is reached. This technique establishes contact with the client, introduces relaxation, and gets him into a regular deep-breathing pattern.

You should be standing directly behind the center of the client's back. Keep your arms outstretched with just a slight bend in the elbows, back straight, head erect, moving from the pelvis in a lunge position. If you are using the heels of the hands, the wrists will be significantly extended. If pressure applied with the heels of the hands creates discomfort in your wrists, then switch to a loosely clenched fist. Using a loose fist to apply compression keeps the wrist straight as you apply pressure with the proximal phalanges.

Repeat the above pattern using loosely clenched fists but with a circular deep-friction stroke. Make four to eight circles with each hand, working simultaneously down and up the sides of the spine. If massaging in circles with both hands at the same time is too difficult or tiresome, you may choose to switch to cross-fiber or longitudinal friction. Apply four friction strokes medial to lateral over the paraspinal muscles, then four friction strokes superior to inferior, and then move a hand width and repeat.

Every few minutes, ask the client how he is perceiving the pressure, using the guidelines discussed in the adaptive professional communications section in this chapter.

Grasp the upper trapezius muscle using a pincerlike grip on each side of the neck (Fig. 25–6). Roll the muscle between the thumb and fingers (petrissage). Work laterally to the acromion process, then work medially to the neck as far superior on the neck as you can, isolating the trapezius fibers. When tender areas or trigger points are encountered, stop and maintain the pressure for 8 to 12 seconds. If your pressure is appropriate for the person, he will feel it relax within 12 seconds; if he does not, you are applying too much pressure. Slowly release the pressure and move to another area, returning to the tender area in about a minute. It is common for trigger points in the upper fibers of the trapezius to refer to the back of the head and up to the temple area.

You may now move to the side of the client in the chair and grasp and petrissage the back of his neck. Work all the way up to the occipital bone and back down to the shoulder. Because the thumb is more sensitive and powerful, you may choose to go to the other side and repeat this step. This decision is based on the sensitivity found in the tissues the first time over them and the client's main complaint. If the main complaint is the neck and shoulders, you will want to be very thorough in this area. If the main complaint is in the lower back, less time will be spent in the cervical region.

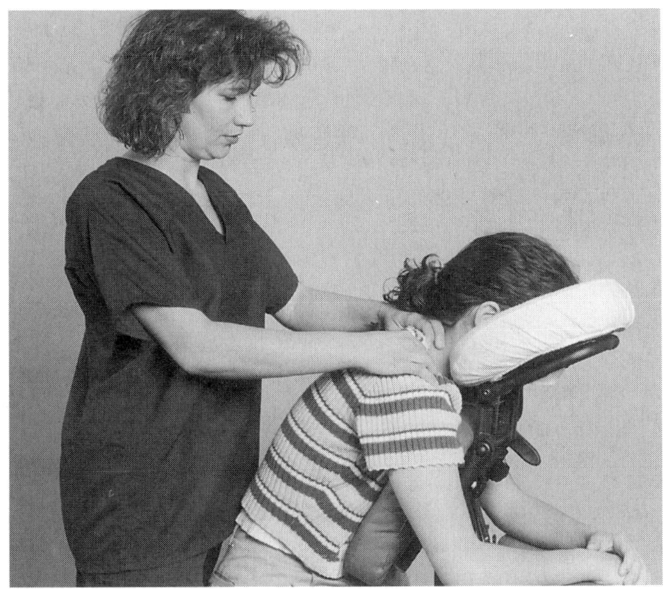

Figure 25•6 Trapezius petrissage technique.

If the client complains of a stiff neck or headache, examine the suboccipital muscles; these are involved in rocking, tilting, and rotation of the head and are often the victims of whiplash. Injury or chronic overload from head forward postures can cause a trigger point to develop that refers into the head and behind the eyes. The suboccipital muscles are very accessible in the seated position.

Tilt the face cradle forward to place the head and neck in 45 degrees of flexion. While standing at the side of the client, use the thumb and second finger of one hand to apply deep friction in a lateral-medial direction to the tissues between the occiput and C2. Work from lateral to medial and back. These tissues can be very tender and ischemic, so be sure to check with the client about appropriate pressures when working this area.

Using the heel of the hand or fingertips, examine the rhomboid muscles and the posterior surface of the scapula with deep circular friction. When massaging the posterior region of the scapula, support the anterior aspect of the shoulder with the other hand. If this area is the client's primary complaint, a more specific examination of these tissues can be done with the thumbs or a guided elbow. When this area is complete, move lateral to the shoulder joint, and treat the rotator cuff tendons with circular friction.

Apply circular friction to the area below the scapulas using the heels of the hands, working both sides of the spine at once. This will address the latissimus dorsi muscle and the paraspinal muscles in the midback.

Lower Back

Moving your hand inferiorly, use circular friction to relax the lower back. The quadratus lumborum muscle can be examined and treated very effectively in the seated position. This muscle is responsible for many complaints of low back pain. Trigger points in the quadratus lumborum often mimic hip and sciatic nerve pain. Palpate the client's waistline, being careful not to elicit a tickle response. After locating the lateral end of the 12th rib, apply deep friction with your thumbs in a medial to lateral direction along the inferior surface. As you move medially, you will encounter a hard structure; this is the spine and is often more lateral than expected. Change directions of pressure to 45 degrees medial-anterior. Using circular friction, ex-

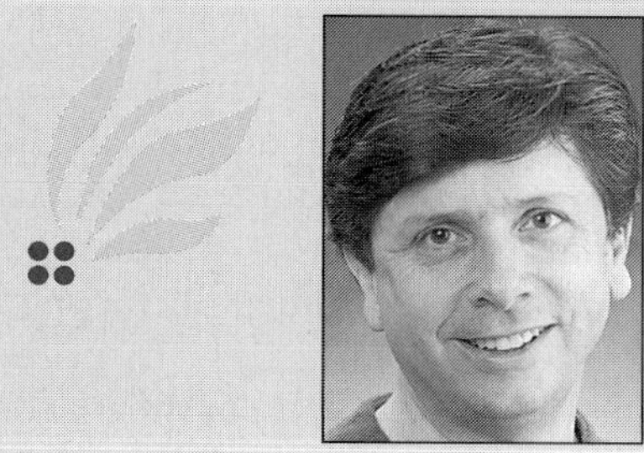

David Palmer

Born: November 27, 1948

"My vision is to make touch a positive social value in our culture."

The topic of chair massage can hardly be discussed without the name David Palmer surfacing at least once. Read any article on the subject and you will soon discover that he is the "father of chair massage." The story of how he came to earn such a title is fascinating yet somewhat obscure.

His career in massage began in 1980. Considering his previous profession of 10 years as an administrator of social service programs for nonprofit agencies in Chicago and San Francisco, it seemed only natural that he would focus his sight on a field in which he could have a great effect on the mental well-being of people through the art of touch. He first encountered massage in his early 20s, during a Rolfing session. He had been suffering from chronic shoulder pain and the Rolfing combined with tai chi and stretching gave him a feeling of being back inside his body. It was this experience that led him to explore massage.

After he received a massage in a spa in San Francisco, a series of events over a 3-year period led to his position as director of a massage institute specializing in the Japanese art of amma. After only a short period of teaching he realized that there was a serious gap between the people who wanted to give and people who wanted to receive professional massage. After a little investigating, he came to the conclusion that there was a significant packaging problem in the massage industry. Palmer says, "The package that the mainstream massage community was selling to the general public was a package that the general public was not interested in buying." It was very hard to convince most people to accept an idea that required going into a private room, removing clothing, lying on a table, and being rubbed with oils by a stranger for a costly fee on a regular basis. The whole idea was just too "scary" for the average individual. It was then that he gave massage a hard look from a marketing point of view. He says, "They [mainstream massage community] were selling a graduate level understanding of the field of touch to a population who had not even begun kindergarten regarding touch."

Palmer's solution to this problem was to make massage less scary and more affordable. The result was his legacy of the seated chair massage. Although this type of massage had been done for thousands of years, as can been seen in ancient Japanese and Chinese woodcuts, Palmer's contribution was to revive its visibility and identity. He felt that it would be very difficult for a massage that is given with the client fully clothed on an open sidewalk in a chair to be perceived as violating.

At the time, the chair massage was being done on a drummer's stool, but in 1983 he decided to create a special chair. He had seen one of the Scandinavian computer chairs called Balance with slanted leg rests and thought "Hey, that would be perfect if only it had some sort of head rest and chest support." He hired a French cabinetmaker named Serge Bouyssou to be his design partner and after 2 years the chair was introduced to the national market. The year was 1986 and chair massage was now viewed as being significant enough to have its own physical product.

Vision has clearly been an important factor in David Palmer's career. From the very beginning he saw a challenge and immediately acted on it. Chair massage has given so many people the opportunity to experience the wonderful benefits of massage and so much more. It allows the client to safely experience the much needed sense of touch. "We're so touch phobic that you can't grow up in this culture without having some serious issues about touch. Parents are afraid to touch their kids; teachers can't touch their students; it's crazy out there. My feeling is that we need to shift that around, and massage is a vehicle for doing that because it provides structured touch," says Palmer. Although he fully appreciates the

Continued

many wonderful benefits of massage, it's not his main interest. He states, "My vision is to make touch a positive social value in our culture." He admits that this is what primarily motivates his professional life.

The most important thing he feels that students can do in massage school is first learn how to touch and how to be touched. He confesses, "I'm one of those unreformed 60's brats who thinks it's still possible to change the world." If his previous record is any reflection on his future, he just might succeed. It's a big job for one man, but as future touch professionals, we can all do our part in our own small way and conquer a huge task. After all, Palmer says, "The reason I am in this profession is because I think it has the best people in the world."

amine the edge of the lumbar spine in the area of the transverse processes. Then using deep circular friction, massage this area in thumb-width increments from L1 inferior to the ilium bone. Change the direction of pressure to inferior-anterior and treat the superior surface of the ilium laterally to the midline of the body.

The paraspinal muscles can now be examined more thoroughly using fingertips, thumbs, or a guided elbow. Treat one side at a time with deep circular or cross-fiber friction, using sustained pressure on tender areas and trigger points. Apply friction on this area from medial to lateral, allowing the client to rock slightly in the chair. This is very effective and relaxing.

Arm

Because there is no surface against which to compress the biceps and triceps during seated massage, the therapist is limited to petrissage, rolling, jostling, or squeezing the tissues of the upper arm with one or two hands.

Facing the front of the chair, slightly to one side, place the forearm with the palm down on the arm rest to treat the forearm muscles. Apply compression to the extensor muscle group using the heel of the hand, working from wrist to elbow. Repeat this sequence three times, then rotate the arm, palm up, and apply three sets of compression to the flexor muscles.

Roll the hand over, palm down, and instead of compression repeat this pattern using circular friction applied with the heel of the hand, with your fingers pointed toward the elbow of the client. Work from wrist to elbow in 1- or 2-inch intervals, making five to ten circles on each spot. Repeat this sequence three times. Rotate the arm, palm up, and repeat the circular friction moves on the flexor muscles (Fig. 25–7).

Apply circular friction to all sides of the wrist capsule using the thumbs. Grasp the client's hand, and shake out the arm and return it to the arm rest.

Repeat this sequence on the other arm.

Face and Scalp

Facial and scalp massage feels great while in a chair; however, many people do not want their hair or makeup messed up; be considerate, ask first. Apply circular friction to the temples, jaw, face, and scalp (Fig. 25–8). During scalp massage, the tissue can be shifted back and forth across the cranium using deep friction. Tapping style tapotement also works well on the scalp, especially as part of the general finishing strokes. Tapotement on the cranium is not appropriate if someone has a significant headache.

Stretches

Stretches are very useful in seated massage. Because most individuals spend much of their time in a flexed position, the anterior cervical region and pectoral regions of the body are typically contracted. Most cli-

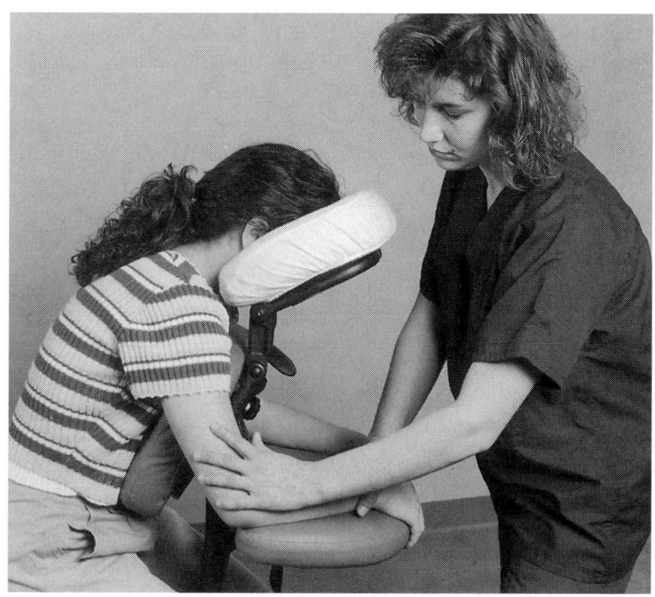

Figure 25•7 A nerve stroke of the arms.

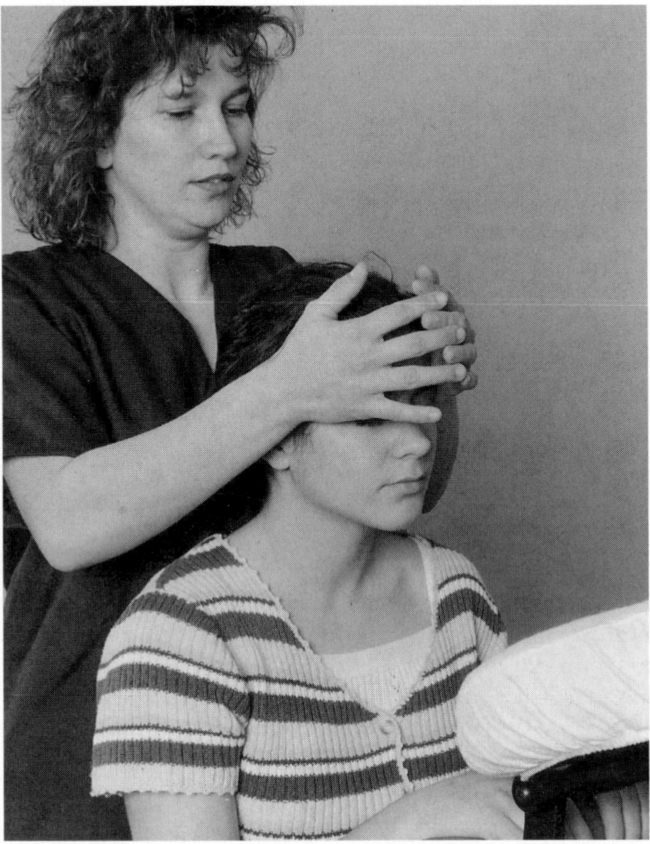

Figure 25•8 Circular friction to the temples.

ents also have chronically internally rotated shoulders. Static, PNF, and active-assisted stretches can relax and lengthen these habitually contracted tissues (Fig. 25–9). Massage therapists should use only those systems of stretching they are trained in and must always be careful not to overstretch the client's soft tissue and to avoid bouncy (ballistic) or prolonged stretching.

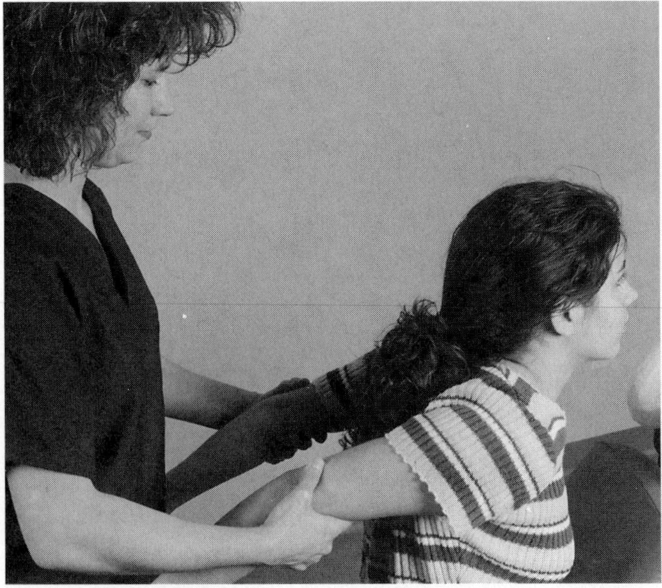

Figure 25•9 A pectoralis stretch.

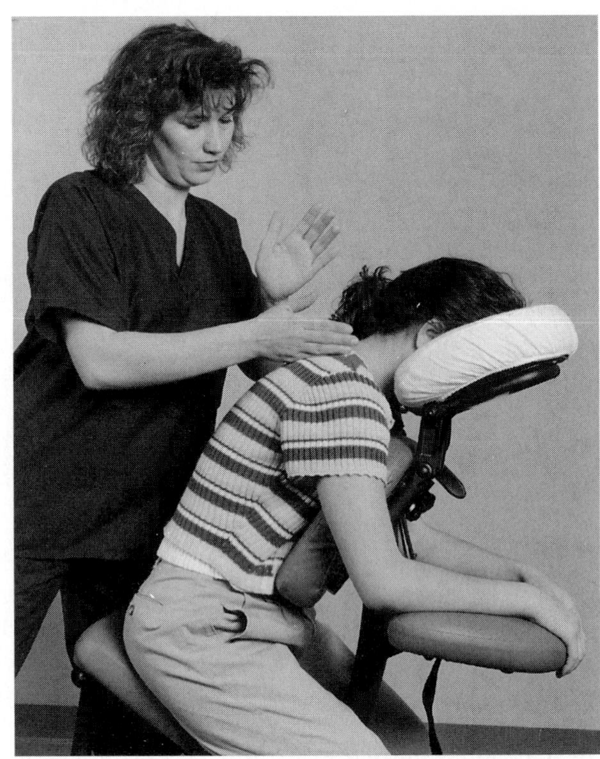

Figure 25•10 Tapotement to back and shoulders.

Conclusion

As the seated massage session draws to a close, the therapist returns to general strokes. If the goal is to leave the client very relaxed and sedated, finish with some effleurage and slow nerve strokes on the back and shoulders. If the client is returning to work and needs to be more alert, finish with tapotement, superficial (palmar) friction, and faster nerve strokes. Tapping on the head, hacking on the shoulders and back, and beating on the hips is a more stimulating way to finish the massage (Fig. 25–10).

When the treatment is complete, tell the client, and ask her to get off the chair slowly. Remain close by because many people, especially senior citizens, may feel unsteady for a few moments. Some people actually doze off during the seated massage and may need time to become fully oriented. Be prepared to assist your client as needed.

Always have your schedule book handy to reschedule appointments as well as business cards to distribute. As you collect your fee from the client or just say thank you and goodbye, suggest that the client book another appointment. It is also appropriate to mention that if he liked your work, he should tell others.

Upon completion of all transactions with the client, clean your hands, disinfect the chair, write your case notes, take a few deep breaths, and get ready for the next client.

SUMMARY

Seated massage is a very important specialty area in the profession of massage therapy. It allows the therapist to reach a different group of clients who may not be available for traditional table massage. Usually done in a special portable chair, seated techniques can be used onsite at the client's location or at the therapist's office. Seated massage sessions tend to be shorter, ranging from 5 to 30 minutes. The work is done through the clothes without lubricants. Seated massage is used for promoting the therapist's private practice or as a complete practice in itself. The portable massage chair has made massage as accessible to the general public as a haircut and has become a valuable adjunct to any therapist's practice.

SELF-TEST

Multiple Choice • Write the letter of the best answer in the space provided.

_______ 1. In North America, seated massage came to prominence due to the efforts of

A. George Washington C. Pehr Ling
B. David Palmer D. Jack Meagher

_______ 2. Palmer's routines for seated massage were adapted from a traditional Japanese system of massage called

A. amma C. akido
B. tai chi D. shiatsu

_______ 3. During seated massage, the client does not disrobe and

A. a special massage cream is used
B. lubricant is applied to the face
C. oils or lotions are not used
D. ear plugs are offered to the client

_______ 4. Research published by Dr. Tiffany Field found that

A. individuals who received seated massage twice a week showed increased cognitive ability, performed better in math, and increased test accuracy and speed
B. premature babies bonded with the individuals who massaged them
C. baby monkeys preferred cloth surrogate mothers over wire surrogate mothers
D. individuals who receive seated massage like it better than table massage

_______ 5. In choosing a massage chair, the following is important *except*

A. it should be lightweight because you may be moving it from location to location
B. the more adjustments, the more comfortable the client will be
C. it should be sturdy and strong
D. buying from a manufacturer who is well established

_______ 6. Because onsite massage locations occasionally do *not* have easy access to a restroom for handwashing

A. the therapist must wash her hands before leaving the office
B. the client must sign a release form
C. antimicrobial disposable towels replace handwashing
D. you can omit handwashing because you are massaging through clothes

_______ 7. Before you set up your massage chair

A. wash your hands
B. collect your fees
C. select an area near a restroom and an exit
D. select an area allowing you to move around the chair during the massage

_______ 8. The chair massage therapist works in the

A. horse stance C. bow stance
B. lunge position D. sitz position

_______ 9. Seated massage routines use Swedish as well as ancillary massage strokes. Which stroke is *not* used in seated massage?

A. compression and sustained pressure
B. petrissage, effleurage, and tapotement
C. deep and superficial friction
D. effleurage, using lubricants

_______ 10. Because eye contact is impossible when the client is in the face cradle

A. a method of communication is established before beginning the treatment
B. cue cards are used for communication
C. communication with the client is before and after the treatment only
D. communication is not important; let your fingers do the talking

_______ 11. During the initial interview, the client agrees to

A. tell you if an area is tender
B. tell you if the area is referring pain
C. tell you if the pressure is too hard
D. all of the above

_______ 12. During onsite massage, the massage area may be noisy, making it difficult to hear the client. In this case, ask the client to

A. ignore the noisy environment
B. communicate by raising his hand if he is in pain
C. wear headphones and enjoy relaxing music
D. wear disposable ear plugs

_______ 13. You can always tell when you are working too hard when the client

A. begins to pull away from you
B. unconsciously contracts muscles to limit your access into the tissues
C. tenses up, squirms, or pulls away
D. all of the above

_______ 14. During the initial interview process, the following information is important to obtain from the client *except*

A. eye conditions that could be affected by the face cradle
B. any medical conditions for which she is being treated
C. the last time she received a massage
D. her primary and secondary complaints

_______ 15. If this is your client's first time to sit in the massage chair,

A. adjust the massage chair before she sits down
B. explain and demonstrate how to sit in the chair properly
C. use guided imagery to relax the client and describe how to sit in the chair
D. show her a photograph or illustration of someone sitting in the chair

_______ 16. Once the chair is completely adjusted to the client, the therapist should ask

A. Is that all right?
B. Does your face feel too smashed?
C. Would you like a breath mint?
D. If you could change anything, what would it be?

References

Mattes, Aaron. *Active Isolated Stretching.* Published by Aaron Mattes, Sarasota, FL, 1995.

Palmer, David. *How to Market On-Site Massage.* Santa Rosa, CA: Living Earth Crafts, 1986.

Palmer, David. *The Bodywork Entrepreneur.* San Francisco, CA: Thumb Press, 1990.

Stephens, Ralph R. *Seated Therapeutic Massage Videos.* Volumes I–III. Cedar Rapids, IA: Helping Hands Seminar, 1996.

Travell, Janet G. and David G. Simons. *Myofascial Pain and Dysfunction, The Trigger Point Manual.* Baltimore: Williams & Wilkins, Vol I 1983, Vol II 1992.

Learning is experience. Everything else is just information.
—Albert Einstein

Michael Loomis

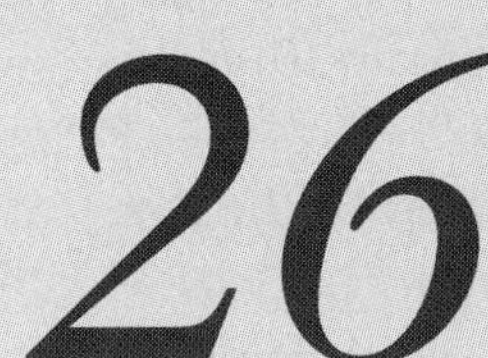

26 Sports Massage

Student Objectives

After completing this chapter, the student should be able to:

- List the components of sports massage
- Identify sport-specific soreness patterns for running, cycling, and swimming
- Recognize the difference between eccentric and concentric muscle contractions
- Recognize the three different types of tissue damage using the injury recognition chart
- Identify general time frames for healing various types of tissue damage
- Explain the three steps of the repair response for tissue damage
- Explain the factors to consider when scheduling various types of sports massage for an athlete
- Demonstrate the tracking response while working on a variety of participants at an athletic event
- Demonstrate massage techniques commonly used in postevent, recovery, and maintenance massage formats
- Outline the recovery tools available to an athlete who is experiencing muscle soreness
- Discuss the different tissue pathologies that occur in muscles, tendons, ligaments, and fascia
- List the factors that predispose an athlete to injury
- Explain the relationship between microtrauma, spasm, adhesion, trigger point, and lesion as they apply to rapid- and gradual-onset injuries

INTRODUCTION

Sports massage is one of the most visible specialties in massage therapy today. Reducing muscle soreness and recovery time, providing prevention and treatment of athletic injuries, and enhancing performance are but a few of the most commonly acknowledged benefits of sports massage.

Sports massage is the specific application of *purposefully timed* massage techniques, hydrotherapy protocol, range of motion/flexibility procedures, and strength/endurance training principles for athletes in competitive and recreational settings.

Advanced practitioners of sports massage possess the expertise to provide a broad base of comprehensive therapies. The effective sports massage therapist combines highly refined palpation skills with orthopedic assessment, injury rehabilitation/prevention strategies, and an understanding of the essentials of sports biomechanics.

Both amateur and professional athletes may seek services from the massage therapist. Endurance sports such as running, biking, and swimming involve thousands of daily repetitive movements that produce fatigued, sore muscles and aching joints. Sudden stops, starts, and twisting motions in tennis, baseball, and basketball, for example, stress muscles, tendons, ligaments, and fascial components in particular patterns that are unique to each sport.

These repetitive movements manifest as predictable, highly palpable, well-defined textural patterns in an athlete's tissue (Figs. 26–1 and 26–2). As with other forms of massage therapy, hands-on experience is the final teacher. By palpating these similar patterns, you develop a sense of what is familiar, which breeds knowledge, confidence, and skill.

Integrating specific knowledge (see the definition of sports massage at the beginning of this chapter) with hands-on experience is a building block in developing expertise. Through additional training, knowledge, and more experience, the practitioner paves the road toward mastery.

The components of sports massage are: understanding when and when not to petrissage a sore muscle, what specific techniques to use to treat tendinitis (and how to prevent its return), why delayed muscle soreness occurs, when to schedule a session for an athlete who works out 10 to 12 times per week, and where to look for adhesions, trigger points, or other ischemic pockets that are particular to a given sport.

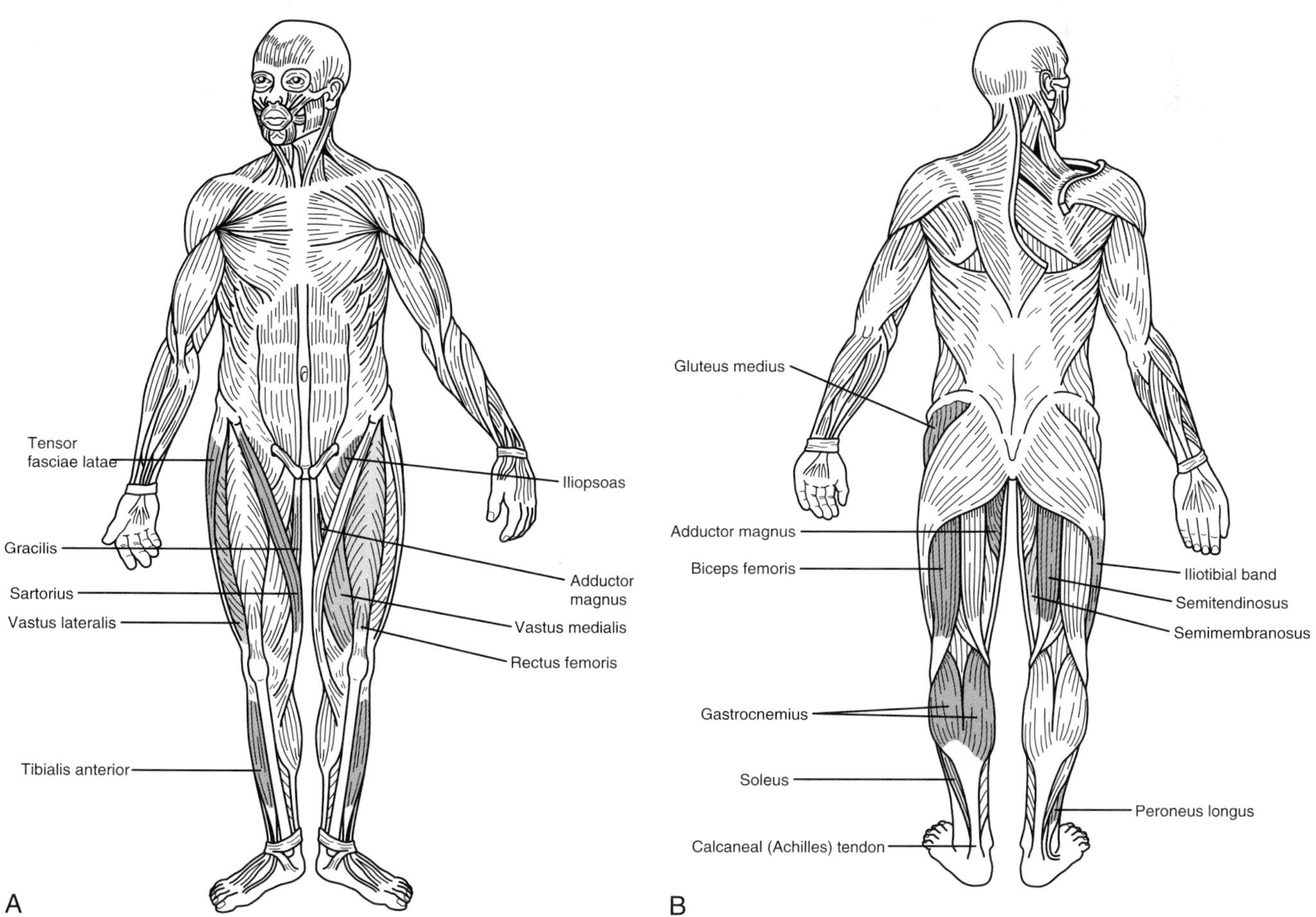

Figure 26•1 Common areas of soreness—runner. *A*, anterior view; *B*, posterior view.

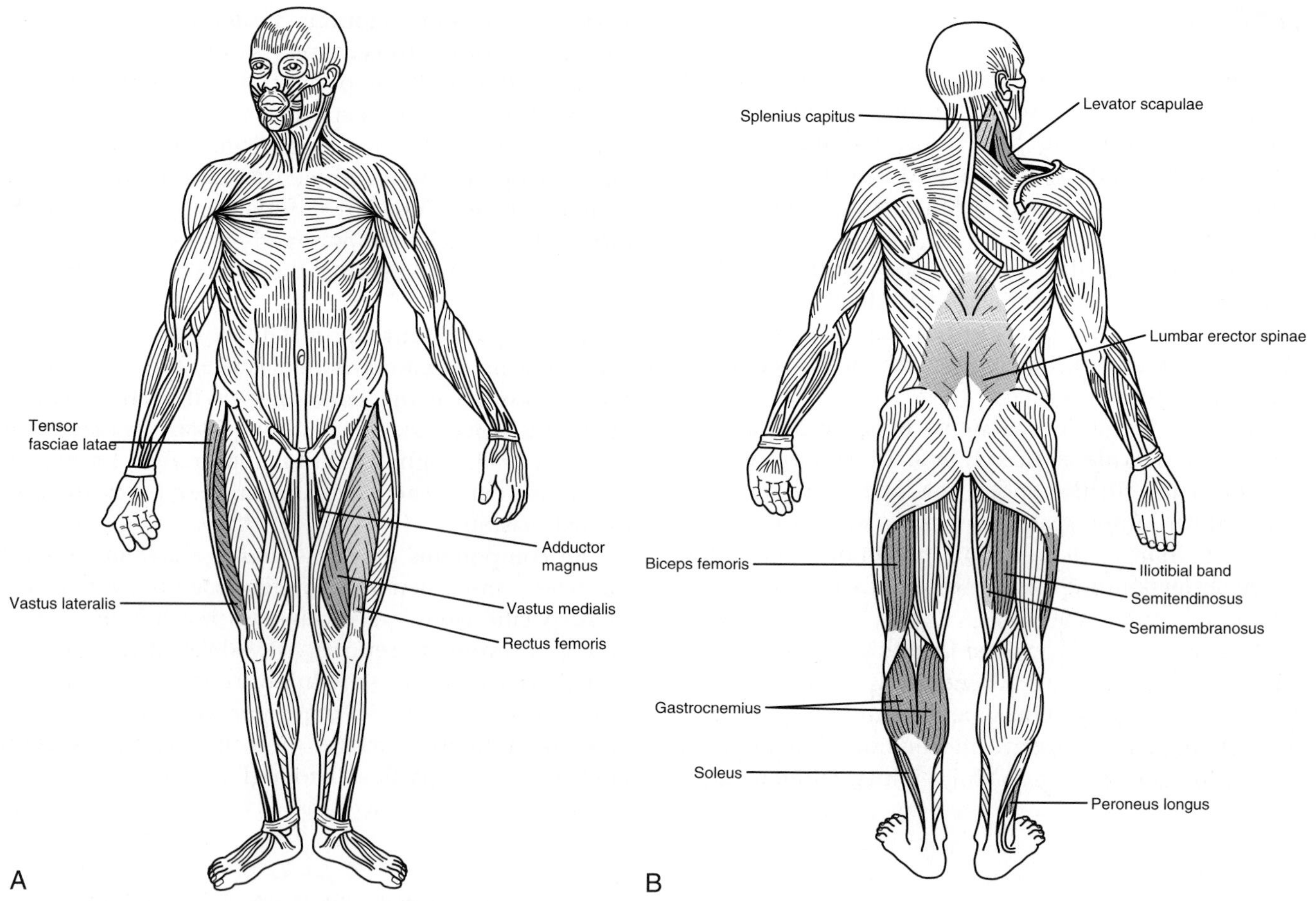

Figure 26•2 Common areas of soreness—cyclist. *A*, anterior view; *B*, posterior view.

Being an excellent massage therapist is an obvious prerequisite for doing good sports massage, but that is only one part of the process. If you do not know the when, where, and why that are particular to athletics, the optimal sports massage treatment may be a hit or miss experience. There is artistry not only in the doing but in the deciding as well. The tools of deciding are listening, questioning, palpating, recognizing patterns, and making judgments based on knowledge and experience.

PHYSIOLOGY FOR ATHLETICS

There are two simple mechanisms that all humans are dependent upon to stay alive: (1) we ingest and burn fuel for energy; and (2) we eliminate waste that results from burning (metabolizing) this fuel. The efficiency of this process has a direct impact on how healthy we are. The efficiency of this process *for an athlete* is critical for performance and for recovery to occur normally.

Oxygen Transport

The body's primary fuel is oxygen. Wilmore and Costill note that oxygen is transported from the external environment to the muscles where it is consumed by specialized components of cells that release the energy needed to produce movement, strength, power, and endurance. Our cardiovascular system (blood flow) nourishes muscle tissue with oxygen and, along with the lymphatic system, removes waste products. Training these systems to work more efficiently is a central task for some athletes—especially when endurance is a critical factor in their sport.

Water As the Medium

The key component of both systems is water. Healthy muscle tissue is well hydrated and vascularized. When athletes push themselves, oxygen becomes limited. When glycogen, the muscles' fuel, is metabolized without oxygen, certain metabolites (such as lactic acid) accumulate in the blood and muscles, causing fatigue, soreness, and pain. Soreness and pain stimulate nerve activity, which frequently results in muscle spasm. Kresge indicates that muscle spasms hinder the free flow of fluids in the tissue. *Uninterrupted* spasm significantly limits blood flow and oxygen to the tissue, bringing additional soreness, pain, and increased spasm.

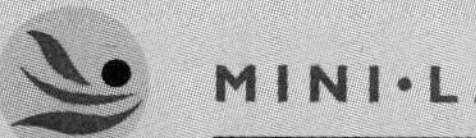

MINI•LAB

Arrange a massage session with an athlete who is experiencing some discomfort. Make it clear that your intention is to practice your massage skills. Now, as you glide across the muscle belly, focus your palpation skills as you trace the fibers tapering into tendon. Notice how the tendon thins and splays into bone. Concentrate on the fluid content of the tissues as you reexamine them. The distribution of blood and lymph should be uniform throughout a healthy muscle. Ask yourself the following questions: Are the tissues consistently hydrated and vascularized? Are there ischemic pockets or localized areas that feel dehydrated? Does a sense of fluidity return with repeated stroking, wringing, or more focused, specific manipulation? Or does a more granular, sticky consistency remain? As your palpation focus deepens, you may become aware of areas that are generally congested or hypertoned. Note whether these areas are resistant to lengthening, broadening, and the other textural suggestions that normally relax a client's muscles.

Locating and treating these congested, hypertoned areas of spasm and the associated ischemic pockets can be the key to unlocking soreness and pain. Remember, reducing soreness and pain for an athlete can mean speeding up her recovery process, thus allowing her to train harder and more frequently.

Ischemia, a localized, temporary anemic condition associated with uninterrupted muscle spasms, is also a contributing factor in exercise-related muscle soreness, and in acute and chronic pain (see Pain-Spasm-Pain Cycle Chapter 19). An effective sports massage therapist skillfully locates and relaxes these spasms, ensuring the free flow of fluids, thereby diminishing soreness and pain.

KINESIOLOGY FOR ATHLETICS

Kinesiology is the study of the muscles and joints of human body and their movements. For the purposes of this chapter we will focus briefly on biomechanical and musculoskeletal principles as they pertain to movements in sports. A frequent biomechanical focus in sports is the human gait as it applies to running.

Running consists of different phases of movement. Stand with both feet firmly planted, ready to move forward. Focus on the right thigh from the moment the right foot leaves the ground. Stanton indicates that the forward swing phase is initiated (as the right thigh swings forward) by the flexors of the thigh at the hip, primarily the rectus femoris, tensor fasciae latae, and iliopsoas muscles. These muscles are activated in a *concentric contraction,* and they shorten as they contract. These same muscles are also known as *accelerators* or *spurt* muscles as they organize force and provide accelerated momentum via concentric contraction. As the thigh flexes forward out of neutral, the hamstrings begin to lengthen and continue to lengthen until the end of the forward swing phase.

The contraction of the hamstrings as they continue to lengthen through the last few degrees of the forward swing phase actually decelerates this rapid, forceful forward swinging of the thigh. The hamstrings are activated in an *eccentric contraction;* they are lengthening as they contract. In this particular motion the hamstrings are known as *decelerators* or *shunt* muscles, as they put the brakes on the powerful swinging of the thigh in flexion at the hip. Unless the body compensates with some corrective braking action, the runner would tear tissue or twist out of control. The faster an athlete runs, the more force is generated and the more contractile energy needed to brake the action.

Injury prevention and performance enhancement goals often rest on your knowledge of the sports-specific demands placed on your client. If you are working with someone who sprints, for example (baseball, football, soccer, basketball, track), an obvious focus in your work needs to be the strength, flexibility, and healthy tonus of the hamstrings. Other decelerators that function in an eccentric mode in athletics are the calf musculature when jumping rope, the posterior shoulder muscles (part of the rotator cuff) in throwing, the forearm extensors at the end of a forehand swing in tennis and the hip adductors at the height of a kick in karate.

Benjamin, Noakes, Stanton, and Weineck are good

MINI•LAB

Find a piece of rope that is long enough to jump rope with. Swing the rope and jump up and down from foot to foot. Can you feel the plantar flexors in the back of your calves working to lift you off the ground each time you jump? Now pay attention to the calf muscle as you land on the ball of your foot. Can you feel it lengthen as you land on that foot? The muscle contracts and lengthens to absorb the shock of the weight of your body upon impact. This is an eccentric contraction. The muscle quickly shifts to contracting and shortening, concentrically propelling you upward once more.

Please consult your physician before attempting any strenuous exercise.

sources for more information about how biomechanical forces impact athletics.

ATHLETIC INJURIES—TRAINING AND TISSUE DAMAGE

Most strenuous activity will challenge the integrity of our body's soft tissues. Varying levels of discomfort, soreness, or pain are normal day-to-day manifestations of most athletes' schedules. To improve performance, Sleamaker notes that athletes may employ a proven training technique known as overloading. The *overload principle* has two components: (1) *regularly stress the body,* which stimulates cardiovascular efficiency, muscular strength, or increased speed, and (2) *allow an adequate amount of rest for recovery and adaptation to occur.*

Problems often arise because there is a fine line between an optimal overload and overtraining. *Overtraining* is defined as "too much, too soon," and happens in one of two ways. Sometimes athletes just do too much in a workout, and they pay for it with varying levels of discomfort afterward, or they work previously stressed muscle groups that have not fully recovered from the last workout. The tissues suffer additional stress and damage, often resulting in uninterrupted soreness and chronic inflammation. When tissue is traumatized in either of these ways, it is known as an *overuse injury.*

It is extremely common for active people not to allow enough rest time for recovery and adaptation. Personal limits change frequently. Each athlete has a different training goal and pain threshold. In endurance sports, as much as 75 to 80 percent of all injuries can be attributed to training mistakes. Tissue damage is inevitable. The body's soft tissues are injured in one of three different ways: microtrauma and soreness, fiber separation and lesions, and contusions.

Microtrauma and Soreness. Greene notes that microtrauma results from microscopically small amounts of strain spread over time. These stresses can create spasm and build tension, eventually pulling and extending the tissue until fatigue and failure occurs. This kind of damage is cumulative, usually traumatizing a few fibers at a time and only at microscopic levels.

Endurance athletes such as runners, swimmers (Fig. 26–3), and skill sports such as tennis or soccer are susceptible to microtrauma. Symptoms include general soreness or mild pain, which usually dissipates within 24 to 72 hours. With adequate rest and recovery, there is no loss of ROM or strength, and activity can continue with little disruption. Massage techniques that

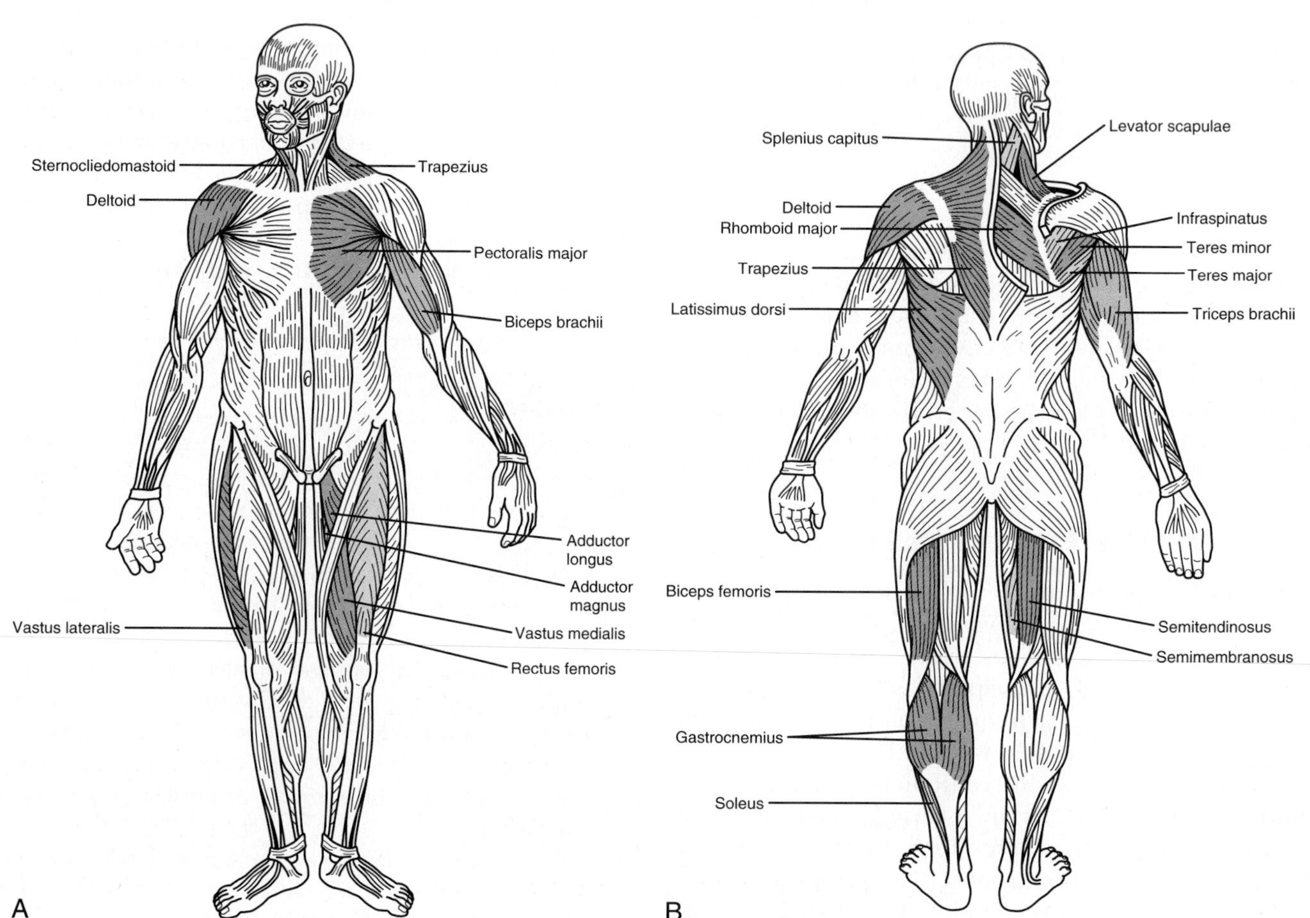

Figure 26•3 Common areas of soreness—swimmer. *A,* anterior view; *B,* posterior view.

reduce spasm and stimulate circulation, such as the ones described in the postevent and recovery sections, are appropriate for this kind of tissue damage.

Fiber Separation and Lesion. A **lesion** is an injury that involves disruption of an anatomic structure. There is usually a significant amount of fiber separation and tensional tearing that can result in a loss of strength and ROM. Lesions in muscle and tendon are referred to as *strains,* in ligaments as *sprains* and are categorized (grades 1, 2, or 3) by the amount of tissue torn. In grade 1 lesions up to 10 percent of the tissue is torn, grade 2 involves up to 50 percent, and grade 3 is a complete rupture of the structure.

These injuries frequently occur in sports in which explosive movements are common, such as sprinting. An athlete who is sprinting after a ball, or around a track can tear hamstring fibers, creating a lesion. Ankle sprains in soccer, basketball, or football involve lesions in tendons or ligaments. Tissue tearing that happens suddenly is a rapid onset injury.

Chronic, long-term overuse injuries (those that start as soreness and microtrauma) can slowly develop cumulative damage and can become a grade 1 or 2 lesion. Patellar tendinitis (runner's knee), lateral epicondylitis (tennis elbow), and shin splints are examples of chronic overuse injuries that form lesions and scar tissue. Tissue tearing that evolves slowly and progressively over time is called a gradual onset injury. Transverse friction massage can be a valuable technique for the scarring that forms in response to these injuries. Please refer to the maintenance section for more information and treatment suggestions regarding muscle, tendon, and ligament lesions.

Contusions are a crush injury from a blow or a fall and are common in contact sports such as football, hockey, rugby, or martial arts. Initially, massage therapy will be of minimal assistance with these injuries. Ice and a progressive, *pain-free* active and passive stretching regimen will be much more productive. See Figure 26–4 for a chart outlining injury recognition skills for the beginning massage therapist.

Soft-Tissue Repair: Homeostasis in Action

Homeostasis is the body's constant migration toward physiological balance, a state of relative constancy and equilibrium. When we are hungry we eat, thirsty we drink, tired we rest, and when we are stressed we seek relaxation. Regardless of how much tissue is damaged, Greene indicates that our body's cellular mechanisms immediately go to work to equalize the trauma, then begin repair, and finally regain tissue integrity. This three-phase healing process is known as the repair response: The first phase is inflammation, the second is regeneration, and the third is remodeling.

1. **Inflammation.** Symptoms can include local heat, swelling, redness, pain, and possibly decreased function. This phase is designed to prevent infection by eliminating debris and dead tissue from the wound. After the acute phase, general draining strokes that

Injury Recognition for the Beginning Massage Therapist

Factors to consider:	MUSCLE SORENESS (micro trauma)	LESION (strain/sprain)	CONTUSION (crush injury)
1. Location of complaint:	General, nonspecific complaint—client moves hands over large area	Specific location Client points to a specific spot	Specific location Client points to a specific area
2. Quality of sensation:	General achiness, soreness or tenderness	Mild to intense Sharp, throbbing or piercing pain Muscle guarding	Early on = intense throbbing or stabbing pain Later = dull pain that lingers Muscle guarding
3. History/Chronology A. Onset:	Associated with specific activity in the last 48 hours (Usually new activity or eccentric work)	Rapid = felt a snap or pop Gradual = chronic inflammation or an initial "twinge"... either could build into specific pain over several days or weeks. Muscle guarding	Rapid from a sudden blow or fall
B. Frequency:	Comes and goes with frequency of activity	Constant, unless low grade 1 then possibly intermittent	Constant, unless in latter stages of healing

Figure 26•4 Injury recognition skills for the beginning massage therapist. (Copyright M. Loomis 1990; Sports Massage Certification Training, Florida School of Massage.)

push edema toward the groin and armpits are indicated.

2. **Regeneration.** Heat, swelling, and pain have decreased; the cleansing process (inflammation phase) is ending. Cellular activity results in the growth of new capillaries (stimulates the nutrition/waste exchange) and begins to produce collagen, which is carefully constructed into a matrix of scar tissue. Massage strokes that address secondary spasms and flushing techniques that stimulate blood and lymph flow are indicated in this phase.
3. **Remodeling.** In this final phase, collagen is produced, broken down, and built up again. Properly applied transverse friction massage can assist in influencing randomly matted collagen fibers into an organized pattern of scar tissue. Repeating pain-free movement patterns (with and/or without weight) can stimulate the design and strength of collagen growth, and scar tissue can then be woven along the direction of stress or line of pull. A strong, mobile, pain-free scar marks the end of this phase. If tissue damage is moderate (microtrauma and general soreness), *this entire three-phase process can occur in 24 to 72 hours.*

When more serious tissue damage has occurred (grades 2 and 3 strains), the repair process can take much longer to resolve. These time frames depend on (1) the extent of the injury, (2) the frequency and efficacy of treatment, and (3) the client's compliance regarding self care.

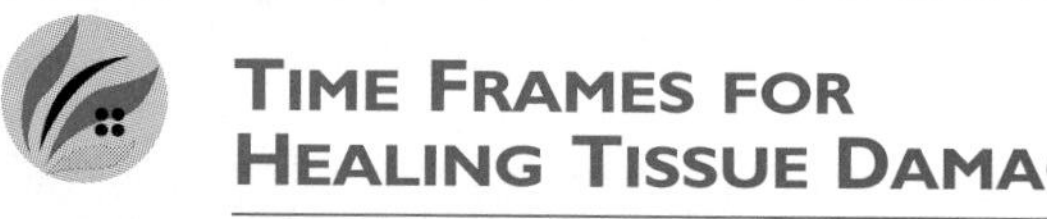

Time Frames for Healing Tissue Damage

- General muscle soreness = 24-72 hours
- Grade I and 2 lesions, mild contusions = 4-8 weeks
- Severe grade 2 and grade 3 lesions, more severe contusions = 2-6 months

Muscle Soreness

Sports massage can be a tremendously effective tool for addressing postexercise discomfort. If you have been involved in any rigorous activity, you know what it feels like to have sore muscles. Muscle soreness is by far the most frequent complaint that athletes bring to a sports massage therapist.

There are two kinds of soreness: immediate and delayed. The first is immediate soreness, which is experienced during or immediately after activity. Usually disappearing as soon as exercise stops and blood flow returns to normal, immediate muscle soreness is caused by a buildup of metabolic wastes and ischemia.

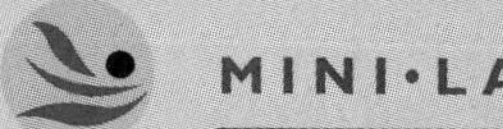

MINI•LAB

Stand with your arms outstretched in front of you. If any of the following suggested movements bring you pain, stop the activity immediately. Now, with your feet firmly planted, slowly begin to lower yourself into a deep-knee bend, keeping your gaze straight ahead of you and your back straight. Lower until your thighs are as close to parallel to the floor as possible, and hold this position. Notice where you start to feel discomfort (not pain) and maintain this position for a few moments.

Usually you will feel a burn in your thigh and/or shoulder muscles after a short period. Note how long it takes for this burning sensation to disappear after you stand normally again. As soon as the stress on your muscles stops, blood flow normalizes, and the sensation should dissipate. This is immediate muscle soreness.

Delayed Muscle Soreness

The second kind of muscle soreness, known as delayed soreness, is usually not felt until 24 to 48 hours after activity. The cause of delayed soreness is still debated. Abraham has outlined three well-recognized scientific theories.

1. **Damaged Muscle.** Abraham explains Hough's torn muscle tissue hypotheses (1902) stating that an untrained muscle group subjected to a prolonged period of work can be damaged. Microscopic tears in muscle tissue are a source of pain that lead to inflammation and increased discomfort.
2. **Pain-Spasm-Pain Cycle.** Abraham notes De Vries (1966) found that as waste products and ischemia increase with exercise, these changes irritate nerve endings, causing pain, which in turn brings a muscle into spasm. Additional pain and spasm continue to reduce blood flow to the tissues, decreasing available oxygen and increasing metabolic by-products. This chain reaction of increased waste, ischemia, pain, and spasm becomes a continuous cycle in the body.
3. **Connective Tissue Damage.** Abraham (1979) established a direct relationship (through urinalysis studies) between delayed soreness (24 to 72 hours after exercise) and connective tissue damage. It has also been found that eccentric contractions (a muscle lengthens rather than shortens as it contracts) are primarily responsible for connective tissue damage. Eccentric movements are also known as negative work in weight training.

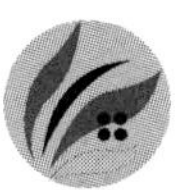

Conditions That Will Cause Muscle Soreness

- New activities that your body is not used to. This is especially true if you push your limits.
- Using the same muscles or joints for an extended time.
- Repeating movements that involve jerking, bouncing, or twisting.
- Activities that include eccentric movements such as jumping rope (calf), running downhill (shins or quads), lowering heavy weights slowly (biceps or hamstring curl), leg press (quads), or seated calf raises.

Depending upon individual circumstances, varying combinations of each of these three physiological explanations can be responsible for delayed soreness.

Recovery Tools for Sore Athletes

Combine any of the following for soreness reduction and breaking the pain-spasm-pain cycle.

1. **Sports Massage**
2. **Stretching**
3. **Absolute or endurance rest**
4. **Cold (Hydrotherapy chapter)**
5. **Gentle movements in a pool**
6. **Hot and cold (Hydrotherapy chapter)**

SPORTS MASSAGE: TIMING AND TECHNIQUE SELECTION

Decisions about *when* sports massage is provided, *how long* the sessions will last, and *which techniques* will be used are dependent upon the following factors:

How long before or after rigorous activity will the massage be administered? The closer to a period of physical exertion, the less intrusive the massage should be. There are two reasons for this: inflammation and neurological familiarity.

Inflammation. Vigorous, powerful, repetitive movements often have an inflammatory effect on an athlete's tissues, frequently leaving them sore and tender to touch. As therapists providing recovery massage, you want to be careful not to reinflame or further traumatize the tissue with prematurely applied deep or specific pressure. Intrusive massage administered too soon after exercise may actually *increase* levels of postexercise inflammation and soreness, thereby increasing rather than decreasing the amount of time needed for recovery. You want to support the forward movement of the repair response rather than slow it down or reverse it.

Also, when working with an athlete before a game, event, or training session, you need to be attentive to levels of depth and specificity. Inflammation and soreness that is the direct and immediate result of massage can adversely affect performance. This is an obvious concern when providing **pre-event massage** sessions.

Neurological Familiarity. Deep massage just before exercise can change familiar tensional systems that an athlete relies on for responsiveness, coordination, or precision movements. This could be a special concern for sprinters, dancers, gymnasts, or springboard divers. Deep massage immediately after exertion can so radically change the current tonus/spindle setting in the musculature that an athlete may suddenly cramp in response to attempts at such vigorous, rapid change. During **postevent massage** at marathons, a runner's calf can cramp quickly if the currently entrenched neuromuscular patterns are prematurely challenged with incorrectly applied massage. After thousands of broadening plantar flexion contractions that often last for several hours in a marathon, the unfamiliar twisting motions of postevent petrissage can quickly stimulate a violent calf cramp.

Other Factors to Consider

The Amount of Massage Experience the Athlete Has Had. Athletes who work extremely hard sometimes find the initial relaxation response to their first few massages to be so overwhelming that they feel sluggish during their next workouts; they feel as if they have relaxed too much. Others have difficulty letting go, cramp, or respond with muscle guarding, repeatedly tensing to the work. Experiment with the best combination of invigorating, brisk technique and more specific tactics. A successful sports massage therapist strives to refine each athlete's internal kinesthetic experience of transitioning from exertion to relaxation.

Familiarity Between the Athlete and the Therapist. Trust is the medium for relaxing in ways that hold the potential to be completely restorative. Working together weekly for several months can create this kind of bond. Being an athlete and a therapist is almost always an edge, especially if you are involved in the same sport as your client. Runners trust runners and surfers trust surfers to know the aches and pains that are particular to their sport.

The Competitive versus the Recreational Athlete. An athlete's training schedule will influence the detail and intensity of her massage. Some athletes have invested tremendous amounts of time and energy in pursuit of championships, medals, and personal excellence. A more conservative massage approach may be prudent with this population especially if this is her first attempt to use sports massage as a training tool.

Recreational athletes, weekend warriors, and general fitness enthusiasts obviously have less demanding and usually more flexible schedules. If so, there is more freedom for both you and your athletic client to experiment with the strategic placement of sports massage appointments in ways that meet your client's goals. See Figure 26–5 for a chart illustrating sports massage timing and technique.

Ask These Questions at Every Session

- Were you sore after the last session? If so, for how long and did it adversely affect your training or performance?
- Was the combination of general and specific work in the last session an agreeable mixture for you?
- Any suggestions for changes this time?
- Given your current training schedule, do you feel the day of the week we are scheduling your sports massage is optimal for you?

Author's Note

When working with athletes who are new to sports massage, we have found that the best time to initially explore possible reactions to combining sports massage with athletics is before or after a training session, rather than immediately before competition. This guideline is true for both recreational and competitive athletes.

SPORTS MASSAGE TIMING AND TECHNIQUE

(all times are approximate)

(these times can vary greatly depending upon the individual athlete)

Before... **ACTIVITY or COMPETITION** ...After

MAINTENANCE	PRE-RECOVERY	PRE-EVENT			POST-EVENT	POST-RECOVERY	MAINTENANCE
48 HR	6 HR	2 HR	30 MIN		15–30 MIN	6 HR	48 HR
Length of Massage (Minutes)	25	20	8–10		15	25–60	45–75
Type of Massage	Full Body-Flush	Invigorating strokes (tapot; jostle; compr.; vibration)			Flush sport specific areas	Full Body-Flush	Full Body-specific work where necessary, add stretching & ROM
Intent	Invigorate Develop mental readiness	Invigorate Develop mental readiness			Begin recovery	Recovery	Address specific problems; Prevent injuries Enhance performance
Guidelines	*Be positive *Use caution with deep or specific work *Don't dwell on or point out problem areas	*Be positive *No deep work *Don't linger on one area *Minimal relaxation			*General; Non-specific *Begin recovery	*General; more specific attention *Deeper relaxation *Used in many team scenarios	*Full recovery *Increase body awareness

Variables to consider
*Amount of massage experience athlete has had
*Familiarity between the athlete and the therapist
*Competitive athlete vs. recreational
*Individual responsiveness to various techniques

INTERCOMPETITION
*Combination of Pre/Post-Event
*Used when athlete competes more than once a day
*Recover and invigorate

Remember...
*The closer to a period of physical exertion, the less intrusive the massage should be

Figure 26•5 Sports massage timing and technique. (Copyright M. Loomis 1990; Sports Certification Training, Florida School of Massage.)

POSTEVENT MASSAGE

Time: 30 minutes to 6 hours after athletic activity (training or competition); sessions are approximately 10 to 20 minutes long

Setting: This kind of work is often provided for a group of athletes (after a triathlon, soccer match, or karate tournament, for example) as part of massage school learning so that students can gain more hands-on experience. In some communities groups of licensed therapists form a sports massage team to provide postevent massage for a fee.

These events are generally part of a fun filled, high-energy atmosphere; sometimes they are fund-raisers. Generally you cannot go wrong when you offer massage to a group of athletes after a long bike ride, a crew regatta, a swimming practice session, or softball tournament. People love the way massage feels after they have worked really hard and are especially thrilled if you are waiting with a group of tables and well-trained therapists on site! The ease and convenience of receiving massage without extra logistics make it a treat for the active person who may be continually challenged with a busy schedule.

Technique Application

The Art of Tracking. Good **tracking skills** are an essential foundation for all massage therapists. Tracking is the ability to notice and respond to changes that a client experiences as you work with them. Observe your client's facial expressions as you work, watching for changes in breath (in the belly when supine or the lumbar region when prone) or a subtle flinch from a technique that is applied too forcefully or quickly; listen for modulations in voice tone or cadence. With each new technique that you introduce, can you palpate whether the muscles are tightening or relaxing? Do you have a sense of whether your pressure is adequate or perhaps too strong? Watch for obvious cues such as a squint, a grimace, or the hands or feet being clenched.

The Tracking Response. The **tracking response** combines careful observation of a client's moment-to-moment responses to technique with your willingness to adjust and change your work accordingly. Developing tracking competency can be summed up by asking yourself, "What can I do, in this moment, to bring my client into a deeper state of relaxation?" Critical to this process is paying attention, continually cultivating concentration that refines your observation and palpation skills. This allows us to stay present, engaging our clients in a way that finds them feeling nurtured.

Maintaining tracking focus in a postevent massage environment can be particularly challenging. If you are at a large event, your table may be one of many. Your client may be joking with friends or family members while you provide postevent sports massage. She might be "talking shop" with an athlete at an adjoining table. A local radio station may be blasting loud music from its sound truck. Sudden, loud cheers from spectators, dogs barking, a strong gust of wind, or the noise of the starter's gun can tug incessantly at your focus (Fig. 26–6).

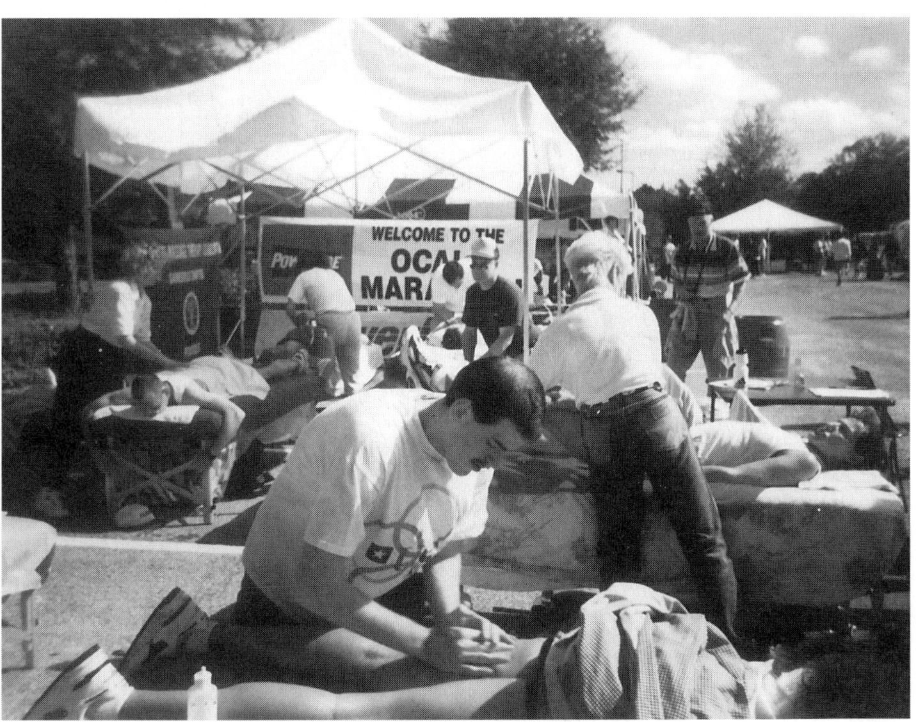

Figure 26•6 Postevent massage: concentration in a sea of distractions.

In 1989, at the Gasparilla 15K run in Tampa, Florida (a local event that has thousands of participants annually), I was supervising postevent massage for approximately 75 therapists. A runner approached me with ambivalence about receiving sports massage. He told me that the only other postevent session that he had received (after a run in his hometown elsewhere in Florida) was very painful. He said, "Sports massage is like going to the dentist. I know it's going to hurt, but I know it's good for me."

Think about your work and the person you are working with as being at the center of your experience; everything else is peripheral. Each athlete's level of satisfaction will be directly proportional to your ability to concentrate on who she is and what she is needing in the moment.

When an athlete experiences pain in a postevent massage, we know that too much pressure is being applied too soon after exercise. This kind of massage adds additional stress and does *not* facilitate recovery. Massage that is continuously painful produces muscle guarding and additional spasms rather than relaxation. Instead of increasing circulation, blood flow decreases when a client endures sustained, painful pressure. If there is pain, the athlete does not gain.

Techniques for the Lower Extremity

"Loosen and Liquefy." These techniques are done briskly to relax and invigorate. The work is general, because it is too soon after activity to challenge specific tissues (exceptions to this rule include individual athletes with whom you have worked privately). Without prior knowledge of individual responsiveness, a general, conservative approach is best.

Even though these techniques are described for the hamstrings, they are appropriate for all the major muscle groups of the thigh and leg except lifting and jostling on the anterior shin. Athletes often comment that they have much less postexercise soreness after receiving a good postevent sports massage. The order of the following techniques is completely interchangeable; an easy way to remember them is to repeat the saying **Every (effleurage) Body (broadening) Can (compression) Love (lifting) Jam (jostling).**

Alternating Hand Effleurage: Hamstrings. Lightly and briskly begin short effleurage strokes at the knee, alternating left and right hands, progressively moving up toward the hip and ischial tuberosity. As you complete your last stroke in the pelvic region with one hand, quickly shift your contact back down at the knee with your other hand, and repeat the same sequence moving up the hamstrings once again. Take care to transfer your weight forward, as your left and right

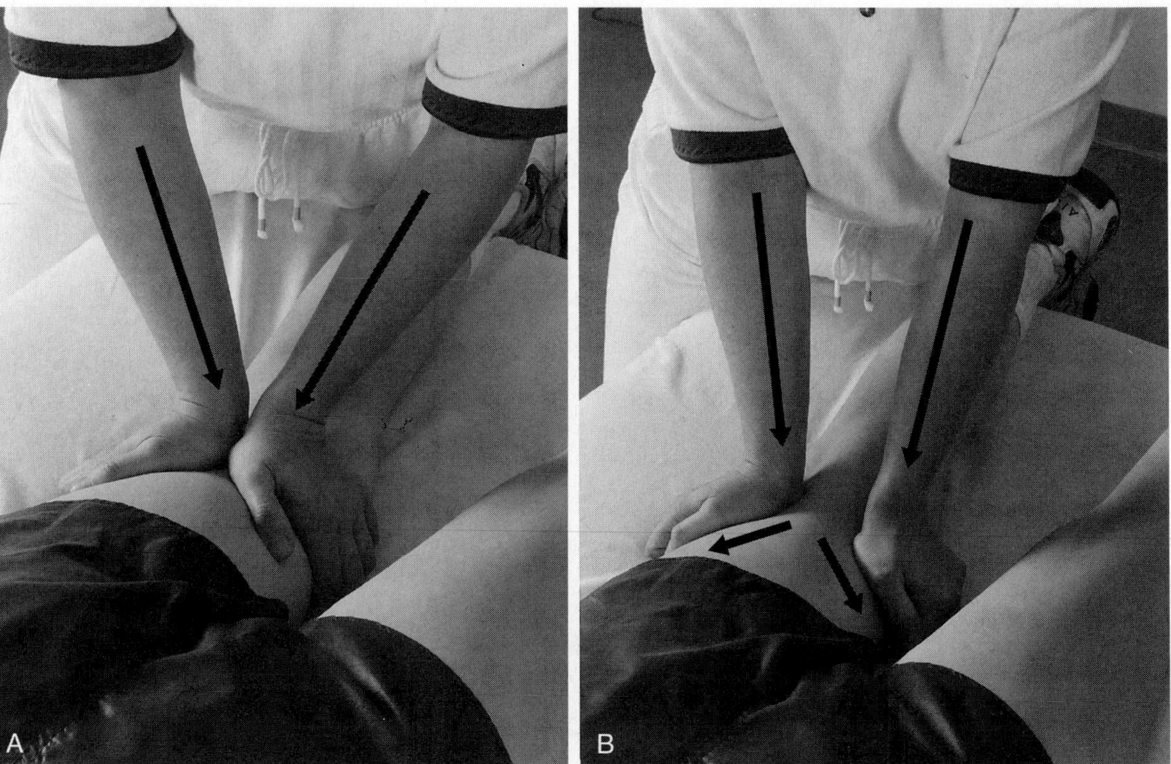

Figure 26•7 Two-handed broadening: hamstrings.

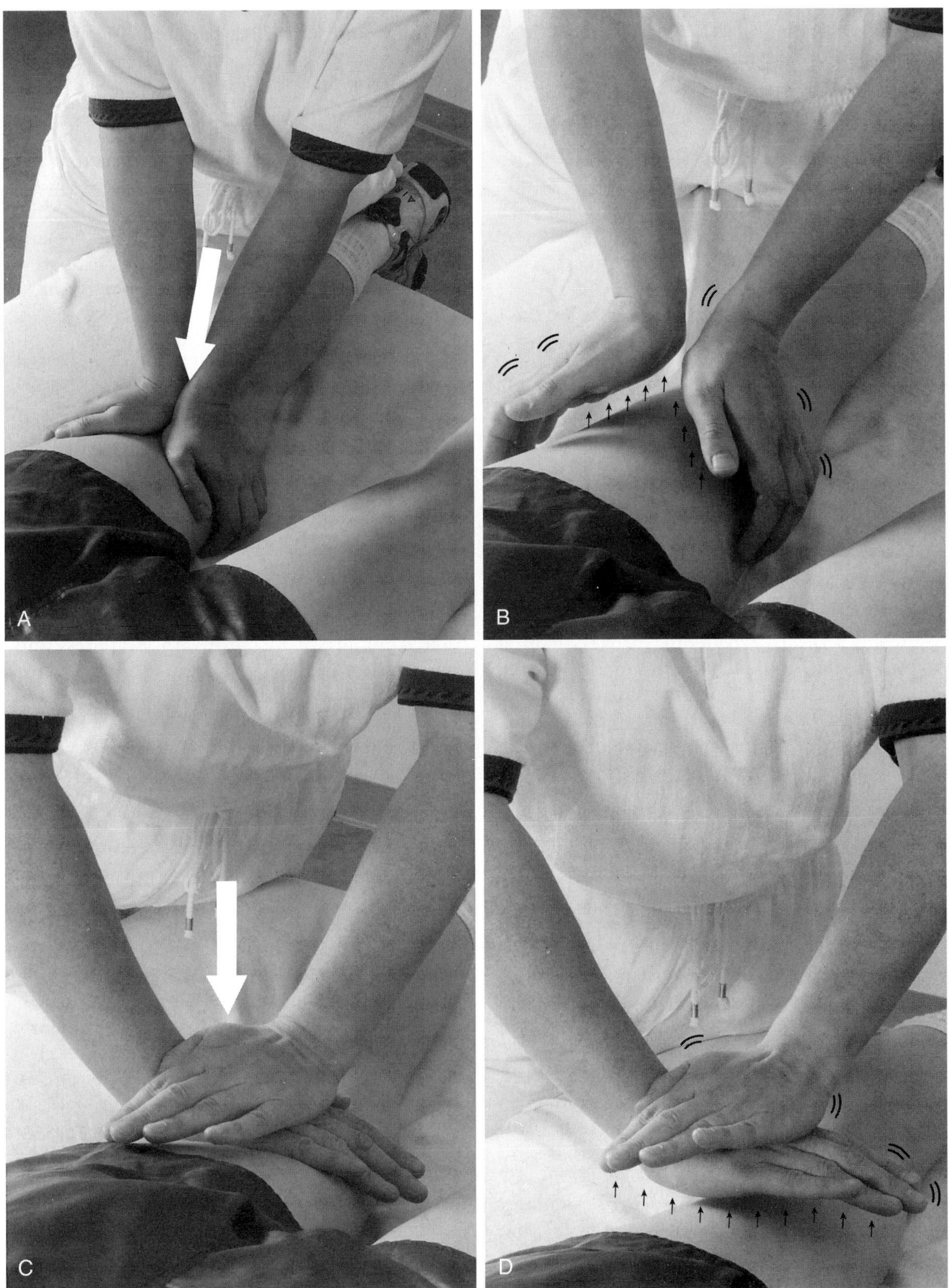

Figure 26•8 Rhythmic compression: hamstrings/gluteals.

hands advance quickly and energetically in a proximal direction.

Two-Handed Broadening (Fulling): Hamstrings. Place the heels of both hands, palms down, wrist to wrist on the belly of the hamstring muscles just superior to the popliteal area of the knee. The fingers of each hand are pointing medially and laterally respectively. Sink into the pressure by bending your knees slightly and transferring your weight into your hands. The heels of your hands broaden out away from each other, separately molding to your client's thigh and traveling perpendicular to the muscle fibers (Fig. 26–7).

Broaden through all the fibers until the stroke ends as each heel of the hand reaches the table. Remember, *broadening mimics the movement of a muscle when it contracts,* which qualifies this technique as one of the most neurologically familiar techniques in a sports massage session. Repeat the stroke again and again in an overlapping fashion, starting each new stroke almost a full hand width superior to the last stroke. Finish your last broadening stroke at the ischial tuberosity (the site of the common tendinous attachment of all three hamstrings), being careful to maintain approximately one full hand's width distance from your client's groin.

Now begin this series of broadening strokes again at the place you started originally (just superior to the knee). Repeat the sequence from the knee to the ischial tuberosity two or three times, carefully tracking your client's responses to the massage. Can you palpate one particular area where the texture of the tissue feels tighter, more congested, or less resilient to the repeated challenge of broadening?

Compression: Hamstrings/Gluteals. Compression is a powerful, rhythmic mechanical pumping of muscle over bone. It is a quick and relatively simple way to bring extra blood to a localized area of the body; extra blood means extra oxygen to tissue that needs optimal nutrition for full recovery. This technique can also be an excellent method for diminishing tension or spasm in large muscles.

Compression is applied with the palms of both hands resting next to each other (the same position as when beginning to broaden the hamstrings) or with one palm on top of the other (for support and extra pressure). Occasionally a therapist will use a fist or forearm, although you may be limited in the amount of palpation detail you receive, which will inhibit the tracking response.

Bend your arms slightly at the elbows. Begin by compressing the distal hamstring fibers into the shaft of the femur. Lean into the muscle with the heel(s) of your hand(s). As you sink into the muscle, try to land softly yet firmly like a cat; after a very brief moment spring back up and out of the muscle fibers. Avoid punching the muscle. Focus on a rhythmic sinking, landing, and springing back out of the muscle (Fig. 26–8).

The most important aspect of this technique is that pressure is a direct result of transferring the weight of your body into your hands. Sink with your entire body, bending your knees as you work, so that each downstroke of compression is as effortless as possible. Table height is a critical item in compression technique. Experiment with your pace, sensing and seeking a relaxing rhythm; move proximally up through the hamstrings toward the ischial tuberosity. From this bony landmark, continue up into the body of the gluteal muscles. Compress all of the musculature of the iliac fossa region, taking special care to mobilize and liquefy the sacroiliac joints.

If this technique bothers your wrists, step slightly back away from the body so that the angle of your hand at your wrist is decreased. Since compression is extremely direct and can be more potentially painful to your athletic clients than other techniques, it should be offered cautiously with extra care given to tracking each athlete's response to pressure, especially in a postevent setting where levels of soreness may be higher.

It is important to move with awareness and sensitivity. Track carefully with your hands and your eyes. Avoid compressing directly on a bone. If you vigorously compress a skier's or a cyclist's quadriceps, a body builder's sore pectoralis muscle, or a runner's calves an hour after a hard workout or competition, this technique may be quite painful. When this is the case, other postevent techniques may be a better choice to reduce your athlete's soreness.

Lifting: Hamstrings. Start just superior to your client's knee with your hands gently cupped around the lateral and medial edges of the hamstrings. Point your fingers toward the ceiling; the heel of each hand provides opposing pressure. Now simultaneously lift the heels of both hands skyward so that as much muscle as possible is lifted off the shaft of the femur but without lifting the thigh itself off the table (Fig. 26–9). A carefully measured balance of pressure is needed to achieve this.

Lift completely up through the most posterior fibers of both the medial and lateral thigh. Return to the starting position again with the heels of your hands opposing each other, slightly proximal to their original placement; you can somewhat overlap the portion of tissue covered in the last stroke. Repeat the movement, lifting again with the opposing pressure of the heels of both hands.

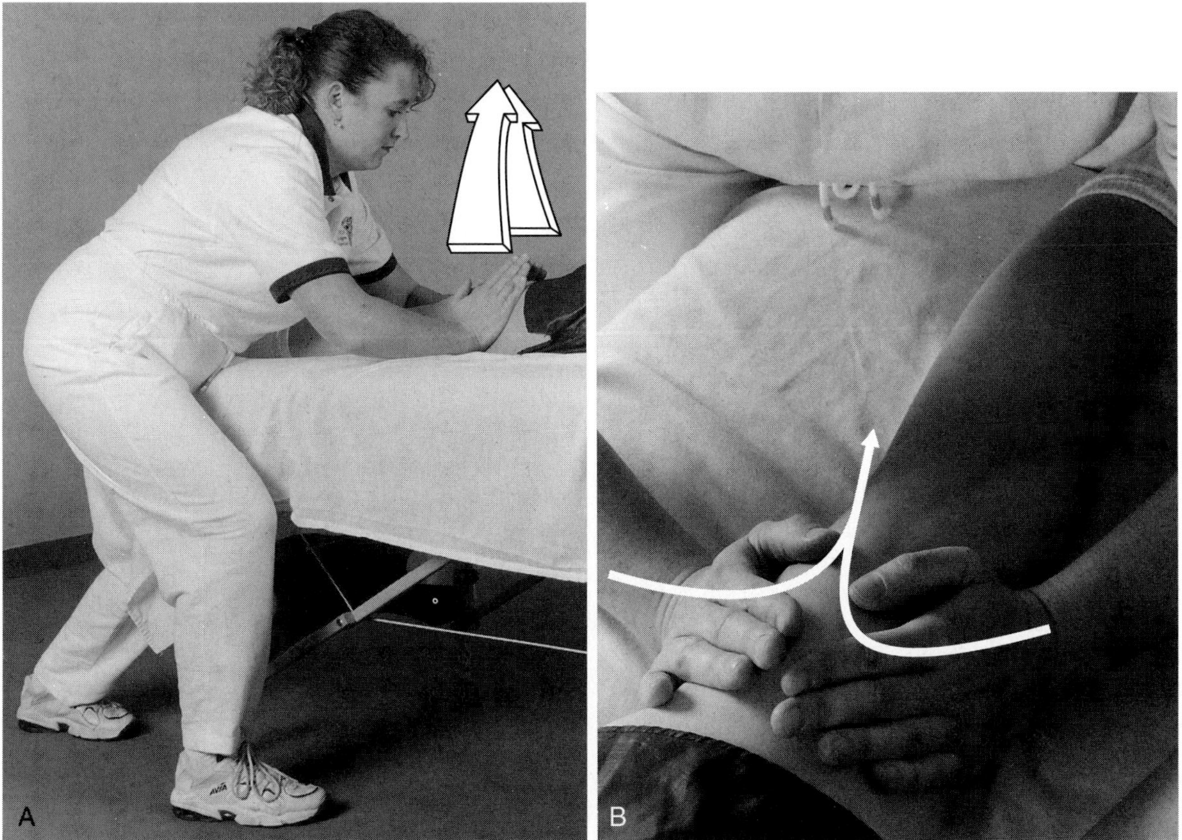

Figure 26•9 Lifting: hamstrings.

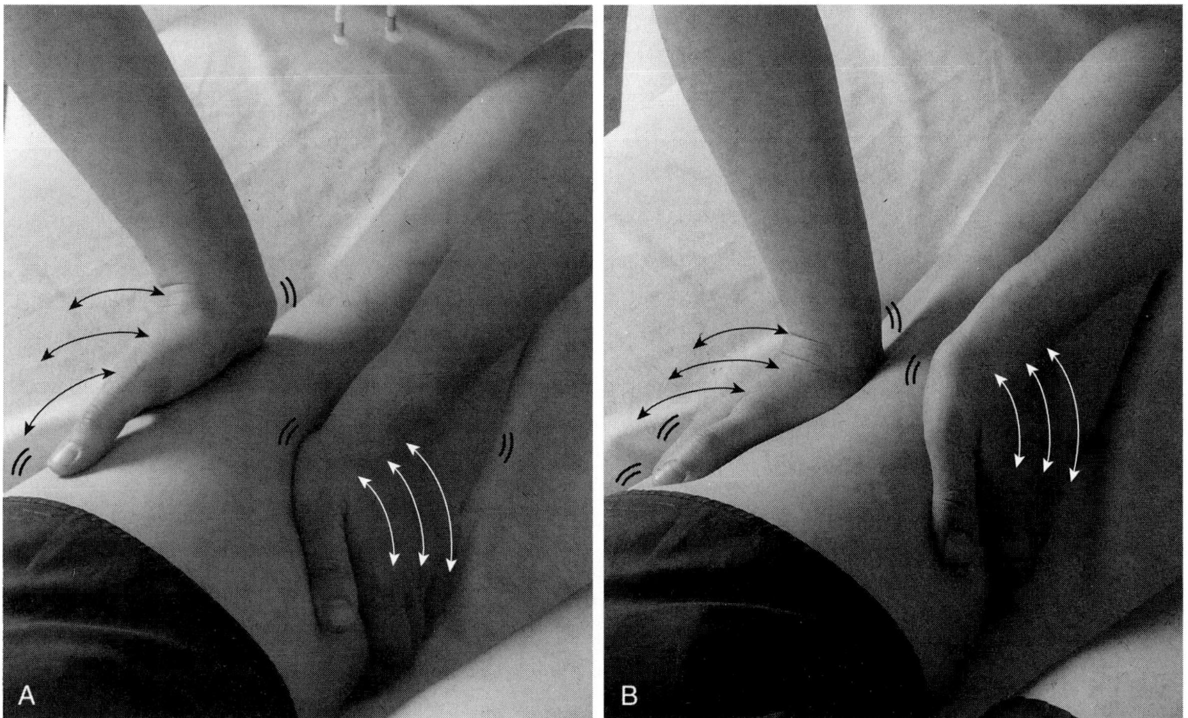

Figure 26•10 Jostling: hamstrings.

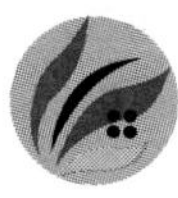

POSTEVENT MASSAGE—SAMPLE TECHNIQUE LIST

Posterior Thigh	*Posterior Leg*	*Anterior Thigh*	*Anterior Leg*
effleurage	effleurage	effleurage	effleurage
broadening	broadening	broadening	broadening
compression	compression	compression	compression
lifting	lifting	lifting	
jostling	jostling	jostling	

Repeat this overlapping stroke sequence one to three more times, finishing with a lifting stroke that is approximately one palm's width from your client's groin. Return to just above your client's knee and repeat the entire sequence one or two more times. Work briskly and rhythmically. The mechanics of this stroke may feel awkward to you when you first try it, so take your time getting a feel for it. Slow it down in the beginning, and the rhythm will come with time and practice.

A modified bow stance (outside foot up near the client's hip and the inside foot down near his knee) is essential for this stroke to be done comfortably. Your knees are slightly bent, back relatively straight, and you lean into the stroke with your entire body. Transfer the momentum of your torso into your hands, staying behind your work as you rhythmically rock forward and back, knees repetitively bending and slightly straightening. If your legs do the work, little arm strength is needed.

Jostling (Vibration): Hamstrings. Gently grip the posterior thigh a few inches above the knee with the palms and fingers of both hands as if you are beginning another broadening stroke. Begin alternately leaning and rocking the heels of your left and right hands down into the belly of the hamstring fibers. Keep your contact loose and relaxed, focusing your pressure on each downstroke of your palm (Fig. 26–10). Keep your fingers relaxed, and avoid pulling up on the tissue with them since this will tire you more quickly. As you jostle the hamstring bellies, gradually increase the speed of the technique, being careful to establish a pace that allows you to maintain control.

Continue jostling and begin to move proximally with your work toward the hip. Stay over your work with your upper torso so that you can transfer the weight of your body into the downstroke of each palm in a way that finds you exerting minimal effort with your shoulder girdle muscles. Experiment with the pace and rhythm of this technique, paying close attention to your client's reactions as you jostle, especially when you change the pace. Continue to work up and down the thigh, seeking out tighter, more congested areas. You will know you are proficient at this stroke when you can comfortably sustain it for 15 to 20 seconds, changing pressure, rhythm, direction, and pace with minimal effort.

TRAINING INFORMATION FOR SPORTS MASSAGE

After you have provided a postevent session for an athlete, she may want to know when a good time would be to schedule a session, how frequently you recommend "receiving sports massage," and what the content of the session will be. The answers to these questions will depend on an athlete's training schedule and your knowledge of different training techniques, terminology, and scheduling strategies. Knowing more about strength and/or endurance training principles can be essential to meeting the needs of athletic clients. Noakes, Sleamaker, and Sudy suggest the following considerations.

Identify Your Athlete's Goals

Some people exercise because it's fun, and they want to increase the quality and length of their lives. Other people work out to decrease weight, and still others exercise as a way to socialize. Competitive athletes will usually bring a sport-specific purpose to your massage practice. Tailor your sessions to support individual needs and goals.

Frequency and Duration of Exercise

An average, healthy schedule is a minimum of three and a maximum of six workouts per week. At least 30 minutes three times per week is the minimum recommended for some level of healthy change to occur from exercise. Some athletes will train as much as 3 to 5 hours per day, 7 days a week. But more is not always better: The quality of a workout can be more important than quantity. At least one rest day per week is a healthy choice. Many athletes choose their rest day to receive their weekly massage.

Any athlete who wants to apply the overload principle must develop a training base or foundation. This takes 2 to 3 months (depending upon previous fitness levels), and consists of low-intensity, high-volume workouts. When developing a training base, variety comes from activity, distance, and the like rather than from adding intensity. You will see athletes whose specific complaints are a result of not developing a solid training base. Encourage them to be patient, and educate them to proper training techniques.

Intensity

A training approach that incorporates more difficult workouts into a given week is the concept of hard/easy. Hard workouts use the overload principle to stress an athlete's body, stimulating increased speed, strength, coordination, or cardiovascular fitness. Teach your athlete to establish a solid training base before attempting to stress his body with a strenuous workout.

Hard workouts come in a variety of forms and usually occur only once or twice per week. Intervals are fast repeats on the track, road (cycling), or in the pool, with a short rest between each interval. Tempo workouts are medium-length workouts in which you pick up the pace during the middle of the training session. Many athletes are sore after hard workouts and some clients do not do well if they receive maintenance work on the same day. Deep, specific maintenance massage techniques may actually increase soreness levels for these athletes.

Easy/rest days are *essential* to a successful training program. This is a time for the body to replace energy stores and to adapt to the stresses placed upon it. Absolute rest is a day of no workouts, and may include hydrotherapy (soaking in a tub or ice massage), stretching, massage therapy, and extra sleep. Endurance rest means a day of easy exercise, but this is a relative term. For an elite runner who logs 110 miles and three hard workouts per week, endurance rest might mean a 7-mile "jog" at a 7-minute-mile pace. The average fitness enthusiast might walk, lightly jog, take an easy spin on the bike, or use light weights for a gym routine. A day of endurance rest is a good day to schedule a maintenance session.

Enforced rest means a lengthy rest period (weeks or months) that occurs as a result of significant injury. Some athletes lose perspective, pushing themselves until they get injured or burn out from overtraining.

The warning signs of overtraining are

- Mild, *persistent* soreness
- Insomnia
- Decreased performance
- Lowered resistance
- Inability to relax, irritability
- Elevated pulse in the morning
- Fatigue, lethargy, depression
- Higher frequency of colds and flu

Type of Exercise

Each activity or sport places different demands on muscles, joints, and the body in general. It is a good idea for serious athletes to employ the cross-training principle. This involves alternating their sport of choice with other activities that are fun, support their primary activity, add variety to their routine, and reduce the risk of injury from overtraining. Runners can swim to support cardiorespiratory fitness, or a tennis player might spend time on a rowing machine to increase muscular endurance. Cross-training can be a fun, creative tool to introduce into an athlete's training schedule.

Other Factors to Consider

Age, developmental level, motivation, nutrition, overall stress levels, and genetics can affect an athlete's training process. Learn all you can about your client's training choices and patterns to help prevent injuries. In some sports, up to 75 percent of chronic injuries can be attributed to training mistakes.

PRE- AND POSTRECOVERY (FLUSH) MASSAGE

Time: 6 to 24 hours before or after athletic activity (training or competition). Remember: These times are an approximation to help offer a general sense of timing. Sessions are usually 30 to 60 minutes long.

Setting: These sessions can be done in a private clinic as part of your athletic clientele's recovery process. A 30-minute, full-body "flush massage" can be an economical and time-efficient method for recovering from competition or midweek hard workouts. A 60-minute, Friday afternoon appointment is a perfect training tool to help an athlete fully recover from the week's workouts and develop mental readiness for Saturday's competition. This is also an optimal form of recovery work to offer a team of athletes once or twice a week. Therapists often set up at the track, on the pool deck, or in a local training facility.

Recovery Techniques for the Lower Extremity

"Loosen and Liquefy." The previously described postevent techniques can serve as a base for a longer recovery session. These techniques are also very easily adapted to the arms, shoulders, and back. Your primary focus is to reduce muscle soreness by addressing localized spasms and by manually flushing metabolic wastes toward the lymph nodes in the groin or armpits. Recovery work maintains a general focus with a special caution regarding deep or specific massage if you are working with an athlete who will compete in 24 hours or less.

Effleurage, broadening, compression, lifting, and jostling are effective in softening tension and revascularizing any palpable ischemic pockets. The following techniques are ways to further address specific areas of residual tension without leaving your athlete inflamed,

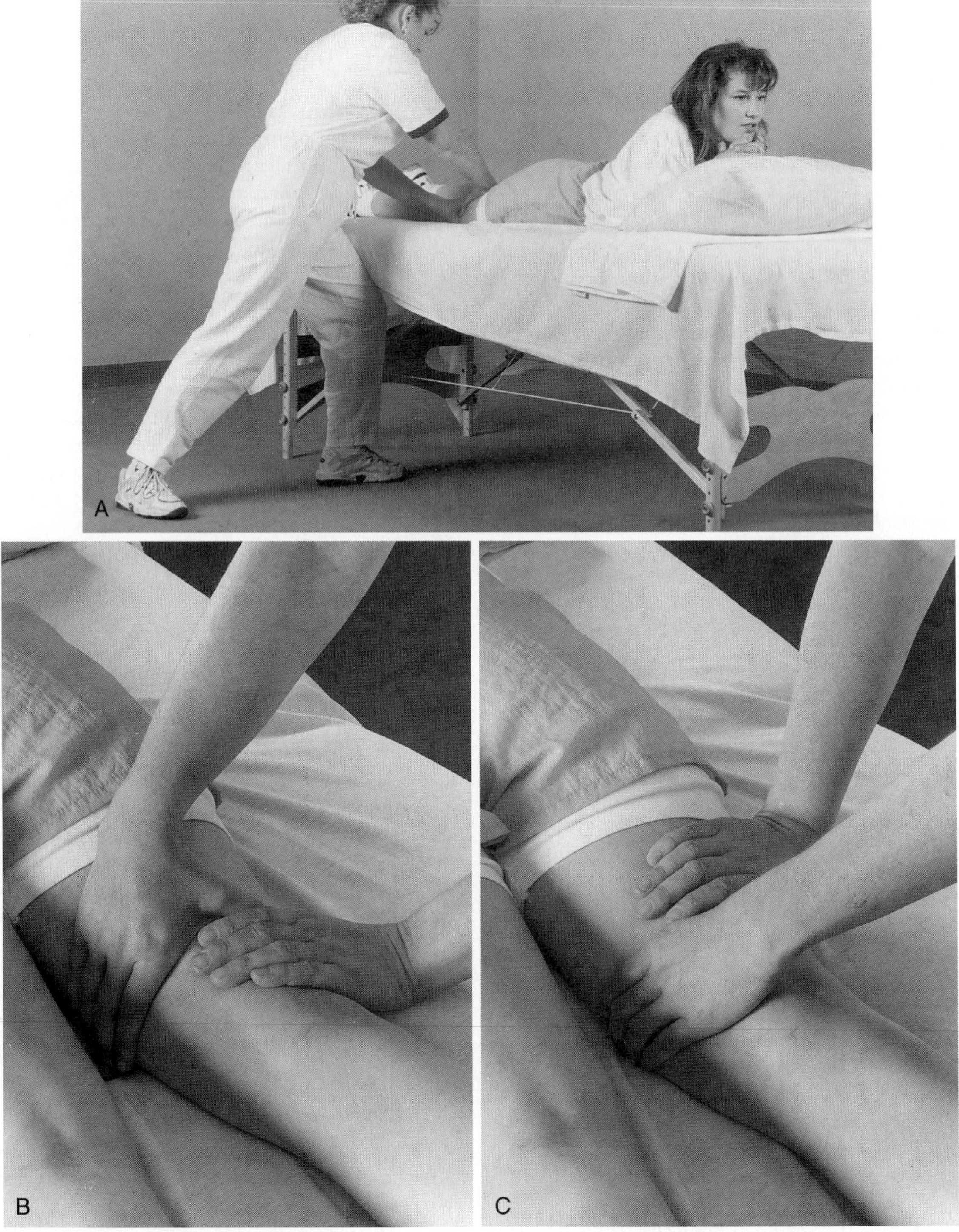

Figure 26•11 Opposing heel of hand wringing (petrissage) on posterior thigh.

sore, or concerned about his "problem areas" for tomorrow's competition or training session.

Opposing Heel of Hand Wringing (Petrissage) on Posterior Thigh

Stand facing your client's lateral lower extremity and grasp the thigh with the index fingers of both hands immediately adjacent to each other. With a firm grip, allow both of your hands to mold to the thigh as you begin wringing your hands in opposite directions. Keep both of your index fingers in constant contact as you grip and twist in a fashion that produces a mild amount of opposing traction between your left and right hands. Leaning in with your body weight, apply enough pressure to generate tissue differentiation and spasm reduction without creating discomfort (Fig. 26–11).

Continue this wringing traction as you glide up toward the hip and down toward the knee. Try repeating a few extra wringing movements in areas that are particularly sore or that feel more congested. Generate additional relief by repeating a few well-chosen postevent techniques on areas that need them, then return to the opposing wringing movements. Opposing wringing is also an effective recovery technique for the quadriceps, calves, or the triceps when a client is prone with his arms off the sides of the table.

Two-Handed Drain (Effleurage): Calf

Use draining techniques to push fluid out of the tissue. With the client prone, kneel on the table so that as you flex the person's knee, you can comfortably return his leg to a resting position on your thigh. Grasp the ankle just proximal to the malleoli with both of your hands so that your fingers are underneath and your thumbs create a broad flat bar on the posterior surface of the calf muscle. Grip with moderate to firm pressure as you slowly glide proximally through the Achilles tendon, the soleus, and gastrocnemius muscles all the way to the knee (Fig. 26–12). Repeat this two or three times, maintaining a constant pressure throughout the stroke. Avoid using thumb tips; the broad, flat portion of your thumb offers a more comfortable, less specific form of pressure to an athlete's sore muscle bellies. Check with your client regarding pressure and speed. You want to go slowly enough to allow your client to respond without flinching, while generating enough momentum to move a significant volume of lymphatic fluid and to assist in venous return.

As with opposing wringing, draining strokes combine well with various postevent techniques. Draining can be a wonderful way to help alleviate the feeling of fullness and heaviness that athletes often report if there is an excessive buildup of tension and waste products in a sport-specific major muscle group. Drain-

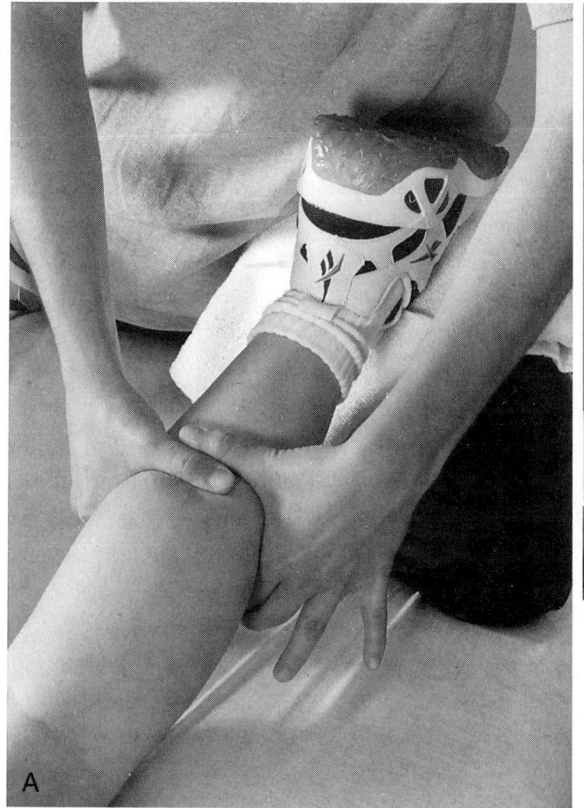

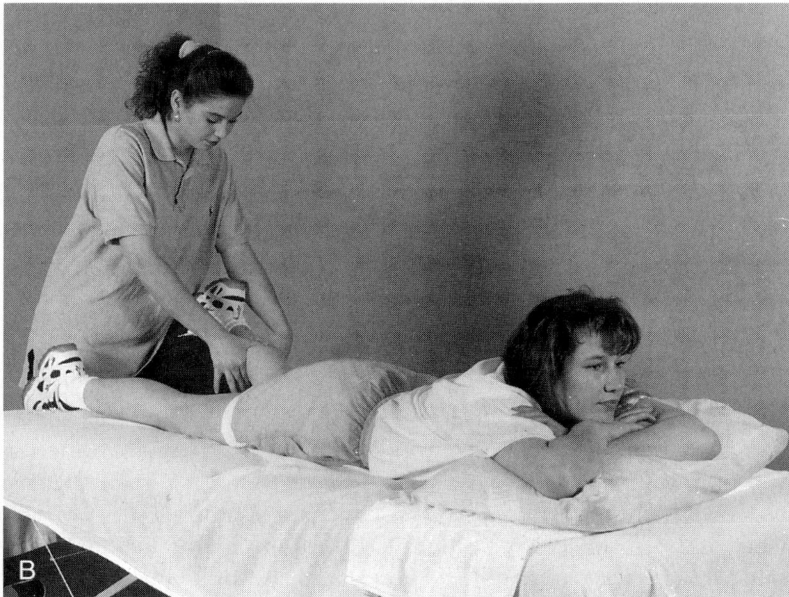

Figure 26•12 Two-handed drain (effleurage): calf.

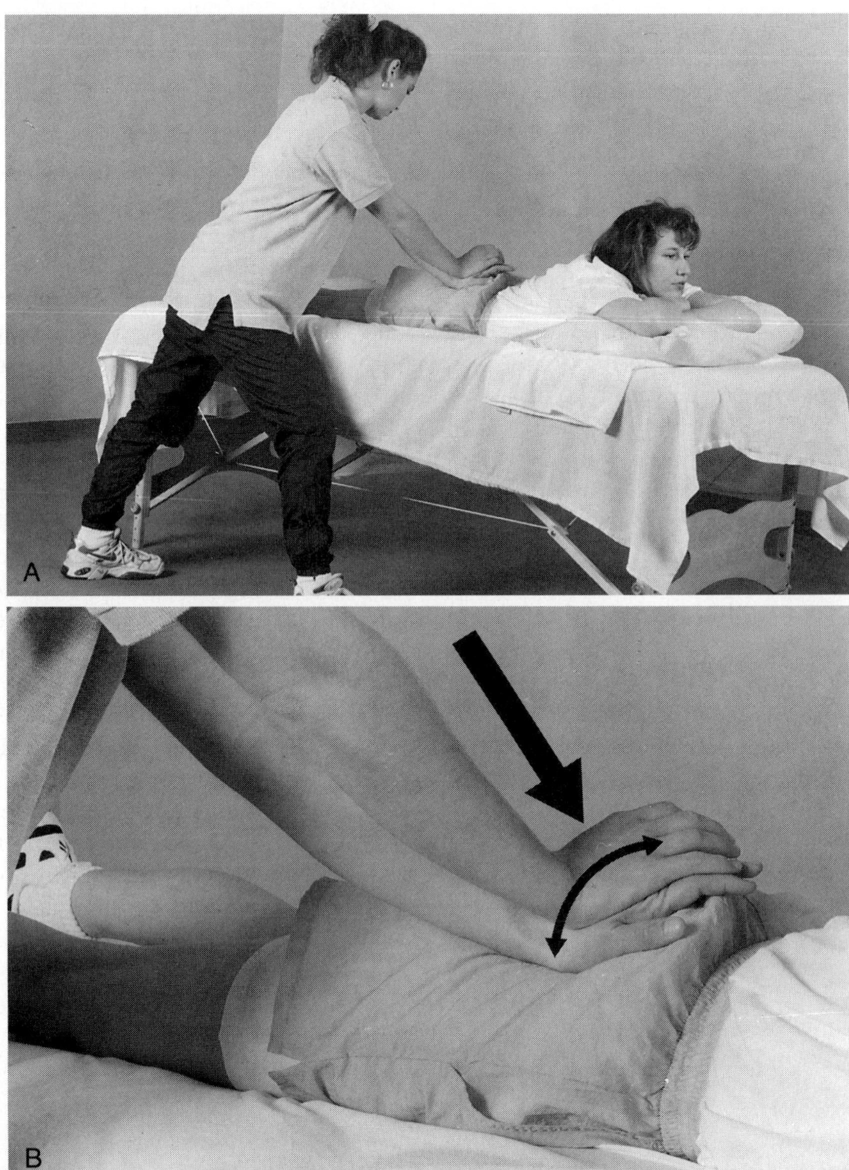

Figure 26•13 Heel of hand friction: buttock.

ing strokes are easily applied on the quadriceps in the supine position with the leg bent at the knee or on a forearm that is flexed at the elbow.

Heel of Hand Friction: Buttock

As you rhythmically compress your client's buttock/iliac fossa, you encounter a bundled portion of muscle tissue that feels resistant to change, and as you compress deeply, you sense a wincing reaction from your client. When you ask, she acknowledges that the area feels mildly sore to the touch. Heel of hand friction offers a therapist the perfect tool to bridge the gap between staying general and offering just enough specific attention to generate healthy change in the muscle tissue.

Place the heel of your hand over the gluteus medius muscle, and leaning in with your body weight, begin to friction back and forth across the grain of the muscle fibers (Fig. 26–13). Track your client carefully as you settle into a pace and depth that relaxes her. Be attentive to palpation that reveals particular patterns in the tissue that need more specific diagonal friction; you can also use lateral or medial frictioning to create increased freedom in the tissue. Sometimes a clockwise or counterclockwise circular frictioning will help your client relax more completely.

ANATOMY FOR ATHLETICS: ADDING SPECIFICITY TO THE WORK

Developing precision with your massage skills begins with a solid understanding of anatomy. Repeated opportunities to palpate and compare structures that undergo similar daily stresses can strengthen your hands-on anatomy skills immensely. Palpatory repetition can cultivate a kinesthetic comprehension of what is normal and abnormal.

The abnormalities that you encounter in an athletic population most often manifest in the form of muscle spasms, adhesions, trigger points, and lesions. Muscle spasms are an increase in tension due to excessive, sustained motor nerve activity, increased waste products, and ischemia; the previously described postevent and recovery techniques are superb tools for reducing spasm.

Successful maintenance massage begins with a capacity to recognize and palpate limitations in the soft-tissue matrix of muscle, fascia, ligament, and tendon. Your palpation skills are the foundation for successfully assessing and treating the more complex, interrelated soft-tissue pathologies that are addressed in a maintenance massage session.

Muscle Tissue

Muscle fibers broaden when they contract. When individual fibers adhere to each other or to neighboring structures (another muscle or fascia), full contractile energy and power are limited, which will increase fatigue and inhibit performance.

When portions of muscle tissue are stressed, microscopic damage and inflammation result. Greene notes that during the early stages of an inflammatory response, cellular mechanisms (vasoconstriction and clotting) are set in motion that are designed to localize the extent of the injury. Clotting agents in the blood exude fibrinous matter that forms adhesions. An **adhesion** is newly introduced fibrous tissue that forms an abnormal union between two previously separate structures.

Muscles fatigue more quickly when they are adhered and cannot function independently of each other. Long-distance runners will often have adhesions between the iliotibial band and vastus lateralis, cyclists between the soleus and peroneus longus, and sprinters between the proximal portions of adductor magnus and semimembranosus. These areas will produce sensations that vary from a dull ache to soreness, tenderness, or pain.

Adhesions that are not addressed become firmly established and will often repetitively strain and repair, creating a cycle of inflammation and pain. In response to this pain, secondary spasms develop in the surrounding musculature. Unless these spasms are resolved, they continue to *support* the inflammation by inhibiting the natural, healing flow of fluids through the adhered tissues. If spasms persist, they may become a breeding ground for trigger points.

Trigger Points

Trigger points, localized areas of hypersensitivity in a muscle, will refer pain. With athletes, trigger points are often found in areas of biomechanical stress. The musculotendinous junction is the place where tendon and muscle join and is a site of biomechanical stress for some athletes. For example, highly charged trigger points that refer pain to the ankle will sometimes be found in the soleus/Achilles junction of sprinters (Fig. 26–14). The musculotendinous junction of the common forearm flexors or extensors of weight lifters, golfers, or tennis players when triggered, will commonly refer pain distally to the wrist or hand.

Regions that have the potential to develop trigger points will often exhibit levels of increased spasm in the tissue. If you work with a client weekly, pay attention to these changes. These localized areas of hypersensitivity will feel knotted, progressively more congested, or ropy. When normal pressure on these painful points creates referred sensation, this is a warning sign for you and your client that changes need to be made in the consistency and focus of her massage sessions, in her self-care programs, training schedule, equipment choices, or biomechanical patterns. When regarded in this way, sports massage becomes an invaluable biofeedback tool to help your athletic client train in a healthy and pain-free way. Relaxing localized spasms, separating adhered structures, and locating and treating any offending trigger points are the goals for performance enhancement and injury prevention.

The real object of education is to have man in the condition of continually asking questions.

—Bishop Creighton

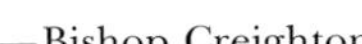

Tendons

Tendons are tightly woven, tough fibrous bands that link muscle to bone. They do not stretch or contract the way muscles do. Tendinitis (inflammation of the tendon) is extremely common in athletes. A tendon's blood supply is limited so it usually does not heal quickly or easily. One of the most common scenarios athletes regularly report is that a tendon will hurt (patellar or Achilles is common) when they first start their activity, but the pain subsides once the tissue is warmed up and extra blood is flowing freely to the tendon. This particular history is the gradual onset of an overuse injury, an early warning sign that a minor injury could become more serious. When pain shifts from an intermittent status to one that is more constant, microtrauma is slowly building, accumulating inflammation to the point that a lesion may form in the tendon.

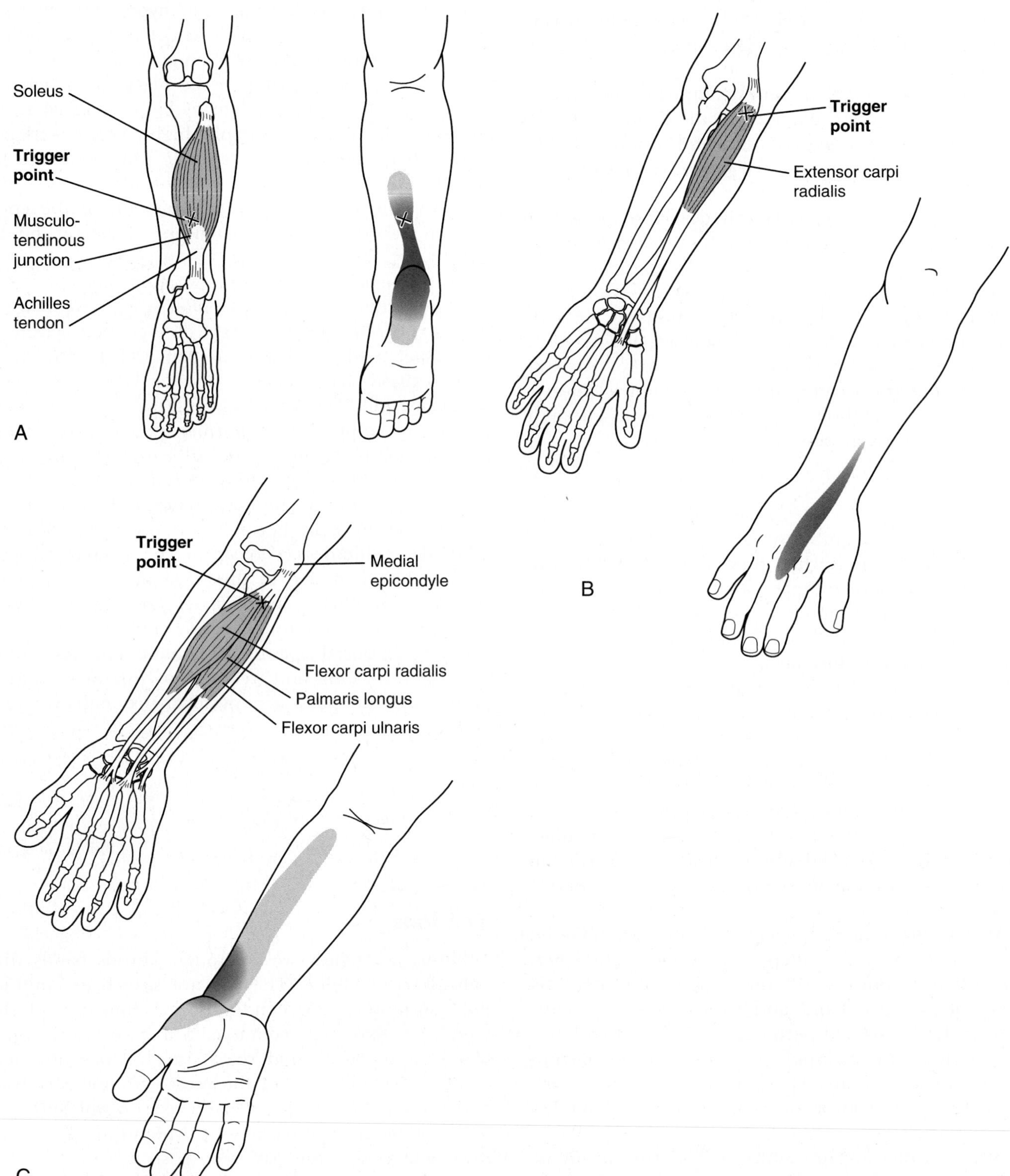

Figure 26•14 Common musculotendinous junction trigger points in athletics. (Pain radiates distally depending on severity.) *A*, musculotendinous junction—soleus trigger point (running and jumping activities); *B*, Musculotendinous junction—forearm extensor trigger point (racket sports, weight training, golf); *C*, Musculotendinous junction—forearm flexor trigger point (racket sports, weight training, golf).

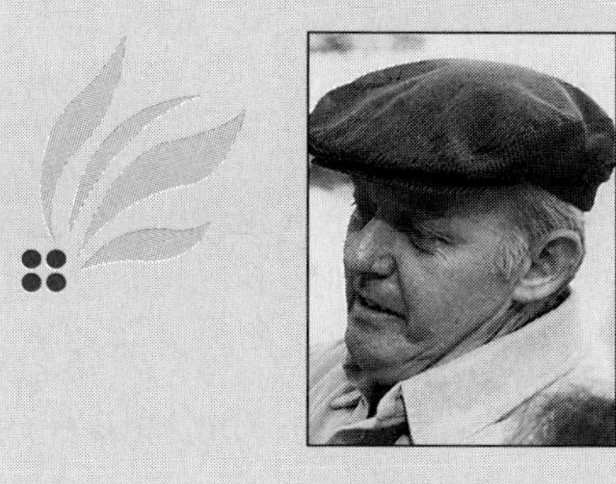

Jack Meagher

Born: July 6, 1923

"Massage is the study of anatomy in Braille."

He is the father of sports massage, a man of 74 with cancer at the time of this interview, yet he radiates the energy and demonstrates the quick wit rarely encountered in men half his age. Jack Meagher was the only child of a wonderful mother and a father who was a "genius with machines."

Before enlisting as an army medic for four years, Meagher took a course in Swedish massage, hoping eventually to get into physical therapy. It was while he was in Epernay, France, that he experienced a different type of massage than he had learned back home. This massage, performed by a German POW, made Meager move markedly better on the baseball field.

After his discharge, he was signed by the Boston Braves as a pitcher, but a wartime shoulder injury threw him a curve that landed him in physical therapy unable to continue a baseball career. That sent him looking for the same kind of massage he'd received in France. Finally, he found another German therapist, this time an instructor at the Viennese Massage School in Connecticut, who relieved his pain to the extent that Meagher was able to play semipro ball in his hometown of Gloucester, Massachusetts.

The success of his therapy did more than put Meagher's body into motion again, it got him to thinking. The result was sports massage, the massage that can enhance athletic performance. Just as Swedish massage uses specific strokes, sports massage strokes were classified by Meagher as direct pressure, friction, compression, and percussion. When called for, he also recommends effleurage and kneading.

"It took me 15 years of putting it together," says Meagher. "I was at a YMCA working on professional athletes and people for whom exercise was a way of life. The sports massage helped them do more before they faded. A loose body uses less energy."

Soon Meagher discovered that what made man go farther and faster could also help horses. That's when sports massage really took off. "In the '76 Olympics, the horses I'd worked on took two golds and a silver," remembers Meagher. "I was written up and asked to do a book. Then the American Massage Therapy Association became interested and I was invited to speak at one of their conferences," he adds.

The classic sports massage text is *Sports Massage, A Complete Program for Increasing Performance and Endurance in Fifteen Popular Sports.* Reading it does more than introduce you to a specific massage. It gives you glimpse into a man who is warm and dedicated, yet extremely results-oriented, a man with a sharp mind who understands the intricate biomechanics of the body, but is able to break it down into simple steps in order to make his life's work accessible to weekend warriors and professional athletes alike.

Meagher also has a wonderful sense of humor. Only he would write the book titled, *Never Goose an Appaloosa.* He is ticklish himself, so he doesn't receive Swedish massage. About the horses he massages, Meagher says: "I would not get on a horse, but I do get along with horses. I've never been kicked. Horses understand when you're trying to help them." He is still helping them, massaging 40 to 50 horses per week, an astounding number it seems, until he tells you what his workload was in his prime: "I used to do 55 people and 30 horses a week."

When asked what characteristics should be present in a successful massage therapist, he cites "the desire to help people, the ability to know how to use their hands, and he or she should possess the education that can help put it all together."

Jack Meagher, the father of sports massage, has four children and six grandchildren—"all successful in their own right," he says proudly. If he

continued on page 586

Continued

Jack Meagher

had it to do all over again? "I wouldn't do anything differently. It's taken years of hard work. One time a chief of orthopedics told me I had a real gift and I had to disagree. Gifts come easily. What I do is not a gift. I work hard. I developed my instincts through my failures and my successes. I've gone to the Olympics and I've made six trips abroad."

In his book, *Sports Massage,* he writes: "At your fingertips you have—once you learn to use it—the most powerful of all the therapeutic modalities."

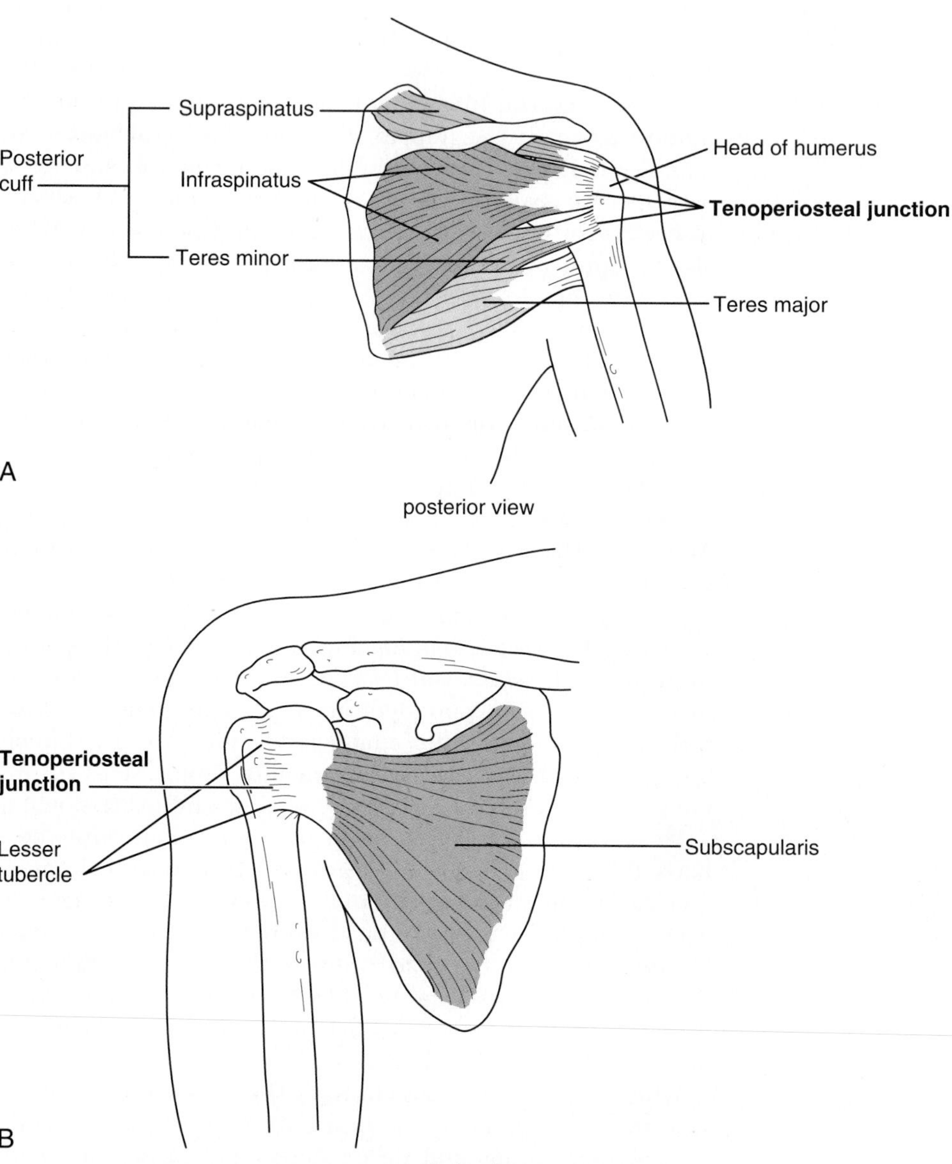

Figure 26•15 Common tendon injuries (lesions) at the tenoperiostial junction—rotator cuff. (Pain will refer to a variety of locations in the shoulder with rotator cuff lesions.) *A,* Posterior rotator cuff (throwing, tennis serve, weight training); *B,* Subscapularis (throwing, weight training, swimming).

Without proper treatment and rest, tendinitis can be a source of chronic pain that can last for years. Properly applied transverse friction massage can be an effective technique for healing tendon injuries. The corresponding muscle bellies of the injured tendon should be thoroughly massaged and stretched. Tension, spasms, adhesions, and trigger points with their resultant lack of flexibility in the musculature are often significant contributing factors in the onset of tendinitis. In addition, ice and a carefully planned program of strengthening is indicated. Duration of healing is dependent upon the amount of damage, consistency of treatment, and client compliance.

Tendon injuries commonly occur in two different portions of the muscle/tendon complex. The **tenoperiostial junction** is the place where the tendon joins the periosteum of the bone. This is the most common injury site for the rotator cuff of the shoulder (Fig. 26–15) and for the flexor and extensor tendons of the elbow (Fig. 26–16). Sometimes fibers are torn in the body of the tendon itself. This can happen in the common proximal tendon of the hamstrings, the patellar tendon, and in the Achilles and peroneal tendons of the ankle (Fig. 26–17).

Ligaments

Ligaments are strong, fibrous, somewhat elastic tissues that are usually cordlike in nature. Their attachments to various skeletal components help to maintain the bones in correct relationship to one another, stabilizing the joints. When torn, usually because of a collision or violent motion, ligaments heal slowly due to a poor blood supply.

Common ligament sprains that you will encounter include the anterior talofibular and calcaneofibular ligaments in lateral ankle sprains, collaterals in knee injuries, and sacrotuberous ligament sprains between the sacrum and the ischial tuberosity (Fig. 26–18). With specific training, a therapist may use transverse friction on ligament scarring to increase blood flow, promote healthy repatterning, and prevent external adhesions from forming.

Fascia

Fascia consists of fibrous connective tissue that envelops certain muscles and that forms partitions for others. When these cellophane-like sheets become adhered to neighboring muscle tissue, efficiency and function can be significantly diminished. There are two locations where fascia functions as a strong, supportive fibrous band: the iliotibial band that supports the knee, and the plantar fascia that supports the arch of the foot. Iliotibial band friction syndrome (lateral knee pain) and plantar fasciitis (heel or arch pain) are common problems brought on by overuse and/or biomechanical imbalances. You will often find both of

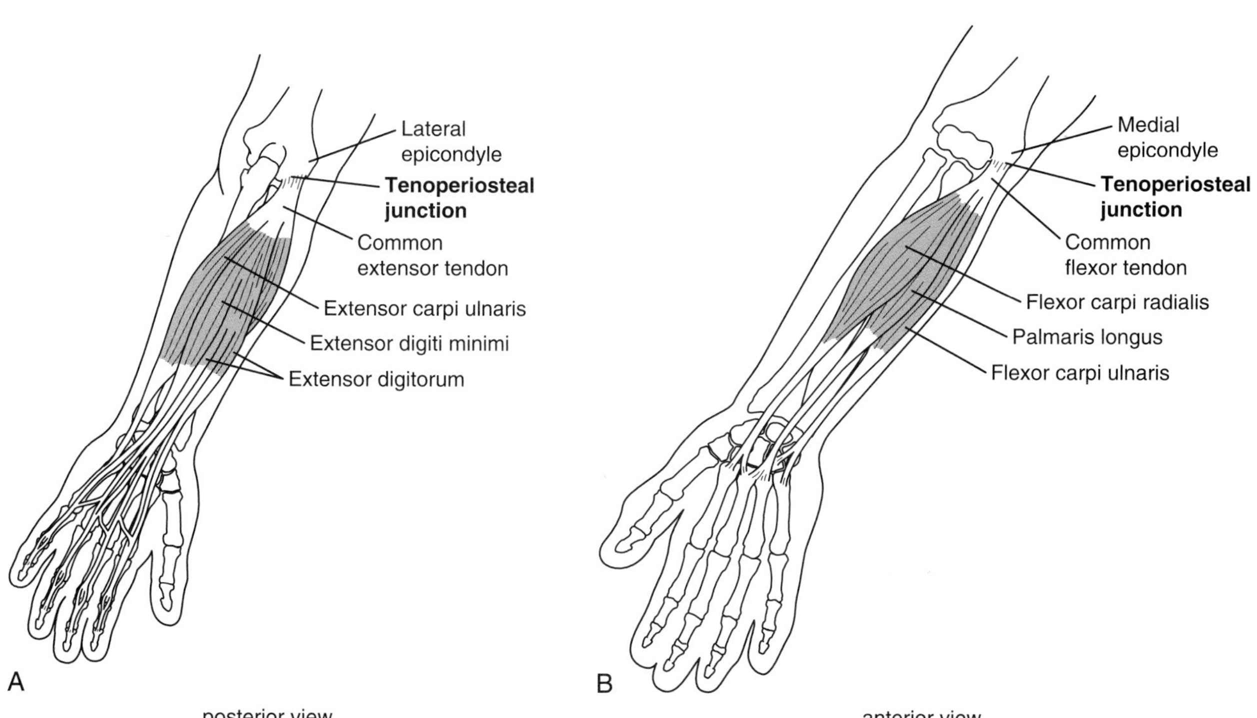

Figure 26•16 Common tendon injuries (lesions) at the tenoperiostial junction—epicondylitis (racket sports, weight training, golf). *A*, Common extensor tendon at the lateral epicondyle; *B*, Common flexor tendon at the medial epicondyle.

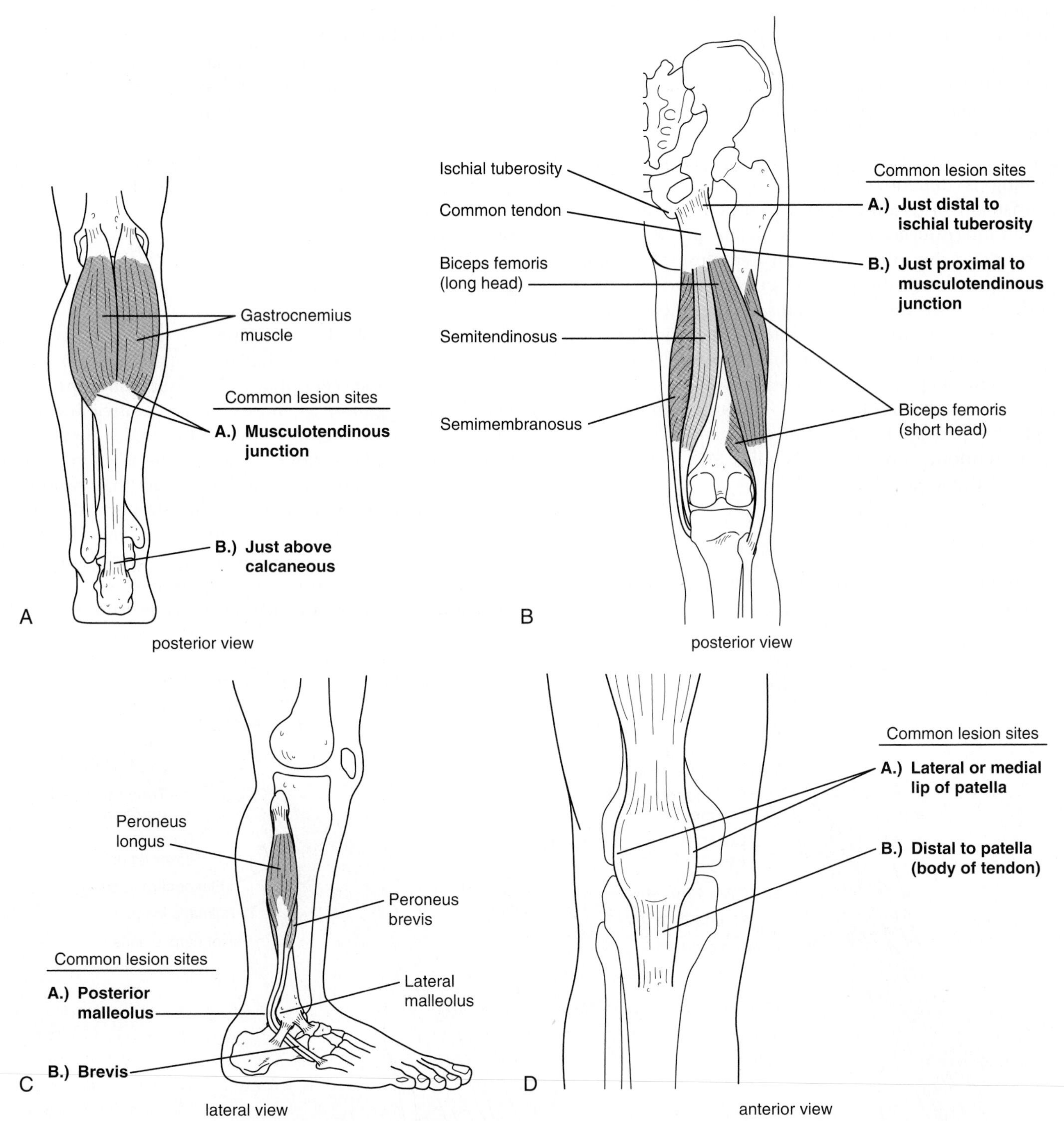

Figure 26•17 Common tendon injuries (lesions) in the body of the tendon. *A,* Achilles tendinitis (runners, basketball, volleyball); *B,* Hamstring tendinitis (sprinting); *C,* Peroneal tendinitis (often results from lateral ankle sprains); *D,* Patellar tendinitis (basketball, volleyball, running).

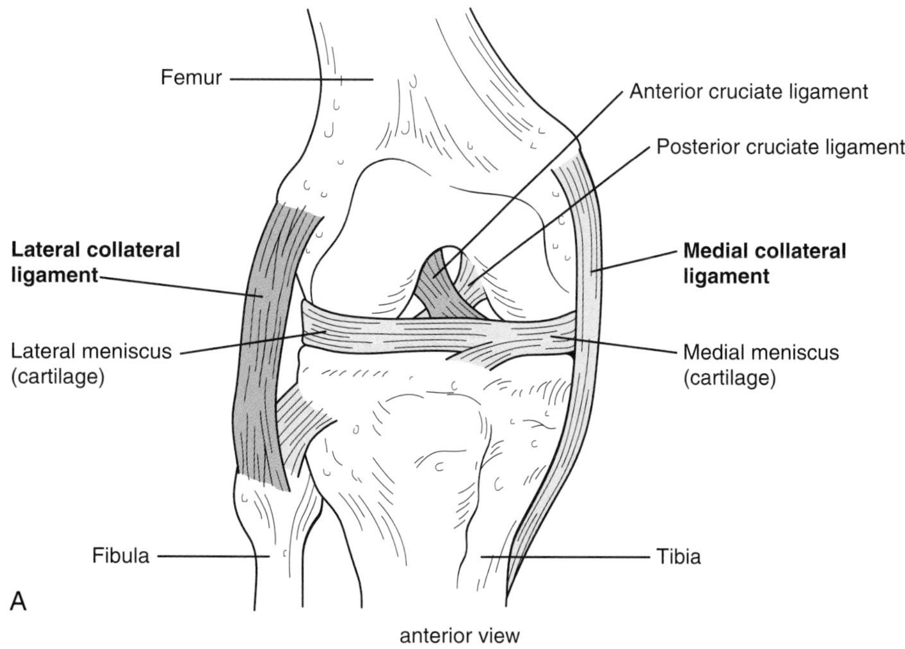

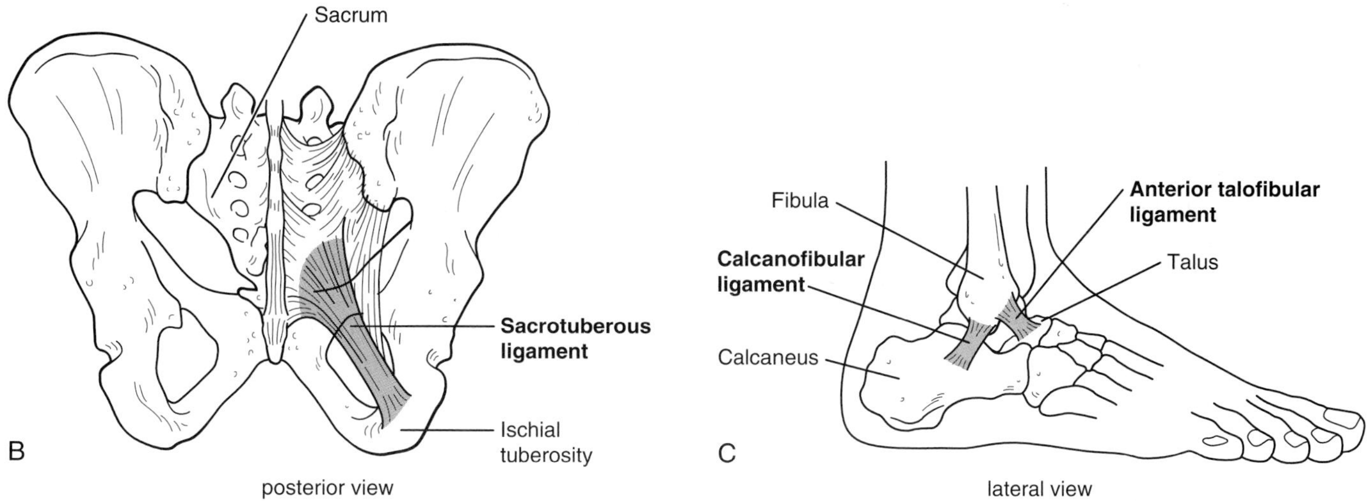

Figure 26•18 Commonly injured ligaments in athletics. (Can be treated with transverse friction massage.) *A,* Collateral ligament sprains—knee (football, skiing, soccer) (pain felt at the site of the lesion, medial = swelling, lateral generally does not); *B,* Sacrotuberous ligament sprain (sprinting, dancing, distance running) (pain can be felt locally or occasionally radiates down posterior thigh); *C,* Lateral ankle sprains (football, basketball, volleyball) (pain felt at the site of the lesion—localized puffiness and swelling common).

these structures enduring repetitive strain that produces inflammation, which results in adhesion to adjacent muscle tissue (Fig. 26–19).

MAINTENANCE MASSAGE

Time: *Approximately* 48 hours before or after activity/competition.

Setting: In a clinic or training facility where there are *no distractions.* Create a safe environment where athletes can completely relax. **Maintenance massage** sessions are a blend of general soreness reduction massage and more specific therapeutic work. The frequency and content of maintenance sessions are determined by an athlete's training schedule because *the closer to a period of physical exertion, the less intrusive the massage should be.*

The Intent of Maintenance Massage Is:

- To bring about full recovery and promote healthy tissue consistency by addressing common tension patterns, chronic areas of spasm, soreness, or pain.

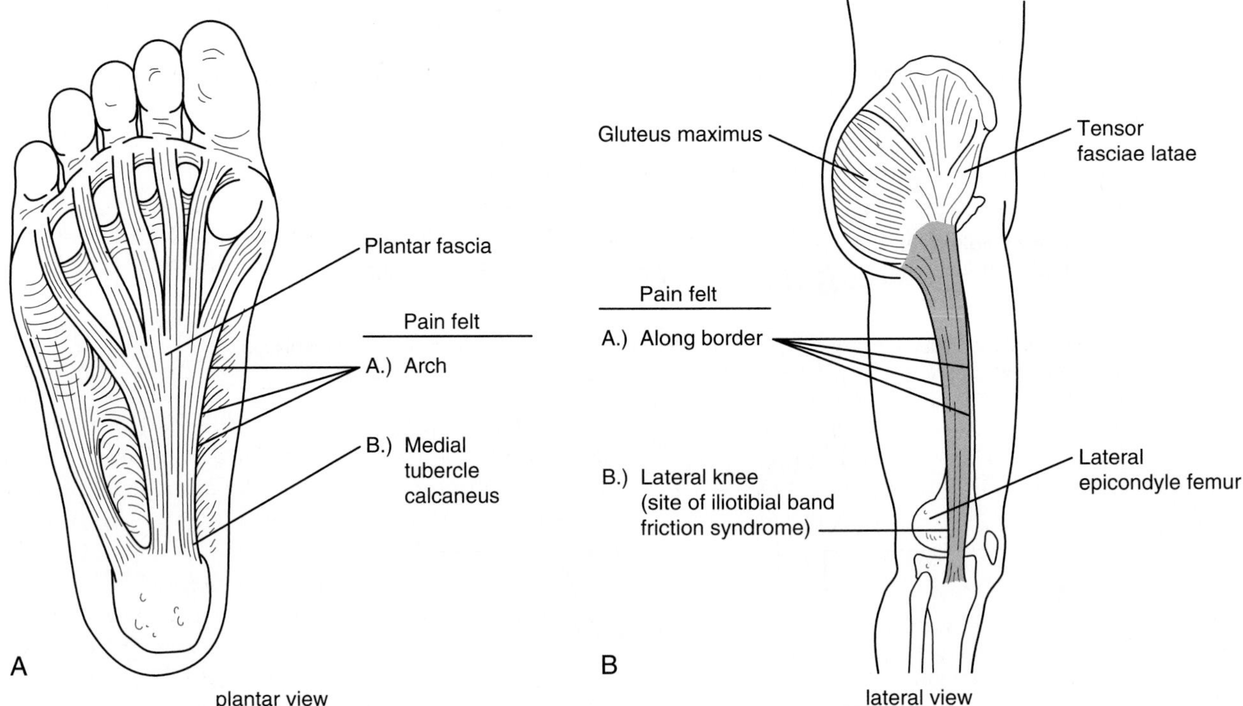

Figure 26•19 Commonly injured fascial bands (overuse injuries). *A*, Plantar fascitis (running and jumping sports); *B*, Iliotibial band (cycling, running, martial arts, fencing).

- To increase the athlete's awareness of use patterns and potential problem areas.
- To implement self-care programs that facilitate independence and support sports massage goals.
- To prevent injuries before they occur by eliminating spasms, separating adhered contractile structures, and treating trigger points.
- To create effective injury rehabilitation and prevention programs.
- To address structural problems.
- To enhance performance.

In the maintenance format, soreness reduction techniques can be effectively combined with a number of other approaches. Maintenance is the forum in which you can creatively combine all of the skills and techniques you have studied, practiced, and mastered. Each client has a unique blend of sport specific needs, massage experiences, and personal preferences. Swedish, shiatsu, sports techniques, energy work, trigger point approaches, deep-tissue applications, and structural therapies are all appropriate and can be successfully integrated. Deep-tissue applications combined with trigger point therapy will define the maintenance technique focus for this chapter.

A variety of flexibility systems improve range of motion and are also available to be combined with the hands-on work. Proprioceptive neuromuscular facilitation (Voss), Active-assisted stretching (Mattes or Wharton), and Muscle Energy Technique (Chaitow) can integrate well with the aforementioned massage applications. Each of these range of motion systems can also provide a rich base of self-care tools.

It is important to know your limits and when to refer clients to a more appropriate healthcare professional. As you gain more experience, you will develop a growing sense of when to refer to an athletic trainer, acupuncturist, chiropractor, physical therapist, or perhaps a more qualified massage therapist. Sports massage therapist Benny Vaughn has an appropriate saying for those times when you are not sure what to do: "When in doubt, don't." A good healthcare practitioner knows that you can never have enough training; there is always more to learn.

Author's Note

You will be faced with many choices as you develop your own style of therapy. If you work with athletes, take a moment to reflect on the following question: Who takes responsibility for what happens in the context of the therapy? Consider the following example as an opportunity to define this issue.

"Can I continue to train through the pain?" This is a question that many athletes will ask you. It is generally not a good idea to tell an athlete who is in pain to stop running, swimming, throwing, weight training, or playing a sport she loves. In many cases, this will

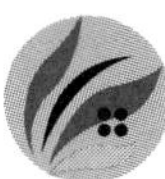

General Guide to Technique Selection

- Warm up the tissue with postevent recovery techniques or other appropriate strokes.
- Identify and work specific areas. Locate and treat muscle spasms, adhesions, trigger points, and any other tissue pathologies that prevent full recovery or hinder performance.
- Use your knowledge of sport-specific needs, your client's preferences, and your palpation skills to guide you.
- Track changes and use good communication skills.
- Invite deeper breathing to facilitate an increased depth of focus and deeper relaxation.
- Return to general recovery strokes to flush the area of metabolic waste and tissue debris.
- Revisit localized specific areas with increased anatomical precision and a deepening focus.
- Carefully track your client's tolerance for increased depth and specificity.
- Flush the area a final time with strokes that relax and invigorate.

be a virtual guarantee that she will find another therapist to continue to work with her.

Explain to the athlete that each time she trains with pain, more tissue is being damaged. Let her know that increased damage increases the length of time it takes to heal the injury and that experiencing pain during exercise may actually mean a tendinitis or muscle strain is getting worse.

From this point on in your therapy, training in pain can be presented as a choice that she makes on her own. Step back and let her decide, from day to day whether to choose to train in pain. Take this opportunity to teach her to be more aware of her own body. If your primary objective is to educate, facilitate, and motivate healthy change, then the nature of your work will encourage your client's independence, rather than her dependence on you.

Tissue Pathologies and Treatment Options

Treating Adhesions. One of the most common locations for adhesions to form is where the iliotibial band (ITB) overlies the vastus lateralis muscle on the lateral thigh. Cyclists and runners are especially prone to adhesions here. Place your client on his side and warm up the area using recovery massage techniques (Fig. 26–20). Address any local spasms, paying close attention to areas that are particularly sensitive immediately anterior or posterior to the band. Identify a 1 to 3 inch section that is the most tender. Remove 80 to 90 percent of the lubricant and anchor three or four supported fingers immediately above or below the adhesion.

With your elbow straight and your arm extended from your shoulder, slowly lean your body weight into your fingertip pressure. The speed at which you increase pressure can be critical to having the client "allow you in" to the space between the vastus and the ITB. The slower you go, the deeper you will be able to go without having the client respond with reflexive guarding and splinting. Then *very slowly* sink and glide through the fibrotic formation that adheres the ITB to the vastus lateralis muscle. Be attentive to areas that feel especially crystallized or resistant to pressure.

Developing "Kinesthetic Acuity" with Your Fingertips. Adhesions are built over time, individually and precisely constructed by repeated use patterns that ripple through overused, ischemic, inflamed tissues. These fibrotic formations will progressively prohibit normal contractile separation. Once the foundation of an adhesion has been palpated and assessed by your fingertips, subsequent techniques can unfold *from within the tissues you are working,* rather than from a list on a page.

Standard treatment options might include a simple, singular form of sustained digital pressure that evolves into transverse or circular friction. Pay close attention to what you feel as you move against the grain of the fibers in different directions. You might find that digital friction or a slow deep glide with a thumb or a supported fingertip contributes to a feeling of in-

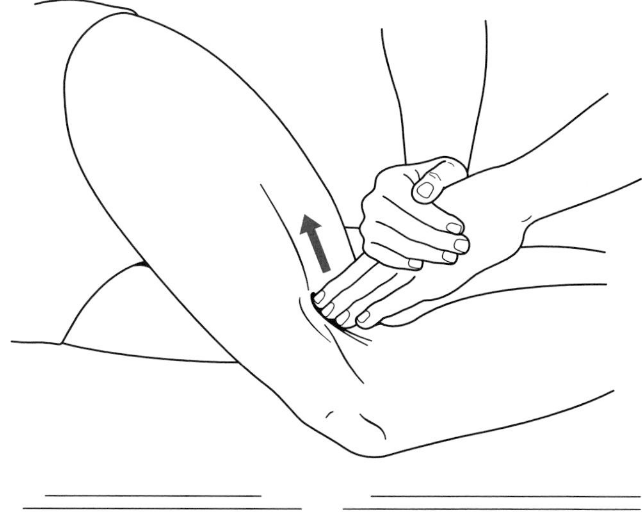

Figure 26•20 Supported fingertip glide—differentiating adhered structures (ITB/vastus lateralis).

creased freedom in the surrounding tissue. Enter and reenter these areas sensing their "architectural nature" in ways that offer clues to undoing them. You may create techniques you have never seen or used before!

It is essential that you slow down, your work occasionally arriving at stillness, sensing the energy in your hands (both need to be in contact) and in the person on the table. What you sense when you slow down like this can help to dictate a comfortable, healing pace for the session. Tearing down old adhesions has the potential to be very uncomfortable. Slowing down can help to generate the kind of trust that allows clients to let go into the work, instead of guarding and splinting *against* your pressure.

Remember to give your client (and your hands) a break from this deep, potentially challenging work by occasionally returning to recovery strokes to flush the area of metabolic waste. Generally you will find that each time you revisit the localized adhered area, your levels of specificity and precision will increase. Your goal is to decrease spasms and to increase differentiation between adhered structures.

Locating and Treating Trigger Points

During postevent and recovery work, you may encounter hypersensitive tender, ropy, and knotted areas. If a particular site refers pain when specific pressure is applied, you have located a trigger point. Quite often a generalized area may feel much cooler to the touch due to vasoconstriction. When a client's condition becomes entrenched, overlying skin might also feel dry, tight, thickened, or waxy.

When you apply pressure that re-creates the pain that an athlete has been experiencing during or after training, you know you are on the right spot. Referrals from gluteus medius into the low back or from points in the tibialis anterior to the ankle are very common in athletics. It is not at all unusual to find trigger points that an athlete had no previous awareness of; focus on these points to ensure injury prevention.

Another effective method for locating trigger points is to familiarize yourself with the common referral pat-

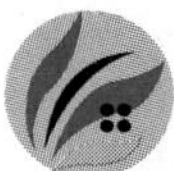

When Treating Trigger Points . . .

- Avoid treating during the acute stages of an injury (first 24 to 48 hours).
- Remember that trigger points refer sensation distally. The farther the sensation refers the more "active" the trigger point is and the more it needs work. Trigger points that refer *during* exercise are generally more active than those that refer only *after* exercise.
- Warm up the tissue first before treating trigger points. Areas where trigger points are located are often ischemic and need manual assistance to increase blood flow and tissue temperature. Encourage client feedback as you are working.
- Always work *with* the client. Look for a pressure that allows the client to let go. Be attentive to the client guarding or tensing in response to the work. Encourage deeper breathing, and, when it is appropriate, offer visualizations that suggest softening, a sense of ease, melting or releasing.
- Once an area has been treated, return to relaxing techniques for at least three to five minutes before re-treating. One to three treatments per area per session is recommended.
- Be aware that residual soreness in the area that has been treated is not unusual. Inform your clients that they may be sore for up to 48 hours after trigger-point work. Ice and stretching are recommended to diminish this time. If the client is sore for more than 48 hours, the work may have been too deep or the area may have been worked too long. Be especially careful in soft tissue that is adjacent to major organs (e.g., quadratus lumborum [kidneys] or iliopsoas [colon]).
- Remember, if weekly sessions do not begin to help the chronic pain dissipate, a treatment sequence that is spaced in 3 to 5 day intervals is necessary.
- Keep in mind that athletes will often exhibit trigger points in areas of biomechanical stress that are directly related to their sport. For athletes in heavy training (twice per day 6 to 7 days per week), completely eliminating trigger points is not always possible. In these cases, we can usually serve athletes best by helping them to monitor these areas, making sure that trigger points do not *increase* in severity.

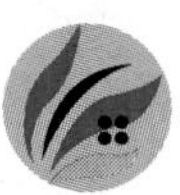

Typical Locations for Adhesions in Athletes

- trapezius/supraspinatus
- erector spinae/thoracolumbar fascia
- trapezius/levator scapula
- gluteus maximus, medius, and minimus
- pectoralis major/minor
- rectus femoris to underlying quadriceps
- latissimus/teres major and minor
- semimembranosus/adductor magnus
- extensors and/or flexors of the forearm
- soleus/peroneus longus

terns that can be found in a variety of charts and books. Janet Travell's two volumes (upper and lower body) of *Myofascial Pain and Dysfunction, The Trigger Point Manual* are an excellent addition to your personal library. When an athlete complains of pain in a particular area, study the charts and look for points in the body part that might be responsible for the pain referral. Receiving additional training in this approach from experienced practitioners is a very good idea.

Locating and Treating Lesions: Using Transverse Friction

Identifying and treating lesions can be a valuable addition to your sports massage skills. When a muscle, tendon, or ligament is torn, lesions of varying sizes (grades 1 through 3) and dimensions occur in the tissue. The body's need to regain tissue integrity stimulates the repair response. During the regeneration and remodeling phases, fibroblasts are busy producing and laying down collagen for wound repair, forming a randomly knit, fragile scar. This new, vulnerable scar tissue is easily strained with movements that prematurely stress the injured tissues. With repeated strain and repair, the site of a lesion often develops into a weak, poorly woven scar. Without proper treatment, this site can become the source of chronic pain that can last for years.

Transverse friction is a precise form of medical massage developed by Dr. James Cyriax. It can be a useful tool for helping muscle, tendon, and ligament lesions heal quickly and more completely. It stimulates blood flow to the injured area, decreases newly formed adhesions at the injury site, thereby increasing tissue mobility, and, assists in the repatterning of scar tissue itself. All of this adds up to decreased chances for reinjury. Identifying the exact site of a lesion is critical for the proper treatment of this specific tissue damage. Many lesions, especially in their initial stages, are no more than ⅛ inch square!

In some cases, transverse friction that is *sustained* for more than 60 seconds on a site other than a lesion can *create* scar tissue that was not there originally. Ligaments or tendons in the areas immediately surrounding the joints of the shoulder, knee, ankle, or the cervical and lumbar spine are especially vulnerable.

Sustained transverse friction is not recommended unless you are certain you are on the site of the lesion. Look for sports massage workshops that teach injury evaluation and treatment skills. Without proper training, transverse friction can be a brutal technique that leaves athletes more wounded than they were before treatment. A well organized program of highly refined palpation and orthopedic skills that is taught by staff with years of teaching and practical experience is best and highly recommended.

Understanding and Treating Tissue Pathologies: Getting Results

If you want to develop the skills to achieve consistent results when a client is in need of relief from chronic pain, locate and treat *the source* of the pain. For example, for discomfort in a client's calf muscle, ask questions regarding the type of exercise, duration, and frequency of training. Are adhesions between the soleus and peroneus longus responsible for that nagging calf pain? Where does the client point when you ask her to show you the location of the discomfort? Are there trigger points in the calf tissue? Can you find tender points that refer pain distally in a pattern that is familiar to your athlete? Use your injury recognition chart if you need help with assessment.

Take a thorough step by step history of your client's experience of pain. Prolonged spasm, inflammation, and pain will often give rise to adhesions. These limitations may produce additional stress that finds trigger points forming. Established trigger points can restrict movement and flexibility of internal tissues, creating a condition that could eventually develop into a grade 1 or 2 lesion. When soft-tissue conditions unfold in a progression similar to those previously described, your athlete has developed a gradual onset injury.

In rapid onset injuries, explosive movements suddenly tear tissue and form lesions. Hamstring strains often occur in this way in track and field, baseball, or basketball. Spasms, trigger points, or adhesions may form as a secondary response to the initial tearing and usually compound or prolong the life of a lesion.

Remember that homeostasis is at work regardless of the nature or the amount of damage. Support the momentum of the repair response with your massage choices and self-care recommendations. Use the sports massage and timing guidelines to schedule sessions appropriately. Review your anatomy so that you are absolutely clear about what you are palpating. Look over the training information, and make sure your client is not overtraining or making other training-related mistakes. Keep the big picture in mind. Use the following list of factors that predispose athletes to injury as a checklist for considering other contributing components to your client's pain profile. Seek out advanced classes in injury evaluation and treatment skills if you want to be proficient at alleviating chronic pain. If you are seeing someone who is in pain and you are unsure about how to help her, refer her to a therapist who has the necessary knowledge and experience.

Factors That Predispose Athletes to Injury

If the techniques that have been outlined in this chapter do not bring your clients *complete* relief, it is important to consider other factors that may contribute to an athlete's condition. Ask questions to identify other missing links and teach your client to initiate the necessary changes.

- ***Lack of Warm-up.*** Some athletes stress their bodies prematurely and simply need to spend extra time heating up and sufficiently vascularizing key sport-specific structures before they begin working hard.
- ***Poor Flexibility.*** Putting more energy into a stretching routine will sometimes be the key that unlocks the door to chronic, puzzling, and painful symptoms. Some athletes unknowingly perform stretches that actually aggravate a chronic condition. Review stretching routines with your clients, and recommend any needed changes in technique.
- ***Muscle Imbalance.*** Shin splints are a classic example. A runner's calf muscles can be inordinately strong compared with a weak, tired, sore, and achy tibialis anterior that repeatedly struggles to produce adequate dorsiflexion against overpowering plantar flexors.
- ***Lack of Strength.*** Forceful repetitive motions require strength. Because of the eccentric stress on a sprinter's hamstrings, a pitcher's posterior shoulder, or the forearm extensor muscles of a tennis player, you must focus on strength to maintain healthy tonus.
- ***Improper Training.*** Failure to develop an adequate base, planning too many hard workouts per week, or not getting enough rest can lead to increased levels of soreness, pain, and decreased performance.
- ***Improper Equipment.*** Worn-out shoes, a bicycle seat that is too high or low, or weight-training equipment that is an incorrect size for your client's body are just a few of the many equipment issues that can contribute to unexplained soreness and pain.
- ***Other Factors to Consider.*** Poor nutrition, lack of hydration, emotional stress, structural abnormalities (e.g., leg length discrepancies or scoliosis), and unsafe conditions such as extreme temperatures.

SUMMARY

Though knowledge hones the knife of your skills, experience dresses the edge and is the finishing touch. Start offering postevent massages at athletic events in your community. Volunteer to provide recovery massages for a local team. Your tracking and palpation skills, hands-on knowledge of anatomy, and your ability to recognize problems in the tissues will improve with each athlete you massage.

Everything in our bodies occurs in a water medium. The free flow of fluids carries oxygen in and metabolic wastes out of the tissue. This process depends on healthy tonus in the musculature. Uninterrupted muscle spasms inhibit the flow of blood and lymph in the tissue spaces, contributing to an ongoing cycle of increased waste, pain, and ischemia. Athletes who train regularly have varying levels of muscle spasm and ischemic areas that respond favorably to sports massage.

Muscles that work eccentrically (lengthen as they contract) are the decelerators that are sore 24 to 48 hours after exercise. This is known as delayed muscle soreness. These tissues are the most commonly injured in sports where repetitive eccentric contractions occur. Massage and stretching will help to promote healthy tonus, and a specific focus on strengthening these tissues will also help to improve performance and prevent injury.

To improve performance, an athlete will often use the overload principle in his training process. This well-recognized training approach involves stressing the body to stimulate desired changes in strength, speed, efficiency, or endurance and then resting so that recovery and adaptation can occur. Too much stress and inadequate time for rest and recovery can result in an overuse injury. There is a fine line between optimal overload and overtraining.

When athletes stress their bodies to improve physical abilities, varying amounts of tissue damage are inevitable. Minor damage that produces soreness is known as microtrauma. Lesions are strains (muscle/tendon) or sprains (ligaments) that involve more significant disruption. A contusion is tissue that is crushed due to a blow or a fall. Whenever tissue damage occurs, internal cellular mechanisms (the repair response) immediately react in an effort to regain integrity. Duration of healing depends upon the extent of the injury, the frequency of treatment, and client compliance.

Frequency, length of sports massage sessions, and technique selection depend upon an athlete's training cycle. Your primary guidelines are to be attentive to varying levels of inflammation and stay within what is neurologically familiar for your athlete client. You will want to consider the amount of massage experience the athlete has had, familiarity between the athlete and the therapist, and levels of competitiveness. Ongoing palpation and verbal assessment refine this process.

Postevent massage is provided soon after an event or training session. Nonspecific techniques are used to relax spasms and reduce soreness. Two kinds of muscle soreness are common to athletes: immediate and delayed. Delayed soreness may not appear until 48 hours after activity. A well-educated athlete knows how to use massage, stretching, rest and hydrotherapy as effective recovery tools to reduce muscle soreness.

Pre- and postrecovery massages can further reduce localized spasms and flush exercise-related metabolic wastes out of the tissues. Techniques are more general than specific. Maintenance massage is a combination of general soreness reduction techniques and specific work that addresses sports-specific patterns.

Providing skilled maintenance massage sessions requires knowledge of anatomy and physiology as they apply to athletics. The effective sports massage therapist understands common problems that can occur in muscles, tendons, ligaments, and fascial structures as they are stressed from sport to sport. Being able to recognize, palpate, and treat spasms, adhesions, and trigger points are essential ingredients for providing effective maintenance massage. Basic knowledge of strength and endurance training principles can help you meet the needs of an athletic clientele.

Teaching your clients to pay attention to the changes in their training choices and the effects these choices have on their bodies is the beginning of a healthy therapeutic relationship. You can empower your clients by helping them become more aware of their own bodies. A therapist who chooses to educate, facilitate, and motivate can encourage a relationship that is based on independence rather than on dependence.

Educate your client athletes about scheduling work-outs and the best timing for massage. Encourage them to make their own scheduling decisions. As you regularly massage and palpate your clients, teach them the difference between spasms, trigger points, and adhesions and help them understand the origins of these problems in their training process, from the list of factors that predispose athletes to injury or from other lifestyle choices. Teach your clients about approximate time frames for tissue healing, encouraging patience and positive self-regard during the healing of soft-tissue injury. Use the list of recovery tools as a base for self-care information. Movement, stretching, and hydrotherapy can be useful at this time. Inspire hope, offer reassurance, and be positive about even the smallest amounts of self-care progress. Be careful to avoid the role of someone who stands over your client shaking the dreaded "should" finger.

Offer this approach in a caring way. People can tell when you truly care. Your intentions are clear and their trust in you will grow. Be spontaneous with your sense of humor, have fun with people, and express a genuine excitement for the work and all of its incredible possibilities.

SELF-TEST

Multiple Choice • Write the letter of the best answer in the space provided.

_______ 1. Cross-training refers to

A. training activities that stress muscles across the grain of the fibers
B. alternating your sport of choice with other activities that are fun and add variety
C. alternating your rest day
D. running in crossing patterns that are designed to increase speed

_______ 2. Maintenance massage is

A. quick, brisk work
B. light, general massage
C. a blend of soreness reduction and more specific therapeutic work
D. trigger point massage

_______ 3. The most frequent complaint that athletes bring to a massage therapist is

A. lesions
B. adhesions
C. muscle soreness
D. muscle imbalances

_______ 4. Which of the following is *not* a warning sign of overtraining?

A. insomnia
B. elevated pulse in the morning
C. increased flexibility
D. lowered resistance

_______ 5. Sports massage sessions should be tailored to meet the specific needs of the

A. athlete
B. therapist
C. coach
D. athletic trainer

_______ 6. The tracking response is

A. the ability to find tender areas and thoroughly work them
B. finding bands of tension that inhibit performance
C. combined observation of a client's reaction to technique with a therapist's willingness to adjust the work accordingly
D. what happens when an athlete overtrains

_______ 7. Which statement is false?

A. spasms and trigger points can create an environment in which lesions are more likely to occur
B. the closer to a period of physical exertion, the less intrusive the massage should be
C. compression is designed to create ischemia
D. the repair response in the soft tissues of the body is an example of homeostasis

_______ 8. Adhesions commonly form between

A. two ligaments
B. nerves and blood vessels
C. two bones
D. muscle and fascia

_______ 9. Given appropriate therapy and client compliance, grades 1 and 2 lesions usually heal in about

A. 4 to 8 weeks
B. 24 to 72 hours
C. 6 months
D. not until all trigger points and spasms are diminished

_______ 10. An overuse injury

A. always involves trigger points
B. can be the result of working previously stressed muscle groups that have not fully recovered from the last workout
C. is best treated with heel of hand friction
D. is an example of neurological familiarity

_______ 11. Which of the following is *not* appropriate for postevent massage?

A. broadening
B. compression
C. trigger point work
D. jostling

_______ 12. The most commonly strained muscle group in athletics is the

A. quadriceps
B. rotator cuff
C. calf muscles
D. hamstrings

_______ 13. Shunt muscles

A. are decelerators
B. are contusions
C. always exhibit delayed muscle soreness
D. are found only in the upper extremity

_______ 14. The repair response involves all but one of the following

A. rapid onset
B. inflammation
C. remodeling
D. regeneration

_______ 15. The tendons that are most commonly injured at the tenoperiostial junction are

A. rotator cuff tendons of the shoulder and extensor tendons of the elbow
B. Achilles and patellar tendons
C. tendons of the wrist
D. gluteus minimus and medius

_______ 16. The intent of maintenance massage is to

A. enhance performance
B. seek out and prevent injuries before they occur
C. implement self-care programs that facilitate independence
D. all of the above

_______ 17. The speed at which tissue repair occurs depends upon

A. the client's compliance regarding self-care
B. the extent of the injury
C. the frequency and nature of the treatment
D. all of the above

_______ 18. Which of the following is *not* a factor to consider when determining scheduling and technique selection for sports massage?

A. the amount of massage experience the athlete has had
B. familiarity between the athlete and the therapist
C. what the athlete ate for her last meal
D. individual responsiveness to various approaches and techniques

_______ 19. Which of the following is an important factor to consider when you examine an athlete's training program?

A. the intensity of his workout
B. frequency and duration of exercise
C. identifying your athlete's goals
D. all of the above

_______ 20. Which of the following is *not* a cause of delayed muscle soreness?

A. pain-spasm-pain
B. connective tissue damage
C. adhesions
D. damaged muscle tissue

_______ 21. A major focus for performance enhancement and injury prevention is

A. always use heel of hand friction
B. take lots of naps
C. relax localized spasms, separate adhered structures, locate and treat any offending trigger points
D. eat lots of costly supplements

_______ 22. One of the most common chronological scenarios that athletes regularly report is

A. a tendon will hurt when they first start their activity, but the pain subsides once the tissue is warmed up
B. they sleep better if they do not exercise
C. when they eat bananas, delayed soreness is reduced
D. they notice decreased flexibility when not properly hydrated

References

Abraham, William M. "Exercise-Induced Muscle Soreness." *The Physician and Sports Medicine* 7. Oct. 1979: 57–60.

Benjamin, Ben. *Listen to Your Pain.* New York: Penguin, 1984.

Chaitow, Leon. *Muscle Energy Techniques.* New York: Churchill Livingstone, 1996.

Greene, Elliot. "Tissue Healing and Massage Therapy." *Massage Therapy Journal* 26. Fall 1987: 22–24, 48–51.

Kresge, Carol A. "Benefits of Sports Massage." *Sports Medicine: Fitness, Training, Injuries.* Otto Appenzeller (Ed.). Baltimore: Urban and Schwarzenberg, 1988. pp. 419–30.

Mattes, Aaron L. *Active Isolated Stretching.* Sarasota, FL: Mattes, 1995.

Mattes, Aaron L. *Flexibility—Active and Assisted Stretching.* Sarasota, FL: Mattes, 1995.

Noakes, Tim. *Lore of Running.* New York: Leisure Press, 1991.

Sleamaker, Robert. *Serious Training for Serious Athletes.* Champaign, IL: Leisure Press, 1989.

Stanton, Peter, and Craig Purdam. "Hamstring Injuries in Sprinting—The Role of Eccentric Exercise." *The Journal of Orthopaedic and Sports Physical Therapy* 10. March 1989: 343–48.

Sudy, Mitchell, ed. *Personal Trainer Manual: The Resource for Fitness Instructors.* Boston: Reebok University Press, 1991.

Travell, Janet G., and David G. Simons. *Myofascial Pain and Dysfunction.* Baltimore: Williams & Wilkins, 1983.

Voss, Margaret. *Proprioceptive Neuromuscular Facilitation, Patterns and Techniques,* 2nd ed. New York: Harper, 1968.

Weineck, Jurgen. *Functional Anatomy in Sports.* Chicago: Year Book Medical Publishers, 1986.

Wharton, Jim, and Phil Wharton. *The Whartons' Stretch Book.* New York: Times Books–Random House, 1996.

Wilmore, Jack H, and David L. Costill. "Cardiovascular Regulation." *Training for Sport and Activity: The Physiological Basis of the Conditioning Process,* 3rd ed. Dubuque: William C. Brown Pub., 1988. pp. 61–81.

A baby is born with a need to be loved—and never outgrows it.
—Frank A. Clark

Maria Mathias

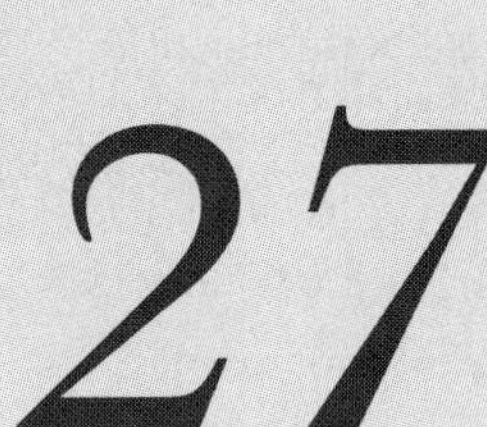

27

Infant Massage

Student Objectives

After completing this chapter, the student should be able to:

- Define infant massage
- List the benefits of infant massage for mothers or caregivers and babies
- Discuss the importance of bonding for infants and caregivers
- Name the elements that contribute to parent-infant bonding
- List the benefits of infant massage for parents and caregivers
- Describe the environmental and biomechanical considerations of infant massage
- State the groups, organizations, or agencies that could be approached to lecture or teach infant massage
- Describe ways to handle crying babies in class-room settings

INTRODUCTION

Infant massage is a parenting tradition of loving touch that parents of many cultures have been using for centuries. First introduced as a parenting tool in the United States in the mid-1970s, infant massage has since gained an increasingly large and active following; both parents' and professionals' hearts have been drawn to the powerful experience of the deep bonding of parents and babies (Fig. 27–1).

The most significant early step in infant massage popularity in the United States came in 1979 with the publishing of Vimala Schneider McClure's groundbreaking book *Infant Massage—A Handbook for Loving Parents.* Since then, many well-trained infant massage instructors have participated in teaching this gentle craft. Scientific research has helped verify the benefits, and today many professional groups, both medical and nonmedical, are embracing infant massage. It is written about in journals and magazines and is often mentioned on television. With certified instructors in more than 32 countries, infant massage is commonly recognized by parents and professionals as a viable parenting modality and as a useful intervention for infants with special needs.

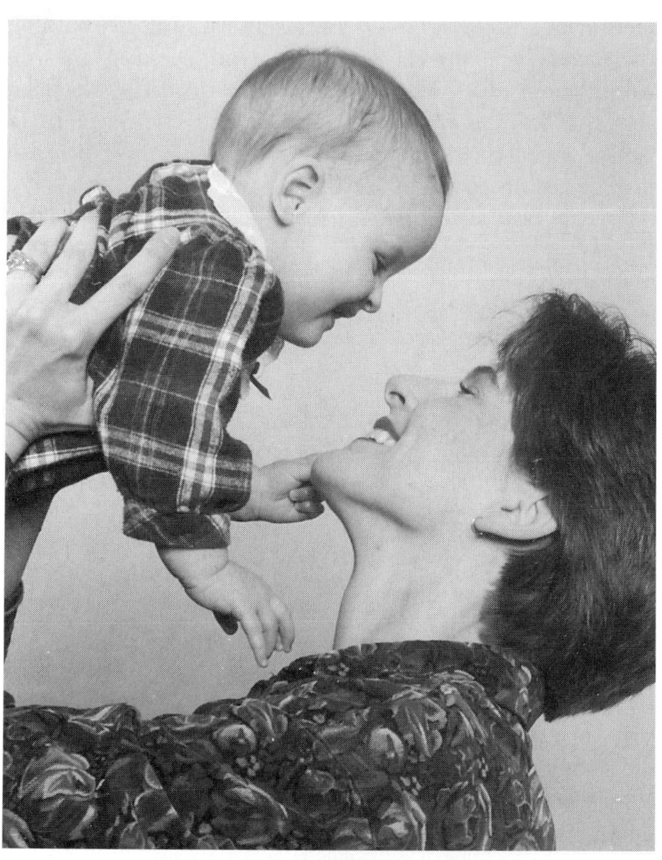

Figure 27•1 Mother and child.

MASSAGE BENEFITS FOR BABIES AND CHILDREN

According to Ross Campbell, author of *How to Really Love Your Child,* many children think they are loved, but most *do not feel loved.* Infant massage is a very powerful demonstration of unconditional love and support that is deeply experienced on many levels of the baby's being and is held as a tactile memory in the baby's body. If the deep message of the massage experience for the baby is "I am cherished . . . I'm okay . . . I'm enough . . . I am loved," then continuity of the massage verifies and reinforces these beliefs. Other benefits of infant massage for the baby may include the following:

- It helps to foster parent-infant bonding due to the intimate interaction time between parent and baby.
- It relieves discomfort from teething, congestion, gas, and colic.
- Infant massage promotes digestion by activating the relaxation response.
- It stimulates the nervous system through the stimulation of the skin, while speeding myelination of the nerves and enhancing neurological development.
- It increases blood flow, ensuring that oxygen and nutrients reach the infant's cells and tissues.
- Infant massage slows and deepens respiration rate.
- It improves muscle tone through activation of sensory and motor neurons.
- It encourages midline orientation and sensory awareness due to tactile stimulation.
- It increases vocalization, thus assisting in speech and language development.
- Infant massage promotes deeper and longer sleep for the baby.
- It provides a special time for communicating with parents.

THE IMPORTANCE OF BONDING

Bonding is a reciprocal relationship that goes from the caregiver to the infant and from the infant to the caregiver. According to Drs. Marshall Klaus and John Kennell, bonding is a "solid connection between the parent and child that nourishes the infant on a core level; the process that attaches the infant to reality." Bonding occurs when certain elements are in place soon after the baby's birth. These elements include skin-to-skin contact, odor or scent, high-pitched voice, prolonged eye contact, warmth, and the reestablishment of biorhythmic activity that existed between the mother and baby in utero. Infant massage is especially unique in providing a vehicle for all of the necessary elements for parent-infant bonding, a process that builds trust and intimacy, calls forth the innate protective and nurturing instincts in parents, and sets the tone for long-term quality of the parent-child relationship.

BENEFITS FOR PARENTS AND CAREGIVERS

Parents can also benefit from massaging their infants. Bonding is a reciprocal process; parents bond to their babies while babies bond to their parents. A brief list of parental benefits follows.

- Infant massage assists parents in acquiring self-confidence and self-esteem in their parenting roles.
- It enhances and reinforces parental skills and validates the parental role.
- It helps to ease the stress of a working parent by reinstating the connection with the infant.
- Infant massage offers parents a time to relax by providing focused time and attention with their infant.
- It increases the parent's ability to help relax the child in times of stress.
- It helps to release the pituitary hormone prolactin in both mothers and fathers. In females prolactin is involved in milk production and may help to foster maternal feelings. In males it is believed that prolactin stimulates the desire to protect and nurture the infant.
- Infant massage enhances communication between the parent and infant and builds mutual respect.
- It provides a special time for intimacy between fathers and their children.
- It helps teach parents to read infant cues.

Author's Note

A social worker in a hospital once told me that she overheard a nurse say that she (rather than the mom) had massaged a particular baby for the first week due to his fragile medical condition. The mother happened to be present and replied respectfully, "Why? Aren't I good enough to massage my own baby?"

There were volumes left unsaid within that last statement, but the baby's mother recognized her impulse to touch her own baby and to express the attachment process that was emerging from within. When a fragile baby cannot tolerate massage stroking, yet can handle a containment or touch-hold, who better to provide that tactile assurance and support than the mother or father? Deep bonding (or the impulse preceding it) awakens a parent's desire to protect the baby. In medical settings where baby John Doe can become lost in the hustle and bustle, a parent advocate is a guardian angel who, learning to advocate for his child as an infant, is empowered to actively support and protect the child throughout his life.

When the infant massage instructor, as a parent advocate, provides gentle intervention that supports and empowers the parent or caregiver, these continual life-giving experiences for the infant are more likely to occur (Fig. 27–2). This is precisely why infant massage instructors are encouraged to avoid seeking to empower themselves by actually doing successful massage with the baby; it may lower the parent's self-esteem in the process (because parents may feel they do not have the skills to do as well as the instructors).

Parents and caregivers must have success in order

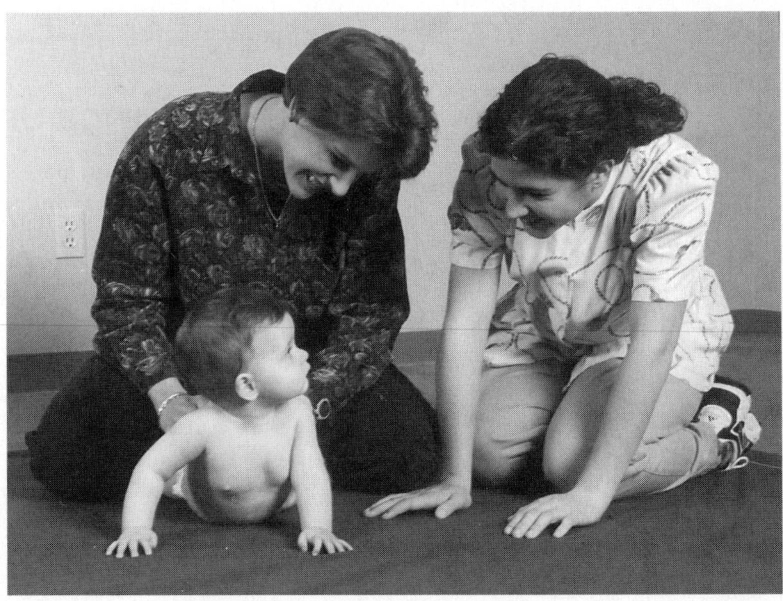

Figure 27•2 Mom, baby, and instructor.

for infant massage to become a family tradition that will serve as ongoing physical and emotional nourishment for the baby. To really be a baby advocate, we need to ensure that the baby's caregiver becomes adept at parenting skills. An infant massage instructor must therefore be a parent advocate who endeavors to help parents become increasingly more competent and eventually outgrow their need for the instructor's expertise. The instructor's obsolescence is the optimum side effect of this process.

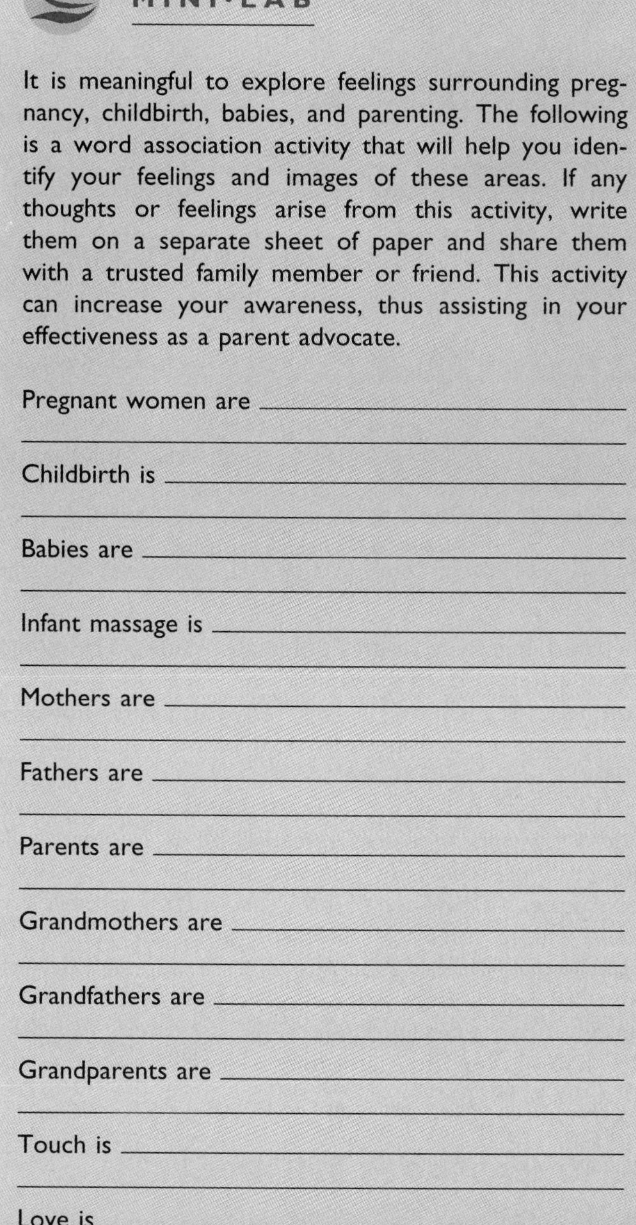
MINI•LAB

It is meaningful to explore feelings surrounding pregnancy, childbirth, babies, and parenting. The following is a word association activity that will help you identify your feelings and images of these areas. If any thoughts or feelings arise from this activity, write them on a separate sheet of paper and share them with a trusted family member or friend. This activity can increase your awareness, thus assisting in your effectiveness as a parent advocate.

Pregnant women are ______________________

Childbirth is ______________________

Babies are ______________________

Infant massage is ______________________

Mothers are ______________________

Fathers are ______________________

Parents are ______________________

Grandmothers are ______________________

Grandfathers are ______________________

Grandparents are ______________________

Touch is ______________________

Love is ______________________

Excerpted from *Pregnant Feelings*, Copyright © by Rahima Baldwin and Terra Palmatini. Reprinted by permission of Celestial Arts, PO Box 7123, Berkeley, CA 94707.

This same perspective holds true for the entire family support system of the baby. If an infant massage instructor is truly functioning as an advocate for the baby, she must endeavor to be a parent advocate as suggested previously, and ultimately as a family advocate to promote a family chemistry that offers support for the baby's well-being.

CREATING THE SETTING FOR INFANT MASSAGE

When a parent or caregiver is being taught in the home, the first thing you might ask is where they (baby and caregiver) like to spend time together. This is where they will be most comfortable in introducing a new experience of massage into their daily routine. For years, infant massage has been taught on the floor where the baby is stable and where parents can get good back support and make eye contact with the baby. This has worked well for most families; however, not all families gather on the floor. A family's familiar and cozy "power spot" is the most inviting place to massage the baby.

It is important that you teach the caregiver how to remain comfortable. This will make the massage experience more enjoyable for the caregiver and ensure continuity for many years. Another challenge the infant massage instructor has is to find ways to help make the massage successful by supporting the baby appropriately. Parents are encouraged to be thoughtful in creating support so the baby stays comfortable during the massage. An example is forming a small nesting border around the baby with towels or sheets to give a sense of boundary and to provide physical organization and comfort.

Massaging on a person's lap can work if the baby is a newborn. However, it can be difficult as the child grows (and the lap seems to get smaller) because the caregiver is then responsible for providing support under the infant as well as focusing on the massage. Environmental considerations include the following points:

1. The environment needs to be warm and without drafts. Massage oil will wick heat off the baby's body, so the room temperature should be about 10° warmer than usual. Babies are calmer in warmer temperatures.
2. Keep the environment free from distractions such as ringing telephones, television, or radio noise. However, some households are active with other children, so you may need to be accommodating with this rule.
3. Parents need back support without having to lean over too far to look at the baby during the massage. Parental positioning is as crucial as that of the baby.
4. The baby's positioning will vary from baby to baby, according to what works best. The position initially

used in the massage will change as the massage progresses and as the baby grows and develops.

5. The most preferred type of oil to use is cold-pressed or pure-pressed vegetable, fruit, or nut oil. Avoid mineral oils because they clog the skin's pores and are not digestible if swallowed. Also avoid scented oils—they may cause an allergic reaction in a sensitive baby. However, if a family cannot afford a cold-pressed oil, parents can use whatever oil they may have in their house; the massage will still be wonderful.
6. Soft background music can assist the parent in creating the rhythm for the massage as well as promote the relaxation response. The *best* music is when the parents sing their own lullabies to their baby, so that the sound of the lullaby becomes associated with the relaxing, nurturing touch.

NEWBORNS AND THEIR BEHAVIORAL STATES

In the 1970s, researchers found that infants exhibit predictable behavioral states that cycle in times of both sleeping and wakefulness. Being aware of these behavioral states can help caregivers choose the best time to massage their baby.

1. **Quiet Sleep.** The baby's eyes are firmly closed and still. There is little or no motor response observed. The respiration can be seen primarily in the abdominal region.
2. **Active Sleep.** During sleep, the eyes remain closed, but they may twitch and move, showing signs of rapid eye movement (REM), or dream sleep. Facial movements can be observed, such as smiling, frowning, and sucking. The baby may even make sounds such as crying and laughing. Motor activity (i.e., stretching, twitching, and writhing) may occur.
3. **Drowsy.** Appearing dazed, the baby usually lies very still, with her eyes partially open.
4. **Alert Inactivity or Quiet Alert.** Motor activity and facial expression are relaxed and relatively inactive. Babies' eyes are open, and they appear bright, interested, observant, and alert (Fig. 27–3).
5. **Waking Activity.** The baby appears very active: crying, grunting, moaning, fussing, and laughing. There is no sustained crying. Respiration is irregular and fluctuates between costal and abdominal breathing.
6. **Crying.** The baby appears unhappy or in pain, and respiration is deep and uneven.

It is important to identify these states and to be able to point them out to parents. Encourage parents to observe their babies at home, noting which behavioral state the baby may be experiencing. Observation will give valuable insight to the caregivers and help them to discover the best massage time for their baby. The most appropriate behavioral state for infant massage is the alert inactivity or the quiet alert state. The baby's natural tendency is to follow the cycle as previously outlined, regardless of his environment; however, states can be activated by external stimuli such as noise, activity, or massage.

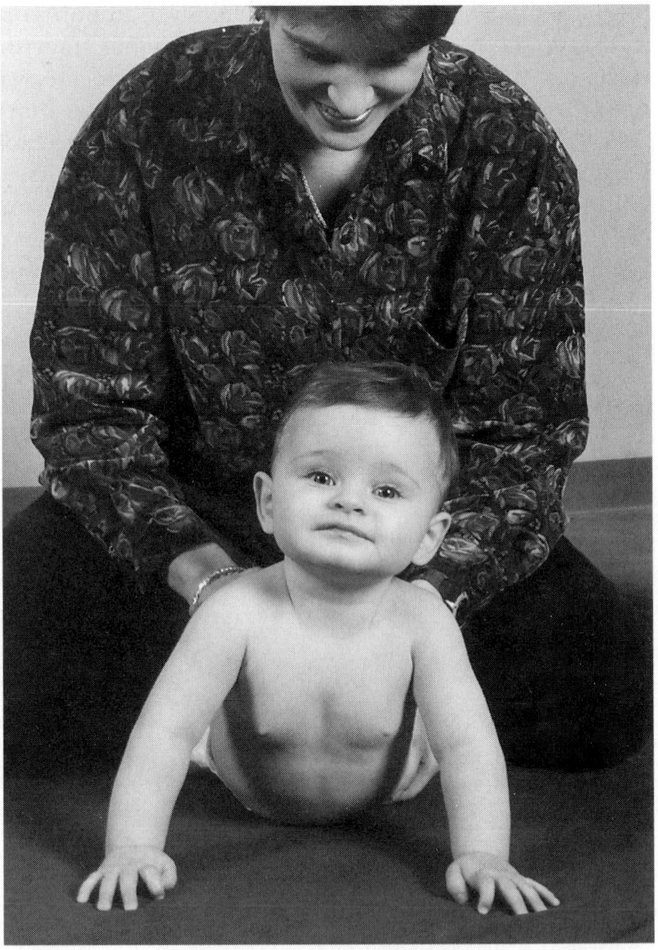

Figure 27•3 An alert baby.

The list also has its share of limitations. The baby who is crying vigorously because he is hungry or in pain will probably not respond as eagerly to massage techniques. Drowsiness that the infant experiences while falling asleep is different from drowsiness she experiences while waking up after a nap; try to time your infant massage accordingly. As you are teaching caregivers to massage their baby, ask them to notice the baby going into and out of waking activity and drowsiness.

WHO MASSAGES THE BABY?

Massage belongs, first of all, to the family—whoever loves the baby is a candidate to massage the baby.

The obvious people to massage the baby are the baby's parents, although the touch of grandparents, aunts, or even a sibling can also be welcoming and nurturing.

If a massage therapist (rather than a family member or a caregiver) regularly massages a baby, the benefits of the massage experience are short term and the parents are denied deepening the all-important core attachment that is a baby's immediate lifeline and springboard for a satisfying journey through life. The unspoken statement from a therapist to the parent may be that "You are not skilled enough to give your baby what a professional can." In most cases this is untrue and represents yet another parental discouragement. Subtle, covert messages such as this can strip power from the caregiver and have a negative impact on the long-term well-being of the infant.

If an instructor massages someone's baby and has success (which can easily happen after an instructor has become experienced) and later the parent massages the baby and does not have success, the parent will likely feel incompetent and may never massage the baby again. Thus a great opportunity for enriching baby's life and deepening the relationship with the parent is lost. Infant massage strengthens parent-infant and parent-child relationships and builds positive communication skills and family bonds. It is truly a treasure for many families and should not be taken away by an instructor's thoughtlessness in this area.

It's difficult to define success because the boundaries of such a definition would have to be infinitely flexible to accommodate the infinite experiences of the infant massage process. However, most caregivers feel successful if the baby and caregiver truly engage, and that the relational sharing of the event includes the caregiver honoring the infant's communication cues by responding supportively, and thereby deepening the engagement even more. There usually is a sense of satisfaction by both parties, which is followed by experiencing one or more of the benefits previously discussed.

One way to address a parent if she asks you to massage her baby during a class is to say, "Oh, my baby (which is a doll) would be hurt if I do not massage him, so you need to massage your own baby." The subtle message for parents is that infant massage belongs to parents and babies.

THE INFANT MASSAGE ROUTINE

It is important to remember that infant massage is an interaction that is done *with* the baby rather than *to* him. It is a dance defined by the quality and intention of touch that is transformed into a shared experience of timeless presence. The parent or caregiver begins the massage by asking the baby for permission. This demonstrates a sense of respect. Initially the baby will not know what is being asked or what to expect but in a short time will understand what is to come when the bottle of massage oil appears. It is empowering for a baby to be able to say yes or no to being touched. This early lesson teaches a child to set his own touch boundaries that are comfortable and controlled by him. Babies as young as 6 months can communicate no to a massage, and of course refusal is always respected by the caregiver.

An infant massage routine is composed of basic, fun, and easily applied strokes geared for the well baby—a combination of Swedish and Indian massage, with some reflexology (Figs. 27–4 and 27–5). Infants who are biologically and environmentally at risk or children with special needs will require touch adaptations that may be quite different from the well-baby stroke format. Adaptations should be used to fine-tune the mas-

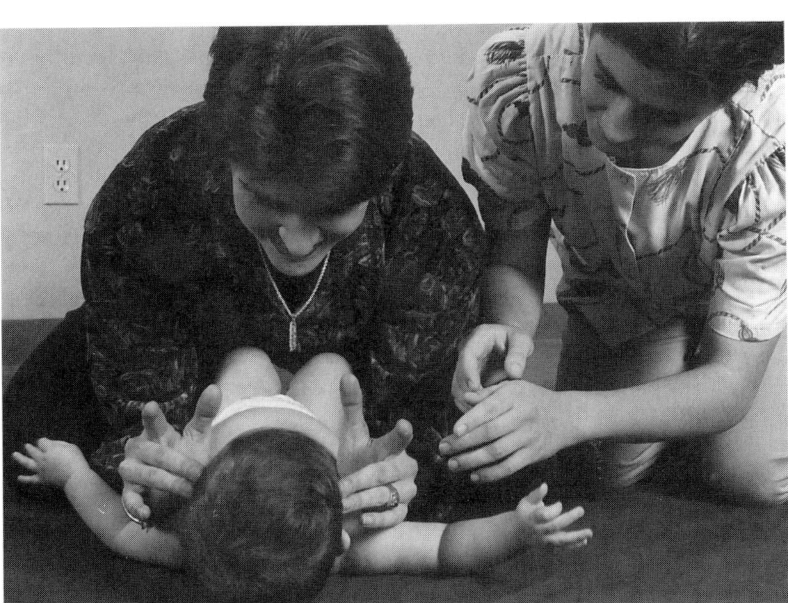

Figure 27•4 Mom massaging baby's temples.

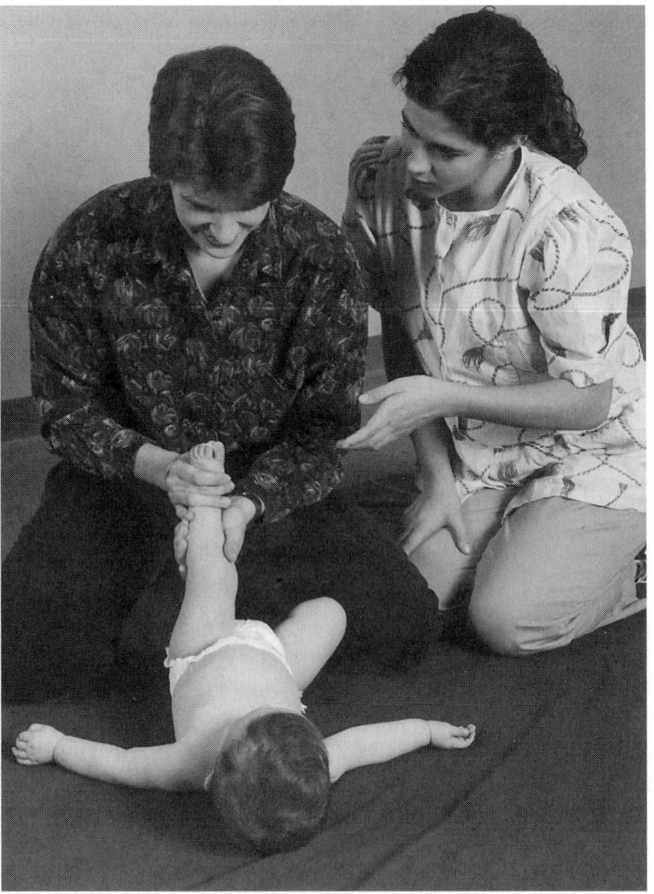

Figure 27•5 Mom massaging baby's leg.

sage for each child. The focus is to teach the parent to use rhythm and pressure that works for the child. Books and videos show these standard strokes in detail.

Because it is a mutual exchange, both parent and baby should to be able to enjoy and focus on the interaction. Alert inactivity or the quiet alert state is the most preferred for the baby because more touch can usually be tolerated. A parent can massage a baby when she is drowsy or fussy, but often it may be too much for the baby to handle. There is no set time frame for how long the massage should last—parents need to be flexible and willing to stop if they are not really in the mood or when the infant communicates that he has had enough. If the baby can initially only tolerate 5 to 10 minutes of massage, frustration can occur when a parent is enthusiastic about enjoying this new experience and wants to continue.

For an infant to receive the massage, a parent needs to be attentive—to read the baby's cues and respond in a respectful way to establish a tolerable level of intimacy and safety for the baby. Attention to and respect for these cues will ensure that the baby's tolerance will gradually increase until a complete massage can be received (Fig. 27–6).

If an adult becomes overstimulated during a massage, he may show time-out cues of sleeping or random talking. By contrast, infants can become overstimulated at any given moment, but they have not developed the adult's coping mechanisms. Also, their bodies have not yet developed the numbing body armor that many adults use. The baby can only respond with clear expressions and postures that say, "No more!"

According to information adapted in large part from the *Nursing Child Assessment Satellite Training (NCAST) Learner's Manual,* University of Washington School of Nursing, by Dr. Kathryn Barnard, we can generally group cues as indicators of an infant's need or openness for engagement or disengagement. Attentiveness to these cues translates into a very deep level of empathy and communication and ultimately the ability to attend to a baby's needs in a very refined and appropriate way.

There are clinically more than 108 known infant communication cues that parents can learn to recognize so that in each moment the touch approach can be adapted to fit the baby. An infant may present a stress cue (for example, yawning) but may still be able to stay organized and stable while the parent continues the massage. However, if an infant presents a cluster of stress cues, such as yawning, sneezing, gaze aversion, and skin mottling, then it may be necessary for

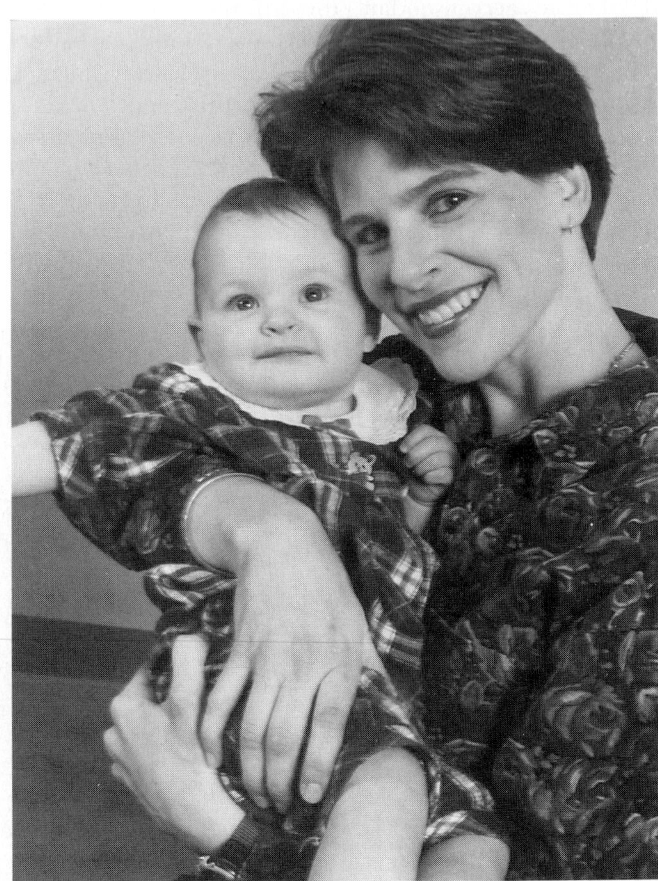

Figure 27•6 This mother and her child enjoy each other after massage.

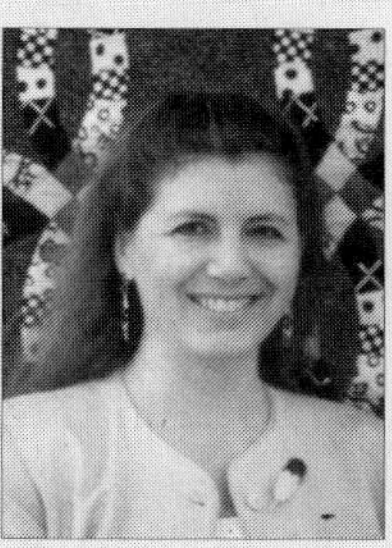

Vimala Schneider McClure

Born: June 7, 1952

"Do all the good you can in all the ways you can, for all the people you can for long as ever you can."
P. R. Sarkar

Vimala Schneider McClure, the pioneer of infant massage in the United States, always had the feeling that she was put here to fulfill a specific purpose. At age 21, the starry-eyed humanitarian sold everything she had and took off for India. "I was terrified," she confided, "but my sense of purpose was so strong it was worth putting myself in harm's way."

In India she studied with Yogi Master P. R. Sarkar until a bout with malaria cut her trip short and landed her in a New York hospital for a couple of weeks.

She had recurrences for years afterward, but her health has never been perfect. McClure is a diethylstilbestrol (DES) (a drug given to prevent miscarriages now proved to have adverse effects) daughter. As a child she had open-heart surgery. She's had 11 operations and has lost "every expendable organ." Today she suffers from severe fibromyalgia.

Somewhat recovered from the malaria, she returned to India and worked in an orphanage. It was there she learned the art of infant massage from an assistant. Out of necessity, the nun who ran the orphanage spent much of her time begging money for its support, so McClure was left to care for the children along with two Indian girls. "They couldn't speak my language and I couldn't speak theirs," she remembers. In the evenings, when the courtyard cooled off to 90°, she learned traditional Indian baby massage.

"They've done it in India for 10,000 years or more," she explains. Mothers massage their infants and pass along the skill to their daughters. "I began to see how relaxed these children were . . . how different from American children. They were easier with each other and less aggressive. Boys and girls alike walk around with their arms around each other. Then it began to click. I began to see massage as something that could change lives. A good analogy is that we're like a cup and the more love that goes into that cup—until it is overflowing—the more you can give. If your cup didn't get filled as a child, then you're always looking for someone to fill it up."

McClure points out that every mammal species licks their young, which isn't just for cleaning. It's a bonding process that stimulates the whole system. Without this stage, mothers kill their offspring. Or, offspring are affected down the road in the same way that abused children may perpetuate abuse.

McClure returned to the States and in 1976 became pregnant with her first of two children. In addition to everything about massage and yoga she'd learned in India, she asked friends to teach her some Swedish massage techniques to develop a routine for her newborn. In *Infant Massage, A Handbook for Loving Parents,* she writes: "This joyful blend provided my son with a wonderful balance of outgoing and incoming energy, of tension release, and stimulation. Additionally it seemed to relieve the painful gas he had been experiencing that first month."

McClure began to keep copious notes. Eventually she invited mothers over to show them what she was doing. During these sessions she distributed a small hand-made flyer.

One of McClure's tiny flyers fell into the right hands and she was invited to speak at a childbirth education conference. It was there that she met the owner of a baby products company, who asked, "Have you ever thought about writing a book? Write one and I'll publish it."

She had already done so, and *Infant Massage, A Handbook for Loving Parents* became and still is, the definitive work on infant massage. Pressed by others to begin an organization, the International Association of Infant Massage is worldwide now, but she receives no money for her pioneering

continued on page 606

Continued

Vimala Schneider McClure

training, except royalties from the book. "I was zero percent motivated by money at the time. I didn't think about how much profit I could make. I didn't think of my work as a business venture. At this point in my life, I'm not so sure how smart that was," she confesses.

Her advice to beginning massage therapists regarding infant massage is to start with a very different mindset because what happens between parent and child is different from what happens during a therapeutic massage. McClure says, "It's the act of bonding and impacting a lifetime. That's why I trained instructors to train parents rather than training massage therapists to massage infants. As an instructor, you have to allow parents to develop their own style. Even if they don't apply strokes in an expert manner, the message comes through. You have to empower parents and not allow them to turn over their power to the instructor as the expert."

McClure considers the rearing of her two children her main mission in life. Asked how she'd respond if her daughter said she was off to some Third World country to find her purpose, Schneider admits: "I'd try to talk her out of it. I'm too much a mom. But if it was something she positively had to do, I'd give her my blessing." Schneider continues to write and to help parents develop closer, more meaningful relationships with their children. Her other works include *The Tao of Motherhood, A Woman's Guide to Tantric Yoga,* and her current book, *The Path of Parenting: Twelve Principles to Guide Your Journey.*

the parent to take a comfort break so the infant can get organized again or to end the massage because the infant has become overstimulated.

Put a significant effort into educating parents in understanding the baby's cues because it is vitally important for deepening and refining infant massage skills. It gives parents confidence to learn to understand their baby's cues and to know what to do. Although stress cues indicate that the infant does not want any more massage, engagement cues such as eye contact or hand to mouth indicate that the child is ready to interact. Regard for these communications ensures that as the child grows and becomes verbal she will openly volunteer whether she wants the massage.

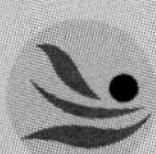

MINI•LAB

As an experiential task that will possibly trigger some memory or empathy of what it was like to be a baby, allow yourself to "take on" the following disengagement postures: splayed fingers, averted gaze, arched back; do them all together. Then very mindfully ask yourself, "What is this like? What is the quality of my inner world when I'm experiencing these positions?" Also, ask yourself what it might feel like if someone forced you to make contact or picked you up when you feel like this.

Next take on the postures of bright and wide eyes, hands open with fingers slightly flexed, and smiling; again ask yourself "What is the quality of my inner world when I am experiencing these positions?" And what might it feel like if someone picked me up when I am feeling like this?

Author's Note

Once I was working with a mother and her infant, and I began singing a lullaby during the massage to help the baby stay calm so that the mother could feel successful. Instead, the baby was relaxing and the mother thought it was because the baby liked hearing my singing. Sensing that she was attributing her success to me, I stopped singing and we did 10 or 15 more minutes of massage so that Mom could see that it was through her own efforts and loving touch that the baby relaxed.

ORGANIZING CLASSES IN YOUR COMMUNITY

If your geographical area has had little exposure to infant massage, volunteer your services. Conducting demonstration classes with parent groups, such as La Leche League, parents' church groups, parenting classes for special populations, and teen parents can all be helpful in popularizing infant massage.

Many opportunities have been opening up during the past 5 years. Given its current popularity in this country, infant massage may soon be part of nearly every agency and program that serves families. Infant massage instructors are being hired through county health department grants to serve families at risk and through local parenting programs. Many massage therapists are teaching in health clubs, churches, shelters, jails, hospitals, continuing education at local universities, as adjuncts to midwifery postpartum care, in private practices, and in home healthcare, providing individual instruction in home visit environments. There is a growing need for infant massage instructors who are strong advocates for families, parents, and infants.

CONDUCTING CLASSES

Two decades ago infant massage was presented to our society as a parenting modality broadly geared to the well-baby population. Over time, this basic system of nurturing strokes has expanded to become a parent-empowering paradigm utilized by highly sensitive, skilled, and committed instructors working in a wide range of settings. Requiring educational and experiential training, competency in infant massage instruction suggests that beyond the acquisition of knowledge is the attainment of a significant level of maturity, compassion, and wisdom. The Chinese proverb is fitting: "When the sage is at work, the people will say, 'We did it ourselves.'"

Orchestrating the class, while modeling for parents the many skills that comprise infant massage, is truly an art form. Often a parent has no massage experience and may even harbor some negative bias around the issue of touch. Basic handling, positioning skills, awareness of infant development, and understanding infant crying must be modeled in a positive but often chaotic environment. As an instructor, you must maintain sensitivity and regard for the parents' self-esteem and accept where they are in their parenting process. This is especially true for the new parent, but even the experienced parent learns some lessons with each child. Include adaptations for any infants, children, or parents who have special needs in order to facilitate a successful massage experience for them.

Fortunately these challenges are taken in stride by instructors who are functioning in partnership with the family. The teacher may receive the rare gift of occasionally witnessing time standing still—wonderful work in this often disconnected world where parenting skills are not always as effective as we hope. Training helps to familiarize an infant massage instructor with the parent-infant world and provides strategies (shared from the experiences of other instructors and professionals) to empower caregivers to engage with infants in what might seem like impossible circumstances. Providing the space for the opening of the hearts of both parents and infants, even in a chaotic environment of fussy, screaming babies, is a privilege.

Empowering parents requires a very different perspective than that of a therapist. Whereas a therapist actually massages a baby, an infant massage instructor uses a doll to model both the strokes and the relational dynamics of the massage. The doll is used to demonstrate strokes for parents and to model how to respond—not react—to the baby during the massage. Of course there are pitfalls with dolls: A new instructor turned her doll over to demonstrate the back strokes, and the doll's head fell off! So much for modeling.

Since the caregiver (parent) is the one who is massaging the baby, success is attributed to his or her competence rather than to the manual skills of either a therapist or the instructor. Parental success will ensure the continuity of infant massage in the family, thereby sustaining or deepening the attachment and the quality of the family's life.

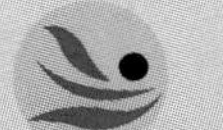

MINI•LAB

Reading aloud to others and being read to are both enjoyable experiences. Gather your classmates or your family together, and read *Love You Forever* by Robert Munsch (published by Firefly Books). This book is wonderful for exploring parental love and bonding and should be required reading if you are going to teach infant massage to parents. Enjoy!

P.S. Stock up on tissues first!

WHAT ABOUT THOSE CRYING BABIES?

Occasionally, facilitators have commented about the headaches they get if there is very much crying in the classes. Over years of facilitating infant massage with parents and their babies, you will witness a variety of cries undoubtedly triggered by a wide range of distresses. One such instructor experienced a 180-degree shift in her attitude about this very natural and necessary expression. Her current approach to crying during the massage is that when it is happening, it is *the happening*. Whatever personal agenda (like completing the massage) is driving either the instructor or the caregiver has to be dropped so that the baby's process is allowed to set the course.

If a parent is uncomfortable or hesitant about listening to her baby during this process, the instructor should make it okay to comfort her baby. A mother's intuition with her baby should always be respected even if your own instinct is to support the baby's expression instead. With more massage experience comes greater skill in really listening to one's baby.

In public, whenever you are around a baby who is crying, you should automatically tune in to the sound and ask yourself, "What kind of cry is this? What is this cry expressing?" Of course there are "I'm hungry" cries, "Change my diaper" cries, and "I've got gas pain" cries. But there are also release cries that simply say "Hear my grief" and "Hear my rage!" Another dimension of crying is that of releasing stress or "talk-crying." You may witness very young babies looking right into their caregiver's eyes and expressing their feelings of frustration, anger, or grief. When asked if the parent knows what the baby seems to be saying, sometimes he knows and sometimes he does not. Because of the intimate connection with the baby, often additional tears will come from the caregiver. The release cry is a way for the baby to communicate and it is hoped the parent will respond by listening and acknowledging, and thereby initiating healing. Obviously, rather than trying to figure out a way to get the crying to stop, it is healthier to allow it to happen, and therefore expression of the feeling is complete.

By supporting the spontaneous expression of the crying infant with intuitive listening, by helping to position the baby however he seems to be trying to position himself, and by maintaining a welcoming presence for the emerging expression, we open the door to a baby's discovery of himself and the world around him. You do not massage a baby during a stress release. As a facilitator, resist the impulse to stop the crying just to relieve yourself of any discomfort you may be experiencing through your own empathy. Not really knowing what is going on with this process, but supporting the natural unfolding of infant release, allows for deep healing and reorganizing.

Reports by parents of magical changes in their baby by simply allowing this natural process to unfold are very common. Some parents have expressed this as follows. "It's like I have a new baby, like lights have been turned on inside him; he's so different!" "After going through his process together, I feel like our souls have touched each other and a real opening has happened. He is so much more present and available."

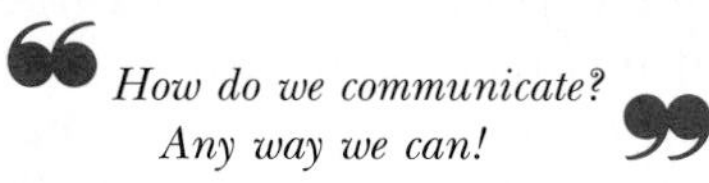

How do we communicate?
Any way we can!

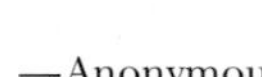

—Anonymous

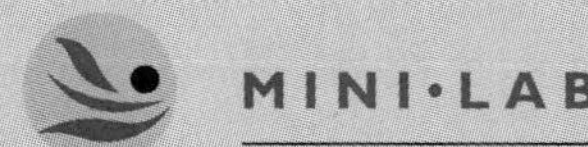

MINI•LAB

It is not absolutely necessary to be in touch with your own infant experiences to be an instructor, but it does help. To assist in your understanding of what a baby's experience is like, try the following exercise.

1. Imagine yourself as an infant and that you are being massaged by your mother. Take a few minutes to experience what this is like.
2. In your journal, record for each stage of your life what your experience would have been like if you had had this nurturing interaction with your mother.
   - infancy
   - toddlerhood
   - preschool age
   - school age
   - adolescence
3. Explore the same exercise concerning your father. It is important and eye-opening to start at infancy and go through each developmental phase.

   If this exercise stirs up strong feelings, get support from a friend or family member who can be a sensitive listening partner. If this is not possible, take some time just to be with yourself and with whatever feelings you experience, whether they be tears of release or joyful memories. Be gentle with yourself.
4. Finally, in your journal, write how your adulthood would be different if you had been lovingly massaged as an infant and throughout your growing-up years.
   - How might your relationships be different?
   - How might your profession be different?
   - How might it have affected your interests? Goals? Dreams?
   - Might it affect how you cope with adversity?
   - Might it affect the level of intimacy in your life as an adult?

SUMMARY

This chapter has provided you with a brief vicarious experience of the world of an infant massage instructor. It is a field that absolutely requires a deep connection with parents and babies. It does make a difference, a huge difference in many cases, and changes the lives not only of parents and babies but of the infant massage instructors as well. I have received so many letters over the years from instructors who say, "This work has deeply changed my life." I can only respond with a knowing smile and a nod of agreement.

SELF-TEST

Multiple Choice • Write the letter of the best answer in the space provided.

_______ 1. Infant massage is a
A. parenting tradition of loving touch that parents of many cultures have been using for centuries
B. very powerful demonstration of unconditional love and support that is deeply experienced on many levels of the baby's being and held as a tactile memory in the baby's body
C. dance defined by the quality and intention of touch that is transformed into a shared experience of timeless presence
D. all of the above

_______ 2. Infant massage was first introduced as a parenting tool in the United States around the
A. mid-1790s
B. mid-1960s
C. mid-1970s
D. mid-1980s

_______ 3. Which of the following is *not* a benefit of infant massage for babies and children?
A. helps the parent to feel more competent and confident
B. it can relieve discomfort from teething, gas, and colic
C. the baby sleeps deeper and longer after infant massage
D. frequent infant massage assists in increased vocalization

_______ 4. According to Drs. Marshall Klaus and John Kennell, bonding is a
A. type of adhesive agent
B. reciprocal relationship between parents
C. solid connection between the parent and child that nourishes the baby on a core level
D. reciprocal relationship between siblings

_______ 5. Which is an important vehicle for parent-infant bonding?
A. formula feeding
B. piggyback rides
C. infant massage
D. trips to Disneyland

_______ 6. Deep bonding (or the impulse preceding it) awakens a parent's
A. love for the spouse
B. need for further education
C. desire to protect the baby
D. desire to own a dog or cat

_______ 7. When massaging the baby, parents need
A. bright overhead lights
B. a pillow
C. good back support and eye contact with the baby
D. a pacifier

_______ 8. The location for the caregiver to massage the baby is
A. in the baby's nursery
B. only in the presence of the massage therapist
C. on a couch or a bed
D. on the floor in front of the television so the baby is distracted

_______ 9. The most preferred type of oil to use is
A. cold-pressed or pure-pressed vegetable oil
B. commercial aromatherapy massage oil
C. mineral oil
D. commercial baby oil

_______ 10. If a massage therapist (rather than a caregiver) massages a baby, the massage experience is
A. long term
B. short term
C. significant
D. cathartic

_______ 11. Infant massage teaches a child to
A. use oil on her skin frequently
B. set her own comfortable touch boundaries that she controls
C. massage the ones you love
D. relax when the caregiver enters the room

_______ 12. Infant massage is a combination of
A. Swedish and Indian massage with some reflexology
B. Rolfing and reflexology
C. Sports massage and shiatsu
D. Trager and shiatsu

_______ 13. Infants who are biologically and environmentally at risk or children with special needs will require

A. a doctor's referral
B. touch adaptation that may be quite different from the well-baby format
C. extra pillows and blankets
D. the massage to be given by a professional only

_______ 14. The most preferred behavioral state for the baby to receive the massage is the

A. quiet sleep state
B. quiet alert state
C. drowsy state
D. crying state

_______ 15. Infant cues such as yawning, sneezing, gaze aversion, and skin mottling indicate that it may be necessary for the parent to

A. change his diaper
B. turn up the lighting
C. be ready to interact
D. take a comfort break

_______ 16. Infant cues such as eye contact or hand to mouth indicate that the child is ready to

A. have his diaper changed
B. have more lighting in the room
C. interact
D. take a comfort break

_______ 17. Conducting demonstration classes is helpful in popularizing infant massage and can be offered in

A. La Leche League, parent church groups, and parenting classes for special populations
B. teen parents' groups, health clubs, shelters, jails, and hospitals
C. continuing education at local universities and in-services at medical agencies
D. all of the above

_______ 18. As an infant massage instructor, you must maintain sensitivity and regard for the parents' self-esteem and

A. take parenting classes yourself
B. offer healthy snacks at the classes
C. accept where they are in their parenting process
D. never let the class last more than 1 hour

_______ 19. To model both the strokes and the relational dynamics of the massage, the infant massage instructor uses

A. a doll
B. a stuffed animal
C. one of the parent's children
D. imagery

References

Baldwin, Rahima and Terra Palmarini. *Pregnant Feelings.* Berkeley, CA: Celestial Arts, 1986.

Brazelton, T. Berry, M.D., Steven Parker, M.D. and Barry S. Zuckerman, M.D. "Importance of Behavioral Assessment of the Neonate." *Current Problems in Pediatrics.* December, 1976.

Klaus, Marshall H., John H. Kennell, and Phylis H. Klaus, *Bonding: Building the Foundations of Secure Attachment and Independence.* Addison-Wesley, 1983.

Leboyer, Fredrick. *Loving Hands.* New York: Alfred A. Knopf, 1987.

McClure, Vimala Scheider. *Infant Massage: A Handbook for Loving Parents.* New York: Bantam Books, 1982.

McClure, Vimala Scheider. *Infant Massage Instructor Handbook.* Boulder, CO: Self-published manuscript, 1997.

Wolff, Peter H. *"The Causes, Controls, and Organization of Behavior in the Neonate." Psychological Issues,* Vol. 5, No. 1, Monograph 17.

U N I T   F I V E

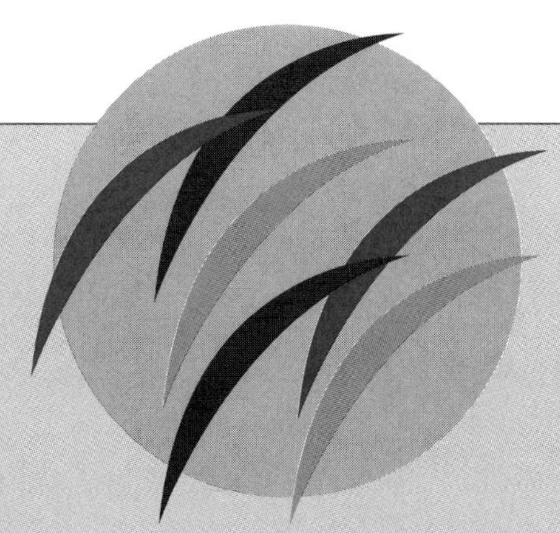

The Business of Bodywork

To accomplish great things we must not only act, but also dream; not only plan, but also believe.
—Anonymous

28 Business Practices

Student Objectives

After completing this chapter, the student should be able to:

- Identify what is valued in life
- Write a mission statement
- Discuss how professional image relates to success as a massage therapist
- Set goals for a practice
- Complete a business plan and use it to evaluate and modify goals
- Develop skills in telephone communication
- Create a curriculum vitae
- Describe various promotional activities and advertising appropriate for a practice
- List five business resources
- Describe how you will grow and evolve in the field of massage therapy

INTRODUCTION

■ *"If I had really wanted to do all this damned secretarial work, I'd have gone to a secretarial school."* ■

—S. Devillier

Many people go into business for themselves without ever really knowing the first thing about it. They love their craft, and they are good at it, but professional knowledge, technical skills, and experience are almost never the cause of a failed business venture but rather the lack of business skills and capital. The purpose of this chapter is to provide the new therapist with basic business practices: from the "work" done before opening the doors to the practical knowledge of operating a business and creating opportunities. This material can also be used for "seasoned" therapists who would like to reevaluate themselves and their practices.

Most basic business plans for a massage business are built on your personal beliefs, values, goals, and professional image. Often, writing a mission statement (defining, on paper, what you value), declaring a mission statement, and answering questions that lead to a business plan are cornerstones of your business.

Once your plan is mapped out, acquire business permits and determine start-up costs. Once these essential elements have been established, you need to master the art of telephone etiquette, advertise and promote your business, write contracts and proposals, locate resources, plan career advancement, diversify your income, and return something to the community through volunteering. Finally you will learn how to manage or avoid discouragement and burn-out.

WHAT DO YOU VALUE?

Your massage practice must reflect who you are. If your work is not an extension of yourself, the person you are deep inside, you may experience an internal tug-of-war. You will find that a big part of success is imbedded in your personal and spiritual philosophy.

How you behave in your personal, professional, and spiritual life typically comes from your needs, attitudes, and beliefs. The following activity will help you identify these important elements of yourself. On the lines provided, list 15 to 20 things or concepts you value—a bit like "soul searching." The items can range from basic needs (such as adventure, creativity, self-expression, health, independence, and fun) to more complex needs such as your spiritual life, family life, protecting the environment, and world peace.

1. ____________________
2. ____________________
3. ____________________
4. ____________________
5. ____________________
6. ____________________
7. ____________________
8. ____________________
9. ____________________
10. ____________________
11. ____________________
12. ____________________
13. ____________________
14. ____________________
15. ____________________
16. ____________________
17. ____________________
18. ____________________
19. ____________________
20. ____________________

Next, read over your list and circle the five most important items, (i.e., the five most important things in your life). This exercise is often liberating because you will discover that once you have identified your five most important values, it is easier to make decisions involving your energy and your time, which are two of your most valuable assets! List the five most important things in your life in order of priority (Your list may change to reflect your changing needs).

1. ____________________
2. ____________________
3. ____________________
4. ____________________
5. ____________________

Copy the list on several sheets of paper, and tape it where you can see your priorities—the bathroom mirror, the refrigerator, the dashboard of your car. This is also a beneficial activity to teach clients for stress reduction. If your clients feel overwhelmed, ask them to go through this process, and help them identify what is important to them. As Goethe said, "Things which matter most must never be at the mercy of the things which matter least."

Mission Statement

Once you have identified your values and needs, the next step is to write a **mission statement** (statement of purpose); this is comparable to a time and thought organizer. Like the five most important things in your life, your mission statement will reflect your ideals, values, attitude, beliefs, or your essence. The Constitution of the United States can be viewed as a mission statement. Taking time to write your mission statement will help you define where you would like to be once your craft is mastered and may answer the question, "What on earth am I doing here?"

There are a few guidelines for writing a mission statement. First, it must be short; if not, you are probably not going to remember it or read it often; it's a good idea to be able to recite it by memory. Next, it must begin with the words, "My lifework." Third, it must focus on the needs of other people and not your own! Every successful massage therapist will tell you the same thing; When your focus is serving humanity, opportunities are never in short supply. Last, your mission statement must be totally compatible with your most important values; it will evolve as you evolve, so it must be flexible and revised as needed. Your birthday or New Year's Day may be a good time to reevaluate it.

My life work ______________________________

____

____

____

____

For example: "My life work is, through touch, to assist others in removing their physiological and psychological restrictions and limitations."

YOUR PROFESSIONAL IMAGE

First impressions of you and your business are formed within 30 to 60 seconds. Within 3 to 6 minutes, most clients have decided whether they will schedule a massage. Because your initial contact with a client is so important, take a few minutes to write down a 30-second introduction, including your name, your title, and the name of your business. Rehearse what you will say to your clients about your practice. Remember that most clients will repeat what you say to others, so let it be positive.

What images do you want to instill in your community about massage? Is it an oasis of relaxation or a means of managing pain and discomfort? You cannot be all things to all people. Once you state your position (who you are and what you represent in the massage profession), your professional direction will be clearer (Fig. 28–1).

Your **professional image** is often an instantaneous impression or picture of you when your name is spoken or read. Professional image comes from a variety of sources: your personal and academic background, relationships, community affiliations, and general impressions that people have of you. This image can be flattering or unfavorable, depending on how you handle life's challenges. You cannot buy a favorable professional image; it must be earned and maintained daily. A favorable professional image is beyond price and is built on integrity. Consider the meaning of the word "integrity." It comes from the word "integer," to integrate. **Integrity** is the condition of being whole and undivided. To have a character with integrity, you must deal honestly with yourself and with others. In dealing with yourself, profess to a value system and adhere to it. Your integrity is yours alone; others can know your reputation only by demonstration of your integrity.

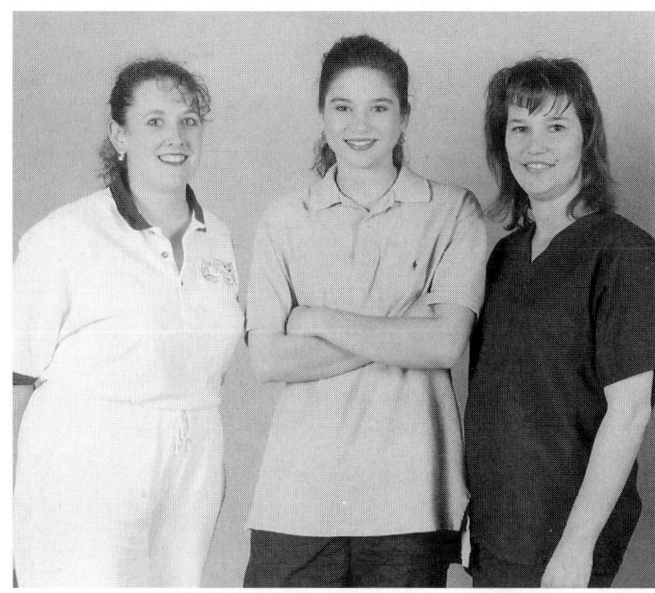

Figure 28•1 Three professionals.

In business, a good image comes from demanding and giving nothing but your best. The way you carry yourself, your appearance, your business card, your establishment, how you conduct your business will all promote your image.

GOAL SETTING

Goal setting is essential to the success of any project. Without a goal, your life may be like a ship floating aimlessly in the wind. Goals give you something to reach for; a dream to embrace. It is important to ask yourself, "What do I want?" We encourage clients to set treatment goals, so why not use the same strategy in our own lives? Set goals for all the areas of your life: financial, academic and educational, personal and familial, and spiritual. Your goals ideally expand your mission statement and give you a target to shoot for. It is easier to get to your destination if you have a map (Fig. 28–2).

To chart your map, spend some time identifying your goals, so make them as specific as possible. For-

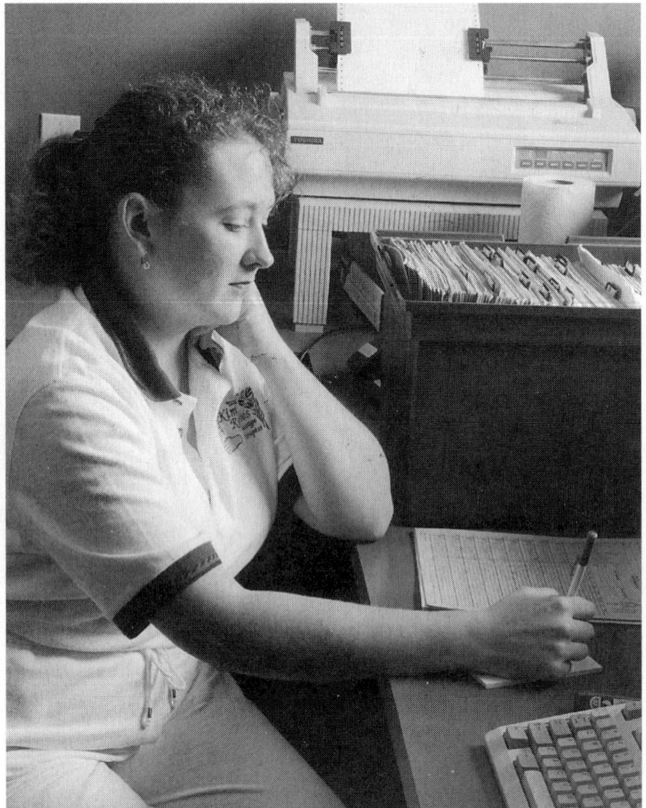

Figure 28•2 Goal setting.

mulate them in the present tense; when appropriate, reflect a positive quality about yourself. Rather than a general "I want to be a better massage therapist," specify, "I attend two 3-day workshops a year to enhance my skills as a massage therapist."

Once you have identified your goals, write them down. The act of writing will add an element of commitment and reinforcement, and the written goals will serve as reminders of your focus. Writing is the first step in turning abstract ideas or concepts into realities. Be aware that before goals can be realized and achieved, you need both personal commitment and faith. Wanting the goal and having faith in your abilities, combined with a goal, gives focused direction to your effort. Without desire and faith, the discipline that it takes to achieve a goal will not be forthcoming. Goals are first realized in the mind (imagined) before they can be realized (obtained).

The next step is to identify your resources. There are areas in your life or aspects of your character that you can draw upon for support. Resources may be financial and familial or may include your abilities to take time off to attend a workshop as well as your own personal discipline and determination. To give you a broader perspective, refer to the section on locating your resources in this chapter.

Once you have mapped out specific goals, consider strategies to narrow your focus. You can set goals to be reached within a specific time frame: short range (daily, weekly, or monthly); midrange (6 months to 1 year); and long-range goals (3 to 5 years). Short-range goals are attained more quickly than long-range goals and are important to build confidence when they are achieved. Use a method that you can live with. By setting and achieving your goals, you will be able to manage your time, your career, and your life more efficiently. Post your goals in a place where you will read them often; evaluate them often, and modify them when needed. Be flexible enough to learn from mistakes in goal setting, but be persistent enough to keep striving. Goals are not cast in stone.

The last step is to develop a plan of action by dividing the goal into smaller, more manageable pieces, then using your resources to accomplish each smaller goal. For instance, if you want to enhance your skills as a massage therapist by attending workshops, determine your weak skills and survey your clientele to find out what kind of massage skills they need, such as myofascial release or pregnancy massage. Then locate the workshop, register for it, make your travel plans, and mark those days on your calendar. Your plan of action may also include raising money for the workshop if you do not have a surplus.

If your plans do not work, try others. This is where many massage therapists panic; it is hard for some people to shuffle the deck and to deal themselves a new hand. Temporary setbacks only mean that there are details that need attention.

BUSINESS DEVELOPMENT THROUGH A BUSINESS PLAN

Once you have gotten to know more about yourself, learn more about your practice. Answering the following questions to the best of your ability will help you to identify your business parameters and to develop a better understanding of the business side of your massage practice.

Many therapists shudder when you mention the word "business" to them. Conducting your massage practice in a businesslike manner does not make you any less a therapist. In fact, doing so will enhance your abilities as a therapist because you will develop a sense of direction and purpose. A good business plan not only includes your current values but also helps you grasp a view of the future. Many answers to the questions of the business plan are only assumptions, but they will guide you to purposeful action in meeting present and future goals.

Part of a business plan is the marketing, which begins with a description of your business and special marketing concepts (e.g., advertising, competition analysis, location, operations, personnel). A marketing plan can help you discover the promotional activities that will be the most effective and enjoyable. The components of basic business and marketing plans are personal information, a general description of your business, services, fees and pricing, marketing, advertising, competition, your location and operations, management and personnel, and your insurance needs.

Personal Information

1. Why will you be successful in this business?
2. What is your experience in this business, if any?
3. What are your weaknesses, and what are your strengths and resources?
4. Project a sense of what you expect to accomplish in 5 years.

General Description of Business

1. Write your mission statement. Does it reflect your 5-year projection?
2. How do you define your business? What business are you in, and what do you offer?
3. Describe your services.
4. For what purpose will people generally buy your service?
5. Are you willing to change what you offer, to some extent, to meet your client's changing needs?
6. What will be the opening date of your business?
7. What hours of the day and days of the week will you be in operation?
8. What will your fee schedule look like? How have you determined your fees?

Marketing

1. What do you want people to say to others about your services? What do you want your brief message or "identity" to be? Describe the image you would like to project. Remember, *you never get a second chance to make a first impression.*
2. To what groups of clients (target market) will you sell your services? Identify the primary beneficiaries of your work by describing important characteristics such as age, gender, occupation, income, and so on.
3. How can you get the attention of the people you want to reach?
4. What unique features or talents can you bring to your service?

Marketing: Advertising

1. What media are appropriate for your business image and targeted clients? **Media** are methods of mass communication such as newspapers, magazines, radio, and television.
2. What other channel(s) will you use to reach your market?
3. How can you discover which promotion is working and which isn't?
4. Plan an advertising budget for 6 months. Include specific media you will use and the cost of each.

Marketing: Competition

1. Who else provides a similar service? In order of their strength in the market, list your five closest competitors by name and address. Next, describe each competitor's business strengths and weaknesses.
2. How are you different in ways that matter to potential clients?
3. How will you distinguish yourself from the competition? What advantages do you have over competitors that will allow you better to serve clients? Referring to your image as stated in the first part of the chapter, what unique qualities will you bring to the field of massage therapy?
4. How will you make your operation the best in the business? Be specific.

Marketing: Location/Operations

1. What type of location does your business require? Describe the type of building your business needs. Include space for a reception room, bathroom, hydrotherapy area (if appropriate), parking, security needs, proximity to other businesses for added traffic and exposure, and so on.
2. Where do you plan to locate your business? Is this location right for your business?
3. Why have you chosen your present location? Is there a better location in your market area?
4. Describe the geographic area your business will serve. Are there sufficient numbers of potential clients located there?
5. What types of operations are needed for your business? Include layout for waiting room, restroom, hydrotherapy room, retail, inventory, and gift certificate sales.

Management/Personnel

1. What is your management experience? Include experience in the business field and elsewhere.
2. What is the legal structure of your business? Examples of legal structures are sole proprietorship, partnership, limited liability partnership, corporation, and limited liability corporation. Contact an accountant to set up bookkeeping and enlist an attorney to discuss with you the pros and cons of different legal structures and to draw up proper legal documents.
3. Who will be the other key figures in your business? Include an organizational chart, list of duties/back-

Choice of Business Entity

Business enterprises may take many forms. Common choices in for-profit entities include **proprietorships, corporations, partnerships,** and **limited liability companies.** Not-for-profit businesses may organize as **membership** or **stock nonprofit corporations** or **trusts.** The choice of format has compliance, tax, and liability consequences that call for consultation with lawyers, accountants, and other experts; however, some insight into these matters can make a consultation more efficient and beneficial. Most massage therapists organize their businesses as for-profit entities, so this will be our primary focus.

Proprietorship, or sole proprietorship, has a single owner. It is the simplest and least expensive to open. The owner provides all the capital and receives all the profits. Legally there is no distinction between the business and the owner. Creditors of the proprietorship may look to the owner's personal assets, as well as to business assets, to satisfy their claims. Also, people injured by an employee of the proprietorship during the course of employment may pursue a claim against the owner of the proprietorship. In the case of a proprietorship that uses a different name than that of the owner, the proprietor often must make a filing under local statutes to protect the use of the assumed name. The profits or losses of the business are reported on the owner's personal tax return, in most cases on schedule C to a 1040 federal individual tax return. A sole proprietorship is recommended for the small-business person who is just getting started. Other benefits of sole proprietorship are that the owner has complete control and that the business may be easily terminated.

Corporations. The Internal Revenue Code divides for-profit corporations into two categories: C and S corporations. C corporations pay federal taxes on their income. Subject to many complex exceptions, the income or loss of S corporations flows to those holding their shares. A properly organized and operated corporation of either type may limit the owner's liability. Limiting liability is the principal reason most small-business owners organize in the corporate format. Apart from filing tax returns, corporations must pay fees and give certain notices to state government periodically. Where corporations have more than one shareholder, issues of corporate governance require careful thought. Shareholders elect directors, who in turn govern the corporation. The manner of casting and counting those votes can differ markedly from corporation to corporation. Questions that organizers may wish to discuss with their attorneys include: (1) What happens if the shareholders disagree on a fundamental issue? (2) If a death or divorce changes share ownership, will the remaining shareholders have a right to purchase and, if so, at what price? (3) What happens if a shareholder working in the business becomes disabled?

Partnerships act much like S corporations in that they have the characteristic of flow-through taxation. Partners generally reflect partnership income and losses on their schedule E to form 1040 from information included in a K-1. Partnerships are easier to form than corporations, and investment expense is shared among the partners; however, authority is divided, and the partners must all have good personal chemistry. Partnerships can have *general partners* who have shared responsibility for decisions, share in the profits, and share in personal liability. *Limited partners* do not actively participate in the management of the partnership, but still receive a profit and are only liable up to the amount of their personal investment.

Limited liability companies have appeared fairly recently as organizational choices. As a consequence of the "check the box" regulations, the owner of a one-member company can treat the business for tax purposes as a corporation or report any income and expense on the owner's 1040, schedule C. A limited liability company with two or more members may elect corporate or partnership taxation. Members can generally limit their liability to their equity in the company. However, as a practical matter, banks, landlords and other significant trade creditors may require the members to personally guarantee some of the company's obligations. Limited liability companies contrast with limited partnerships in that a member can retain protection against the company's general creditors while actively participating in the business. The laws of most jurisdictions permit the owners of limited liability companies to conduct most of their affairs in private.

Nonprofit Organizations provide employment for many therapists. Occasionally the therapists are instrumental in their organization. The organizers and management of nonprofit entities can receive reasonable compensation for their services, but as the name implies no profits are earned and divided. Nonprofit organizations employing therapists usually fall into the classification of private operating foundations or publicly supported charities. These organizations pay no income tax and thus may reinvest their earnings without depletion for taxes in additional equipment and services for those they serve. On the other hand, the organizers do not build equity.

grounds of key individuals, outside consultants/advisers, and board of directors.
4. How will your services be provided? Will you use employees or contract labor?
5. Describe the types of support your business requires. This list can include child care, janitorial service, lawn and garden care, bookkeeping and accounting.
6. Describe the wages you will pay each type of employee.

Insurance Needs

What types of insurance do you have? What types of insurance will you need to operate your business? How much coverage do you need?

Insurance needs vary from person to person and from time to time. A reputable insurance agent should be contacted to discuss your individual insurance needs. Some of your insurance needs can be obtained through professional massage organizations.

Professional Liability

Also referred to as malpractice insurance and errors and omission insurance, professional liability covers liability costs rising from your professional activities. Massage therapists are accountable for their actions and may be held liable for any mistakes made while performing that service. Most affordable professional liability policies are available through the major massage and bodywork professional associations.

General Liability

Also referred to as premise liability, general liability takes care of liability costs that are a result from bodily injury, property damage, and personal injury incurred when the client is on your premises.

Business Personal Property

This type of insurance covers the cost of business property, such as a desk, massage table, chairs, and stereo equipment in your business location.

Automobile

Some states require that you have an automobile policy that is rated for business use if you travel to a client's home or office.

Disability Insurance

If you need income protection, you may want to obtain disability insurance. This type of insurance provides you with disability income in the event that you cannot work due to illness or injury.

SETTING UP YOUR PRACTICE: LICENSING AND PERMITS

The following is a list of licenses and permits that may be required before starting your massage therapy business. Each state, county/parish, and municipality is different in how these licenses and permits are issued. Please contact your local city hall for the proper procedure. The local small-business administration may be of assistance as well.

Find Out What the Prelicensing Requirements Are in Your State

If you do not know whether your state has a massage licensing board, contact your state attorney's office or the secretary of state. If there is *not* a massage board or a state licensing program for massage, it is recommended that you contact the National Certification Board for Therapeutic Massage and Bodywork (NCBTMB; 800-296-0664) and request an application for certification. You may want to do this anyway, for the prestige of being nationally certified, even if your state does have a licensing board.

If your state *does* have a licensing board, request by mail or by phone an information packet, an application, and a list of upcoming testing dates. Carefully read the state requirements, and be sure the program you choose meets or exceeds the state standards. Preparation for certification may include successfully completing an approved course of study and an internship program. Some states require not only a minimum number of hours but also how many hours are required in each subject area. It may also be helpful to get a copy of your state's massage therapy laws. Many massage therapy boards will *not* provide them for you, so you may have to check at the local library.

Obtaining Your Massage Therapy State License

Once you have graduated from a reputable massage therapy program, take the state exam or become nationally certified. Obtain an application form from the state or national board, and fill it out completely; an incomplete application may delay or void your testing date and may cost you a resubmission fee.

If your application is approved, you may be able to apply for a temporary license while you are waiting for the exam date and your test scores. If not, do not practice massage until you have received verification that you have successfully passed your state exam. In some states you may have passed your exam but you cannot legally practice until you receive your state license. This procedure varies from state to state, so be sure you obtain specific licensing instructions from your state board.

Your state board of massage therapy exists to protect the public. It is *not* its responsibility to inform you of proposed or current changes in the law. It is up to each massage therapist to keep abreast of changes in the state law, by attending open board meetings or local massage therapy association meetings.

Obtain Your Business/Occupational License

In most cities, you must acquire a business (occupational) license to operate any kind of business. Contact the clerk of court or the city planning department or appropriate public office in your area. Typically, part of the procedure of obtaining your business license is to have your business location approved through the city zoning department and the fire marshall. This process includes a home, or "cottage," business. All business licenses and permits should be displayed in a public place.

Apply for a Sales Tax Permit

Some states tax services. Most states collect taxes on goods sold. If either one of these scenarios applies to you, obtain a sales tax permit through state or county/parish taxing authorities. You will receive a gross receipts tax payer identification number and instructions on how to pay your sales tax, which usually involves monthly, quarterly, or twice yearly tax payments. You are usually allowed to choose a payment schedule when you apply for your sales tax number.

How to Register Your Business Name

If you have a business name (other than your name), you must register it with the city clerk's office or appropriate state office. Also known as a fictitious name, a "trade name," or a "doing business as" (DBA) name, the statement filed with the clerk's office will protect you from other businesses using your name and will ensure that you are not using a name currently registered by someone else.

Federal Tax Identification Number

Also known as an employer identification number (EIN), a federal tax identification number is issued to a business if you have employees or are incorporated. If your business falls into either of these categories, apply for a EIN number by filling out form SS-4, available at your local Internal Revenue Service (IRS) office. Your EIN number will usually begin with the prefix "72." All other business can operate using your social security number.

SETTING UP YOUR PRACTICE: DETERMINING START-UP COST

Your start-up costs will vary from person to person and from one geographical region to the next, but you need to take a realistic look at how much money you will need to open your doors. This section assumes that you will be working for yourself. Once you have made your initial calculations, you can make adjustments before purchases are made if you find that the figures are high. For example, you may decide that it will be more advantageous financially to ask another therapist to share certain expenses with you. High overhead and an office are risky when you are just starting out and do not have any clients. Some of these cost items, such as advertising and printing costs, will eventually have to be repeated. This worksheet will help you clarify your one-time start-up costs.

Equipment and machinery (massage tables, stereo, phone)	______
Room furnishings (shelves, lamp, chair)	______
Initial licenses and permits	______
Professional services (accountant, attorney)	______
Remodeling	______
Beginning inventory (cream, linens)	______
Initial office supplies (appointment book, stapler, pens)	______
Insurance prepayments	______
Rent prepayments	______
Advertising and promotion	______
Printing cost (business cards, gift certificates, stationery, forms)	______
Utility deposits and installation costs	______
Petty cash	______
Miscellaneous	______
Total	______

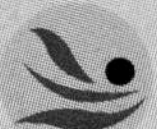

MINI•LAB

In your own words, discuss how you think massage can be used in our society today. You may include your own particular vision and how you plan to market yourself. Please include some facts on massage that you have learned in lecture or your own reading.

YOUR BUSINESS PHONE AND TELEPHONE ETIQUETTE

The telephone is the second contact between the client and the therapist. The first is your promotional advertising, such as a business card, brochure, or word of mouth. Due to the importance of the business phone, it makes good sense to spend time learning how to manage incoming calls and telephone communications. *Telephone etiquette* is the telephone behavior that is observed and used by people in social or professional life.

When answering your phone or recording your outgoing message on your answering machine, always speak slowly and clearly. Begin with "Good morning," "Good afternoon," or "Good evening," followed by your name, the name of your establishment, and an inquiry. For example, "Good afternoon. This is Jane Smith at the Nest. How may I help you?" Use a pleasant but expressive tone of voice. Smile as you are talking; most people can "hear" a smile. Avoid eating or chewing while on the phone as it is impolite (Fig. 28–3).

Find out the caller's name, and use it as you speak to him. Give him your undivided attention; listen carefully to what he is asking. Do not carry on two conversations at once. Be courteous and use words like "please," "thank you," and "you're welcome."

If you must place the caller on hold, ask permission and wait for a reply. For example, "May I put you on hold?" If he concurs, do not leave the caller on hold for more than 1 minute. If it appears that the caller will be on hold longer than that, offer to return the call. Always thank the caller for holding.

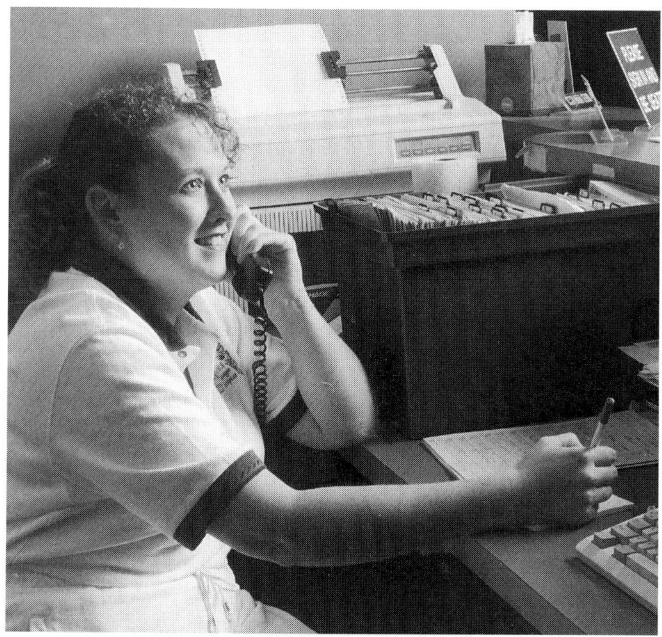

Figure 28•3 Telephone etiquette.

As quickly as possible, assess the caller's general needs, such as what kind of massage she is looking for (inquiry and listening are two important communication skills). If the caller wants basic information, have your answers ready and rehearsed. In the section of professional image, you were asked to take a few minutes to write down a 30-second introduction. Use this carefully thought out introduction during telephone inquires. It is often helpful to walk around as you talk on the phone. This may allow ideas to flow. If appropriate, give your professional background and licenses.

If the caller decides to schedule an appointment, your next task is to prepare her for the session. Inform her of the cost and the length of the session. If you have several options, give her that information so she can make an informed decision. If possible, prescreen the client for medical conditions that may contraindicate massage. Recommend that she not eat or eat only lightly 1 hour before the scheduled session and, if she comes from work, she might elect to bring clothes to wear home afterward. If you require that the client bring special items, such as shorts, a swimsuit, or a towel, tell her now. For best results, let the client know to schedule "downtime," or time to relax, after the session. If you have a cancellation policy, let her know when the appointment is scheduled. Give her directions to your establishment and any other information that you deem necessary. Last, ask if she has any questions.

Use a notebook-type pad to keep a record of incoming messages, including the date of the call, the agency and/or person who called, phone number and extension, why the person called, and the result of the call.

Be accurate and complete when writing messages. Repeat all the information back and check for accuracy before hanging up. When appropriate, tell the caller when to expect a return call. When ending the conversation, thank the caller for his interest and wait until he hangs up before you do. As soon as possible, give the message to the proper person. *Keep your promises, and return phone calls within 24 hours.*

Many massage therapists rely on answering machines, or "electronic secretaries," for their incoming calls, but in this ever changing world of technology, opinions differ about the benefits and liabilities of hi-tech devices. If you use an answering machine, keep the outgoing message short, and set the machine to pick up before the third ring. Many people do *not* like large voice mail systems, usually because they are time consuming. Voice mail is the choice of those who share large practices or who want every caller to have access to information such as location, hours, prices, and services offered. Although voice mail systems can be used, they must be used wisely by giving regular callers a "shortcut" code to get straight to your mailbox. Many answering machines have this option as well; pressing the "#" key may abort the outgoing message, sound the tone, and begin recording the caller's message. Other voice mail strategies are to begin the voice mail by telling the caller that he can leave a message at any time by pressing zero.

Another extension of your phone business may be your pager. Some therapists prefer to use a beeper that has voice mail capabilities, giving callers a personalized outgoing message when they dial your beeper. They then have the choice of keying in their phone number, which is transferred directly to your pager's display, or they may leave a short voice message.

Most pagers have two settings to alert the wearer to an incoming message; one is an audible "chirp" or beep, the other is a relatively silent vibration. It is recommended that massage therapists leave their pagers on vibrate and out of the massage room during a massage so as not to disturb the client.

Author's Note

A satisfied client will tell on average 3 other people how happy she was with the treatment she received.
A dissatisfied client will tell 11.

EMPLOYMENT OPPORTUNITIES

A career in massage therapy offers many employment opportunities for working with people in the healthcare industry. As a massage therapist, your personal practice may cover a wide range of services, from specific corrective massage and trigger point work to relaxation therapy.

As the medical community shifts its focus from sickness to wellness, the demand for massage therapy is on the rise. A variety of settings is available for massage therapists:

- Nursing homes
- Day spas
- Chiropractic clinics
- Acupuncturists
- Airports
- Truck stops
- Hospitals
- Cruise lines
- Resorts
- Casinos
- Hotels
- Psychiatric treatment centers
- Pain-reduction clinics
- Physical therapy and sports medicine clinics
- Athletic teams and dance companies
- Golf, tennis, and country clubs
- Gyms and health clubs
- Facial, nail, and beauty salons
- Corporate wellness programs
- Veterinarians (animal massage)
- Onsite massage in offices or shopping malls
- Private practice (in office or out-call)

Author's Note

Professional success often depends upon an integration of technical skills, anatomical knowledge, intuition, communication skills, business strategy, and tableside manner.

EMPLOYEES AND INDEPENDENT CONTRACTORS

Massage therapists often associate with each other and other businesses as common law employees or independent contractors. These classifications have extensive legal and tax consequences.

An employer usually sets the hours and place for employee massage services. Employers generally provide employees with the tools and materials required to perform the work and exercise and at least a measure of control and supervision over how the employees go about their tasks. The employment relationship typically involves a single employer and continues for an indefinite period (i.e., term of employment). Independent contractors, in most cases, receive a fee based on completion of the task. They usually have special skills, training, or licensure that allows operation without detailed supervision by others. Independent contractors often provide their own tools, equipment, or work area. They generally determine the precise time for performing services and work for more than one party.

Contracting parties occasionally attempt to characterize employees as independent contractors. This temptation may arise from an employer's responsibility to withhold income taxes on wages, contribute to social security, pay unemployment compensation insurance, and obtain workman's compensation coverage. These are significant compliance and financial burdens, particularly when the employer lacks bookkeepers and other associates adept at handling the necessary paperwork.

However, a mischaracterization can expose an employer to interest and penalties for missing tax payments. A common law employee treated as an independent contractor may take legal action for gaps in social security and unemployment compensation coverage. Even worse, if the employee has failed to pay income taxes due, the employer may have to pay the employee's taxes to the extent of the tax withholding shortfall. A massage therapist considering an independent contractor relationship should obtain tax advice from a lawyer or accountant to confirm that a proper characterization of the relationship exists.

YOUR CURRICULUM VITAE OR RÉSUMÉ

A **curriculum vitae** (CV), also known as a résumé, is an autobiographical sketch that documents all your achievements: occupational, avocational, academic, and personal information that you wish to disclose to a prospective employer or business contact. Even if you are self-employed, your CV will help you in business meetings, in developing business relationships, and in acquiring a referral base. A well-written CV will let your business contacts know who you are and what you can offer their employers, members, clients, or patients. A well-written and properly distributed CV will help you advance your practice.

Before you sit down to write your CV, take time to reflect on your life. What accomplishments are you proud of? What are the things that have brought you the most joy? Your list of accomplishments may include acting in a community play or assisting with a political campaign. Next, study the list. You might notice a pattern of personal strengths or interests emerging. You may find that you are a natural leader or that you work best with groups of people. This information will help you write your personal data section.

Now it's time to begin organizing and writing your CV. The most widely used format is the reverse chronological format, which emphasizes your education and work experience. Begin by writing your name, address, and phone number at the top center of the page, making them larger than the rest of the text. Use the following headings to organize your CV or use the format provided in Figure 28–4.

Education

List all your academic achievements in reverse chronological order. If you did not attend college, list your high school; if you did attend college, omit your high school in this section. Your education section should include the name of the educational institution, any college degrees, postgraduate degrees, certificates, or any awards or honors. Also include the dates you attended school and any major and minor courses that have helped you as a massage therapist (e.g., psychology, anatomy and physiology, or kinesiology). If you have attended any postgraduate workshops, list them after your formal educational achievements.

Work Experience

Starting with the present or most recent, list all the jobs held within the past 5 to 7 years. Include the names of your employers, the titles or positions held, job description, and the starting and termination dates. If you do not have any work experience in the job you are applying for, focus on your field experience while you were at school. Did you provide sports massage for athletes? Did you massage residents in a nursing home? Select the activities that will enhance your qualifications, such as hobbies, sports, and professional affiliations.

Personal Data

Although not necessary, this section is your opportunity to let an employer know about you. List your marital status, number and ages of your children, your general health status, and, if you are a nonsmoker, you may even list that. Include your date of birth. Use only the personal information what will help you project the positive image that you began to formulate in the preceding sections. You might even mention that you like to coach baseball or that you enjoy playing chess. This may create a pleasant image in someone's eyes.

Once your curriculum vitae is organized, type it on 8½″ × 11″ white bond paper. Keep your writing style simple. After you have proofread it once, let three other people proofread it for you. This is a good system for reducing grammar and spelling errors. Typos in a professional CV are taboo.

If you have a specific employer in mind, send him your CV along with a well-written cover letter addressed to a specific person in the company or organization. Avoid phrases such as "Dear Sir" or "To Whom It May Concern." Spell his or her name properly, and use his full name. If you are invited to an interview or a business meeting, call the day before to confirm. Arrive 15 minutes before the meeting begins. Within a week, send him a thank-you note, and mention how much you enjoyed the opportunity to share ideas.

ADVERTISING AND PROMOTIONAL STRATEGIES FOR THE MASSAGE THERAPIST

Advertising will let people know who you are and about your services. General advertising announces or reminds the public about your product or service, as well as creating a professional image for you. Specific advertising may be geared toward gift certificate sales or increasing the purchase of a new or existent service (i.e., reflexology). By determining your target group in the business plan, you can decide what advertising and promotional strategies are most effective because the most effective ads target a specific population.

Massage therapists should always consider a variety of means to get information to potential clients. Word of mouth—newspaper, radio, or television interviews—and community service have little direct cost, whereas professional brochures, business cards, news-

Resume of
James Michael Brown

- **James Michael Brown**
  555 Seoul Drive
  Middleton, LA 77777
  315.555.1212

Massage Therapy Work Experience

- **Owner and Operator** of The Body Shoppe-Massage Therapy by James Michael Brown and Associates, 1987-Present.
  Gulf Coast Physical Therapy, **Primary Massage Therapist,** 1987-1989.
  Middleton Hospital, **Outpatient Massage Therapist,** 1989-1990.
  Gulf Coast Chiropractic Clinic, **Primary Massage Therapist,** 1989-1994.

Education

- **Gulf Coast Academy of Massage Therapy,** Middleton, LA, 1987.
  Gulf Coast State University, Middleton, LA, Associate Degree in History, 1989.

Massage Therapy Certification Credentials

- Gulf Coast Academy of Massage Therapy, **Certified Massage Therapist,** 1987.
  Texas Department of Health and Hospitals, **Registered Massage Therapist,** 1990.
  Louisiana Board of Massage Therapy, **Licensed Massage Therapist,** 1992.
  National Certification Board for Therapeutic Massage and Bodywork, **National Certification,** 1993.
  Infant Massage Instructor Certification, **Certified Instructor,** 1990.
  Neuromuscular Guild of America, **Neuromuscular Therapy Certification,** 1995.

Continuing Education Credentials

- Aromatherapy for Massage, Gulf Coast Academy of Massage Therapy, 1988.
  Massage for the Expectant Mother, IMICA, 1989.
  Infant Massage Instructor Certification, IMICA, 1990.
  Sportsmassage I, Connecticut College of Massage, 1991.
  Sportsmassage II, Connecticut College of Massage, 1992.
  Anatomy Refresher for Massage Therapists, Gulf Coast Academy of Massage Therapy, 1993.
  The Cadaver Dissection Experience, Connecticut College of Massage, 1994.
  Insurance Billing and the Massage Professional, Connecticut College of Massage, 1996.
  Advanced Hydrotherapy Workshop, Gulf Coast Academy of Massage Therapy, 1996.

Professional Activities

- Member, American Association of Massage Practitioners, 1987-Present.
  Member, AAMP's National Sports Massage Team, 1987-Present.
  Captain, AAMP's National Sports Massage Team, 1992.
  Assistant Convention Coordinator, Texas Chapter of the AAMP, 1991.
  Member, AAMP's Texas Sports Massage Team, 1992-Present.
  Leisure Learning Program, Middleton, LA, 1988-Present.

Awards and Achievements

- Eagle Award for Small Business Achievement, 1996.
  Olympic Games, Sportsmassage Therapist, Gymnastic Venue, Atlanta, GA, 1996.

Publications

- "Massage and Sports Injuries," *Sportsguide Magazine* Fall 1990.
  "Ice and Tennis Elbow," *Sportsguide Magazine* Winter 1990.
  "The Runner's Survival Kit-Massage Included," *Sportsguide Magazine* Spring 1991.
  "Not for Humans Only-Massaging Your Horse" *Sportsguide Magazine* Summer 1991.
  "When Hamstrings Hurt...," *Sportsguide Magazine* Fall 1991.
  "The Shoulder Injuries of Duck Season," *Sportsguide Magazine* Winter 1991.
  "And you Don't Even Need a Prescription...," *Sportsguide Magazine* Sprint 1992.
  The Relaxation Vacation-a Guide to Massage When Traveling, Lifetime Publishing, Middleton, LA, 1995.

Hobbies and Interests

- Big Brothers/Big Sisters of the Gulf Coast, Volunteer Big Brother
  Travel
  Singing

Figure 28•4 A sample résumé.

paper, and radio are moderately expensive (television is fairly expensive). Most media that sell advertising can offer you a media kit. When looking at all the forms of advertising, you must consider not only the price but also the audience and timing. When an ad comes out is as important as what the ad looks like and what it says (Fig. 28–5). Let's look at a few promotional ideas:

1. Natural selling (your enthusiasm)
2. Word of mouth
3. Referrals from other professionals
4. Community service
5. Public speaking such as giving talks, speeches, or lectures
6. Teaching classes or workshops
7. Writing for newspapers, magazines, or newsletters
8. Direct mail—expect a low return (1 to 7 percent)
9. Booths—have dates for upcoming classes confirmed; give away lots, not just one big gift; for visuals, videos are eye-catching and memorable
10. Yellow Pages
11. Newspaper
12. Radio
13. Television

Some therapists use an advertising agency, which can help you make decisions about how, when, and where to advertise. Once you have a better understanding of the choices available to you, evaluate the ones you might like to use by asking these questions.

1. How much does it cost?
2. What kind of return will I get and when?
3. Will this form of advertising continue to bring a return or will I have to keep doing it over and over again?
4. Will it display my natural strengths and abilities?
5. Will it enhance my image and position?
6. Will it be something that I enjoy doing?
7. Does it reach my target market?
8. Does it contribute to my goals?

Business Cards

Also known as calling cards, business cards project a favorable image and let the public know how to contact you. Your card should be well spaced and not crowded with words or graphics. If you have a logo, use it on your business card as well as on every other piece of printed material. Make sure the type style is clear and easy to read and the phone number (including area code) is easy to locate by a larger and/or bolder type. Be sure to proofread all information before it goes to print. These guidelines are helpful for any type of printed media.

The appearance of the cards and where you place them will help determine who responds to them. For example, if your card has a waterfall or flowers on it, it will appeal to a certain type of client. If it has an illustration of a group of muscles identifying a group

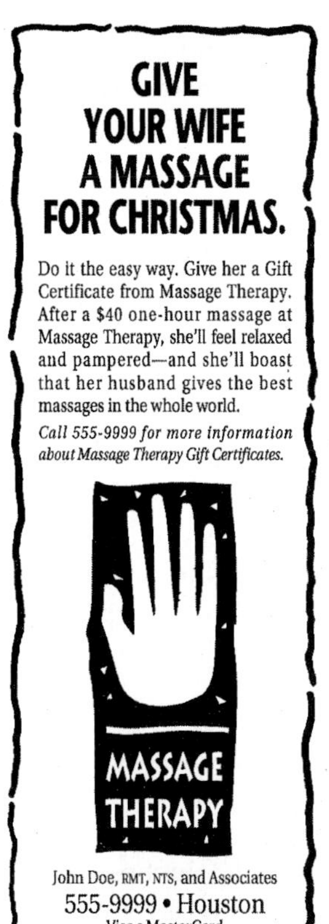

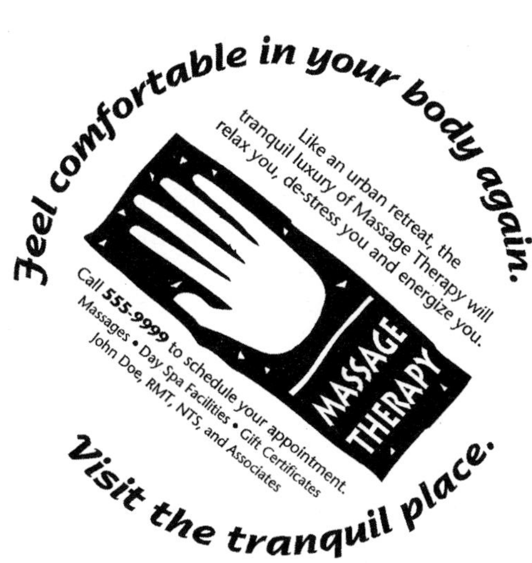

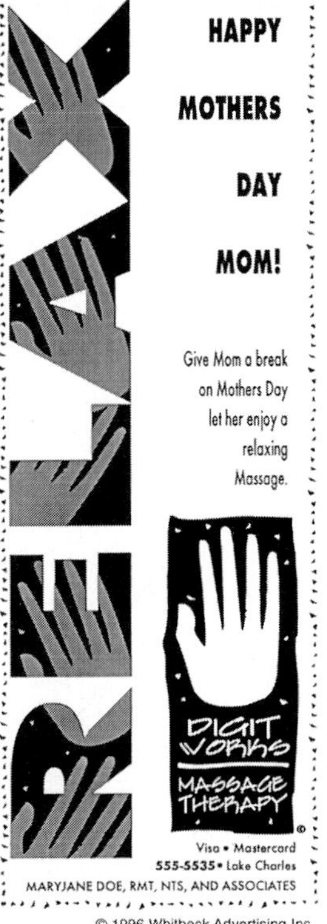

Figure 28•5 There are various ways to advertise a massage therapy practice.

of trigger points, it will also attract a different group of clients. Another idea for business cards is to have only have your name and phone number printed on them. When you hand them to a current or prospective client, she will already know who you are and what you do. This will help you develop an exclusive clientele. If you have an office in your home, you may choose to specify your geographical area (e.g., the Garden District) but not your home address.

Hand your card to people as you introduce yourself. Business cards may also be used for appointment cards. You may even use your business card as part of an incentive program by writing something like "$10 off next massage." Be creative and have fun, but remember, this is your "face."

Writing an Effective Brochure

The purpose of a brochure is to explain to prospective clients in some detail about you and your services. Professionally printed brochures are more expensive than business cards but, because of space, can be very effective in promoting your business. If you have an adequate computer, printer, and computer program, you can print your own. The most popular format is a trifold double-sided 8½″ × 11″ sheet of paper. This size can also be used as a mailer.

Begin your brochure with an attention grabber, perhaps a statement that conveys some benefit of massage, such as "Feel comfortable in your body again." Then describe the benefits people often experience (in your clients' words). Next, describe what you actually do, and give a brief autobiography. In your autobiography, give a brief description of your qualifications and, if appropriate, your years of experience. Be sure your phone number is large and readable at the end of the brochure. Close with a statement that may provoke action such as "Call now." Use vivid language, appealing to vision, hearing, and emotion-movement-touch (e.g., "One part therapy, one part luxury" or "Visit the tranquil place"). Note that you do not have to say things directly. For example, "Feel comfortable in your body again" or "Must be experienced to be fully understood." What mental images come to mind when you read those words! A brochure will read more easily if you use bullets and attractive graphics instead of paragraphs of text.

If you include your fees and menu of services in your brochure, you will have to reprint it every time you adjust your fees or add or delete a service. It is better to have a price sheet that slips into your brochure as an insert for this additional information. Avoid dating your flyer, for example, put "practicing since 1987" instead of "10 years of experience." Use fax machines and electronic mail to send out your brochure when someone calls you with an inquiry.

Once you have a rough draft, give it to three trusted friends and ask for feedback. Revise it as often as needed. Be sure that after reading your brochure, the potential client knows what needs you fill, and how you are different from others providing a similar service.

Author's Note

After graduation, throw a massage party. It is similar to a Tupperware party. Have one of your friends sponsor you. You give a small lecture, answer any questions, and give a demonstration (on a guest, of course). As a door prize, give away several massages. This is also a promotional idea once you are an established practitioner.

HOW TO WRITE A PRESS RELEASE

Part of your promotional strategy might include publicity writing and submitting press releases to newspapers as a way of letting people know what you are doing. Each workshop you attend, each office you hold, each lecture you give should be announced in the newspaper as a noteworthy event. This provides a subtle reminder of who you are and gives the message that you are active in your community and your profession. A press release is not an advertisement. If yours sounds like an advertisement, the editor of the newspaper will not print it.

Begin your press release with something that a newspaper will consider interesting and newsworthy. Keep it simple, and use a writing style that is direct and delivers a clear and concise message.

When writing your press release, use short words, short sentences, short paragraphs, and write in the present tense as much as possible. Make sure your press release answers the questions Who? What? When? Where? Why? How? Use the "funnel approach" of publicity writing. Place the most important information in the beginning of the press release and less important information in each subsequent paragraph. Then, if the editor has to cut the size of the release, important information located at the beginning of the release will not be eliminated (most editors cut from the bottom of the release). Last, and most important, proofread your work and ask at least three other objective people to proofread it as well (Fig. 28–6).

The following guidelines are helpful:

1. Type a press release on 8½″ × 11″ white bond paper.
2. Leave a 2-inch margin on the top and bottom of the press release; side margins are 1½ inches.
3. Date it and identify it as a press release by typing the words "Press Release" at the top center of the page followed by the phrase "For Immediate Re-

PRESS RELEASE

Contact Person: James M. Brown

Release Date: February 29, 1999

Phone: (318) 555-1212

TRIATHLETES RECEIVE MASSAGES: February brought to Metropolis the tenth annual Super-Man Triathlon.

The morning was surprisingly cold and windy. One would think the only people bold enough to brave the weather would be the triathletes...well, think again.

At 6:45AM, a group of people started transporting massage tables and equipment to the race site. These dedicated individuals were staff and students of the Gulf Coast Academy of Massage Therapy in nearby Middleton. School owners Ann and Barry McDonald coordinated the event in association with the Greater Metropolitan Runners Association and the Orthopedic Clinic of Dr. Cary Ellender, the event sponsor. The massage students and faculty volunteered their time to assist athletes before and after the event. The 22 massage tables were never vacant. Of the 230 entrants in the event, approximately 178 received complimentary sportsmassage. "I give the massage therapists an A+," commented the winner of this year's event, William Saunders.

"The massage is what I look forward to after the race," said another participant. Many people received their first massage during the event and expressed their desire to incorporate massage into their fitness and training routine.

Gulf Coast Academy of Massage Therapy students traveled from all over Louisiana and Texas to participate in this year's event. The students participating included: Laura Ardoin, Connie Bertrand, James Brown, Sehoya Butterworth, Geoffrey Curtis, Jamie Dubus, Charlie Duhon, Robbie Byrd, Charmaine Clement, Edward Griffin, Lanette Hidalgo, Clark Kent, Jill Maggiore, Faye Morvant, Debra O'Sonnier, Sam Parker, Martin Sheila, Jackie Short, Bo Scroggins, Sara Smith, Moxie Sporl, and Gert Verrett. Ernie Ogg, Susan Cormier, Cheryl Lavergne, Ann Gott, Tony Chapman, and Ken Duhon, school alumni, also donated their time and expertise for the event.

For additional information about sportsmassage or the Gulf Coast Academy of Massage Therapy, call 318-555-1212.

# # #

Figure 28•6 A sample press release.

lease." A specific date can be substituted if the release should be delayed.

4. At the upper left-hand corner of the page, identify yourself (or the appropriate person) as the "Contact Person," and include an address and daytime phone number.
5. Type only the lead sentence in capital letters; it should be action-oriented.
6. Double space the text if the press release is for print and triple space the release if it is for broadcast. Confine the release to one page (if possible), and type on only one side of the paper. If the press release is more than one page, write "More" at the bottom of page one. End the press release with either -30- or these symbols:

###

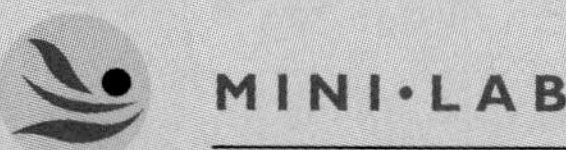

MINI•LAB

Using the guidelines outlined in this chapter, write a press release.

WRITING CONTRACTS AND PROPOSALS

When embarking on a new business venture, you may be asked to write a business contract or proposal.

A **contract** is a written agreement between two or more parties, that outlines expectations, duties, and responsibilities; it is enforceable by law. Begin with your ideas concerning the working relationship you wish to establish. A contract is more formal and more legally binding than a proposal and should not be taken lightly. In most cases, the other party will prepare the contract. If you are doing so, use your proposal to create a first draft of the contract, adding the following elements. Regardless of which party prepares the final draft of the contract, have your attorney look over it to point out possible problems. And remember, everything is negotiable, but negotiate *before* signing.

1. Clarify the business relationship of each party (e.g., lessor, lessee, employer, employee, partner, independent contractor, etc.).
2. The duration of the contract (e.g., 6 months, 1 year, etc.).
3. On what grounds the contract can be terminated, if before the previously agreed time.

A **proposal** is a written idea put forward for consideration, discussion, or adoption. By telling another your ideas, you make your intentions known. Many massage therapists entering the field will have the opportunity to approach businesses that do not offer massage therapy and to create a position for themselves or other therapists. The following are a list of proposal elements that can be used when addressing a sports group, nursing home, or any other business endeavor where you wish to be hired or to volunteer your services.

Title Page or Letter of Introduction

The title page should include your name (name of person submitting the proposal), title, address, and your telephone number. This page should also include the title of the project, and a 25-word summary introducing your concept of the proposed massage therapy services.

Purpose or Objective

This broad statement should embody the goal and/or expected results of the project, for example, "by providing stress reduction services to the employees of said corporation and to enhance employee productivity and reduce absenteeism." Next, the objective describes whom the project will serve and the geographic location. Then, discuss the significance and need for this project; compare your project with other projects in the same field and/or geographic locations (when applicable).

Logistics

Logistics (managing details of the operation) is the what, when, and where section of the proposal. If you are familiar with the facility, you may recommend a specific location where massage services will be provided. Briefly discuss physical arrangements such as room dimensions, bathroom location, lighting, equipment, and supplies. Mention which of these items you are willing to provide. State when your services would be offered. Are you proposing full-time or part-time work? Will massage services be available during the day, evenings, or weekends? One idea is to propose a part-time availability and to increase your hours as demand increases. Within what time frame would you conduct the proposed massage services, or what hours of the day will massage services be offered and who will pay for them?

Qualifications

This section will introduce you as a healthcare professional. Include a brief curriculum vitae of your training and experience. If you do not have postgraduate experience, focus on the field experience you acquired while you were in school. Introduce other people (such as staff or volunteers) that are key to the project, and give their training and backgrounds. Mention any professional affiliations such as the AMTA, NCBTMB, ABMP, IMA, and if the participating massage therapists are insured.

Approach

List and describe the modality of massage that will be used as well as its documented benefits. Include your justification for the chosen approach and specific outcomes anticipated. When appropriate, include a method of evaluating and reporting your anticipated results.

Communication

Outlined in this section is who is contacted as ideas are developed and as problems arise. State which person in their company will be responsible for managing the project, and define your organization's contact person, if different from the person negotiating the proposal. Specify how you can be reached. Include pager, mobile, daytime, and evening numbers. Also include a mutually agreed upon mediator (or third party) to help settle disputes if irreconcilable problems arise.

Funding and Budget

This important section outlines the projected budget for the project and includes the amount you are contributing (if any), the names (and amounts) of funds received from other participants, and the amount you are requesting from the agency or corporation. If needed, suggest plans for additional fund-raising. The budget should include both expenses and revenues for the entire proposed project. If revenue is to be generated by this project, outline who will benefit financially. This section should also include payment schedules and payment method.

Concluding Remarks

Your closing remarks, which will summarize your proposal, should convey a sense of warmth, camaraderie, confidence, and willingness to be of service in this project.

Brief Synopsis

This section is optional but useful during the meeting in which your proposal is presented before the board members. List all the elements in your proposal and "outline" their contents. Do not use complete sentences but rather a rough description of what each element entails.

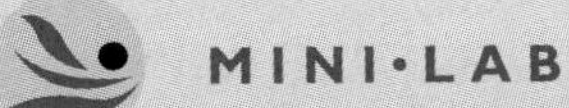

Using the guidelines outlined in this chapter, write a proposal and a contract.

INSURANCE BILLING

Another aspect of expanding your practice and increasing your income may be to incorporate insurance billing for your clients. There are advantages and corresponding risks in doing so. Because of the effectiveness of massage in treating musculoskeletal and myofascial pain, more and more doctors are referring to massage therapists. More physical therapists are hiring massage therapists to work in their offices. When the time-consuming work of massage is handled by massage therapists, the physical therapist becomes free to perform the more technically demanding tasks of evaluations, assigning exercise protocols, iontophoresis, and so on. Chiropractors also are taking advantage of the success of massage therapy by employing therapists within their practices and billing insurance for massage services.

In most cases, the requirements for reimbursable massage therapy services are that a medical or chiropractic physician write a prescription for treatment and that massage therapy helps the client to regain function. The usual reimbursable treatments are myofascial release, soft-tissue mobilization, massage, and hydrotherapy. In some states, these procedures can also be performed and billed to worker's compensation insurance following an on-the-job injury, to automedical insurance following a vehicular accident, and even to many common major medical insurance policies.

There are positive aspects of insurance reimbursement:

1. Fee repayments set by the insurance company are competitive with industry standards.
2. Treatment times are shorter, generally 15 to 30 minutes, allowing more clients to be seen in a day.
3. There is greater professional respect by networking with physicians and attorneys.
4. There is an ability to reach a larger percentage of the population for services.
5. Some clients respond better and make faster and more complete recoveries to massage than other treatment modalities.

The drawbacks of insurance reimbursement are specific:

1. A possible loss of money when litigation is involved
2. Time delay in receipt of reimbursement
3. Increased paperwork on each client

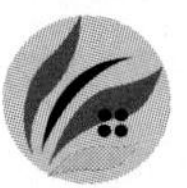

How to Handle a Nonsufficient Funds (NSF) Check

When you receive a nonsufficient funds (NSF) check, call the client and politely explain the situation. Tell him that you are mailing him a letter to serve as official notification and ask him for a specific time and date that he can deliver or mail payment. Write this information down. It is best to receive payment in a certified check, cash, or money order. Be sure to collect any NSF check fees. Send two copies of the letter: one by certified mail with return receipt requested and one by regular mail.

If you have not received payment within 10 days after you have received verification that the certified letter was claimed or if your certified letter was not picked up or refused, contact your local district attorney's office. Do not open the certified letter if it is returned to you. The district attorney's office may require a copy of the certified letter, your returned receipt card, or the unopened returned certified letter before collection can be pursued.

If you accepted a postdated check and it was returned, you have accepted a check knowing the person did not have money in her bank account. In this case, the district attorney's office may not be able to help you.

In any case, be pleasant, patient, and understanding. For your convenience, a sample letter to be used in these circumstances follows below.

Sample Letter

Your Letterhead with name, logo, address and phone number

Personalize the words in bold type to fit your specific situation.

Name
Address
City, State, Zip
Date

Dear **Name,**

The check we received from you in the amount of **fifty dollars ($50.00)** dated **August 15, 1998,** was returned.

We understand that occasionally these mishaps occur as a result of mathematical errors, mistakes on the bank's behalf, or sometimes a deposit not being credited to your account. These situations are often embarrassing but be assured that we are willing to work with you.

Please bring the above mentioned amount plus a twenty-dollar ($20.00) NSF check charge (total amount **$70.00**) to our offices as soon as possible. This payment must be made in cash, money order, or certified check. If you cannot come by our office, we will give you 10 days from receipt of this letter to mail your payment to us at the above address. Please do not send cash through the mail.

We are happy to provide you with massage therapy services and try to keep all collection attempts inside our office.

Please note the following office policies:

1. Payment is due at the time of service.
2. Should a check or credit card fail to clear, a notice (this letter) is sent to the client.
3. Failure to comply by making payment of original amount and NSF fees within the designated time frame will result in filing the check with the district attorney's office.
4. We reserve the right to place any client whose check or credit card has failed to clear on a cash-only basis.

Please contact us so that we can take care of this matter.

Sincerely,

Terry Pist, L.M.T.
1 copy certified mail
1 copy regular mail
1 copy to file

4. Increased accounting costs for handling billing and updating accounts

Special workshops are offered to prepare you to handle insurance clients. If you are still unsure about expanding your practice by working with insurance clients after taking the training, a part-time job with a physical therapist, doctor, or chiropractor can give you invaluable experience. You can also boost your in-

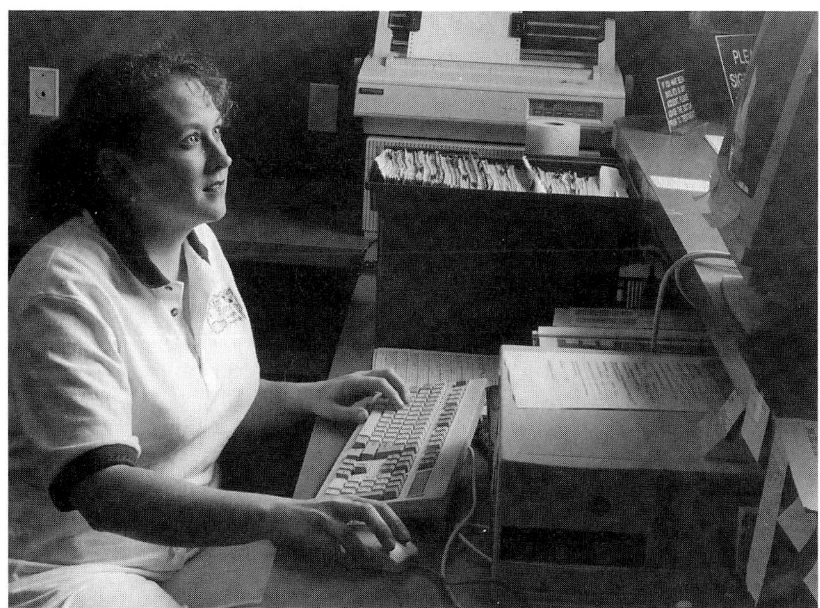

Figure 28•7 Filing insurance.

come, and you may even receive employment benefits. After you have become comfortable with insurance cases, you may want to work them into your own practice.

MINI•LAB

In your own words, define the following concepts.

For me, success is ______________________________

____

____

____

____

____

____

For me, security is ______________________________

____

____

____

____

____

____

LOCATING RESOURCES WHEN YOU NEED THEM

Another approach to business practice is to reach out to others. There are several good methods for doing this. The first involves finding a mentor, someone whom you can look up to in the business world and ask for professional advice. Your mentor may be an established massage therapist, a chiropractor, a physical therapist, a banker, or an experienced self-employed person. These people can act as a sounding board if you need perspective and can help in making decisions. The keys to finding and keeping a successful mentor relationship are clear.

1. Find someone you admire.
2. Find someone who is successful.
3. Find someone who is willing to be a mentor.
4. Be willing to learn from his mistakes.
5. Give back something to him. Money is probably not appropriate in this circumstance, but find a service that he needs such as cooking or baby-sitting or give a gift such as flowers, a book, or a massage. Show as well as tell him how much he is appreciated.
6. Remember that no matter what advice is offered the decision and the responsibility are ultimately your own.

The next method involves **networking,** developing business relationships with vast groups of people who are looking for the same thing you are—promoting their businesses. Ask someone who owns a local gift shop to sell your gift certificates. By sending prospective clients there, it generates traffic in her place of business and exposes her clients to *your* business. Work out a commission for every gift certificate she sells (suggested commission is 5 percent of the sale). Trade business cards with a popular hairdresser and manicurist, and agree to refer to them. Networking can be done through civic groups and business organizations such as your local chamber of commerce and the Rotary Club. It can be through informal luncheons with other business people.

Other important business resources include a variety of business and civic organizations such as your public library, the Small Business Association (SBA), and the Service Corps of Retired Executives (SCORE). Most major hospitals have medical librarians who can help you locate important information. Often your secretary of state can put you in touch with these resource organizations.

Furthermore, do not be afraid to approach people you want to learn from. These individuals are often pleased and flattered that you are asking them for their guidance. Membership in a professional bodywork organization is a very important resource and networking tool. Belonging to a massage association helps you to keep up with current trends, to exchange ideas with the only people who truly understand your problems, and to support actively your industry as a whole. Attend massage conferences and conventions often. There is nothing quite as inspiring as thousands of people gathered together who share a common experience.

If you are fortunate to live in the vicinity of a college or university, you will be able to develop resources on campus. Most colleges and universities have a business and marketing department. Volunteer your business as a project for graduate students who must analyze and prepare local businesses. The college library, which typically has more scientific resources available, is also a wealth of information and generally includes large periodical indexes, as well as an *Index Medicus*.

It isn't what you know when you start, but what you learn when you get out there. ❞

—Carol Kresge

CAREER ADVANCEMENT

Most people have several reasons for learning massage therapy such as personal success as a massage client, the personal fulfillment of helping others, financial reward, flexible hours, or being your own boss. But once you have worked in the massage field for a few years, what are the opportunities for career advancement? In short, where can you go from here?

The answer to this question is perhaps as complex as the question itself. First, look back at the beginning of this chapter to the section on goal setting. What does career advancement mean to you? Greater income? More free time without loss of income? Personal recognition? Travel? A line of work as you approach retirement? Before exploring these questions let's look at how you can improve your chances for success.

The pyramid approach is one of the keys to success in career advancement. The pyramid is a very stable geometric shape if placed upon its base. If you try to stand the pyramid on its tip, it is very unstable. When we build our careers, we need a wide base—the broader the base, the more stable the career pyramid. In this case, the secret is to become overqualified as a massage therapist. Thus, an essential element of your base is a massage school diploma (a college degree in *any* field is always helpful). Your base may include any combination of the following:

1. Your massage school diploma
2. Continuing education massage courses
3. A degree from a college or university
4. Postgraduate courses
5. A knowledge of computers
6. A course in business
7. Vocational experience and life experience
8. Red Cross or American Heart Association certification for first aid and CPR

Once your base is established, add more onto the pyramid and build it higher. Ask yourself, what are the five most important things in my life? Where do I want to go from here? What do I want to accomplish in my work? What skills do I want to develop? These goals represent the apex of the pyramid. Span the gap between the base and the apex by carefully choosing strategies that will enable you to achieve your chosen goals.

Here are some practical examples. Let's say that your goal is personal fame and notoriety. To you fame might mean a great reputation as a therapist and expertise in your field. Next, let's look at the cost. In this case, the price tag is patience. No one gets famous overnight (you could run through a convenience store with a chain saw to become famous, but this will not make you reputable).

After you have some initial experience in massage therapy, write a column for a local paper or magazine. Write about anything you are experienced with, and tie it back into massage. Stress and stress reduction are always good topics. If you like sports, write about ways to manage common sports injuries. Teach classes at the local massage school. Teach leisure learning classes to the public. Engage in public relations activities such as free massages for firefighters at a nearby station, and write a press release on it. Wear professional attire with a name tag or monogrammed shirt. Not only will you be promoting massage, personal recognition will come as more and more people recognize your name. In the words of Joan Rivers, "It took me seven years to achieve overnight success." There is truth to that statement because success takes time.

Perhaps your goal is to work in a certain aspect of

massage therapy because you enjoy it. Let's assume sports massage is your forte. Attend classes or learn how to play a certain sport, and practice, practice, practice. Once you become sore, you will know first-hand what areas to target because you will have a better biomechanical understanding of the sport. Give free sports massage sessions to players and coaches at your local high schools, colleges, and to professional teams.

If your goal is greater income, define what that is. If your goal is to make $50,000 a year, you are going to have to work hard and work smart. First we need to establish a formula. For the sake of making the arithmetic easier, let's say that you will take 2 weeks of vacation every year, giving you 50 workweeks per year, and that you will work 5 days a week or 250 days per year. Divide $50,000 by 250, and you make $200 per day. If you can do four massages a day at $50 per massage, you can make $50,000 per year *gross.*

Is more free time your goal? Once you have built a clientele base, hire an associate to help you keep volume high while you take time off. Realistically, you should decide how much income you need to live on, and then begin to limit the hours of your practice. Start by taking weekends off, then take either Fridays or Mondays off, to create a long weekend. You can even limit the times of day you work such as mornings off, and working noon to 7:00 P.M. or 2:00 P.M. to 9:00 P.M. One creative therapist works 3 days a week doing ten clients a day and takes 4 days off per week. If more time off is your goal, find creative ways to make it a reality.

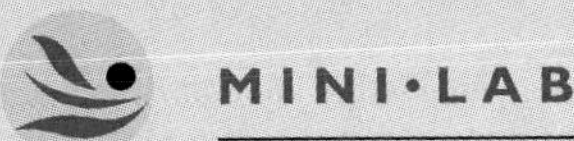

MINI•LAB

Design your own business card, and let it reflect your area of specialty.

DIVERSIFYING YOUR INCOME

The business world is often referred to as a jungle and the law of the jungle is survival of the fittest. One way for massage therapists to survive in the ever changing business environment is by diversifying their income. Diversity helps take financial stress off while you are building a clientele. The idea of diversity follows the same idea as financial investments: Do not put all the eggs in one basket. It is easier to find ten places to scrape up $1,000 each year than to find one place that provides $10,000. Diversify your income by using different strategies for producing revenue. Here are a few ideas to protect you from extinction.

Retail sales can bring in extra money. Clients may choose to buy individual containers of massage cream; massage tools; relaxation music on cassette tapes or compact disks; aromatherapy oils, candles, bath salts; and eye, neck, and back pillows. If you are going to sell retail, make sure that you have the proper license requirements. You must also collect and pay sales tax regularly. There are several things to consider when engaging in retail sales.

1. Make sure that the items you retail are affordable. Many clients will buy a $5 item, but only a few will buy a $100 item.
2. Have a significant markup. Common markups are between 50 to 100 percent.
3. The items should be related to massage or relaxation. Do not sell candy and cigarettes.
4. Do not tie up your money in a large inventory.
5. Sell what you use yourself or what you recommend.

Expand your services by offering clients a variety of treatment options. Some salons offer whirlpool baths, steam rooms, saunas, salt exfoliations, facials, and other services. Make sure that the services offered do not take away from the atmosphere of the massage environment. The sound of hair dryers and the smell of nail polish and acetone are usually not conducive to relaxation.

Specialized training is a good way to attract new business and expand your client base. Most states, as well as NCBTMB, require massage therapists to earn continuing education units (CEUs) each year. It may be worthwhile to take a training that will help you develop a new area of expertise. Learn an approach or technique that is unique to your community—something that will fill a gap in the existing market. For example, if you practice relaxation massage, attend a workshop in hydrotherapy, give some experience in the field, and develop a day spa facility.

Work in more than one location. This is especially true if you are self-employed. Locate part-time work a couple of afternoons a week for a chiropractor. Offer chair massage at the local health food store, a busy office building, or anywhere else there is high traffic. Practice foot reflexology treatments anywhere there is a shoeshine booth and split the proceeds with the owner. Take a new technique you learned and teach it at the local massage school. Offer a low-cost "leisure learning" class in massage or relaxation techniques at your local university for those who want to learn massage.

VOLUNTEERISM

Almost any massage therapist can tell you that this profession has it all. Almost everyone loves massage. Our work is personally satisfying, knowing that you helped someone each day. There are a variety of career opportunities open to massage therapists and many ways to express ourselves creatively. As blessed as we are by our profession, we should consider ways to return this good fortune to our communities. Perhaps the best way to accomplish this is through becoming a volunteer. A **volunteer** is someone who renders aid or performs a service without direct monetary gain. It is done of her own free will, usually with a sense of charity.

Virtually every known religion or philosophy is concerned with some form of volunteerism or charity. Volunteerism is a vital component of our success in the massage profession because it involves service; it's how we give back to the community that supports our practice. Massage has the ability to make a tremendous impact on our communities.

Virtually all great people perform acts of charity out of their regard for humanity. Some people may never receive massage because of economical factors. It may just be too expensive for them to make it a priority in their lives. Through the donation of your time and talents, massage can touch their lives. There are many ideas for volunteering such as doing postevent sports massage at local athletic events or donating gift certificates to civic and church groups as door prizes or auction items for fund-raisers. Get a group of therapists together, and support your local police and fire departments by giving free foot rubs or massages to each officer or firefighter. Donate time at retirement homes. Work with hospice programs to make the terminally ill more comfortable with massage. Donate gift certificates to schools for teacher appreciation week. The possibilities are limited only by your imagination.

Author's Note

Remember the ripple effect of the pebble tossed into the pond. I once donated a gift certificate to a local auction benefiting AIDS patients. The auction raised more than four times what the massage was worth. The eventual winner was a local doctor's spouse. She was so pleased with the session that she tipped me very generously and has been a regular client ever since. Additionally, she recommended me to her other friends, and my practice grew. Also, her influence was instrumental in getting two local surgeons to refer their clients for massage therapy.

OPTIMIZE YOUR SCHEDULE

When you arrive at the office, get there early enough to call your first few clients to verify their appointments. This not only cuts down on no-shows but gives you time to fill any slots that may be canceled. When returning calls to make appointments, always try to book your open slots of the current day first. Offer the client whatever slots you have open today and pause for his response. If he can't make it in with short notice, book him for a future time. But any client you can squeeze into today is an open slot that you may also be able to fill tomorrow.

As a last resort for those unfilled slots in the schedule, have a sign-up sheet posted on a clipboard for clients who wish to be called for cancellations and no-show slots. Go down this list and call each client, offering her the slot(s) you have open for the day. Keep

EXAMPLES OF TAX DEDUCTIONS

1. Accounting and bookkeeping fees
2. Legal, consulting, and professional services
3. Advertising and promotion
4. Bank service charges and card merchant fees
5. Interest on business and investment loans; business bank card interest and annual fees incurred
6. Books and periodicals
7. Mileage (cents per mile or deduct actual cost); keep a mileage log
8. Depreciation on major purchases
9. Conventions and conferences of business and trade organizations
10. Continuing education and professional development
11. Gifts to and entertaining current or prospective clients
12. Business-related insurance
13. Laundry and cleaning services
14. All license fees
15. Postage and shipping
16. Printing and duplication
17. Office supplies (including lubricants)
18. Rent (home office; use a ratio of either office space to total square footage or number of office rooms to total number of rooms)
19. Repairs to office or equipment
20. Uniforms and protective clothing
21. Utilities and phone (home office; use a percentage of utilities; should be the same percentage as #18; cannot deduct personal phone line, but can deduct business-related long distance calls)
22. Accounting courses (may be deductible as continuing education)

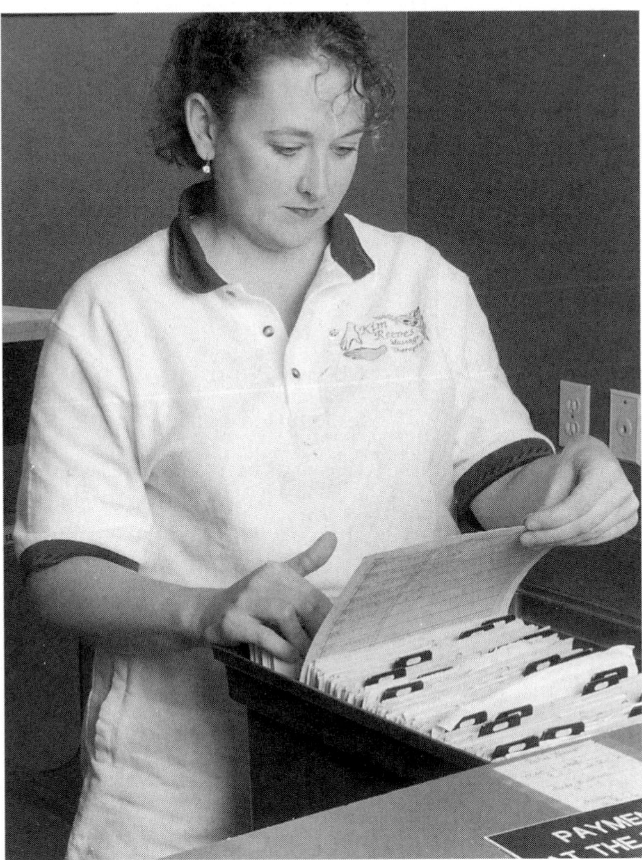

Figure 28•8 Optimize your schedule.

notes of who you called so that you start at the next name the following day. In this way you can maximize your schedule loading (Fig. 28–8).

For clients who canceled or failed to arrive for their appointment, call them and reschedule the missed session.

HOW TO PREVENT BURN-OUT

Burn-out is the condition of being tired of or unhappy with one's work. It does not discriminate against any race, gender, religion, or age and is not specific to one type of profession. It affects everyone from ditch diggers to neurosurgeons and leaves calamity in its wake. Symptoms of burn-out can range from simple disinterest in the job at hand to outright hatred of a job or employer. It can include boredom, depression, lack of productivity, increased tardiness, increased absenteeism, decline of social skills, workaholism, and a decline in professional boundaries. The added stress can also affect your health.

Burn-out affects people for different reasons. Many massage therapists are entrepreneurs and are highly motivated, hardworking people. Many self-employed people have difficulty setting limits on their professional time. Since there is no one to delineate a 40-hour week, self-employed people may overwork. If burn-out is due to overwork, it is possible that the therapist is mad at herself. The inherent danger with this type of burn-out is that at times this anger may come out "sideways" toward the client. The strategies for dealing with it are varied and depend upon the type of problem. Here are some scenarios and a few suggestions.

1. Exercise. This will help reduce stress and keep you fit.
2. It is extremely important that massage professionals schedule a certain amount of time off for themselves *every week*. Be flexible: If your massage days are Monday through Friday, take off Saturday and Sunday, or if everyone wants Saturday massages, take off Sunday and Monday. Remember that you cannot give away what you do not have and that it is necessary to recharge your own batteries.
3. It is important for a therapist to book some time off for himself on a *daily* basis. For example, if you know that you do not function well without food, schedule a lunch as well as a snack break every day.
4. Make sure you take a vacation every year. Get away from the office, especially if you work out of your home. Better yet, get out of town. Most therapists who have a home practice have a hard time refraining from answering the phone, doing paperwork, or booking massages.
5. Some therapists burn out from the boredom of repetitious routines and not being challenged. That's what continuing education is for! Take a class in something interesting and outrageous, not just massage technique and anatomy. Workshops also bring you together with your colleagues.
6. Go back, and reread the section in this chapter on values and goal setting. This will help remind you why you are doing massage.
7. Get massages yourself! Regular massages are a necessity due to the tremendous physical requirements of our work. The recommended minimum is one massage per month. There is no maximum number of massages you can receive, just make sure you can afford the time and the money, or just trade off massages with your colleagues (Fig. 28–9).

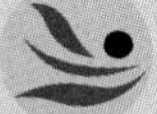

MINI•LAB

List ten things you like to do, and how long it has been since you have done them. When you feel excessively stressed, pick one of your favorite things and do it. This is also a great stress-reduction activity for your clients.

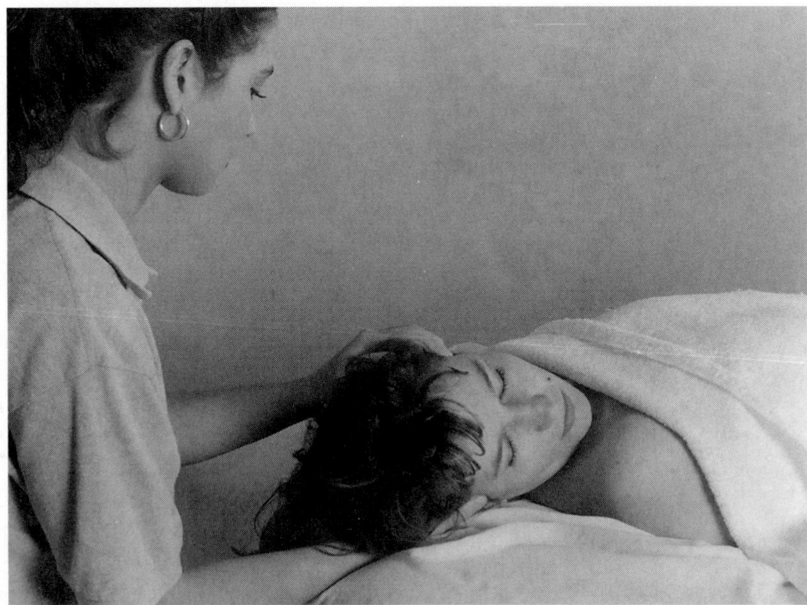

Figure 28•9 Get massages yourself.

SUMMARY

Basic business consists of two phases, the preparatory work and the actual business operation. The preparatory work includes the development of a business plan. To design properly an appropriate plan, take your personal values, goals, and professional image into consideration. Business plans will include details of services offered, hours, fees, marketing, protecting yourself with insurance, determining start-up costs, and obtaining licenses and permits. Once this is accomplished, you can open your doors.

It's been said that anyone can open a business, but keeping it open is the hard part. Staying in business depends upon how we treat our clients, how we advertise and promote ourselves, upon locating resources, career advancement, and diversifying our incomes.

If you find all this business thinking helpful, realize that this is just the tip of the iceberg. There are many ways to learn more about business. Your public library has more books about promotion, publicity, advertising, marketing, and selling than you ever dreamed of! Your local massage schools and professional organizations offer continuing education courses in business.

SELF-TEST

Multiple Choice • Write the letter of the best answer in the space provided.

_______ 1. Before you begin practicing massage therapy, it is essential that you examine

A. yourself
B. your market
C. your business
D. all of the above

_______ 2. How you behave in your personal, professional, and spiritual life typically comes from your

A. parents
B. needs, attitudes, and beliefs
C. neighbors and friends
D. health and academic background

_______ 3. What is a mission statement?

A. a statement of purpose
B. a bill of therapist's rights
C. the title of your house or car
D. your code of ethics

_______ 4. The guidelines for writing a mission statement are

A. shortness in length and in accord with your values
B. to begin with "My life work" and focus on the needs of other people
C. approved by someone you respect
D. A and B

_______ 5. Most potential clients have decided whether they will schedule a massage within

A. 5 to 10 seconds
B. 30 seconds
C. 30 minutes
D. 3 to 6 minutes

_______ 6. In this chapter, image is referred to as a

A. mental and emotional portrayal of you in the public eye
B. an instantaneous impression or picture of you when your name is thought of, spoken, or read
C. an illustration or photograph of yourself
D. A and B

_______ 7. Having integrity is

A. the condition of being whole and undivided
B. dealing honestly with yourself and with others
C. subscribing to a value system and adhering to it
D. all of the above

_______ 8. Which of the following is *not* involved in goal setting?

A. identifying your goals
B. writing these goals down
C. limiting your resources
D. developing a plan of action

_______ 9. Media are

A. midrange points of business
B. the middlemen in a business transaction
C. methods of mass communication, such as newspapers, magazines, radio, or television
D. business supplies used when making a brochure

_______ 10. Which of the following types of insurance provides you with income in the event that you cannot work due to illness or injury?

A. professional liability
B. general liability
C. business personal property
D. disability insurance

_______ 11. Also referred to as premise liability, this type of insurance takes care of liability costs that are a result from bodily injury, property damage, and personal injury.

A. professional liability
B. general liability
C. business personal property
D. disability insurance

_______ 12. This type of insurance is also referred to as malpractice insurance and errors and omission insurance and covers liability costs rising from your professional activities.

A. professional liability
B. general liability
C. business personal property
D. disability insurance

_______ 13. One-time start-up costs do *not* include which of the following?

A. salaries
B. equipment and machinery
C. room furnishings
D. utility deposits

_______ 14. The second contact between the client and the therapist is the
A. telephone
B. word of mouth
C. handshake
D. actual massage

_______ 15. Managing incoming calls and telephone communications is called
A. secretarial work
B. telephone etiquette
C. electronic secretary
D. office etiquette

_______ 16. Which of the following is *not* recommended when managing phone calls?
A. pick up by the third ring
B. find out the caller's name and use it as you speak to him
C. chew gum to keep your jaw in motion
D. verbally prepare him for the session

_______ 17. Which of the following is a written idea put forward for consideration, discussion, or adoption?
A. curriculum vitae (CV)
B. contract
C. proposal
D. opportunity

_______ 18. A proposal does *not* include a
A. title page and objective
B. background and education
C. qualifications and approach
D. funding and budget

_______ 19. A written agreement between two or more parties that outlines expectations, duties, and responsibilities and is enforceable by law is
A. a curriculum vitae (CV)
B. a contract
C. a proposal
D. an opportunity

_______ 20. Part of your promotional strategy might include publicity writing and submitting _______ to newspapers as a way of letting people know what you are doing.
A. short stories
B. press releases
C. novels
D. poetry

_______ 21. Some of the positive aspects of insurance reimbursement are
A. fee repayments set by the insurance company that are competitive with industry standards
B. time delay in receipt of reimbursement
C. greater professional respect by networking with physicians and attorneys
D. A and C

_______ 22. Networking generally means to
A. develop business relationships with vast groups of people who are looking for a larger clientele base
B. to take a course in basket weaving
C. to use methods of mass communication such as newspapers, magazines, radio, or television
D. to prepare written ideas and to put them forward for consideration, discussion, or adoption

_______ 23. Important business resources include a variety of business and civic organizations such as the
A. public library
B. Service Core of Retired Executives
C. Small Business Association
D. all are important resources

_______ 24. A _______ is someone who renders aid or performs a service without direct monetary gain. It is done of his or her own free will, usually with a sense of charity.
A. therapist
B. client
C. volunteer
D. consumer

_______ 25. Which one of the following is *not* important in preventing burn-out?
A. schedule time off frequently
B. attend continuing education classes
C. exercise
D. all are important

References

Ashley, Martin. *Massage: A Career at Your Fingertips,* 2nd ed. Mahopac Falls, NY: Enterprise Publishing, 1995.
Barnhart, Tod. *The Five Rituals of Wealth: Proven Strategies for Turning the Little You Have Into More Than Enough.* New York, NY: HarperCollins, 1996.
Beck, Mark F. *Theory and Practice of Therapeutic Massage,* 2nd ed. Albany, NY: Milady Publishing Company, 1994.
Boldt, Laurence G. *Zen and the Art of Making a Living: A Practical Guide to Creative Career Design.* New York, NY: Penguin Books USA, Inc., 1993.

Fritz, Sandy. *Fundamentals of Therapeutic Massage.* St. Louis, MO: Mosby–Year Book, Inc., 1995.

Gaedeke, Ralph, and Dennis Tootelian. *Small Business Management,* 3rd ed. Needham Heights, MA: Simon and Schuster, Inc., 1991.

Harrison, Bhanu Joy. *Business Practices: A Guide to Starting Your Massage Therapy Practice in New Mexico.* A self-published manuscript.

Palmer, David, A. *The Bodywork Entrepreneur.* San Francisco, CA: Thumb Press, 1990.

Peter O'Carroll Advertising. Lake Charles, LA.

Sohnen-Moe, Cherie. *Business Mastery: Business Guide for Creating a Fulfulling, Thriving Business and Keeping It Successful,* 2nd ed. Tucson, AZ: Sohnen-Moe Associates, 1991.

Whitbeck Advertising. Lake Charles, LA.

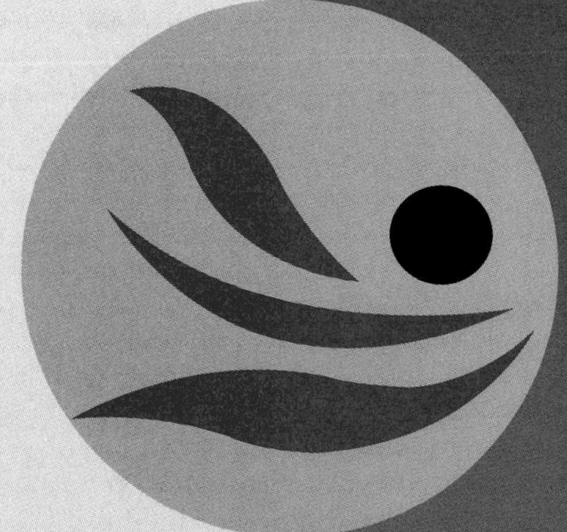

Appendices

Appendix 1. STATEMENT OF CLIENT RIGHTS AND RESPONSIBILITIES

1. I understand that, as the client, I have the right to request and require that any procedure or technique be modified, changed, stopped, or simply not performed.
2. I understand that I have the right to decline a particular procedure during a massage for any reason, including, but not limited to the fact that the procedure will or may cause me pain or physical discomfort or may make me feel uncomfortable or intrude on my sense of modesty and personal privacy. In short, I can "veto" any procedure at any time.
3. I understand that the relationship between the client and the massage therapist is a confidential one and that all information provided to the therapist and all statements made to the therapist are to be kept confidential by the therapist.
4. I understand that I have the right to present any grievances concerning the massage therapy or the therapist to the state board of massage therapy and a professional massage therapy association.
5. I understand that the massage is being given solely for the purpose of therapeutic massage and that the massage therapist also has the right to be free from any unwanted, harmful, offensive, and/or abusive physical contact or behavior.
6. I understand that the massage therapist reserves the right to end a session at any time, at the therapist's sole discretion. I understand that if the therapist ends a session in this fashion, an appropriate adjustment to and/or waiver of the charges for the session may be made if warranted under the circumstances.

Appendix 2. ABBREVIATIONS

Common Abbreviations and Symbols Related to Prescriptive Directions and Patient Charting

Abbreviation	*Meaning*
Tx	Treatment, therapy
Rx	Prescription, drug, or medication
OTC	Over-the-counter Rx
Dx	Diagnosis
Eval	Evaluate
Ex	Exam, examination
PRN	As needed; necessary or required
q	Every, each
qd/od	Every day
qod	Every other day
qwk	Once a week
#	Number
×	Times
per, /	Through, or by
qs	As much as required; sufficient amount
sos	Once only if needed
stat	immediately
Ø	No, none
c; w	With
s; w/o	Without
a; pre	Before
p; post	After
↑	Increase, above
↓	Decrease, below
→	Through, causes to results in
2°	Secondary to
Δ	Change
$\not\Delta$	No change
>	Greater than
<	Less than, caused by
+	Plus, positive, present
−	Minus, negative, absent

Symptoms

Abbreviation	*Meaning*
HA	Headache
P	Pain
P&B	Pain and burning
T/TEN	Tender, tension
NV/N&V	Nausea and vomiting

Symptoms commonly used by massage therapists that may not be approved by the Joint Commission on Accreditation of Healthcare Organizations and may therefore not be understood by all healthcare professionals:

TP	Trigger point
tp	Tender point
SP	Spasm
HT	Hypertonus
N/T; N&T	Numbness and tingling
ADH	Adhesion, fibrosis
L	Lesion
MFW	Myofascial web, continuous fascial planes
CON	Congested
ISC	Ischemic
M; ms	Muscle, musculoskeletal
INFLAM	Inflammation

Pathologies

Abbreviation	*Meaning*
HBP	High blood pressure
FX	Fracture
TOS	Thoracic outlet syndrome
CTS	Carpal tunnel syndrome
LBP	Low back pain
str.	Strain
spr.	Sprain
OA	Osteoarthritis
RA	Rheumatoid arthritis
CVA	Cerebral vascular accident, stroke
CHF	Congestive heart failure
TMD	Temporomandibular joint dysfunction

Massage Techniques and Modalities

Abbreviation	*Meaning*
~	Approximately
@	At
○—<	Recumbent supine position
⚲	Standing
⚲	Sitting
L	Left
R	Right
BIL	Bilateral
SUP	Superior, supination
INF	Inferior
ANT	Anterior
PRO	Promotion
LAT	Lateral, left anterior thigh
CAUD	Caudal
CEPH	Cephalic
PROX	Proximal
dist.	Distal
INT	Internal
EXT	External, extension
inver	Inversion
ever	Eversion
DEV	Deviation
ROM	Range of motion
PAROM	Passive-assisted ROM
PROM	Passive ROM
AROM	Active ROM
Pas Ex	Passive exercise
WNL	Within normal limits
Add/ADD	Adduction
Abd/ABD	Abductor, abdomen
int. rot.	Internal rotation
ext. rot.	External rotation
FLEX	Flexion
Hx	History
Px	Prognosis, physical exam
c/o	Complains of
PAT; PT; pt	Patient, physical therapy
DOB	Date of birth
DOI	Date of injury
MVA	Motor vehicle accident
NA	Non applicable
ADL	Activities of daily living

Abbreviated List

Abbreviation	*Meaning*
XFF	Cross-fiber friction
DP	Direct pressure
MLD	Manual lymphatic drainage
SwM	Swedish massage
M	Massage, general inclusive term
MET	Muscle energy technique
SCS	Strain, counterstrain
PNF	Proprioceptive neuromuscular facilitation
MFR	Myofasical release
STM	Soft-tissue mobilization
NMT	Neuromuscular therapy
CST	Craniosacral therapy
Ther-X	Therapeutic exercise, or procedure

Abbreviations Denoting Location and Specific Muscles

Abbreviation	*Meaning*
C1->7	Cervical vertebrae, spine
T1->12	Thoracic vertebrae, spine
L1->5	Lumbar vertebrae, spine
S1->5	Sacral vertebrae, sacrum
ITB	Iliotibial band
SI	Sacroiliac
LB	Low back
QL	Quadratus lumborum
SCM	Sternocleidomastoid
LATS	Latissimus dorsi
TRAPS	Trapezius
PEC Mm	Pectoralis major, minor
LEV	Levator scapulae
Gastroc	Gastrocnemius
TMJ	Temporomandibular joint

Appendix 3. UNITED STATES MASSAGE THERAPY BOARDS

Alabama
Board of Massage Therapy
300 N. Dean Road, Suite 5115
Auburn, AL 36830
Phone: (334) 826-3842

Arkansas
State Board of Massage Therapy
P.O. Box 34163
Little Rock, AR 72203
Phone: (501) 623-0444

Connecticut
Department of Public Health & Addiction Services
Massage Therapy Licensure
150 Washington Street
Hartford, CT 06106
Phone: (203) 509-7566

Delaware
Department of Administrative Services
Division of Professional Regulation
Commission on Massage & Bodywork Practitioners
Margaret O'Neill Building
P.O. Box 1401
Dover, DE 19903
Phone: (302) 739-4522, x205

Florida
Department of Professional Regulation
Board of Massage
1940 North Monroe Street
Tallahassee, FL 32399-0774
Phone: (850) 488-0595
Fax: (904) 922-2918

Hawaii
Department of Commerce & Consumer Affairs State Board of Massage
P.O. Box 3469
1010 Richards Street
Honolulu, HI 96801
Phone: (808) 586-3000

Iowa
Iowa State Department of Public Health Massage Therapy Advisory Board
Lucas State Office Building
321 E. 12th Street, 4th Floor
Des Moines, IA 50319-0075
Phone: (515) 242-5937
Fax: (515) 281-4958

Louisiana
Louisiana Board of Massage Therapy
P.O. Box 1279
Zachary, LA 70791
Phone: (504) 658-8941

Maine
Department of Professional & Financial Regulation Division of Licensing & Enforcement
Massage Therapist
State House Station #35
Augusta, ME 04333
Phone: (207) 624-9603

Maryland
Board of Chiropractic Examiners
4201 Patterson Avenue
Baltimore, MD 21215-2299
Phone: (410) 764-4726

Nebraska
Department of Health
Bureau of Examining
Board of Massage
State Office Building
P.O. Box 95007
Lincoln, NE 68509-5007
Phone: (402) 471-2117

New Hampshire
Department of Health
Bureau of Health Facilities Administration
Hazen Drive
Concord, NH 03301-6527
Phone: (603) 271-4592

New Mexico
State of New Mexico
Massage Therapy Board
P.O. Box 25101
Santa Fe, NM 87504
Phone: (505) 827-7013

New York
Board of Massage
Cultural Education Center
Room 3041
Albany, NY 12230
Phone: (518) 474-3817

North Dakota
State Board of Massage
P.O. Box 701
Dickinson, ND 58601
Phone: (701) 225-3906

Ohio
State Medical Board
Massage Licensing Division
77 South High Street, 17th Floor
Columbus, OH 43266-0315
Phone: (614) 466-3934
Fax: (614) 466-4670

Oregon
Oregon Board of Massage
800 NE Oregon Street #21, Suite 407
Portland, OR 97232
Phone: (503) 731-4064
Fax: (503) 731-4207

Rhode Island
Department of Health
Division of Professional Regulation
3 Capitol Hill, Room 104
Providence, RI 02908-5097
Phone: (401) 277-2827

South Carolina
Division of Professional Licensing
110 Center View
P.O. Box 11329
Columbia, SC 29211-1329
Phone/Fax: (803) 896-4494

Tennessee
Massage Licensure Board
Cordell Hull Bldg., First Floor
426 5th Avenue, North
Nashville, TN 37247-1010
Phone: (615) 532-5096
Fax: (615) 532-5164

Texas
Department of Health/Professional Licensing Massage Therapy Program
1100 West 49th Street
Austin, TX 78756-3183
Phone: (512) 834-6616
Fax: (512) 834-6677

Utah
Division of Occupational & Professional Licensing Board of Massage
P.O. Box 45805
Salt Lake City, UT 84145-0805
Phone: (801) 530-6551

Virginia
Department of Health Professions
Board of Nursing
6606 W Broad St., Fourth Floor
Richmond, VA 23230-1717
Phone: (804) 662-9909
Fax: (804) 662-9943

Washington
State of Washington Department of Health/Health Professions
Quality Assurance Division
P.O. Box 47869
Olympia, WA 98504-7869
Phone: (360) 586-6351
Fax: (360) 586-7774

Appendix 4. BUSINESS FORMS

(Permission is hereby granted to reproduce these forms in their entirety, including the copyright notices, for commercial or instructional use but not for resale.)

Daily Income Log for: Month ______ Year______

Page _____ of ____

No.	Date	Client Name	Fees Paid	Tips Paid	Payment Method (check one): Cash	Check	Charge	Gift Cert	Comp	Comments
1										
2										
3										
4										
5										
6										
7										
8										
9										
10										
11										
12										
13										
14										
15										
16										
17										
18										
19										
20										
21										
22										
23										
24										
25										
26										
	← Total no. of clients seen this period									
	Total Fees for this page →				← Total Tips for this page					
	Total Income for this page (fees + tips) →				← Cumulative Gross Monthly Income					

Yearly Business Expenses by Quarter for the ________ Calendar Year

Category	First Quarter		Second Quarter		Third Quarter		Fourth Quarter	
Advertising								
Auto Expense								
Bank Service Charges								
Books and Periodicals								
Childcare								
Continuing Education								
Donations								
Entertainment and Gifts								
Furniture and Fixtures								
Insurance								
License Fees								
Miscellaneous								
Office Supplies								
Postage and Shipping								
Printing and Duplicating								
Prof. Asso. Memberships								
Prof. Services (legal, acct.)								
Refunds								
Rent								
Repairs								
Retail Merchandise								
Taxes								
Telephone								
Travel								
Utilities								
Wages-Contract Labor								
Wages-Salary								
Wages-Owner's Draw								

Totals								
Grand Total →								

Gift Certificate Sales Log for: Month ______ Year______ Page ____ of ____

No.	Date Issued	Certificate Number	Client Name on Certificate	Name of Purchaser	Purchaser's Telephone	Certificate Value	Method of Payment	Date Redeemed
Ex.	01/02/99	1000	John Jacobs	Sherrie Jacobs	555-1212	$45.00	check	Jan. 23,1999
1								
2								
3								
4								
5								
6								
7								
8								
9								
10								
11								
12								
13								
14								
15								
16								
17								
18								
19								
20								
21								
22								
23								
24								
25								
26								
27								
28								
29								
30								

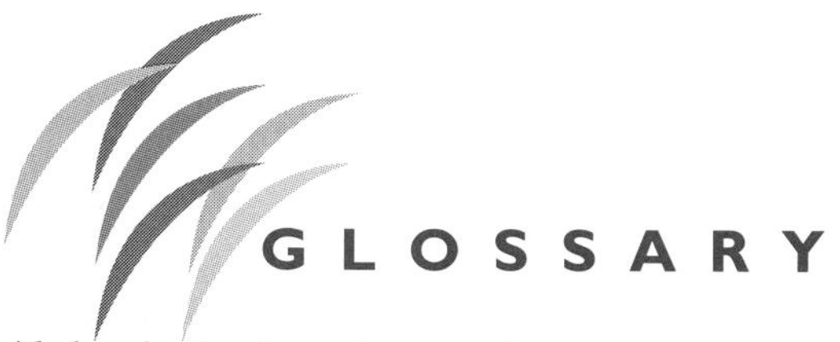

GLOSSARY

Abdominal Anterior trunk.

Absolute contraindications Conditions in which massage is inappropriate, is not indicated, and in which it may be harmful.

Absorption The processes by which the products of digestion move into the bloodstream or lymph vessels and then into the body's cells.

Acetylcholine A chemical stored in vesicles at the axon terminal located at the end of the motor neuron. It mediates nerve activity to the skeletal muscles.

Achalasia Failure of the lower esophageal sphincter to relax normally to allow food to enter the stomach.

Acid mantle A chemical barrier provided by the skin's acidic secretions that inhibits the growth of some foreign agents.

Acne vulgaris An infection of the sebaceous glands and hair follicles, caused by bacteria.

Acquired immunodeficiency syndrome AIDS is a disease caused by the human immunodeficiency virus (HIV).

Acromegaly Caused by the overproduction of growth hormone characterized by an elongation and enlargement of the bones of the extremities, face, and jaw.

Actin A thin myofilament. Actin is pulled over myosin filaments to produce the muscular contraction.

Action potential or **action current** A measurement of electrical difference between the charge inside the cell and the charge outside a neural cell membrane.

Active-assisted stretching Stretching in which the client contracts the agonist to stretch the antagonist while outside forces assist the lengthening action.

Active resisted stretches or **isometric movements** Stretches that involve the therapist applying gentle resistance while the client is actively engaging in the stretch.

Active stretches Client-instructed stretches or the therapist describing or demonstrating the stretch while the client actively follows along.

Active transport The movement of important atoms and molecules such as ions against the concentration gradient from low levels to high levels in order to maintain such vital processes as nerve conduction.

Acute Refers to those conditions that last for a short time, usually a few days to a few weeks.

Adaptation A decrease in sensitivity to a prolonged stimulus.

Addison's disease Caused by partial or complete failure of adrenal functions, often resulting from an autoimmune disease, local or general infection, or adrenal hemorrhage.

Adhesion Newly introduced fibrous tissue that forms an abnormal union between two previously separate structures.

Adipose tissue Another type of loose connective tissue, specialized for fat storage. This connective tissue also insulates the body against heat loss, provides fuel reserves for energy, and provides a cushion around certain structures (e.g., heart, kidneys, and some joints).

Adrenal glands or **suprarenals** These important glands are located superior to each kidney and are among the most vascular organs in the body. They are divided into two regions and, like the pituitary gland, possess two types of tissue, each producing different hormones.

Adrenocorticotropic hormone A hormone that regulates the endocrine activity of the adrenal cortex, especially cortisol secretion.

Afferent lymphatic vessels Lymphatic vessels that bring the lymph into the lymph node to be filtered and cleaned.

Agonist The muscle that is most responsible for causing desired joint action.

Aldosterone A hormone produced by the adrenal cortex. This hormone causes the kidneys to retain sodium, which stimulates the reabsorption of more water back into the blood plasma. The plasma volume of the blood increases, and blood pressure rises correspondingly.

Alimentary canal A mostly coiled, muscular passageway leading from mouth to anus.

All-or-none response Each individual muscle fiber, when sufficiently stimulated, will contract to its fullest extent. Likewise, in the absence of sufficient stimuli, each muscle fiber relaxes to its full resting length. This refers to nerve impulses as well.

Allergies Hypersensitivity and overreaction to otherwise harmless agents.

Alveolar sacs Two or more alveoli that share a common opening.

Alveolus Tiny sacs attached to the bronchioles. They are made of a single layer of epithelial tissue blended with elastic tissue.

Amino acids The building blocks of protein. There are 22 identified amino acids vital for proper growth, development, and maintenance of health.

Amphiarthrotic These joints are slightly movable (only a few millimeters).

Anal canal The final portion of the colon located between the rectum and the anus.

Anatomical position A standard body position; the body is erect and facing forward, the arms are at the side, the palms are facing forward with the thumbs to the side, and feet are slightly apart with toes pointing forward.

Anatomy The study of the structures and shape of the human body and their positional relationship to one another.

Ancillary Something that is auxiliary or supplementary to a standard.

Androgens A group of hormones that maintain male sexual characteristics.

Anemia A condition in which the oxygen-carrying capacity of the blood is decreased due to a decrease in red blood cells or a decrease in the amount of functional hemoglobin in the blood.

Aneurysm A weakness and dilation of a wall of a blood vessel.

Angina pectoris Often felt as chest pain, angina pectoris is frequently caused by constriction of coronary arteries and myocardial anoxia (lack of oxygen in the heart muscle).

Angiotensin II A powerful stimulant that has two major effects. First, it works directly on the blood vessels by causing vasoconstriction, which raises the blood pressure; second, it stimulates the adrenal cortex to release aldosterone.

Ankylosing spondylitis This is an inflammatory disease leading to calcification and fusion of the joints between the vertebrae and the sacroiliac joint.

Anorexia nervosa The prolonged avoidance of eating.

Anothomia Work written by Mondino dei Luzzi in 1316. Considered to be the first modern treatise on human anatomy.

Antagonist The opposing muscle that must resist, or yield, to the joint motion initiated by the agonist.

Antebrachium Pertains to the forearm; between the wrist and elbow.

Antecubital Space in front of the elbow or at the bend of the elbow.

Anterior or **ventral** Pertaining more to the front of a structure.

Anterior ramus The anterior branching of the spinal cord that innervates the extremities, the lateral and anterior trunk, and the superficial muscles of the back.

Antidiuretic hormone or **vasopressin** Decreases urine output by stimulating the kidneys to reabsorb water into the blood.

Antigens Substances, usually proteins, that stimulate production of antibodies.

Antiseptic An agent that retards pathogenic growth and removes pathogenic organisms from the tissues of the skin's surface and mucosa without damaging or destroying the tissues.

Anus The terminal end of the anal canal.

Aortic semilunar valve The semilunar valve between the left ventricle and the aorta.

Apnea A temporary cessation or absence of spontaneous respiration, typically 15 seconds in duration.

Apocrine gland A type of sweat gland attached to the hair follicles that is located in the axilla, the groin, and the areola surrounding the nipples.

Aponeurosis A broad, flat tendon that attaches skeletal muscle to bone, to another muscle, or to the skin.

Appendicitis An inflammation of the vermiform appendix often detected by acute pain in the lower right quadrant of the abdomen, vomiting, fever, and elevated white blood cell count.

Arachnoid The middle layer of the meninges of the brain that possesses many threadlike strands, giving it a cobwebbed appearance.

Areolar connective tissue One of the most widely distributed types of connective tissue. It has several types of cells: macrophages, fibroblasts, mast cells, plasma cells, adipocytes, and a few white blood cells.

Arrector pili The muscles of the hair that allow them to stand upright.

Arterial pulse The expansion effect that occurs when the left ventricle contracts, producing a wave of blood that surges through and expands the arterial walls.

Arteries Blood vessels that move blood away from the heart.

Arterioles Smaller, thinner branches of arteries.

Arteriosclerosis Narrowing of arteries due to the accumulation of hard lipid plaques in their walls, reducing blood flow, especially to the heart and brain.

Arthritis Several chronic diseases characterized by inflammation, swelling, and pain in the joints.

Asclepiades Founder of the group of ancient Greek physicians known as the Methodists.

Aseptic protocol Methods used to eliminate pathogenic microorganisms.

Association, connecting, interneuron, or **internuncial neurons** These neurons connect sensory to motor neurons and vice versa.

Asthma A chronic, inflammatory disorder in which the smooth muscles in the walls of the smaller bronchi and bronchioles spasm to close or partially close the respiratory passageways.

Atherosclerosis An arterial disorder associated with a buildup of plaque (made of lipids) in the blood vessels.

Athlete's foot A superficial fungal infection of the foot characterized by discoloration of the skin, a ring, or ridge of red tissue.

Atrioventricular bundle or **bundle of His** A bundle of conducting fibers arising from the distal portion of the atrioventricular (AV) node; it quickly branches into a right and left bundle, which run in the interventricular septum to the right and left ventricle. The AV bundle regulates the heart rate.

Atrioventricular node The node in the interventricular septum that is designed to work at a slower rate than the sinoatrial node in order to give the atria plenty of time to empty of blood.

Atrioventricular valves The heart valves separating the atria from the ventricles.

Atrium The superior heart chambers that receive blood from the body through large veins.

Aulus Celsus Ancient Roman writer, considered to be the first important medical historian.

Autoimmune diseases Part of a large group of diseases characterized by an alteration of immune functions. These disorders result from an attack by the body's own immune system.

Autonomic or **involuntary nervous system** Supplies impulses to smooth muscles, cardiac (heart) muscle, skin, special senses, some proprioceptors, organs, and glands.

Avicenna (980–1037) Name by which Persian physician Abu-Ali al-Husayn ibn-Sina was known in the West. He authored over 100 books that compiled all the theoretical and practical medical knowledge of his time, and was thus greatly influenced by the works of Galen of Pergamon.

Axillary Armpit; pyramid-shaped area formed by the underside of the anterior and posterior aspects of the shoulder.

Axillary nodes Lymph nodes located in the axillary region.

Axon or **efferent processes** A single cylindrical extension of the neural cell that transmits impulses away from the cell body.

Axon terminal or **telodendron** Fine filament-like terminal extension of the axon.

Æsculapius (Asclepius) A legendary physician who became the Greek god of medicine and healing.

Bacteria Unicellular microorganisms, most of which are not pathogenic or require living tissue for survival.

Balance The ability of the muscles, joints, and nerves to maintain static and dynamic stability while having the capacity to adapt to change.

Ball-and-socket joint Also referred to as a spheroid or a triaxial joint, this type of joint permits all movements and offers the greatest range of motion, such as the hip (iliofemoral joint) and shoulder (glenohumeral joint).

Ballistic stretching High-velocity, forceful, and sometimes dangerous repetition of a bouncing or bobbing motion. Each successive bounce increases the extension of the muscle.

Baroreceptors Pressure-sensitive receptor cells that affect blood pressure by sending impulses to the cardiac center and to the vasomotor center in the medulla oblongata.

Basal cell carcinoma A slow-growing skin cancer characterized by lesions that begin as small raised nodules that ulcerate.

Basement membrane The attaching surface of epithelial tissue.

Basilar membrane A membrane within the cochlea, containing sensory cells.

Belly of a muscle or **gaster** The central portion or bulk of the muscle.

Benign A condition that is not cancerous or life threatening.

Bicuspid or **mitral valve** The left atrioventricular valve containing two flaps or cusps.

Bile Produced from the hemoglobin in worn-out red blood cells, bile is not an enzyme but an *emulsifier.* It physically breaks apart large fat globules in the gastrointestinal (GI) tract into smaller ones and provides a larger surface area for the fat-digesting enzymes to work.

Biogenic amines These are the simplest hormone molecules and are derived from amino acids, like peptide hormones. These substances regulate blood pressure, elimination of waste, body temperature, and many other functions.

Bipolar neurons Neurons possessing two extensions from the cell body, one dendrite and one axon.

Blisters A collection of fluid below the epidermis sometimes caused by pressure or friction.

Blood pressure The pressure exerted by blood on an arterial wall during the contraction of the left ventricle.

Blood-brain barrier A very selective semipermeable membrane that controls which substances are allowed into the brain.

Body mechanics The proper use of postural techniques to deliver massage therapy with the utmost efficiency and with minimum trauma to the practitioner. Also known as biomechanics.

Bolus A ball-like, masticated lump of swallowed food.

Bonding A reciprocal relationship that goes from the caregiver to the infant and from the infant to the caregiver. According to Drs. Marshall Klaus and John Kennell, bonding is a "solid connection between the parent-child that nourishes the infant on a core level; the process that attaches the infant to reality."

Bone The hardest and most solid of all connective tissue, bone consists of compact tissue, a spongy cancellous tissue, collagenous fibers (for strength), and mineral salts (for hardness).

Borelli, Giovanni Alfonso (1608–79) Italian anatomist who carried out extensive anatomical dissections and analyzed the phenomenon of muscular contraction.

Boundaries The limits we establish between ourselves and others regarding various aspects of our lives.

Bow stance A foot stance used in massage therapy when applying any gliding stroke where length may be important. The feet are placed on the floor in a 90-degree angle, one pointing straight (sagittal plane) and one pointing toward the side (coronal plane).

Brachial Refers to the upper arm; between the shoulder and the elbow.

Bradycardia Slow heart rate (under 50–60 beats per minute).

Brain One of the largest organs in the body containing an estimated 9 to 15 billion neurons. The brain is divided into four major regions: *cerebrum, diencephalon, cerebellum,* and *brain stem.*

Brain stem The inferior part of the brain that contains three main structures: *midbrain, pons,* and *medulla oblongata.*

Bright, Timothy (c. 1551–1615) British Renaissance-era physician who taught and published on the use of baths, exercise, and massage to restore health.

Broca's area An area located in the frontal lobe (typically left hemisphere only) that regulates speech production.

Bronchi The large air-conduction passageways leading to each lung. Each tubelike structure is reinforced with hyaline cartilage to keep it open.

Bronchioles Smaller divisions of the bronchi.

Bronchitis An inflammation of the bronchial mucosa that causes the bronchial tubes to swell and extra mucus to be produced.

Bronchogenic carcinoma Also known as lung cancer, this condition is caused by a long-term irritant such as air pollution, cigarette smoke, asbestos, and coal dust.

Brunner's or **duodenal glands** Intestinal glands that secrete alkaline mucus.

Buccal Pertaining to the cheek area.

Bulimia Characterized by overeating (bingeing) and self-induced vomiting (purging).

Bunions Abnormal medial tilting and enlargement of the joint between the first metatarsal of the great toe and the associated proximal phalanx.

Burn-out The concept of burn-out is a familiar one for almost every profession. Simply put, burn-out is the condition of being tired of or unhappy with one's work. It does not discriminate against any race, sex, religion, or age.

Bursae A collapsed saclike structure with a synovial membrane that contains synovial fluid.

Bursitis Acute or chronic inflammation of the bursae is called bursitis. It is caused by infection, trauma, disease, or excessive friction or pressure in the joint.

Business personal property insurance This type of insurance covers the cost of business property, such as a desk, massage table, chairs, and stereo equipment in your business location.

Calcitonin Decreases blood calcium and phosphorus by stimulating osteoblasts (bone-forming cells) to make bone matrix. This causes calcium and phosphorus to be deposited in the bones.

Calf or **sural** Pertaining to the calf area of the lower leg.

Calyx A small expanded duct located at the apex of the renal pyramid. Note that there are *minor* and *major calyces.*

Capillaries Blood vessels with thin, permeable membranes for efficient gas exchange.

Capillary beds A collection of capillaries.

Capillary exchange The process by which nutrients and oxygen are provided to tissues and waste from cells is removed.

Carbohydrates Also known as starches and sugars, carbohydrates are classified according to molecular structure as mono-, di-, tri-, and polysaccharides.

Carbon monoxide poisoning A toxic, often lethal condition that is caused by the absorption of carbon monoxide through inhalation.

Carcinogenic Cancer-causing agent.

Cardiac arrest The sudden and complete cessation of the heartbeat, stopping all cardiac output, including pulmonary and systemic circulation.

Cardiac cycle The cycle of events occurring with each alternating contraction and relaxation of the heart muscle, coordinated by the conducting system.

Cardiac muscle A type of involuntary striated muscle found in the heart.

Cardiac or **cardioesophageal sphincter** The superior sphincter, found at the junction between the esophagus and the stomach.

Carpal tunnel syndrome A painful repetitive strain injury of the hand and wrist caused by compression of the median nerve.

Cartilage An avascular, tough, protective tissue capable of withstanding repeated stress. Cartilage is the slowest tissue to heal since it has no direct blood supply.

Cauda equina The ends of the spinal cord which fan out like a horse's tail.

Cecum The first section of the colon that is a small saclike structure located in the right lower quadrant of the abdomen.

Cell body, cyton or **soma** Part of the neuron that contains the nucleus and other standard equipment (i.e., organelles) of the cell.

Cell or **plasma, membrane** Separates the cytoplasm (intracellular) from the surrounding external environment (extracellular).

Cell The fundamental unit of all living organisms and the simplest form of life that can exist as an independent self-sustaining unit. Cells are the building blocks of the human body.

Centering A mental, emotional, and physical state of the therapist that is calm, yet responsive.

Central nervous system Part of the nervous system that occupies a central or medial position in the body. It is primarily concerned with interpreting incoming sensory information and with issuing instructions in the form of motor response. The major components of the CNS include the brain (cerebrum, cerebellum, diencephalon, brain stem), meninges, cerebrospinal fluid, and spinal cord.

Central Pertaining to or situated at a center of the body; it is often referred to as *deep.*

Centrioles Rod-shaped paired structures that appear as tiny cylinders positioned at right angles to each other and are associated with cell division.

Centripetally Toward the center.

Centrosome Dense areas located near the nucleus.

Cerebellar cortex The thin outer layer of the cerebellum.

Cerebellum A cauliflower-shaped structure located posterior and inferior to the cerebrum. The cerebellum is concerned with muscle tone, coordinates skeletal muscles and balance (posture integration and equilibrium), and controls fine and gross motor movements.

Cerebral cortex A thin gray layer covering the outer portion of the cerebrum.

Cerebral palsy A group of motor disorders resulting in muscular incoordination and loss of muscle control.

Cerebrospinal fluid A clear, colorless fluid circulating around the brain and spinal cord; it functions as a shock absorber and provides a medium for nutrient exchange and waste removal.

Cerebrovascular accident Also known as a stroke, a CVA is an occlusion of cerebral blood vessels by an embolus or thrombus, or cerebrovascular hemorrhage.

Cerebrum The largest part of the brain that governs all higher functions (i.e., language, memory, reasoning, and some aspects of personality).

Cervical Pertaining to the neck area.

Cervical nodes Lymph nodes located at the cervical region.

Chemoreceptors Sensory receptors activated by chemical stimuli that detect smells, tastes, and chemistry changes in the blood.

Chen-chiu ta-ch'eng Sixteenth-century Chinese work, written by Yang Chi-chou, that contains a discussion about pediatric massage.

Chief or **zymogenic cell** Another type of exocrine cell in the stomach, that produces the gastric enzyme pepsinogen, which is a precursor of pepsin.

Cholinesterase A chemical stored in vesicles at the axon terminal that enters the sarcoplasmic reticulum and neutralizes the effects of acetylcholine.

Chromatin A threadlike mass of chromosomes (genetic material) present in a nondividing cell.

Chronic Refers to conditions that have a long duration, in some cases, a lifetime.

Chronic illness A condition of the body for which there is no known cure.

Chyme A thin viscous fluid that is formed as food is blended and digested.

Cilia Projections on the outer surfaces of certain cells that can produce movement of particles or fluids.

Cirrhosis A chronic degenerative disease of the liver in which the hepatic cells are destroyed and replaced with fibrous connective tissue, giving the liver a yellow-orange color.

Cisterna chyli A large collecting chamber that gathers drained fluids from the lower extremities and from the digestive organs.

Client abuse Physical or emotional harm sustained by the client due to *deliberate* acts of the therapist. An abusive therapist is one who makes a conscious decision to take advantage of a client physically, sexually, financially, or emotionally.

Client incident report A report documenting an unusual occurrence.

Client neglect Physical or emotional harm sustained by the client due to lack of knowledge or sensitivity on the therapist's behalf.

Coagulation The ability of blood to clot.

Cochlea A coiled, fluid-filled cavity of the inner ear.

Code of ethics A set of guiding moral principles that governs one's course of action.

Cold mitten friction An application of cold accompanied by friction movements generated at a force of 5 to 10 pounds of pressure.

Cold or **ice immersion, baths** Soaking an affected area in a container of icy water. This method is ideal for hands and feet.

Colitis An inflammation of the mucosa of the large intestine and rectum characterized by weight loss, intestinal ulcerations, diarrhea, and bleeding of the colon wall.

Collagen An insoluble, fibrous protein that constitutes about 70 percent of the dermis and offers support to the nerves, blood vessels, hair follicles, and glands.

Compression massage Rhythmic pumping on a muscle belly to create a sustained increase in circulation and muscle relaxation.

Concentric, shortening, or **positive contractions** This type of isotonic contraction occurs as the muscle shortens, pulling on a bone to produce movement.

Conduction Involves the exchange of thermal energy while the body's surface is in direct contact with the thermal agent (e.g., hot packs).

Cones Photoreceptors of color vision. They are shorter and thicker than rods with short, blunt projections.

Confidentiality The nondisclosure of privileged information; that is, it may not be divulged to a third party without the client's permission.

Congestive heart failure In CHF, the heart is a failing pump. Causes include coronary artery disease, long-term hypertension, and myocardial infarct (areas of dead heart tissue from a previous heart attack).

Connective tissue The most abundant and ubiquitous tissue of the body. Some connective tissue types serve as nutrient transport systems, some defend the body against disease, some possess clotting mechanisms; other connective tissue acts as a supportive framework and provides protection for vital organs.

Constipation Infrequent or difficult passing of stools.

Contagious/Communicable Transmitted from one person to another, either directly or indirectly.

Contamination A process that occurs when an infectious, or causative, agent enters an organism (e.g. airborne, fluid-borne, direct contact). Once the organism is contaminated, the next phase is infection.

Continuity The uninterrupted succession or flow of strokes and the unbroken transition from one stroke to the next.

Contract A written agreement between two or more parties, that outlines expectations, duties, and responsibilities; it is enforceable by law.

Contracture An abnormal, usually permanent condition of a joint in which the muscle is fixed in a flexed position.

Contralateral Related to opposite sides of the body.

Contrast method or **contrast bath** The combined use of ice and heat. There are two variations: the alternate contrast method and simultaneous contrast method.

Contusion An injury resulting from a direct, blunt blow to soft tissues. A contusion is commonly called a bruise. The discoloration comes from blood escaping from the blood vessels that were broken or damaged during the blow.

Convection A more rapid process than conduction that involves the body's surface contacting heat energy through a fluid or gaseous medium (e.g., whirlpool bath or steam bath).

Coronary artery disease In coronary artery disease the coronary arteries are narrowed so that there is a reduced blood flow to the heart. The three main causes are atherosclerosis, coronary artery spasm, and blood clots.

Corpus callosum Large fibrous bundles of transverse fibers that provide a communicative pathway for impulses to move from one hemisphere to another.

Corpus Hippocraticum Collection of ancient Greek works that summarized much that was known about disease and medicine in the ancient world. Compiled by Hippocrates and his followers.

Corpus luteum Within the ovaries, a structure called the corpus luteum produces the hormones estrogen, progesterone, and relaxin.

Cortisol Affects carbohydrate, protein, fat metabolism, and when needed, produces an anti-inflammatory response.

Costal Referring to the ribs; the space near a rib or on a side close to a rib.

Coulter, John S. American physician who, in 1926, became the first full-time academic physician in the field of physical medicine, which became known as physiatry.

Countertransference An emotional reaction of the therapist that is generally a reflection of the therapist's inner needs and conflicts; it may be a reaction to the client's behavior. The projected feelings may be affectionate, which results in a positive countertransference, or they may be feelings of hostility or animosity, which creates a negative countertransference.

Cranial nerves Nerves originating from the brain.

Crepitus A noise produced by the body.

Cretinism A congenital deficiency of the thyroid hormones characterized by a lack of physical and mental development.

Crohn's disease A progressive inflammatory disease of the colon and/or ileum.

Cross-contamination The passing of microorganisms from one person to another.

Cryokinetics The application of cold, followed by full range of motion of the affected area.

Cryotherapy Refers to the application of cold on the body. It may include ice, icy water, frozen gel, or chemical cold packs.

Cubital Pertains to the elbow.

Curriculum vitae Also known as a résumé, curriculum vitae is an autobiographical sketch that documents all your achievements: the important occupational, avocational, academic, and personal information that you wish to disclose to a prospective employer or business contact.

Cushing's disease Classified as a metabolic disorder caused by an overproduction of adrenocortical steroids.

Cyanosis The presentation of bluish or dark purplish skin due to reduced blood flow, oxygen deficiency, and an increase in carbon dioxide.

Cystic fibrosis A genetic disorder involving the pancreas and the respiratory system.

Cystitis An inflammation of the urinary bladder and/or ureters caused by a bacterial infection from neighboring organs such as the kidney, prostate, or urethra.

Cytoplasm The gel-like intracellular fluid within the boundaries of the cell membrane.

Cytoplasmic organelles Small cellular structures that provide special functions such as reproduction, storage, and metabolism. Types of organelles are the nucleus, ribosomes, endoplasmic reticulum, Golgi apparatus, mitochondria, lysosomes, and centrioles.

De Arte Gymnastica Work written by Girolamo Mercuriale (1569) that is considered to be the first book written in the field of sports medicine.

De Humani Corporis Fabrica Written by Andreas Vesalius in 1543, the work is considered one of the most important studies in the history of medicine.

De Medicina Medical text written by Aulus Celsus that

bridged the gap between the Roman medical writers and the earlier Greek *Corpus Hippocraticum.*

Decompression sickness The unusual absorption of nitrogen, carbon dioxide, and oxygen in the body's tissues that impairs normal tissue oxygenation.

Decubitus or **trophic ulcers** Ulcers caused by constant deficiency of blood to tissues that have been subjected to prolonged pressure.

Defecation The process of eliminating indigestible or unabsorbed material from the body.

Deficiency diseases Caused by a lack of an essential vitamin or nutrient, typically interfere with the body's growth and development or help to establish metabolic diseases such as *scurvy* (deficiency of ascorbic acid or vitamin C), *rickets* (deficiency of vitamin D), and *beriberi* (deficiency of thiamine, or B_1). Deficiency diseases are not contagious.

Deglutition Swallowing.

Deltoid Curve of the shoulder and upper arm formed by the large deltoid muscle.

Dendrites or **afferent processes** Typically short, narrow, and highly branched neural extensions that receive and transmit stimuli toward the cell body.

Dense fibrous connective tissue Densely packed, strong collagenous fibers with fewer cells than loose connective tissue. This connective tissue type is not very vascular and so is slow to heal.

Dense irregular connective tissue Possesses collagen fibers that are ordinarily irregularly arranged. It can resist pulling forces in several directions.

Dense regular connective tissue Possesses bundles of collagen fibers in an orderly parallel arrangement that gives great strength and can resist pulling forces in one direction.

Depth The spatial distance into the body's tissue that is achieved through pressure application.

Dermis or **corium** Region of skin under the epidermis that contains adipose tissue, many blood vessels, and nerve endings.

Diabetes A family of metabolic disorders that alter the fluid balance of the body characterized by *polyuria,* an excessive excretion of urine, and *polydipsia,* or excessive thirst.

Diabetes insipidus Caused by a posterior pituitary gland dysfunction that results in deficient production of antidiuretic hormone.

Diabetes mellitus A group of disorders that lead to elevated blood glucose levels (hyperglycemia).

Diagnosis The identification or naming of a disease or illness by a scientific evaluation by a qualified practitioner or healthcare provider.

Diaphysis The shaft of a long bone.

Diarrhea Frequent passing of unformed, loose, watery stools.

Diarthrotic Also known as synovial joints, these are freely movable joints, allowing movement in one, two, or three dimensions.

Diastole The static pressure against the arterial wall during the rest or pause phase between ventricular contractions.

Diencephalon Located approximately in the center of the brain; houses two primary structures: *thalamus* and *hypothalamus.*

Diffusion The movement of dissolved substances from a region of higher concentration to a region of lower concentration.

Digestion The mechanical and chemical processes that occur as food is mixed with digestive enzymes and converted into an absorbable state.

Digital Pertaining to a digit; fingers or toes.

Disability insurance This type of insurance provides you with disability income in the event that you cannot work due to illness or injury.

Disassociation A coping mechanism to deal with traumatic events in which the person "leaves the body," does not feel, or believes that the abuse is happening to someone else.

Disinfection The process of removal of pathogenic microorganisms or their toxins from surfaces by a chemical or mechanical agent.

Dislocation Occurs when bones are forced out of their normal position in the joint cavity.

Distal Farther from the point of reference, usually away from the midline or a central point.

Diuretic Any substance that promotes the formation and excretion of urine.

Diverticulosis Pouchlike herniations of the colon wall where the muscle has become weak.

Documentation Information that is recorded on paper.

Dorsal cavity Located on the back, or posterior, aspect of the body; it is further divided into the cranial cavity (containing the brain) and the spinal, or vertebral, cavity (containing the spinal cord).

Draping Covering the client with a drape during the massage to promote warmth and a professional atmosphere that supports the client's need for emotional privacy (modesty) and comfort.

Duodenum The first section in the small intestine. It is between 10 and 12 inches long.

Dura mater The outermost meningeal layer, which is thick, durable, and lies up against the bone.

Duration The length of time spent on an area or the length of time of a massage.

Eccentric, lengthening, or **negative contractions** A type of isotonic contraction when the muscle lengthens during a muscle contraction.

Eccrine glands A type of sweat gland found in largest concentration in the palms of the hands, soles of the feet, and the forehead, and are absent in the nail beds, the tympanic membrane (ear drum), and parts of the external genitalia.

Ectoderm The outermost of the three cell layers that gives rise to the structures of the nervous system, the mucosa of the mouth and anus, the epidermis of skin, and epidermal tissues.

Eczema An acute or chronic superficial inflammation of the skin characterized by redness, watery discharge, crusting, scaling, itching, and burning.

Efferent lymphatic vessels Lymphatic vessels that take lymph from lymph nodes.

Effleurage An application of purposeful, gliding movements that follow the contour of the client's body.

Eicosanoids Also called local or tissue hormones, eicosanoids are produced by almost every cell in the body. They work on the cells that produce them or on nearby cells.

Elastic cartilage Is soft and more pliable than hyaline or fibrocartilage and gives shape to the external nose and ears and to internal structures, such as the epiglottis and the auditory tubes.

Elastic connective tissue Has an abundance of elastic fibers. It can be stretched and restored to its natural shape. It is found in vocal cords and in the ligaments connecting adjacent vertebrae.

Elastin Pliable fibers within the collagen fibers that give skin its elasticity, and resilience.

Electrocardiogram A device that records the electrical changes in the heartbeat as the impulse travels through the heart.

Ellipsoidal joints Also referred to as a condyloid joint, or a biaxial joint, ellipsoidal joints are essentially a reduced ball-and-socket joint. Ellipsoidal joints allow flexion, extension, abduction, and adduction, but rotation is not permitted (e.g., radiocarpal joints located in the wrist).

Embolus A blood clot, bubble of air, or any piece of debris transported by the bloodstream.

Emphysema Destruction of the alveoli, producing abnormally large air spaces that remain filled with air during expiration.

Empirical Something that is measurable and verifiable by use of the senses.

Encephalitis Inflammation of the brain typically transmitted by the bite of an infected mosquito.

Endangerment sites Areas of the body that contain certain anatomical structures that are susceptible to injury.

Endocardium The thin, inner lining of the heart that is continuous with the endothelial lining of the heart chambers and blood vessels, as well as with the valves of the heart.

Endocrine glands Glands with cells that produce secretions called hormones that diffuse directly into the bloodstream. Also known as "ductless glands," endocrine glands empty their products directly in the bloodstream, which carries the hormones to the sites of action.

Endocytosis A process that moves large particles across the cell membrane into the cell. The two main types of endocytosis are *phagocytosis* and *pinocytosis*.

Endoderm The innermost cell layer that gives rise to the lining of the alimentary canal, lining of the respiratory passages, and all tissues of the organs and glands.

Endomysium The protective covering that encloses each muscle fiber.

Endoplasmic reticulum A complex network of membranous channels within the cytoplasm.

Enzyme A catalyst that accelerates chemical reactions.

Epicardium Also called the visceral pericardium, it is the thin outer layer of serous membrane surrounding the heart. This protective layer possesses adipose tissue and the blood vessels that nourish the heart.

Epidermis or **cuticle skin** The superficial region of the skin that consists of four or five layers. Composed solely of epithelial tissue, the epidermis does not contain blood vessels. All oxygen and nutrients reach the epidermal cells by diffusion of tissue fluids from the underlying dermis.

Epiglottis One of the single laryngeal cartilages that closes the trachea during swallowing, preventing food from entering the inferior respiratory passageways.

Epilepsy The presence of abnormal and irregular discharges of cerebral electrical activity.

Epimysium The tough and thick fascial layer that wraps the entire muscle.

Epinephrine or **adrenaline** An adrenal hormone that increases blood pressure by stimulating vasoconstriction, rather than by affecting cardiac output.

Epiphyseal plate A flat plate of hyaline cartilage between the diaphysis and epiphysis of growing bones.

Epiphysis One or more shaft endings of a long bone.

Epithelial tissue or **epithelium** Tissue that lines or covers the internal and the external organs of the body, lines blood vessels and body cavities, and lines the digestive, respiratory, urinary, and reproductive tracts. The functions of this tissue include protection, absorption, filtration, secretion, excretion, and diffusion.

Eponychium or **cuticle** The tough ridge of epidermis (stratum corneum) that grows out over the nail from the proximal nail fold.

Ergonomics The scientific study of individual anatomy, physiology, and psychology as it relates to humans' work; adjusting the environment and equipment to support the alignment and balance of the body in its daily activities.

Erythrocytes Red blood cells, or red corpuscles.

Esophagus The muscular tube that connects the pharynx to the stomach. The esophageal lining secretes mucus to aid in the transport of food.

Estrogen Promotes the development of secondary sex characteristics in females. It is also known as the "feminizing" hormone, because it is responsible for female secondary sex characteristics. During the menstrual cycle, estrogen triggers the preparation of the female genital tract for fertilization and implantation of the early embryo.

Eustachian tube, auditory canal, or **auditory tube** This structure opens into the pharynx from the ear canal.

Excursion The distance traversed on the client's body or the length of a massage stroke.

Exocrine glands Glands containing cells that produce glandular secretions and use ducts to transport their products to the site of action.

Exocytosis The movement of large particles to the outside of the cell.

Expiration or **exhalation** A process that occurs when the diaphragm relaxes and ascends back up toward the thoracic cavity. Air is forced out of the lungs.

External Nearest the outside of a body cavity.

External or **pulmonary respiration** Gas exchange in the lungs between blood and air in the alveoli that came from the external environment.

Fasciculus A small bundle of myofibrils; can refer to bundles of tendons or nerve fibers.

Fast twitch A Type of fatigue-resistant fiber that is intermediate in diameter. It contains large amounts of myoglobin, many mitochondria, and numerous capillaries, but breaks down ATP quickly.

Fast twitch B or **white muscle** Rapidly fatigable fibers. They possess the largest diameters, have the lowest amount of myoglobin, few mitochondria, and few capillaries.

Fats Fats are composed of lipids or fatty acids and can range in consistency from a solid to a liquid.

Femoral or **crural** Pertaining to the femur or the thigh area; between the hip and the knee.

Fibrinogen One of the solutes in plasma that functions in blood clotting. When necessary, fibrinogen is converted to an insoluble fibrin, forming the foundations of a blood clot.

Fibrocartilage It has the greatest tensile strength of all three cartilage types. Fibrocartilage is found in the intervertebral disks, in the meniscus of the knee joint, and between the pubic bones (pubic symphysis).

Fibromyalgia A chronic inflammatory disease that affects muscle and related connective tissues.

Fibroplasia The process by which the traumatized tissue is repaired or rebuilt, following the clean-up of the trauma site.

Fibrosis or **scar formation** A process in which the original tissue type is replaced with a different kind of tissue. Fibrosis occurs when the damage is so severe that there are not enough healthy cells to reproduce the tissue required or when the damaged tissue does not have the ability to readily reproduce itself. The scar tissue formed by fibrosis is usually stronger than the original tissue.

Filtrate The term used to refer to the filtered fluids once it has crossed from the glomerulus into the glomerular capsule.

Filtration The movement of particles across the cellular membrane due to pressure.

Filum terminale The threadlike lower end of the spinal cord.

Fixators or **stabilizers** Specialized synergists that stabilize the joint over which the prime mover exerts its action. This allows the prime mover to perform a motion more efficiently.

Flaccid Muscles lacking normal tone that appear flattened rather than rounded.

Flexibility The ability of the muscles, joints, and soft tissues to bend and not break.

Flexor withdrawal reflex The reflex most commonly associated with pain by contracting a skeletal muscle and withdrawing the body part from the painful stimulus.

Follicle-stimulating hormone Stimulates oogenesis, or egg development, in the ovaries. It also stimulates estrogen production by the ovaries. In men, FSH stimulates sperm production, or spermatogenesis in the testes.

Fomite An inanimate object.

Foot reflexology A system of therapy based on the theory that our entire body, including organs, glands, and body parts, has reflex points located on the feet. Through applied pressure, one can release blockages around the corresponding body part and rebalance the entire body.

Fractures A fracture is a break, chip, crack, or rupture in a bone.

Free nerve endings or **nociceptors** Bare nerve endings that detect pain.

Friction A brisk, often heat-producing compression stroke that may be delivered either superficially to the skin or to deeper tissue layers of muscle, depending upon the intention of the therapist.

Frontal or **coronal plane** The plane passing through the body from side to side to create anterior (ventral) and posterior (dorsal) sections.

Fungus A microorganism that requires an external carbon source; multicellular fungi reproduce by spore formation. Fungal agents include molds and yeast, and their growth is promoted by warm, moist environments. Only a few fungal varieties are pathogenic.

Furunculus A boil or an abscess caused by the staphylococcal bacteria resulting in necrosis (death) of a hair follicle.

G Cells Endocrine glands located in the gastric mucosa that secrete the hormone *gastrin,* which initiates the production and secretion of gastric juice and stimulates bile and pancreatic enzyme emission into the small intestines.

Gait Refers to a person's walking pattern.

Galen of Pergamon (c. 130–200) Roman physician who synthesized and unified Greek medical knowledge. His works dominated Western medicine for over 1,500 years.

Gallbladder A pear-shaped sac located in a depression on the inferior surface of the liver that stores bile manufactured by the liver.

Gallstones The result from the fusion of cholesterol crystals in bile.

Ganglion A cluster of nerve cell bodies located in the peripheral nervous system.

Gastric rugae Longitudinal folds in the stomach to permit expansion.

General liability insurance Also referred to as premise liability, general liability takes care of liability costs that are a result from bodily injury, property damage, and personal injury.

Genetic diseases Caused by an imperfect genetic code in the chromosomes (structures found in the nucleus of every cell of the body). Examples of genetic diseases are Down's syndrome, cystic fibrosis, sickle cell anemia, and hemophilia. These genetic disorders are not contagious, but may be passed down from generation to generation.

Geriatric Refers to elderly clients who are 70 years of age and older.

Gestational diabetes mellitus May occur in women in the second and third trimesters of pregnancy. Hormones secreted by the placenta disturb the function of insulin, causing expectant mothers to become glucose intolerant.

Glandular epithelium A specialized type of epithelium that produces and secretes substances the body needs. These tissue cells lie below the surface of a gland, usually in clusters, and secrete their products either into ducts (exocrine glands) or directly into the bloodstream (endocrine glands).

Glaucoma A condition of elevated pressure within an eye due to an obstructed outflow of aqueous humor.

Gliding joints Also referred to as arthrodia or biaxial joints, these joints permit movements limited to gliding in flexion, extension, abduction, and adduction (intercarpal and intertarsal joints).

Glomerular capsule or **Bowman's capsule** The section of the nephron where urine formation begins.

Glomerulonephritis Also known as Bright's disease, glomerulonephritis is an inflammation of the glomeruli and is often characterized by blood in the urine, edema, and hypertension.

Glomerulus or **glomeruli** Loops of minute blood vessels contained within the glomerular capsule.

Glucagon Secreted by the pancreatic alpha cells of the pancreatic islets of Langerhans, it increases blood glucose levels, producing hyperglycemic effects.

Gluteal Curve of the buttocks formed by the large gluteal muscles.

Goblet cells Cells that produce mucus in the nasal cavity, which moistens the air and traps incoming foreign particles.

Goiter An enlarged thyroid gland associated with hyperthyroidism, hypothyroidism, inflammation, infection, or lack of iodine in the diet.

Golgi apparatus or **complex** A series of four to six horizontal membranous sacs typically located near the nucleus and attached to the endoplasmic reticulum, for the purpose of altering proteins and lipids.

Golgi tendon organs Receptors that are stimulated by both tension and excessive stretch and are located at the musculotendinous boundary of skeletal muscles. This protective mechanism helps to ensure that muscles do not become excessively stretched or do not contract too strongly and damage their tendons.

Goniometer An instrument used to measure the range of motion of a joint.

Gout A condition characterized by high levels of uric acid in the blood due to the inability of the kidneys to excrete this substance.

Gouty arthritis Abnormal accumulation of uric acid in the body, settling in the soft tissue around joints, typically the feet and toes, causing irritation, pain, and swelling.

Graham, Douglas O. American physician and Swedish massage practitioner who authored several works on the history of massage.

Graves' disease Caused by hyperthyroidism and characterized by related anxiety, fatigue, tremors of the hands, loss of appetite, and increased metabolic rate. An enlarged thyroid (goiter) and enlarged lymph nodes as well as an unusual protrusion of the eyeballs often accompany this condition.

Greater omentum A double-layered structure that attaches from the greater curvature of the stomach and the duodenum, draping down over the coils of the small intestine, to the transverse colon.

Groin or **inguinal** Area where the thigh meets the abdomen.

Gross or **macroscopic anatomy** The study of larger body structures, such as bones, muscle, nerves, blood vessels, visceral organs, and glands.

Grounding See **Centering**.

Gustatory organs The chemoreceptors nestled in spheric pockets on the superior and lateral surface of the tongue that detect the primary tastes of sweet, sour, bitter, and salty.

Gyri Elevations of the cerebral cortex.

Hair follicle Pouchlike depressions in the skin that enclose the hair shaft.

Hair follicle receptors Nerve receptors that respond briefly to hair movement.

Hara or **Tan tein** An ancient "center of gravity" that is a topographical *and* meditative point of reference. This area has been known for thousands of years in many cultures as the center of balance, both physically and spiritually.

Harvey, William (1578–1657) British anatomist who demonstrated that blood circulation in animals is caused by the beat of the heart.

Haustra A series of pouches created as "gathers" or "tucks" along the length of the colon.

Haversian canals Minute vascular canals found in osseous tissue that run longitudinally through the bone.

Heart The hollow organ, located in the mediastinal region of the thoracic cavity, that pumps blood.

Heartburn Failure of the lower esophageal sphincter to close normally after food has entered the stomach.

Hemocytoblast A matrix blood cell from which almost all types of blood cells are formed.

Hemocytopoiesis or **hemocytogenesis** The process of blood formation occurring primarily in the red bone marrow of long, flat, and irregular bones.

Hemoglobin A red respiratory pigment in erythrocytes.

Hemophilia A genetically determined condition in which a clotting factor is missing in the blood, making it difficult or impossible for the blood to clot.

Hemopoiesis The formation of blood cells.

Hemorrhage Excessive bleeding, either internally (from blood vessels into tissues) or externally (from blood vessels directly to the surface of the body).

Hemorrhoids or **piles** Varicosities of the rectal veins.

Hemostasis The cessation of vascular bleeding by either mechanical (i.e., pressure) or chemical (vitamin K) means or by the coagulation process of the body.

Hepatic portal system A pathway of blood that starts and ends with veins; it collects blood and nutrients from the digestive organs (stomach, intestines, gallbladder, spleen, and pancreas) and delivers it to the liver for storage.

Hepatitis An inflammation of the liver.

Hernia A protrusion of an organ or part of an organ through its surrounding connective tissue membranes or cavity wall.

Herpes simplex A viral infection that has the ability to lie dormant for extended periods without expressing any signs or symptoms of disease.

Hilton's law The nerve trunk that supplies innervation to a joint in the body also supplies enervation to the muscle of that joint and to the skin and connective tissue surrounding the muscles.

Hilus or **hilum** A depression in a lymph node.

Hinge joints Also referred to as a ginglymus or a monaxial joint, movements are limited to flexion and extension (elbow, knee, and interphalangeal joints).

Hippocrates of Cos (c. 460–375 B.C.) Greek physician; generally considered the "father of modern Western medicine."

Histamines A compound, found in all cells, that is released in allergic, inflammatory reactions, causing dilatation of capillaries, decreased blood pressure, and constriction of smooth muscles of the bronchi.

Histology The study of tissues.

Hodgkin's disease Cancer of the lymph nodes.

Homeostasis A relatively stable condition of the body's internal environment within a very limited range.

Homolateral or **ipsilateral** Related to the same side of the body.

Hormonal control system A system whereby hormones themselves trigger the release of other hormones in the endocrine system. One hormone can stimulate or inhibit the release of another through the hormonal control system.

Hormones Internal secretions that are the "chemical messengers" of the endocrine system. They act as catalysts in biochemical reactions and regulate the physiological activity of other cells in the body.

Horse stance A foot stance used in massage therapy when applying massage strokes that traverse relatively short distances, such as petrissage and certain friction strokes. Both feet are placed on the floor, toes pointing forward (in the sagittal plane) a little more than hip distance apart.

Hot pack Moist heat applications used for pain relief; also called hydrocollator packs, fomentation packs, hot compresses, and hot dressings.

Huang-ti nei-ching Chinese medical text that served as the classic on traditional Chinese medicine. The work contained descriptions of therapeutic touch procedures and their uses. Written sometime around 2,600 B.C.

Hubbard tank When warm water immersion is combined with light exercise; often in rehabilitation clinics because the buoyancy of the water allows easier movement and produces a soothing sensation.

Human growth hormone, somatotropin or **somatogrowth hormone** Stimulates protein synthesis for maintenance of muscle and bone growth. It also plays a role in metabolism.

Hunting response An up-and-down cycle of vasoconstriction and vasodilation that occurs if the initial ice application continues more than 9 to 16 minutes. One cycle of vasoconstriction and vasodilation may take from 15 to 30 minutes.

Hyaline cartilage An elastic, rubbery, smooth type of cartilage that covers the ends of bones (epiphysis), connects the ribs to the sternum (costal cartilage), is part of the larynx and the nose, and forms the C-shaped rings of the trachea.

Hydrolysis Chemical breakdown in the presence of water.

Hydrotherapy The external therapeutic use of water

and complementary agents, such as soap and salt, at temperatures no more than 8° from normal body temperature.

Hydrotherapy tubs or **spas** Similar to immersion baths and whirlpool baths, but the water is treated to remain clean and sanitary for multiuse.

Hygiene The collective principles of health preservation.

Hyperemia The observable reddened skin that results from increased blood flow.

Hypertension A common, often asymptomatic disorder of elevated blood pressure; 140/90 mmHg is regarded as the threshold of hypertension, and 160/95 is classified as serious hypertension.

Hypertrophy An increase in the size and diameter of muscle fibers without cell division.

Hypodermis, subcutaneous layer, or **superficial fascia** A layer of tissue under the dermis.

Hypoglycemia An excessive loss in blood glucose levels that can result in a variety of symptoms including weakness, lightheadedness, headaches, excessive hunger, visual disturbances, anxiety, and sudden changes in personality.

Hyponychium The thickened layer of the epidermis below the distal area of the nail.

Hypothalamus Governs many important homeostatic functions such as regulating the autonomic nervous system and the endocrine system by governing the pituitary gland, controlling hunger, thirst, temperature, anger, aggression, release of hormones, sexual behavior, sleep patterns, and consciousness.

Hypoxia A decrease in the amount of oxygen in the blood.

Ice massage Combining the use of cryotherapy with circular friction.

Ice packs Plastic or cloth bags filled with ice or icy water and placed on an affected area.

Ileocecal sphincter or **valve** Sphincter located between the ileum of the small intestine and the cecum of the large intestine.

Ileum The final division of the small intestine; it is approximately 9 feet long.

Impetigo An inflammatory skin infection caused by staphylococcal or streptococcal bacteria.

Infant massage A parenting tradition of loving touch that parents of many cultures have been using for centuries.

Infectious diseases Highly contagious diseases caused by a biological agent, like a virus or a bacterium. Examples are the flu, measles, and tuberculosis.

Inferior or **caudal** Situated below or toward the tail end.

Inflammation The body's immediate reaction to soft-tissue injury. Inflammation is a protective mechanism, and its purpose is to stabilize and prepare the damaged tissue for repair. The primary symptoms of inflammation are local heat, swelling, redness, pain, and decreased function or range of motion.

Ingestion The process of orally taking materials into the body.

Inguinal nodes Lymph nodes located in the inguinal region.

Initial evaluation A report that is written from your SOAP notes of the first session.

Insensible perspiration The constant evaporative cooling that occurs as microscopic beads of perspiration evaporate from the skin's surface

Insertion The insertion, usually located laterally or distally, is the muscle attachment undergoing the greatest movement.

Inspiration or **inhalation** The flow of air into the lungs that occurs when the diaphragm contracts and descends into the abdominal cavity, and when the external intercostal muscles contract to raise the ribs.

Insulin Secreted by pancreatic beta cells, decreasing blood glucose levels by enhancing the uptake of glucose into the cells.

Integrity The condition of being whole and undivided; the firm adherence to a code of moral or artistic values.

Intention A clearly formulated plan of action, generally based upon the needs the client has stated and the subjective information provided in the client intake.

Internal Nearer the inside (within) of a body cavity.

Internal or **tissue respiration** The gas exchange between blood and tissues throughout the body.

Interosseous membrane A tough membrane that interconnects select bones (i.e., the ulna and radius) by attaching to their periosteum. This is also referred to as the *interosseous ligament* because it connects bone to bone.

Interstitial cells of Leydig Within the testis these groups of specialized cells produce and secrete androgens, namely testosterone.

Intestinal tonsils or **Peyer's patches** Groups of lymphatic nodules found in the mucous membrane of the small intestine that combat pathogens we ingest.

Intimacy An innermost sensual (meaning an experience of the senses) bond to another in which the following elements exist: choice, mutuality, reciprocity, trust, and delight.

Invasive medical procedures Medical practices that involve puncturing or penetrating body tissues or entering a body cavity.

Inverse stretch reflex or **autogenic inhibition** The stretch reflex is mediated by the Golgi tendon organs. When Golgi tendon organs are stimulated by slow, low-force stretches, they inhibit regular muscle contraction, which relaxes the entire muscle and allows maximum stretching.

Irritable bowel syndrome A condition of the large intestine characterized by abnormal muscular contraction and excessive mucus in stools.

Ischemia A reduction of oxygenated blood to a body organ or part, often marked by pain and tissue dysfunction.

Islets of Langerhans or **pancreatic islets** Groups of specialized cells within the pancreas. The pancreas contains over a million islets, each consisting of alpha cells and beta cells.

Isometric contractions The muscle increases in tension by contraction, but does not change its length or angle of the joint.

Isotonic or **dynamic contractions** Contractions in which the muscle changes length against resistance, and movement occurs.

Jejunum The intermediate portion of the small intestine that joins the duodenum with the ileum and is approximately 6 feet long.

Jump sign A spontaneous reaction of pain or discomfort that may cause a client to wince, jump, or verbalize upon application of pressure.

Juxtaglomerular apparatus A mechanism monitoring the blood pressure consisting of two specialized groups of cells; the macula densa and juxtaglomerular cells.

Juxtaglomerular cells Cells that monitor changes in blood pressure in the afferent arteriole.

Kellogg, John Harvey (1852–1943) American popularizer of health concerns. Kellogg wrote numerous articles and books on massage that brought the issue to the general populace.

Keratin A cordlike protein that provides protection by waterproofing the skin's surface (it is insoluble in water).

Kidneys Paired organs located bilaterally in the upper lumbar region of the spine. They are bean-shaped, (convex laterally and concave medially, like a kidney bean) and are slightly smaller than a fist.

Kinesiology The study of the body's muscles, joints, and their movements.

Korsakoff's syndrome A syndrome caused by thiamine and other B vitamin deficiencies.

Krause's end bulbs Although the operating mechanism of Krause's end bulbs is not exactly known, they are believed to be stimulated by lowering temperatures.

Kupffer's cells Phagocytic cells that line the sinusoids of the liver and filter bacteria and other foreign material out of the blood before sending it through the hepatic vein.

Lacteals The lymph capillaries in the villi that assist in the absorption of fat.

Large intestine or **colon** The final path undigested and unabsorbed food takes before it is eliminated by the body.

Laryngitis Inflammation of the larynx that often results in loss of voice often caused by respiratory infections or irritants such as cigarette smoke.

Larynx or **voice box** Formed by three single and three paired pieces of cartilage. The single cartilages are the epiglottis, the cricoid, and the thyroid (laryngeal prominence or Adam's apple), which is the largest, especially in men. The three paired cartilages are arytenoid, corniculate, and the cuneiform; they attach to and support the vocal folds.

Lateral Oriented farther away from the midline of the body.

Law of facilitation This neurological law states that once an impulse has traveled a certain nerve pathway, it tends to "imprint" or "facilitate" the pathway; therefore, it will take the same path on future occasions.

Lesion An injury that involves disruption of an anatomic structure.

Lesser or **gastrohepatic omentum** A fatty, membranous extension of the peritoneum that attaches from the right side of stomach and first section of the duodenum to the liver.

Leukemia Also called "cancer of the blood," leukemia is a cancer of white blood cells.

Leukocytes White blood cells or white corpuscles.

Ligaments Connective tissues that connect bone to bone. Functionally, ligaments are an extension of the bone to allow lightness, flexibility, and added strength.

Ling, Pehr Henrik (1776–1839) Swedish physiologist and gymnastics instructor. Ling is considered the "father of Swedish massage." He developed his own system of medical gymnastics and exercise, known by several different names—the Ling System, Swedish Movements, or the Swedish Movement Cure. An important part of the Ling System was a particular style of massage, known today as Swedish massage.

Liniments Alcoholic, oily, or soapy agents used in massage to create the sensation of heat.

Liquid connective tissue Also known as hemopoietic tissue, vascular tissue, or blood.

Liver The largest internal organ of the body located in the upper right quadrant of the abdominal cavity.

Lobes Regions of the cerebrum named for the bone each lies beneath: the frontal, parietal, temporal, and occipital lobes.

Local twitch response An involuntary firing or twitching in a muscle (a reflex motor output) in response to the sensory stimulation (pressure) on the trigger point.

Logistics (managing details of the operation) is the what, when, and where section of a business proposal. If you are familiar with the facility, you may recommend a specific location where massage services will be provided.

Longitudinal muscle fiber arrangement Longitudinal muscles have fibers aligned parallel to a long axis. Types of longitudinal muscles are quadrilateral, triangular, or fan-shaped, and fusiform, or spindle-shaped.

Loose connective tissue Regarded as the packing material of the body, it attaches the skin to underlying structures, serves to wrap and support the body cells, fills in the spaces between structures (i.e., organs, muscles), and helps to keep them in their proper places.

Lucas-Championniere, Just (1843–1913) French physician who advocated the use of massage and passive-motion exercises after certain injuries.

Lumbar Pertaining to the area of the back between the ribs of the thorax and hips of the pelvis.

Lumen The open space within the blood vessel.

Lungs The highly elastic, paired organs of respiration.

Luteinizing hormone Stimulates ovulation in women. It also stimulates the production of estrogen and progesterone by the ovaries; it also stimulates testosterone secretion by the testes in men.

Lyme disease A recurrent form of arthritis caused by the bacterium *Borrelia burgdorferi,* which is transmitted by a tick bite.

Lymph capillaries Lymph vessels that are larger, more irregular, and more permeable than blood vessels.

Lymph nodes Bean-shaped structures located along lymph vessels that collect and filter lymph. These are powerful defense stations that help to protect the body from unwanted invaders.

Lymph The fluid of the lymph system.

Lymphatic trunks Large vessels in the lymphatic system. These trunks join to form one of two lymphatic ducts: the right lymphatic duct and the thoracic duct.

Lymphedema An accumulation of interstitial fluid (swelling) in the soft tissues due to local or general inflammation, obstruction, or removal of lymph vessels.

Lysosomes Membrane-bound organelles containing various digestive enzymes.

Macula Special receptors in the wall of the inner ear that help determine orientation with respect to gravity. Each macula contains a membrane with groups of modified hair cells, or cilia, that are attached to sensory nerves.

Macula densa Cells located in the ascending limb of the loop of Henle that monitor filtrate concentration.

Maintenance massage A blend of general soreness-reduction and specific therapeutic massage between events or training sessions.

Major duodenal papilla A dilation that is formed by the juncture of the pancreatic and bile ducts as they open into the small intestines. It is also referred to as *hepatopancreatic ampulla* and the *ampulla of Vater.*

Malignant A condition that worsens and causes death if not treated.

Malignant melanoma Cancer of the melanocytes in the skin, which begins as a raised dark lesion with irregular borders and appears uneven in color.

Manav Dharma Shastra Ancient Hindu work (c. 300 B.C.) that mentions the use of therapeutic massage.

Massage The systematic and scientific manipulation of the soft tissues of the body for the purpose of improving and maintaining health; it can also be defined as organized, intentional touch.

Mastication Chewing.

Meatus Creaselike passageways that subdivide the three nasal conchae.

Mechanical responses A physiological response of the body to direct response brought on by force or pressure; tissue being pulled, lifted, rubbed, compressed, and manipulated.

Mechanoreceptors Sensory receptors that respond to mechanical stimuli and are located in the skin, ears, muscles, tendons, joints, and fascia. They detect sensations such as touch, pressure, vibration, stretching, muscular contraction, proprioception, sound, and equilibrium.

Media Methods of mass communication such as newspapers, magazines, radio, or television.

Medial Oriented more toward or near the midline of the body.

Mediastinum A portion of the thoracic cavity occupying the area between the lungs.

Medical asepsis The combination of water, friction, and soap or other disinfecting agents to eliminate the presence of pathogenic microorganisms. This can be accomplished chemically and/or mechanically.

Medical gymnastics Gymnastics style concerned with the treatment of ailments that have arisen through abnormal conditions.

Medulla oblongata The most inferior portion of the brain stem that is often considered the most vital part of the brain; it contains the respiratory center, the cardiac center, and the vasomotor center. The medulla also controls gastric secretions and reflexes, such as sweating, sneezing, swallowing, and vomiting.

Meissner's corpuscles Receptors for light touch, responding to both the actual movement and the length of the movement across the skin. More specifically, Meissner's corpuscles monitor low-frequency vibration (the onset and removal of pressure), and adapt slowly.

Melanin Skin pigment that contributes to the color of the skin but is also found in the hair and in the iris of the eye. Melanin granules serve to protect the underlying cells from ultraviolet radiation.

Melanocyte-stimulating hormone It stimulates the distribution of melanin granules, therefore increasing skin pigmentation.

Melanocytes Specialized cells in the stratum germinativum and the stratum spinosum, where the yellow, brown, or black skin pigment, or melanin, is synthesized.

Melatonin A hormone that may be involved in the control of circadian rhythm, or diurnal cycles (occurring daily, such as sleeping and eating) and in the growth and development of sexual organs. When injected into the body, melatonin produces drowsiness.

Membranes Thin, soft, pliable sheets of tissue that cover the body, line tubes or body cavities, cover organs, and separate one part of a cavity from another.

Meninges Special connective tissue membranes that envelop the entire central nervous system (brain and spinal cord); it contains three layers: the pia mater, the arachnoid, and the dura mater.

Meningitis An infection or inflammation of the meninges often characterized by a sudden severe headache, vertigo, stiff neck, and severe irritability.

Mercuriale, Girolamo (1530–1606) Italian Renaissance–era physician who synthesized ancient medical writings. He wrote *De Arte Gymnastica,* considered to be the first book written in the field of sports medicine.

Merkel's disks Receptors that respond to skin displacement, somewhat like the Meissner's and Pacinian's corpuscles, but Merkel's disks have the capacity for a longer or more continuous response.

Mesentery A large, fan-shaped section of the peritoneum, connecting the small intestine to the posterior abdominal wall.

Mesoderm The midlayer of the three germ layers that becomes the muscles and connective tissues of the body, as well as vascular and lymphatic tissue.

Metabolic diseases Involve abnormal activities of cells and/or tissues like diabetes, cardiovascular conditions, and jaundice. Metabolic diseases are not contagious, but may have originated from a contagious disease, such as hepatitis, which can lead to jaundice or vice versa.

Metabolism The total of all the physical and chemical processes that occur in a given organism (i.e., those that are considered to be signs of life).

Metastasis The process of cancerous cells spreading to distant parts of the body, usually through the bloodstream or the lymphatic circulation.

Metazoa These are parasites (organisms obtaining nourishment from other living organisms) that can produce diseases in the bodies of their living hosts.

Methodists Term used to refer to a group of ancient Greek physicians who supported a simplistic view of healing and generally restricted their treatments to bathing, diet, massage, and a few drugs.

Mezger, Johann (1839–1909) Dutch physician who is generally given credit for making massage a fundamental component of physical rehabilitation. He is also credited for the introduction of French terminology into the massage profession.

Microscopic anatomy The study of the smaller structures of the body, such as cells and tissues, that make up larger structures.

Microtrauma Tissue trauma that results from microscopically small amounts of strain spread over a period of time.

Microvilli Tiny projections of a cell to increase surface area.

Micturition or **voiding** Also known as urination, micturition is the act of emptying the bladder by passing urine out of the body through the urethra.

Midbrain or **mesencephalon** The most superior structure of the brain stem that houses voluntary motor tracts descending from the cerebral cortex to the spinal cord.

Midsagittal or **median plane** A plane that runs longitudinally, or vertically, down the body, anterior to posterior, dividing the organism into right and left sections. This plane creates a right lateral and a left lateral portion of the body.

Minerals Minerals are essential nonorganic compounds found in nature and used by the body to aid enzymatic actions.

Mission Statement A statement of purpose.

Mitochondrion An oval-shaped organelle lying within the cytoplasm; considered the cell's "power plant" because it is a site for cellular respiration, which provides most of a cell's adenosine triphosphate supply.

Modality A general term used to denote any technique, procedure, or product used to produce a positive response for the client.

Mononucleosis An acute viral infection caused by the Epstein-Barr virus (EBV).

Motor end plate An expansion at the end of some motor nerves.

Motor neurons Neurons responsible for carrying messages of contraction (or in some cases, inhibiting contraction) to a muscle or gland.

Motor or **efferent nerves** Nerves that carry messages from the brain or spinal cord.

Motor unit A single motor neuron and all its associated skeletal muscle fibers. A single muscle is composed of many motor units.

Mucous membranes or **mucosae** Membranes that line openings to the outside of the body. This type of membrane is found in the respiratory, digestive, reproductive, and urinary tracts. Mucous membranes secrete a viscous, slippery fluid called mucus.

Multiple sclerosis The progressive destruction of myelin sheaths in the central nervous system.

Multipolar neurons Neurons that contain many dendrites and only one axon.

Mumps An acute viral disease caused by a Paramyxovirus (an airborne member of the herpes family).

Muscle cramp An acute, painful contraction of a single muscle or group of muscles.

Muscle fatigue The inability of a muscle to contract even though it is still being stimulated.

Muscle or **neuromuscular spindles** Stretch-sensitive receptors wrapped around intrafusal muscle fibers (striated muscle fiber within a muscle spindle) that monitor changes in the length of a muscle and the rate of this change.

Muscle spasm An increase in muscle tension with or without shortening, due to excessive motor nerve activity.

Muscle tissue Extremely elastic, this tissue is very vascular and has the unique ability to shorten (contract) and to elongate to produce movement.

Muscular atrophy A decrease in the size of muscle fibers or a wasting away of muscles from poor nutrition, lack of use, motor unit dysfunction, or lack of motor nerve impulses.

Muscular dystrophy A collection of genetically transmitted diseases, muscular dystrophy is characterized by the progressive atrophy of skeletal muscles without any indication of neural degeneration or damage.

Myasthenia gravis A weakness in the muscles characterized by chronic fatigability.

Myelin sheath A fatty material around most axons that electrically insulates the neuron and increases the speed of nerve impulse conduction.

Myocardial infarction A heart attack followed by death (necrosis) of myocardial tissue due to an interrupted coronary blood supply.

Myocardium The thick muscular layer that makes up the bulk of the heart wall.

Myofibril The simplest unit of a muscle fiber. Groups of these cells are organized into tissues.

Myofilaments Bundles of smaller structures called actin and myosin that comprise a myofibril.

Myoglobin or **myohemoglobin** A chemical similar to the hemoglobin molecule present in red blood cells.

Myosin heads Ball-like structures on myosin fibers.

Myosin The thicker myofilament.

Myotatic stretch reflex The reflex activated when a muscle is pulled and there is a resultant contraction of the muscle.

Narrative report A type of progress report that may include many sessions and prescriptive periods. Usually the initial baseline session and the latest session are chosen as the measures to show improvement. The application of therapy and the client's responses are discussed in detail.

Nasal conchae The nasal cavity leads to the nasal conchae. The superior, middle, and inferior nasal conchae are the ridges that extend out of each lateral wall of the nasal cavity.

Nausea A sensation that often leads to vomiting. Common causes of nausea are motion sickness, severe pain, food poisoning, infection, first trimester pregnancy (due to hormonal changes), and irritants such as spicy foods, toxins, bacteria, and certain medications.

Necessary care Therapy that helps a client regain function (i.e., able to do more of his daily living activities).

Negative feedback system A process of the endocrine system that triggers the negative, or opposite, response; this process may or may not involve the nervous system.

Nei Ching *See* ***Huang-ti nei-ching.***

Nephrogenic diabetes insipidus Much the same as diabetes insipidus, except that the cause is due to kidney dysfunction, often a result of disease or damage.

Nephrons The basic filtering unit of the kidney responsible for filtering waste products from the blood.

Nerve A group of impulse-carrying fibers connecting the brain and the spinal cord with other parts of the body.

Nerve compression Also known as nerve impingement, this compression is similar to a nerve entrapment except that the pressure against the nerve is due to contact with hard tissues such as bone or cartilage.

Nerve entrapment Also known as entrapment neuropathy, this refers to dysfunction of a nerve as a result of pressure against it by adjacent soft tissues such as muscle, tendon, fascia, and ligaments.

Nerve stroke A light fingertip tracing over the surface of the skin in order to signal psychologically the end of the massage session to the client. This ancillary stroke is often classified as light effleurage.

Nervous tissue Oddly shaped cells that can pick up and transmit electrical signals by converting stimuli into nerve impulses. Located in the brain, spinal cord, and peripheral nerves, nervous tissue possesses characteristics of excitability and conductability.

Networking To develop business relationships with vast groups of people who are looking for the same thing you are—promoting their businesses.

Neural control system Hormones secreted due to direct nerve stimulation. The neural control system has a much faster response time than the negative feedback or the hormonal control systems.

Neurilemma or **sheath of Schwann** A layer of one or more Schwann's cells enclosing the myelin sheath; it plays an important role in the regeneration of peripheral nervous system nerve fibers.

Neuroglia or **glial cells** Connective tissues that support, nourish, protect, insulate, and organize the neurons.

Neurology The study of the functions and disorders of the nervous system.

Neuromuscular or **myoneural junction** A fluid-filled space between nerve endings and muscle fibers.

Neurons The basic impulse-conducting cell. These cells possess two major properties: excitability and conductability.

Neuropathy Decrease or change in sensation in the hands and feet.

Neurotransmitters A collective term for a vast range of chemicals that facilitate, arouse, or inhibit the transmission of nerve impulses between synapses.

Nissen, Hartvig Prominent early practitioner of Swedish massage (created by Pehr Ling) in the United States. He helped popularize Ling's methods with his numerous publications.

Nociceptor Receptors for detecting pain.

Nodes of Ranvier Gaps located at certain intervals along an axon; during neural activity, impulses jump from one node to another, resulting in an increased rate of conduction.

Nonverbal communication Involves the transmission of messages by means other than the spoken word.

Norepinephrine or **noradrenaline** Hormones that help the body to maintain the stress response. The effects of norepinephrine are increased heart rate, blood pressure, and blood glucose levels, and dilation of the small passageways of the lungs.

Normal reflex arc This is the pathway that is responsible for normal body functions in response to stimuli.

Nucleoli Clusters of protein, DNA and RNA, and chromatin within the nucleus.

Nucleus The largest organelle in the cytoplasm; the control center of the cell.

Obesity Abnormal increase in subcutaneous fat tissue, primarily in visceral regions of the body.

Occipital Posterior surface of the head; situated near the occipital bone.

Occlusion Any clogged vessel or passage of the body.

Olfaction Olfaction refers to the sense of smell.

Oligodendrocytes Cells in the central nervous system that produce myelin.

Oral cavity Also known as the mouth, the oral cavity contains the tongue, teeth, gums, and openings from the salivary ducts. Digestion begins in the oral cavity.

Oral Pertaining to the mouth.

Orbital or **ophthalmic** Pertaining to the eye area.

Origin The tendinous attachment of the muscle that is relatively fixed during the muscle's action.

Osmosis A process that depends upon the concentration of dissolved elements that lie in the solutions on each side of the cell membrane. The fluid from the less concentrated solution (usually water) moves across the cell membrane. Osmotic movement of water is always from lowest concentration (most dilute) to highest concentration (least dilute). This action continues until the two concentrations equalize.

Ossification The process by which bone develops.

Osteoarthritis Progressive erosion of the articular cartilage due to chronic inflammation of the joints.

Osteoblasts Bone-forming cells found in the periosteum.

Osteoclasts Bone-destroying cells that help maintain homeostasis and repair bone.

Osteocytes Mature osteoblasts that soon become embedded in bone matrix.

Osteoporosis Decreased bone mass and increased susceptibility to fractures.

Otoliths Calcium carbonate particles floating above the macula of the ear that shift position as the body moves; when this occurs, the cilia are disturbed, which initiates a nerve impulse.

Outcome The client's response to therapy and progress toward short- or long-term goals.

Oval window The ear membrane that covers the opening of the cochlea.

Ovaries Functioning both as endocrine and exocrine glands, the ovaries are located in the abdominopelvic region of the female body.

Oxytocin Hormone involved in milk expression from the mammary glands and uterine muscular contraction. Oxytocin's function in men is unknown.

Pacinian's or **laminated corpuscles** Pressure-sensitive receptors that respond to skin displacement and high-frequency vibration, adapting quickly to all external stimuli.

Palliative care Therapy that eases or reduces pain or other symptoms.

Palmar Refers to the anterior surface or the palm of the hand.

Palpatory assessment Assessment through touching, with purpose and intent.

Pancreas Both an endocrine and an exocrine gland, the retroperitoneal pancreas is a carrot-shaped organ located inferior and posterior to the greater curvature of the stomach.

Pancreatitis An inflammation of the pancreas, usually the result of trauma, alcohol abuse, infection, or certain medications.

Papillae Projections on the tongue.

Papule A small, round, firm, elevated area in the skin, varying in size from a pinpoint to that of a small pea.

Paracelsus (1493–1541) Name by which Philippus Aureolus Theophrastus Bombastus von Hohenheim was generally known. Paracelsus was a Swiss physician and chemist who promoted chemically prepared medicines instead of herbal remedies.

Paraffin bath Involves the use of a petroleum-based waxy mixture that is white and odorless. Paraffin wax treatments are used to apply heat energy to the tissues and are particularly useful with injuries to the more angular bony areas.

Paralysis Loss of muscle function and/or the loss of sensation.

Parasympathetic nervous system or **craniosacral outflow** An anabolic system that conserves the body's energy resources.

Parathyroid glands The tiny, usually four, parathyroid glands are located on the posterolateral surface of the thyroid lobes.

Parathyroid hormone Increases blood calcium levels by stimulating osteoclast (bone-destroying cells) activity, and breaks down bone tissue. The liberated calcium is released in the bloodstream, and blood calcium levels increase. PTH also increases calcium reabsorption from urine and the intestines back into the blood.

Paré, Ambroise (c. 1510–90) French military surgeon. In addition to inventing several surgical instruments, he was among the earliest modern physicians to discuss the therapeutic effects of massage, especially in orthopedic surgery cases.

Parietal or **oxyntic cells** One type of exocrine cell in the stomach. They produce intrinsic factor, a substance required for the absorption of vitamin B_{12} from the small intestine to the bloodstream. They also produce hydrochloric acid, a component of gastric juice, which breaks down protein and activates many gastric enzymes.

Parietal Referring to the walls of a cavity or an organ.

Parkinson's disease A progressive, degenerative, neurological disorder marked by the destruction of certain areas of the brain (specifically, dopamine-producing neurons) and depletion of the neurotransmitter dopamine.

Partial or **relative contraindications** Conditions or situations that merit caution and adaptive measures to ensure that the massage is safe and that the client is comfortable.

Passive stretching Stretches in which the client remains relaxed (or passive) and makes no contribution while the therapist applies the stretch.

Pathogen or **pathogenic agent** A living biological agent capable of causing disease.

Paul of Aegina (625–690) Greek physician who was one of the most important medical men of his time and one of the last of the Greek compilers.

Pectoral Pertaining to the thorax or chest area.

Pedal Referring to the foot.

Pediatric Young people between 3 to 18 years of age.

Pelvic Inferior region of the abdominopelvic cavity.

Penniform muscle fiber arrangement Penniform muscles are arranged with a central tendon and muscle fibers extending from the tendon diagonally, giving the muscle a featherlike appearance.

Peptide hormones Peptide or protein hormones are derivatives of amino acid chains. These hormones are water soluble. They attach to the cell membrane and introduce a series of chemical reactions to alter the cell's metabolism.

Peptides Smaller chains of amino acids.

Percussion or **tapotement** Involves repetitive staccato striking movements of the hands, simultaneously or alternately, with loose wrists and fingers, for the purpose of stimulating the underlying tissues.

Pericarditis An inflammation of the parietal pericardium that may be due to trauma or infectious disease.

Pericardium or **pericardial sac** The tissue layers surrounding the heart.

Perimysium A fascial layer within the muscle that binds together fasciculi.

Perineal Region between the anus and the genitals; inferior pelvic cavity.

Periosteum Fibrous, dense, vascular connective tissue sheath around the bone that penetrates the bone like nails, anchoring itself to the bone.

Peripheral nervous system Part of the nervous system composed of the nerves emerging from the central nervous system.

Peripheral Pertaining to the outside surface, periphery, or surrounding external area of a structure; often referred to as superficial.

Peripheral vascular disease An abnormal condition that decreases circulation in the hands and feet. This involves the flow of blood and lymph.

Peritoneum The largest serous membrane in the body that envelops the entire abdominal wall. Sections of the peritoneum include the mesenteries, the parietal and visceral peritoneum, and the greater and lesser omentum.

Peritonitis An acute inflammation of the peritoneum produced by bacteria or irritating substances that gain access into the abdominal cavity.

Peritubular capillaries A second network of blood vessels branching off before the glomerulus that is interwoven with corresponding renal tubules.

Petrissage A cycle of rhythmic lifting of the muscle tissues away from the bone or underlying structures, followed by firmly kneading or squeezing the muscle, ending with a release of the tissue.

Phagocytosis Phagocytosis, or "cell eating," is the process by which specialized cells engulf harmful microorganisms and cellular debris, break them down, and expel the harmless remains back into the body.

Pharynx Also called the throat, the tubular structure that transports food, liquid, and air to their respective destinations. In the digestive system, the pharynx takes food from the oral cavity to the esophagus during deglutition.

Phlebitis An inflammation of the veins, frequently accompanied by a thrombus (blood clot).

Photoreceptors Sensory receptors that are sensitive to light stimuli. There are two types: rods and cones.

Physical fitness The ability to carry out daily tasks efficiently with enough energy left over to enjoy leisure pursuits and to meet unforeseen emergencies.

Physiology The study of how the whole body and its individual parts function in normal body processes.

Physiopathological reflex arc This is the nerve pathway taken when strong afferent stimuli to the central nervous system produce a strong efferent motor impulse; the opposite of a normal reflex arc. The increased motor stimuli may cause vasoconstriction, a decrease in visceral function, an increase in muscular tonus, and an increase in intrajoint pressure.

Pia mater The innermost meningeal layer; it is thin, vascular, and lies close to the brain.

Pinched nerve A phrase used to refer to a broad spectrum of nervous conditions: sciatica; thoracic outlet syndrome; Bell's palsy; ruptured disks; slipped disks; vertebral subluxations; carpal tunnel syndrome; paresthesia; symptoms of radiating pain, numbness, or weakness in the extremities; and a host of other symptoms.

Pineal gland The pineal gland, or epiphysis cerebri, is a pinecone-shaped structure in the brain, attached to the roof of the third ventricle and inferior to the corpus callosum. Although its function is not clear, the pineal gland produces and secretes the hormone melatonin.

Pinocytosis Or "cell drinking," is almost identical to phagocytosis except that the targeted object is liquid.

Pitch The quality of a tone or sound, which is dependent on the relative rapidity of the vibrations.

Pituitary gland The bilobed pituitary gland, or hypophysis, is located in the sella turcica of the sphenoid bone and extends from the hypothalamus by a stalklike structure known as the infundibulum.

Pivot joints Also known as a trochoid or a monaxial joint, these joints allow movements that are limited to rotation (e.g., atlantoaxial and proximal radioulnar joints).

Plantar Pertaining to the bottom surface of the foot.

Plasma A straw-colored liquid that is left when the formed elements are removed from the blood.

Platelet plug The process by which platelets enlarge, become sticky, and clump together, forming a plug, which helps to seal the damaged vessel.

Pleurisy Inflammation and/or adhesion of the pleural membranes characterized by stabbing pain during breathing.

Plexus A network of intersecting nerves.

Plicae circulares Circular folds in the lumen of the small intestine.

Pneumonia An infection or inflammation of the alveoli due to the bacterium *Streptococcus pneumoniae,* but other infectious agents such as bacteria, protozoans, viruses, and fungi may be responsible.

Poliomyelitis Polio is an infectious disease transmitted through fecal contamination or nasal secretions caused by one of three polioviruses.

Pons The large rounded area below the midbrain that relays messages from cerebral cortex to the spinal cord.

Popliteal Area located on the posterior aspect of the knee.

Postevent massage Massage provided soon after an event or training session.

Posterior or **dorsal** Pertaining more to the back of a structure.

Posterior ramus The posterior branching of the spinal cord that innervates the skin and deep muscles of the back.

Posture The position of the body in space, such as sitting, standing, lying supine, and lying prone.

Pre-event massage Massage provided before an event or training session.

Prescription A written order by a licensed healthcare provider that literally means "take thou this."

Pressure The application of force (or thrust) exerted by the massage therapist on the client's body.

Professional communication An interaction between the massage therapist and the client (or agents of the client) for the collection, recording, and transmission of data for therapeutic purposes.

Professional image A mental and emotional portrayal of yourself in the public eye. It is often an instantaneous impression or picture of you when your name is evoked, spoken, or read.

Professional liability insurance Also referred to as malpractice insurance and errors and omission insurance, professional liability covers liability costs rising from your professional activities. Massage therapists are accountable for their actions and may be held liable for any mistakes made while performing that service.

Progesterone Hormone that prepares the endometrium for pregnancy and helps to maintain the corpus luteum once conception and implantation occur. One cause of spontaneous abortion (miscarriage) is a drop in progesterone levels.

Progress report A progress report summarizes the client's progress to date.

Prolactin lactogenic hormone Stimulates the mammary glands to create milk production in women. Prolactin's role in men is not known.

Prone Lying face or belly down in a horizontal, recumbent position.

Proposal A written idea put forward for consideration, discussion, or adoption. By telling another your ideas, you make your intentions known.

Proprioceptive neuromuscular facilitation Also known as contract-relax technique, it is based on the neurological phenomenon of reciprocal inhibition. PNF involves stretching a muscle through active participation of the client and a 6-second sustained isometric contraction by the attending therapist. Then the muscle is further stretched and its action is resisted.

Proprioceptor A special type of mechanoreceptor detecting stimuli within the body itself. Examples of proprioceptors are muscle spindles, Golgi tendon bodies, and baroreceptors.

Proteins Naturally occurring organic compounds that contain large combinations of amino acids.

Protozoa These single-celled organisms are considered the lowest form of animal life; pathogenic protozoa can only survive in a living subject and are commonly transmitted through contaminated food, water, and feces.

Proximal Nearer to the point of reference, usually toward the trunk of the body.

Pruritus Severe itching of the skin caused by dryness, sweat retention on the skin, kidney failure, allergic reactions, fungi, or parasitic agents such as scabies or body lice.

Pseudostratified columnar epithelium This tissue has the appearance of being stratified, but it is actually a single layer of tissue. The cells possess different heights, and not all cells reach the free surface. This type of epithelium is found in portions of the respiratory tract and the male reproductive tract.

Psoriasis Distinct, red, flaky skin elevations marked by periods of remission and exacerbation.

Pubic Pertaining to the region of the pubic symphysis or the genital area.

Pulmonary circuit The pathway of blood from the heart to the lungs and back.

Pulmonary edema A condition involving an excessive amount of blood and interstitial fluid in the lungs.

Pulmonary semilunar valve The semilunar valve between the right ventricle and the pulmonary trunk.

Purkinje fibers or **conduction myofibers** Conducting fibers from the bundle of His that spread an impulse throughout the myocardium, causing the ventricles to simultaneously contract and expelling the blood from the ventricles to the arteries.

Pustule A small raised elevation of the skin often with a "head" containing lymph or pus.

Pyloric sphincter The sphincter located between the stomach and the small intestine.

Rabies An acute infection, often fatal, caused by the rabies virus usually transmitted by animals (dogs, cats, bats, raccoons, and skunks) to people by infected blood, tissue, or, most commonly, saliva.

Radiation The transfer of heat energy in electromagnetic rays through a conducting medium like air (e.g., infrared lamps).

Range of motion A measure of possible joint movement from the least to the greatest by a particular joint. Active ROM measures the client's movement using his voluntary muscles; passive ROM measures movement while the client assists by relaxing or disengaging voluntary muscle control.

Raynaud's phenomenon Periodic attacks of vasospasm of blood vessels in the body's extremities, especially the most distal parts, such as the toes, fingers, ears, and nose.

Recidivism Relapse into the previous condition such as substance abuse.

Recruitment The process of motor unit activation based upon need of strength.

Rectum The lower end of the colon that usually contains three circular folds that overlap when empty and grow in size as the rectum fills with "ready to excrete" wastes. The main function of the rectum is storage.

Referred pain Pain (e.g., pain, tingling, numbness, itching, aching, heat, cold) experienced at a site different from that of an injured or diseased part of the body.

Reflex An instantaneous, involuntary response to a stimulus originating from either inside or outside the body.

Reflex arc Two or more neurons; one of which is sensory and one of which is a motor neuron innervating a muscle, gland, or organ; the functional component of the nervous system.

Reflex sympathetic dystrophy A complex disorder or group of disorders affecting the muscles and nerves of limbs that may develop as a result of trauma (accident, repetitive motion, or surgery).

Reflexive responses A physiological response of the body due to reaction of a stimulus, frequently due to mechanical stimulation of nerve receptors.

Regeneration A method of tissue repair, the damaged tissue is replaced with new tissue of the same type. Often the open wound becomes sealed with a scab, and the surrounding healthy epithelial cells divide until the skin beneath the scab has been reproduced completely.

Relaxin Hormone that softens the connective tissue in the body of a pregnant woman, which is helpful for loosening up the body's connective tissue, especially the pelvic ligaments, for fetal delivery. It also helps to dilate the cervix during labor and delivery.

Remodeling or **scar maturation phase** The process by which collagen fibers in the scar tissue are formed randomly. At this time the body is continually restructuring the scar tissue by a simultaneous destruction and creation of new collagen fibers.

Renaissance The intellectual and artistic movement (a "rebirth") beginning in northern Italy in the 14th century and extending throughout much of Europe by the 17th century.

Renal dialysis The process of using a mechanical kidney to remove substances from the blood in an attempt to restore its electrolyte and acid-base balance.

Renal failure The inability of the kidneys to perform their essential functions (i.e., filtering the blood, collecting and secreting wastes, retaining essential elements).

Renal hilus/hilum or **renal sinus** The indentation located in the medial concave region of the kidney;

here is where the renal arteries, renal veins, and the ureters attach.

Renal or **medullary pyramids** The term used to describe the bundles of renal tubules in the renal medulla. Each kidney, composed of 8 to 18 renal pyramids, contains many straight collecting tubules, which gives each pyramid a striated appearance.

Renal pelvis The funnel-shaped origin of the ureters located in the interior compartment of the renal hilus.

Renal tubules A urine-routing vessel.

Renin An enzyme secreted by the juxtaglomerular apparatus in response to a drop in blood pressure and a drop in the chloride ion concentration of the filtrate. This enzyme serves as a catalyst to change inactive angiotensin into active angiotensin II.

Rennin An enzyme found in the gastric juices of infants.

Repetitive motion injuries Also known as repetitive strain injuries, repetitive motion injuries are caused by the repeated flexing and extending of a joint.

Resolution Normal replacement of damaged tissue when the trauma is mild and when the tissue has the ability to replicate itself by mitosis.

Respiratory diaphragm or **thoracoabdominal diaphragm** A dome-shaped muscular partition that separates thoracic cavity from abdominal cavity. It is the main muscle of respiration.

Respiratory distress syndrome An acute infantile lung disease characterized by inelastic lungs, respiration rate of more than 60 per minute, and nasal flaring.

Respiratory pump Pressure changes in the thorax and abdomen during breathing that assist lymph flow and blood moving back to the heart.

Reticular connective tissue A type of loose connective tissue; it forms the framework of certain organs as well as provides support.

Retina A delicate nervous tissue membrane of the eye, which is continuous with the optic nerve.

Retinaculum Bandagelike retaining bands of connective tissue found at the ankles and wrists to keep tendons and tendon sheaths in place.

Retroperitoneal Refers to structures located behind the peritoneum.

Rh factor The presence or absence of the Rh protein on the erythrocyte membrane. There are two types: Rh-positive (about 85 percent of the population) and Rh-negative (about 15 percent of the population).

Rhazes (c. 850–932) Name by which Persian physician Abu Bakr Muhammad ibn-Zakariya al-Razi was known in the West. He was a noted physician of his time and the first important Arab medical writer.

Rheumatoid arthritis Systemic arthritis that destroys the synovial membranes of joints characterized by flare-ups and remissions.

Rhythm An ordered repetition of strong and weak elements in the delivery of the massage strokes.

Rhythmic or **peristaltic contractions** Wavelike involuntary contractions that mix and propel materials in the gastrointestinal tract.

Ribosomes Small granules of RNA and protein in the cytoplasm.

Rickettsia Rickettsia are intracellular parasites that share characteristics of both bacteria and viruses. They are similar to viruses in that they require living cells for growth and replication, yet similar to bacteria in susceptibility to antibiotics.

Right lymphatic duct One of the two main lymphatic ducts which move lymph from the right arm and the right side of the head and the right half of the thorax and enter the right subclavian vein.

Ringworm A group of fungal diseases characterized by itching, scaling, and sometimes painful lesions manifested as a raised red-ringed patch.

Rods Thin cellular structures with slender rodlike projections that are very sensitive to dim light (night vision) and to shades of black, white, and gray.

Rubefacient An agent that reddens the skin. This color change is due to the counterirritation caused by the ingredients in the liniment.

Ruffini's end organs These bodies alert us when the skin comes into contact with deep or continuous pressure. Some references indicate that these receptors detect the increased sensation of heat.

Russian bath A steam cabinet that allows the head to be exposed.

Sacral Pertaining to the sacrum or sacral area of the spinal column.

Saddle joints Also known as sellar or biaxial joints, these joints allow all movements, but rotation is limited (carpometacarpal of the thumb and the great toe to the first metatarsal).

Sagittal plane A plane that passes through the body parallel to the midsagittal or median plane.

Salt rubs or **salt glows** The rubbing application of wet salt on the skin.

Saliva A clear, nondigestible, viscous fluid secreted by the salivary and mucous glands in the mouth.

San-tsai-tou-hoei Japanese publication (c. 1610) that mentions both passive and active massage procedures.

Sanitation The application of measures to promote a healthful, disease-free environment.

Sarcolemma The cell membrane that envelopes each individual muscle fiber.

Sarcomere The functional contractile unit of a muscle.

Sarcoplasm The cellular fluid that is contained in each skeletal muscle fiber.

Sarcoplasmic reticulum Fluid-filled system of cavities encircling each sarcomere that stores and releases calcium ions.

Satellite trigger point A tender area that lies within the referred pain zone of the primary trigger point.

Sauna bath A hot-air bath with temperatures ranging from 160° to 180°F in 6 to 8 percent humidity.

Scapular Referring to the shoulder blade.

Schwann's cells Cells in the peripheral nervous system that produce the myelin sheaths on axons.

Sciatica Inflammation of the sciatic nerve often experienced as a dull pain and tenderness in the buttock region with sharper radiating pain or numbness down the leg.

Scleroderma An autoimmune disorder affecting blood vessels and connective tissue.

Scope of practice This is often derived from the legal definition of massage and defines the working parameters of a particular profession; it is solely a matter of state law, which may vary from state to state.

Seated position Also known as the chair position, it describes a massage given while the client is sitting in an ordinary chair or a chair that has been specially designed for client comfort and accessibility to major tension areas of the body.

Sebaceous or **oil glands** Glands that possess ducts (exocrine) and are attached to the hair follicle. Sebaceous glands secrete sebum.

Seborrhea A topical disease of the sebaceous glands, marked by an increase in the amount of oily secretions.

Sebum A mixture of fats, cholesterol, proteins, and inorganic salts secreted by sebaceous glands; it is mildly antibacterial, antifungal, and lubricates both the hair and the epidermis.

Self-disclosure When the speaker reveals honestly his thoughts and feelings.

Self-report form A form that describes the client's perception of his symptoms. This form contains simple pictures of a body (front and back) for the client to mark or circle areas in which there is discomfort.

Semilunar valves Heart valves between both ventricles and their adjacent arteries.

Senile lentigo Tan or brown patches found on the skin of older people, especially those who have been exposed excessively to the sun.

Sensory or **afferent nerves** Nerves that carry impulses from nerve receptors to the brain or spinal cord.

Separation A separation is almost the same as a dislocation, but the joint structure is simply pulled and stretched; the bone is not displaced out of the joint capsule.

Sequence A succession of strokes.

Serous membranes Membranes that line closed body cavities that do not open to the outside of the body. These membranes consist of two layers: parietal and visceral. Serous membranes secrete a thin, serous fluid, between the parietal and visceral layers, which lubricates organs and reduces friction between the organs in the thoracic or abdominopelvic cavities.

Shingles An acute infection of the peripheral nervous system caused by the reactivation of the latent herpes zoster (chickenpox) virus.

Sickle cell anemia An inherited type of severe, chronic anemia in which red blood cells are "sickled." This shape greatly reduces the amount of oxygen that can be supplied to the tissues.

Side-lying position Lying on one's side. Also known as the lateral position or lateral recumbent position.

Simple columnar epithelium A single layer of cells that are taller than wide, in which the nuclei are located toward the bottom portion of the epithelial cells (near the basement membrane). This tissue offers some protection to underlying structures and is found in stomach and intestines. The free surface typically possesses tiny projections called microvilli.

Simple cuboidal epithelium A single layer of cube-shaped cells possessing more volume, as well as more cytoplasmic organelles, than simple squamous epithelium. This type of tissue is well suited for secretion and absorption and is found in the ovaries, kidney tubules, thyroid gland, pancreas, and salivary glands.

Simple squamous epithelium Also called pavement epithelium, this is a single layer of thin, flat cells that are close together, attaching at their edges. This tissue type is well suited for cellular processes such as diffusion and filtration (e.g., alveoli of lungs, areas of the kidney, and capillary walls).

Sinoatrial node The node that lies within the right atrium and initiates the cardiac impulse, stimulating both the right and left atria to contract.

Sinusoids Specialized venous channels located in the liver.

Sitz bath A sitting bath with the water covering the hips and coming up to the navel. The bath chamber is usually designed so the legs can remain out of the water.

Skeletal or **voluntary muscle** Muscle that attaches to bones and their membranes, fascia, and other muscles. Skeletal muscles must be stimulated by a nerve impulse to contract.

Skin pallor This term refers to an unnatural paleness or lack of skin color.

Sliding filament theory The theory that discusses how muscle filaments slide past each other in order to change muscle length.

Slow twitch or **red muscle** Fatigue-resistant fibers that are small in diameter and have copious amounts of a red respiratory pigment called myoglobin.

Small intestines The small intestine is actually the longest section of the alimentary canal and is situated in the central abdomen, framed by the large intestine. This muscular tube is bound at both ends by the pyloric sphincter (at the stomach) and the ileocecal sphincter (at the large intestine).

Smooth visceral or **involuntary muscle** Muscle that forms the walls of hollow organs and tubes like the stomach, bladder, uterus, and blood vessels. These muscle fibers are adapted for long, sustained contraction and consume very little energy.

Snoring Audible breathing during sleep due to vibration of the uvula and soft palate.

SOAP format An acronym that denotes categories of information included in documenting the health plan. **Subjective** assessment information; **Objective** assessment information; **Application** of massage or therapy and response; and **Plan.**

Sodium-potassium pump A mechanism that actively transports ions (sodium and potassium) across a cell membrane against an opposing concentration gradient.

Solutes Substances dissolved in a solution.

Somatic or **voluntary nervous system** Supplies impulses from the central nervous system to the skeletal muscles.

Somatic reflexes Reflexes responsible for the contraction of skeletal muscle, such as when the doctor taps your patellar tendon with a rubber hammer (knee-jerk or patella reflex).

Spasticity Increased muscle tone and stiffness associated with an increase in tendon reflexes.

Speed The rate of motion or how fast or slow a massage movement is being executed.

Sphincter A ring of muscle fibers that regulates movement of materials from one compartment of the gastrointestinal tract to another.

Sphincter of Oddi Sphincter that regulates the flow of secretions from the pancreas, liver, and gallbladder.

Sphygmomanometer The instrument used to measure blood pressure, most often in the brachial artery.

Spina bifida A congenital defect characterized by a lack of osseous development in the lamina (posterior vertebral arch).

Spinal cord Located in the vertebral canal of the vertebral column, it is an extension of the brain stem from the foramen magnum to the region of L2.

Spinal nerves Nerves originating from the spinal cord.

Spinal pack A long, narrow fomentation pack applied directly on the spine.

Spleen The lymphatic organ that lies within the left lateral rib cage (between ribs 9 and 11) just posterior to the stomach. The functions of the spleen appear to be defense (destroys bacteria), hemocytopoiesis, destruction of red blood cells and platelets, storage of these destroyed and worn-out blood cells, and returning these blood cells to the liver for bile production.

Spondylolisthesis Spondylolisthesis is an anteriorly displaced vertebra, usually the fifth lumbar vertebra over the first sacral vertebra.

Spores The reproductive units of a microorganism.

Sprain Joint trauma that stretches or tears the ligamentous attachments, causing pain and possible temporary disability.

Squamous cell carcinoma A type of skin cancer that arises from the epidermis, beginning as a scaly pigmented area that may develop into a ulcerated crater.

Stamina Endurance, vigor, constitutional energy, and strength.

State-dependent memory This type of memory is triggered by duplicating the original position of a client, location or amount of pressure, body movements, emotions, and nervous system activation at the time the experience occurred.

Static stretching Slow, held stretches that consist of bringing a muscle to full extension and then maintaining the pressure necessary to keep the muscle in extension for 1 to 30 seconds, depending on the stretching ideology involved.

Status report A type of progress report that describes how the client is doing at a point in time or over a short duration of time, such as a prescriptive period. It is brief and concise, using the last SOAP note with an estimate of progress to date or since the last progress report.

Steam baths or **wet sauna** Hot vapor baths given in specially designed chambers where temperatures are maintained at 105° to 130°F at 100 percent humidity.

Sterilization A technique for destroying microorganisms using heat, water, chemicals, or gases.

Steroid hormones Steroid hormones are derived from cholesterol and alter a cell's activity by turning genes on or off.

Stimuli Any change in the internal or external environment.

Stomach The stomach is a J-shaped organ that is essentially an enlargement of the gastrointestinal tract bound at both ends by sphincters.

Strain A muscle or tendon injury due to a violent contraction, forced stretching, or synergistic failure.

Stratified squamous epithelial cells Epithelial cells that are packed closely together and arranged in layers over the external surface of the body and line most of the hollow structures (e.g., oral cavity). Cells in the lower layers undergo cell division and are soon pushed toward the free surface. As the cells approach the exterior, they become thinner, die, and are sloughed off.

Stratum corneum The outermost layer of the skin.

Stratum germinativum Also known as the basal layer, this is the innermost or the matrix layer of the epidermis. The stratum germinativum undergoes continuous cell division and produces all other layers.

Stratum granulosum A layer of cells containing an

accumulation of keratohyalin granules distinguishing it from other skin layers under a microscope. This layer is three to five cells deep, depending on the thickness of the skin.

Stratum lucidum The translucent layer between the stratum corneum and the stratum granulosum. In thin skin, the stratum lucidum is absent.

Stratum spinosum The stratum spinosum, or "prickly layer," is a bonding and transitional layer between the stratum granulosum and the stratum germinativum, because it possesses cells of both these layers.

Strength Intensity or power.

Stretching Involves elongating or extending the muscle tissue to its full length.

Striae Silvery to white stretch marks characterized by linear scars.

Stroke volume The amount of blood ejected from the left ventricle during each contraction of the heart.

Subthreshold stimulus A stimulus below the neural threshold.

Sudoriferous or **sweat glands** Exocrine glands located in the dermis that secrete sweat, or perspiration. The primary functions of sudoriferous glands are to regulate body temperature and to eliminate waste products.

Sulci Grooves or depressions of the cerebral cortex.

Summation Occurs when a subthreshold stimulus is repeated in succession and cumulatively creates a nerve impulse.

Superior, cranial, or **cephalic** Situated above or toward the head.

Supine Lying face up or belly up in a horizontal, recumbent position.

Surfactants Phospholipids made by the cells forming the alveoli that assist the exchange of gas in the alveoli, reduce surface tension, and contribute to the elasticity of pulmonary tissue.

Swedish gymnastics A system of active, passive, and resisted movements of the body's various joints and muscles. Most often, Swedish gymnastics include the artful and fluid presentation of passive range of motion. Swedish gymnastics are also known as Swedish movements, remedial gymnastics, table stretches, joint mobilizations, and range of motion exercises.

Swedish shampoo or **body shampoo** Involves brushing the body with a brush dipped in warm soapy water.

Sydenham, Thomas (1624–89) English physician who emphasized clinical observation rather than theory.

Sympathetic nervous system or **thoracolumbar outflow** A catabolic system that is involved with spending body resources and with preparing the body for emergency situations.

Symptom Anything the client notices as unusual and uncomfortable.

Synapse A junction between two neurons, or between a neuron and a muscle or gland, where they connect to transmit information.

Synaptic end or **terminal bulbs** Bulblike structures at the end of axon terminals.

Synaptic transmission The electrochemical method by which the nerve impulse from one neuron bridges the synaptic gap to convey the nerve impulse to the next neuron. This is a one-way nerve impulse conduction from the axon of one cell to the dendrite of another.

Synaptic vesicles Sacs located at synaptic end bulbs, storing chemicals called neurotransmitters.

Synarthrotic A type of joint in which movement is absent or extremely limited.

Synergist Aids the prime movers by causing the same movement.

Synovial fluid Viscous fluid found in joints, bursae sacs, and synovial sheaths.

Synovial membranes Lines the joint cavities of freely moving joints (e.g., shoulder, hip, and knee). These membranes secrete synovial fluid, a viscous liquid that provides nutrition and lubrication to the joint so it can move freely without friction.

Systemic circuit The pathway blood from the left ventricle of the heart through numerous arteries into the capillaries back to the heart through the veins to the right atrium of the heart.

Systemic lupus erythematosus An autoimmune, inflammatory disease of connective tissue that occurs mostly in young women.

Systole The pressure exerted on the arterial wall during active ventricular contraction.

Table mechanics The positioning, bolstering, and draping of the client as well as table considerations (e.g., height of the massage table).

Tachycardia Rapid heart rate (more than 100 beats per minute).

Taenia coli Thick, longitudinal bands located in the tunica muscularis of the large intestine that resemble thread gathering fabric.

Target cells Cells that contain receptor sites, which are chemically compatible to join with their corresponding hormone.

Taylor, Charles Fayette American physician, who along with his brother George Henry Taylor, introduced the Swedish movement system (created by Pehr Ling) into the United States; he helped popularize Ling's methods with his publications.

Taylor, George Henry American physician, who along with his brother Charles Fayette Taylor, introduced the Swedish movement system (created by Pehr Ling) into the United States; he helped popularize Ling's methods with his publications.

Techne Iatriche Term used to refer to the ancient Greek knowledge that comprised their philosophy of a "healing science."

Tender point If an area is locally sensitive, but stimulation of the site causes no referred sensations, it is not a trigger point but a tender point.

Tendon A cord of tough fibrous connective tissue that anchors the ends of muscle to bone, fascia, or other connective tissue structures.

Tendon sheaths Tubular-shaped structures found where tendons cross multiple joints (e.g., hands and feet), and are lined with synovial membrane.

Tendinitis Inflammation of the tendon, accompanied by pain and swelling.

Tenoperiostial junction Where the tendon joins the periosteum of the bone.

Terminal illness A type of chronic illness, in the sense that there is no cure, but the client is expected to die as a result of this illness.

Testes The testes are the reproductive glands that function both as endocrine and exocrine glands and are located in the male scrotum.

Testosterone An androgenic hormone that promotes secondary male sex characteristics, as well as libido (sex drive), and sperm production.

Thalamus A relay station and interpretation center of the brain for all sensory impulses except olfaction.

Thermoreceptors Receptors sensitive to temperature changes located immediately under the skin.

Thermotherapy The external application of heat modalities in their various forms to the body. Thermotherapy includes the use of whirlpools, moist heat packs, and steam baths as well as paraffin baths, saunas, and steam baths.

Thoracic duct The lymphatic duct that drains lymph from the parts of the body not drained by the right lymphatic duct.

Thoracic The chest area; between the neck and the respiratory diaphragm.

Threshold stimulus Occurs when the stimulus is of sufficient intensity to generate a nerve impulse.

Thrombocytes or **platelets** Blood cell fragments from megakaryoblasts/megakaryocytes that help repair leaks in the blood vessels through various clotting mechanisms.

Thrombosis An abnormal vascular condition characterized by thrombus (blood clot) formation in an unbroken blood vessel.

Thymopoietin Both thymosin and thymopoietin are immunologic hormones that play a role in the body's growth and development, in sexual maturation, and in the growth and maturation of antibodies, namely T cells.

Thymosin See **Thymopoietin.**

Thymus gland The thymus gland is a bilobed gland posterior to the sternum in the mediastinal region of the thorax. It is large in infants, reaches its maximum size at puberty, then atrophies and is replaced by adipose tissue in adults.

Thyroid gland Located at the base of the neck, posterior and inferior to the larynx, is the butterfly-shaped thyroid gland; a bilobed gland connected in the center by a mass of tissue known as the isthmus.

Thyroid-stimulating hormone Stimulates the thyroid gland to produce and secrete triiodothyronine (T_3) and thyroxine (T_4).

Thyroxine or **T_4** Both triiodothyronine and thyroxine regulate growth and development as well as influence mental, physical, and metabolic activities. These hormones consist of a small peptide molecule bound to iodine.

Tissot, Simon André (1728–97) French hygienist who was an important figure in physical therapy. He published several works on gymnastics and massage.

Tissues A group of similar cells that act together to perform a specific function.

Tonic contractions Sustained contractions that occur in sphincter muscles.

Tonsils A group of large specialized lymph tissues embedded in the mucous membranes in the throat.

Tonus A state of continuous, partial muscle contraction.

Topical Pertaining to the surface.

Touch Laying the hands on the skin without movement.

Trachea A tube from the larynx to the upper chest. Located anterior to the esophagus, it measures about 5 inches long and consists of 16 to 20 half-ring hyaline cartilages.

Tracking response Combining careful observation of a client's responses to technique with a willingness on the therapist's part to adjust and change the treatment accordingly.

Tracking skills The ability to notice and respond to changes that a client experiences during treatment (i.e., facial expressions, changes in breath, a subtle flinch).

Tract A bundle of nerve fibers running down the spinal cord in columns.

Transference The unconscious tendency to assign to others feelings and attitudes associated with significant persons in a client's early life, especially the client's transfer to the therapist of feelings associated with a parent.

Transient ischemic attack An event of temporary cerebral dysfunction caused by ischemia or reduced blood circulation.

Transitional epithelium A type of stratified squamous epithelium that can stretch in response to pressure. The appearance of transitional epithelium varies depending on whether it is relaxed or expanded.

Transverse or **horizontal plane** The plane that passes through the body and creates superior (cephalic, or cranial) and inferior (caudal) sections.

Transverse or **T tubules** Extensions in the sarcolemma within a muscle.

Treatment protocol A form that describes the steps used to form the therapy plan.

Treatment record A journal of treatment or therapy sessions. It contains the client's information and responses to therapy in SOAP format for each session.

Trepanation Surgical procedure involving the removal of a skull segment.

Tricuspid valve The right atrioventricular valve containing three flaps or cusps.

Trigger point work Sustained digital pressure applied to trigger points to relieve pain and discomfort.

Trigger points Hypersensitive areas in muscles, fascia, tendons, and ligaments that refer pain to distal regions of the body.

Triiodothyronine or $\mathbf{T_3}$ See **Thyroxine.**

Tropic hormones Hormones that regulate the growth and secretory activity of other endocrine glands.

Troponin and **Tropomyosin** Protein molecules present on actin molecules. These protein molecules mark the sites of attachment of the myosin filament during contraction.

Tuberculosis A chronic lung infection caused by the bacterium *Mycobacterium tuberculosis.*

Tunica adventitia or **externa** The outermost layer of arteries and veins.

Tunica intima The innermost layer of both arteries and veins.

Tunica media The middle layer of arteries and veins.

Tunics The layers of the alimentary canal; the mucosa, the submucosa, the muscularis, and the serosa.

Turkish shampoo Essentially the same thing as a Swedish shampoo, with one exception: after the 105°F pail pour, it concludes with a 90°F pail pour.

Tympanic membrane The eardrum, which separates the outer ear from the middle ear.

Ulcer A lesion in a membrane, usually in parts of the digestive tract exposed to acidic gastric juice.

Umbilical Referring to the area of the midabdomen or navel.

Unipolar neurons Neurons possessing one extension from the cell body, split into two portions. One portion of the neural extension functions as a dendrite and another functions as an axon.

Universal donor The term used to describe blood type O people; their blood will not react to any other blood types.

Universal precautions A system of preserving health that may include any combination of the following: mandatory handwashing, vinyl gloves, protective eyewear, nose-face masks, protective clothing, laundering of linens and uniforms, cleaning of disinfecting equipment, and proper methods for disposing used medical supplies and biological material.

Universal recipient The term used to describe blood type AB people; they can receive all other blood types.

Uremia A toxic level of urea and other nitrogenous waste products in the blood due to a renal insufficiency and abnormal retention of these waste products normally removed by the kidneys.

Ureters Two slender hollow tubes that transport urine formed by the kidneys to the urinary bladder. The ureters are located bilaterally; there is one ureter for each kidney.

Urethra A small tubular structure that transports urine from the urinary bladder out of the body during micturition (urination).

Urinalysis The microscopic, chemical, or physical examination of urine.

Urinary bladder A hollow muscular organ located in the pelvis behind the symphysis pubis that provides temporary storage for urine.

Urinary incontinence The inability to control micturition.

Urinary tract infections An infection of one or more structures of the urinary system often caused by bacteria.

Varicose veins Dilated veins possessing incompetent valves.

Vascular spasm Occurs when the smooth muscle in the broken blood vessel begins to spasm; this may reduce blood flow for up to 30 minutes.

Vasoconstriction When the diameter of a blood vessel becomes narrower.

Vasodilation When the diameter of a blood vessel enlarges.

Veins Blood vessels that drain the tissues and organs and return blood back to the heart and lungs.

Venous pump The one-way valve system to prevent backflow, together with the pumping action of muscular contraction in the limbs.

Ventral cavity Located anteriorally to the dorsal cavity; it is further divided into the thoracic cavity and the abdominopelvic cavity. The thoracic cavity contains the right and left pleural cavities and the mediastinum. The abdominopelvic cavity is further divided into the abdominal cavity and the pelvic cavity.

Ventricles The inferior heart chambers that pump blood to the body's organs and tissues.

Venules Smaller, thin branches of veins.

Vermiform appendix A worm-shaped lymph gland, 3 to 6 inches long, suspended from and opening into the inferior portion of the cecum. It helps fight pathogens.

Vermis The midsection of the cerebellum.

Verruca A mass of cutaneous elevations caused by a contagious virus, papillomavirus.

Vertebral Pertaining to one or more vertebrae of the vertebral or spinal column.

Vesalius, Andreas (1514–64) Flemish physician. His *De Humani Corporis Fabrica* (1543) is considered one of the most important studies in the history of medicine.

Vibration A rapid shaking, trembling, or oscillating movement, which is applied with full hands, fingertips, or a mechanical device for the purpose of inducing relaxation.

Villi Fingerlike projections housing blood and lymph capillaries located in the lining of the small intestines.

Viruses Viruses are considered to be nonliving entities because they do not carry out independent metabolic activities. They can only replicate themselves within the cell nucleus of a living plant or animal host.

Visceral or **autonomic reflexes** Homeostatic reflexes such as coughing, sneezing, blinking, and corrections to heart rate, respiratory rate, and blood pressure.

Visceral Pertaining to the outer coverings of a body cavity or hollow organ.

Vital capacity The total amount that can be forcibly inspired and expired from the lungs in one breath.

Vitamins Vitamins are organic compounds that are essential for normal physiologic and metabolic functioning of the body.

Vocal folds Bands of elastic ligaments that are attached to the rigid cartilage of the larynx by skeletal muscle. There is a space between the folds and when air passes over the folds, they vibrate and produce sound. The tighter the skeletal muscles pull the vocal folds, the higher the pitch of the voice.

Volkmann's canals Osseous canals that connect Haversian canals.

Volume The loudness of sound.

Volunteer A volunteer is someone who renders aid or performs a service without monetary gain. It is done of his or her own free will, usually with a sense of charity.

Vomiting Reverse peristalsis of the upper gastrointestinal tract accomplished by contraction of the abdominal muscles to squeeze the stomach against the diaphragm.

Warm immersion bath or **whirlpool baths** Tubs for soaking or for receiving jets of water against the skin; water is drained after each use.

Wernicke's area An area located in the temporal lobe (typically left hemisphere only) crucial to language comprehension.

Zones In foot reflexology, energy pathways are called zones. There are ten zones in the body, five on each foot.

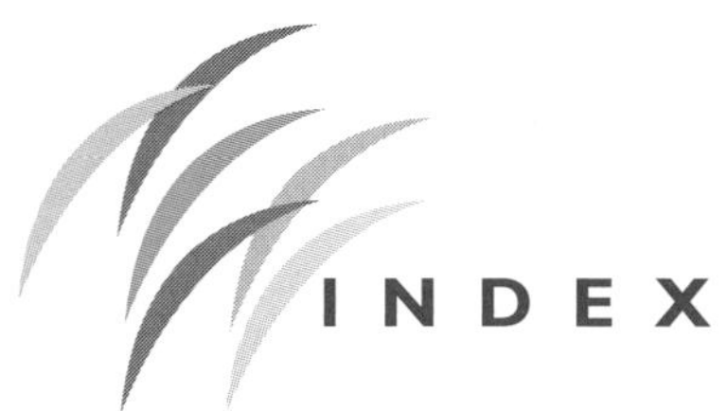

INDEX

Page numbers in *italics* refer to illustrations; page numbers followed by *t* refer to tables.

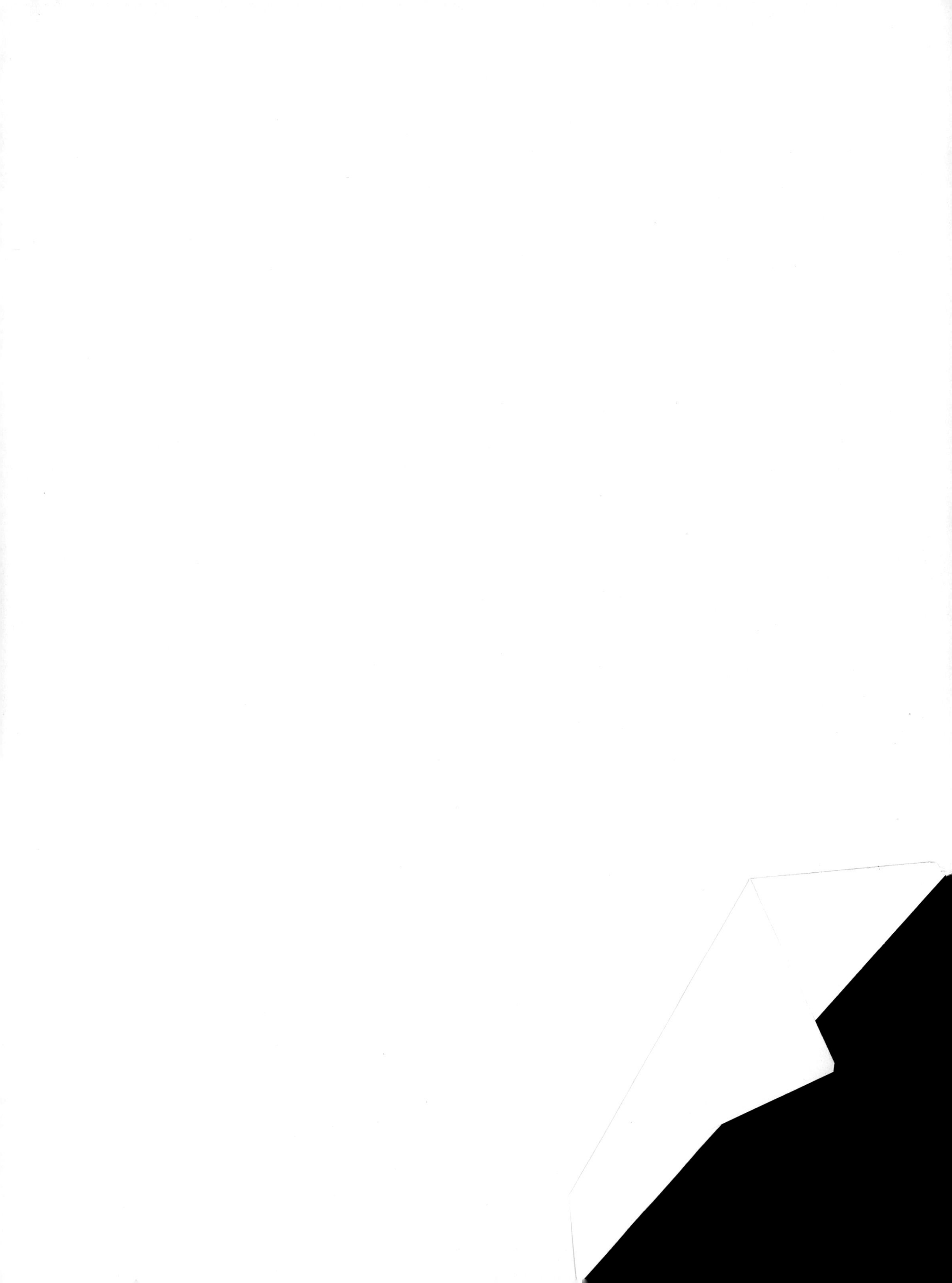